Problem Solving in

CHEST IMAGING

Problem Solving in

CHEST IMAGING

Subba R. Digumarthy, MD
Radiologist
Massachusetts General Hospital;
Assistant Professor of Radiology
Harvard Medical School
Boston, Massachusetts

Suhny Abbara, MD
Chief, Cardiothoracic Imaging Division
Professor, Department of Radiology
UT Southwestern Medical Center
Dallas, Texas

Jonathan H. Chung, MD
Section Chief, Thoracic Radiology
Associate Professor
The University of Chicago Medicine
Chicago, Illinois

ELSEVIER

PROBLEM SOLVING IN CHEST IMAGING ISBN: 978-0-323-04132-4

Library of Congress Control Number: 2018959607

Publisher: Russell Gabbedy
Content Development Specialist: Caroline Dorey-Stein
Publishing Services Manager: Catherine Jackson
Book Production Specialist: Kristine Feeherty
Design Direction: Bridget Hoette

Printed in China

Last digit is the print number: 9 8 7 6 5 4 3 2 1

ELSEVIER

1600 John F. Kennedy Blvd.
Ste 1600
Philadelphia, PA 19103-2899

To our families:

To my dear wife Nagamani and lovely daughter Reethika for their constant support and encouragement. — S.R.D.

To Cory, Tyler, and Amanda; and Mona, Susu, Marlene, and Yasser, with deep gratitude for your friendship, love, and support. — S.A.

To Aimee and Alexandra: Thank you for your endless love and support. — J.H.C.

And to all the residents, fellows, colleagues, mentors, and patients for their questions and intellectual curiosity, which perpetually makes us think and learn.

Contributors

Suhny Abbara, MD
Chief, Cardiothoracic Imaging Division, Professor, Department of Radiology, UT Southwestern Medical Center, Dallas, TX
Normal Anatomy of the Lungs
Mediastinum, Chest Wall, and Diaphragm
Imaging Anatomy of the Heart and Thoracic Great Vessels
Introduction to Terminology
Acquired Diseases of the Aorta
Cardiac and Vascular Tumors

Gerald F. Abbott, MD
Associate Radiologist, Department of Imaging, Massachusetts General Hospital, Boston, MA
The Pleura

Jeanne B. Ackman, AB, MD, FACR
Assistant Professor, Harvard Medical School; Radiologist, Massachusetts General Hospital, Boston, MA
Problem Solving in the Mediastinum

Saurabh Agarwal, MD
Assistant Professor, Department of Diagnostic Imaging, The Warren Alpert Medical School of Brown University, Providence, RI
Imaging of Thoracic Trauma

Mukta D. Agrawal, MD
Assistant Professor of Radiology, Oklahoma University Hospital Medical Sciences, Oklahoma City, OK
Introduction to Terminology

Tami J. Bang, MD
Assistant Professor, Department of Radiology, University of Colorado School of Medicine, Aurora, CO
Acquired Diseases of the Aorta

Dhiraj Baruah, MD
Assistant Professor and Chief, Cardiothoracic Radiology; Program Director, Scanlon Cardiothoracic Fellowship; Co-Director, Cardiac MRI; Medical Director, Emergency Radiology, Medical College of Wisconsin, Milwaukee, WI
Radiographic Techniques

Kiran Batra, MD
Assistant Professor, Department of Radiology, UT Southwestern Medical Center, Dallas, TX
Normal Anatomy of the Lungs

Adam Bernheim, MD
Assistant Professor of Radiology, Icahn School of Medicine at Mount Sinai, New York, NY; Adjunct Assistant Professor of Radiology, Emory University School of Medicine, Atlanta, GA
Differential Diagnosis Based on Imaging Findings

Sanjeev Bhalla, MD
Professor of Radiology, Mallinckrodt Institute of Radiology, St. Louis, MO
Imaging of Thoracic Trauma

Michael Bolen, MD
Cardiothoracic Radiology, Cleveland Clinic, Cleveland, OH
Step-by-Step Analysis of Cardiac Chambers in CT
Cardiac Valves

Christopher G. Brown, MD
Research Analyst, Department of Diagnostic Radiology, University of Maryland Medical Center, Baltimore, MD
Cardiac CT for the Evaluation of Acute Coronary Syndrome in the Emergency Department

Julia Capobianco, MD
Chest Radiologist, Fleury Group, São Paulo, Brazil
Collagen Vascular Diseases and Vasculitis

Brett W. Carter, MD
Diagnostic Radiology, University of Texas MD Anderson Cancer Center, Houston, TX
Neoplasms of the Lung and Airways

Nihara Chakrala, MD
Formerly of the Department of Radiology, Beth Israel Deaconess Medical Center, Boston, MA
Trachea and Bronchi

Jay Champlin, MD
Resident, Department of Radiology, University of Washington, Seattle, WA
Hypersensitivity Pneumonitis

Thanissara Chansakul, MD
Neuroradiology Fellow, Radiology, Brigham and Women's Hospital/Harvard Medical School, Boston, MA
Cystic Lung Disease

Jonathan H. Chung, MD
Section Chief, Thoracic Radiology, Associate Professor, The University of Chicago Medicine, Chicago, IL
Interstitial Lung Disease
Acquired Diseases of the Aorta

Pierluigi Ciet, MD, PhD
Thoracic Radiologist and Postdoc at Radiology-Nuclear Medicine and Pediatric Pulmonology Departments of the Erasmus Medical Center, Rotterdam, Netherlands
Trachea and Bronchi

Christian W. Cox, MD
Department of Radiology, Mayo Clinic, Rochester, MN
Occupational and Inhalational Lung Diseases

Subba R. Digumarthy, MD
Radiologist, Massachusetts General Hospital; Assistant Professor of Radiology, Harvard Medical School, Boston, MA
Differential Diagnosis Based on Imaging Findings
Infection
The Pleura

Sharmila Dorbala, MD, MPH, FACC, FASNC
Associate Professor, Radiology, Harvard Medical School; Director, Nuclear Cardiology, Division of Nuclear Medicine and Molecular Imaging, Department of Radiology, Division of Cardiology, Department of Medicine, Brigham and Women's Hospital, Boston, MA
Problem-Oriented Radionuclide Myocardial Perfusion Imaging

Rachel Edwards, MD
Assistant Professor, Diagnostic Radiology, University of Washington, Seattle, WA
Cardiovascular CT
Cardiac MRI

Brett M. Elicker, MD
Professor of Clinical Radiology, Department of Radiology and Biomedical Imaging, University of California, San Francisco, San Francisco, CA
Lung and Heart Transplantation

Ahmed H. El-Sherief, MD
Health Sciences Associate Clinical Professor, David Geffen School of Medicine at UCLA; Division of Cardiothoracic Imaging, Veterans Administration Greater Los Angeles Healthcare System, Los Angeles, CA
Step-by-Step Analysis of Cardiac Chambers in CT
Cardiac Valves

Tony Hany Fattouch, MD
Assistant Professor, Department of Radiology, University of Cincinnati, Cincinnati, OH
Congenital Heart and Vascular Disease

Florian J. Fintelmann, MD, Dr. med.
Assistant Professor of Radiology, Harvard Medical School; Staff Radiologist, Department of Radiology, Division of Thoracic Imaging and Intervention, Massachusetts General Hospital, Boston, MA
Thoracic Interventions

Stephen Fisher, MD
Fellow, Department of Radiology, UT Southwestern Medical Center, Dallas, TX
Normal Anatomy of the Lungs
Mediastinum, Chest Wall, and Diaphragm

Christopher J. François, MD
Professor, Department of Radiology, University of Wisconsin–Madison, Madison, WI
Pulmonary, Mediastinal, Vascular, and Chest Wall MRI

Brian B. Ghoshhajra, MD, MBA
Service Chief, Cardiovascular Imaging, Department of Radiology, Massachusetts General Hospital, Harvard Medical School, Boston, MA
Imaging of Cardiomyopathy and Myocarditis

Matthew Gilman, MD
Division of Thoracic Imaging and Intervention, Massachusetts General Hospital, Boston, MA
Congenital and Developmental Diseases of the Lungs and Airways

Lawrence R. Goodman, MD, FACR
Professor, Department of Radiology, Medical College of Wisconsin, Milwaukee, WI
Radiographic Techniques

Cameron Hassani, MD
Assistant Professor, Department of Radiology, Keck Hospital of the University of Southern California, Los Angeles, CA
Diaphragm and Chest Wall

Sandeep S. Hedgire, MD
Instructor of Radiology, Massachusetts General Hospital, Boston, MA
Introduction to Terminology

Benedikt H. Heidinger, MD
Resident in Radiology, Department of Biomedical Imaging and Image-guided Therapy, Vienna General Hospital, Medical University of Vienna, Vienna, Austria
Trachea and Bronchi

Travis S. Henry, MD
Associate Professor of Clinical Radiology, Department of Radiology and Biomedical Imaging, University of California San Francisco, San Francisco, CA
Radiation, Medication, and Illicit Drug–Related Lung Disease

Stephen B. Hobbs, MD, FSCCT
Assistant Professor, Department of Radiology, University of Kentucky, Lexington, KY
Smoking-Related Lung Diseases

Bruno Hochhegger, MD, PhD
Thoracic Radiologist and Professor of Radiology, Pontifical Catholic University, Rio de Janeiro, Brazil
Collagen Vascular Diseases and Vasculitis

Jared Isaacson, MD
Resident, Department of Radiology, UT Southwestern Medical Center, Dallas, TX
Mediastinum, Chest Wall, and Diaphragm

Daniel Jeong, MD, MS
Assistant Member, Department of Radiology, Moffitt Cancer Center, Tampa, FL
Pulmonary, Mediastinal, Vascular, and Chest Wall MRI

Robert Joodi, MD
Faculty Radiologist, M&S Radiology Associates Pa, San Antonio, TX
Introduction to Terminology

Kirk Jordan, MS, MD
Department of Radiology, UT Southwestern Medical Center, Dallas, TX
Normal Anatomy of the Lungs

Mannudeep K. Kalra, MBBS, MD, DNB
Radiologist, Division of Thoracic and Cardiac Imaging, Massachusetts General Hospital; Professor, Harvard Medical School, Boston, MA
Pulmonary CT: The Scanner, the Protocol, and the Dose

Sanjeeva P. Kalva, MD, RPVI, FSIR
Chief, Interventional Radiology; Professor, Department of Radiology, UT Southwestern Medical Center, Dallas, TX
Angiography and Interventions

Jeffrey P. Kanne, MD
Professor, Department of Radiology, University of Wisconsin School of Medicine and Public Health, Madison, WI
Eosinophilic Lung Disease
Collagen Vascular Diseases and Vasculitis

Gregory A. Kicska, MD, PhD
Associate Professor, Department of Radiology, University of Washington, Seattle, WA
Cardiovascular CT
Cardiac MRI

Seth Kligerman, MD
Associate Professor, Division Chief of Cardiothoracic Imaging, Department of Diagnostic Radiology, University of California, San Diego, La Jolla, CA
Imaging of the Pericardium

Jerry Kovoor, MD
Associate Professor of Clinical Radiology, Indiana University, Indianapolis, IN
Angiography and Interventions

Christopher Lee, MD
Associate Professor, Department of Radiology, Keck School of Medicine of USC, Los Angeles, CA
Interstitial Lung Disease
Diaphragm and Chest Wall

Marie-Helene Levesque, MD, FRCP
Clinical Fellow in Cardiothoracic Imaging, Department of Radiology, Division of Cardiac Imaging, Massachusetts General Hospital, Harvard Medical School, Boston, MA
Imaging of Cardiomyopathy and Myocarditis

Diana Litmanovich, MD
Associate Professor, Radiology, Harvard Medical School; Attending, Department of Radiology, Beth Israel Deaconess Medical Center, Boston, MA
Trachea and Bronchi

Brent P. Little, MD
Radiologist, Department of Radiology, Division of Thoracic Imaging and Intervention, Massachusetts General Hospital, Boston, MA
Diffuse Lung Disease With Calcification and Lipid

Michael T. Lu, MD, MPH
Assistant Professor of Radiology, Harvard Medical School; Director of Research, Division of Cardiovascular Imaging, Massachusetts General Hospital, Boston, MA
Pulmonary Vascular Diseases

Rachna Madan, MD
Associate Radiologist and Instructor, Radiology, Harvard Medical School; Thoracic Imaging, Brigham and Women's Hospital, Boston, MA
Cystic Lung Disease

Nagina Malguria, MD
Assistant Professor, Department of Radiology, Johns Hopkins University, Baltimore, MD
Cardiac and Vascular Tumors

Gustavo Meirelles, MD, PhD
Medical Manager and Head of Thoracic Imaging, Radiology, Fleury Group, São Paulo, Brazil
Collagen Vascular Diseases and Vasculitis

Matthew P. Moy, MD
Clinical Assistant, Department of Radiology, Massachusetts General Hospital, Boston, MA
The Pleura

Venkatesh Arumugam Murugan, MD
Radiology Resident, University of Massachusetts Medical School, Worcester, MA
Pulmonary CT: The Scanner, the Protocol, and the Dose

Scott K. Nagle, MD, PhD
Associate Professor, Department of Radiology, University of Wisconsin–Madison, Madison, WI
Pulmonary, Mediastinal, Vascular, and Chest Wall MRI

Prashant Nagpal, MD
Clinical Assistant Professor, Co-Director Cardiac CT, Department of Radiology, Division of Cardiovascular and Thoracic Radiology, University of Iowa Hospitals and Clinics, Iowa City, IA
Imaging Anatomy of the Heart and Thoracic Great Vessels

Karen Ordovas, MD, MAS
Professor in Residence, Department of Radiology and Biomedical Imaging, University of California, San Francisco, San Francisco, CA
Lung and Heart Transplantation

Atul Padole, MD
Research Fellow, Department of Radiology, Massachusetts General Hospital, Boston, MA
Pulmonary CT: The Scanner, the Protocol, and the Dose

Anil K. Pillai, MD, FRCR
Associate Professor of Radiology, University of Texas Health Science Center, Houston, TX
Angiography and Interventions

Sudhakar Pipavath, MBBS, MD
Professor of Radiology, Cardiothoracic Imaging Section, Department of Radiology, University of Washington Medical Center, Seattle, WA
Hypersensitivity Pneumonitis

Prabhakar Rajiah, MBBS, MD, FRCR
Associate Professor of Radiology, Associate Director of Cardiac CT and MRI, Department of Radiology, Division of Cardiothoracic Imaging, UT Southwestern Medical Center, Dallas, TX
Imaging Anatomy of the Heart and Thoracic Great Vessels

Rishi Ramakrishna, MD
McHenry Radiologists and Imaging Associates, S.C., McHenry, IL
Intensive Care Imaging

Constantine Raptis, MD
Associate Professor of Radiology, Mallinckrodt Institute of Radiology, St. Louis, MO
Imaging of Thoracic Trauma

Guatham P. Reddy, MD, MPH
Professor of Radiology and Vice Chair for Education, Department of Radiology, University of Washington School of Medicine, Seattle, WA
Cardiovascular CT
Cardiac MRI

Rahul Renapurkar, MD
Cardiothoracic Radiology, Cleveland Clinic, Cleveland, Ohio
Cardiac Valves

Carlos A. Rojas, MD
Cardiothoracic Section, Department of Radiology, Mayo Clinic Florida, Jacksonville, FL
Step-by-Step Analysis of Cardiac Chambers in CT
Congenital Heart and Vascular Disease

Sachin S. Saboo, MD, FRCR
Associate Professor of Radiology, UT Health Science Center, San Antonio, TX
Imaging Anatomy of the Heart and Thoracic Great Vessels
Introduction to Terminology

Mohammad Sarwar, MD, FACR
Associate Professor of Radiology, Cardiothoracic Division, UT Southwestern Medical Center, Dallas, TX
Mediastinum, Chest Wall, and Diaphragm

U. Joseph Schoepf, MD, FACR, FAHA, FNASCI, FSCBT-MR, FSCCT
Professor of Radiology, Medicine, and Pediatrics, Director, Division of Cardiovascular Imaging, Vice Chair for Research Development, Department of Radiology and Radiological Science, Medical University of South Carolina, Charleston, SC
Ischemic Cardiac Disease

Kaushik Shahir, MD
Associate Professor, Cardiothoracic Radiology, University of South Florida, Tampa, FL
Radiographic Techniques

Amita Sharma, MD
Assistant Professor of Radiology, Harvard Medical School; Staff Radiologist, Department of Radiology, Division of Thoracic Imaging and Intervention, Massachusetts General Hospital, Boston, MA
Thoracic Interventions

Jo-Anne O. Shepard, MD
Professor of Radiology, Harvard Medical School; Director, Thoracic Imaging and Intervention, Massachusetts General Hospital, Boston, MA
Thoracic Interventions

Girish S. Shroff, MD
Diagnostic Radiology, University of Texas MD Anderson Cancer Center, Houston, TX
Neoplasms of the Lung and Airways

Arlene Sirajuddin, MD
National Institutes of Health, National Heart, Lung, and Blood Institute, Bethesda, MD
Eosinophilic Lung Disease

Pedro Vinícius Staziaki, MD
Research Fellow, Department of Radiology, Cardiac MR PET CT Program, Massachusetts General Hospital, Harvard University; Radiology Resident, Department of Radiology, Boston Medical Center, Boston University School of Medicine, Boston, MA
Pulmonary Vascular Diseases
Imaging of Cardiomyopathy and Myocarditis

Pal Spruill Suranyi, MD, PhD
Associate Professor of Radiology and Medicine/Cardiology, Department of Radiology and Radiological Science, Division of Cardiovascular Imaging and Department of Medicine, Division of Cardiology, Medical University of South Carolina, Charleston, SC
Ischemic Cardiac Disease

Azadeh Tabari, MD
Research Fellow, Department of Radiology, Massachusetts General Hospital, Boston, MA
Pulmonary CT: The Scanner, the Protocol, and the Dose

Attila Tóth, MD
Radiologist and Cardiac MR Specialist, Heart and Vascular Center, Semmelweis University, Budapest, Hungary
Cardiac and Vascular Tumors

Hsiang-Jer Tseng, MD
Assistant Professor, Department of Radiology, Advent Health Medical Group, University of Central Florida College of Medicine, Orlando, FL
Diffuse Lung Disease With Calcification and Lipid

Akos Varga-Szemes, MD, PhD
Assistant Professor, Division of Cardiovascular Imaging, Department of Radiology and Radiological Science, Medical University of South Carolina, Charleston, SC
Ischemic Cardiac Disease

Vikas Veeranna, MD
Director of Cardiac Imaging, Division of Cardiology, Department of Medicine, Berkshire Health Systems, Pittsfield, MA
Problem-Oriented Radionuclide Myocardial Perfusion Imaging

Paul von Herrmann, MD
Lauderdale Radiology Group, Florence, AL
Smoking-Related Lung Diseases

Christopher M. Walker, MD
Associate Professor of Radiology, Department of Radiology, The University of Kansas Medical Center, Kansas City, KS
Infection

Lara A. Walkoff, MD
Department of Radiology, Mayo Clinic, Rochester, MN
Occupational and Inhalational Lung Diseases

Yingbing Wang, MD
Radiologist, Department of Radiology, Massachusetts General Hospital, Boston, MA
Thoracic Nuclear Imaging

Charles S. White, MD
Department of Diagnostic Radiology and Nuclear Medicine, University of Maryland School of Medicine, Baltimore, MD
Cardiac CT for the Evaluation of Acute Coronary Syndrome in the Emergency Department

Julian L. Wichmann, MD
Visiting Instructor, Division of Cardiovascular Imaging, Medical University of South Carolina, Charleston, SC, United States; Resident, Department of Diagnostic and Interventional Radiology, University Hospital Frankfurt, Frankfurt, Germany
Ischemic Cardiac Disease

Lindsay E. Wright, MD
Assistant Professor, Department of Radiology, The Ohio State University Wexner Medical Center, Columbus, OH
Smoking-Related Lung Diseases

Carol C. Wu, MD
Associate Professor, Diagnostic Radiology, University of Texas MD Anderson Cancer Center, Houston, TX
Differential Diagnosis Based on Imaging Findings
Neoplasms of the Lung and Airways

Steven Zangan, MD
Associate Professor of Radiology, University of Chicago, Chicago, IL
Intensive Care Imaging

Evan James Zucker, MD
Clinical Assistant Professor of Radiology, Department of Radiology, Stanford University School of Medicine, Stanford, CA
Pulmonary Vascular Diseases

Preface

We are honored to be the editors of the cardiothoracic imaging textbook in the *Problem Solving* series in a field that has undergone a substantial evolution in recent years. The current-day chest radiologist should have a robust understanding of the anatomy and pathology—as well as insight to the management strategies—of diseases affecting the lungs, pleura, heart, mediastinum, vessels, diaphragm, and chest wall. This knowledge then should be applied across various imaging techniques ranging from radiography, CT, MRI, nuclear medicine, and interventional techniques to guide management in the most effective way. Chest imaging has witnessed transformative developments that are quickly adapted into clinical practice, such as dual energy CT and rapid MRI, and newer interventional techniques such as ablation of thoracic tumors. Many newer treatment techniques such as endoluminal aortic stent graft repair, pulmonary vein isolation, transcatheter aortic and mitral valve implantation, and bronchial valve placement are heavily dependent on precise imaging. The diagnosis and management of patients with interstitial lung diseases and neoplasms are mostly determined by imaging findings.

The content is organized to provide incremental knowledge to the reader on the basics in anatomy, imaging techniques, terminology used in chest imaging, and differential diagnosis based on common imaging patterns, and then finally leading to discussions based on pathology and interventions. After disease-specific discussion, we also cover new topics that are becoming common such as cardiac CT in the emergency setting.

We have had the privilege to be able to call upon many of the top experts within their respective fields in cardiac or thoracic imaging to develop the content of this textbook. We are very grateful to the many submissions, recognizing that they meant time away from family, patients, and other academic pursuits of our colleagues. Thank you!

We hope that this text will be useful in the care of patients with cardiothoracic disease and provide a useful reference source for trainees, practicing radiologists, clinicians, and scientists with an interest in cardiothoracic diseases and imaging. We truly hope that you enjoy reading this text and find it helpful.

Subba R. Digumarthy, MD
Suhny Abbara, MD
Jonathan H. Chung, MD

Contents

SECTION 1

Anatomy

CHAPTER 1
Normal Anatomy of the Lungs

Kiran Batra, Kirk Jordan, Stephen Fisher, and Suhny Abbara

CHAPTER OUTLINE

Introduction

The lungs incorporate the parenchyma, vasculature, bronchial tree (trachea, bronchi, and bronchioles), and a network of investing connective tissue that supports and connects the structures to one another. The human lungs are a pair of large spongy organs for gas exchange between blood and the air. The lungs are covered by a serous membrane called the *visceral pleura,* and the surrounding cavity formed between the lungs and the surrounding chest wall and mediastinum, covered by parietal pleura, is called the *pleural cavity*. Understanding diseases of the chest requires the radiologist to have a sound knowledge of the normal lung anatomy. This chapter describes the gross and radiologic anatomy of the lungs. Although imaging with computed tomography (CT) is commonplace, most chest imaging is still done with plain chest radiography.

Surfaces

There are three surfaces of each lung—the costal, mediastinal, and diaphragmatic surfaces. The costal surface is the outer smooth and convex surface, which faces the ribs and the vertebrae. The mediastinal surface abuts the mediastinum. The mediastinal surface of the right lung carries the impression of the right subclavian artery, superior vena cava (SVC), and paratracheal soft tissues, including the esophagus, the azygous vein, the right atrium, and the inferior vena cava (IVC). The left lung carries the impression of the left subclavian artery, thoracic aorta, and the left atrium and ventricle. The diaphragmatic surface, also called the *base of the lung,* rests on the thoracic diaphragm (Fig. 1.1).

Hilum

The hilum of the lung (also called the *root of the lung*) is formed by the principal bronchi, the central pulmonary arteries and veins, the bronchial nerves and vessels, and the lymphatics, which enter and leave the lung from the mediastinum (Fig. 1.2). The root of the right lung lies behind the SVC, the superior part of the right atrium, and below the azygos vein. The root of left lung lies beneath the aortic arch and in front of the descending aorta.

Lobes

The interlobar fissures are deep clefts in the lungs, lined by visceral pleura, which divide each lung into lobes. The right lung is divided into three lobes—the upper, middle, and lower lobes, separated by two fissures. The oblique fissure (major) separates the lower lobe from the middle and upper lobes; the horizontal fissure (minor) separates the upper from the middle lobe. The left lung is comparatively smaller and has only one oblique fissure, which divides it into two lobes, the upper and the lower. Fissures are frequently incomplete, allowing for collateral air drift and the spread of disease between lobes.

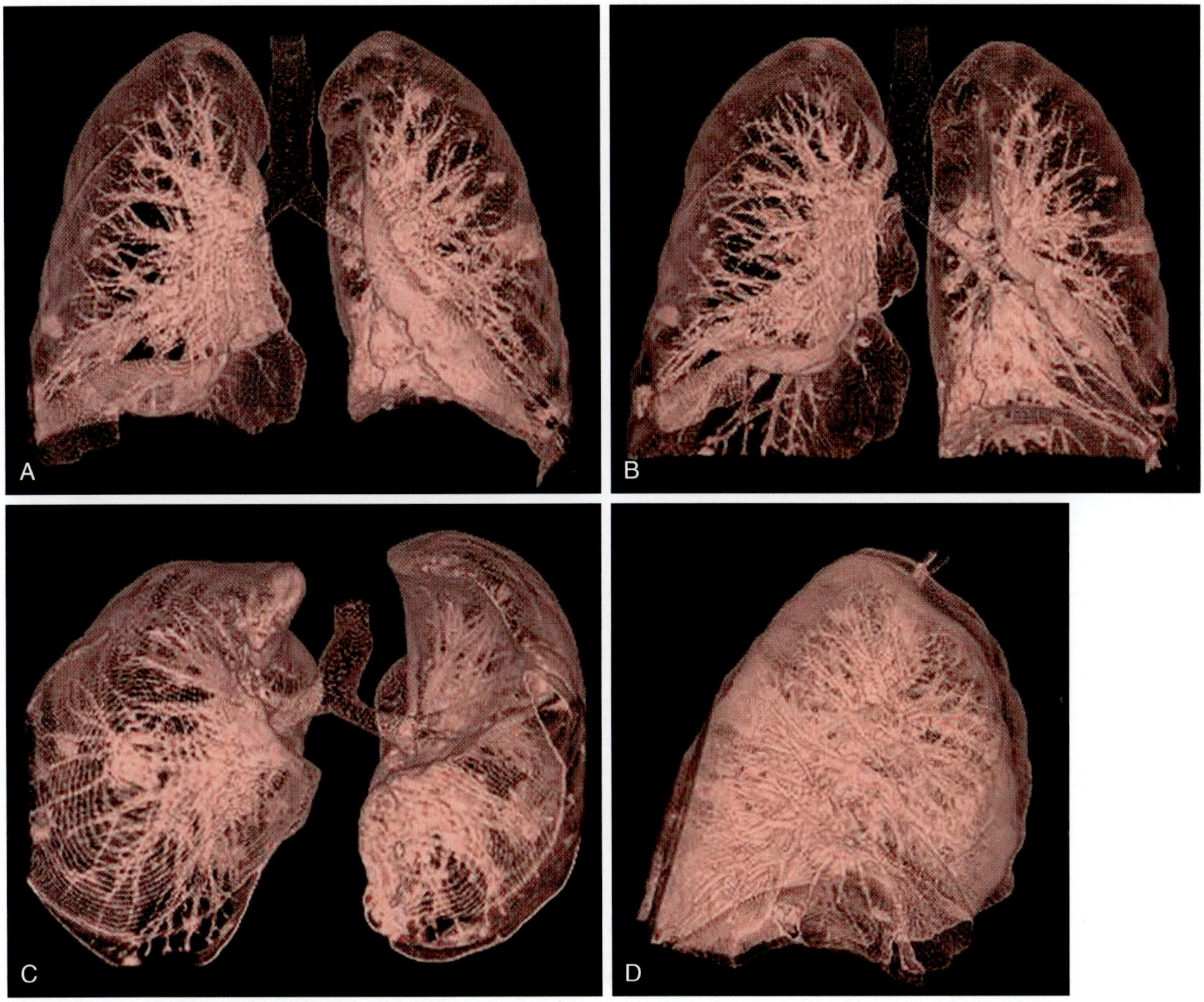

Figure 1.1 Three-dimensional CT volumetric images demonstrate visceral surfaces of the lung. Frontal (A) and shallow left posterior oblique (B) images demonstrating the left mediastinal; caudal (C) shows diaphragmatic, and right lateral projection (D) shows costal surfaces. Pulmonary nodules are secondary to colon metastases.

■ Bronchopulmonary Segments

The bronchopulmonary segment is a smaller division of each lobe, supplied by a tertiary bronchus and its own segmental artery. The significance of such compartmentalization is that each segment is functionally and anatomically discrete, and thus can be removed surgically without affecting the neighboring segments. The veins and lymphatics run along the edges of the segments. There are typically 10 bronchopulmonary segments in the right lung (three, upper lobe; two, middle lobe; five, lower lobe) and eight segments in the left lung (four, upper lobe; four, lower lobe). Table 1.1 lists the typical segmental anatomy (Fig. 1.3). The branching pattern at the segmental level is relatively constant, with the largest variations occurring in the lower lobes. The most common variation occurs in the left lower lobe (LLL), with 4% to 10% of the lobes demonstrating separate origins of the anterior and medial basal segments, similar to the right lower lobe (RLL). On CT, one can define these segments based on the fissures and bronchovascular anatomy. Knowledge of segmental anatomy for the bronchoscopist is important for localization, for the surgeons, because the segments are considered surgical units and can be resected with conservation of adjacent lung, and for the clinician, because many disease processes are segmental in distribution, such as bronchopneumonia, mycobacterial infections, tumor, aspiration, pulmonary infarction, and sequestration.

■ Pulmonary Interstitium: Skeleton of the Lung

The pulmonary interstitial fibers are a network of connective tissues that provide support to the airways. The

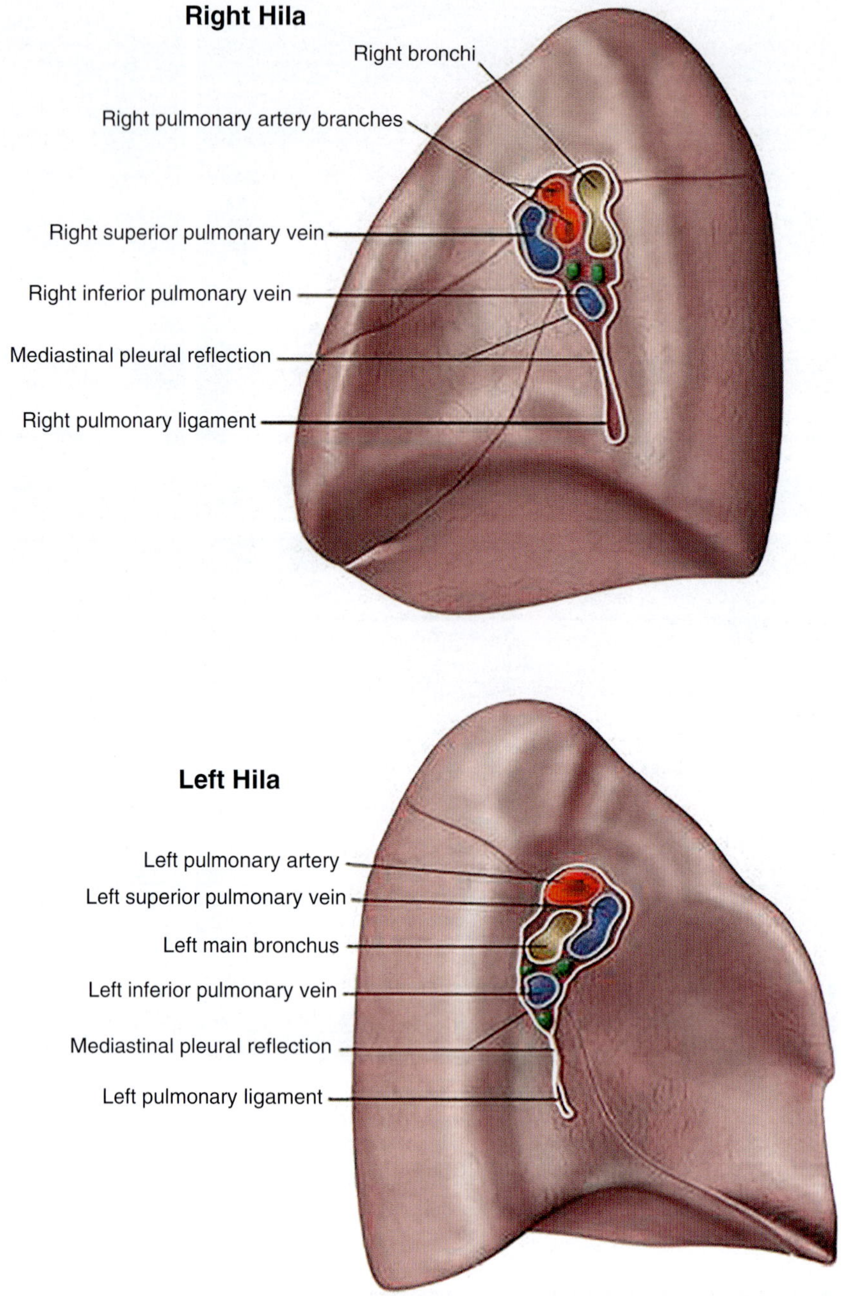

Figure 1.2 Drawings of the root of the right and left lungs show the principal bronchi, the main trunks of the pulmonary arteries, and the pulmonary veins. Note the relationship of the right epiarterial and left hyparterial bronchi.

pulmonary interstitium is divided into two communicating compartments consisting of the axial or bronchovascular interstitium and the peripheral or subpleural interstitium. The axial interstitium extends from the hilum toward the periphery of the lung and surrounds the bronchovascular bundles. The axial interstitium is contiguous with the centrilobular interstitium, which surrounds the centrilobular arteriole and bronchiole within the secondary pulmonary lobule (SPL). The subpleural or peripheral interstitium lies beneath the visceral pleura and forms the borders of the SPL (interlobular septa). Extending between the centrilobular interstitium of the lobular core and the interlobular septa is a fine network of connective fibers known as the *intralobular, parenchymal,* or *alveolar interstitium* (Fig. 1.4). The pulmonary gas exchange units, including the respiratory ducts, alveolar ducts, and alveoli, lie in close relation to the interlobular septa.

It is important to understand these different networks of interstitial fibers so that one can localize the interstitial disease processes and differentiate and diagnose interstitial lung diseases accurately. On radiographs, the interstitium is not well seen, and the diagnosis of the interstitial lung disease is frequently delayed. On high-resolution CT (HRCT), the interstitium is well seen, both centrally and peripherally. Therefore it is the modality of choice for interstitial lung diseases. The bronchovascular margins are smooth, and one should look for marginal blurring (edema, inflammation, and lymphangiectasia), irregularity (fibrosing conditions), and nodularity (granulomatous conditions and malignancy).

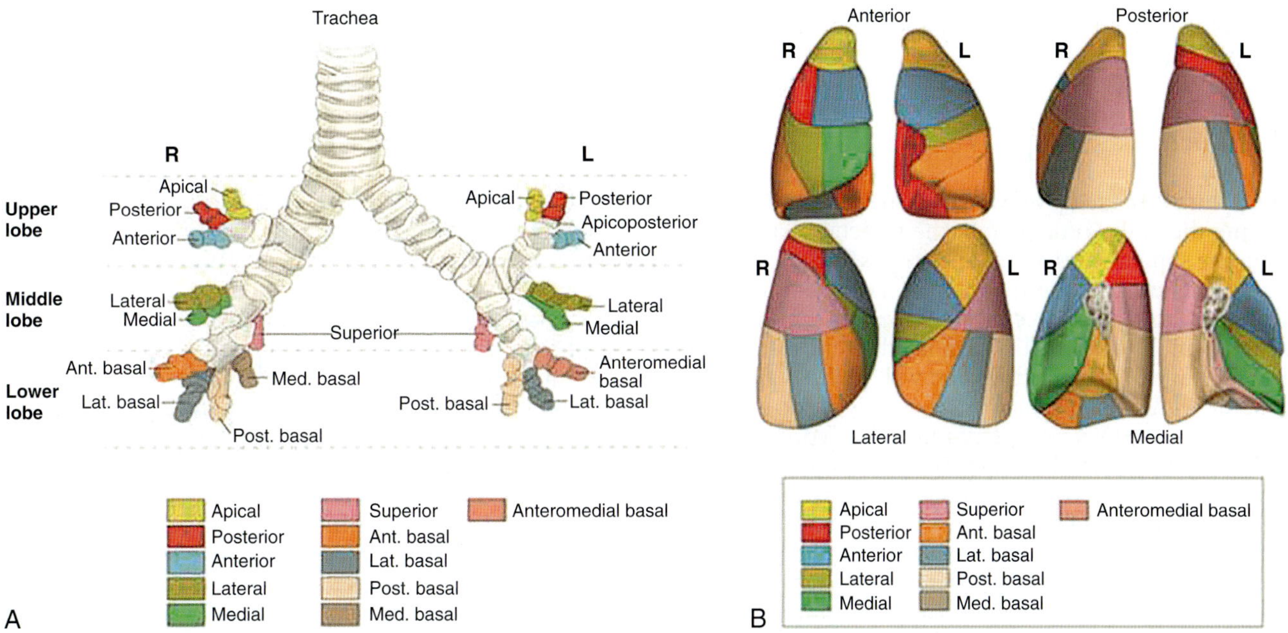

Figure 1.3 (A) Typical 10 and 8 bronchopulmonary segments of the right and left lung, respectively. (B) Lobar and segmental volumetric anatomy for both lungs is illustrated in various projections.

TABLE 1.1 Nomenclature of Pulmonary Segments

RIGHT LUNG	LEFT LUNG
Upper Lobe	
Apical	Apicoposterior
Anterior	Anterior
Posterior	Superior segment (lingula) Inferior segment (lingula)
Middle Lobe	
Lateral	
Medial	
Lower Lobe	
Superior	Superior
Anterior	Anteromedial
Medial	
Lateral	Lateral
Posterior	Posterior

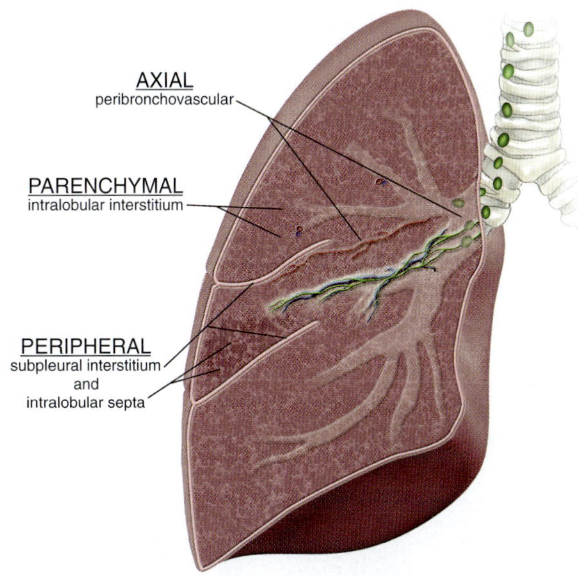

Figure 1.4 Illustration of the axial and peripheral interstitium. The axial interstitium, which surrounds the bronchovascular bundles, is contiguous with the centrilobular interstitium, which surrounds the core structures of the secondary pulmonary lobule. The peripheral interstitium forms the interlobular septa. The parenchymal or intralobar interstitium is the connective tissue support between the centrilobular interstitium and interlobular septa.

Blood Supply and Bronchovascular Anatomy

The connective tissues, bronchi, and pleura are supplied in a dual fashion, in small part by the pulmonary arteries and veins and to a larger degree by the bronchial arteries and veins. The bronchial arteries arise from the aorta, are variable in number (more on the right side), and accompany the airways. Their branching pattern is similar to the bronchial tree. There is extensive anastomosis between the bronchial and pulmonary arteries under the pleura and adjacent to the small bronchi. They can be enlarged, and many chronic conditions are visible on CT, such as cystic fibrosis, bronchopulmonary aspergillosis, and tuberculosis. The bronchial veins drain via the pulmonary veins to the left atrium and the mediastinal veins, which later join the vena cava. The lymphatics drain the loose connective tissue below the pleura, arising from the interlobular septa and periarterial-peribronchial connective tissue. The lymphatics channel the lymph to the tracheal-bronchial, tracheal, and mediastinal lymph nodes.

Pleura

The pleura is made up of two layers, parietal and visceral. During the embryonic period, the parietal pleura arises from the somatic mesoderm and the visceral pleura from the splanchnic mesoderm. The parietal pleura measures about 0.1 mm; the visceral pleura measures about 0.1 to 0.2 mm. The visceral pleura is adherent to the lung and the parietal pleura to the chest wall. There is a negative pressure within the pleural cavity, which is a space between the parietal and visceral pleura normally containing 10 to 20 mL of a plasma-like fluid. The parietal pleura courses along the cervical, costal, diaphragmatic, and mediastinal lung surfaces and reflects to constitute the costodiaphragmatic and costomediastinal recesses. The parietal pleura is supplied by the intercostal neurovascular bundles. Additional innervation comes from the phrenic nerve. The parietal pleura, in contrast to the visceral pleura, is exquisitely sensitive to the sensation of pain. However, the visceral pleura does receive autonomic innervation from the vagus nerve and is involved in some pulmonary reflexes. The visceral pleura receives blood supply from bronchial arteries, and its drainage is via the pulmonary veins; 25 to 75 mL of pleural fluid is necessary to be detectable on a lateral or decubitus examination, whereas 100 to 200 mL is required for the detection of an effusion on a posteroanterior (PA) radiograph.

Lung Fissures

The major and minor fissures are composed of two adjacent layers of visceral pleura and divide the pulmonary parenchyma into different lobes. Other additional fissures are present. The inferior accessory fissure of the lower lobe is the most common accessory fissure and is present in 40% to 50% of pathologic specimens. The fissures' depth and extent are variable but complete in 13% of lower lobes. The inferior accessory fissure can infrequently be identified on both the frontal and lateral chest radiographs and is best identified on CT scans, separating the medial basal segment from the other basal segments. With upper lobe collapse or post–upper lobectomy, the lower lobe expands, and the inferior accessory fissure moves laterally. The origin of the fissure adjacent to the diaphragm is frequently accentuated, forming a juxtaphrenic peak (Fig. 1.5). A superior accessory fissure separates the superior segment from the basal segments. The superior accessory fissure is more common on the right than on the left and, when it is seen on the lateral radiograph, the position is posterior to the major fissure, with a slight caudal inclination at or below the minor fissure. Infrequently, a left minor fissure and other accessory fissures of the upper lobes can be identified (Fig. 1.6). The azygos lobe is a normal variant, with an incidence of 0.4% to 1.0%, and is seen as a pleural line that crosses the right lung apex. The azygos vein is contained within this fissure and, although its position is variable within the fissure, it is usually seen in the lowermost aspect as a teardrop-shaped structure. The azygos lobe is formed when the right posterior cardinal vein, the embryologic precursor to the azygos vein, courses through the right upper lobe (RUL) instead of migrating medially. The azygos fissure is unique, except for its less frequent counterpart in the left upper lobe (LUL), in that it contains four layers of pleura instead of the usual two layers of visceral pleura. The inferior pulmonary ligaments contain a double layer of visceral pleura that tethers the mediastinum to the lungs and extends inferiorly from the pulmonary hila to the diaphragm; it may contain systemic vessels, nerves, and lymphatics. On axial CT, the inferior pulmonary ligament is visible in 40%

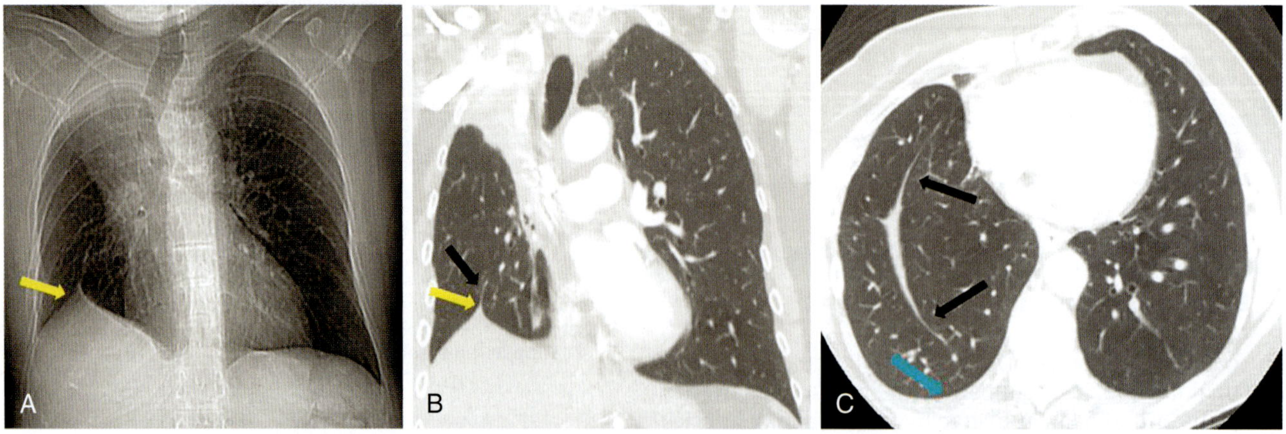

Figure 1.5 This 65-year-old woman had underlying lung carcinoma treated with radiation therapy. (A) Frontal scout film and associated CT images (B, C) show volume loss in the right upper lobe, with an elevated right hemidiaphragm and juxtaphrenic peak *(yellow arrow)*. (B) Coronal multiplanar reconstruction image demonstrates the inferior accessory fissure *(black arrow)* displaced laterally, with a juxtaphrenic peak *(yellow arrow)* that contains pleural fluid and extrapleural fat. (C) Axial CT image demonstrates the curvilinear appearance of the inferior accessory fissure *(black arrows)*, with fluid in it, and the relative expansion of the medial basal segment of the right lower lobe. Note the small posterior pleural effusion *(blue arrow)*.

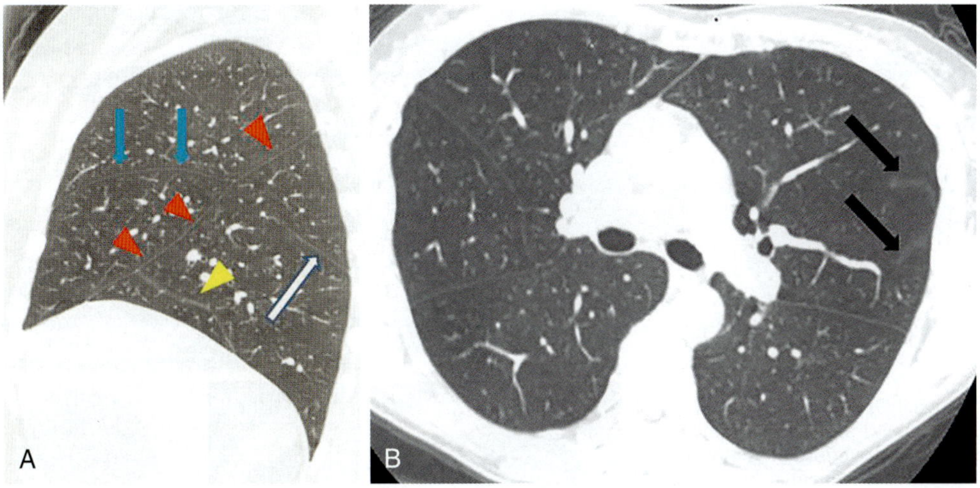

Figure 1.6 (A) Superior accessory fissure of the right lower lobe (RLL) seen on a sagittal multiplanar reconstruction image. A superior accessory fissure *(white arrow)* of the RLL separates the superior segment from the basal segments of the lower lobe and resides posterior to the major fissure *(red arrowheads)* on the lateral and inferior to the minor fissure *(blue arrows)* when present. An inferior accessory fissure is seen inferiorly *(yellow arrowhead)*. (B) Left upper lobe accessory fissure *(arrows)* on an axial CT image are seen as a curvilinear band, with an adjacent avascular zone. The right minor and major fissures can be seen in the contralateral lung.

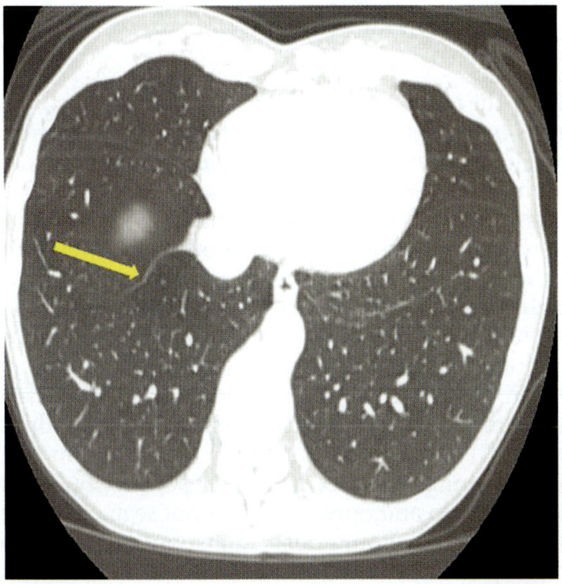

Figure 1.7 Axial CT image shows the pleural reflection *(yellow arrow)* over the right phrenic nerve, lateral to the inferior vena cava.

to 70% of the general population. It is seen as a triangular opacity just inferior to the inferior pulmonary veins and is extrapulmonary in location. Thin linear and curvilinear densities are sometimes seen anterior to the inferior pulmonary ligaments and represent pleural reflections over the phrenic nerve (Fig. 1.7).

Fissures are best seen on CT because the x-ray beam may not be perpendicular to the fissure on the radiographs (Fig. 1.8). Because the major fissures are oriented obliquely relative to the scan plane, their appearance may vary depending on the slice thickness and effects of volume averaging. An avascular band is associated with the fissures due to the small size of the vessels located in the peripheral lung on either side of the fissure (Fig. 1.9). A few small dots in relation to the fissures or at the pleural surface may be seen in normal subjects, reflecting the presence of subpleural veins or points of intersection of interlobular septa with the pleural surfaces.

Radiology

Normal Chest X-Ray

Plain chest radiography is a cost-effective, high-yield examination of the entire thorax. The three most common views of the chest are the upright PA, lateral, and anteroposterior (AP) views. The preferred examination is in the radiology department PA and lateral views. Approximately 25% of the lung volume and 40% of the pleural surface reside in relative blind areas on the frontal radiograph, behind the mediastinal silhouette in the retrocardiac space and behind the diaphragms in the costophrenic angles. The lateral view helps identify abnormalities in the retrocardiac region, within the mediastinum, paraspinal location, and costophrenic angles. Single-view, bedside portal AP examinations account for approximately one-half of all plain chest radiographs. On the AP view, the cardiomediastinal silhouette appears about 15% wider than on the PA view and can lead to a higher incidence of reported false-positives of cardiomegaly. In addition to magnification issues, AP portable radiography frequently is plagued by technical issues related to patient positioning and a lower energy technique.

The mediastinal silhouette on the PA view consists of the heart, hila, fat, and great vessels. Mediastinal border-forming structures on the frontal radiograph with the adjacent lung include the innominate and subclavian

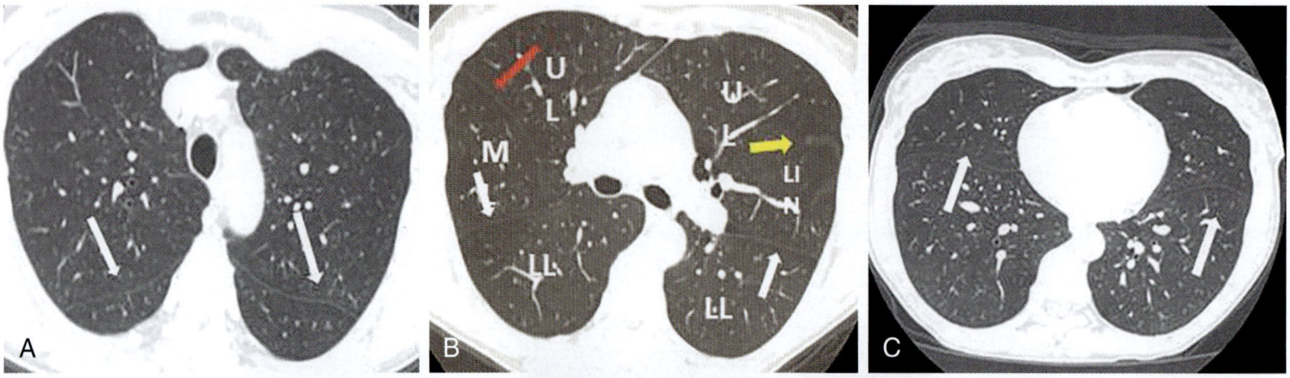

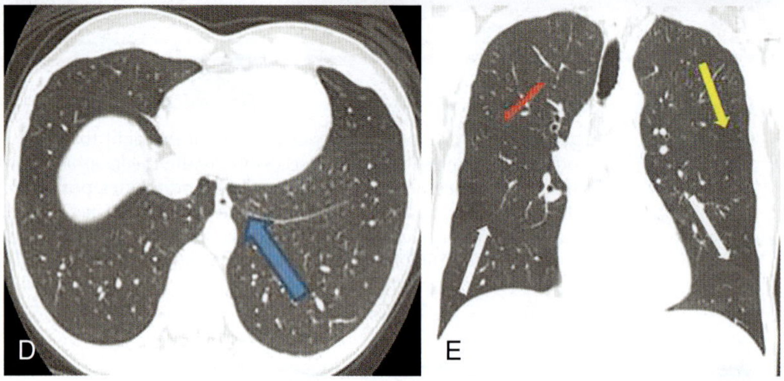

Figure 1.8 (A–D) Axial CT images show both oblique fissures *(white arrows)* in the right and left lungs as thin lines moving posterior to anterior as the fissures move caudally on sequential images. Also note the minor fissure *(red arrows)* extending from medial to lateral in the right lung. (B) The fissures demarcate the upper *(U)*, middle *(M)*, and lower *(L)* lobes on the right. Incidental note is also made of an incomplete left minor fissure *(yellow arrow)* in (B) and (E) delineating the lingula from the remainder of the left upper lobe. (D) The inferior pulmonary ligament (IPL) is seen as a triangular structure *(blue arrow)* lateral to the esophagus; the pleural reflections extend outward from the IPL.

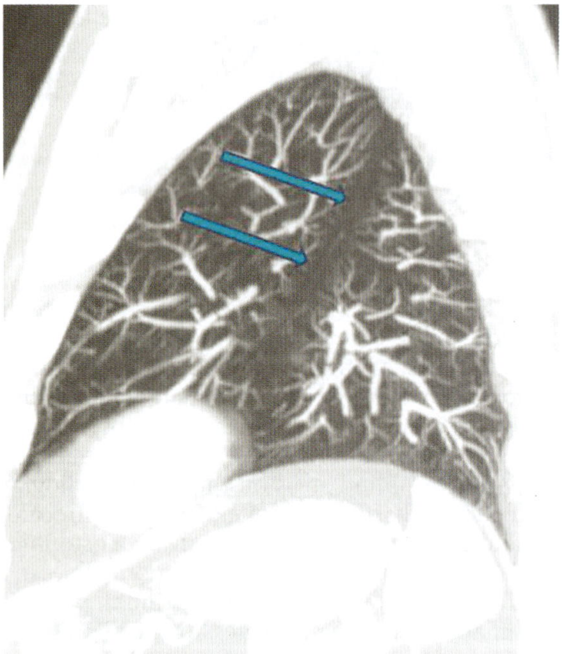

Figure 1.9 Sagittal maximum intensity projection image shows an avascular zone along the left oblique fissure *(blue arrows)*.

vessels, aorta, SVC–right paratracheal soft tissues, azygos arch, left main pulmonary artery and both hila, right atrium, left atrial appendage, and left ventricle (Fig. 1.10A). Mediastinal border-forming structures on the lateral film include the right ventricle, pulmonary outflow tract, aorta, retrotracheal stripe (posterior wall of the trachea and esophagus), left atrium, left ventricle, and IVC (see Fig. 1.10B). The pulmonary arteries and accompanying bronchi are the major contributors to the hila on both the frontal and lateral chest radiographs. The density of the hila and their size are nearly symmetric, with concave lateral margins. The left hilum sits cephalad to the right hilum. The hilar angle, whose apex points medially, is formed by the junction of the superior pulmonary vein and interlobar pulmonary artery. The superior aspect of the right hilum on the frontal view is formed by the truncus anterior and superior pulmonary vein, with the inferior portion consisting of the interlobar pulmonary artery ($\leq$16 mm) and the bronchus intermedius medially (see Fig. 1.10C). The superior margin of the left hilum on the frontal examination is formed by the superior pulmonary artery and vein and upper lobe anterior segmental artery, with the interlobar pulmonary artery forming the inferior margin (see Fig. 1.10C). The superior pulmonary veins on the frontal radiograph are positioned medially and are frequently difficult to recognize as distinct structures, whereas the inferior pulmonary veins are posterior and reside behind the cardiac silhouette on the frontal view; these are the major component of the structures posterior and inferior to the infrahilar window on the lateral view. Lymph nodes are infrequently identified on plain radiographs unless they are enlarged (e.g., bulging contour, increased density, or exhibit mass effect) and thus, when identified, are considered abnormal. The pulmonary arteries are parabronchocentric. The right pulmonary artery (epiarterial bronchus) and left pulmonary artery (hyparterial bronchus) can be localized relative to the right upper bronchus and bronchus intermedius and left main stem bronchus, respectively, on the lateral view (Fig. 1.11). The posterior wall of the bronchus intermedius should be no thicker than 3 mm.

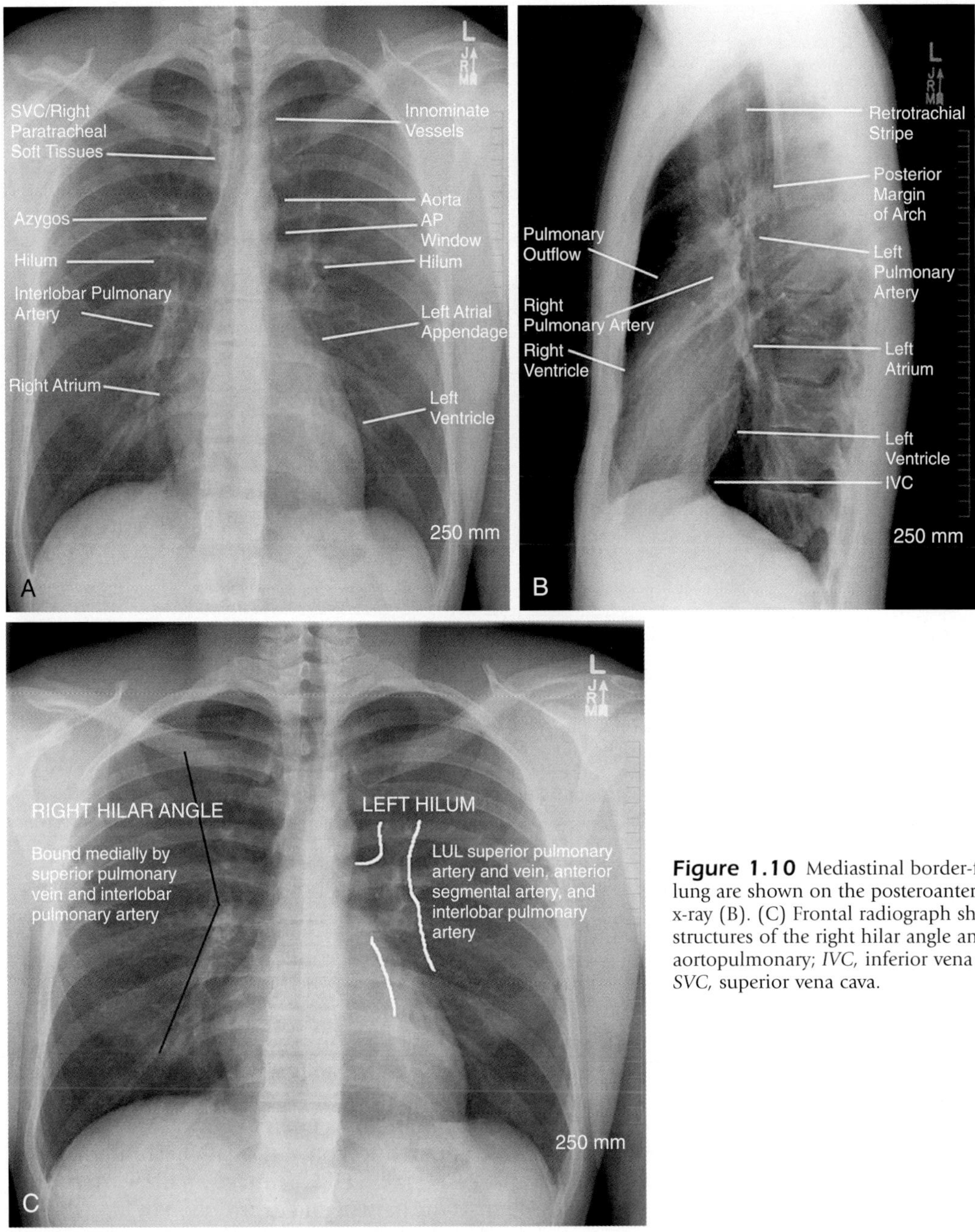

Figure 1.10 Mediastinal border-forming structures with the lung are shown on the posteroanterior (A) and lateral chest x-ray (B). (C) Frontal radiograph shows border-forming structures of the right hilar angle and left hilum. *AP,* aortopulmonary; *IVC,* inferior vena cava; *LUL,* left upper lobe; *SVC,* superior vena cava.

Localization of pathology within the lungs is most easily determined relative to the lobar or segmental anatomy. Lobar anatomy on a plain chest radiograph can be determined relative to the pleural fissures. The right minor fissure (horizontal) separates the RUL from the right middle lobe (RML) and can often be seen on both the frontal and lateral views. The major fissure (oblique) separates the lower lobes from the other lobes and can best be seen on the lateral view. The major fissures can be differentiated on the lateral view by the intersection of the minor fissure with the right major fissure, the left major fissure by its interface with the left hemidiaphragm and cardiac apex (being obscured when it comes in contact with the mediastinum), and the relative position of the fissures, with the major right fissure frequently being seen more caudal in location posteriorly over the spine and having a more horizontal course (Fig. 1.12).

Computed Tomography

Noncontrast and contrast-enhanced spiral CT are used to evaluate the pulmonary parenchyma and airways and to characterize mediastinal, vascular, and lung masses, respectively. The dataset is collected as a volume and can easily be used to create maximum intensity projection image for vascular evaluation and lung nodule detection, and minimum intensity projection images to evaluate air trapping, emphysema, and tracheobronchial lesions; multiplanar reconstruction images are routinely used for

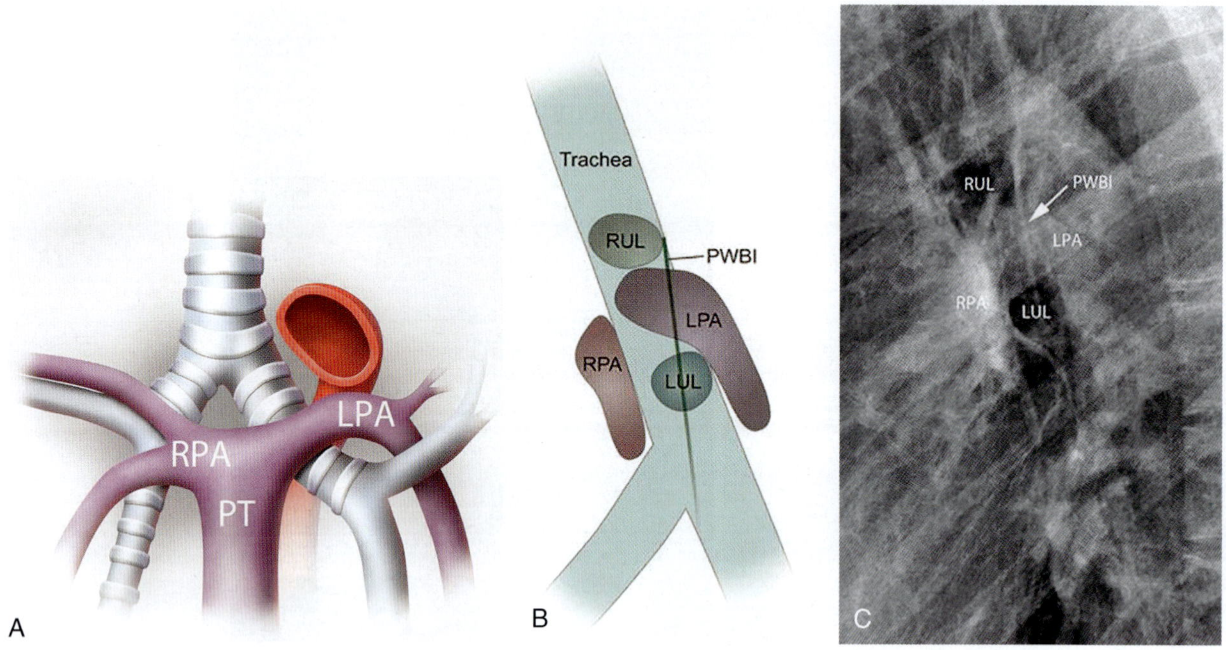

Figure 1.11 (A) Frontal and (B) lateral drawings show the relationship of the pulmonary arteries to the trachea, upper lobe bronchi, and bronchus intermedius. The right pulmonary artery runs anterior and adjacent to the right main stem bronchus, right upper lobe *(RUL)* bronchus, and bronchus intermedius. The right main stem bronchus is referred to as the *epiarterial bronchus*. The left pulmonary artery crosses over and then posterior to the left main stem bronchus. This airway is referred to as the *hyparterial bronchus*. This anatomic arrangement defines a right and a left lung. On (B) and (C), the left-sided hypoarterial main stem bronchus is seen inferior to the left main pulmonary artery and right main pulmonary artery, and the right interlobar pulmonary artery is seen adjacent to the bronchus intermedius. (C) Targeted lateral image demonstrates the anatomic relationship of both hila on a lateral chest radiograph. On a nonrotated image, the posterior wall of the bronchus intermedius typically bisects the lucent area of the left upper lobe *(LUL)* bronchus seen on end. *BI*, Bronchus intermedius; *LPA*, left pulmonary artery; *PT*, pulmonary trunk; *PWBI*, posterior wall of bronchus intermedius; *RPA*, right pulmonary artery.

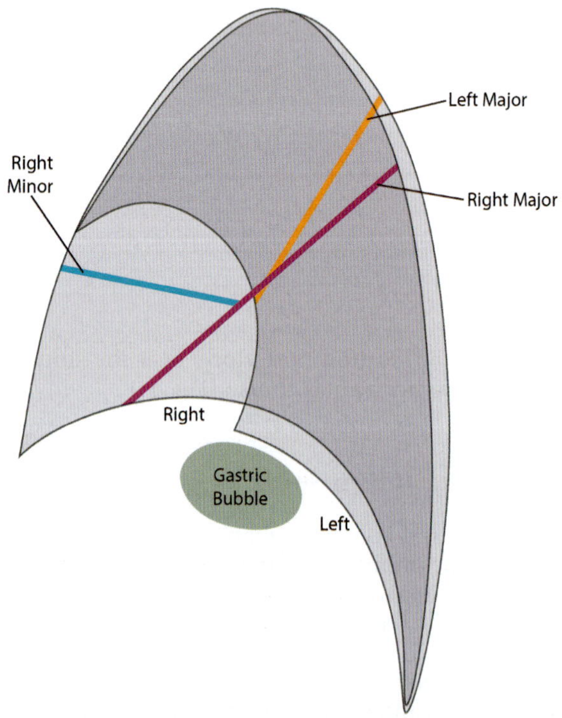

Figure 1.12 Drawing showing the relationship of the major and minor fissures to each other and to the mediastinum.

sagittal and coronal projections for localization and image interpretation (Fig. 1.13).

Thin section (1–1.25 mm) reconstructions and a high spatial frequency algorithm are used to obtain HRCT images and to evaluate patients with known or suspected interstitial lung disease, vascular related perfusion abnormalities, and small airway disease.

When compared to conventional chest radiographs, CT scans—especially HRCT images—allow improved assessment of the pattern and distribution of lung disease in relation to the lobar and interstitial anatomy, as well as provide an accurate delineation of the extent of pulmonary parenchymal abnormalities.

The pulmonary artery and adjacent bronchi are usually of similar size throughout the lung. However, the vessels can be larger in the dependent lung due to the gravitationally increased blood flow. In normal patients, the outer walls of the arteries exhibit a sharp interface with the surrounding lung, and the walls of the bronchi should appear smooth and uniform in thickness. Bronchi can be traced to approximately 1 cm from the pleural margin.

Computed Tomography of the Hilar Bronchi

The appearance of the bronchi, vessels, and nodes and their relationship vary between the hila and are described

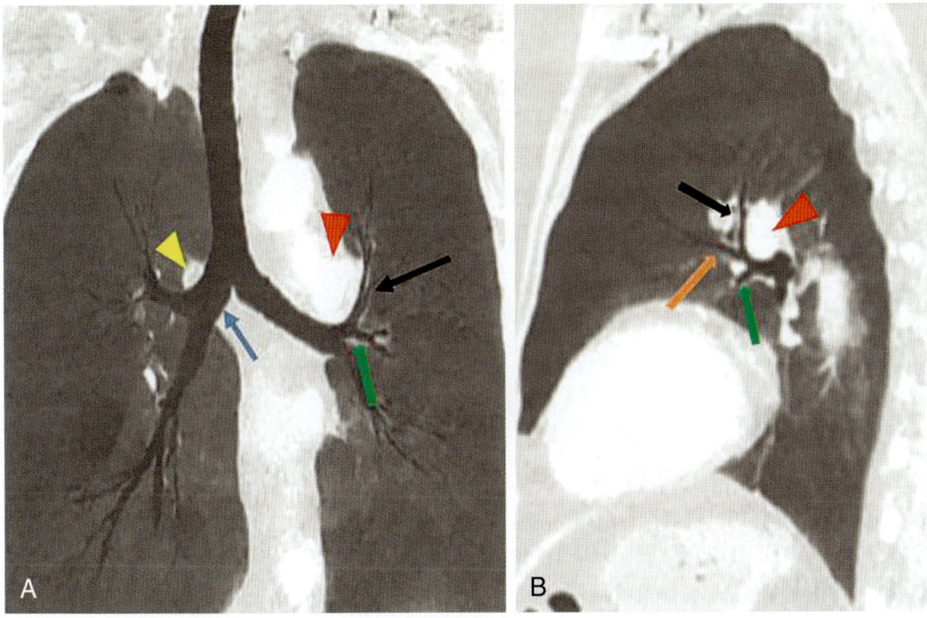

Figure 1.13 Bronchial anatomy on minimum intensity projection images. (A) Paracoronal and (B) sagittal images of the lung demonstrate the normal bronchia. The right main bronchus *(blue arrow)* is shorter than the left main bronchus. The left main bronchus gives rise to the left upper lobe (LUL) and lower lobe bronchus. The LUL bronchus divides into the superior trunk, which divides into the apicoposterior *(long black arrow)* and anterior segment *(orange arrow)*, and the lingular trunk *(green arrow)* divides into the superior and inferior segmental branches. The azygous vein is seen as an elliptic structure overt the right main bronchus *(yellow arrowhead)* in (A). The left pulmonary artery *(red arrowhead)* is seen to course superior to the left bronchus in (B). Medium and long arrows show the anterior and apicoposterior segmental bronchus, respectively.

in the following section. On spiral CT, all lobar and segmental bronchi should be visible, with a slice thickness of 3 to 5 mm.

The bronchi seen in the long axis on axial scans include the following:

1. RUL bronchus, including its anterior and posterior segmental bronchi
2. LUL bronchus, including its anterior segmental bronchus
3. Portion of RML bronchus
4. Superior segmental bronchi of both lower lobes

Bronchi seen in the short axis as round structures on axial scans include the following:

1. Apical segmental bronchus of the RUL
2. Apicoposterior segmental bronchus of the LUL
3. Proximal portions of both lower lobe bronchi
4. Medial and posterior basal lower lobe segmental bronchi

The remaining bronchi appear elliptic.

Bronchial Anatomy

Right Bronchial Anatomy

The right main stem bronchus is relatively short in length and divides into the RUL bronchus and bronchus intermedius. The apical, anterior, and posterior segmental bronchi arise from the upper lobe bronchus. The origin of the apical segmental bronchus can be superimposed on the distal RUL bronchus at or immediately superior to the origin of the anterior and posterior segmental bronchi. The tracheal bronchus (bronchus suis) is an uncommon accessory bronchus that comes directly from the trachea (Fig. 1.14A). The bronchus intermedius originates distal to the origin of the RUL bronchus and measures about 3 to 4 cm in length; therefore it can be seen in consecutive scans in cross section, with a thin sharp posterior wall usually measuring between 0.5 and 2.0 mm. The upper limit of normal is 3 mm (see Fig. 1.14B). The accessory cardiac bronchus is an anomalous bronchus that can originate from the medial bronchus intermedius or lower lobe bronchus, and it courses medially (see Fig. 1.14C). It may supply a portion of aerated or nonaerated (nonfunctional) lung anatomy. The bronchus intermedius divides into an RML bronchus and RLL bronchus. The RML is short (1–2 cm), with the medial and lateral segments being similar in size in most cases. However, the medial segmental bronchus is larger in 40% of cases. Both bronchi traverse inferiorly and are visible as elliptic structures.

The RLL bronchus is a very short bronchus, with the superior segmental bronchus arising shortly after its origin; distal to this, it divides into the four basal segments of the RLL. The superior segmental bronchus is 1 cm in length and arises posteriorly. Distally, the medial, anterior, lateral, and posterior basal segments are arranged medially to laterally in a counterclockwise direction (Fig. 1.15).

Left Bronchial Anatomy

The LUL bronchus is 2 to 3 cm in length and branches into a superior segment and lingular bronchus. The superior trunk is about 1 cm in length and gives rise to the anterior and apicoposterior segmental bronchus (Fig. 1.16A and B). In about 25% of the general population, the LUL bronchus trifurcates into the apicoposterior segmental bronchus, and anterior and lingular bronchi. The left main and upper lobe bronchi are outlined by the lung and show a very thin retrobronchial stripe. In about 10% of the general population, this stripe is not visualized—the left lung does not contact the bronchial wall because the descending pulmonary artery is positioned more medially. Thickening of the retrobronchial stripe is concerning for hilar or airway pathology. The anterior segment bronchus of the LUL lies longitudinally

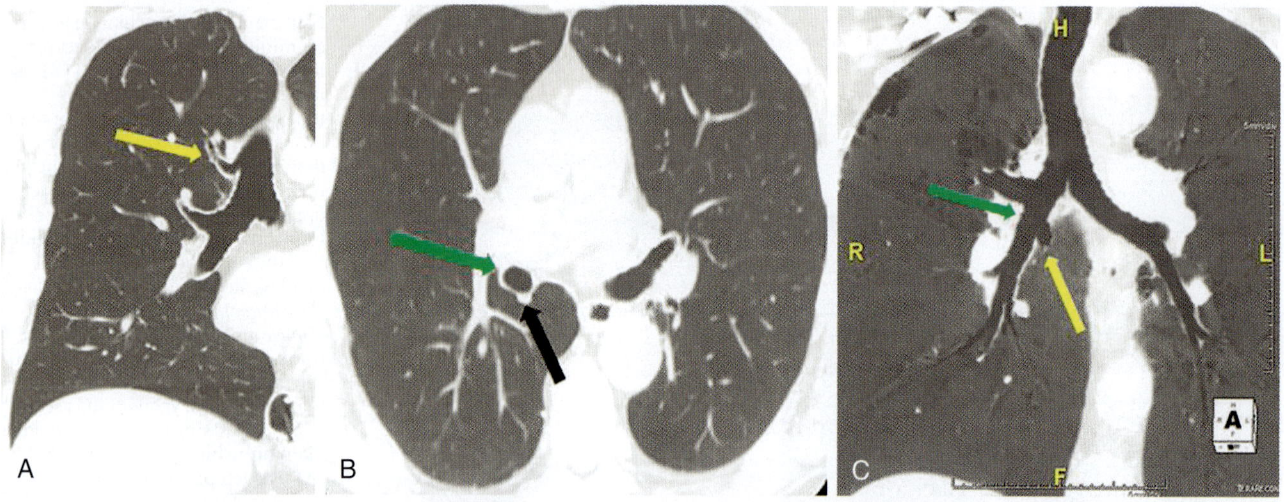

Figure 1.14 (A) Bronchus suis *(yellow arrow)* shown on coronal multiplanar reconstruction image of the right hemothorax as a short bronchus connecting the medial right upper lobe directly to the trachea. The bronchus intermedius (*green arrow* in B) may have a small anomalous pulmonary vein positioned behind it. (B) When present, this vein usually drains the posterior right upper lobe. Cardiac bronchus *(yellow arrow)* on paracoronal minimum intensity projection is shown arising from the bronchus intermedius with abrupt termination (C). Note emphysematous changes in the lungs in (C).

in the axial plane, whereas the apicoposterior segmental bronchus is seen in cross section. The lingular bronchus courses obliquely from the inferior aspect of the upper lobe bronchus and appears elliptic on axial images (see Fig. 1.16C). It measures 2 to 3 cm in length before dividing into superior and inferior segmental branches. Typically, the LLL bronchus branches into three basal segments. The medial and anterior basilar bronchi form a common trunk; the other two are the lateral and posterior basal segments (see Fig. 1.16E).

Computed Tomography of Hilar Vessels

The hilar vessels usually have a fixed relationship with respect to the bronchi. The greatest variation is in the pulmonary venous drainage. This anatomic arrangement helps in their identification.

Right Side

The truncus anterior is the first major branch of the right main pulmonary artery and is similar in size to the right main stem bronchus. At the carina, the apical segmental artery typically lies medially to the bronchus, and the later branch of the superior pulmonary vein lies laterally to the bronchus (Fig. 1.17A). The lateral branch of the right superior pulmonary vein lies in the angle formed by the bifurcation of the anterior and posterior RUL bronchi. At the level of the bronchus intermedius, the interlobar pulmonary artery lies anterior and lateral to the bronchus. The lower lobe pulmonary artery is lateral to the middle and lower lobe bronchi. The RML arteries parallel the corresponding RML bronchi. The lower lobe pulmonary artery divides into two branches, which terminate into four basilar segmental pulmonary arteries. These travel posterolaterally to the proximal basilar segmental bronchi. The right superior pulmonary vein is anterior to the right interlobar pulmonary artery and passes anteriorly and medially to the middle and lower lobe bronchi (see Fig. 1.17B). The inferior pulmonary veins travel posteriorly to the lower lobe bronchi and arteries before draining into the lower left atrium.

Left Side

The anatomic variation on the left is far more common than on the right. At the level of the upper lobe segmental bronchi, the artery supplying the anterior segment of the LUL is medial to the anterior segment bronchus. At the level of the LUL bronchus, the interlobar left pulmonary artery produces a posterior bulging margin to the hilum, whereas the superior pulmonary vein forms the anterior bulging margin. At the lingular bronchus level, the left interlobar pulmonary artery is lateral to the lower lobe bronchi, immediately posterolateral to the lingular bronchus. The superior pulmonary vein runs anteriorly and medially to the bronchi to enter the left hilum (see Fig. 1.17C). The superior pulmonary veins course obliquely in an inferomedial direction as they approach the hilum, whereas the inferior pulmonary veins have a more horizontal course in the periphery before they take a vertical course. The veins pass anteroinferior to the pulmonary arteries, forming a short intrapericardial segment that drains into the left atrium.

Computed Tomography of the Hilar Lymph Nodes

In normal subjects, it is common to see unenhanced soft tissue composed of small nodes and fat, ranging in size up to 1.5 cm at the level of the bifurcation of the main pulmonary artery, anterolateral to the bronchus intermedius and medial to the superior pulmonary vein. Normal nodes measure up to 3 mm in size, except in the following locations:

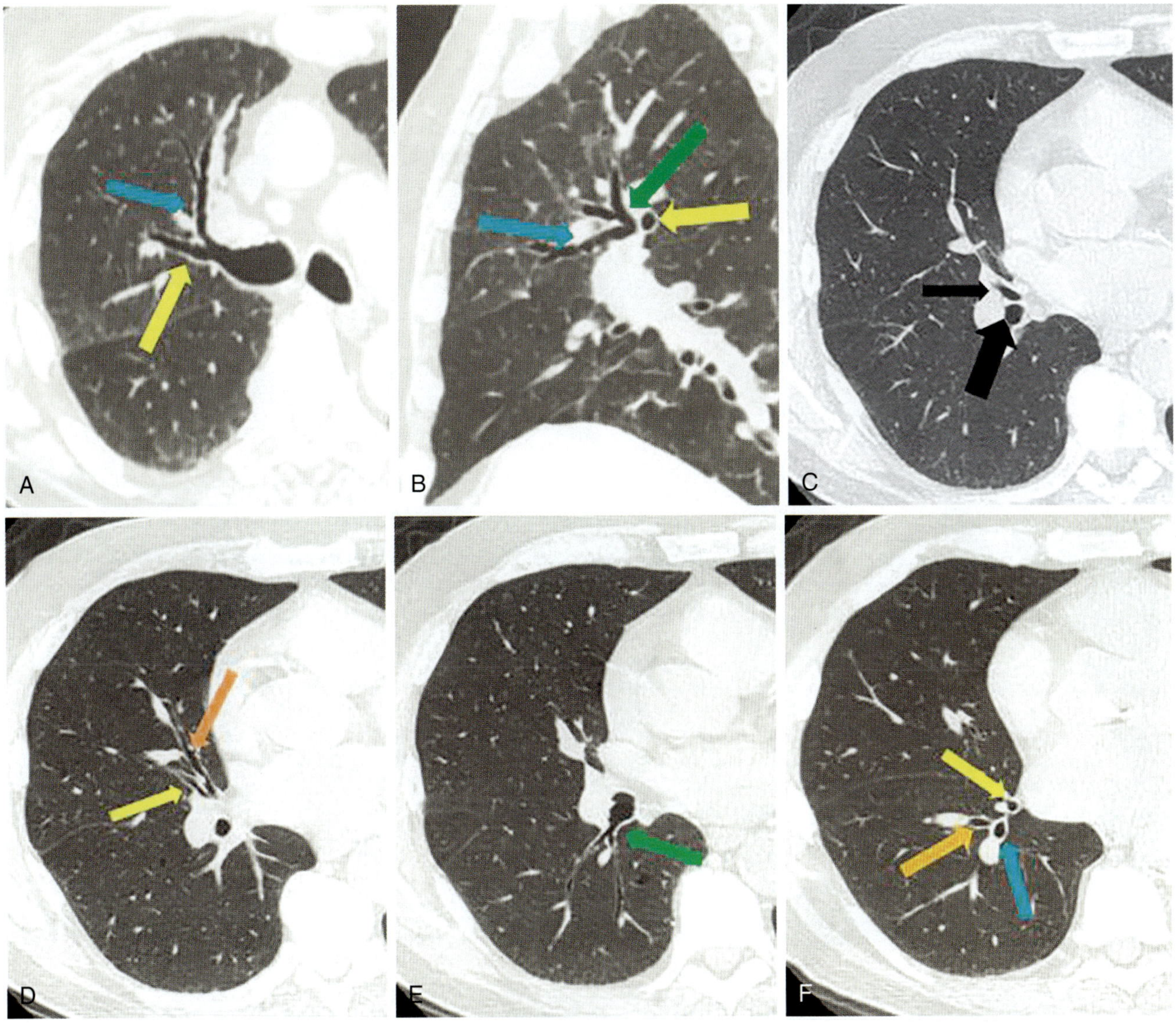

Figure 1.15 Axial and coronal images showing the segmental bronchial anatomy to the right lung. Right upper lobe (RUL) segmental bronchial anatomy shown on images (A) and (B). (A) At the level of the RUL bronchus shows the anterior segmental *(blue arrow)* and posterior segmental *(yellow arrow)* bronchi to the RUL. (B) The posterior segmental bronchus to the RUL on end *(yellow arrow)* and segmental and subsegmental bronchi to the apical *(green arrow)* and anterior *(blue arrow)* segments are shown. (C) This view, just caudal to the bronchus intermedius, shows the lobar bronchi to the right middle lobe (RML) *(thin arrow)* and right lower lobe (RLL) *(thick arrow)*. (D) The lateral *(yellow arrow)* and medial *(orange arrow)* segmental bronchi to the RML are shown. (E) The superior segmental bronchus *(green arrow)* to the RLL is seen originating in a posterolateral direction from the RLL lobar bronchus. (F) Distal to that, in a counterclockwise rotation, the medial segmental bronchus *(yellow arrow)*, anterior basal segmental bronchus *(orange arrow)*, and a common trunk to the posterior and lateral basal segments *(blue arrow)* are seen.

1. At the bifurcation of the right pulmonary artery and bronchus intermedius, where nodes can measure up to 1.5 cm
2. Adjacent to the RML bronchus, up to 1 cm
3. Adjacent to the LUL and lingular bronchi, up to 1 cm

Bronchoarterial Ratio and Bronchial Wall Thickness

The bronchoarterial (BA) ratio is defined as the endoluminal diameter of the bronchus divided by the diameter of the adjacent pulmonary artery. A normal value ranges from 0.65 to 0.70; a BA ratio greater than 1 is usually considered to be the cutoff point to suggest bronchiectasis. However, a ratio greater than 1 can be seen with increasing age and in patients who live at a high altitude. The bronchial wall thickness-to-diameter (TD) ratio averages about 20% and is best measured on lung windows (Fig. 1.18). The visibility of airways depends on their size and the CT imaging technique being used. Smaller caliber airways are more easily seen with HRCT. There is a subpleural radiolucent zone on CT, 5 mm in width, devoid of any vessels, and 10 mm, devoid of any bronchioles.

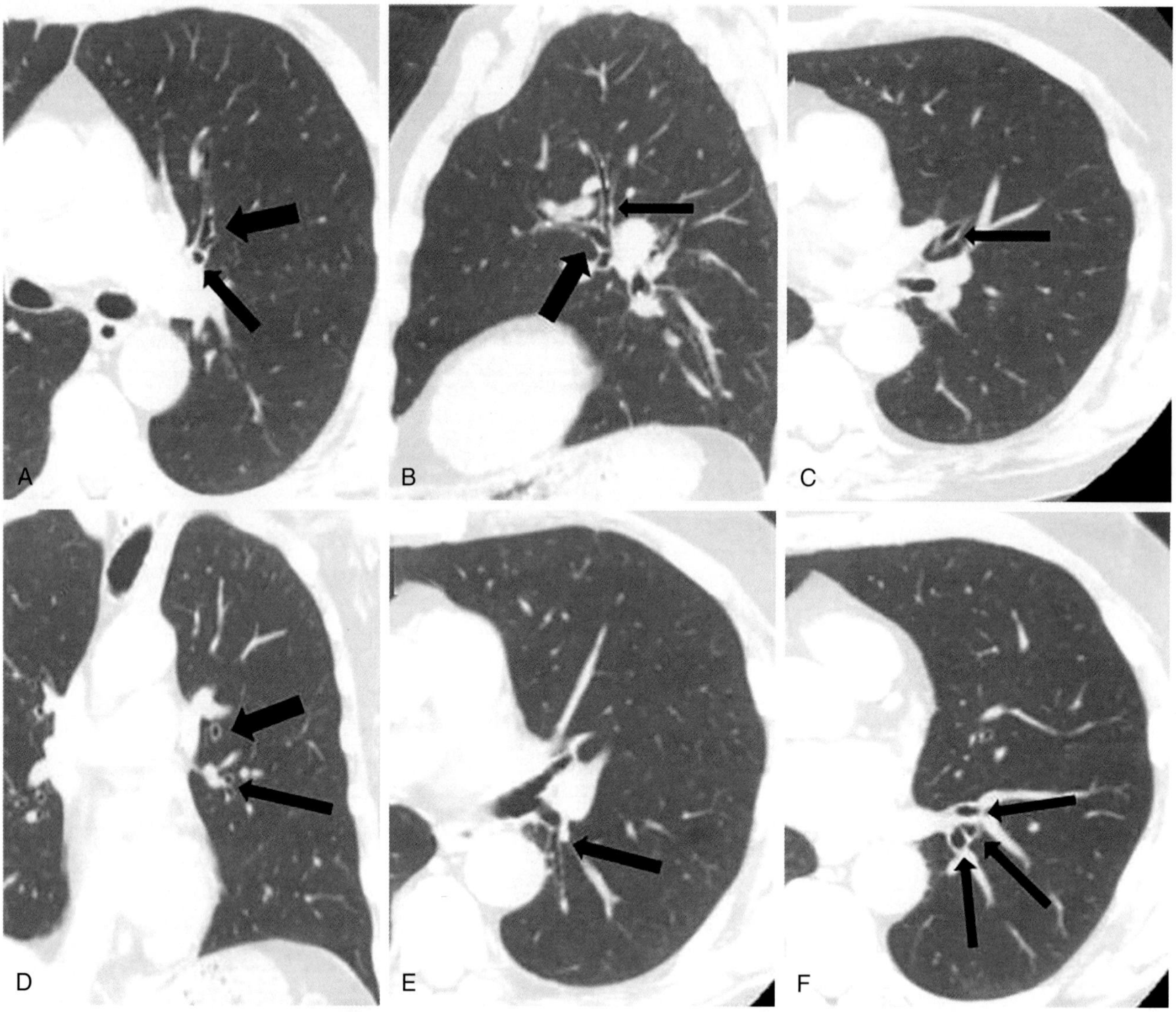

Figure 1.16 Apicoposterior *(thin arrow)* and anterior *(thick arrow)* segmental bronchi of the left upper lobe (LUL) are seen on axial (A) and sagittal (B) images. (C) Axial image shows the lingular bronchus *(arrow)*. (D) The bronchi to the anterior segment LUL *(thick arrow)* and superior segmental bronchus *(arrow)*, just beyond the bifurcation *(arrow)* of the lingular trunk, are seen on this coronal image. (E, F) Axial images at the level of the left lower lobe segmental bronchi show the superior bronchus (*arrow* on E) and anteromedial, lateral, and posterior basal segmental bronchi (clockwise rotation; *arrows* on F).

Normal intralobular bronchioles within the SPL exhibit a wall thickness of less than 0.1 mm and are normally imperceptible. The presence of visible bronchial structures in the lung periphery (within 1 cm of pleura) signifies bronchial wall thickening or ectasia of small airways.

■ Lung Attenuation

The lung parenchyma should appear denser than the air. Inhomogeneous distribution of lung tissue and contained air, as well as hemoglobin in the small vessels, contribute to the varying density of parenchyma. The lung density decreases when lung volume is increased. Due to gravity and increased vascularity in the lower lobes, the lung density is higher in the dependent areas. This attenuation generally increases gradually from anterior to posterior. However, the posterior lingula and superior segments of the lower lobes can appear relatively lucent due to the paucity of bronchovascular bundles. The normal range of pulmonary attenuation on HRCT measures from −700 Hounsfield units (HU) to −860 HU. Mean attenuation values in the posterior third of the lung may differ from the anterior lung by as much as 100 HU, with less variation on deep inspiration.

Expiratory HRCT is used to detect air trapping in patients with small airway obstruction and emphysema. On HRCT, there is a normal reduction in airway size and an increase in lung attenuation, ranging from 80 HU to more than 300 HU on these scans compared to the inspiratory scans. The cross-sectional area of the trachea, main bronchi, and lobar bronchi also decrease with full

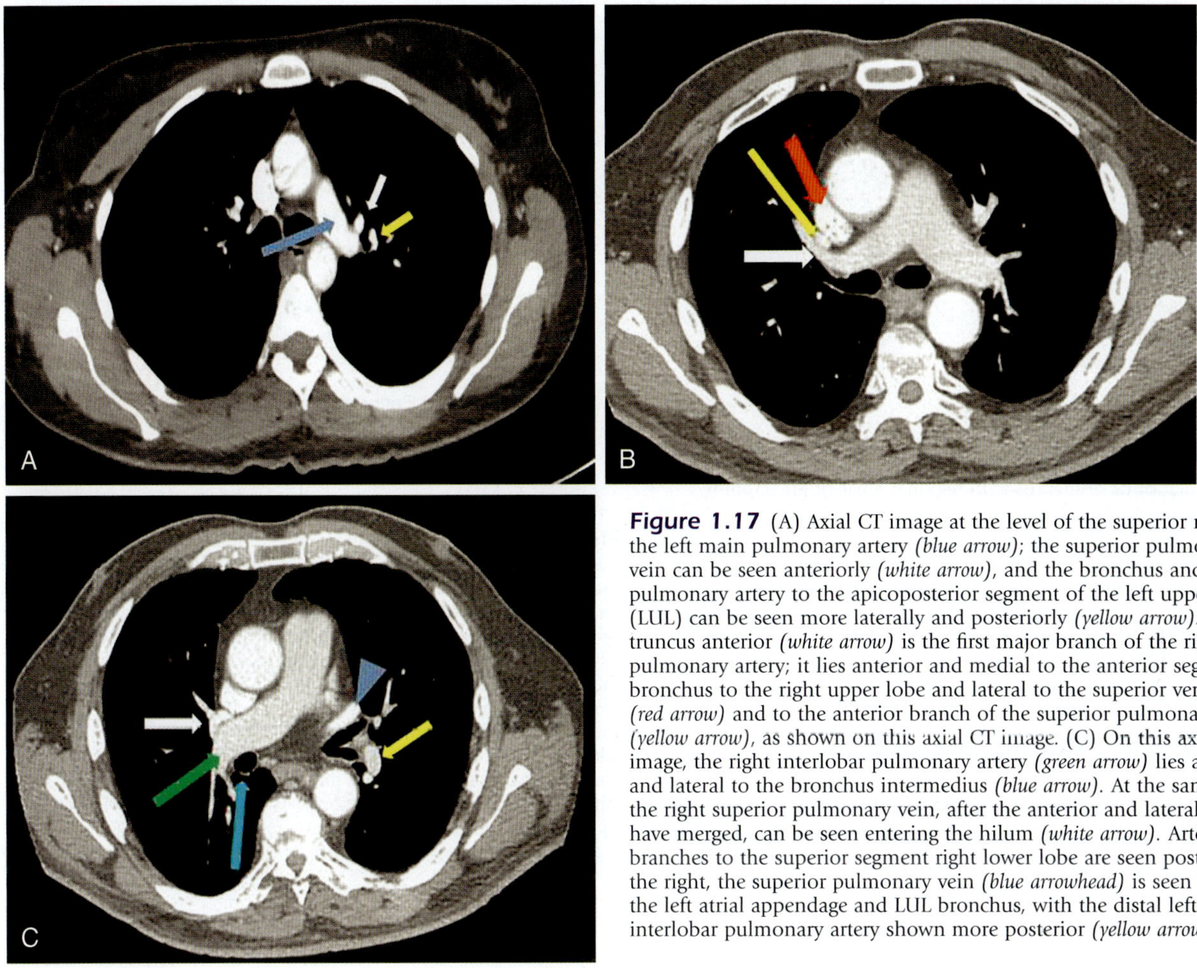

Figure 1.17 (A) Axial CT image at the level of the superior margin of the left main pulmonary artery *(blue arrow)*; the superior pulmonary vein can be seen anteriorly *(white arrow)*, and the bronchus and pulmonary artery to the apicoposterior segment of the left upper lobe (LUL) can be seen more laterally and posteriorly *(yellow arrow)*. (B) The truncus anterior *(white arrow)* is the first major branch of the right main pulmonary artery; it lies anterior and medial to the anterior segmental bronchus to the right upper lobe and lateral to the superior vena cava *(red arrow)* and to the anterior branch of the superior pulmonary vein *(yellow arrow)*, as shown on this axial CT image. (C) On this axial CT image, the right interlobar pulmonary artery *(green arrow)* lies anterior and lateral to the bronchus intermedius *(blue arrow)*. At the same level, the right superior pulmonary vein, after the anterior and lateral branches have merged, can be seen entering the hilum *(white arrow)*. Arterial branches to the superior segment right lower lobe are seen posterior. On the right, the superior pulmonary vein *(blue arrowhead)* is seen between the left atrial appendage and LUL bronchus, with the distal left interlobar pulmonary artery shown more posterior *(yellow arrow)*.

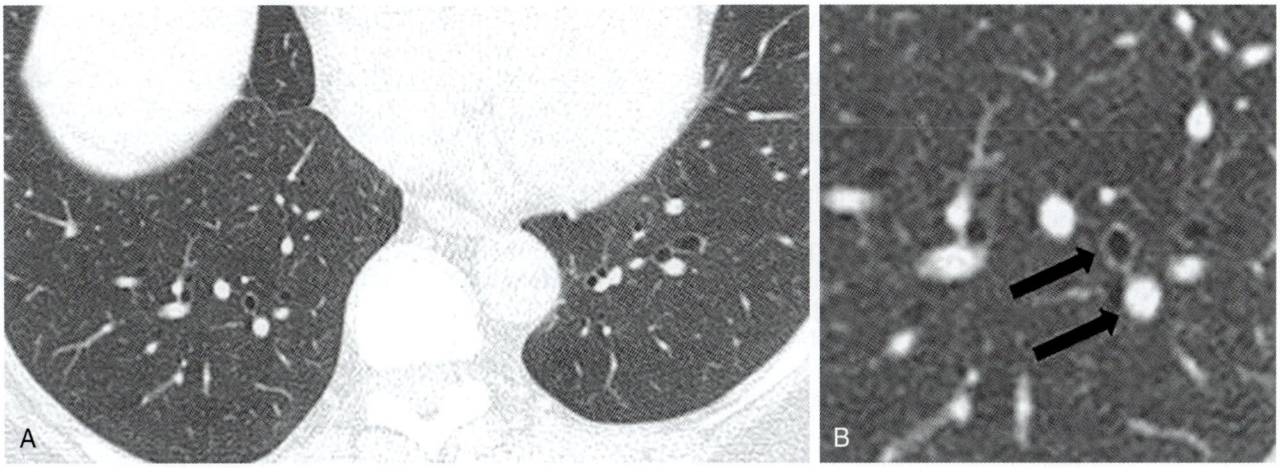

Figure 1.18 (A) The normal bronchoarterial ratio on CT is less than 1, as seen on the axial high-resolution CT image. (B) Magnified image from the posterior basal segment of the right lower lobe shows a normal subsegmental bronchus, with its accompanying artery *(arrows)*.

expiration, with bowing of the posterior wall (Fig. 1.19). There is normally up to less than a 50% decrease in the AP diameter of the trachea on the expiratory scan. Air trapping may result from airway obstruction or abnormal lung compliance. Air trapping is present if the lung parenchyma shows less than a normal increase in lung attenuation on the expiratory images. Insignificant air trapping can be seen in smokers, older adults, and normal patients and is most common in the dependent lung and superior segments of the lower lobes. In normal patients, it should involve no more than 25% of the lungs and is considered significant if it involves three or

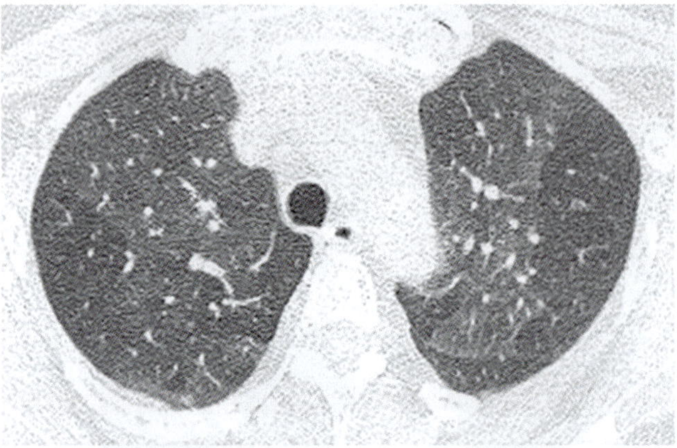

Figure 1.19 Expiratory high-resolution CT axial image at the level of the transverse aortic arch, with underlying mosaic attenuation secondary to bronchiolitis obliterans with regional areas or air trapping.

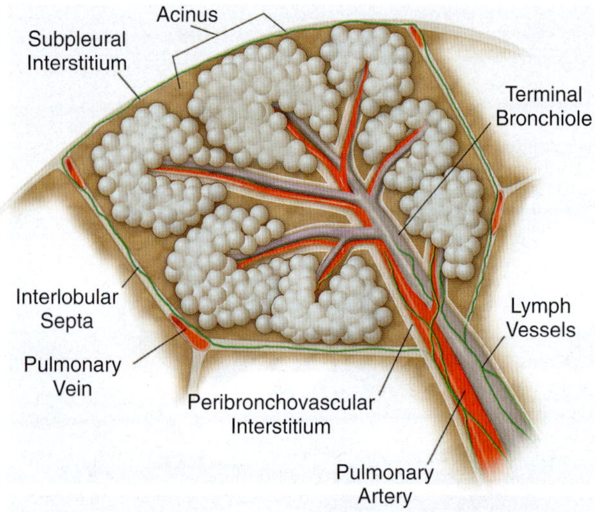

Figure 1.20 Secondary pulmonary lobule (SPL). The subpleural interstitium lies beneath the visceral pleura and forms the borders of the SPL (interlobular septa). The interlobular septum contains venous and lymphatic structures. Air to each SPL is supplied by a terminal bronchus, the smallest purely conducting airway within the lungs. The terminal bronchus and accompanying arterial vessel are supported by the bronchovascular interstitium. Each SPL contains a centrilobular core containing centrilobular arterioles and bronchioles supported by the centrilobular interstitium. Multiple acini are present in each lobule, with each acinus supplied by an individual respiratory bronchiole (largest airway associated with gas exchange). The intralobular interstitium is a fine network that connects the centrilobular interstitium to the subpleural interstitium.

more lobes. Postexpiratory minimum intensity projection images can be useful in the detection of air trapping.

■ Secondary Pulmonary Lobule

The SPL (Fig. 1.20) is the smallest functional and anatomic unit appreciable on a CT chest scan. Its boundaries are formed by the interlobular septa, which are most developed in the peripheral and anteromedial portions of the lungs. It is polygonal in shape and measures approximately 10 to 25 mm in diameter. The SPL is marginated by the interlobular septa, which extend inward perpendicular from the pleural surface, and the septa contains the pulmonary veins and lymphatics. They measure about 0.1 to 0.2 mm in thickness and 1 to 2.5 cm in length. The lobules in the periphery of the lung are cuboidal or pyramidal in shape, whereas they are more hexagonal in the central lung,. The appearance of the septa is affected by the orientation of the lobule in relation to the scan plane. Normally, only a few septa are visible in the lung periphery, usually in the apices, anteriorly and along the mediastinal pleural surface (Fig. 1.21). The septa can also be identified by pulmonary venous branches, occasionally seen as a row or chain of dots as small as 0.5 mm or as branching structures. Small venous branches arise at right angles to the larger main branch.

Each lobule contains 4 to 12 pulmonary acini (each acinus measures 4–8 mm and is supplied by respiratory bronchiole). Secondary lobules are supplied by pulmonary arterial branches and bronchioles. A dotlike opacity or branching structure in the center of a lobule, within 1 cm of the pleural surface, represents the intralobular artery or its branches. The arterial branches supplying the pulmonary acini measure approximately 0.5 mm and can be seen on the HRCT scan. The visibility of the bronchioles in normal subjects depends on their wall thickness rather than diameter. The smallest lobular bronchiole visible on HRCT has a wall thickness of 0.1 mm, measures about 1 mm in diameter, and is visible to within 1 cm of the pleural surface. The terminal and intralobular bronchioles are not normally visible on HRCT.

Intralobular interstitium refers to the connective tissue in the alveolar septa that supports the alveoli and capillary bed and is not normally visible on HRCT. Any abnormality involving the axial, peripheral, and septal interstitium can manifest at the level of the SPL, revealing CT abnormalities. The subpleural interstitium contains small vessels that are involved in the formation of pleural fluid and lymphatic branches. Thus the interstitial lung diseases that affect the interlobular septa often result in abnormalities of the subpleural interstitium.

■ Pleura–Chest Wall Interface

The combined thickness of the pleura and the fluid contained within the pleural space is less than 0.5 cm. The thoracic cavity is lined by endothoracic fascia, which is about 0.25 mm thick. It is separated from the parietal pleura by a layer of loose areolar tissue or extrapleural fat. External to the endothoracic fascia are the innermost intercostal muscles, which pass between the adjacent ribs and do not extend into the paravertebral region. The paravertebral line lies in the paravertebral region, which is grossly visible and represents the combined thickness of the visceral and parietal pleura and endothoracic fascia. Pleural thickening or effusion can be visible as a soft tissue density in the paravertebral region.

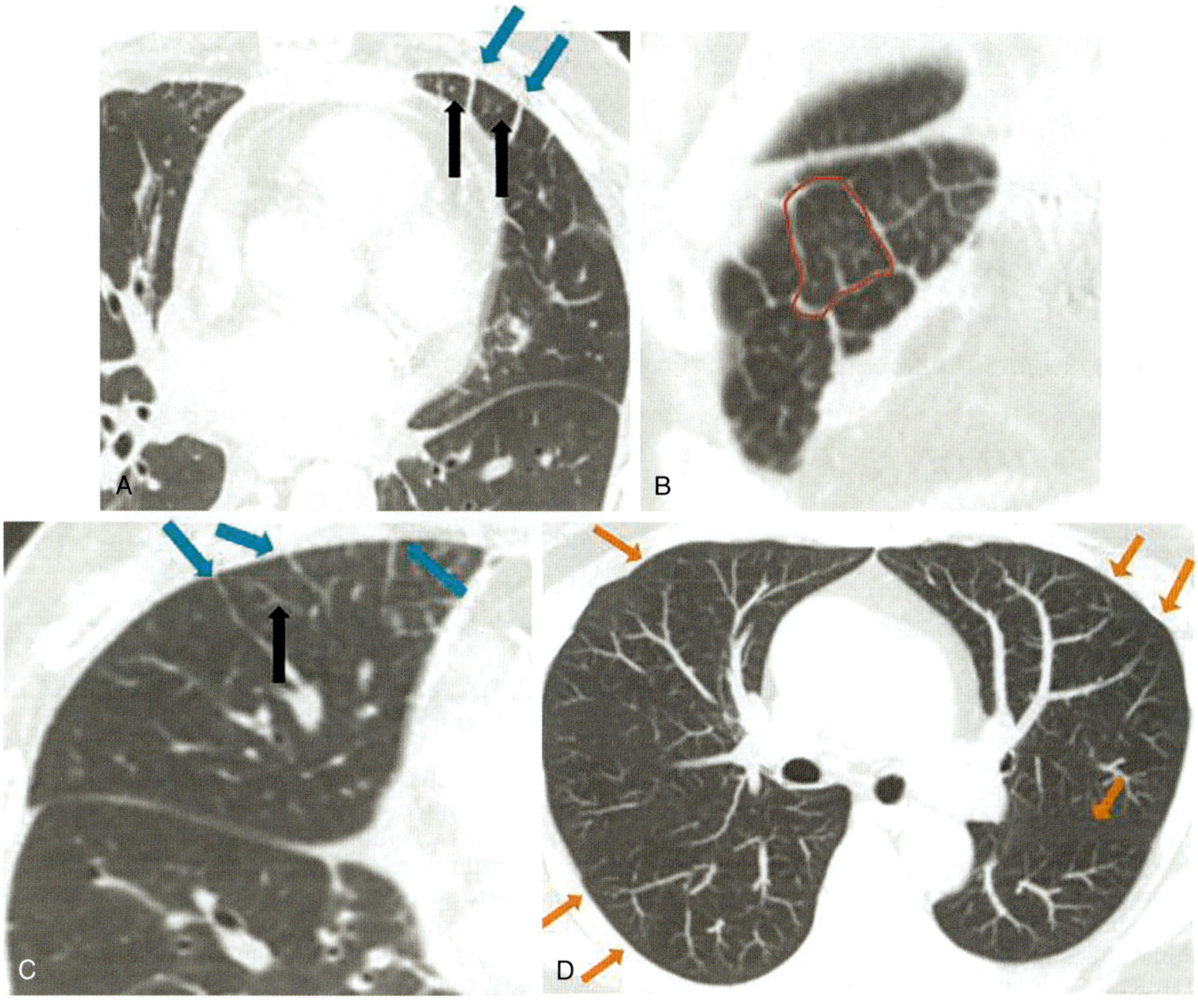

Figure 1.21 Axial (A, C, D) and coronal (B) CT images demonstrate various secondary pulmonary lobules demarcated by thickened interlobular septa *(blue arrows)*. (B) A network of interlobular septa is outlined in red on the coronal image. The centrilobular artery *(black arrow)* runs in the center of the lobule and is seen as a dotlike structure in (A) and as a branching structure in (C). Pulmonary artery branches are visible to within 5 to 10 mm of the pleural surface. (D) Axial CT image shows a subpleural lucent zone up to 5 mm devoid of any vessels, including adjacent to the left major fissures *(orange arrows)*.

Bibliography

Bergin C, Roggli V, Coblentz C, et al. The secondary pulmonary lobule: normal and abnormal CT appearances. *AJR Am J Roentgenol*. 1988;151:21–25.

Berkmen T, Berkmen YM, Austin JH. Accessory fissures of the upper lobes of the left lung: CT and plain film appearance. *AJR Am J Roentgenol*. 1994;162:1287–1293.

Boyden EA. *Segmental Anatomy of the Lungs*. New York: McGraw-Hill; 1955.

Brant WE, Helms CA. *Fundamentals of Diagnostic Radiology*. Philadelphia: Lippincott Williams & Wilkins; 2006.

Froudarakis ME. Diagnostic work-up of pleural effusions. *Respiration*. 2008;75:4–13.

Godwin DJ, Tarver RD. Accessory fissures of the lung. *AJR Am J Roentgenol*. 1985;144:39–47.

Hansell DM. Small-vessel diseases of the lung: CT-pathologic correlates. *Radiology*. 2002;225:639–653.

Jardin M, Remy J. Segment bronchovascular anatomy of the lower lobes. CT analysis. *AJR Am J Roentgenol*. 1986;147:457–468.

Kang EY, Miller RR, Müller NL. Bronchiectasis: comparison of preoperative thin-section CT and pathologic findings in resected specimens. *Radiology*. 1995;195:649–654.

Kattan KR, Eyler WR, Felson B. The juxtaphrenic peak in upper lobe collapse. *Semin Roentgenol*. 1980;15:187–193.

Ketai L, Lofgren R, Meholic A. *Fundamentals of Chest Radiology*. 2nd ed. Philadelphia: Saunders; 2006.

Kim JS, Müller NL, Park CS, et al. Cylindrical bronchiectasis: diagnostic findings on thin-section CT. *AJR Am J Roentgenol*. 1997;168(3):751–764.

Lee KW, Chung SY, Yang I, et al. Correlation of aging and smoking with air trapping at thin-section CT of the lung in asymptomatic subjects. *Radiology*. 2000;214:831–836.

Matsuoka S, Uchiyama K, Shima H, et al. Bronchoarterial ratio and bronchial wall thickness on high-resolution CT in asymptomatic subjects: correlation with age and smoking. *AJR Am J Roentgenol*. 2003;180:513–518.

McGuinness G, Naidich DP, Garay SM, et al. Accessory cardiac bronchus: CT features and clinical significance. *Radiology*. 1993;189(2):563–566.

Otsuji H, Uchida H, Maeda M, et al. Incomplete interlobar fissures: bronchovascular analysis with CT. *Radiology*. 1993;187:541–546.

Raghu R, Collard HR, Egan JJ, et al. The official ATS/ERS/JRS/ALAT statement: idiopathic pulmonary fibrosis: evidence-based guidelines for diagnosis and management. *Am J Respir Crit Care Med*. 2011;183:788–824.

Tanaka N, Matsumoto T, Miura G, et al. Air trapping at CT: high prevalence in asymptomatic subjects with normal pulmonary function. *Radiology*. 2003;227(3):776–785.

Webb WR. High-Resolution CT of the lung parenchyma. *Radiol Clin North Am*. 1989;27(6):1085–1097.

Webb WR, Higgins CB. *Thoracic Imaging: Pulmonary and Cardiovascular Radiology*. Philadelphia: Lippincott Williams & Wilkins; 2010.

Webb WR, Hirji M, Gamsu G. Posterior wall of the bronchus intermedius: radiographic-CT correlation. *AJR Am J Roentgenol*. 1984;141:907–911.

Wittram C, Batt J, Rappaport DC, Hutcheon MA. Inspiratory and expiratory helical CT of normal adults: comparison of thin section scans and minimum intensity projection images. *J Thorac Imaging*. 2002;17:47–52.

Wong CL, Holroyd-Leduc J, Straus SE. Does the patient have a pleural effusion? *JAMA*. 2009;301:309–317.

CHAPTER 2

Mediastinum, Chest Wall, and Diaphragm

Mohammad Sarwar, Jared Isaacson, and Suhny Abbara

CHAPTER OUTLINE

■ Introduction

The mediastinum, chest wall, and diaphragm can be evaluated by multiple imaging modalities, such as radiography, computed tomography (CT), and magnetic resonance imaging (MRI). The chest radiograph is often the initial imaging modality used in the evaluation of these structures and their abnormalities. CT and MRI are important cross-sectional imaging modalities that are useful in the evaluation and characterization of abnormalities in these structures. A thorough understanding of the normal anatomy is essential for the accurate diagnosis of cardiopulmonary disease.

In this chapter, we review the imaging anatomy of the mediastinum, chest wall, and diaphragm.

■ Mediastinum

The mediastinum is the central compartment of the thorax that is bounded by pleura on the right and left, by sternum anteriorly, and by vertebra posteriorly. It contains loose connective tissue and several vital structures, including the heart, great vessels, esophagus, trachea, phrenic and cardiac nerves, thoracic duct, lymph nodes, and thymus. Craniocaudally, it extends from the thoracic inlet superiorly to the diaphragm inferiorly. The mediastinum is divided into compartments based on multiple classification schemes. However, there are no real anatomic boundaries for these compartments; hence, disease processes may extend from one compartment to another. Also, these classification schemes are less relevant with the use of CT and MRI, where the masses can be accurately localized and reasonably characterized.

In the traditional anatomic four-compartment classification, mediastinum is divided into superior and inferior compartments, with the inferior further subdivided into anterior, middle, and posterior compartments. The superior compartment extends from the thoracic inlet to the level of the superior aortic arch—that is, superior to an imaginary line between the manubriosternal angle and the T4–5 intervertebral disk in the lateral radiograph or sagittal tomogram. The inferior mediastinum extends from this level to the diaphragm. The anterior mediastinum is bounded anteriorly by the sternum and posteriorly by the anterior pericardium. This space contains the thymus, lymph nodes, internal mammary artery branches, and fat. The middle mediastinum is located between the anterior and posterior pericardium. The heart, aorta, pulmonary arteries, pulmonary veins, superior vena cava (SVC), inferior vena cava (IVC), phrenic nerve, trachea and proximal bronchi, esophagus, mediastinal fat, and lymph nodes are located in the middle mediastinum. The posterior mediastinum is located posterior to the posterior pericardium and contains vertebral bodies, nerves, fat, and lymph nodes.

There are several three-compartment classifications. The Felson classification is based on lateral radiographs. The anterior mediastinum is located between the sternum and an imaginary line drawn superiorly from the diaphragm along the back of the heart and front of the trachea. The middle mediastinum is located between the above-mentioned line and another imaginary line that is located 1 cm behind the anterior margins of the thoracic vertebra, and the posterior mediastinum is located posterior to this line (Fig. 2.1A). The Zylak classification is also similar, with the middle vascular space containing the pericardium and its contents, anterior aorta with its branches and great veins, an anterior prevascular space containing the thymus, thyroids, and parathyroids, and a posterior postvascular previsceral space containing the trachea, esophagus, descending aorta, and azygos.

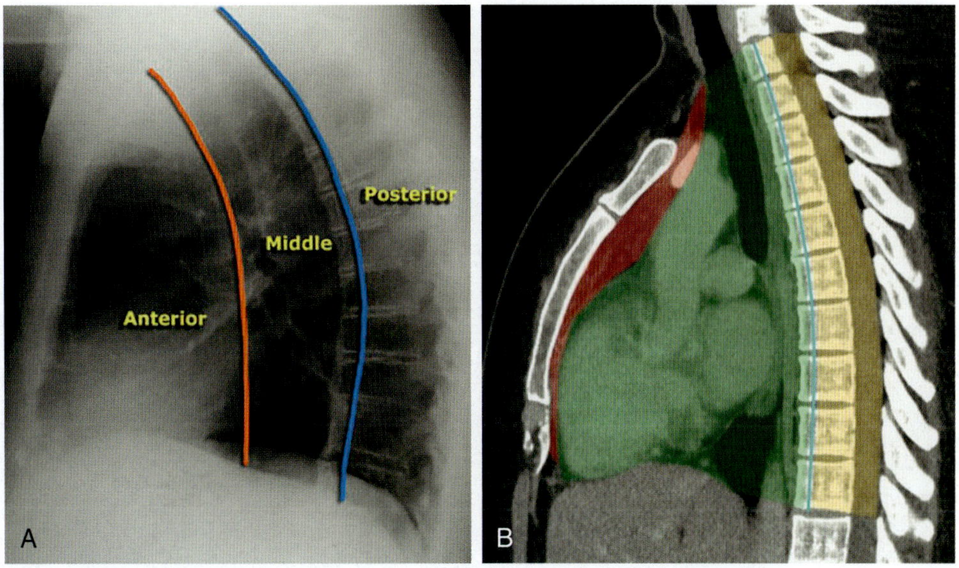

Figure 2.1 Division of the mediastinum. (A) Felson classification of the mediastinum. The anterior mediastinum is located between the sternum, and an imaginary line is drawn superiorly from the diaphragm along the back of the heart and front of the trachea. The middle mediastinum is located between this line. Another imaginary line 1 cm behind the anterior margins of the thoracic vertebra and posterior mediastinum is located posterior to this line. (B) International Thymic Malignancy Interest Group (ITMIG) classification of the mediastinal compartments. The anterior mediastinum is bounded anteriorly by the sternum and posteriorly by the anterior aspect of the pericardium. The middle mediastinum is bounded anteriorly by the anterior pericardium and posteriorly by an imaginary line 1 cm posterior to the anterior border of the vertebral bodies. The posterior mediastinum extends from 1 cm posterior to the anterior vertebral bodies to the posterior paravertebral gutters.

Shield's three-zone classification has a previsceral zone between the sternum and anterior pericardium and great vessels; the visceral zone is between the anterior pericardium and the anterior surface of the spine, and the retrovisceral zone in the paravertebral sulci. In the Whitten classification, the anterior mediastinum is bounded anteriorly by the sternum and posteriorly by the anterior pericardium, aorta, and brachiocephalic vessels. The middle mediastinum is bounded anteriorly by the anterior pericardium and posteriorly by the posterior pericardium and trachea. The posterior mediastinum is bounded anteriorly by the posterior pericardium and posterior trachea and posteriorly by the vertebral column. In the Sone classification, the mediastinum is divided into anterior (precardiovascular) and central (retrocardiovascular) zones, with the latter divided into supracarinal and subcarinal areas. Heitzman (1988) divided the mediastinum into the thoracic inlet, anterior mediastinum, supraaortic area (above the aortic arch), infraaortic area, supraazygos area (above the supraaortic aortic arch), and infraazygos area (below the supraaortic aortic arch). The Japanese Association for Research on Thymus (JART) system classifies the mediastinum into superior, anterior, middle, and posterior based on landmarks in axial cross-sectional images. The International Thymic Malignancy Interest Group (ITMIG) classification is a modification of the JART system; it divides the mediastinum into anterior (prevascular), middle (visceral), and posterior (paravertebral) based on CT landmarks. In this scheme, the boundary between the middle and posterior mediastinum is a vertical line 1 cm posterior to the anterior margin of the spine (see Fig. 2.1B).

The thymus is located in the anterior mediastinum in the thyropericardiac space. There is a wide variation in morphology and size, particularly in children and young adults. The thymus is large at birth, often larger than the heart, and progressively decreases in size with age, with the gland being replaced by fatty infiltration. The thymus is atrophic in the fourth decade but may be seen in less than 50% of those older than 40 years on a CT scan. The normal maximal thickness in those younger than 20 years is 18 mm, and it is 13 mm in older individuals. The normal thymus is a homogeneous bilobulated structure, with the left lobe usually larger than the right. Rarely, there is congenital absence of a lobe. On CT, it has homogeneous soft tissue attenuation (Fig. 2.2A), and on MRI it has intermediate signal intensity (see Fig. 2.2B). However, with age, the T1 signal of the thymus increases due to fat infiltration. On T2 images, the thymus has high signal intensity in all age groups. The normal thymus in patients younger than 20 years typically has diffuse increased fluorodeoxyglucose (FDG) uptake on positron emission tomography (PET). After that age, significant FDG accumulation is less common.

The trachea connects the larynx to the lungs. It extends from the inferior margin of the cricoid cartilage in the neck to the carina, which marks the origin of the main bronchi. It is located in the midline, but it may be located to the right at the level of the aortic arch. The trachea is 10 to 11 cm long in adults, with 6 to 9 cm of this being intrathoracic. However, tracheal length varies with respiration and neck flexion and extension. The normal tracheal lumen is round, oval, or horseshoe-shaped (Fig. 2.3). In men, the tracheal diameter ranges from 13 to 25 mm

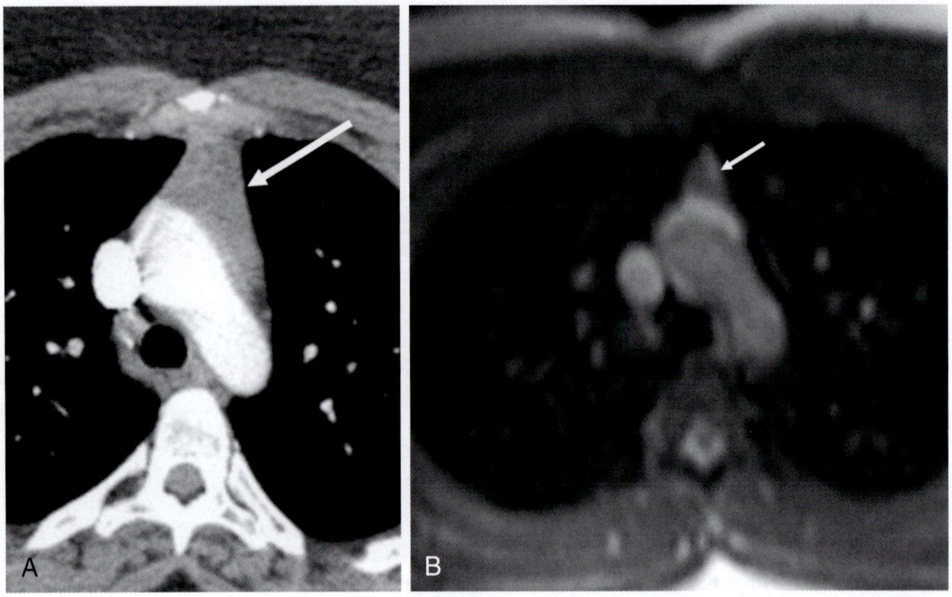

Figure 2.2 Thymus. (A) Axial CT scan showing normal triangular thymic tissue in the anterior mediastinum *(arrow)*. (B) Axial MRI scan showing normal thymic tissue in the anterior mediastinum *(arrow)*.

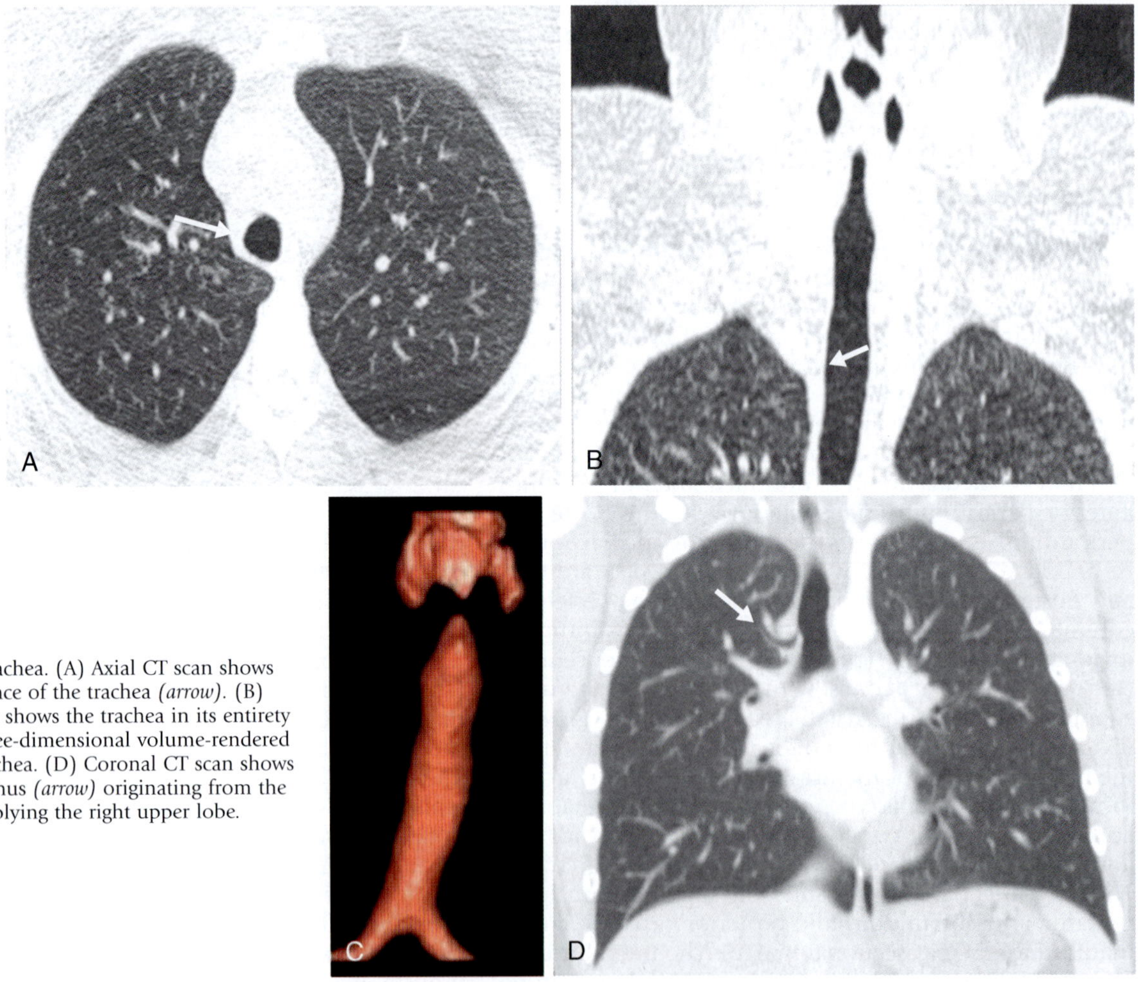

Figure 2.3 Trachea. (A) Axial CT scan shows normal appearance of the trachea *(arrow)*. (B) Coronal CT scan shows the trachea in its entirety *(arrow)*. (C) Three-dimensional volume-rendered image of the trachea. (D) Coronal CT scan shows a tracheal bronchus *(arrow)* originating from the trachea and supplying the right upper lobe.

in the coronal plane and 13 to 27 mm in the sagittal plane; in women, the tracheal diameter ranges from 10 to 21 mm in the coronal plane and 10 to 23 mm in the sagittal plane. The tracheal wall measures 1 to 3 mm on CT and is composed of inner mucosa, submucosa, cartilage and muscle, and outer adventitia. The posterior wall is thinner than the anterior and lateral walls. The trachea has 22 C-shaped cartilages, which are linked longitudinally by annular ligaments of fibrous and connective tissue. The cartilages are connected posteriorly by the membranous tracheal wall, which is supported by the trachealis muscle. With expiration, there is anterior bulging of the posterior membrane, resulting in a decreased anteroposterior dimension of 32%. The main bronchi originate from the trachea at the level of the carina and extend obliquely on the axial plane bilaterally. Normal variants of tracheobrochial tree are rare and are seen in less than 2.3% of cases. They include the tracheal bronchus (see Fig. 2.3D), accessory cardiac bronchus, bronchus hypoplasia, and aplasia. They are relatively more common in males and most often are located on the right side.

The esophagus is a muscular tube that connects the pharynx to the stomach. It is 23 to 37 cm long and has cervical, thoracic, and abdominal portions. The thoracic component extends from the level of T1 to the esophageal hiatus at T10. The esophagus is in close contact with several vital structures in the chest. Posteriorly, it is close to the descending aorta, thoracic duct, hemiazygos, and accessory hemiazygos (Fig. 2.4). Anteriorly, it is close to the trachea, recurrent laryngeal nerve in the tracheo-esophageal groove, left main bronchus, and left atrium. On the right, it is close to the pleura and azygos vein, whereas on the left it is close to the pleura, aorta, left subclavian artery, and thoracic duct. The superior portion of the esophagus is close to the trachea, whereas the lower portion is close to the descending thoracic aorta. The thoracic esophagus is initially located to the left of midline, returns to the midline at T5, and then courses to the left of midline again in the posterior mediastinum. In the inferior aspect of the thorax, it curves anteriorly to exit through the esophageal hiatus. There is a constriction in the thoracic esophagus at the level of the aortic arch at T4–5. When dilated, the esophagus thickness is between 1.9 and 2.7 mm.

Lymph nodes are present at different locations in the mediastinum. As a rule of thumb, normal lymph nodes measure less than 10 mm and have a fatty hilum. It is important to describe the lymph node accurately, particularly in patients with lung cancer, because it is an important component of staging. The International Association for the Study of Lung Cancer (IASLC) has defined a lymph node map that helps in lung cancer staging (Table 2.1; Fig. 2.5). There are 14 lymph node stations:

- 1R: Right low cervical supraclavicular and sternal notch lymph nodes; located between the lower margins of the cricoid superiorly and the upper border of the manubrium and bilateral clavicles inferiorly, on the right.
- 1L: Left low cervical supraclavicular and sternal notch lymph nodes, between the lower margin of the cricoid superiorly and upper border of the manubrium and bilateral clavicles inferiorly, on the left. The tracheal midline is the boundary between 1R and 1L.
- 2R: Right upper paratracheal; its superior boundary is the upper border of the manubrium, apex of the right lung, and pleura, and the lower border is the intersection of the caudal innominate vein with the trachea (Fig. 2.6A).
- 2L: Left upper paratracheal, whose superior border is the upper border of manubrium, apex of the left lung, and pleura, and the lower border is the superior border of the aortic arch. The boundary between 2L and 2R is the left lateral wall of trachea (see Fig. 2.6B).
- 3A: Prevascular superior border, apex of the chest; the lower border is the carina, the anterior border is the posterior aspect of sternum, and the posterior border is the SVC on the right and left carotid artery on the left (see Fig. 2.6C).
- 3P: Retrotracheal, posterior to the trachea; the upper border is the apex of the chest, and the lower border is the carina.
- 4R: Right lower paratracheal; the superior border is the intersection of the caudal margin of the innominate vein with the trachea, and the lower border is the lower border of the azygos vein (see Fig. 2.6D).

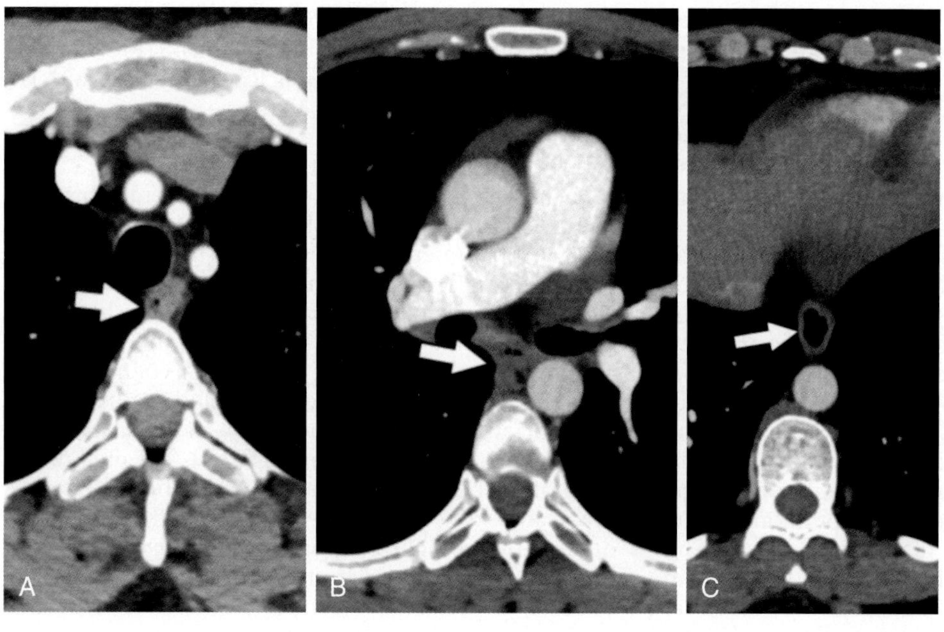

Figure 2.4 Esophagus. (A) Axial CT scan at the level of the aortic arch branch vessels shows the upper thoracic esophagus *(arrow)*. (B) Axial CT scan at the level of the carina shows the midthoracic esophagus *(arrow)*. (C) Axial CT scan at the level of diaphragm shows the lower thoracic esophagus *(arrow)*.

TABLE 2.1 Lymph Nodal Stations in IASLC Lymph Node Map

STATION	LYMPH NODE
1R	Right low cervical, supraclavicular, sternal notch lymph nodes
IL	Left low cervical, supraclavicular, sternal notch lymph nodes
2R	Right upper paratracheal
2L	Left upper paratracheal
3A	Prevascular
3P	Retrotracheal
4R	Right lower paratracheal
4L	Left lower paratracheal
5	Subaortic
6	Paraaortic
7	Subcarinal
8	Paraesophageal
9	Pulmonary ligament
10	Hilar
11	Interlobar
12	Lobar
13	Segmental
14	Subsegmental

IASLC, International Association for the Study of Lung Cancer.

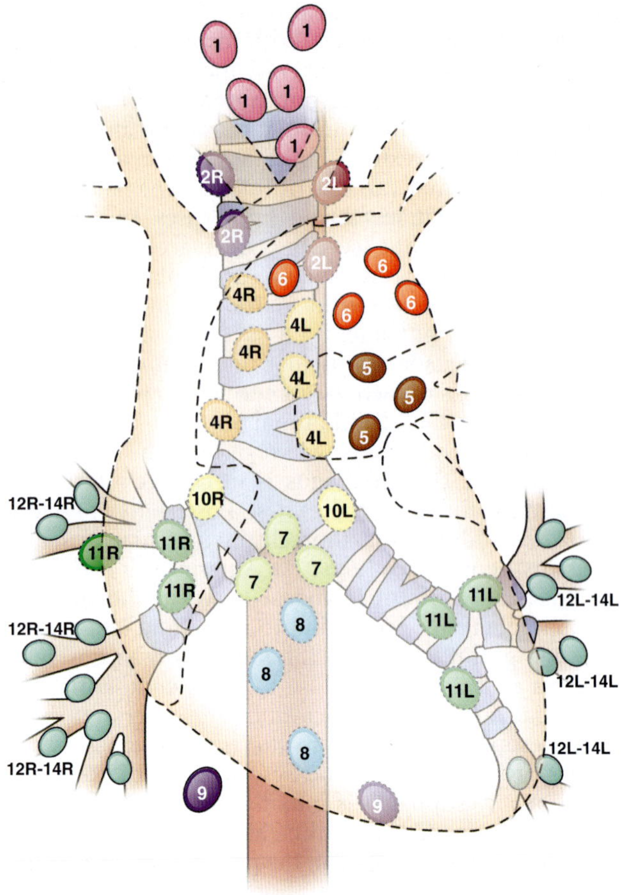

Figure 2.5 The different lymph node stations in the thorax are shown. See text for details.

- 4L: Left lower paratracheal; the superior border is the upper margin of the aortic arch, and the lower border is the superior border of the left pulmonary artery. The boundary between 4L and 4R is the left lateral wall of trachea (see Fig. 2.6E).
- 5: Subaoartic (aortopulmonary window); the upper border is the lower border of the aortic arch, the lower border is the upper rim of the left pulmonary artery, and the medial border is the ligamentum arteriosum (see Fig. 2.6F).
- 6: Paraaortic, anterior and lateral to the ascending aorta and aortic arch; the upper border is a line tangential to the upper border of the aortic arch, and the lower border is the lower border of the aortic arch (see Fig. 2.6G).
- 7: Subcarinal; the upper border is the carina, and the lower border is the upper border of the lower lobe bronchus on the left and the lower border of the bronchus intermedius on the right (see Fig. 2.6H).
- 8: Paraesophageal, adjacent to the esophagus; the upper border is the upper border of the lower lobe bronchus on the left and the bronchus intermedius on the right, and the lower border is the diaphragm (see Fig. 2.6I).
- 9: Pulmonary ligament; within the pulmonary ligament, the upper border is the inferior pulmonary vein, and the lower border is the diaphragm.
- 10: Hilar, adjacent to the hilar vessels and main stem bronchus; the upper border of 10R is the lower border of the azygos vein, the upper border of 10L is the upper border of the left pulmonary artery, and the lower border is the interlobar region bilaterally (see Fig. 2.6B).
- 11: Interlobar, between the origin of the lobar bronchi, 11R on the right (11rs—between the right upper lobe bronchus and bronchus intermedius; 11Ri—between the right middle and lower lobe bronchi), and 11L on the left.
- 12: Lobar, adjacent to the lobar bronchi; 12R on the right and 12L on the left.
- 13: Segmental, adjacent to the segmental bronchi; 13R on the right and 13L on the left.
- 14: Subsegmental, adjacent to the subsegmental bronchi; 14R on the right and 14L on the left.

The thoracic duct is the largest duct in the lymphatic system. It normally begins inferiorly at the level of L2, ascends along the right border of vertebral column, crosses over to the left at the level of T5–6, and drains into the left subclavian vein near the region of the insertion of the left internal jugular vein (Fig. 2.7). The duct drains most of the body, with the exclusion of the right thorax, the head and neck, and the right arm, all of which are drained by the right lymphatic duct. A right-sided chylothorax occurs secondary to an injury below the level of T5–6, whereas a left-sided chylothorax is associated with injury above this level. The amount of lymph drainage that traverses the thoracic duct daily is approximately 4 to 6 L. The average size of the thoracic duct is approximately 5 mm.

Sympathetic ganglia play an important role in the autonomic innervation of the thorax. Numerous ganglia are located deep to the heads of the ribs bilaterally and are covered with costal pleura. Nerves from this autonomic system innervate the aorta and constitute the splanchnic network that supplies the abdominal viscera. The greater and lesser splanchnic nerves descend along the thorax and enter the abdominal cavity, where they join sympathetic ganglia. The greater splanchnic nerve joins the celiac ganglion, the lesser splanchnic nerve joins the aortic renal ganglion, and the lowest splanchnic nerve joins the renal plexus.

■ Chest Wall

The chest wall is composed of bones, muscles, fat, connective tissue, vessels, nerves, and lymph nodes.

Bony Structures

Bony structures in the chest wall include the sternum, ribs, spine, and scapula. The sternum is a cancellous flat bone that plays a key role as a strut on which the rib cage attaches. The sternum is 15 to 20 cm long and has three components—the manubrium, body, and xiphoid process, from top to bottom. The manubrium is a quadrilateral bone, which superiorly has a central suprasternal notch and bilaterally has lateral notches, which articulate with the clavicles. The first rib articulates with the upper lateral manubrium, whereas the second rib articulates with the lower lateral manubrium and upper lateral body. The manubrium joins the body of sternum at the angle of Louis, with fibrocartilage located in between. The body is narrower than the manubrium. The lower portion of the second rib and third to seventh ribs articulate with the lateral margin of the sternal body. The body joins the xiphoid process inferiorly; it has variable size, shape, and length (Fig. 2.8). The sternoclavicular joint is between the lateral manubrial articulation and medial clavicular head. It has a fibrocartilaginous disk and is 2.5 to 4 mm wide.

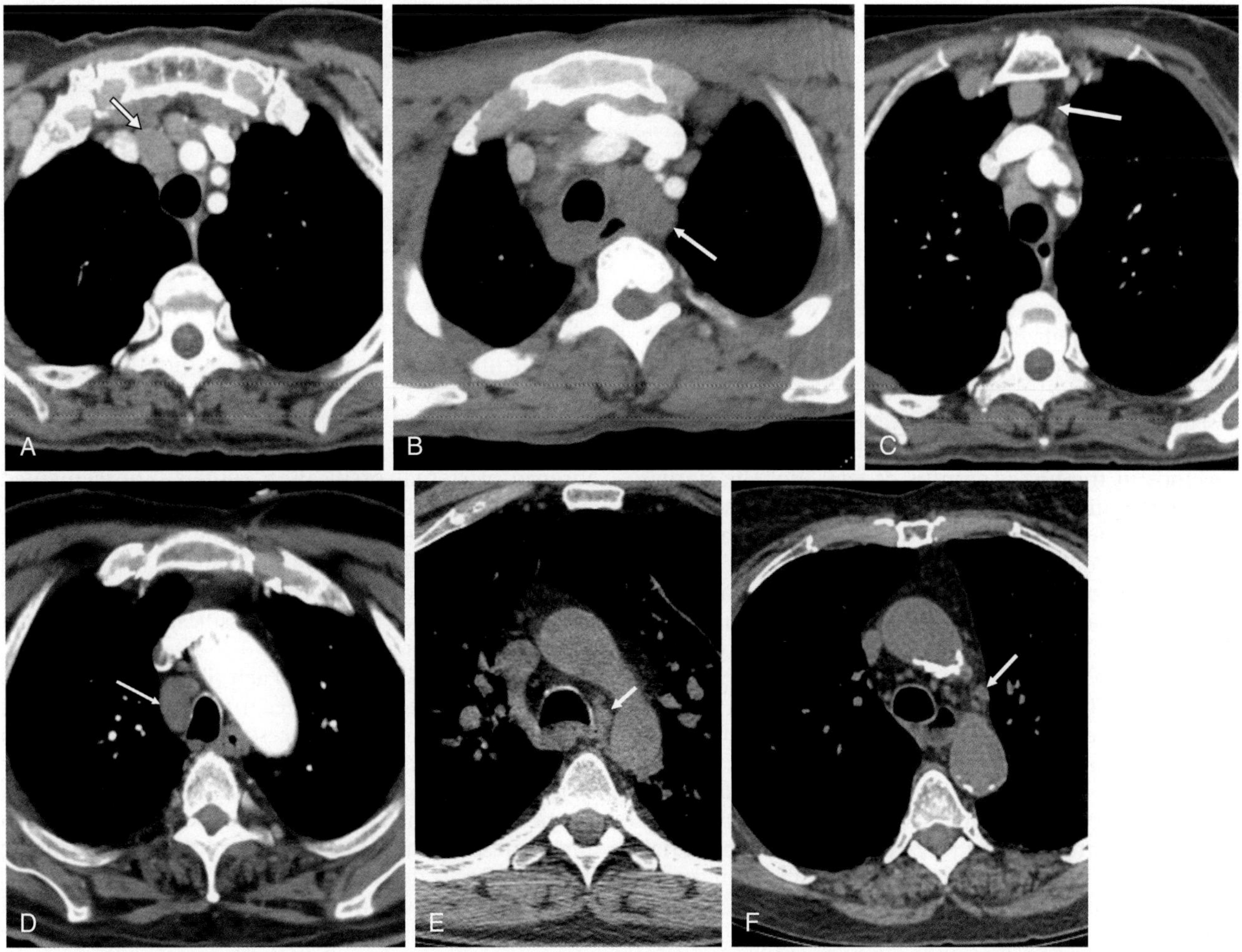

Figure 2.6 Examples of lymph nodes. Multiple axial CT scans at different levels showing the right upper paratracheal (A; *arrow*), left upper paratracheal (B; *arrow*), prevascular (C; *arrow*), right lower paratracheal (D; *arrow*), left lower paratracheal (E; *arrow*), aortopulmonary window (F; *arrow*),

Continued

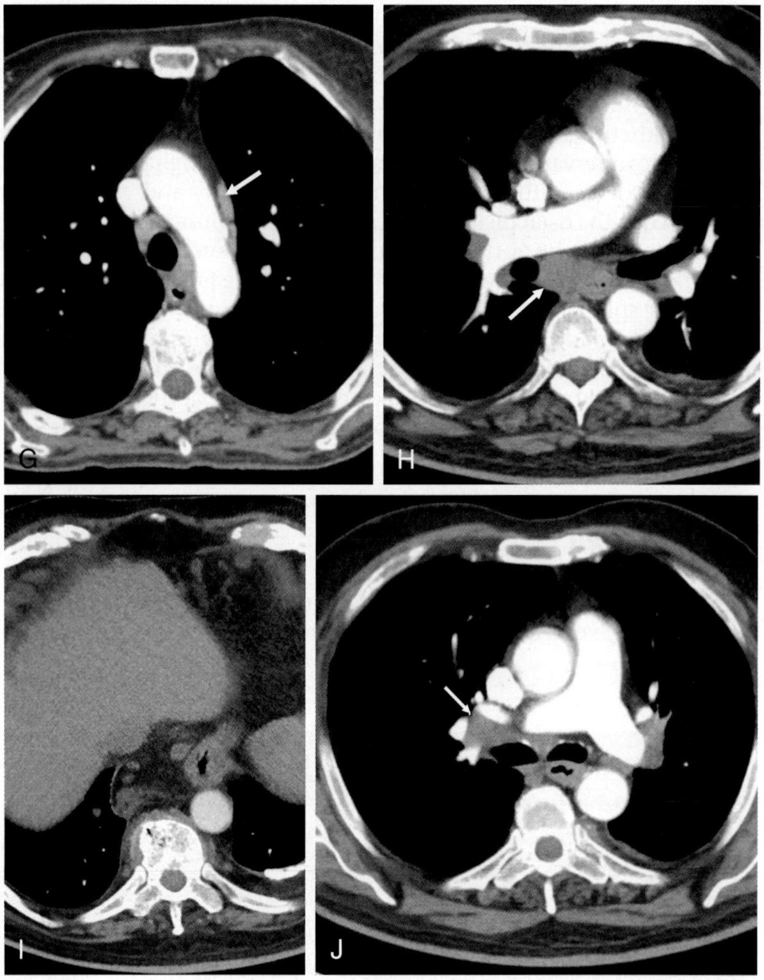

Figure 2.6, cont'd paraaortic (G; *arrow*), subcarinal (H; *arrow*), paraesophageal (I), and right hilar (J; *arrow*) lymph nodes.

Its capsule is stabilized by the sternoclavicular ligaments. The nearby costoclavicular ligament connects the medial first rib and clavicle.

The sternum develops from six ossification centers. The manubrium has a single ossification center that develops in the first 6 months of fetal life. The sternal body has four ossification centers, with the first center developing in the first 6 months of life, the second and third centers developing by the seventh month of fetal life, and the fourth center developing before completion of the first year of life. The xiphoid has one ossification center that ossifies between the fifth and 18th years of life. Accessory sternal and manubrial ossification centers and the developmental absence of ossification centers also occur. The first and second and the second and third sternal ossification centers normally fuse between puberty and the 25th year of life. The third and fourth sternal ossification centers actually fuse earlier in life, typically fusing soon after puberty (see Fig. 2.8). The manubrial ossification center and the first sternal ossification center (at the sternomanubrial joint) rarely join until old age.

Congenital abnormalities result from the failure of fusion of the sternal ossification centers. Midline fusion defects such as a sternal cleft, midline foramina, and bifid xiphoid are occasionally seen. Additional sternal variants include separate or fused suprasternal bones, low manubriosternal junction (at the level of the third rib), ribs articulating alternately to the sternum (rather than pairs), accessory ossification centers, double manubrial ossification centers, congenitally bifid sternum, congenitally bifid sternum with a distal union, developmental absence of sternal ossification centers, nonsegmented sternum, episternal processes, partitioned xiphoid process, and marked anterior flexion of the xiphoid process. Double manubrial ossification centers are associated with Down syndrome. Double ossification centers and the developmental absence of ossification centers can be misinterpreted as fractures.

There are 12 pairs of ribs. Each rib has a head, neck, and shaft. The head articulates through synovial joints, both with the transverse process (costotransverse joint) and vertebral body and both at the level and superior to the level (costovertebral joint) of that particular rib. A tubercle is formed between the neck and shaft of a rib and represents the insertion site of the erector spinae musculature. As described above, the anterior portions of the first through seventh ribs are attached to the lateral sternum. The eighth through tenth ribs join each other and then attach to the anterior cartilaginous portion of the seventh rib to join the sternum. The 11th and 12th ribs are referred to as *floating ribs* because they do not have a bony or cartilaginous attachment anteriorly (Fig. 2.9).

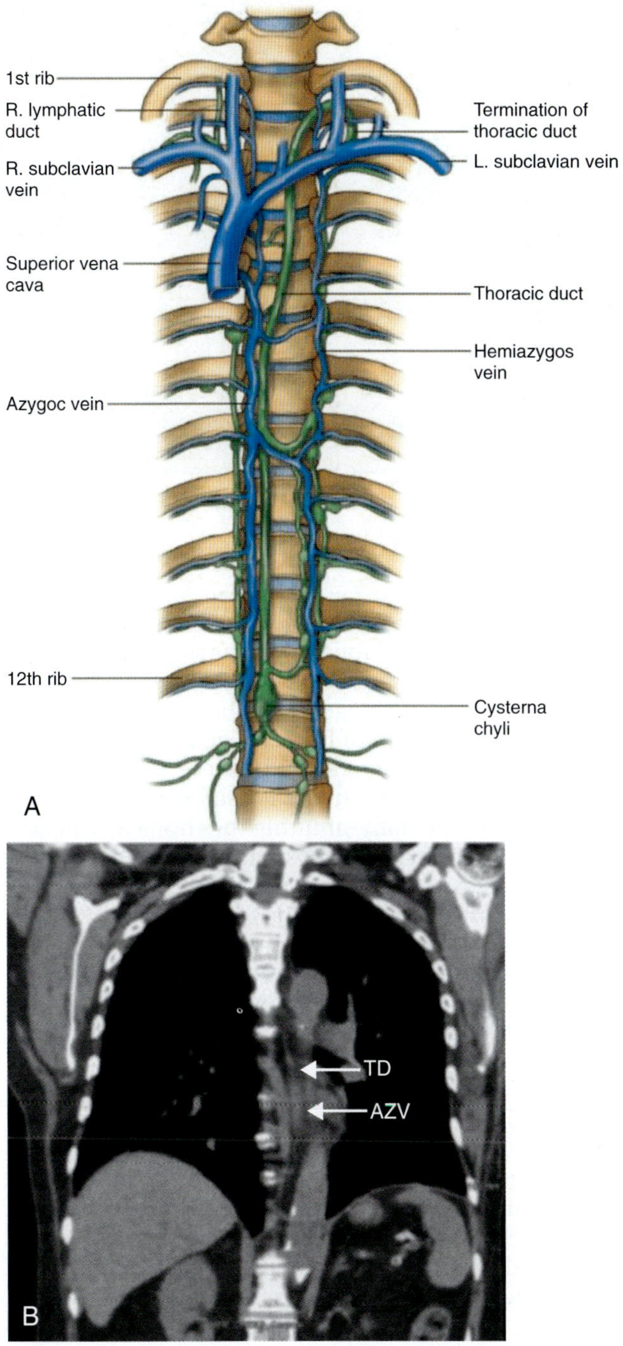

Figure 2.7 Thoracic duct. (A) The thoracic duct, which originates at the level of L2, ascends along the right border of the vertebral column, crosses over to the left at the level of T5–6, and drains into the left subclavian vein. (B) Coronal reconstructed CT image showing the thoracic duct *(TD)* adjacent to the azygos vein *(ASV)*.

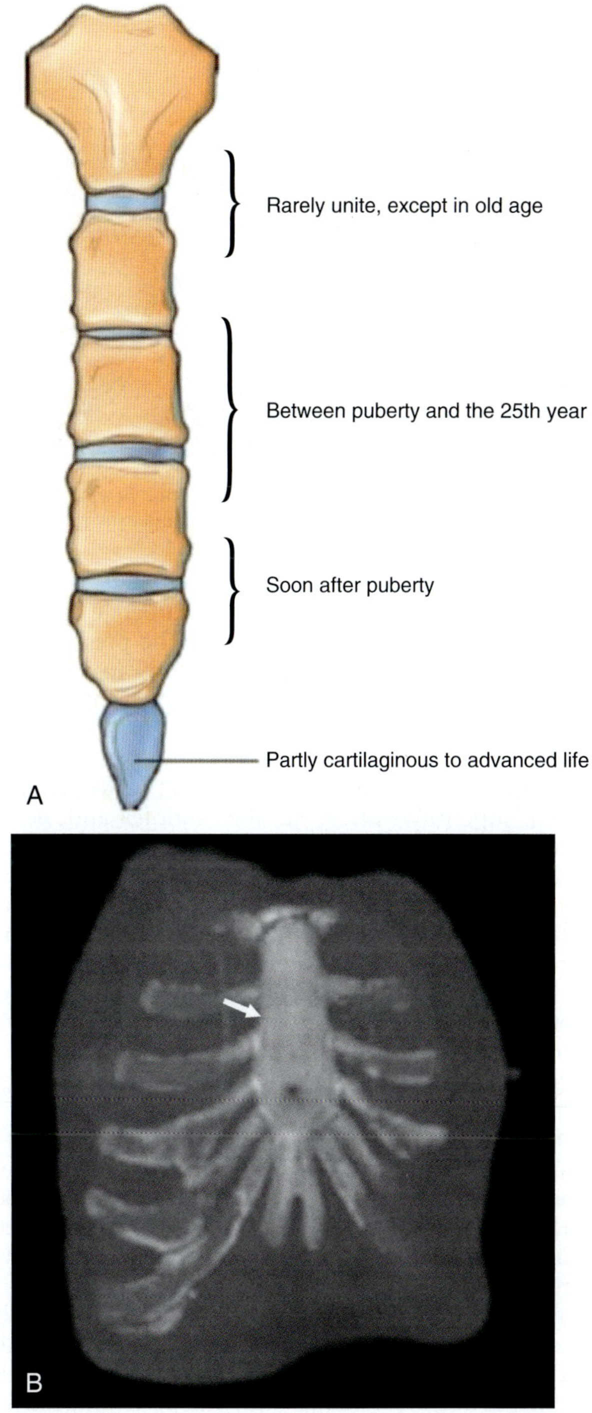

Figure 2.8 Sternum. (A) Sternal ossification centers. (B) Coronal CT image showing the sternal body *(arrow)*.

The ribs are formed via intramembranous ossification. The body has one ossification center, the tubercle has two ossification centers, and the head has one ossification center. The first through tenth ribs have four ossification centers. The first rib usually ossifies at an early age. The second through tenth ribs calcify and rarely ossify later in life. The usual rib variants include supernumerary ribs, which may be found above or below the normal ribs—that is, at C7 or at L1. Variants specific to the first rib include a congenital absence of the first rib and normal areas of lucency in the anterior portions of the first ribs. Additional rib variants include developmental fusion or spurs extending from the first rib toward the second rib, fusion of posterior portions of the ribs, forked or bifid anterior

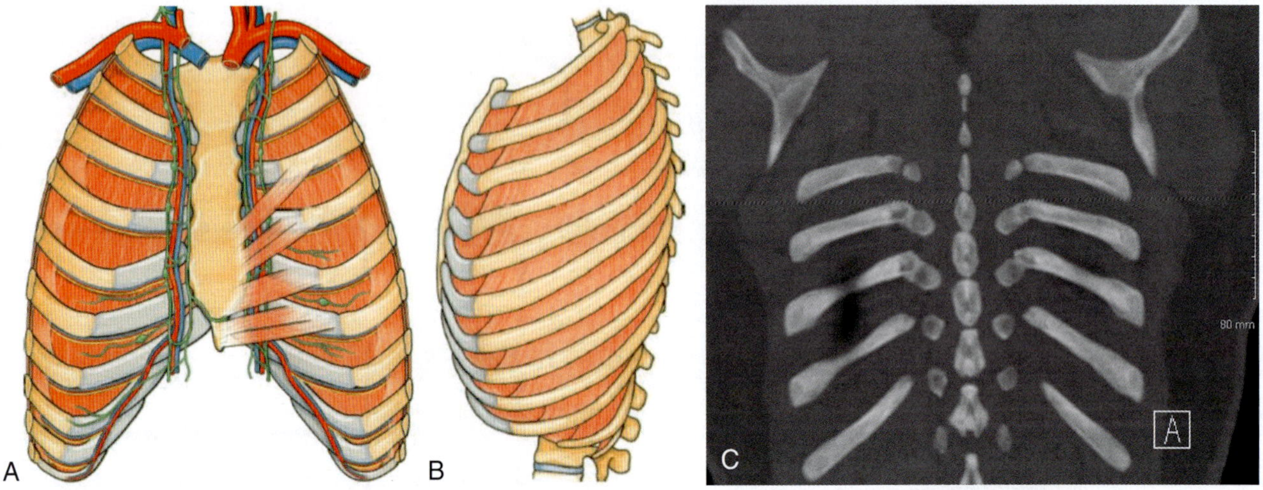

Figure 2.9 Ribs. (A) Anterior view of the 12 pairs of ribs. (B) Oblique view showing the 12 pairs of ribs. (C) Coronal maximum intensity projection image showing the posterior ribs.

portion of a rib, and lucencies in the tubercle of a rib. Occasionally, an intrathoracic rib may be present. The cervical rib (C7) is important because it may cause thoracic outlet syndrome, and it can mimic an upper lobe lesion on radiography.

Neurovascular structures are located along a groove at the inferior and inner surface of a rib, with the *v*ein located superiorly, *a*rtery in the middle, and *n*erve inferiorly (mnemonic: VAN). Hence, interventional procedures are performed with needles entering above the upper margin of the rib. The external and internal intercostal muscles form a superficial shield around the neurovascular structures. Internal to the vessels and intercostal nerves is the innermost intercostal muscle. Anteriorly, the upper six intercostal arteries originate from the internal thoracic artery, and the lower three intercostal arteries originate from the musculophrenic artery, with a branch extending from the distal internal thoracic artery. Posteriorly, there are 12 ribs, and hence there are 11 intercostal spaces. The upper two intercostal arterial branches emerge as branches from the costocervical trunk, which originates from the subclavian artery, and the lower, remaining posterior intercostal branches originate directly from the descending aorta.

The thoracic spine is composed of 12 thoracic vertebrae. Superiorly, T1 articulates with the C7 vertebra and, inferiorly, T12 articulates with the L1 vertebra. Each vertebra has a central vertebral body and posterior pedicles and laminae, which encircle a central spinal canal. Transverse processes project from the lateral aspect of the vertebrae, whereas the posterior spinous process originates from junction of the lamina (Fig. 2.10). Superior and inferior articular processes lie at the lateral angle of lamina and are connected by the pars interarticularis. Facet joints are zygapophyseal joints that connect the superior articular facet of the lower vertebrae with the inferior articular facet of the upper vertebrae. The inferior articular process of the superior vertebrae always lies posterior to the superior facet of the lower vertebrae. Abnormalities of the vertebral body include hemivertebrae, block vertebrae, fused vertebrae, unfused vertebrae, and butterfly vertebrae; variants of the arch include the arcuate foramen, transitional vertebrae such as the cervical rib and lumbar rib, and accessory ossicles.

The scapula is a triangular flat bone that articulates laterally with the head of humerus at the glenohumeral joint and with the lateral end of the clavicle at the acromioclavicular joint. It has a costal surface that faces anteriorly and medially, abutting the thoracic wall, and a dorsal surface that faces posteriorly and laterally. The dorsal surface has the spine of the scapula, which divides the scapula into a smaller supraspinous fossa and larger infraspinous fossa, which are connected by the spinoglenoid notch, which is lateral to the root of the spine. The scapula has two processes: the coracoid process anteriorly and the acromion process posteriorly.

Musculature

Muscles are also an important component of the chest wall. Respiratory muscles include the inspiratory group, which includes the sternocleidomastoid muscles that abut the thorax and help elevate the upper margin of the thorax when the accessory musculature is needed. The expiratory group includes the rectus abdominus and oblique musculature, which increase expiration by reducing the volume of the rib cage during their contraction. The pectoralis major muscle group originates along the medial half of the clavicle, sternum, upper six costal cartilages, and aponeurosis of the external oblique muscle and inserts on the lateral lip of the humeral bicipital groove (Fig. 2.11A). The pectoralis minor originates near the costal cartilages of the third through fifth ribs and inserts upon the coracoid process of the scapula (see Fig. 2.11A). The serratus anterior muscle originates from fleshy slips along the outer surface of the upper eight or nine ribs and inserts along the costal aspect of the medial margin of the scapula (see Fig. 2.11B). As their name suggests, the intercostal muscles extend between the ribs. The 11 external intercostal muscles are located externally and insert on the second through 12th ribs.

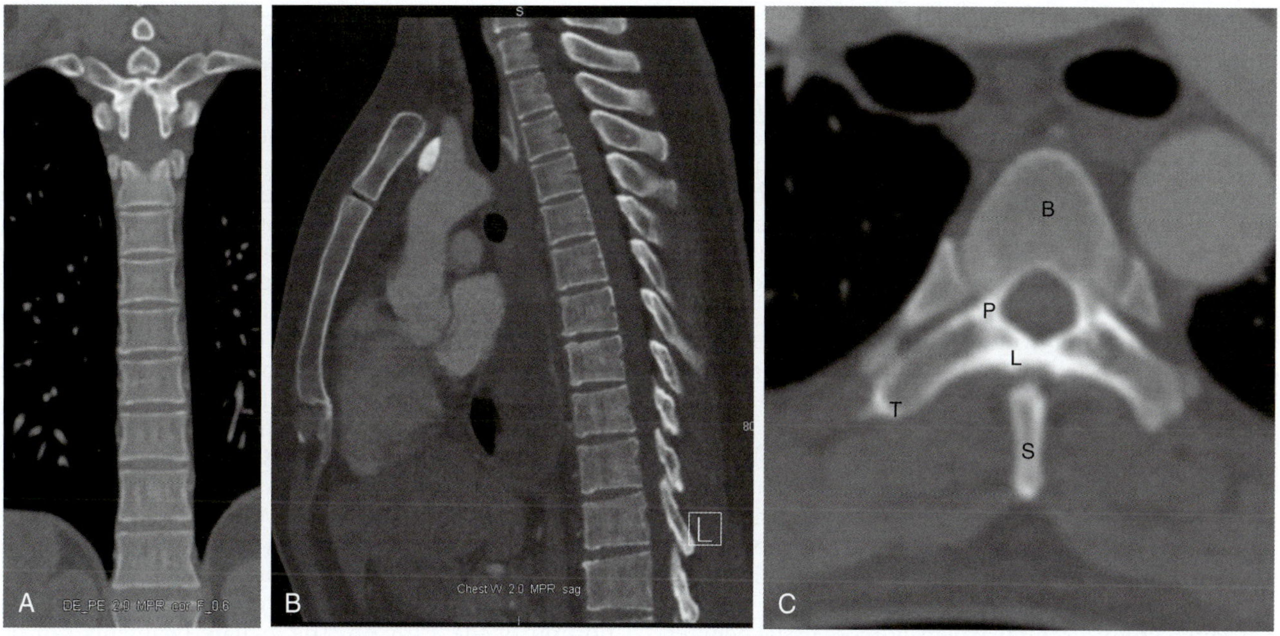

Figure 2.10 Thoracic spine. (A) Coronal reconstruction. (B) Sagittal reconstruction. (C) Axial CT scan showing the vertebral body *(B)*, pedicle *(P)*, lamina *(L)*, transverse process *(T)*, and spinous process *(S)*.

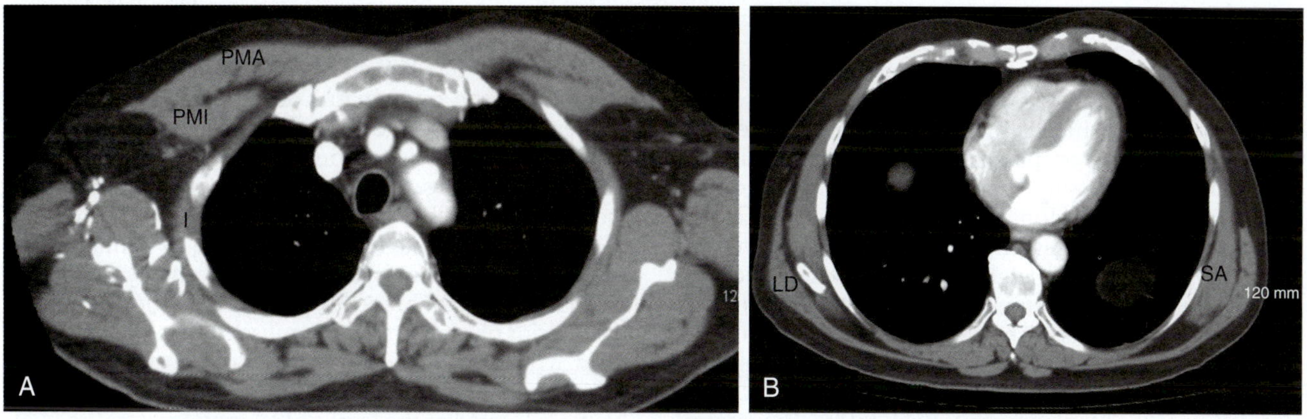

Figure 2.11 Muscles. (A) Axial CT scan at the level of the upper chest showing the pectoralis major *(PMA)*, pectoralis minor *(PMI)*, and intercostal *(I)* muscles. (B) Axial CT scan at a lower level showing the serratus anterior *(SA)* and latissimus dorsi *(LD)* muscles.

The internal intercostal muscles are located internally between the ribs, originate on the second through 12th ribs, and insert on the first through 11th ribs, respectively. The transverse thoracis muscle arises on either side, from the lower third of the posterior surface of the body of the sternum, from the posterior surface of the xiphoid process, and from the sternal margins of the lower three or four true ribs and inserts on the second through sixth ribs.

The posterior superior serratus originates as a thin and broad aponeurosis from the lower portion of the ligamentum nuchae, from the spinous process of the seventh cervical and upper two or three thoracic vertebrae, and from the supraspinal ligament and inserts on four fleshy digitations along the upper borders of the second through fifth ribs. The posterior inferior serratus originates from the T11 through L2 vertebrae and inserts on the lower borders of the ninth through 11th ribs. The latissimus dorsi muscle originates from the spinous processes of T7 through L5, thoracolumbar fascia, iliac crest, and inferior three or four ribs and inferior angle of the scapula and inserts on the floor of the intertubercular portion of the humeral groove (see Fig. 2.11B). The teres major muscle, another posterior chest wall muscle, functions as a medial rotator and adductor. The teres major originates from the posterior aspect of the inferior angle of the scapula and inserts on the medial lip of the humeral intertubercular sulcus. The trapezius muscle is present along the medial neck and upper and mid portions of the posterior thorax. It originates from the external occipital protuberance, nuchal ligament, medial superior nuchal line, and spinous process of vertebrae C7–T12 and inserts on the posterior border of the lateral third of the clavicle, acromion process, and spine of the scapula. The trapezius supports the arm and retracts, medially rotates, and depresses the scapula.

Lymph Nodes

Several lymph nodes are seen in the chest wall. Internal mammary (internal thoracic, parasternal) nodes are located along the internal mammary vessels at the anterior ends of the intercostal spaces (Fig. 2.12A). The posterior intercostal lymph nodes are located near the head and neck of the posterior ribs. The juxtavertebral (prevertebral or paravertebral) nodes are located along the anterior and lateral aspects of vertebral bodies, typically from T8 to T12.

The axillary lymph nodes are also encountered on chest CT scans (see Fig. 2.12B). There are five groups:

1. Lateral or brachial group, located inferomedial to the axillary vein
2. Anterior pectoral group, behind the pectoralis major muscle along the lower border of pectoralis minor, resulting in a chain along the lateral thoracic vessels
3. Posterior subscapular group, along the subscapular vessels in the groove between the teres minor and subscapularis
4. Central group—central axillary adipose tissue between the previously described chains
5. Apical group, seen in the apex of axilla, behind the superior portion and above the pectoralis minor muscle

■ Diaphragm

The diaphragm, which is the primary muscle of respiration, is a dome- or parachute-shaped fibromuscular structure that separates the thorax from the abdomen. The diaphragm develops between 4 and 12 weeks of gestation from the fusion of four major embryologic structures—the paired (right and left) pleuroperitoneal folds, transverse septum, muscular body wall, and esophageal mesentery. The tranverse septum is located anteriorly and fuses with the muscular body wall laterally, posteriorly with the esophageal mesentery, and posterolaterally with the pleuroperitoneal folds. The central tendon of the diaphragm is a noncontractile structure that originates from the transverse septum. A Morgagni hernia results from a defect in fusion of the transverse septum to the lateral body wall, whereas a Bochdalek hernia results from a defect of pleuroperitoneal folds or from the failure of fusion of the pleuroperitoneal folds and transverse septum with the intercostal muscles.

The diaphragm has numerous attachments on the body wall (Fig. 2.13). Anteriorly and laterally, it is attached to the sternum, xiphoid process, lower six ribs, and their costal cartilages. The diaphragmatic slips or muscle bundles are seen in CT attaching to the anterior ribs. Posteriorly, there are two fibrous crura, which are attached to the anterior aspect of the upper lumbar spine and are connected by the fibrous median arcuate ligament. The medial arcuate ligament is another posterior attachment, which extends anterior to the psoas muscle as an attachment (fibrous) between the L1 or L2 vertebral body and L1 transverse process (Fig. 2.14A–C). The lateral arcuate ligament is another posterior attachment, thickened fascial bands anterior to the quadratus lumborum muscle, extending from the T12 transverse process to the mid portion of the 12th rib. The arcuate ligaments can be confused with lymph nodes or peritoneal deposits.

There are three diaphragmatic hiatuses or openings, which allow the passage of structures between the thorax and abdomen (see Fig. 2.14D). The caval hiatus is located at the level of T8, passes through the central tendon, and contains the IVC and right phrenic nerve. With inspiration, the caval hiatus descends and approaches the level of T10. In addition, the hiatus enlarges with inspiration, and thus venous return is increased to the heart. The esophageal hiatus is an oval or elliptic opening located at the level of T10 that passes through the crossing of the right diaphragmatic crus fibers; it contains the esophagus, vagus nerve, branches of the sympathetic plexus, esophageal branches of the left gastric artery, and left inferior phrenic artery. The muscle fibers of this hiatus form a ring around the esophagus, functioning as a sphincter that prevents gastroesophageal reflux. The aortic hiatus is located at the level of T12, posterior and medial to the diaphragmatic crura, and contains the aorta,

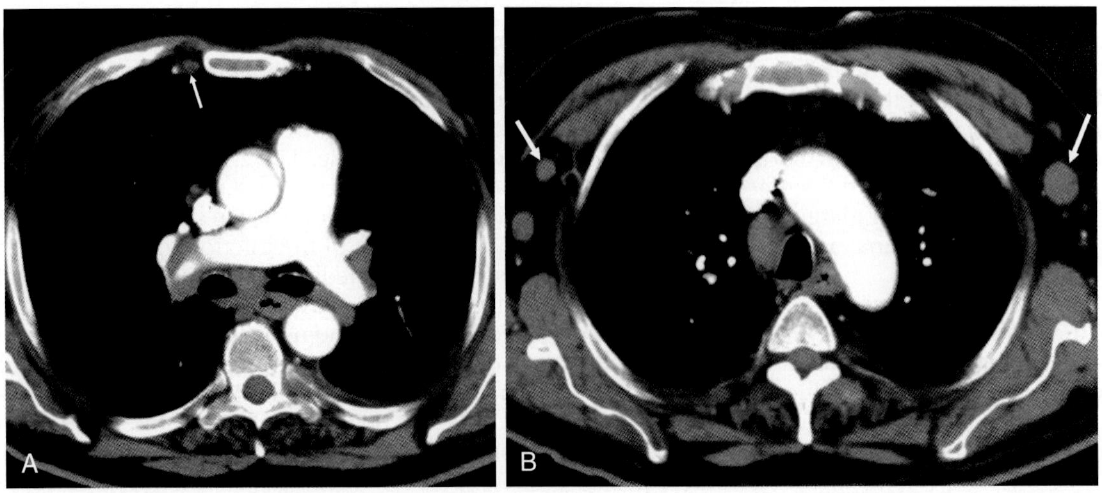

Figure 2.12 (A) Axial CT scan showing enlarged, right internal mammary lymph node *(arrow)*. (B) Axial CT scan showing bilateral enlarged, axillary lymph nodes *(arrows)*.

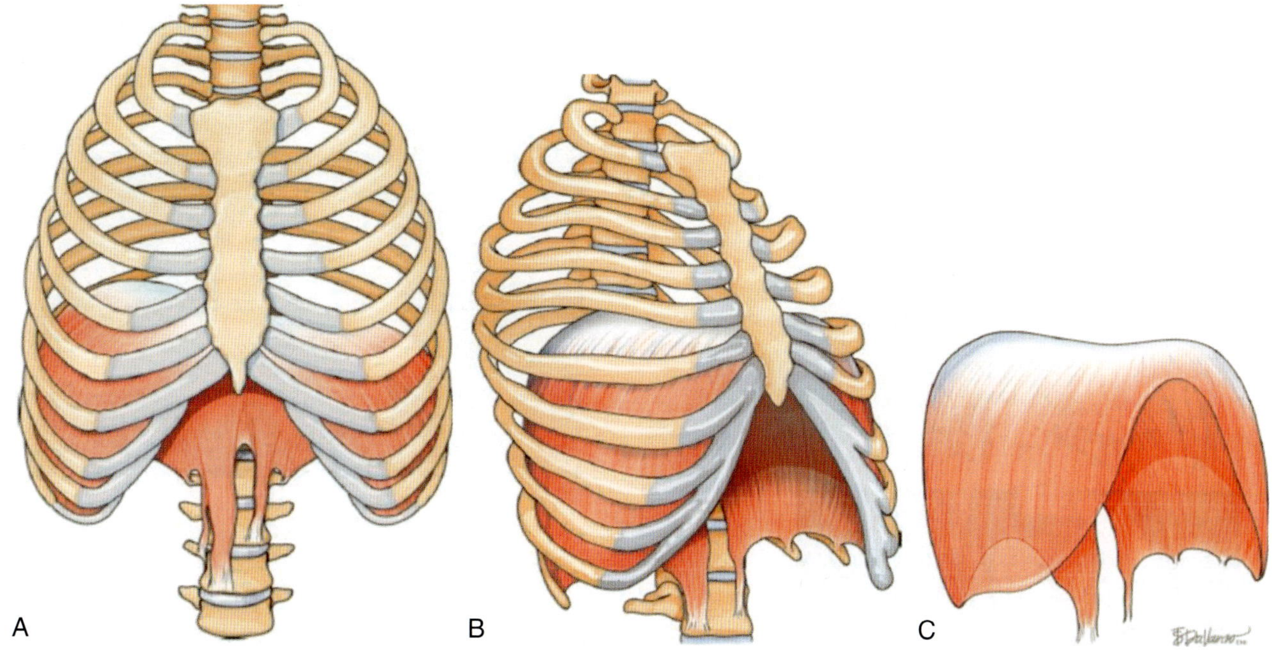

Figure 2.13 Diaphragm. (A) Origin of the diaphragm from the lower ribs and xiphoid process. (B) Origin of the diaphragmatic muscle from the lower ribs and xiphoid process, oblique view. (C) Umbrella dome shape of the diaphragm.

thoracic duct, azygos, hemiazygos veins, lymph nodes, and splanchnic nerves. Because this is located in the retrocrural location, the opening is not affected by diaphragmatic contraction.

The diaphragm is innervated by the right and left phrenic nerves. These nerves originate from the cervical nerves C3–5, extend through the posterior aspect of the lateral compartment of the neck, and extend anteriorly through the thorax and then along the anterior surface of the pericardium to reach the diaphragm, where they branch on the superior and inferior aspects. The phrenic nerves provide afferent sensory and efferent motor branches. The diaphragm is perfused by the pericardiophrenic, musculophrenic, superior phrenic, and inferior phrenic arteries. The pericardiophrenic artery is a branch of the internal thoracic artery that is located close to the phrenic nerve and supplies the superior diaphragm, along with the pericardium. Musculophrenic branches originate from the internal thoracic and superior epigastric arteries and supply the superior portion of the diaphragm. The superior phrenic artery, a branch of the lower thoracic aorta, supplies the posterosuperior portion of the diaphragm. The inferior phrenic artery, a branch of the abdominal aorta, supplies the inferior portion of the diaphragm. The veins of the diaphragm go along with the artery and drain into the azygos vein.

The right dome of the diaphragm is higher than the left dome by one to one-and-a-half intercostal spaces; however, occasionally they can be at the same level as the left or can be higher. On CT and MRI, the diaphragm is smooth and thicker anteriorly and posteriorly and thinner in the center, particularly just above the liver. The average thickness on sagittal CT images is 5 mm, ranging from 7 to 10 mm. The right crus typically measures between 5 and 7 mm in thickness and is thicker than the left. The lower lateral portion of the left hemidiaphragm, which overlies the spleen, often has a scalloped appearance that is not commonly seen with the right hemidiaphragm.

As described above, the diaphragm is the primary respiratory muscle, which during inspiration works in concert with the accessory muscles of inspiration, resulting in expansion of the thoracic cavity and decreased negative intrathoracic pressure, and therefore airflow into the lungs. During relaxation of the diaphragm, the lungs undergo elastic recoil, resulting in exhalation. The normal diaphragmatic excursion, or the expansion that occurs during contraction of the diaphragm for inhalation, ranges from 3 to 5 cm. However, in well-conditioned individuals, such as athletes, the diaphragmatic excursion may increase to 7 to 8 cm. The diaphragm is also used in emesis, urination, and defecation by elevation of intraabdominal pressure. It helps prevents gastroesophageal reflux by contraction of the diaphragmatic hiatus.

There are several lymph nodes located in the superior and central aspects of the diaphragm. The anterior diaphragmatic nodes—cardiophrenic angle, pericardial, paracardiac—are located behind the xiphoid, seventh rib, and costal cartilages, anterior to the pericardium, in the cardiophrenic fat pads. On CT, up to two lymph nodes are seen in normal individuals, typically less than 5 mm. The middle diaphragmatic nodes (juxtaphrenic or lateral group), seen above the diaphragm and medial to the diaphragmatic dome, are commonly seen adjacent to the IVC on the right. These nodes are usually not visible on CT in normal individuals. The posterior diaphragmatic (retrocrural) nodes are located in the inferior aspect of the posterior mediastinum in the retrocrural space, posterior to the crura and anterior to the spine. Normally, these nodes are less than 6 mm.

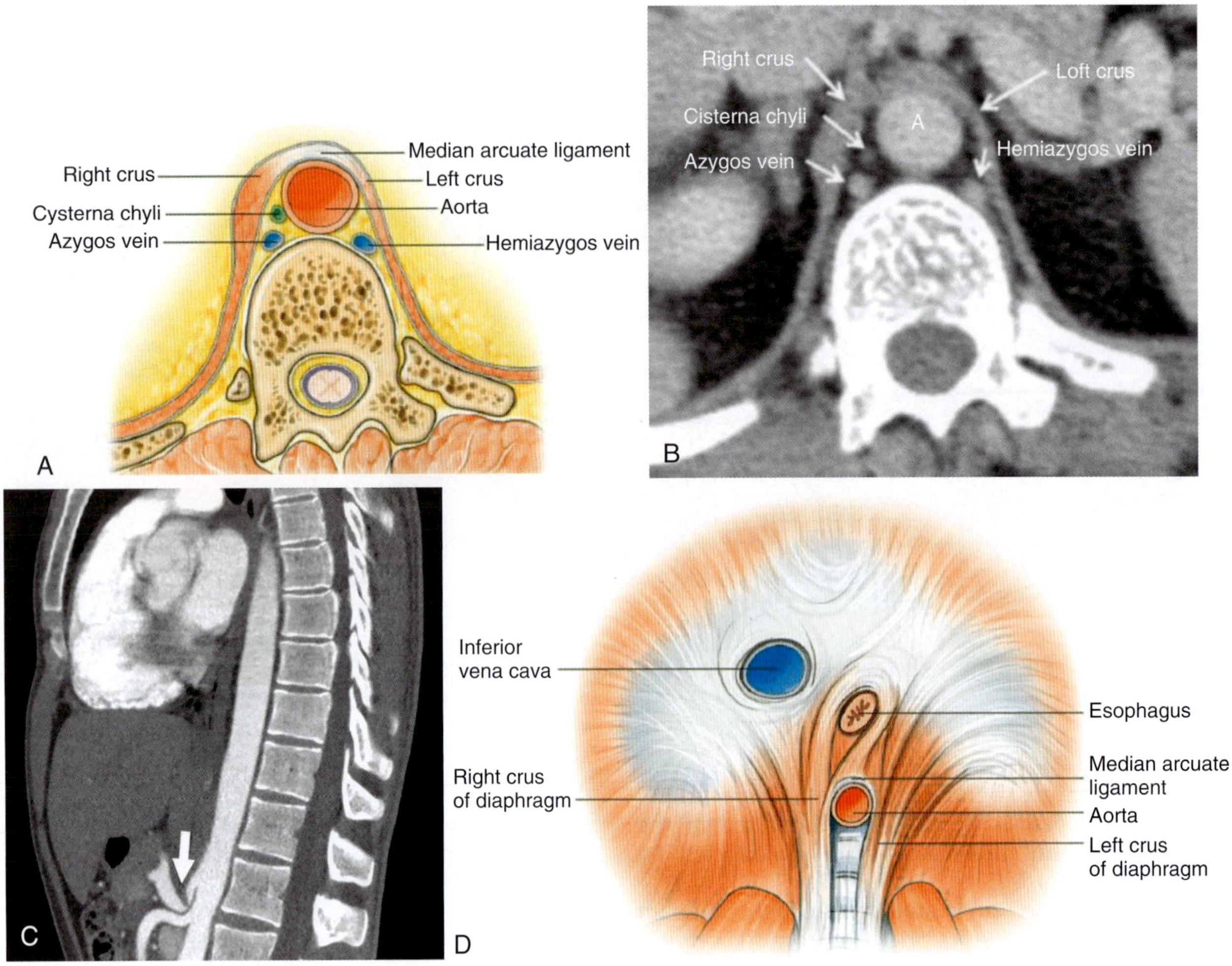

Figure 2.14 Diaphragm. (A) Median arcuate ligament of the diaphragm at the level of the lower thorax, enclosing the retrocrural space, which consists of the azygos vein, hemiazygos vein, and cisterna chyli. (B) Corresponding axial CT scan shows the right and left crus of the diaphragm and retrocrural space containing the azygos vein, hemiazygos vein, and cisterna chyli. (C) Sagittal CT image shows a prominent median arcuate ligament *(arrow)*, which is seen compressing the celiac artery, producing the median arcuate ligament syndrome. (D) Different diaphragmatic hiatuses—caval hiatus at the level of T8, esophageal hiatus at the level of T10, and aortic hiatus at the level of T12.

Conclusion

The mediastinum, chest wall, and diaphragm can be evaluated by multiple imaging modalities. The chest radiograph is often the initial imaging modality used for the evaluation of these structures and their abnormalities. CT and MRI are important cross-sectional imaging modalities that are useful in the evaluation and characterization of abnormalities in these structures. A thorough understanding of the normal anatomy is essential for the accurate diagnosis of cardiopulmonary disease.

Bibliography

Aronberg DJ, Peterson RR, Glazer HS, et al. Superior diaphragmatic lymph nodes: CT assessment. *J Comput Assist Tomogr*. 1986;10:937–941.

Baron RL, Lee JK, Sagel SS, Peterson RR. Computed tomography of the normal thymus. *Radiology*. 1982;142:121–125.

Breatnach E, Abbott GC, Fraser RG. Dimensions of the normal human trachea. *AJR Am J Roentgenol*. 1983;141:903–906.

Carter BW, Tomiyama N, Bora FY, et al. A modern definition of mediastinal compartments. *J Thorac Oncol*. 2014;9(9):S97–S101.

Clemens MW, Evans KK, Mardini S, et al. Introduction to chest wall reconstruction: anatomy and physiology of the chest and indications for chest wall reconstruction. *Semin Plast Surg*. 2011;25(1):5–15.

de Geer G, Webb WR, Gamsu G. Normal thymus: assessment with MR and CT. *Radiology*. 1986;158:313–317.

El-Sherief AH, Lau CT, Wu CC, et al. International Association for the Study of Lung Cancer (IASLC) lymph nodal map: radiologic review with CT illustration. *Radiographics*. 2014;34:1680–1691.

Felson B. The mediastinum. *Semin Roentgenol*. 1969;4(1):41–58.

Ferdinand B, Gupta P, Kramer EL. Spectrum of thymic uptake at 18F-FDG PET. *Radiographics*. 2004;24:1611–1616.

Francis IR, Glazer GM, Bookstein FL, Gross BH. The thymus: reexamination of age-related changes in size and shape. *AJR Am J Roentgenol*. 1985;145:249–254.

Fujimoto K, Hara M, Tomiyama N, et al. Proposal for a new mediastinal compartment classification of transverse plane images according to Japanese Association for Research on Thymus (JART) general rules for the study of mediastinl tumors. *Oncol Rep*. 2014;31(2):565–572.

Gamsu G, Webb WR. Computed tomography of the trachea: normal and abnormal. *AJR Am J Roentgenol*. 1982;139:321–326.

Gatzoulis MA. Mediastinum. In: Standring S, ed. *Gray's Anatomy: The Anatomical Basis of Clinical Practice*. 40th ed. Philadelphia: Churchill Livingstone; 2008:939–957.

Gawande RS, Khurana A, Messing S, et al. Differentiation of normal thymus from anterior mediastinal lymphoma and lymphoma recurrence at pediatric PET/CT. *Radiology*. 2012;262:613–622.

Goldstraw P, Crowley J, Chansky K, et al. The IASLC lung cancer staging project: proposals for the revision of TNM stage group ins in the forthcoming (seventh)

edition of TNM classification of malignant tumors. *J Thorac Oncol.* 2007;2(8):706–714.
Goodman LR, Teplick SK, Kay H. Computed tomography of the normal sternum. *AJR Am J Roentgenol.* 1983;141:219–223.
Guttentag AR, Salwen JK. Keep your eyes on the ribs: the spectrum of normal variants and diseaes that involve the ribs. *Radiographics.* 1999;19(5):1125–1142.
Harisinghani MG. Chest lymph node anatomy. In: Harisinghani MG, ed. *Atlas of Lymph Node Anatomy.* New York: Springer; 2013.
Heitzman ER. *The Mediastinum: Radiologic Correlations With Anatomy and Pathology.* 2nd ed. Berlin/New York: Springer-Verlag; 1988.
Holbert JM, Strollo DC. Imaging of the normal trachea. *J Thorac Imaging.* 1995;10:171–179.
Kuhlman JE, Bouchardy L, Fishman EK, Zerhouni EA. CT and MR imaging evaluation of chest wall disorders. *Radiographics.* 1994;14:571–595.
Liu ME, Branstetter BF, Whetstone J, et al. Normal CT appearance of the distal thoracic duct. *AJR Am J Roentgenol.* 2006;187:1615–1620.
Nason LK, Walker CM, McNeeley ME, et al. Imaging of the diaphragm: anatomy and function. *Radiographics.* 2012;32:E51–E70.
Nasseri F, Eftekhari F. Clinical and radiologic review of the normal and abnormal thymus: pearls and pitfalls. *Radiographics.* 2010;30:413–428.
Noh HM, Fishman EK, Forastiere AA, et al. CT of the esophagus: spectrum of disease with emphasis on esophageal carcinoma. *Radiographics.* 1995;15: 1113–1134.
Shields TW. Primary tumors and cysts of the mediastinum. In: Shields TW, ed. *General Thoracic Surgery.* 1st ed. Philadelphia: Lea and Febiger; 1972:908.
Sone S, HIgashihara T, Morimoto S, et al. Potential spaces of the mediastinum: CT pneumomediastinography. *AJR Am J Roentgenol.* 1982;138(6):1051–1057.
Spritzer C, Gamsu G, Sostman HD. Magnetic resonance imaging of the thorax: techniques, current applications, and future directions. *J Thorac Imaging.* 1989;4:1–18.
Suwatanapongched T, Gierada DS. CT of thoracic lymph nodes. Part I: anatomy and drainage. *Br J Radiol.* 2006;79:922–928.
Taneoue LT. Staging of non-small cell lung cancer. *Semin Respi Crit Case Med.* 2009;29(3):28–260.
Vock P, Spiegel T, Fram EK, Effmann EL. CT assessment of the adult intrathoracic cross section of the trachea. *J Comput Assist Tomogr.* 1984;8:1076–1082.
Whitten CR, Khan S, Munneke GJ, Grubnic S. A diagnostic approach to mediastinal abnormalities. *Radiographics.* 2007;27:657–671.
Wittram C, Fischman AJ, Mark E, Ko J, Shepard JA. Thymic enlargement and FDG uptake in three patients: CT and FDG positron emission tomography correlated with pathology. *AJR Am J Roentgenol.* 2003;180:519–522.
Xia F, Mao J, Ding J, et al. Observation of normal appearance and wall thickness of esophagus on CT images. *Eur J Radiol.* 2009;72(3):406–411.
Zylak CJ, Pallie W, Jackson R. Correlative anatomy and computed tomography; a module on mediastinum. *Radiographics.* 1982;2(4):555–592.

CHAPTER 3

Imaging Anatomy of the Heart and Thoracic Great Vessels

Sachin S. Saboo, Prabhakar Rajiah, Prashant Nagpal, and Suhny Abbara

CHAPTER OUTLINE

Introduction

Various imaging techniques are used in the assessment of the normal anatomy and pathology of the heart and great vessels. Chest radiography is the most commonly used modality and is often the first imaging test used in the assessment of patients with suspected cardiovascular disorders. Advances in cross-sectional imaging, such as computed tomography (CT) and magnetic resonance imaging (MRI), have enabled dedicated and precise assessment of the morphology and function of the heart. The cardiac chambers, coronary vessels, and valves can all be comprehensively imaged with CT and MRI. With the routine use of retrospective electrocardiographic (ECG) gating or prospective triggering and advanced postprocessing techniques, cardiac structures can be assessed without motion artifacts in multiple planes.

Cardiac Anatomy on Conventional Radiography

The use of conventional posteroanterior and lateral chest radiographs enables the assessment of the normal and abnormal cardiovascular structures that have their interface with the lung. On the posteroanterior radiograph, the structures that form the right margin of the cardiomediastinal silhouette from superior to inferior are the right innominate vein, superior vena cava (SVC), right atrial appendage (RAA), right atrium (RA), and inferior vena cava (IVC; Fig. 3.1A). The structures that form the left margin of the cardiomediastinal silhouette, from superior to inferior, are the left subclavian artery, aortic knob, aortopulmonary window, main pulmonary artery (MPA), left atrial appendage (LAA), and left ventricle (LV).

On the lateral radiograph, the anterior margin of the cardiac silhouette is formed by the right ventricle (RV), right ventricular outflow tract (RVOT), and MPA. The upper half of the posterior border of the cardiac silhouette is formed by the left atrium (LA), and the lower half is formed by the posterior wall of the LV. On the lateral radiograph, the right pulmonary artery (RPA) is seen as an oval opacity located immediately anterior to the right upper lobe bronchus, whereas the left pulmonary artery (LPA) is seen above the left upper lobe bronchus (see Fig. 3.1B).

Technical Factors for Cardiac Imaging and the Imaging Planes

ELECTROCARDIOGRAPHIC GATED SCAN

Cardiac motion leads to blurred image borders on CT and MRI. With the use of ECG gating, the image acquisition is timed to the specific phase of the cardiac cycle that provides relatively motionless imaging of the heart, coronary vessels, and proximal aorta. ECG gating can be done retrospectively or prospectively. Retrospective ECG gating is a look-back technique in which images are obtained during the entire cardiac cycle, and the best phases are reconstructed later. In prospective triggering, the data are obtained only during a specific phase of the cardiac cycle that typically is end-diastole, because it is the most motion-free phase of cardiac cycle. The radiation dose to the patient is lower with prospective ECG

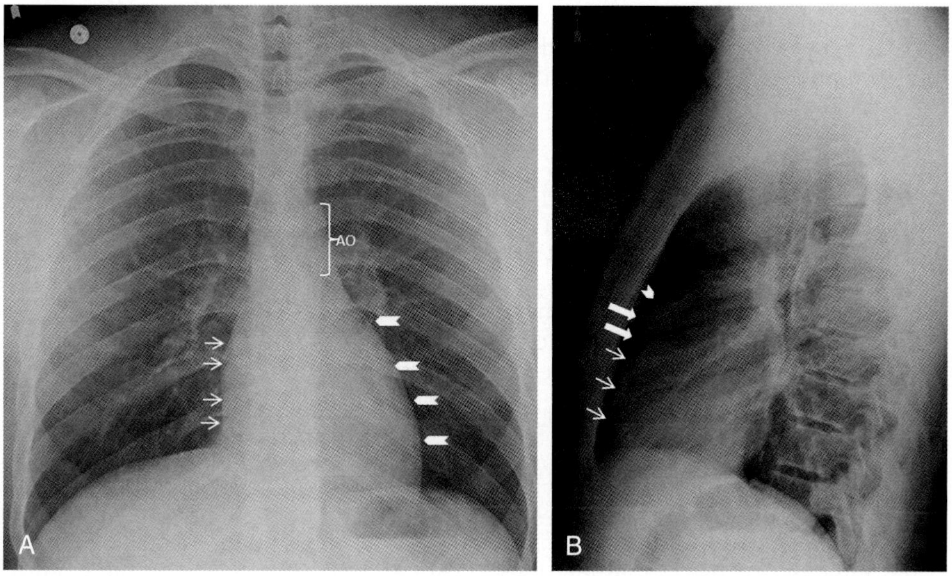

Figure 3.1 Chest radiograph. (A) Posteroanterior radiograph shows that the right border of the cardiomediastinal silhouette is formed by the right innominate vein, superior vena cava, right atrium (RA). and inferior vena cava, from top to bottom. Dilation of the RA *(small arrows)* and inferior vena cava can cause widening of the right cardiac silhouette. The left border of the cardiomediastinal silhouette is formed by the left subclavian artery, aortic knuckle *(AO)*, aortopulmonary window, main pulmonary artery (MPA), left atrial appendage, and left ventricle (LV) *(arrowheads)*. Aortopulmonary (AP) window nodal enlargement and an enlarged MPA are common causes of the convex appearance of the AP window; LV enlargement results in leftward, inferior, or posterior displacement of the left heart border. (B) Lateral radiograph shows that the anterior margin of the cardiac silhouette is formed by the right ventricle (RV; *thin white arrows*), right ventricular outflow tract (RVOT; *white bold arrows*), and the MPA *(arrowhead)*. An enlarged RVOT and RV cause obliteration of retrosternal space on lateral view. The upper half of the posterior border of the cardiac silhouette is formed by the left atrium, and the posterior wall of the LV forms the lower half. Left atrial enlargement causes posterior displacement of the left main bronchus on lateral chest x-ray and a convex appearance of the upper posterior cardiac silhouette.

triggering but, if cine images are required for assessment of left ventricular (LV) wall motion or cardiac valves, retrospective ECG gating is preferred. The images can be reconstructed at specific points during the cardiac cycle for cine imaging. Cine imaging is also required for the assessment of LV wall thickening and determination of quantitative LV functional parameters (e.g., ventricular volumes, stroke volume, ejection fraction).

Cardiac Imaging Planes

Various imaging techniques such as echocardiography, single-photon emission computed tomography (SPECT), positron emission tomography (PET), CT, and MRI have been used to image the heart. To maintain standardization across various techniques, imaging of the heart is displayed along standard orientation planes—short axis, vertical long axis, two chamber, and horizontal long axis, four chamber. These orientation planes also help match various segments of myocardium with their coronary artery supply. The short-axis, horizontal, and vertical long-axis images are obtained at 90 degrees to the long axis of the LV (plane through the apex and center of the mitral valve [MV]).

Although CT images are obtained perpendicular to the long axis of body, four-chamber, three-chamber, and two-chamber planes can be reconstructed from volumetric data due to isotropic resolution of images obtained on newer scanners. The three-dimensional (3D) workstations with cardiac analysis capability can easily produce images in standard planes. These planes can be briefly summarized as below.

Two-Chamber View (Paraseptal View)

The two-chamber or vertical long axis view is an oblique sagittal plane along the LV cavity axis and is best suited for visualization of the left atrial (LA) and LV cavities, MV, and anterior and inferior walls of the LV (Fig. 3.2A).

Three-Chamber View

The three-chamber view is an oblique plane that is useful for the evaluation of the mitral and aortic valves, LA and LV cavities, and aortic root. This plane can be obtained manually on multiplanar images by including three points—the center of the MV, the LV apex, and the center of the aortic valve. Other structures that can be evaluated on this plane include the inferolateral and anteroseptal segments of the LV and the posteromedial papillary muscles, along with its chordae tendineae (see Fig. 3.2B).

Four-Chamber View

The four-chamber view is an oblique plane that displays all four chambers of the heart. This plane can be manually reproduced on multiplanar images by including the center of the MV, the LV apex, and the center of the tricuspid valve (TV). This plane allows for the assessment of cardiac chamber sizes, evaluation of the MV and TV, and LV inferoseptal and anterolateral segments and LV apex (see Fig. 3.2C).

Short-Axis Views

Short-axis views are a stack of oblique planes perpendicular to the long axis of the LV cavity on both the four-chamber and paraseptal long axis views (see Fig. 3.2D). The LV myocardium can be divided into basal, mid, and apical segments in the short-axis planes. Short-axis views are useful for assessing the LV cavity, regional wall motion, and myocardial anatomy based on the 17-segment model (see Fig. 3.2E).

Aortic Valve: Short-Axis View

This plane is used for the evaluation of aortic valvular morphology, stenosis, regurgitation, valve prostheses, or masses. The aortic valve short-axis view is a plane that is orthogonal to the long axis of the LV outflow tract (LVOT) and aortic root on the three-chamber view.

Right Ventricular Inflow-Outflow Plane

This plane is used for the evaluation of the right side chambers and tricuspid and pulmonic valves. It can be manually reconstructed by joining the center of the TV, RV apex, and center of the pulmonic valve (Fig. 3.3A–C).

Bicaval View

The bicaval view is a standard view on echocardiography that helps visualize the SVC and IVC inflow and superior part of the interatrial septum (IAS), mostly needed for the evaluation and treatment planning of ostium secundum atrial septal defect (ASD; see Fig. 3.3D). On CT, this view can be manually reconstructed using multiplanar techniques.

Cardiac Chambers

Right Atrium

The RA forms most of the right heart border on a chest radiograph. The venoatrial junctions form the proximal margin of the RA, and the RA terminates at the fibrofatty tissue plane of the atrioventricular (AV) junction. It can be divided into three parts: (1) venous part; (2) appendage; and (3) vestibule. The RA receives the deoxygenated blood from the SVC and IVC, coronary sinus (CS), Thebesian veins, and anterior cardiac vein. It is morphologically larger than the LA but has a thinner wall, measuring up to 2 mm. The distinct feature of the RA is the presence of an internal ridge called the *crista terminalis* (externally, sulcus terminalis) that divides the smooth-walled venous RA from the rough-walled appendage. It starts from the orifice of the SVC and extends to

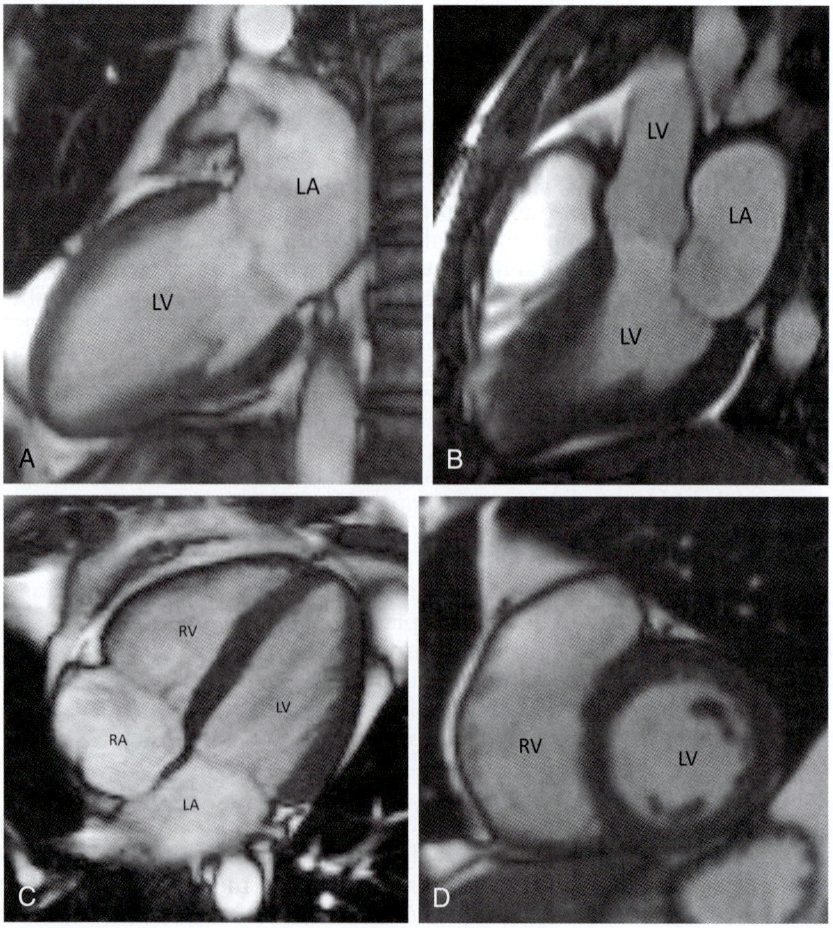

Figure 3.2 Cardiac imaging views. (A) Two-chamber, steady-state free precession (SSFP) view showing the left ventricle *(LV)*, left atrium *(LA)*, and mitral valve (MV). This view helps assess the LV apex and anterior and inferior walls for pathologies, including infarcts and aneurysms. (B) Three-chamber SSFP view shows the LA, LV, and left ventricular outflow tract. The MV and aortic valve are also shown; this is a good view to assess for left atrial enlargement and systolic anterior motion of the MV in hypertrophic cardiomyopathy, in addition to anteroseptal and inferolateral wall abnormalities. (C) Four-chamber SSFP view shows all four cardiac chambers and the mitral and tricuspid valves and is a good view to assess abnormalities of the atrioventricular valves, cardiac chambers, and wall motion abnormalities, including right ventricular free wall dyskinesia in arrhythmogenic right ventricular dysplasia and LV aneurysm. *RA*, Right atrium; *RV*, right ventricle. (D) Short-axis SSFP view shows the LV and RV with the interventricular septum separating them and is a standard view in cine to assess for wall motion abnormalities and cardiac functions.

Continued

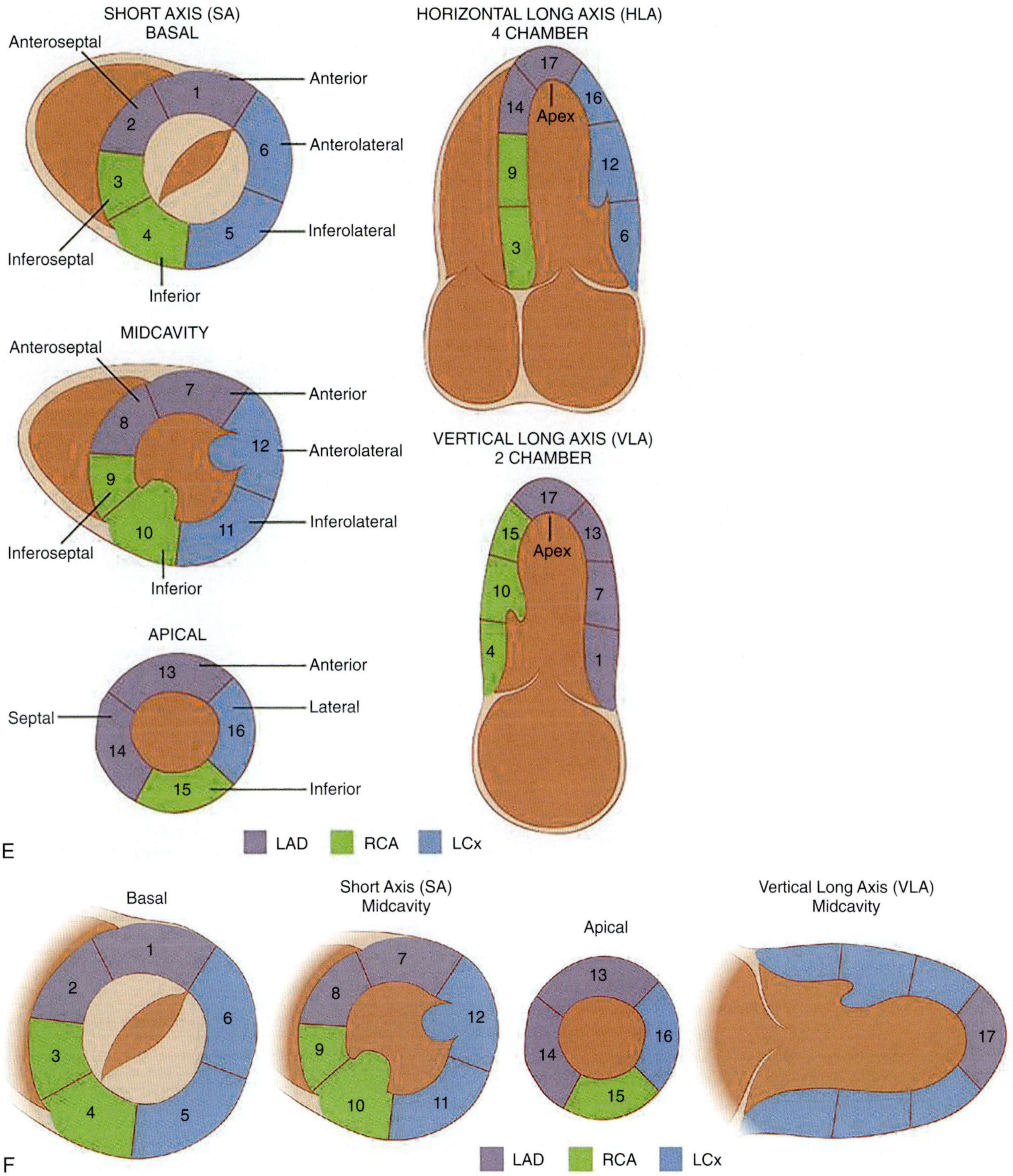

Figure 3.2, cont'd (E) The 17-segment model for two-dimensional transthoracic echocardiography. The ventricle is divided into thirds from base to apex, and then the radial segments are assigned names and numbers at each level. The basal third extends from the mitral annulus to the tip of the papillary muscles at end-diastole, the middle third extends through the papillary muscles, and the apical third is composed of the remaining cavity, distally from the end of the papillary muscle; the true apex is a single segment. *LAD,* Left anterior descending artery; *LCx,* left circumflex artery; *RCA,* right coronary artery. (F) The 17-segmental model for the nuclear stress test. (F from Abbara S, Kalva S. *Problem Solving in Cardiovascular Imaging.* St. Louis: Elsevier; 2012.)

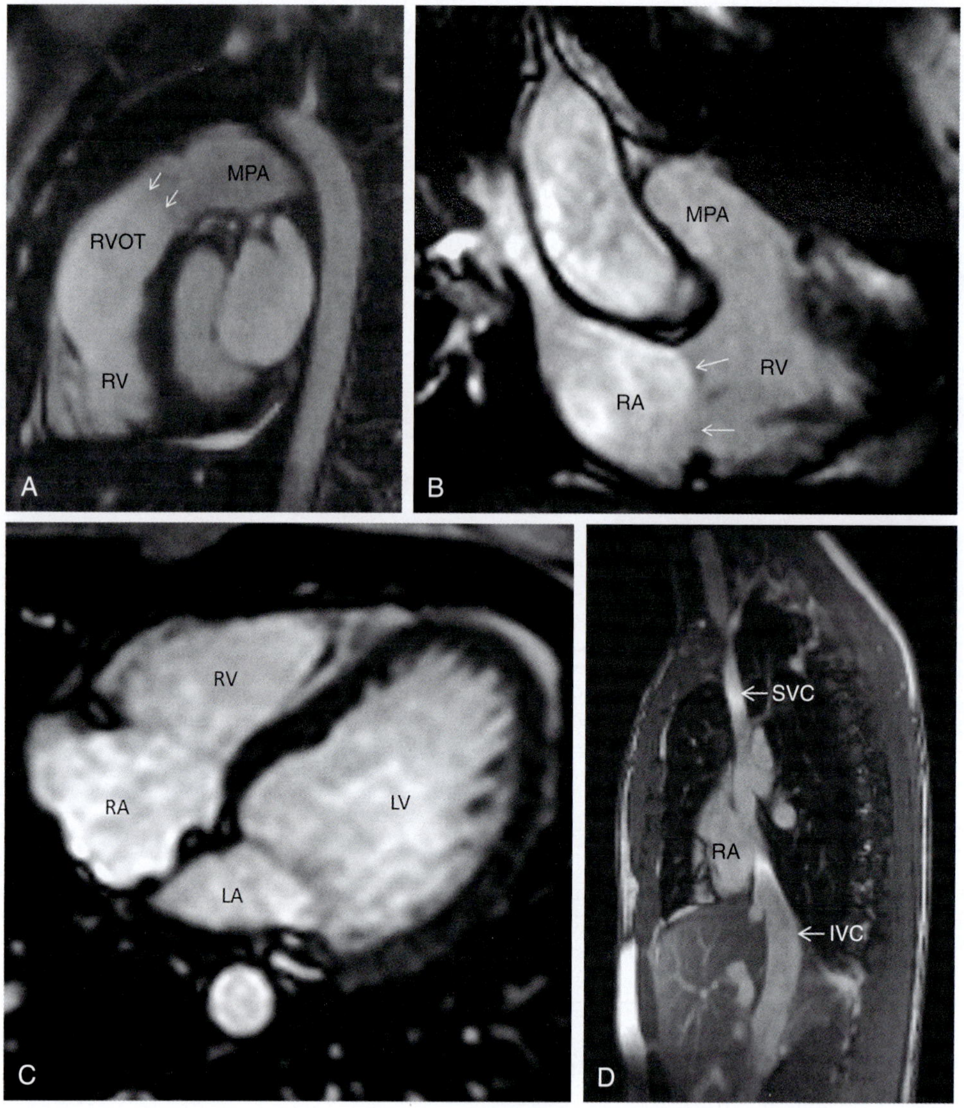

Figure 3.3 Right cardiac chamber imaging views. (A) Right ventricle *(RV)* outflow steady-state free precession view shows the right ventricular outflow tract *(RVOT)*, pulmonic valve *(arrows)*, and main pulmonary artery *(MPA)*. This is useful to assess for RVOT stenosis, pulmonic valve abnormalities, and pulmonary artery dilation and narrowing. (B) RV inflow shows the right atrium *(RA)*, tricuspid valve *(arrows)*, RV, pulmonic valve, and MPA. (C) RV, horizontal long-axis view, shows all four cardiac chambers and the RV free wall anteriorly. *LA*, Left atrium; *LV*, left ventricle. (D) Bicaval view shows both the superior vena cava *(SVC)* and inferior vena cava *(IVC)* draining into the RA and is useful to assess their drainage pattern and filling defects.

the anterior aspect of the IVC orifice. The sinoatrial (SA) node, the pacemaker of the heart, is usually located at the junction of the crista terminalis and SVC. The most accurate assessment of laterality of the cardiac chambers for the determination of situs is based on the extent of the pectinate muscle from the AV junction. The vestibule is the smooth muscular rim adjacent to the tricuspid annulus.

Other important anatomic landmarks within the RA that can be assessed by cross-sectional imaging include the cavotricuspid isthmus and triangle of Koch. The cavotricuspid isthmus is best seen on a coronal view and represents the area between the tricuspid annulus and IVC. This area is a good target for radiofrequency ablation because it aids in the maintenance of reentrant circuits. The triangle of Koch represents the anatomic location of the AV node; it is defined as the area between the tendon of Todaro (fibrous extension from the eustachian valve), septal leaflet of the TV, and orifice of the CS. The morphologic features of the LA and RA are highlighted in Table 3.1.

TABLE 3.1 Morphologic Features of Right and Left Atria

RIGHT ATRIUM	LEFT ATRIUM
1. Larger and more triangular appendage, with a broad junction with smooth part of RA	1. Pointed and finger-like appendage with narrow ostial connection with main LA body
2. Prominent terminal crest between the appendage and smooth venous component	2. Generally on same side as bilobed lung
3. Generally on the same side as trilobed lung	
4. Rule of venoatrial concordance: The chamber receiving the IVC inflow is almost always RA	

IVC, Inferior vena cava; *LA*, left atrial; *RA*, right atrium.

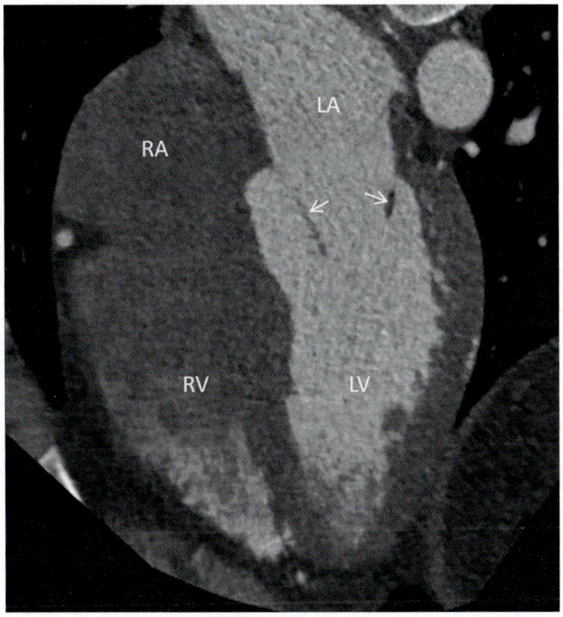

Figure 3.4 CT scan of cardiac chambers. This four-chamber reconstruction shows an expected minimally opacified right atrium *(RA)* and right ventricle *(RV)*, whereas the left atrium *(LA)*, left ventricle *(LV)*, aorta, and coronary arteries are well opacified. Note mitral valve leaflets are well seen *(arrows)*, whereas tricuspid valve leaflets may not be visible, as in this case.

Right Ventricle

The RV is the most anterior chamber of the heart. It has more complex geometry and orientation than the LV. Anatomically, it can be divided into three parts: (1) the inlet, consisting of the TV, chordae tendineae, and papillary muscles; (2) the trabeculated apical myocardium; and (3) the smooth-walled infundibulum–conus arteriosus (also referred to as the RVOT). As compared to the LV, the RV has a thinner wall (measuring ≈3–4 mm) but with significantly more trabeculations. Another distinct feature of the RV is the presence of the moderator band, which is a muscular extension from interventricular septum to the RV free wall, near the RV apex. The moderator band prevents the overdistention of the ventricle and contains the right bundle branch. The RV has three, or sometimes more, papillary muscles (anterior, posterior, and septal) that attach to the respective leaflets of the TV (anterior, posterior, and septal). The anterior papillary muscle is the largest and arises from the anterior free wall of the RV. The septal papillary muscle is the least consistent papillary muscle of the RV and often cannot be distinguished from the ventricular wall. The pulmonary artery arises from the conus of the RV and is positioned anterior and to the left of the aorta. Another feature that helps identify the morphologic RV is that the muscular infundibulum separates the tricuspid and pulmonary valves, with no fibrous continuity among them (Fig. 3.4). The morphologic features of the LV and RV are highlighted in Table 3.2.

Left Atrium

The LA is the most posterior chamber of the heart and is located superior to the RA due to the obliquity of the IAS. It is separated from the RA by the presence of the IAS, which is a thin structure that may be difficult to assess accurately on MRI. Higher spatial resolution of newer multidetector CT (MDCT) scanners allows improved evaluation of the IAS, especially when there is fat deposition in it. It is important to distinguish relatively benign lipomatous hypertrophy of IAS from other fat-containing cardiac masses. The lipomatous hypertrophy of IAS is associated with septal thickening that is usually more than 1.5 cm thick and spares the fossa ovalis, giving rise to the typical dumbbell-hourglass appearance. In-depth knowledge of the LA and its appendage is important because catheter ablation of the LA is being increasingly used for patients with atrial fibrillation.

The transverse pericardial sinus and aortic root lie immediately anterior to the LA, whereas tracheal bifurcation, the esophagus, and the descending thoracic aorta lie immediately posterior to the pericardium lining the outside of the posterior wall of the LA. The wall of the LA is muscular but is smooth on its internal aspect. The wall thickness of the LA varies but is thinnest at the anterior aspect, just behind the aortic root, which is considered the unprotected area and is at a higher risk of perforation. Intervention electrophysiologists are especially interested in the posterior wall of the LA and the relationship of the esophagus relative to the pulmonary vein (PV) orifices due to possible esophageal injury associated with ablation procedures. The LA has a finger-like appendage arising from the anterolateral aspect of the main body, adjacent to the left superior PVs (LSPVs). The main body of the LA can be divided anatomically into the pulmonary venous part, septal part, and vestibule—the portion of the LA adjacent to the MV orifice.

The clinical significance of LA size has been the topic of various studies; it has been shown that an increase in LA size correlates with poor patient prognosis in patients with an acute myocardial infarction, and higher LA size correlates with a higher chance of atrial fibrillation in older populations. The size of the LA is measured at end-ventricular systole, and the LA area and volume can be calculated on 3D workstations by manually drawing the outline along the endocardial border of the LA at the MV and in its superior aspect. The workstation interpolates the endocardial border in between these lines and should

TABLE 3.2 Morphologic Features of Right and Left Ventricles

RIGHT VENTRICLE	LEFT VENTRICLE
1. A septal tricuspid valve leaflet attaches more apically than the matching septal mitral valve leaflet.	1. The trabeculae are thin and delicate, with smooth septal surface.
2. The chamber, including the apex, is coarsely trabeculated and contains the moderator band.	2. Papillary muscles (usually two) attach only to free walls.
3. Papillary muscles (usually three) attach to the free wall and interventricular septum.	3. There is fibrous continuity between the mitral and aortic valves.
4. A muscular infundibulum separates the tricuspid and pulmonic valves.	

exclude PVs and the LAA. The reference limits for the area of the LA are highlighted in Table 3.3.

LEFT ATRIAL APPENDAGE

The LAA is an embryologically distinct part of the LA that arises from the trabeculated primitive LA, as compared to the smooth-walled LA that arises from the pulmonary venous bud. The LAA arises from the superolateral part of the LA and forms part of the left heart border on radiography. The LAA is closely related to the pulmonary trunk superiorly; inferiorly, it is adjacent to the left coronary artery (LCA) in the AV groove and free wall of the LV. Usually, the LAA is directed anterosuperiorly. The LAA is one of the common anatomic sites in the heart to harbor thrombus that may be responsible for an embolic phenomenon. Internally, the LAA contains the pectinate muscles that increase in thickness with age; they are more than 1 mm in thickness in more than 90% of those older than 20 years. These pectinate muscles may be mistaken for thrombus on cross-sectional imaging and echocardiography. Anatomically, the LAA can be further divided into the (1) ostium, (2) neck, and (3) body. Based on its gross appearance, the LAA has been divided into four shape types—cactus, chicken wing, wind sock, and cauliflower (Fig. 3.5). Overall, the chicken wing is the most common subtype and is also associated with the least incidence of embolism in patients with LAA thrombus. The knowledge of various anatomic parameters and their variations is important because it may help guide interventional procedures aimed at closing the LAA to prevent thromboembolism. As compared to the LAA, the RAA has a wider ostium and is more triangular and pyramidal in shape. This distinction may be important in patients with complex congenital heart disease for the determination of situs.

TABLE 3.3 Reference Limits for Left and Right Atrial Areas[a]

LIMIT (cm^2)	SIGNIFICANCE OF FINDINGS
<20	Normal
20–30	Mildly abnormal
30–40	Moderately abnormal
>40	Severely abnormal

[a]For both men and women.

PULMONARY VEINS

Normally, there are four PVs, two on each side, that carry oxygenated blood from either lung to the LA. The knowledge of PV anatomy and its variations is important because the variations in drainage may be symptomatic, and PV ostia are commonly targeted for catheter ablation therapy. The normal configuration of PVs and its ostia is seen in 60% to 70% of the population (Fig. 3.6A). The variations in left side PVs are more common, with the most common variation being the convergence of superior and inferior PVs to drain via a common trunk (short or long; see Fig. 3.6B and C). Variations of the right pulmonary venous system are less common; these include the following: (1) one accessory right middle PV (see Fig .3.6D); (2) two accessory right middle PVs; and (3) one accessory right middle PV and one accessory right upper PV (see Fig. 3.6E).

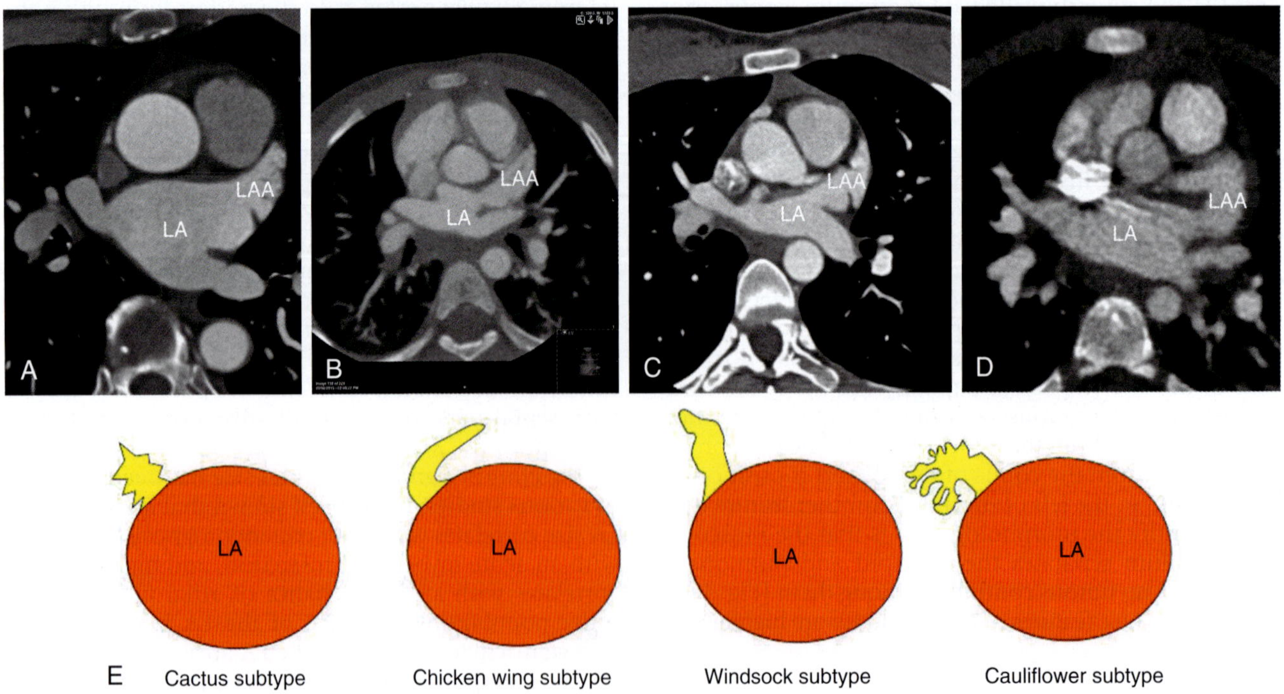

Figure 3.5 Left atrial appendage *(LAA)* morphology types. (A–E) Patients with chicken wing LAA morphology are less likely to develop thromboembolism than patients with non-chicken wing morphology. *LA,* Left atrium.

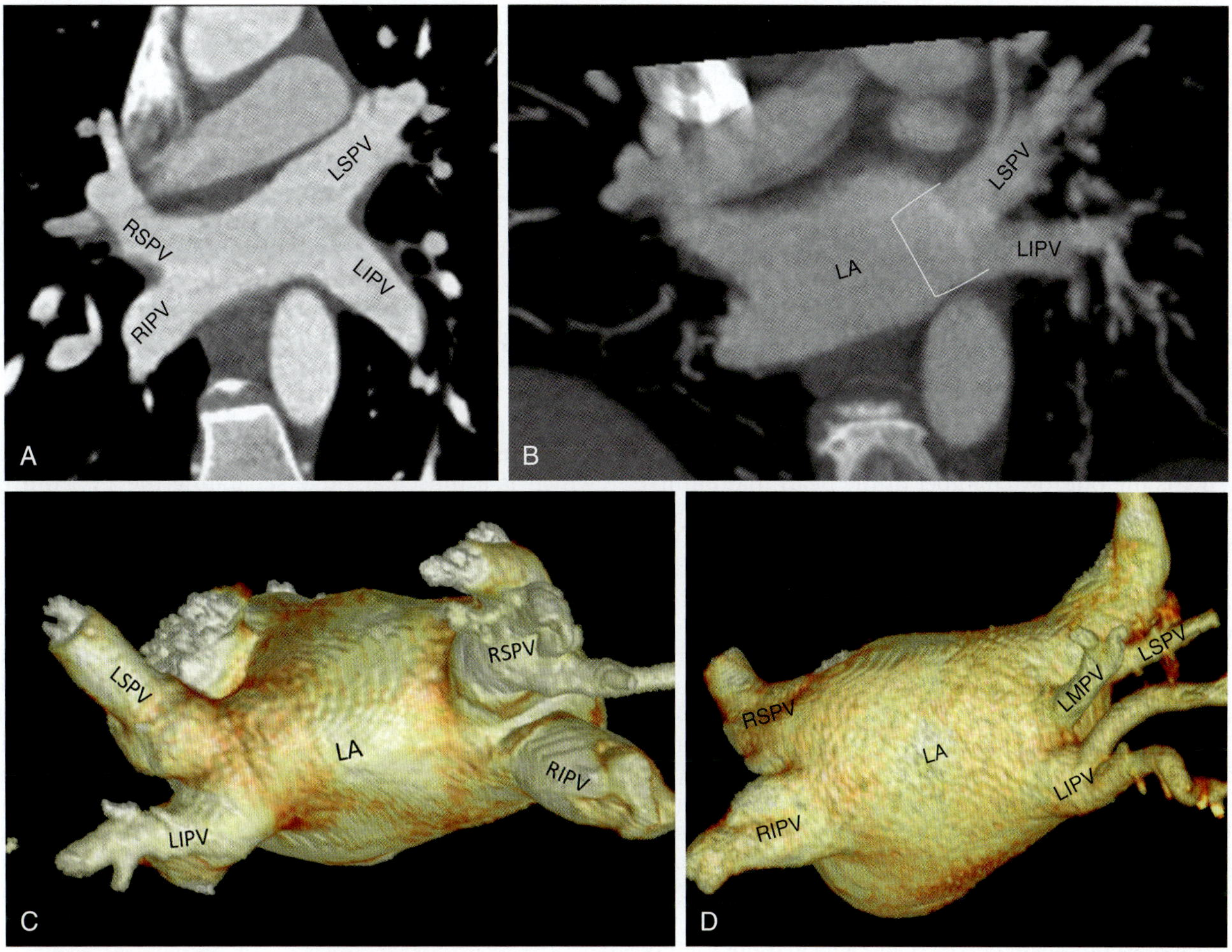

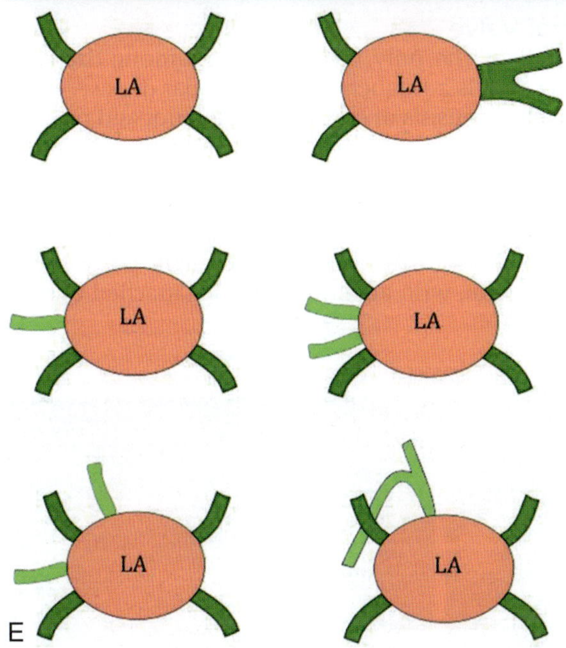

Figure 3.6 Pulmonary venous anatomy. (A) Coronal oblique multiplanar reconstruction (MPR) shows normal pulmonary venous anatomy, with right superior *(RSPV)*, right inferior *(RIPV)*, left superior *(LSPV)*, and left inferior *(LIPV)* pulmonary veins (PVs). (B) Coronal MPR shows common ostium *(boxy arrow)* for the LSPV and LIPV. This represents the most common nonanomalous pulmonary venous variant resulting in a common vein, with only one venoatrial junction on the involved side. (C) Three-dimensional volume-rendered reconstruction of a CT scan shows a common ostium for the LSPV and LIPV. *LA,* Left atrium. (D) Three-dimensional volume-rendered reconstruction shows a separate ostium for the left middle vein, which drains directly into the LA. Note that accessory or supernumerary PVs are more common on the right side, usually the right middle lobe or superior segment of the right lower lobe. *LMPV,* Left middle pulmonary vein. (E) Schematic diagram of PV anatomy and variations. Light green lines connecting to the LA are variant accessory veins, whereas dark green lines connecting to the LA are normally draining PVs. The upper right image shows a normal branching pattern composed of the two PVs on each side. The middle right image shows an accessory right middle PV. The lower right image shows one accessory right middle PV and one accessory right upper PV. The upper left image shows a common trunk formed by the confluence of the left upper and lower PVs. The middle left image shows two accessory right middle PVs. The lower left image shows the right top PV draining separately from the right upper PV into the LA.

The muscular layer of the LA extends into the wall of the distal PVs. The length of extension of the atrial myocardium correlates with the extension of the pericardium along the PVs. The LSPV has the longest intrapericardial course (11–13 mm) and is the focus of atrial fibrillation in most patients. The LSPV is separated from the ostium of the LAA by the presence of a fold of the lateral atrial wall, known as the *left lateral ridge, left tinea terminalis,* or *coumadin ridge*. When prominent, it can be mistaken for a thrombus or mass. It is also important to recognize the anomalous drainage of PVs because it may go undetected until adulthood, when it may present with progressive shortness of breath. Pulmonary venous drainage is defined as anomalous if the PV is draining into any vascular structure other than the LA. If at least one PV drains into the LA, it is called a *partial anomalous pulmonary venous connection*; otherwise, it is called *total anomalous pulmonary venous drainage*. On CT imaging, PV imaging can be obtained without the use of ECG gating but, if CT is being done for radiofrequency ablation planning, ECG gating is preferable (if low-dose acquisition is available), because it helps reproduce accurate epicardial and endoluminal volume-rendered images.

Left Ventricle

The LV is the outflow chamber of the heart that pumps the oxygenated blood into the systemic circulation. With respect to the RV, it lies posteriorly and to the left. The LV has the thickest myocardium among the cardiac chambers, and its inner surface can be distinguished from the RV by the presence of fine trabeculae carneae, giving it a relatively smooth appearance. Fibrous continuity between the mitral and aortic valves also helps distinguish the LV from the RV. Another characteristic feature of the LV is the presence of anterior (lateral) and posterior (medial) papillary muscles, which are attached only to the free wall of the LV. Each papillary muscle receives chordae tendineae from either MV leaflet, which prevents regurgitation of blood into the LA during ventricular systole. The anterolateral papillary muscle has a richer blood supply, derived from the branches of the left anterior descending artery (LAD) and left circumflex artery (LCx). The posteromedial papillary muscle is more prone to necrosis owing to the relatively poor blood supply from the LCx and posterior descending artery (PDA).

Cardiac Valves

Improvement in the temporal and spatial resolutions of CT and MRI has enabled noninvasive evaluation of cardiac valvular structure and function. The valves that are commonly assessed by imaging include the aortic, mitral, pulmonic, and tricuspid valves.

Tricuspid Valve

The TV is composed of three leaflets and separates the RA from the RV. The TV apparatus consists of leaflets, annulus, commissures, chordae tendineae, and papillary muscles. The leaflets are labeled as anterior, posterior, and septal and are connected to a fibrous ring, known as the *annulus*. The three cusps are continuous to each other at their bases, forming the commissures. Due to lower right side pressure, the TV leaflets are usually thinner than the MV leaflets. The chordae tendineae attach to the free margin of the TV leaflets and connect them to the two papillary muscles. One distinguishing feature of the TV is the presence of the crista supraventricularis, which is a muscular ridge separating the TV from the pulmonic valve (Fig. 3.7).

Pulmonic Valve

The pulmonic valve is a tricuspid semilunar valve that separates the RVOT from the pulmonary artery. Its three cusps (or leaflets) are labeled as right, left, and anterior. Anatomically, the pulmonic valve is located superior, anterior, and to the left of the aortic valve (Fig. 3.8). The lack of fibrous continuity with the TV also helps distinguish the pulmonic valve from the aortic valve. The central part of the valve leaflet has a thick central focus, also known as the *nodulus of the semilunar valve*, and a thin lateral free edge margin, known as the *lunula of the semilunar valve*. Normally, the pulmonic valve measures 2.0 cm^2/m^2 of body surface area.

Mitral Valve

The MV is the only bicuspid valve among the cardiac valves that is a frequent site of valvular disease. The MV apparatus consists of two leaflets (anterior and posterior), MV annulus, chordae tendineae, and papillary muscles. The MV allows flow from the LA to the LV during ventricular diastole and prevents any backflow during systole. The mitral annulus is a D-shaped structure, which is the anchor site for MV leaflets. The straight portion of the D is anterior, with an anterior leaflet attached to it. This

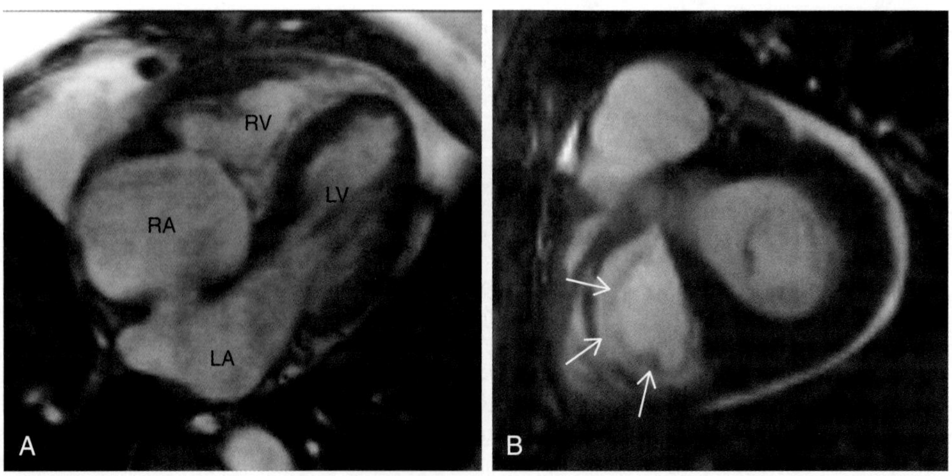

Figure 3.7 Normal tricuspid valve (TV). (A) Four-chamber steady-state free precession MR image shows the three-leaflet morphology of the TV. Note that the septal leaflet hinge point of the normal TV is usually closer to the cardiac apex than the septal leaflet insertion of the mitral valve (usually within ~1 cm). (B) Short-axis steady-state free precession MR image shows the anterior, posterior, and septal leaflets of the TV *(arrows)*. *LA,* Left atrium; *LV,* left ventricle; *RA,* right atrium; *RV,* right ventricle.

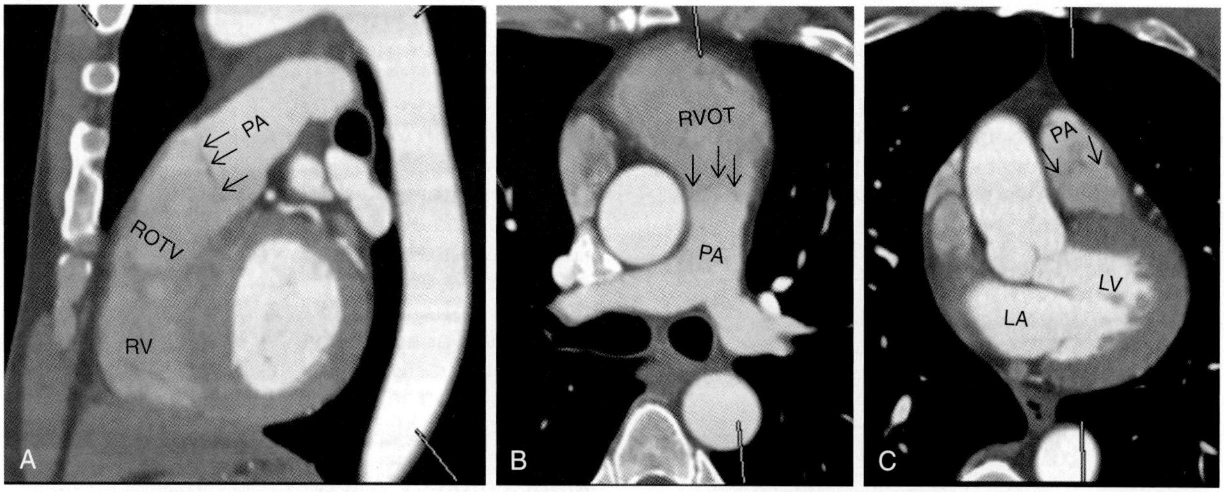

Figure 3.8 Normal trileaflet pulmonic valve. (A) Sagittal reconstructed CT image shows the pulmonic valve *(arrows)* separating the right ventricular outflow tract *(RVOT)* from the pulmonary artery *(PA)*. *RV,* Right ventricle. (B) Axial oblique CT image shows pulmonic valve *(arrows)*. The pulmonary valve level is the most common site for pulmonic stenosis, producing a fibrous, thickened, dome-shaped commisural valve with a fish mouth–shaped narrowing during systole; subvalvular and supravalvular levels are uncommon sites for pulmonic stenosis. (C) Pulmonic valve on an axial image *(arrows)*. *LA,* Left atrium; *LV,* left ventricle.

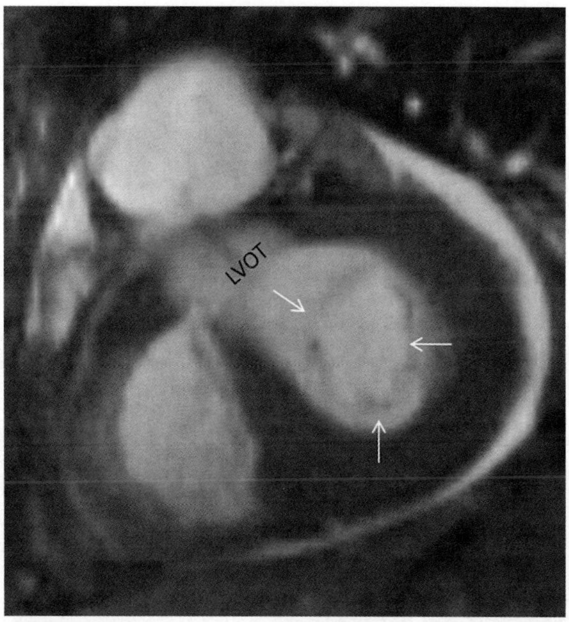

Figure 3.9 Normal mitral valve. This short-axis steady-state free precession MR image shows the normal anterior and posterior leaflets of the open mitral valve *(arrows)* attached to the annulus fibrosus in cross section. *LVOT,* Left ventricular outflow tract.

straight anterior portion of the annulus is responsible for the fibrous continuity between the MV and fibrous skeleton of the heart. Because the anterior (straight) and posterior (curved) portions of the mitral annulus are unequal, the MV leaflets are also unequal in size, with a broader anterior leaflet covering more of the valve area and the narrower posterior leaflet. The anterior and posterior MV leaflets can be subdivided into three segments (scallops)—A1, A2, A3 and P1, P2, and P3, respectively (Fig. 3.9). The most cephalad scallops of the anterior and posterior leaflets are labeled A1 and P1, respectively; the most caudal scallops are labeled A3 and P3, respectively. The MV leaflets are normally less than 5 mm thick, and the valve area is approximately 4 to 6 cm^2. The leaflets are attached to the papillary muscles via multiple chordae tendineae. These papillary muscles contract during the ventricular systole, which is responsible for the close apposition of MV leaflets that prevents prolapse and regurgitation of blood flow. The single blood supply of the posteromedial papillary muscle (vs. dual blood supply of the anterolateral papillary muscle) makes it more prone to ischemia and rupture.

Aortic Valve

The aortic valve separates the LVOT and ascending aorta and is characterized by curvilinear annular attachments to the aortic ring. It has three leaflets; the area where two leaflets come together is known as the *commissure.* The aortic cusps are separated by three aortic commissures that are approximately equidistant around the valve annulus. The aortic valve is sometimes also referred to as the *semilunar valve* because the aortic cusps are half-moon shaped (Fig. 3.10). On the aortic aspect of leaflets, the aortic root has three prominences known as the *sinuses of Valsalva.* The right aortic sinus is most anterior and normally gives off the right coronary artery (RCA). The noncoronary sinus is the most posterior and, as the name signifies, the coronary artery does not normally arise from this sinus. The LCA comes off the left aortic sinus. As opposed to the right side, which has a muscular infundibulum separating the tricuspid and pulmonic valves, there is fibrous continuity between the aortic and mitral valves.

Coronary Arteries

The coronary arteries arise from the aortic sinus of Valsalva and supply various layers of the heart (Fig. 3.11). These arteries are also called *epicardial arteries* because they travel in the epicardial fat of interventricular septum and the AV grooves. Their branches supply the visceral pericardium, myocardium, and endocardium. The RCA and LCA arise from the right and left aortic sinus, respectively. The RCA and its branches almost always supply the RV.

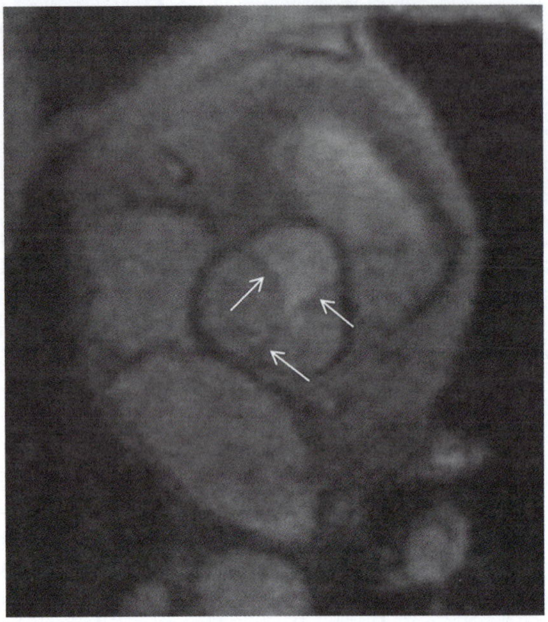

Figure 3.10 Normal aortic valve. This short-axis steady-state free precession MR image viewed through the closed aortic valve shows coaptation of its three normal cusps (*arrows*, right, left, and posterior coronary cusp) forming right, left, and noncoronary sinuses based on the origin of the coronary artery.

Left Coronary Artery

The LCA is also known as the *left main coronary artery* (LMCA). It arises from the left CS and courses behind the RVOT (between the pulmonary trunk and LA) and inferior to the LAA (Fig. 3.12). After coursing in epicardial fat for a variable length (usually <2 cm), the LMCA usually bifurcates into the LAD (Fig. 3.13) and LCx (Fig. 3.14). In approximately 15% of the population, there is an additional third branch between the LAD and LCx, known as the *ramus intermedius* (Fig. 3.15); this supplies the territory typically supplied by the diagonal branch of LAD or the obtuse marginal (OM) branch of the LCx. Unlike other coronary arteries, in which stenosis of 70% or more is considered significant, any stenosis of 50% or more is significant in the LMCA.

Right Coronary Artery

The RCA arises from the right sinus of Valsalva (Fig. 3.16). The RCA courses posterior to the pulmonary artery and inferior to the RAA to travel in the right AV groove. In approximately 50%–60% of cases, the conus branch is the first branch of the RCA that supplies the RVOT and also forms an anastomosis with the LAD circulation (known as the *circle of Vieussens*). In addition to its origin from the RCA, the conus branch arises directly from the aorta in most cases. The next branch of the RCA is the SA nodal artery in approximately 55% of cases. In the rest of the population, the SA nodal branch comes from the LCx. As the name implies, the SA nodal branch supplies the SA node, which is located at the superiormost aspect of the crista terminalis, near the SVC inflow. As the RCA travels in the AV groove toward the diaphragmatic surface of the heart, it gives off branches to the RV

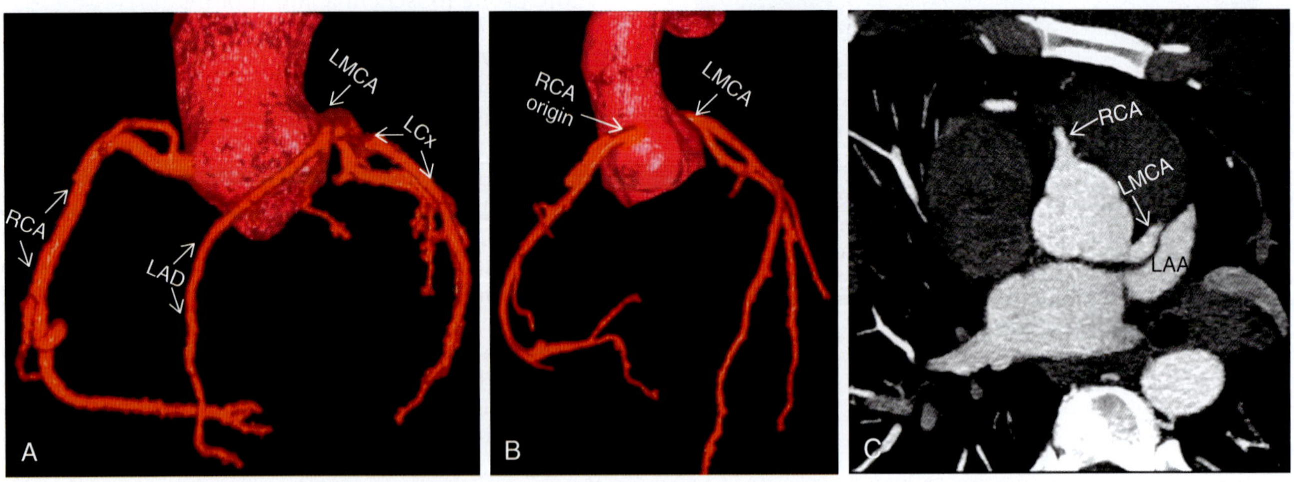

Figure 3.11 Normal coronary artery origin. (A) Three-dimensional volume-rendered coronary CT angiography (CTA) image shows the normal origin, course, branching, and termination of the right *(RCA)* and left *(LCA)* coronary arteries (*arrows*). *LCx,* Left circumflex coronary artery; *LMCA,* left main coronary artery. (B) Oblique three-dimensional volume-rendered reconstructed CTA image shows the origin of the RCA and LCA *(arrows)*. (C) Axial coronary CTA image shows the origin of the RCA and LCA *(arrows)* from the right and left coronary sinuses, respectively, at the aortic root, with no coronary artery originating from the noncoronary cusp, located just anterior to the interatrial septum. Note that coronary artery anomalies are classified as benign or malignant, depending on the anomalous origin and subsequent interarterial course between the aorta and pulmonary artery, with a malignant course presenting as the latter feature. An LCx with an anomalous origin is the most common benign variant, followed by an anomalous origin of the LMCA and RCA; the RCA origin from the left sinus is the most common malignant variant. However, an LCA anomalous origin from the right sinus or RCA has the highest prevalence of sudden death. *LAA,* Left atrial appendage.

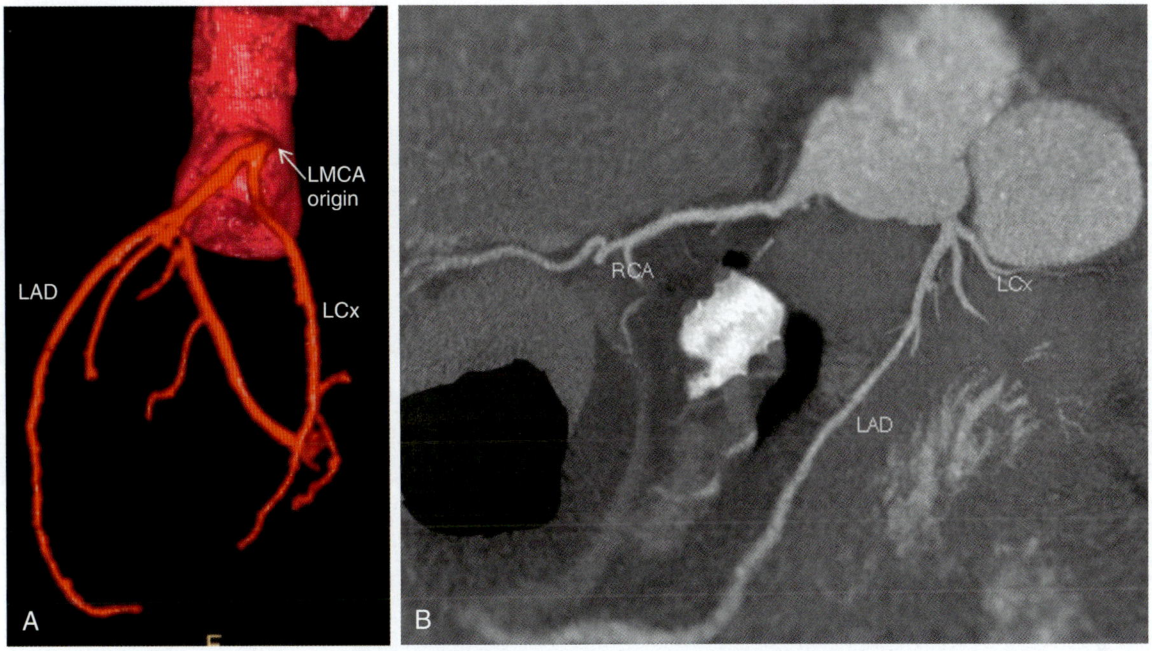

Figure 3.12 Normal left main coronary artery *(LMCA)*. (A) Three-dimensional volume-rendered CT angiography image shows the normal bifurcation of the LMCA into the left anterior descending artery *(LAD)* and left circumflex artery *(LCx)*. (B) Global view of the coronary CT angiography using a maximum intensity projection image shows trifurcation of the LMCA into the LAD, LCx, and ramus intermedius. *RCA*, Right coronary artery.

myocardium, the most prominent of which are RV marginals or acute marginals. The RCA can be divided into proximal, mid, and distal segments, as follows:

1. Proximal RCA: ostium to half the distance to the acute margin of the heart
2. Mid RCA: end of the proximal RCA to the acute margin of the heart
3. Distal RCA: acute margin of the heart to the origin of the PDA

Coronary Dominance

The coronary artery that gives rise to the PDA (Fig. 3.17) and the posterolateral branch (PLB) is labeled as the dominant coronary artery. In about 80%–85% of cases, the coronary circulation is right dominant, meaning that the RCA gives rise to the PDA and PLB, which supply the posterior interventricular septum and the inferoseptal and inferior segments of the LV. In about 15%–20% of cases, the LCx gives off the PDA and PLB, and hence the coronary circulation is left dominant in this scenario. In about 5% of cases, the circulation is codominant, in which the PDA comes off the RCA, and the PLB is a branch of the LCx. Rarely, the LCx is diminutive, and a superdominant RCA also supplies the LCx territory.

Left Anterior Descending Artery

The LAD is usually the larger branch of the LMCA that runs in the anterior AV sulcus, along the interventricular septum. The main branches of the LAD are the diagonal branches and septal perforators. The diagonal branches course over and supply the anterior LV wall. They are numbered sequentially, from proximal to distal, as D1, D2, and D3. The septal perforators supply the anterior two-thirds of the ventricular septum and are also numbered sequentially from proximal to distal. The first septal perforator usually supplies the branches of the AV node and bundle of His. In patients with chronic LAD disease, there may be collaterals to the LAD territory from the RCA via the circle of Vieussens (anastomosis between the conus branch of the RCA and the preinfundibular artery of the LAD) or from the PDA via inferior septal perforators. The LAD can be divided into proximal, mid, and distal segments, as follows:

1. Proximal LAD: from the end of the LMCA to the first large septal or first diagonal, whichever is more prominent
2. Mid LAD: end of the proximal LAD to half the distance to the apex
3. Distal LAD: end of the mid LAD to the termination of the LAD

Left Circumflex Artery

The LCx branches off from the LMCA to run in the left AV groove and gives off branches to supply part of the LA, posterior and lateral free walls of the LV, and anterolateral papillary muscle. In approximately 40% of cases, it gives off a branch to the SA node, but the consistent major branches of the LCx include the OMs, which supply the lateral wall of LV. The OMs are also numbered sequentially, from proximal to distal, as OM1, OM2, and OM3. The nondominant LCx is often diminutive distal to the OM branches, or it terminates as an OM branch. If dominant, the LCx branches into the PDA and PLB. The LCx can be divided as follows:

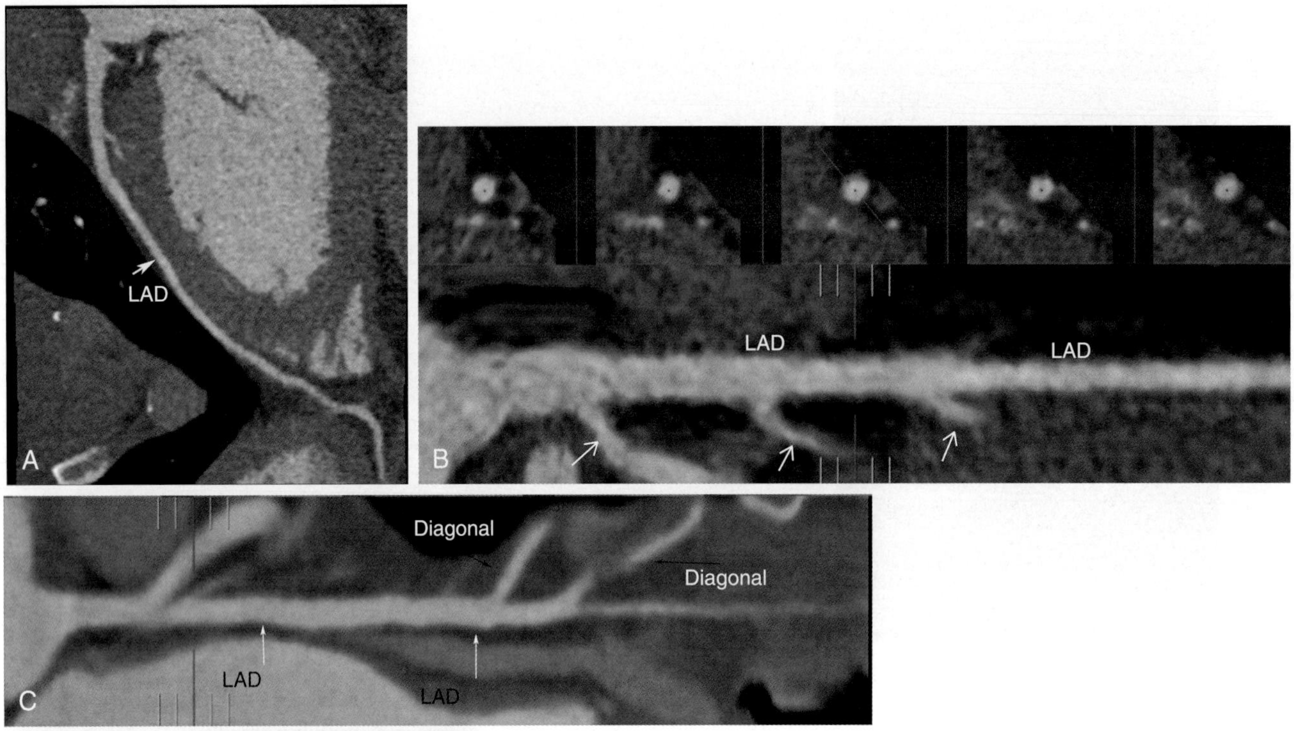

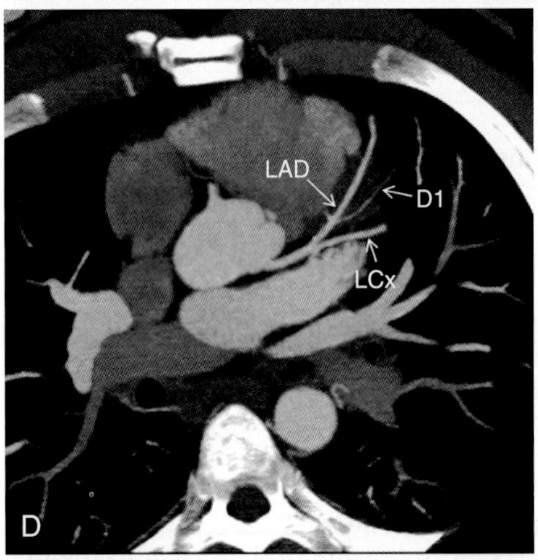

Figure 3.13 Normal left anterior descending artery *(LAD)*. (A) Curved multiplanar reconstruction shows the entire length of the LAD in the epicardial fat of the anterior interventricular groove. (B) Stretched view of LAD showing multiple normal-caliber septal branches *(arrows)*. (C) Stretched view of the LAD artery showing two normal-caliber diagonal branches *(arrows)*. It is important to assess the branch point origin of the diagonal arteries from the LAD artery because atherosclerotic disease in this segment can be overlooked in the absence of proper reconstructions. (D) Axial maximum intensity projection shows the origin of the first diagonal branch *(D1)* from the normal LAD artery. Note the normal proximal portion of the left circumflex artery *(LCx)*.

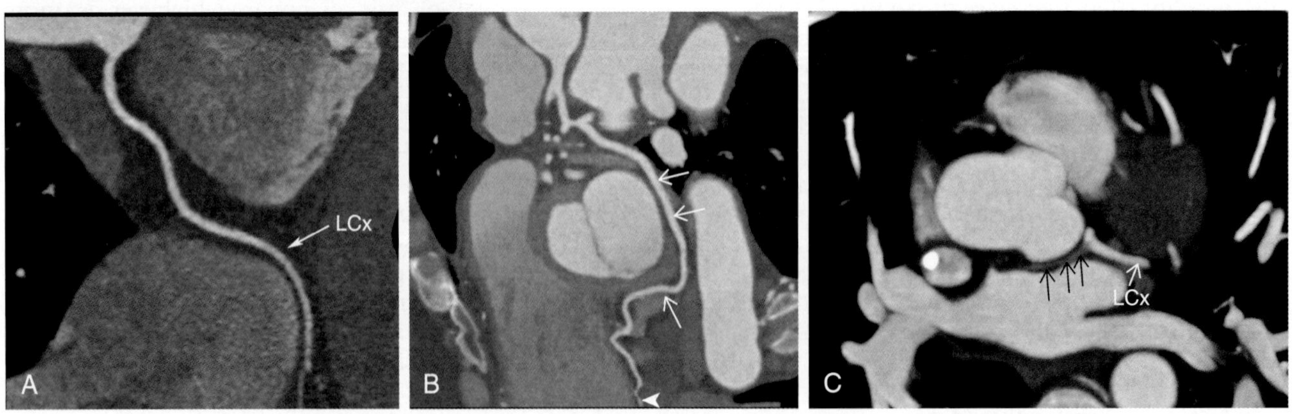

Figure 3.14 (A) Normal left circumflex artery *(LCx)*. Curved multiplanar reconstruction shows the normal course and caliber of the LCx in the epicardial fat of the left atrioventricular groove. (B) Curved multiplanar reconstruction image in a left dominant system shows the LCx *(arrows)* extending along the inferior left atrioventricular groove and giving rise to the posterior descending artery *(arrowhead)*. Conversely, in the usual right dominant system, the LCx is usually a small-caliber artery in its distal course and does not give rise to a posterior descending artery. (C) Axial maximum intensity projection image shows the normal-caliber sinoatrial nodal branch originating from the LCx and coursing in the retroaortic region. A sinoatrial nodal artery can arise from the right coronary artery or LCx; identification of the sinoatrial nodal artery *(black arrows)* is important in patients undergoing a left atrial procedure to prevent its injury.

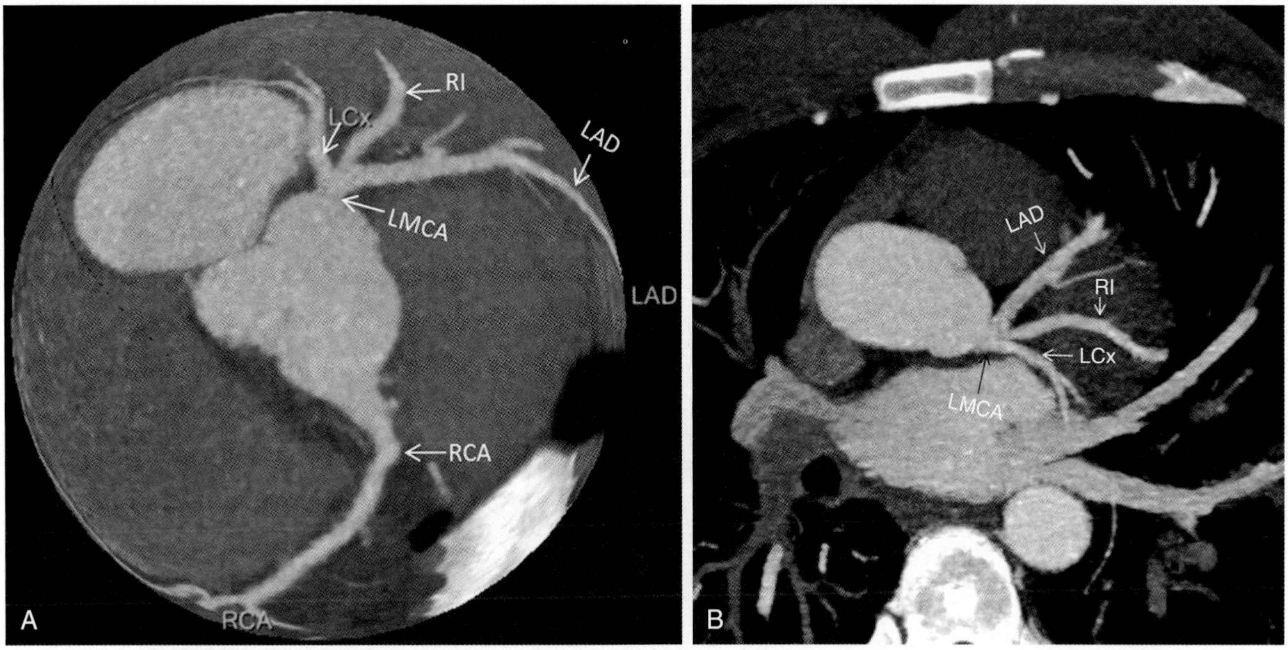

Figure 3.15 Normal ramus intermedius *(RI)*. (A) Global view and (B) axial maximum intensity projection image show the RI artery originating from the left main coronary artery *(LMCA)*, in between the left anterior descending artery *(LAD)* and left circumflex artery *(LCx)*, which supplies the lateral wall of the left ventricle. *RCA*, Right coronary artery.

1. Proximal LCx: from the end of the LMCA to the first OM
2. Mid LCx: end of the proximal LCx to the origin of the second OM
3. Distal LCx: end of the mid-LCx to the termination of the LCx

For reproducible reporting and standardized communication, an 18-segment model has been proposed for the segmentation of the coronary arteries on MDCT by the Society of Cardiovascular Computed Tomography guidelines.

Cardiac Veins

Knowledge of cardiac venous anatomy is important, because imaging is increasingly being used for planning pacemaker and implantable cardioverter-defibrillator lead placement, electrophysiologic procedures, myocardial stem cell therapy, and retrograde cardioplegia. The coronary veins are located in epicardial fat, along with the coronary arteries (Fig. 3.18). These veins carry the deoxygenated blood from the myocardium to the RA. The cardiac veins can be divided into three main subgroups: (1) CS and its tributaries; (2) anterior cardiac veins (which drain the anterior RV and right heart border); and (3) Thebesian veins (which drain the subendocardium directly into either of the ventricles).

The CS is the most consistent structure of the cardiac venous anatomy and is present in nearly 100% of the population. The CS is located at the inferior surface of the heart, within the left AV groove, and drains into the RA, adjacent to the IVC ostium. The CS ostium is guarded by a Thebesian valve, which is thin and fenestrated in most cases. In approximately 15% of cases, the valve may be nonfenestrated, or muscular or fibromuscular; both of these are typically associated with difficult CS cannulation during various procedures. The major tributaries of the CS include the following: (1) anterior interventricular vein; (2) great cardiac vein (GCV); (3) left marginal vein (LMV) and posterior vein of the left ventricle (PVLV); and (4) middle cardiac vein. The anterior interventricular vein accompanies the LAD and continues as the GCV in the anterior left AV groove, along the LCx. The GCV continues in the left AV groove and drains into the CS posteriorly. The LA oblique vein of Marshall marks the external boundary between the CS and GCV; the valve of Vieussens marks the internal boundary. The LA oblique vein is located posterior to the LA, within a fold known as the *ligament of Marshall.* The ligament of Marshall is the developmental remnant of the left SVC. The LMV accompanies the OM branch of the LCx and drains the lateral wall of the LV to terminate in the CS. The LMV is often multiple and may be draining into the GCV. The PVLV drains the lateral wall and diaphragmatic surface of the LV to terminate in the CS (in most cases). There may be considerable variability in the anatomy of the LMV and PVLV, knowledge of which is important because these veins are common targets for the placement of pacemaker leads. The middle cardiac vein, also known as the *posterior interventricular vein,* accompanies the PDA and drains the deoxygenated blood from the posterior aspect of the LV and RV into the CS.

Pericardium

The pericardium is the thin membranous lining that envelops the heart in the middle mediastinum of the chest and anchors the heart to outside structures (the sternum

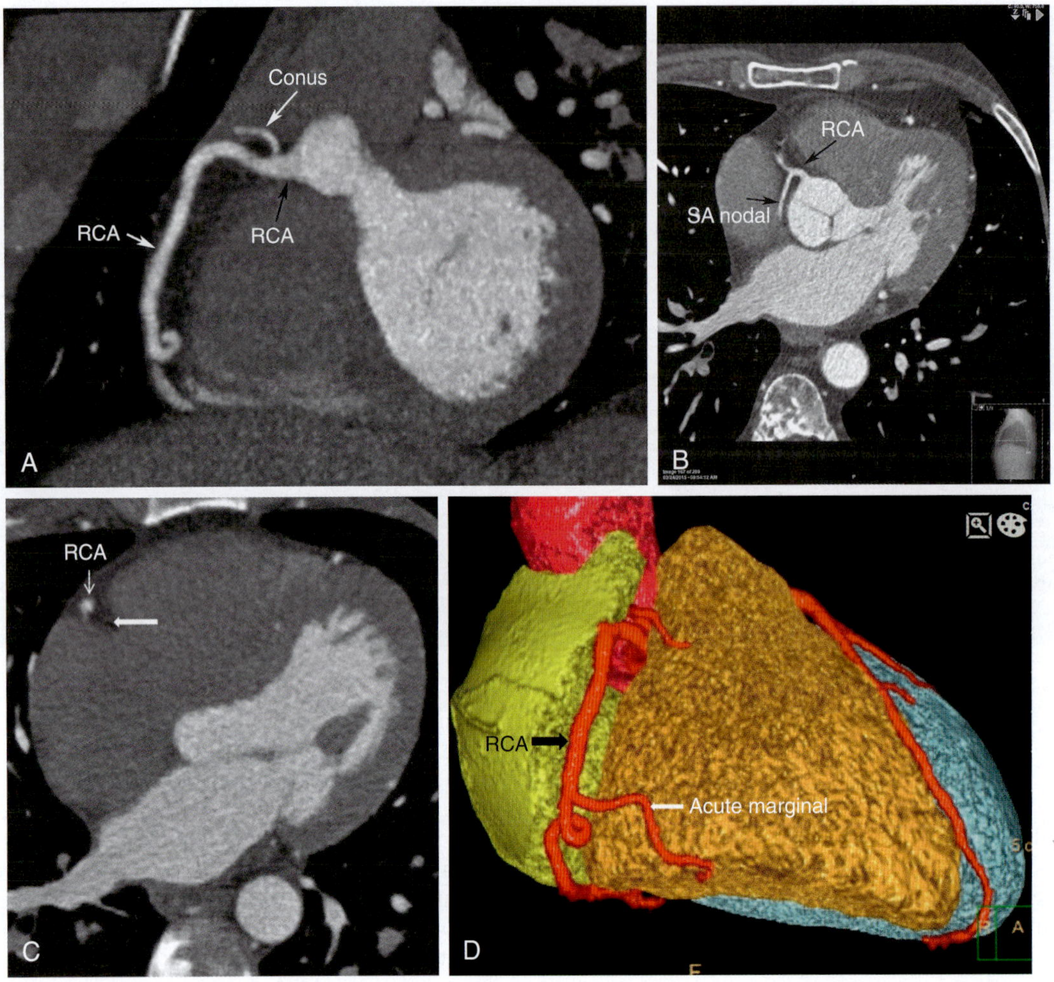

Figure 3.16 Normal right coronary artery *(RCA)*. (A) Coronal oblique multiplanar reconstruction shows a normal RCA origin from the right sinus of Valsalva, with a normal conus branch. (B) Axial reconstructed CT angiography (CTA) image shows the sinoatrial *(SA)* nodal branch originating from the proximal RCA and coursing toward the interatrial septum. (C) Axial CTA image shows a normal RCA in the right atrioventricular groove epicardial fat *(bold arrow)*. (D) Three-dimensional volume-rendered CTA image shows normal-caliber acute marginal branches from the RCA.

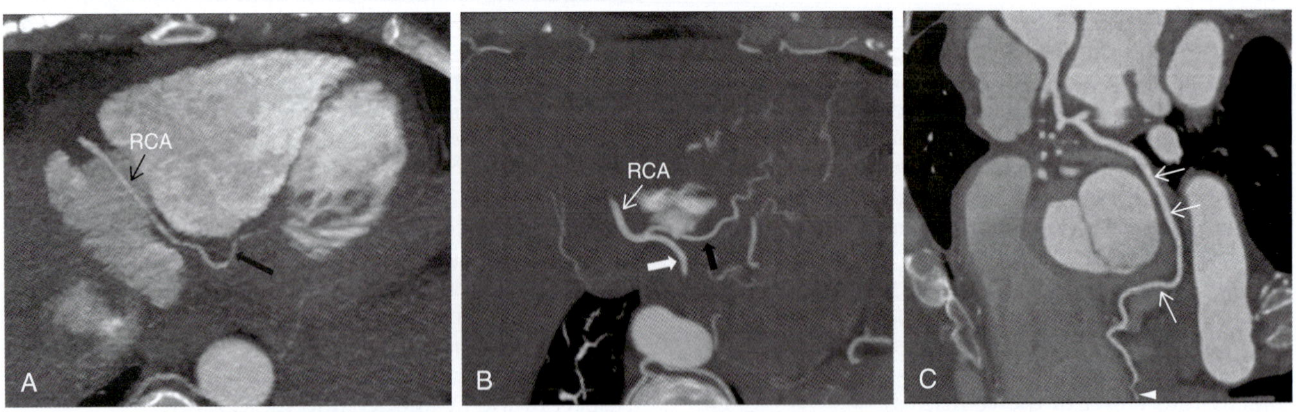

Figure 3.17 Normal posterior descending artery (PDA). (A) Axial maximum intensity projection reconstructed image showing the PDA *(bold arrow)* originating from the right coronary artery *(RCA)* in a right dominant system. (B) Axial maximum intensity projection reconstructed image at the inferior surface of the heart showing PDA *(black bold arrow)* and posterolateral branch *(white bold arrow)* originating from the RCA in a right dominant system. (C) Curved multiplanar reconstruction CT image of the heart showing a normal-caliber PDA *(arrowhead)* originating from the left circumflex artery *(arrows)* in a left dominant system.

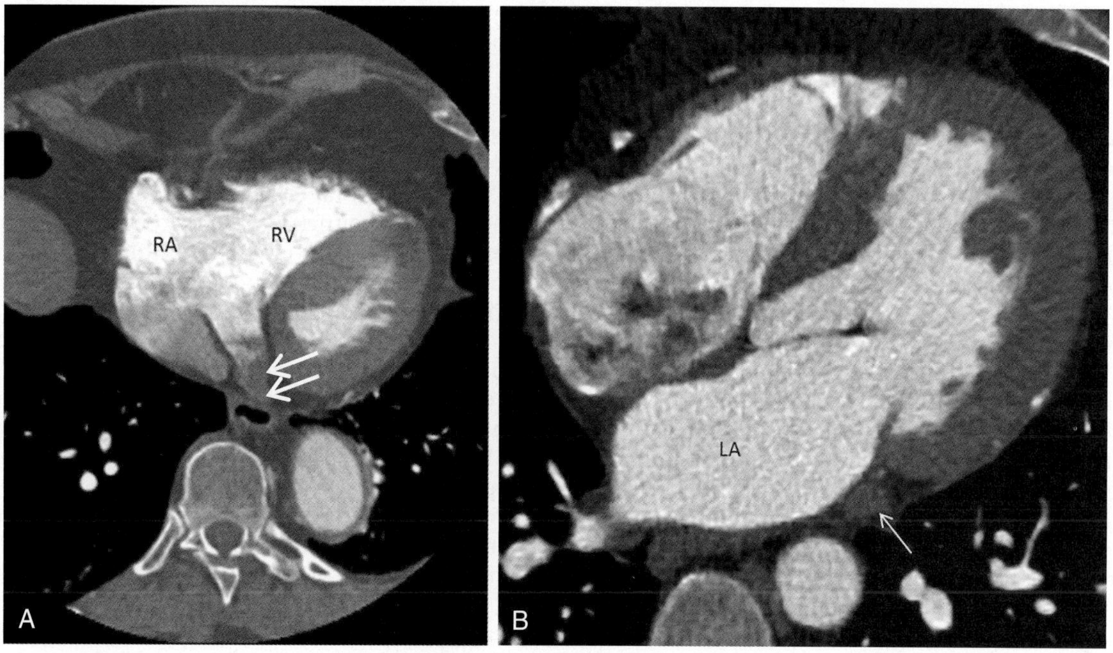

Figure 3.18 Normal cardiac veins. (A) Axial CT image shows a normal-caliber coronary sinus (CS) *(arrows)* draining into the right atrium *(RA)*. Thebesian valves, seen in less than half of patients at the ostium at the termination of the CS in the RA, can interfere with cannulation of the CS. Greater than 11 mm CS dilation, when measured 3 cm proximal to the CS ostium, is considered abnormal. Note that the diagnosis of the hemodynamically significant anomalies of the CS, such as an unroofed CS, anomalous pulmonary venous connection to the CS, and coronary artery–CS fistula require appropriate opacification of the cardiac venous system by timing the acquisition approximately 8 seconds after the coronary arterial phase acquisition. *RV,* Right ventricle. (B) Axial CT image shows a nonopacified great cardiac vein in the left atrioventricular groove *(arrow)* due to arterial phase acquisition of the image. *LA,* Left atrium.

and diaphragm); it also envelops the cardiac chambers and proximal great vessels. It has two components: (1) the outer fibrous pericardium; and (2) a double-layered serous sac (with outer and inner layers; Fig. 3.19). The fibrous pericardium is a connective tissue layer that is anteriorly attached to the sternum. Superiorly, it continues with the adventitia of the great vessels and, inferiorly, it continues with the central tendon of the diaphragm. Just beneath the fibrous layer of the pericardium is the outer layer of the serous sac. In some texts, both these layers together have been simply referred to as *pericardium;* they typically can be measured on imaging and are 2 mm thick together. The pericardial thickening is defined as a thickness more than 3 mm. The inner layer of the serous pericardium (also known as the *visceral pericardium* or *epicardium*) lines the cardiac chambers, attached to the epicardium, great vessels, and venae cavae. There is a potential space between the visceral and parietal pericardium that contains approximately 15 to 50 mL of fluid. Because the fibrous pericardium is a relatively nondistensible layer of pericardium, an acute accumulation of fluid, blood, gas, or pus can lead to compression of the cardiac chambers—cardiac tamponade.

The visceral pericardium encloses two vessel groups—the aorta and pulmonary trunk as one group and the SVC, IVC, and PVs as the other—separately; reflections of the pericardial linings form various pericardial sinuses and recesses. The transverse sinus is the space between the two vascular enclosing groups of visceral pericardium. It is located posterior to the aorta and pulmonary trunk

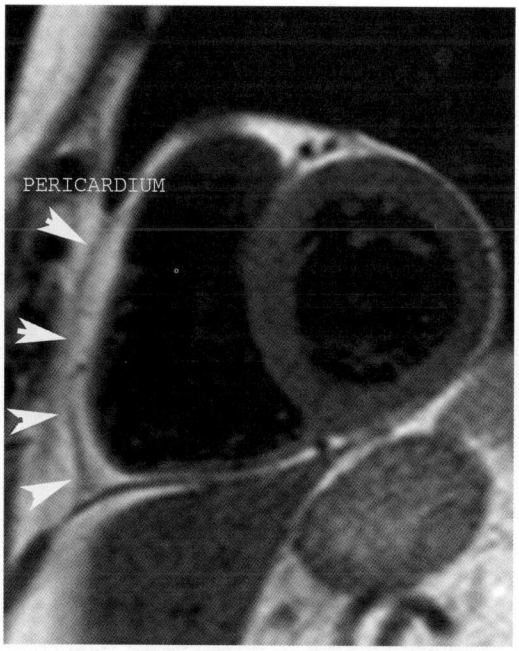

Figure 3.19 Normal pericardium. Short-axis, black blood MR image shows normal, linear, 1–2 mm nonthickened pericardium. Note that a pericardial thickness greater than 4 mm is considered to be abnormally thickened pericardium.

and superior to the LA. The oblique sinus is inferior to the transverse sinus, and its cul-de-sac is located behind the LA and posteromedial to the LSPV. The transverse sinus is further divided into the superior and inferior aortic recesses and the left and right pulmonic recesses. The superior aortic recess is the superior extension of the transverse sinus and covers the posterior aspect of the proximal aorta. The presence of fluid in this recess may mimic intramural hematoma or a thrombosed false lumen of aortic dissection. Sometimes, this recess may extend superiorly into the paratracheal region and, in these cases, fluid within it may mimic a bronchogenic cyst or lymphadenopathy. The inferior aortic recess is located between the ascending aorta and either the inferior portion of the SVC or RA. The right and left pulmonary recesses are lateral extensions of the transverse sinus and are related to the RPA and LPA, respectively. The postcaval recess is a diverticulum of the pericardial cavity proper; it is located lateral to the SVC, at its junction with the RA.

Knowledge of these recesses is important because these potential spaces may have a small amount of physiologic fluid that could mimic lymphadenopathy.

Thoracic Aorta

The aorta is the largest artery in the body; it originates from the LV and extends through the thorax and abdomen. The thoracic aorta can be divided into four segments—the root, ascending aorta, arch, and descending aorta (Fig. 3.20). The root has three components, the annulus, sinus of Valsalva, and sinotubular junction. The annulus is the ring of attachment of the three aortic cusps. The sinuses of Valsalva bulge above the aortic valve. There are three aortic sinuses, the right, left, and noncoronary. The coronary arteries originate from the right and left sinuses. The sinuses then taper and join the ascending aorta at the sinotubular junction. The ascending aorta extends from the sinotubular junction to the origin of the brachiocephalic artery. The arch extends from the brachiocephalic artery origin to the left subclavian artery origin. The arch is divided into proximal and distal segments, with the proximal arch extending from the brachiocephalic origin to the left common carotid origin and the distal arch extending from the left common carotid origin to the left subclavian artery origin. The aortic isthmus is the portion of the aorta just distal to the left subclavian artery origin, at the site of the ductus–ligamentum arteriosum. The descending aorta extends from the level of the ligamentum arteriosum to the diaphragmatic hiatus. The most proximal portion of the descending thoracic aorta appears dilated and is called the *aortic spindle.*

The thoracic aorta can be evaluated and measured using CT or MRI. Measurements of the thoracic aorta (Fig. 3.21) are made in short-axis projections acquired from double oblique views. The diameter is measured from one lumen wall boundary to the other. Maximum intensity projection images should not be used for measurement. For accurate measurement of the aortic root and ascending aorta, CT should be performed with

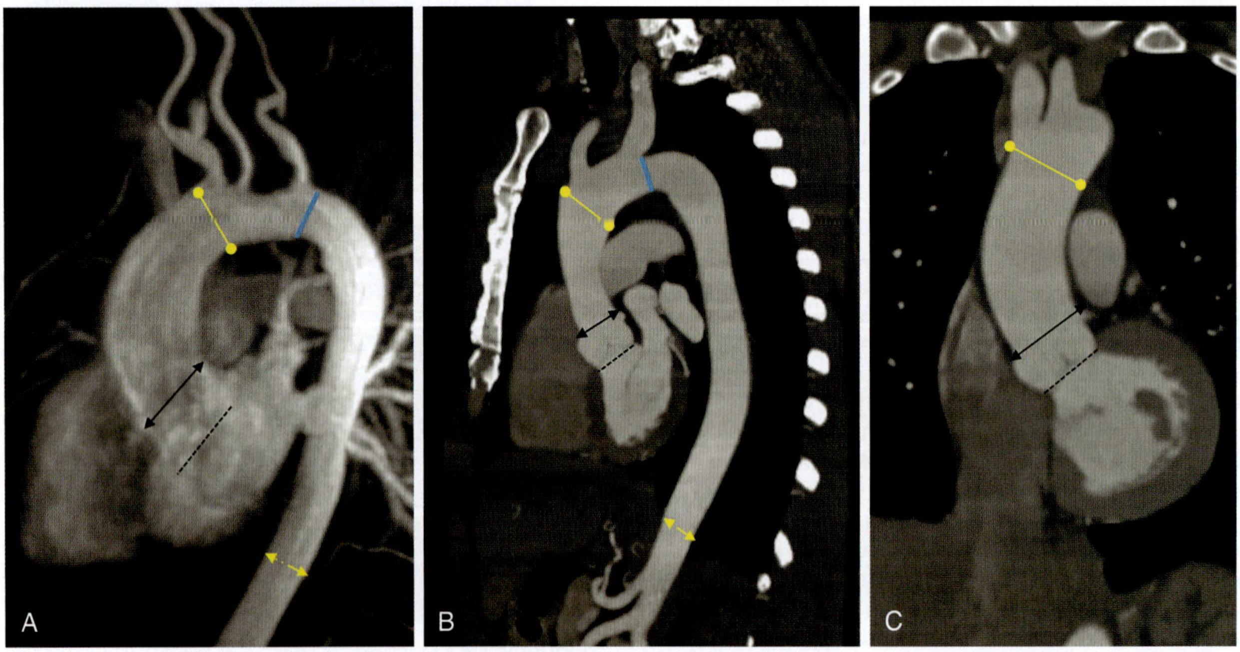

Figure 3.20 Normal thoracic aorta. (A) Sagittal maximum intensity projection reconstructed MR image shows the entire length of the thoracic aorta, including the root (between the *dashed and double-arrowed black lines*), ascending aorta (between the *double-arrowed black and yellow lines*), arch (between the *yellow and blue lines*), isthmus, and descending aorta (between the *blue and dashed double-arrowed black lines*). (B) Sagittal reconstructed CT image also shows the entire thoracic aorta, with labels as in (A). (C) Coronal reconstructed CT image shows the aortic root (between the *dashed and double-arrowed black lines*), sinotubular junction *(double-arrowed black line)*, and ascending aorta (between the *double-arrowed black and yellow lines*).

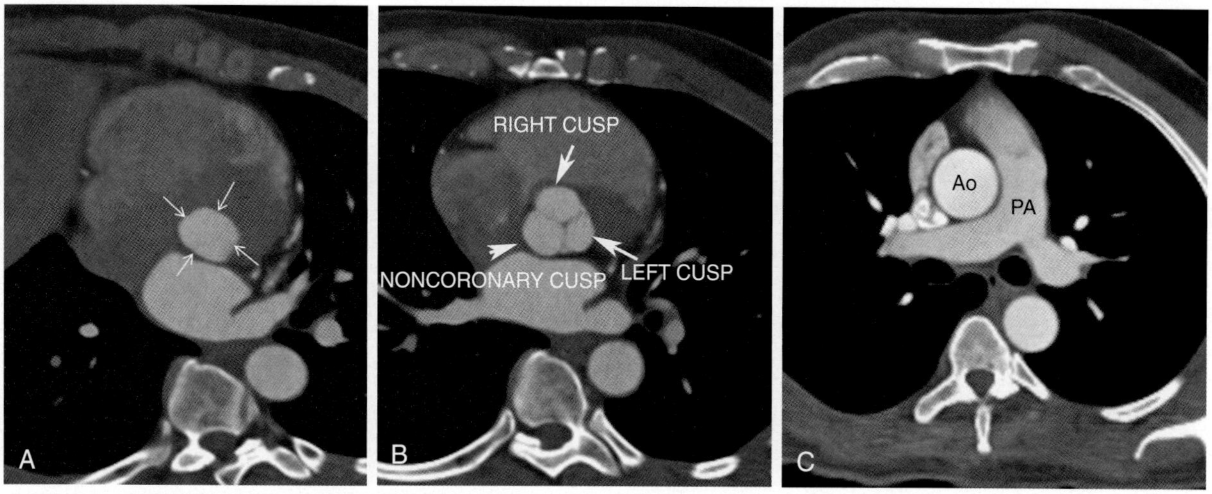

Figure 3.21 Standard planes for measurement of the aortic root and thoracic aorta using short-axis views. (A) Aortic annulus *(arrows)*. This plane is critical for sizing valves prior to transcatheter aortic valve replacement. In this plane, the short- and long-axis diameters, perimeter, and area are measured. (B) Aortic root at the sinus of Valsalva. Three measurements from the commissures to the contralateral sinus are performed. This plane is used to assess for annuloaortic ectasia in Marfan syndrome patients and to evaluate for sinus of a Valsalva aneurysm. (C) Midascending aorta *(Ao)* at the level of the right pulmonary artery *(PA)*. Diameters of the ascending and descending aorta are measured at this level.

ECG gating. The radiation dose is minimized by using prospective ECG gating. In MRI, several sequences are available for measuring the aorta, such as 3D contrast-enhanced MR angiography (CEMRA), noncontrast navigator and ECG-gated 3D, steady-state free precession (SSFP), two-dimensional (2D) cine SSFP, and 2D black blood, T2-weighted images. In a study comparing these sequences, 3D navigator-gated SSFP had the best results, with easy acquisition, good edge profile, and good interobserver correlation. The 3D CEMRA had poor edge sharpness due to lack of ECG gating. Measurements were higher for 3D SSFP and 3D CEMRA and smallest for T2-weighted black blood images.

There is wide variation in the reported normal measurements of thoracic aorta and measurement techniques. The diameter is also affected by multiple factors. One study that analyzed various factors has shown that there is significant linear association between aortic diameter and age, gender, descending aortic diameter, and pulmonary artery diameter, but there was no significant correlation with body surface area, cardiac chamber volumes, and chest diameter. The normal aortic annulus measures 26.3 ± 2.8 mm in the coronal plane and 23.5 + 2.7 mm in the sagittal plane, with no variation between systole and diastole. The normal aortic root and ascending aorta measure up to 3.6 cm in females and 3.8 cm in males. The aortic root diameter can be measured from the cusp to the opposite commissure or from cusp convexity to convexity. Using diastolic SSFP MRI images, the cusp-commissure measurement has been shown to be smaller by 2 to 3 mm but has been shown to correlate better with age, body surface area, echocardiographic measurement, and measurements in the Framingham study. Typically, the average of three measurements across three cusps is used, except in an asymmetric root, when all three measurements are used. In infants, the segments of the arch and isthmus should not exceed 5 mm in length, and the diameters of the proximal arch, distal arch, and isthmus should be at least 60%, 50%, and 40%, respectively, of the diameter of the ascending aorta.

The proximal descending aorta is considered enlarged when it exceeds 2.6 cm, and the distal descending aorta is considered enlarged when it exceeds 2.4 cm. However, for simplicity, the ascending aorta is considered enlarged when it is larger than 4 cm, and the descending aorta is considered enlarged when it is larger than 3 cm. An aneurysm of the ascending aorta is diagnosed when it measures larger than 5 cm and of the descending aorta when it is larger than 4 cm. In children, z-scores are also used to diagnose aortic dilations and aneurysms. The z-score represents the standard deviation from the mean aortic diameter, normalized for the patient's age and body surface area. Normal thoracic aorta wall thickness is 1 to 2 mm.

Branches of the thoracic aorta (Fig. 3.22) are paired and include bronchial, esophageal, pericardial, mediastinal, intercostal, subcostal, and superior phrenic branches. The ductus arteriosus is the structure that normally connects the proximal descending aorta (just distal to the origin of the left subclavian artery) with the proximal LPA (at its junction with the MPA). The ductus arteriosus usually closes functionally within 18 to 24 hours after birth and closes anatomically in 1 month. A patent ductus arteriosus is persistent after 1 month and is seen in 1 of 2000 children.

Arch Vessels

In a normal person, the arch is left-sided. The most common pattern, seen in 70%, is three branches—the right brachiocephalic artery, the left common carotid artery, and the left subclavian artery. The right brachiocephalic artery then divides into right common carotid and right subclavian arteries. There are several variations in the origin of these branch vessels. The most common

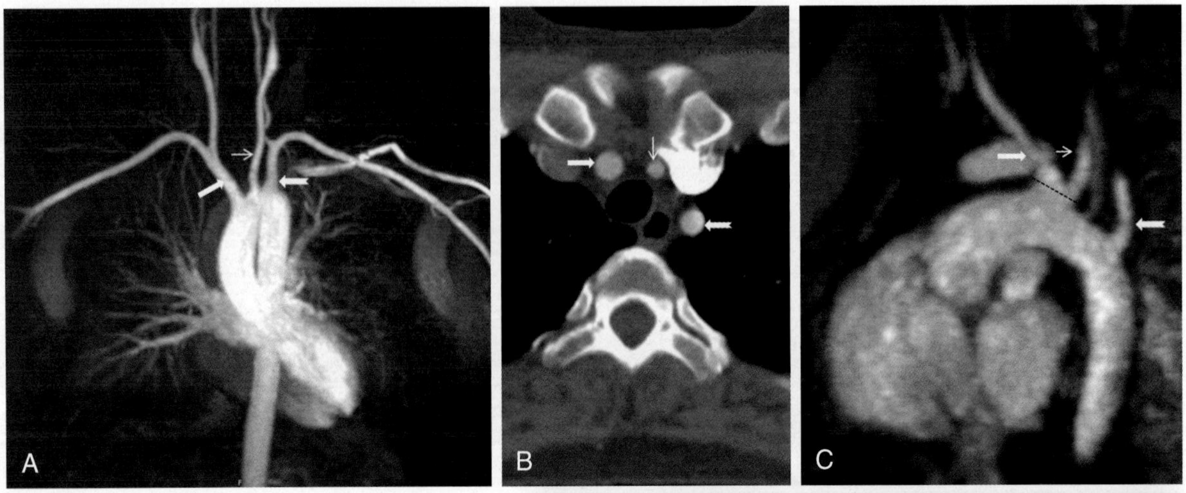

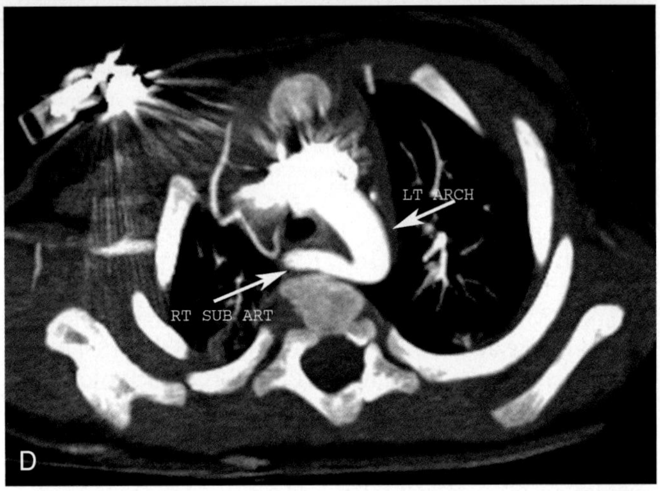

Figure 3.22 Aortic arch branching pattern. (A) Maximum intensity projection (MIP) reconstructed MR image shows a normal, three-vessel branching pattern, with the first branch being the right brachiocephalic artery *(bold arrow on left)*, followed by the left common carotid *(thin arrow in middle)*, and then the left subclavian artery *(bold notched arrow on right)*. (B) Axial CT image above the level of the aortic arch shows the three normal aortic arch branches, with labels as in (A). (C) Oblique sagittal MIP reconstructed MR image shows a bovine arch, consisting of a common trunk *(dashed black line)* for the right brachiocephalic *(bold arrow on left)* and left common carotid arteries *(thin arrow)*, with an incidental left vertebral artery origin between the common trunk and left subclavian artery *(notched arrow on right)*. (D) Axial oblique MIP reconstruction of CT angiogram shows a left-sided aortic arch with an aberrant right subclavian artery originating as the last branch from the arch, the most common arch abnormality. Affected individuals are often asymptomatic but can present with dysphagia due to compression on the posterior wall of the esophagus by the artery. The presence of a diverticulum of Kommerell at the origin of the aberrant artery increases the likelihood of surgical intervention.

variation is a bovine arch (seen in 13%), where the right brachiocephalic and left common carotid arteries have a common origin from the arch. This is more common in African Americans, with 25% prevalence versus 8% in whites. Another variation, truncus bicaroticus, is where the left common carotid artery originates from the proximal 1 to 2.5 cm of the brachiocephalic artery. This is also called *bovine arch* by some authors; it is seen in 9% of the population and is also more common in African Americans (10%) than whites (5%). The term *bovine arch* is a misnomer, because neither of these two patterns is seen in cattle. In cattle, the arch pattern is a single brachiocephalic trunk that trifurcates into bilateral subclavian arteries and a single bicarotid trunk. Another common variant is the left vertebral artery, originating directly from the arch between the left common carotid and left subclavian artery, which is seen in 1% to 3% of the population. The thyroid ima artery may also originate from the arch between the brachiocephalic and left common carotid arteries. Rarely, the right subclavian and right common carotid arteries may originate separately from the arch.

There are also several congenital anomalies that involve the aortic arch due to abnormal development of the aortic arches. In a left arch with an aberrant right subclavian artery, the first aortic branch is the right common carotid artery, followed by the left common carotid artery and then the left subclavian artery. The aberrant right subclavian artery originates as the last branch from the arch and then courses behind the esophagus to reach the right. Other abnormalities include a double aortic arch, where there are two arches, the right and left, with the right giving off the right common carotid and right subclavian arteries and the left giving off the left common carotid and left subclavian arteries. A right-sided aortic arch may present with a mirror image branching pattern, where the first branch is a left brachiocephalic artery, followed by the right common carotid and right subclavian arteries. The left brachiocephalic artery divides into the left subclavian and left common carotid arteries. In a right aortic arch with an aberrant left subclavian artery, the first branch is the left common carotid artery and then the right common carotid and right subclavian arteries; the left subclavian artery originates as the last branch and courses behind the esophagus to reach the left. This is a mirror image of a left-sided aortic arch with an aberrant right subclavian artery.

Pulmonary Arteries

The pulmonary circulation distributes the deoxygenated blood from the right heart to the lungs. The MPA originates from the RV and extends superiorly and posteriorly

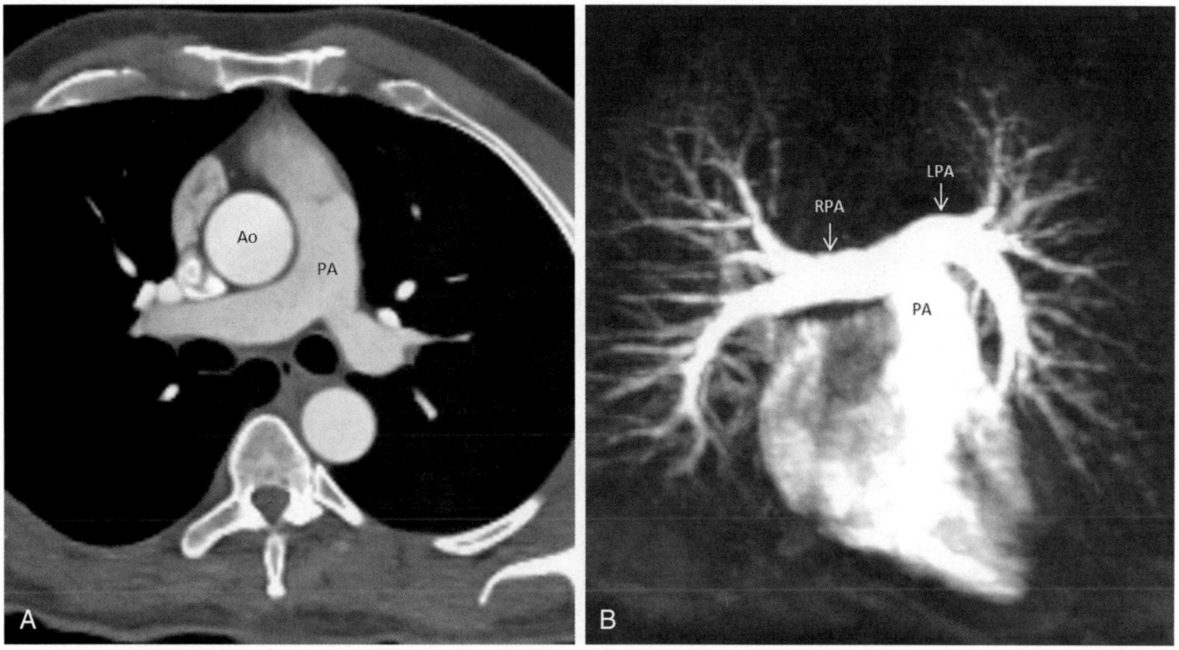

Figure 3.23 Normal pulmonary artery. (A) Axial reconstructed CT image shows a normal-caliber main pulmonary artery *(PA)* giving rise to a right pulmonary artery and a left pulmonary artery. Note that a main pulmonary artery diameter greater than 3 cm or relatively larger caliber than the ascending aorta *(Ao)* is considered as a relatively sensitive and specific finding for pulmonary hypertension. (B) Coronal maximum intensity projection reconstructed MR angiography image shows the normal-caliber main pulmonary artery giving rise to the right pulmonary artery *(RPA)*, left pulmonary artery *(LPA)*, and peripheral branches.

within the pericardium. The MPA bifurcates into the RPA and LPA at the level of T5 (Fig. 3.23). The RPA is longer than the LPA and crosses the mediastinum posteroinferior to the right main bronchus. It then divides into superior and inferior (interlobar) trunks. The superior trunk supplies the right upper lobe, and the interlobar trunk supplies the right middle and lower lobes. The LPA is a continuation of the MPA and extends anterior and superior to the left main bronchus. The LPA divides into the left upper and left interlobar arteries. The lobar branches on both sides give origin to segmental and then subsegmental branches, which are parallel to segmental and subsegmental bronchi, respectively. The segmental arteries are named according to the bronchopulmonary segments.

On CT and MRI, the diameter of a normal pulmonary artery is less than 28 mm. A pulmonary artery diameter more than 29 mm in men and 27 mm in women is considered to be enlargement. Another indicator of pulmonary artery enlargement is if the ratio of the MPA and ascending aorta at the same level is greater than 0.9.

There is no consensus on the best way to measure pulmonary arteries. If the MPA is straight, the axial diameter of MPA is measured along the line that extends from the center of the ascending aorta and is perpendicular to the long axis of the MPA at the level of pulmonary artery bifurcation. If the MPA is not straight, the widest short axis of the MPA in the axial section at the level of MPA bifurcation can be used. Other methods include measurement of the widest short-axis diameter of MPA in the sagittal view and an axial measurement along the line drawn from the center of the ascending aorta to the origin of the LPA. In one study, the first method was shown to have the least interobserver variation.

Bronchial Arteries

Bronchial arteries supply a small amount of blood to the lungs and account for 1% of the systemic cardiac output. They also supply the trachea, airways, bronchovascular bundles, nerves, supporting structures, regional nodes, visceral pleura, esophagus, vasa vasorum of the aorta, and pulmonary arteries and veins. There is anastomosis between pulmonary and bronchial arteries at the capillary level.

The normal bronchial arteries (orthotopic) typically originate from the descending aorta at the T5–6 level (Fig. 3.24). There are four branching patterns of orthotopic bronchial arteries:

- Type 1 (40.6%): two bronchial arteries on the left and one on the right, the intercostobronchial trunk (ICBT)
- Type 2 (21%): one on the left and one ICBT on the right
- Type 3 (20%): two on the left and two on the right (one ICBT and one bronchial)
- Type 4 (9.7%): one on the left and two on the right

The left bronchial artery usually originates from the anterior aspect of the descending aorta and extends toward the left hilum. On the right, the ICBT arises from the

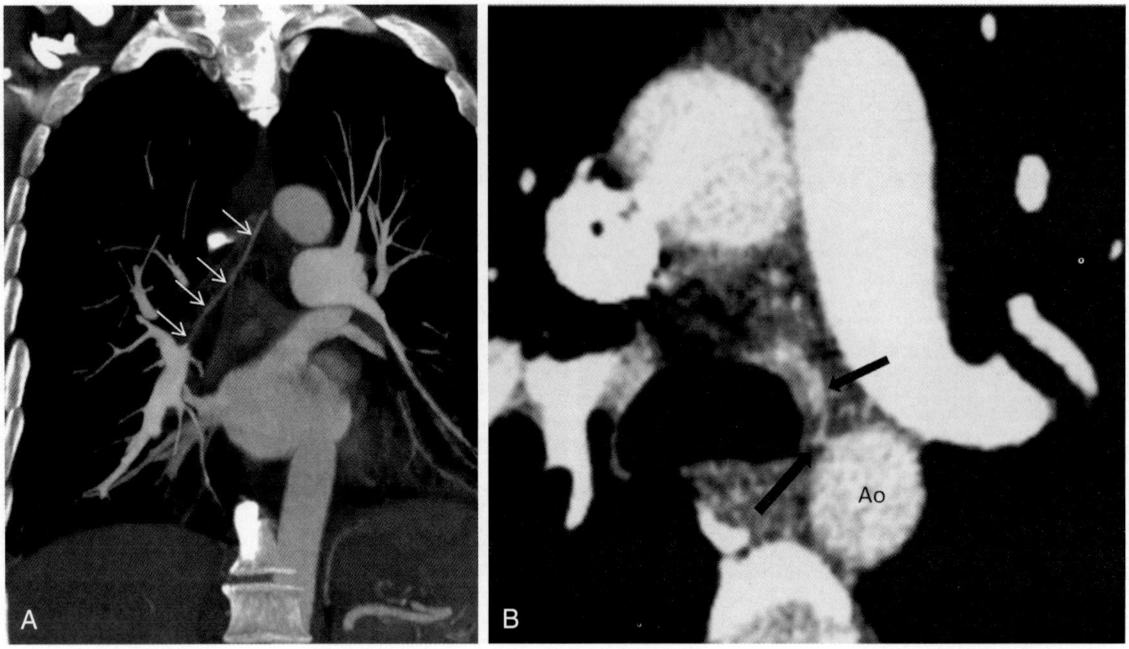

Figure 3.24 Normal bronchial artery pattern. (A) Coronal CT maximum intensity projection image shows a long, normal-caliber right intercostobronchial trunk originating from the descending aorta *(arrows)*. (B) Axial CT image at the level of the carina shows a small bronchial artery *(arrows)* originating from the middescending aorta *(Ao)*. A bronchial artery caliber more than 4 mm is considered to be dilated.

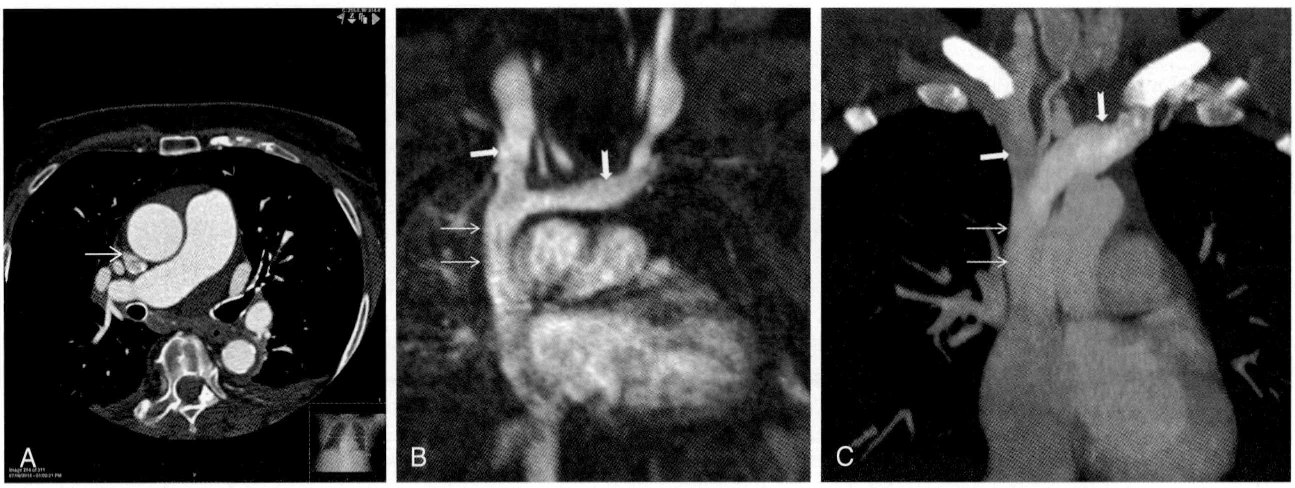

Figure 3.25 Normal right-sided superior vena cava (SVC). (A) Axial CT image shows a normal-caliber SVC *(arrow)* with the usual mixing artifact in the central portion from the nonopacified blood from the azygous vein, mimicking a filling defect. (B) Coronal MR angiography reconstructed image. (C) Coronal reconstructed CT venography image shows a normal SVC *(thin arrows)* formed by the confluence of the right *(bold arrow on left)* and left brachiocephalic veins *(bold notched arrow on right)* draining into the right atrium.

right posteromedial aspect of the thoracic aorta and extends cranially to branch into the intercostal and right bronchial arteries. Then it turns caudally to reach the right main bronchus.

When bronchial arteries originate from an atypical segment of the descending aorta or from aortic branches, they are called *ectopic* or *aberrant*. The most common ectopic sites of origin of the bronchial arteries are from concavity of the aortic arch (74%), ipsilateral or contralateral subclavian artery (10.5%), descending aorta (8.5%), ipsilateral brachiocephalic trunk (2%), ipsilateral internal mammary artery (2.5%), and ipsilateral thyrocervical trunk (2.5%).

Superior Vena Cava

The SVC carries deoxygenated blood from the upper part of the body to the RA. The SVC is formed by the confluence of the right and left brachiocephalic veins on the right side of the superior mediastinum, at the level of the first costal cartilage (Fig. 3.25). The brachiocephalic veins are formed by a confluence of the internal jugular and subclavian veins. The SVC then extends inferiorly and anteromedially and enters the RA at the level of the right third costal cartilage. The SVC is usually 5 to 7 cm long, and the lower half is intrapericardial. The azygos vein and small veins of the pericardium and mediastinum drain into the SVC.

A persistent left SVC (Fig. 3.26) is seen in 0.3% to 0.5% of individuals due to persistence of the left anterior cardinal vein and continuity with the left common cardinal vein. In most patients with a persistent left SVC (80%–90%), the right SVC is also persistent, resulting in a double SVC. This is caused by persistence of the right and left anterior cardinal veins (Fig. 3.27). A bridging vein connecting these two is seen in 35% of the population. In 10% of patients with left SVC, the right SVC is absent due to regression of the right anterior cardinal vein. The left SVC drains into the CS in 80% and into the LA in 20%. A bilateral absence of the SVC is rarely seen. A right SVC may occasionally drain into the LA or both atria (known as the *van Praagh classification*). The left innominate vein may course posterior and inferior to the aortic arch (rather than superoanterior to it) and joins the SVC below the azygos vein. This is usually associated with RVOT in 80% of cases. A retroesophageal left innominate vein and duplicated left innominate vein have also been reported.

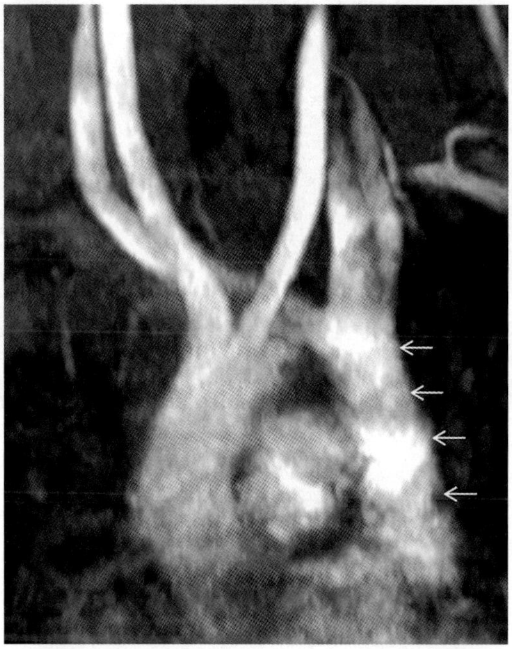

Figure 3.26 Left-sided superior vena cava (SVC). Coronal MR angiography image shows a left-sided SVC *(arrows)* traversing caudally, lateral to the aortic arch, and draining into the right atrium via a dilated coronary sinus (not shown). There is no right-sided SVC. Note that the persistent left SVC may cause difficulty in the placement of pacemakers, implantable cardioverter-defibrillator leads, and Swan-Ganz catheters, whereas the central venous catheter placement in the left SVC may be mistaken for arterial, mediastinal, or pleural placement on a frontal chest radiograph.

Azygos, Hemiazygos, and Accessory Hemiazygos Systems

The azygos system provides the venous drainage pathway for a large portion of the thorax, as well as the abdomen. It is a paired paravertebral venous system in the posterior thorax. The azygos vein originates approximately at the level of T12 by a confluence of the right ascending lumbar and subcostal veins (Fig. 3.28). Other veins that join this system include the intercostal veins, vertebral venous plexus, esophageal veins, pericardial veins, tracheal veins, bronchial veins, and right superior phrenic vein. It enters the thorax through the aortic hiatus and then ascends along the anterolateral surface of the thoracic vertebra.

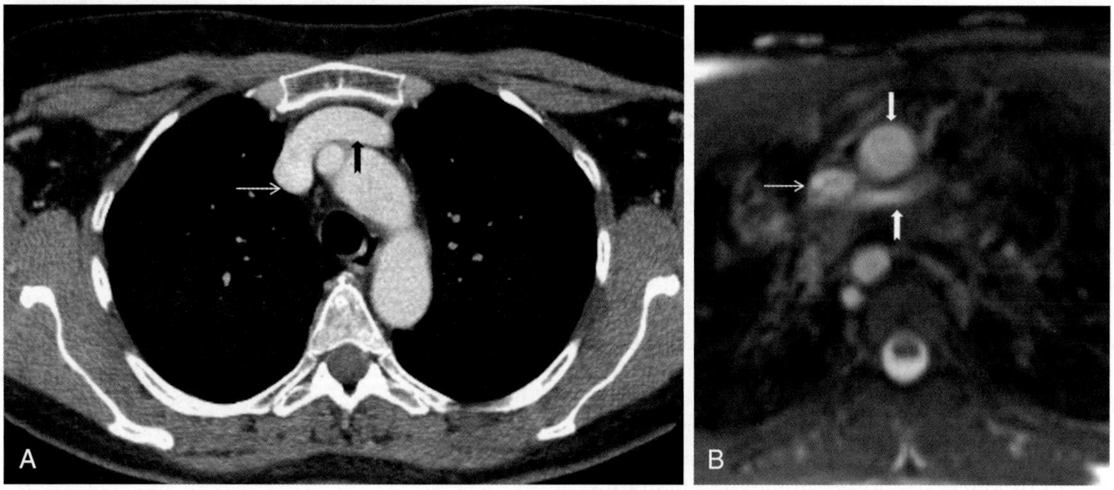

Figure 3.27 Brachiocephalic veins. (A) Axial CT image at the level of aortic arch shows a normal left brachiocephalic *(notched black arrow)* vein anterior to the aortic arch, which joins the right brachiocephalic vein to form the superior vena cava (SVC; *thin white arrow*). (B) Axial MR angiography image at the level of the distal ascending aorta shows a retroaortic left brachiocephalic-innominate vein *(notched arrow on bottom)*, coursing behind the aorta *(bold arrow on top)* to form the SVC *(thin arrow on left)*. Note enhancing signal abnormality in the right upper lobe related to known atelectasis.

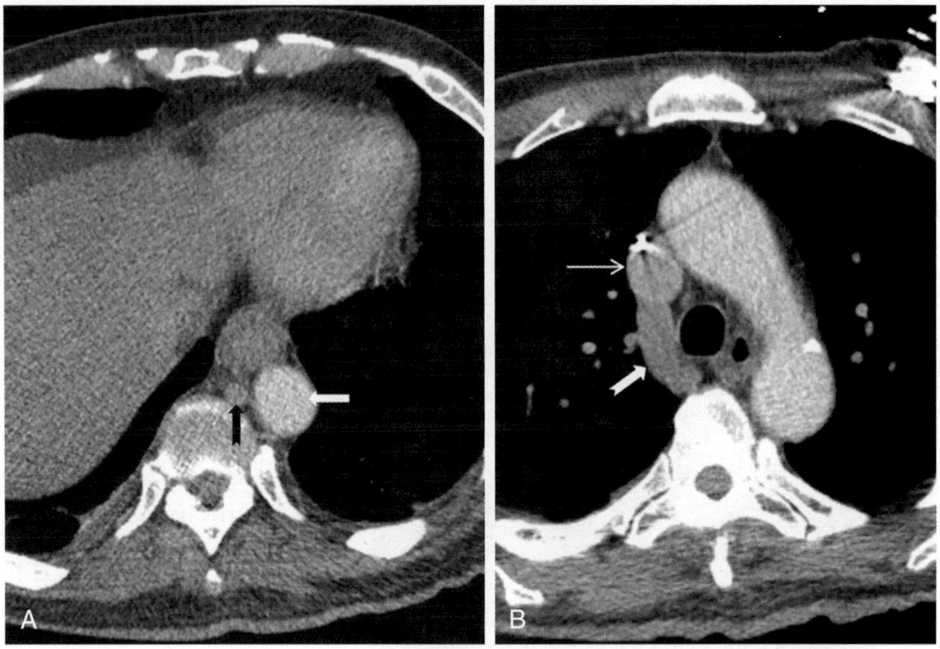

Figure 3.28 Azygos vein. (A) Axial CT image at the level of the lower thorax shows a relatively less well-opacified, normal-caliber azygos vein *(notched black arrow)* on the right anterior border of the thoracic vertebra and to the right of a well-opacified distal descending thoracic aorta *(bold white arrow)*. (B) Axial CT image at a level just above the carina shows the nonopacified normal-caliber azygos venous arch *(notched arrow)*, which is joining the posterior aspect of the distal superior vena cava *(thin arrow)*.

At approximately the level of T5–6, the azygos vein arches anteriorly, just above the right main stem bronchus, and joins the SVC. Occasionally, the azygos vein may demonstrate a variant configuration and join the right brachiocephalic vein, right subclavian vein, intrapericardial SVC, or RA. A variant pulmonary anatomy can occur when the right posterior cardinal vein, the embryologic precursor to the azygos vein, fails to cross over the upper right lobe and involutes in the pleura of the lung instead. This involution leads to the formation of what is known as an *azygos lobe*, which is present in the superomedial right lung in approximately 1% of patients.

The hemiazygos vein (Fig. 3.29) is analogous to the azygos vein but is located in the left paraspinal region. The hemiazygos vein originates at the junction of the left ascending lumbar and left subcostal veins. It receives tributaries from left renal vein and IVC. It ascends along the left anterolateral vertebral bodies. At T8–9, it crosses dorsal to the descending aorta and joins the azygos vein below the level of the azygos arch. From this point, an accessory hemiazygos vein can extend farther cephalad in a left paravertebral position and communicate with the azygos veins at different levels.

Intercostal veins and mediastinal tributaries drain into the azygos, hemiazygos, and accessory hemiazygos veins. The right superior intercostal vein drains the right second through fourth intercostal veins and drains into the azygos vein, just proximal to the azygos arch. The left superior intercostal vein drains the left second through fourth intercostal spaces and communicates with the accessory hemiazygos vein in 75% of patients. Subsequently, it arches ventrally, adjacent to the lateral border of the aortic arch, and drains into the left brachiocephalic vein. This vein produces the aortic nipple in radiographs. The right and left supreme intercostal veins drain the first intercostal spaces and empty into the brachiocephalic veins. These may communicate with the corresponding superior intercostal veins.

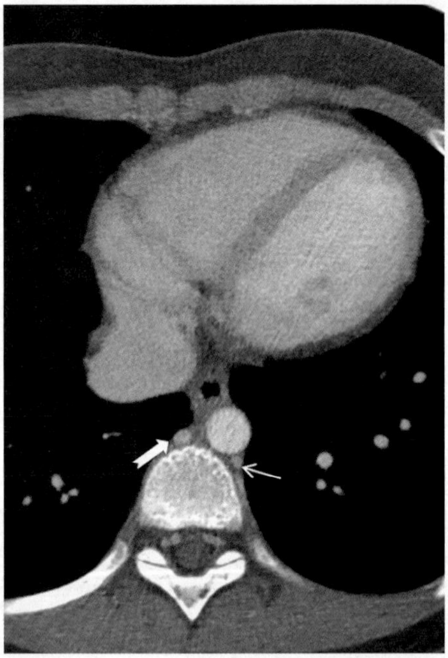

Figure 3.29 Hemiazygos vein. This axial CT image at the level of the lower thorax shows the hemiazygos vein *(thin arrow)* on the left anterior border of the thoracic vertebra and the azygos vein *(thick notched arrow)* on the right anterior border of the thoracic vertebra.

■ Conclusion

This chapter has reviewed the normal and variant anatomies of the heart and great vessels, as depicted by conventional radiography, CT, and MRI.

Bibliography

Abbara S, Cury RC, Nieman K, et al. Noninvasive evaluation of cardiac veins with 16-MDCT angiography. *AJR Am J Roentgenol*. 2005;185:1001–1006.

Agarwal PP, Chugtai A, Matzinger FRK, et al. Multidetector CT of thoracic aortic aneurysms. *Radiographics*. 2009;29:537–552.

Baron MG. The cardiac silhouette. *J Thorac Imaging.* 2000;15:230–242.

Beinart R, Boyko V, Schwammenthal E, et al. Long-term prognostic significance of left atrial volume in acute myocardial infarction. *J Am Coll Cardiol.* 2004;44:327–334.

Bennett CJ, Maleszewski JJ, Araoz PA. CT and MR imaging of the aortic valve: radiologic-pathologic correlation. *Radiographics.* 2012;32:1399–1420.

Bogaert J, Francone M. Pericardial disease: value of CT and MR imaging. *Radiology.* 2013;267:340–356.

Cabrera JA, Saremi F, Sánchez-Quintana D. Left atrial appendage: anatomy and imaging landmarks pertinent to percutaneous transcatheter occlusion. *Heart.* 2014;100:1636–1650.

Cauldwell EW, Siekert RG, Lininger RE, et al. The bronchial arteries: an anatomic study of 105 human cadavers. *Surg Gynecol Obstet.* 1948;86:395–412.

Cerqueira MD, Weissman NJ, Dilsizian V, et al. Standardized myocardial segmentation and nomenclature for tomographic imaging of the heart. A statement for healthcare professionals from the Cardiac Imaging Committee of the Council on Clinical Cardiology of the American Heart Association. *Int J Cardiovasc Imaging.* 2002;18:539–542.

Chen JJ, Manning MA, Frazier AA, Jeudy J, White CS. CT angiography of the cardiac valves: normal, diseased, and postoperative appearances. *Radiographics.* 2009;29:1393–1412.

Dasler EH, Anson BJ. Surgical anatomy of the subclavian artery and its branches. *Surg Gynecol Obstetrics.* 1959;108:149–174.

Demos TC, Posniak HV, Pierce KL, et al. Venous anomalies of the thorax. *AJR Am J Roentgenol.* 2004;182:1139–1150.

Di Biase L, Santangeli P, Anselmino M, et al. Does the left atrial appendage morphology correlate with the risk of stroke in patients with atrial fibrillation? Results from a multicenter study. *J Am Coll Cardiol.* 2012;60:531–538.

Etesami M, Ashwath R, Kanne J, et al. Computed tomography in the evaluation of vascular rings and slings. *Insights Imaging.* 2014;5(4):507–521.

Faletra FF, Muzzarelli S, Dequarti MC, Murzilli R, Bellu R, Ho SY. Imaging-based right-atrial anatomy by computed tomography, magnetic resonance imaging, and three-dimensional transoesophageal echocardiography: correlations with anatomic specimens. *Eur Heart J Cardiovasc Imaging.* 2013;14:1123–1131.

Freman LA, Young PM, Foley TA, et al. CT and MRI assessment of the aortic root and ascending aorta. *AJR Am J Roentgenol.* 2013;200:W581–W592.

Galea N, Carbone I, Cannata D, et al. Right ventricular cardiovascular magnetic resonance imaging: normal anatomy and spectrum of pathological findings. *Insights Imaging.* 2013;4:213–223.

Goo HW, Park IS, Ko JK, et al. CT of congenital heart disease: normal anatomy and typical pathologic conditions. *Radiographics.* 2003;23(Spec No):S147–S165.

Gopalan D. Right heart on multidetector CT. *Br J Radiol.* 2011;84(Spec 3):S306–S323.

Gupta S, Plein S, Greenwood JP. The coumadin ridge: an important example of a left atrial pseudotumour demonstrated by cardiovascular magnetic resonance imaging. *J Radiol Case Rep.* 2009;3:1–5.

Ho SY. Anatomy of the mitral valve. *Heart.* 2002;88(suppl 4):iv5–iv10.

Ho SY, Cabrera JA, Sanchez-Quintana D. Left atrial anatomy revisited. *Circ Arrhythm Electrophysiol.* 2012;5:220–228.

Hoey ET, Ganeshan A. Multi-detector CT angiography of the aortic valve-part 1: anatomy, technique and systematic approach to interpretation. *Quant Imaging Med Surg.* 2014;4:265–272.

Kanmanthareddy A, Reddy YM, Vallakati A, et al. Embryology and anatomy of the left atrial appendage: why does thrombus form? *Interventional Cardiol Clin.* 2014;3:191–202.

Kimura-Hayama ET, Melendez C, Mendizabal AL, et al. Uncommon congenital and acquired aortic diseases: role of multidetector CT angiography. *Radiographics.* 2010;30:79–98.

Kini S, Bis KG, Weaver L. Normal and variant coronary arterial and venous anatomy on high-resolution CT angiography. *AJR Am J Roentgenol.* 2007;188:1665–1674.

Kulkarni S, Jain S, Kasar P, et al. Retroaortic left innominate vein: incidence, association with congenital heart defects, embryology, and clinical significance. *Ann Pediatr Cardiol.* 2008;1(2):131–141.

Lacomis JM, Goitein O, Deible C, Schwartzman D. CT of the pulmonary veins. *J Thorac Imaging.* 2007;22:63–76.

Lacomis JM, Wigginton W, Fuhrman C, Schwartzman D, Armfield DR, Pealer KM. Multi-detector row CT of the left atrium and pulmonary veins before radio-frequency catheter ablation for atrial fibrillation. *Radiographics.* 2003;23(Spec No):S35–S48, discussion S48–S50.

Lang RM, Bierig M, Devereux RB, et al. Recommendations for chamber quantification: a report from the American Society of Echocardiography's Guidelines and Standards Committee and the Chamber Quantification Writing Group, developed in conjunction with the European Association of Echocardiography, a branch of the European Society of Cardiology. *J Am Soc Echocardiogr.* 2005;18:1440–1463.

Layton KF, Kallmes DF, Cloft HJ, et al. Bovine aortic arch variant in humans. Clarification of a common misnomer. *AJNR Am J Neuroradiol.* 2006;27:1541–1542.

Lipton MJ, Boxt LM. How to approach cardiac diagnosis from the chest radiograph. *Radiol Clin North Am.* 2004;42:487–495, v.

Litmanovich D, Bankier AA, Cantin I, et al. CT and MRI in diseases of the aorta. *AJR Am J Roentgenol.* 2009;193(4):928–940.

Mao SS, Ahmadi N, Shah B, et al. Normal thoracic aorta diameter on cardiac computed tomography in healthy asymptomatic adults: impact of age and gender. *Acad Radiol.* 2008;15:827–834.

Ming Z, Ajmin S, Rui H. Evaluation of anomalous retroesophageal left brachiocephalic vein in Chinese children using multidetector CT. *Pediatr Radiol.* 2009;39(4):343–347.

Morris MF, Maleszewski JJ, Suri RM, et al. CT and MR imaging of the mitral valve: radiologic-pathologic correlation. *Radiographics.* 2010;30:1603–1620.

Muhammedi A, Oshmyansky A, Hassoun PM, et al. Pulmonary artery measurements in pulmonary hypertension. The role of computed tomography. *J Thoracic Imaging.* 2013;28(2):96–103.

Nadra I, Dawson D, Schmitz SA, Punjabi PP, Nihoyannopoulos P. Lipomatous hypertrophy of the interatrial septum: a commonly misdiagnosed mass often leading to unnecessary cardiac surgery. *Heart.* 2004;90:e66.

Nagpal P, Khandelwal A, Saboo SS, Bathla G, Steigner ML, Rybicki FJ. Modern imaging techniques: applications in the management of acute aortic pathologies. *Postgrad Med J.* 2015;91:449–462.

Navaratnam V. Design of heart valves: a review. *Clin Anatomy.* 1993;6:327–332.

O'Brien JP, Srichai MB, Hecht EM, Kim DC, Jacobs JE. Anatomy of the heart at multidetector CT: what the radiologist needs to know. *Radiographics.* 2007;27:1569–1582.

Pappone C, Oral H, Santinelli V, et al. Atrio-esophageal fistula as a complication of percutaneous transcatheter ablation of atrial fibrillation. *Circulation.* 2004;109:2724–2726.

Peebles CR, Shambrook JS, Harden SP. Pericardial disease—anatomy and function. *Br J Radiol.* 2011;84(Spec 3):S324–S337.

Porres DV, Morenza OP, Pallisa E, Roque A, Andreu J, Martínez M. Learning from the pulmonary veins. *Radiographics.* 2013;33:999–1022.

Pothast S, Mitsumori L, Stanescu LA, et al. Measuring aortic diameter with different MR techniques: comparison of three-dimensional navigated steady-state free precession (SSFP), 3D contrast enhanced magnetic resonance angiography, 2D T2 black blood and 2D cine SSFP. *J Magn Reson Imaging.* 2010;31(1):177–184.

Povoski SPI, Khabiri H. Persistent left superior vena cava: review of the literature, clinical implications, and relevance of alterations in thoracic ventral venous anatomy as pertaining to the general principles of central venous access device placement and venography in cancer patients. *World J Surg Oncol.* 2011;9:173.

Raff GL, Abidov A, Achenbach S, et al. SCCT guidelines for the interpretation and reporting of coronary computed tomographic angiography. *J Cardiovasc Comput Tomogr.* 2009;3:122–136.

Roberts WC, Cohen LS. Left ventricular papillary muscles. Description of the normal and a survey of conditions causing them to be abnormal. *Circulation.* 1972;46:138–154.

Saboo SS, Hedgire S, Joglar J, Abbara S. Emerging CT Applications in Electrophysiology (EP). 2014 CCT-SAP3. American College of Cardiology Guidelines.

Saboo SS, Juan YH, Khandelwal A, et al. MDCT of congenital coronary artery fistulas. *AJR Am J Roentgenol.* 2014;203(3):W244–W252.

Saremi F, Torrone M, Yashar N. Cardiac conduction system: delineation of anatomic landmarks with multidetector CT. *Indian Pacing Electrophysiol J.* 2009;9:318–333.

Shah SS, Teague SD, Lu JC, Dorfman AL, Kazerooni EA, Agarwal PP. Imaging of the coronary sinus: normal anatomy and congenital abnormalities. *Radiographics.* 2012;32:991–1008.

Shuman WP, Branch KR, May JM, et al. Prospective versus retrospective ECG gating for 64-detector CT of the coronary arteries: comparison of image quality and patient radiation dose. *Radiology.* 2008;248:431–437.

Singh JP, Houser S, Heist EK, Ruskin JN. The coronary venous anatomy: a segmental approach to aid cardiac resynchronization therapy. *J Am Coll Cardiol.* 2005;46:68–74.

Sun Z, Ng KH. Prospective versus retrospective ECG-gated multislice CT coronary angiography: a systematic review of radiation dose and diagnostic accuracy. *Eur J Radiol.* 2012;81:e94–e100.

Tops LF, Wood DA, Delgado V, et al. Non invasive evaluation of aortic root with multi-slice computed tomography. *JACC Cardiovasc Imaging.* 2008;1(3):321–330.

Truong MT, Erasmus JJ, Gladish GW, et al. Anatomy of pericardial recesses on multidetector CT: implications for oncologic imaging. *AJR Am J Roentgenol.* 2003;181:1109–1113.

Truong QA, et al. Reference values for normal pulmonary artery dimensions by non-contrast cardiac computed tomography: the Framingham Heart Study. *Circ Cardiovasc Imaging.* 2012;5(1):147–154.

Tsang TS, Barnes ME, Bailey KR, et al. Left atrial volume: important risk marker of incident atrial fibrillation in 1655 older men and women. *Mayo Clin Proc.* 2001;76:467–475.

Valsangiacomo Buechel ER, Mertens LL. Imaging the right heart: the use of integrated multimodality imaging. *Eur Heart J.* 2012;33:949–960.

Van Praagh S, Geva T, lock JE, et al. Biatrial or left atrial drainage of the right superior vena cava: anatomic, morphogenetic, and surgical considerations-report of three new cases and literature review. *Pediatric Cardiol.* 2003;24(4):350–363.

Veinot JP, Harrity PJ, Gentile F, et al. Anatomy of the normal left atrial appendage: a quantitative study of age-related changes in 500 autopsy hearts: implications for echocardiographic examination. *Circulation.* 1997;96:3112–3115.

Wang ZJ, Reddy GP, Gotway MB, Yeh BM, Hetts SW, Higgins CB. CT and MR imaging of pericardial disease. *Radiographics.* 2003;23(Spec No):S167–S180.

Wu W, Budovec J, Foley WD. Prospective and retrospective ECG gating for thoracic CT angiography: a comparative study. *AJR Am J Roentgenol.* 2009;193:955–963.

Yildiz AE, Anyurek OM, Akpinar E, et al. Multidetector CT of bronchial and non-bronchial systemic arteries. *Diagn Interv Radiol.* 2011;17:10–17.

CHAPTER 4

Step-by-Step Analysis of Cardiac Chambers in CT

Ahmed H. El-Sherief, Michael Bolen, and Carlos A. Rojas

CHAPTER OUTLINE

■ Introduction

Heart disease is a leading cause of morbidity and mortality worldwide. Noninvasive imaging plays a role in the diagnosis, monitoring, and treatment of heart disease. Hence, radiologists can increase the clinical utility of their imaging reports and consultations with basic knowledge of cardiac chamber assessment on computed tomography (CT) for dedicated cardiovascular and conventional thoracic imaging protocols. Although analysis of many CT scans can be performed solely with images oriented in the conventional axial, coronal, and sagittal planes (and, in many cases, images in the axial plane only may suffice), this approach significantly limits the imager in cardiac evaluation.

To analyze cardiac chambers on cross-sectional imaging, the radiologist must first understand cardiac chamber anatomy, as defined by standardized planes that can be obtained from multiplanar reformatted images. Standardized cardiac imaging planes, which include the four-chamber, three-chamber, two-chamber, and short-axis views, are used to assess cardiac morphology, size, and function. These standardized imaging planes, or their approximations, are shared among multiple tomographic imaging modalities. The creation of these planes on CT requires access to multiplanar reconstruction (MPR) software and knowledge of an accurate and reproducible step-by-step approach based on anatomic landmarks.

This chapter will illustrate one such step-by-step approach for creating standardized cardiac imaging planes on CT using MPR software. This chapter will also illustrate how to use these standardized cardiac planes to assess cardiac chamber morphology, size, and function. Knowledge of these imaging planes and the associated anatomy not only sets the stage for the radiologist to analyze cardiac structures on CT scans thoroughly, but also allows the radiologist to begin correlation with other cardiac imaging modalities with shared imaging planes and anatomic vernacular.

■ Standardized Cardiac Imaging Planes

Vertical Long-Axis and True Two-Chamber Views

The vertical long-axis view of the left ventricle is obtained from a plane that passes through the center of the mitral valve and left ventricular apex, parallel to the midportion of the interventricular septum. This view of the left ventricle is a single oblique cardiac imaging plane and is an approximation of the true two-chamber view of the left ventricle. The true paraseptal (parallel to the septum) two-chamber view of the left ventricle is a double-oblique cardiac imaging plane that differs slightly

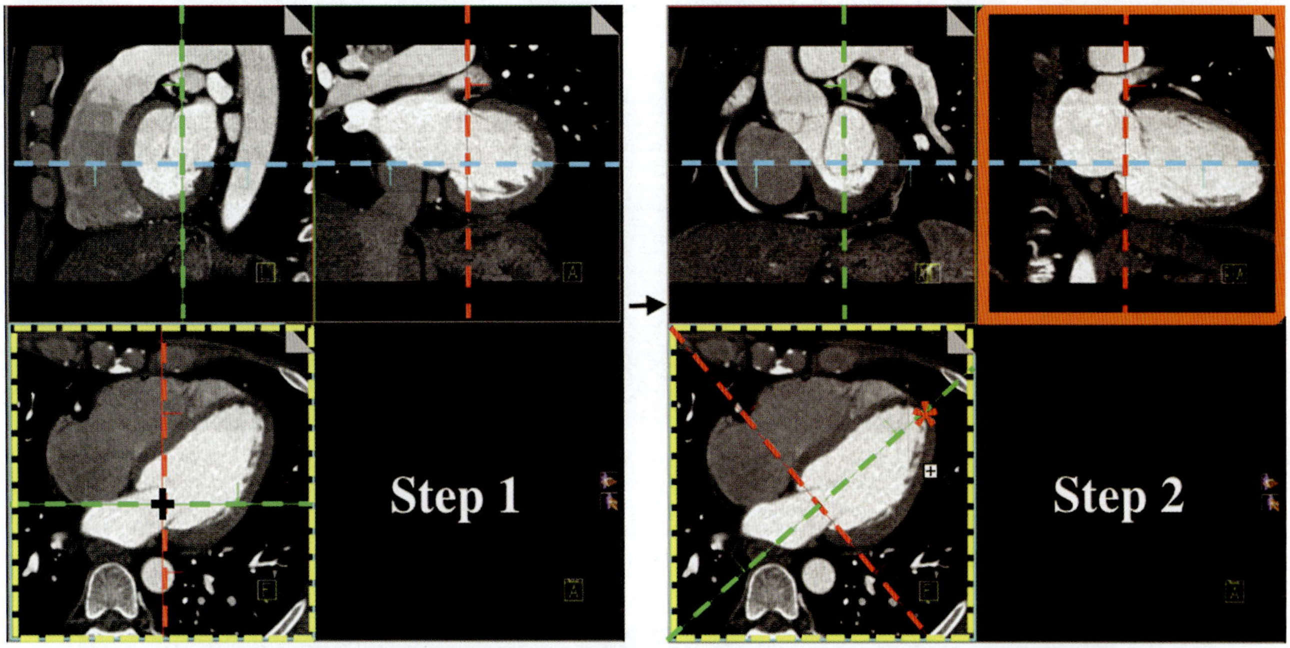

Figure 4.1 Vertical long-axis view of the left ventricle, step-by-step approach. *Step 1.* Open the study in a two-dimensional–three-dimensional multiplanar reconstruction viewer (axial, coronal, and sagittal imaging planes), and scroll to the level of the mitral valve. Identify the axial image *(bottom left-hand image)*, and place the crosshair *(black cross)* through the center of the mitral valve. *Step 2.* With the crosshair fixed, rotate the green line until it is parallel to the interventricular septum and crosses through the left ventricular apex *(red asterisk)*. The top right-hand image has now been transformed into a vertical long-axis view of the left ventricle.

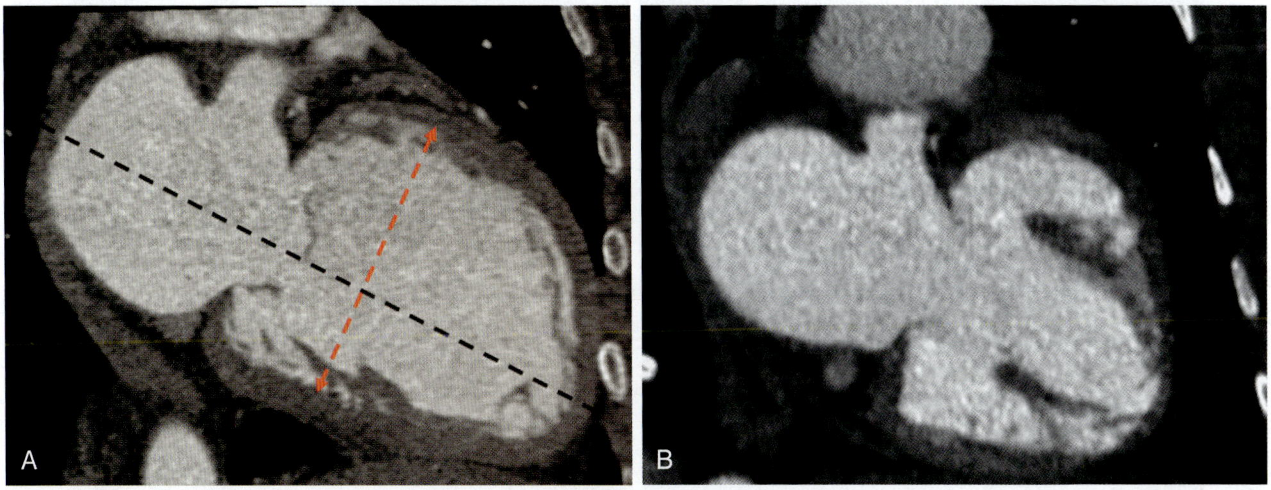

Figure 4.2 Pathologies depicted using the vertical long-axis view of the left ventricle. (A) Left ventricular chamber dilation in the setting of dilated cardiomyopathy. (B) Isolated left ventricular hypoplasia.

from the vertical long-axis view of the left ventricle. It differs by the off-axis tilt from a straight vertical line through the short-axis view. Both of these views can be used to evaluate mitral valve morphology and function; left atrial morphology, size, and function; and left ventricular chamber morphology, size, and function—in particular, the left ventricular anterior and inferior walls on the true two-chamber view, and typically the anterior and inferoseptal walls with the vertical long-axis view.

See Fig. 4.1 for a step-by-step approach for obtaining a vertical long-axis view of the left ventricle. Fig. 4.2 demonstrates sample pathologies that can be depicted with this view.

Short-Axis View

The short-axis view of the left ventricle (a double-oblique cardiac imaging plane) is obtained from a plane that is orthogonal to the vertical long axis of the left ventricle. This view can be used to evaluate global left ventricular function, regional left ventricular wall motion, and left ventricular myocardial wall thickness.

See Fig. 4.3 for a step-by-step approach for obtaining a short-axis view of the left ventricle. Fig. 4.4 demonstrates sample pathologies that could be depicted with this view.

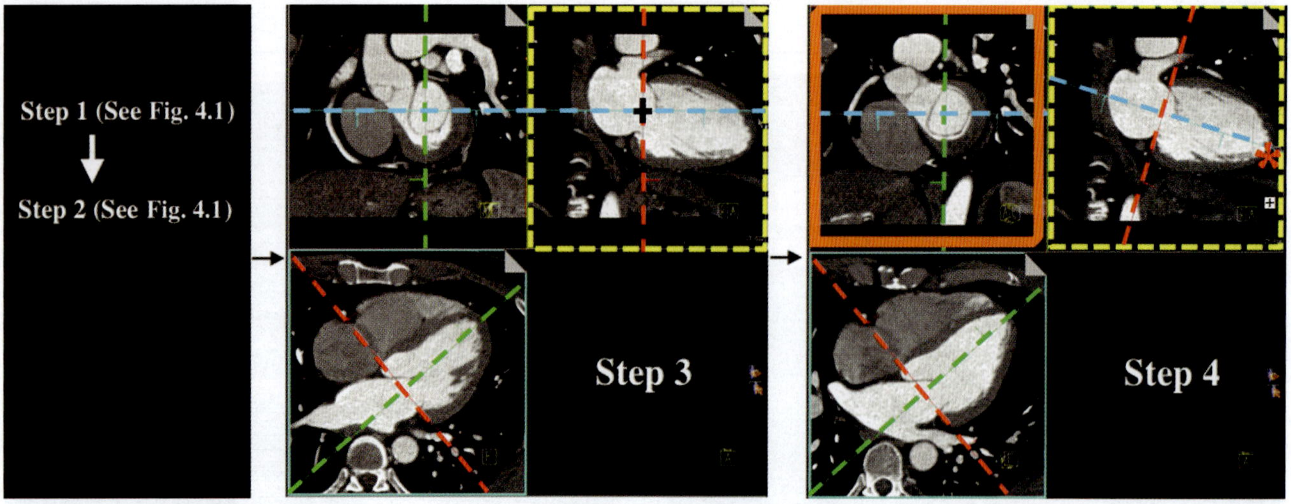

Figure 4.3 Short-axis view of the left ventricle, step-by-step approach. Follow Steps 1 and 2 (see Fig. 4.1). *Step 3.* Identify the resultant vertical log axis view of the left ventricle *(top right-hand image)*, and place the crosshair *(black cross)* through the center of the mitral valve. *Step 4.* With the crosshair fixed, rotate the blue line until it crosses the left ventricular apex *(red asterisk)*. The top left-hand image has now been transformed into a short-axis view of the left ventricle.

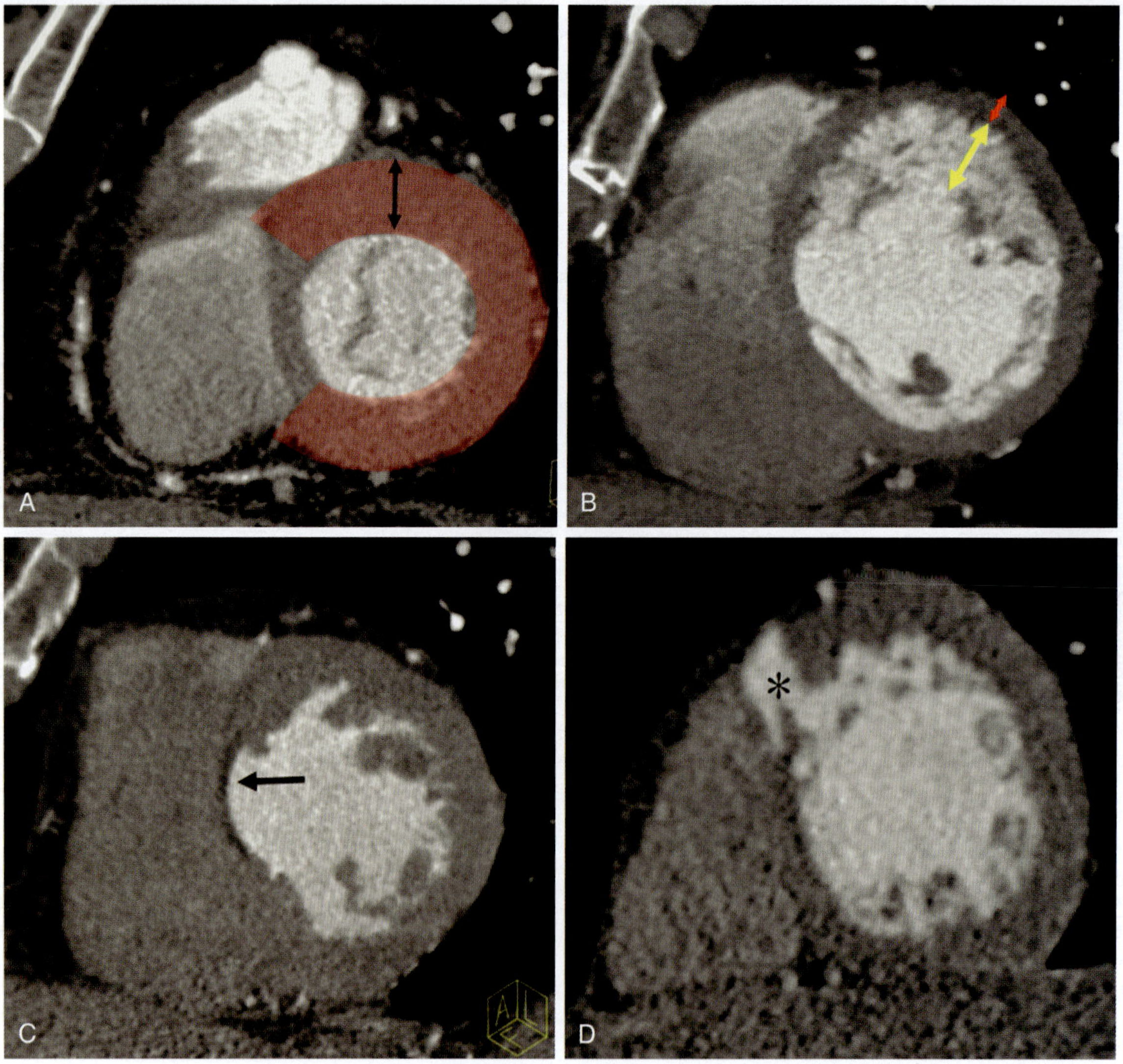

Figure 4.4 Pathologies depicted using the short-axis view of the left ventricle. (A) Hypertrophic cardiomyopathy, with end-diastolic wall thickness exceeding 15 mm in some segments *(double-headed black arrow)*. (B) Noncompaction cardiomyopathy where the ratio of noncompacted *(double-headed yellow arrow)* to compacted *(double-headed red arrow)* myocardium exceeds 2.3 in end-diastole. (C) Septal thinning with fatty replacement and mild aneurysm formation status post remote myocardial infarction. (D) Muscular-type ventricular septal defect *(asterisk)*.

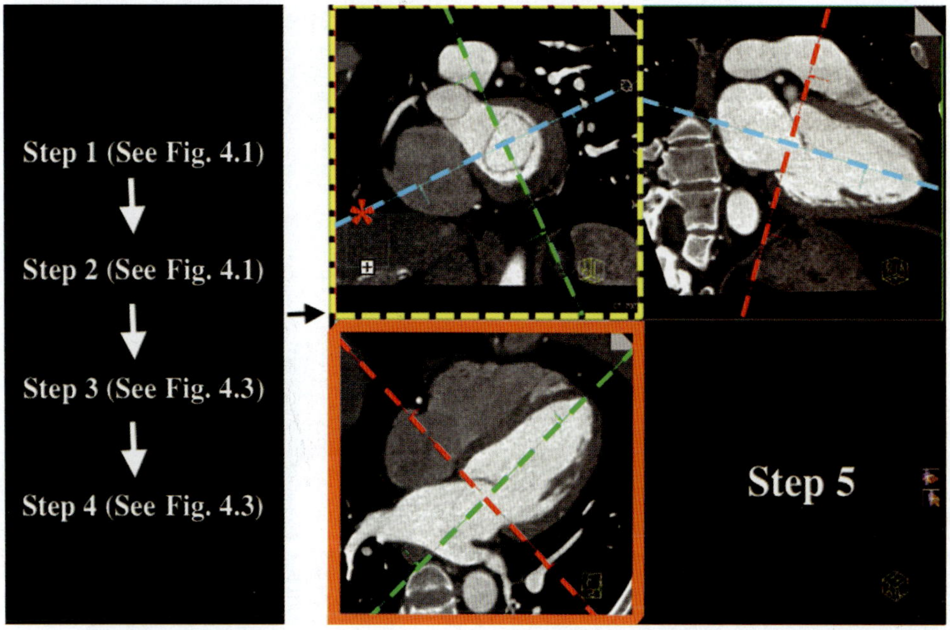

Figure 4.5 Four-chamber view of the left ventricle, step-by-step approach. Follow Steps 1 and 2 (see Fig. 4.1) and Steps 3 and 4 (see Fig. 4.3). *Step 5.* Identify the resultant short-axis view *(top left-hand image)* and, with the crosshair fixed, rotate the blue line so that it transverses the center of the mitral valve and the acute margin of the right ventricle *(red asterisk)*. The bottom left-hand image has now been transformed into a four-chamber view.

Four-Chamber View

The four-chamber view (a double-oblique cardiac imaging plane) is obtained from a plane that slices along the horizontal plane through the short-axis perspective. This view includes both tricuspid and mitral valve planes. The four-chamber view can be used to evaluate interatrial and interventricular septum morphology, cardiac chamber morphology, the left ventricular septal wall, the left ventricular lateral wall, the right ventricular free wall, and the pericardium.

See Fig. 4.5 for a step-by-step approach for obtaining a four-chamber view of the left ventricle. Fig. 4.6 demonstrates sample pathologies that could be depicted with this view.

Three-Chamber View

The three-chamber view of the left ventricle is obtained from a plane that includes the long axis of the left ventricle and the center line through the left ventricular outflow tract and aortic root. This view can be used to evaluate mitral valve morphology and function, left ventricular outflow tract morphology, left ventricular anteroseptal and inferolateral walls, and aortic root morphology, size, and function.

See Fig. 4.7 for a step-by-step approach for obtaining a three-chamber view of the left ventricle. Fig. 4.8 demonstrates sample pathologies that could be depicted with this view.

■ Ventricular Morphology

Ventricles are typically composed of three anatomically distinct components—inlet, apical trabecular, and outlet components. The inlet component extends from the atrioventricular valve to the papillary muscles; the trabecular component extends from the papillary muscles to the ventricular apex; and the outlet component consists of the ventricular portion that leads to the great vessels. The morphologic right and left ventricles demonstrate differences in their inlet, apical trabecular, and outlet components, which allows for their distinction (Fig. 4.9).

In the morphologic right ventricle, the inlet component consists of a three-leaflet (tricuspid) atrioventricular valve. The apical trabecular component consists of coarse trabeculae, and the outlet component (infundibulum) is a smooth muscular structure. The septum contains septal papillary muscle attachments. In the morphologic left ventricle, the inlet component consists of a two-leaflet (bicuspid) atrioventricular valve. The apical trabecular component consists of fine trabeculae in a crisscross pattern, and the outlet component is partly fibrous, secondary to aortic-mitral continuity. The upper septum is relatively smooth compared with the right ventricle, although, in some cases, a few accessory anterior papillary muscle bellies may insert into this region.

■ Standardized Left Ventricular Myocardial Segmentation and Nomenclature

The left ventricular cavity can be divided into 17 segments, thus allowing for standardized nomenclature. The 17-segment model divides the left ventricle into basal, midcavity, and apical thirds (Fig. 4.10). The basal segments extend from the mitral annulus to the tips of the left ventricular papillary muscles and consist of six segments—basal anterior, anteroseptal, inferoseptal, inferior, inferolateral, and anterolateral segments. The midcavity segments extend from the tips of the left ventricular papillary muscles to the base of the left ventricular papillary muscles and consist of six segments—midcavity anterior, anteroseptal, inferoseptal, inferior, inferolateral, and anterolateral segments. The apical segments extend from the base of the left ventricular papillary muscles

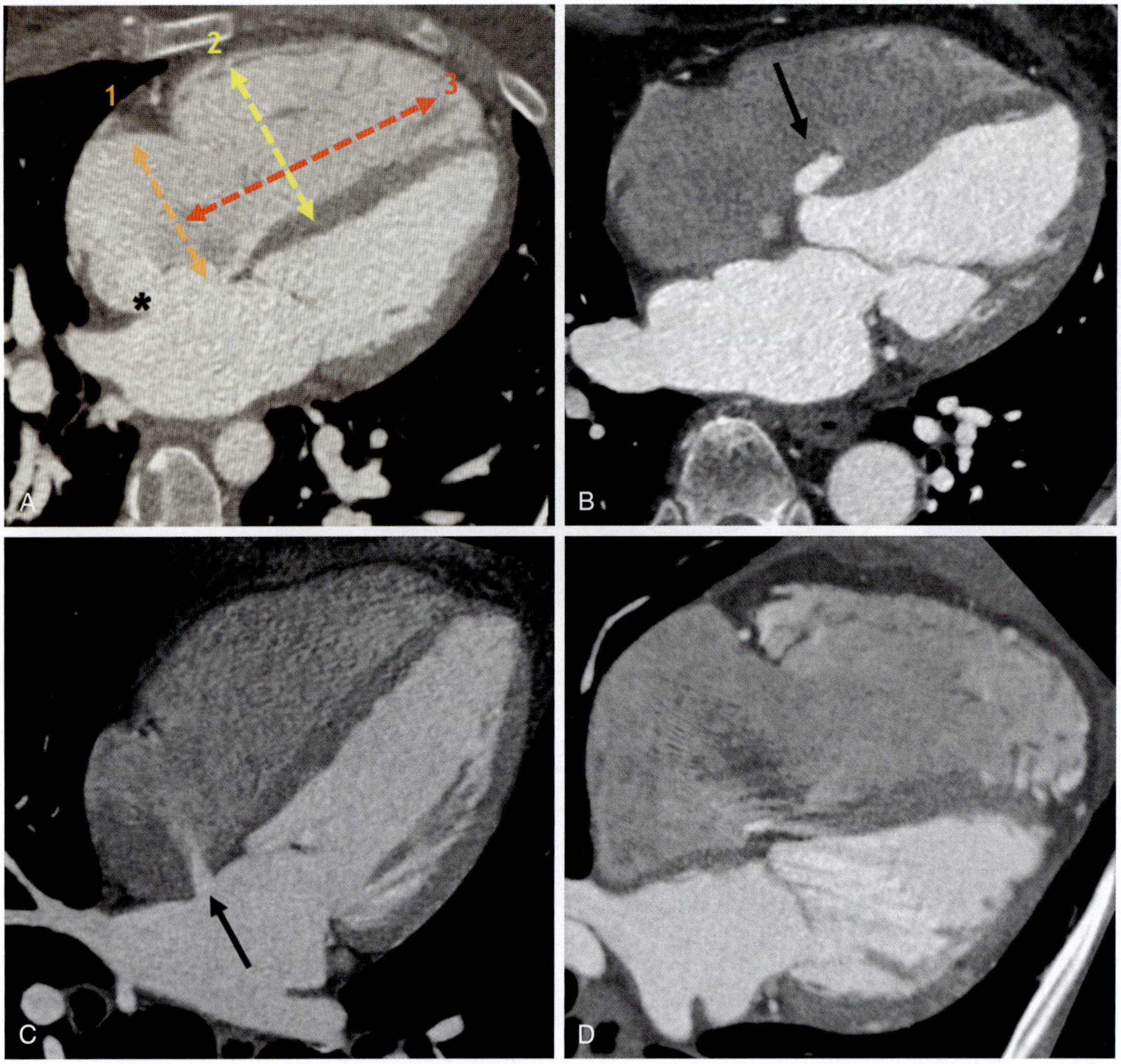

Figure 4.6 Pathologies depicted using the four-chamber view. (A) Right ventricular (RV) dilation in the setting of an atrial septal defect *(asterisk)*. *1*, Basal RV diameter; *2*, mid-RV diameter; *3*, RV base-to-apex length. (B) Membranous ventricular septal aneurysm *(arrow)*. (C) Patent foramen ovale with a left-to-right shunt *(arrow)*. (D) RV chamber dilation in the setting of arrhythmogenic RV dysplasia.

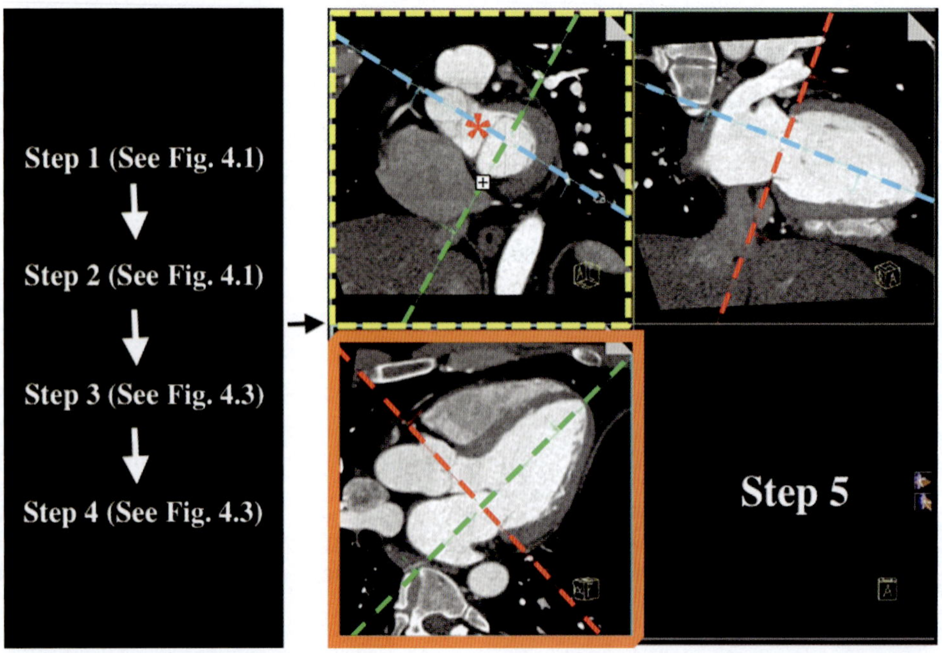

Figure 4.7 Three-chamber view of the left ventricle, step-by-step approach. Follow Steps 1 and 2 (see Fig. 4.1) and Steps 3 and 4 (see Fig. 4.3). *Step 5*. Identify the resultant short-axis view *(top left-hand image)* and, with the crosshair fixed, rotate the blue line until it crosses the left ventricular outflow tract *(red asterisk)*. The bottom left-hand image has now been transformed into a three-chamber view of the left ventricle.

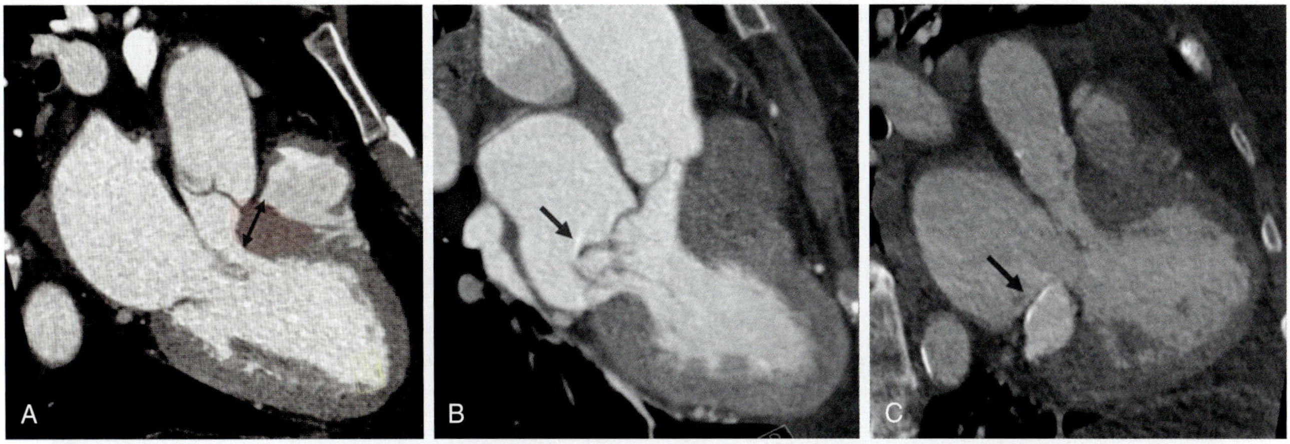

Figure 4.8 Pathologies depicted using the three-chamber view of the left ventricle. (A) Obstructive hypertrophic cardiomyopathy *(double-headed arrow)*. (B) Flail mitral valve prolapse *(arrow)*. (C) Caseous mitral valve annulus calcification *(arrow)*.

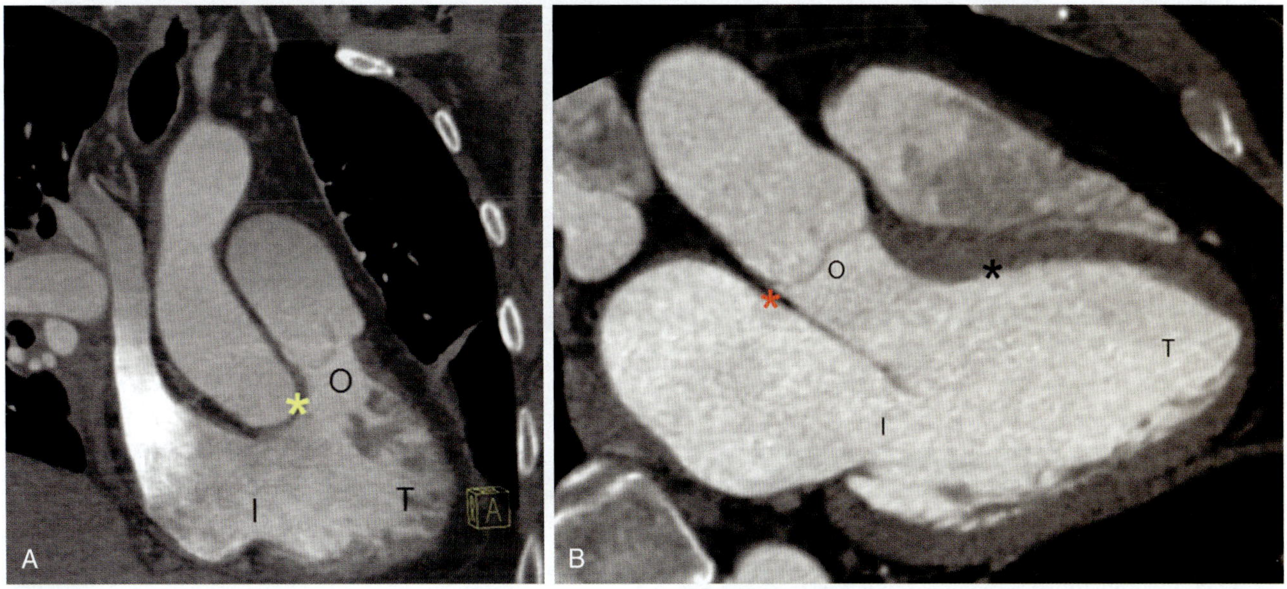

Figure 4.9 Morphologic right ventricle and left ventricle. (A) Three-chamber view of the right ventricle demonstrating a morphologic right ventricle. The inlet *(I)* component consists of a three-leaflet atrioventricular valve, the apical trabecular *(T)* component consists of course trabeculae, and the outlet *(O)* component is a smooth muscular structure. The inlet and outlet components of the right ventricle are not in fibrous continuity; they are separated by a ridge of muscular tissue known as the crista supraventricularis *(yellow asterisk)*. The septum consists of a septal papillary muscle attachment. (B) Three-chamber view of the left ventricle demonstrating a morphologic left ventricle. The I component consists of a two-leaflet atrioventricular valve; the T component consists of fine trabeculae in a crisscross pattern; and the O component is partly fibrous secondary to aortic-mitral fibrous continuity *(red asterisk)*. The upper septum is usually smooth *(black asterisk)*.

to the apex of the left ventricle and consist of four segments—apical anterior, septal, inferior, and lateral segments. The left ventricular apex itself is considered the last of the 17 segments.

■ Atrial Morphology

The morphologic right and left atria demonstrate differences in their appendages. The morphologic right atrium has a broad-based appendage, with abundant pectinate muscles, whereas the morphologic left atrium is a narrow-based tubular appendage, with limited pectinate muscles. In addition to differences in their appendages, the atrium that receives the supradiaphragmatic inferior vena cava or the coronary sinus is usually the morphologic right atrium.

■ Cardiac Chamber Quantification

Quantification of Left Ventricular Chamber Size

Left ventricular chamber size quantification on ECG-gated CT of the thorax may be estimated by a linear

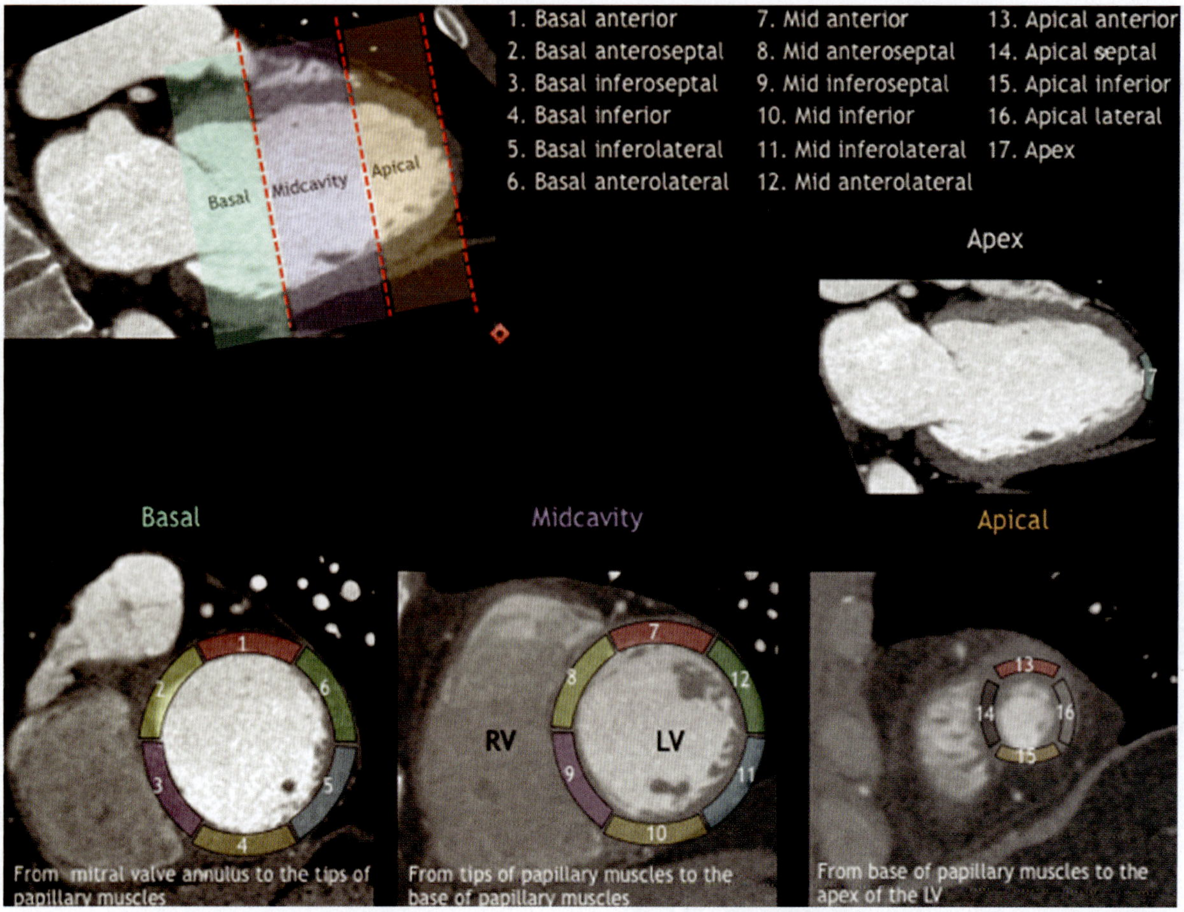

Figure 4.10 Standardized myocardial segmentation and nomenclature. The left ventricle *(LV)* cavity can be divided into 17 segments, allowing for standardized nomenclature. The 17-segment model divides the LV into basal, midcavity, and apical thirds. *RV,* Right ventricle.

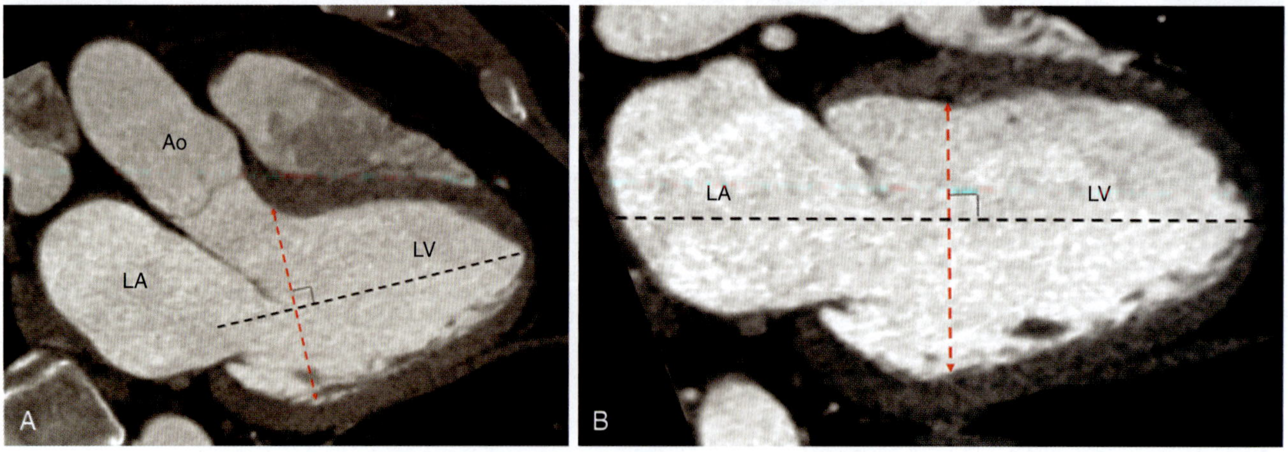

Figure 4.11 Quantification of left ventricle *(LV)* chamber size. LV size may be estimated by a linear measurement known as the LV end-diastolic diameter *(LVEDD;* also known as the LV internal diameter). (A) With the three-chamber view, the LVEDD is measured at the level of the minor axis of the LV, approximately at the mitral chordal-leaflet junction in a line perpendicular to the long axis of the ventricle *(dashed red line).* (B) With the two-chamber view, the LVEDD is measured at the junction of the basal and middle thirds of the long axis in a line perpendicular to the long axis of the ventricle *(dashed red line). Ao,* Aorta; *LA,* left atrium.

measurement known as the *left ventricular end-diastolic diameter* (LVEDD; also known as the *left ventricular internal diameter* [LVID]). Accepted standardized cardiac imaging planes for measuring the LVEDD include the three-chamber and two-chamber views of the left ventricle. With the three-chamber view of the left ventricle, the LVEDD is measured at the level of the minor axis of the left ventricle, approximately at the mitral chordal-leaflet junction in a line perpendicular to the long axis of the ventricle (Fig. 4.11). With the two-chamber view of the left ventricle, the LVEDD is measured at the junction of the basal and middle thirds of the long axis in a line perpendicular to the long axis of the ventricle (see Fig. 4.11). If end-diastolic images are not available (e.g., prospective ECG-gated CT or non–ECG-gated CT of the thorax), and the measured LVEDD is greater than the upper limit of the normal reference value, the left ventricle is enlarged. However, if the measured LVEDD is within normal limits, this does not necessarily mean that the left ventricle is not enlarged because the measurement has not been obtained at end-diastole.

Quantification of Right Ventricular Chamber Size

Right ventricular chamber size on ECG-gated CT of the thorax is usually assessed qualitatively. The right ventricular midcavity diameter in the four-chamber view, in healthy patients, should typically be smaller than that of the left ventricle (given that the reference left ventricle is normal in size to begin with), regardless of the phase of the cardiac cycle. To assess right ventricular chamber size quantitatively requires obtaining three linear measurements from the four-chamber view at the level of the left ventricle papillary muscles at end-diastole: (1) basal right ventricular diameter; (2) mid–right ventricular diameter; and (3) base-to-apex length (Fig. 4.12).

Quantification of Left Atrial Chamber Size

The left atrium is typically measured at end-systole. Linear measurements of the left atrium can be misleading because of inhomogeneous dilation of the left atrial chamber due to constraints of the sternum and a vertebral bony column in the anteroposterior dimension. However, quantifying the left atrial area or left atrial volume on ECG-gated CT of the thorax may be considered cumbersome on routine evaluation. Therefore linear measurements are a rapid, albeit imprecise, way to evaluate left atrial chamber size. Linear measurements include anteroposterior (obtained from the three-chamber view), superoinferior (obtained from the four-chamber view), and mediolateral (obtained from the four-chamber view) dimensions (Fig. 4.13). If end-systolic images are not available (i.e., prospective ECG-gated or non–ECG-gated CT of the thorax) and the measured linear left atrial

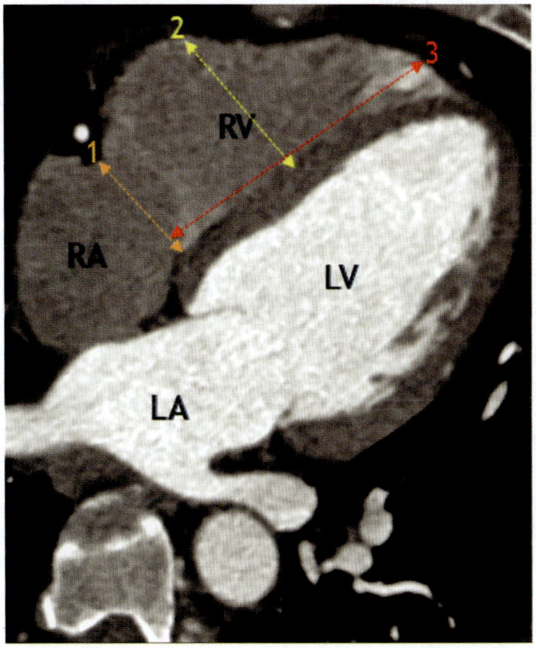

Figure 4.12 Quantification of right ventricle *(RV)* chamber size. RV chamber size may be estimated by three linear measurements from the four-chamber view at the level of the left ventricle *(LV)* papillary muscles at end-diastole: *(1)* basal RV diameter; *(2)* mid-RV diameter; and *(3)* base-to-apex length. *LA*, Left atrium; *RA*, right atrium.

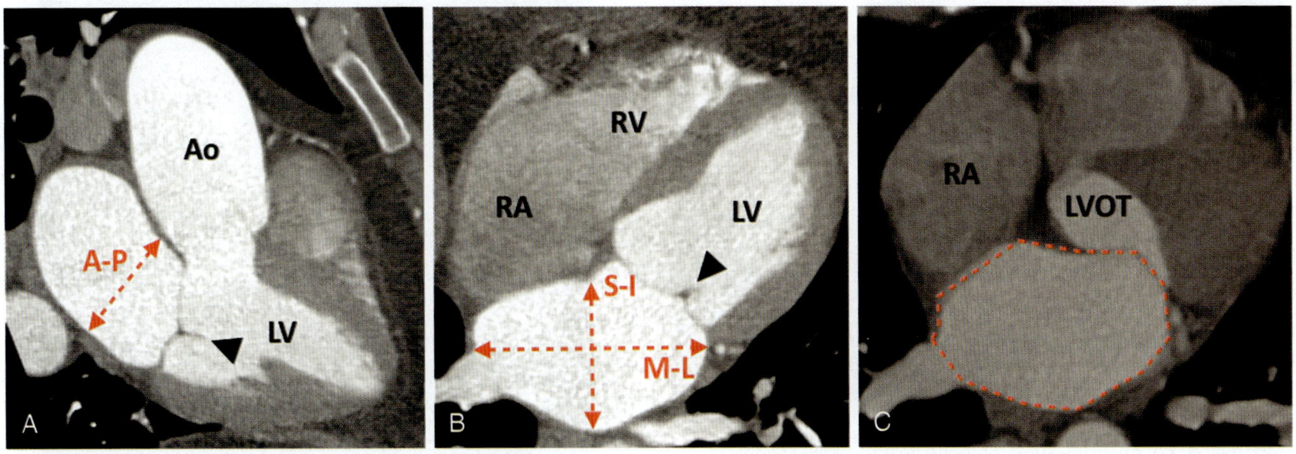

Figure 4.13 Quantification of left atrial chamber size. (A, B) Linear measurements include anteroposterior (*A-P*, obtained from the three-chamber view), superoinferior (*S-I*, obtained from the four-chamber view), and mediolateral (*M-L*, obtained from the four-chamber view) dimensions. Note that the mitral valve is closed *(black arrowhead)*, indicating systole. (C) Measurement of left atrial area on axial images *(dotted red line)* at the level of the left ventricular outflow tract *(LVOT)* and the mitral leaflets. *LV*, Left ventricle; *RA*, right atrium; *RV*, right ventricle.

dimension is greater than the normal reference value, the left atrium is enlarged. However, if the measured linear left atrial dimension is within normal limits, this does not necessarily mean that the left atrium is not enlarged. Some investigators have suggested that measuring the left atrial area on axial images, at the level of the left ventricular outflow tract and the mitral leaflets, is a reproducible approach that offers better correlation with left atrial volume (see Fig. 4.13).

Quantification of Right Atrial Chamber Size

Right atrial chamber size quantification on ECG-gated CT of the thorax is usually assessed qualitatively. The right atrium is considered enlarged if it is larger than the left atrium, assuming that the left atrium is normal in size. Quantitative assessment of the right atrial chamber involves obtaining the right atrial minor axis dimension from the four-chamber view at end-systole. The minor axis of the right atrium is defined as a dimension extending from the lateral border of the right atrium to the interatrial septum perpendicular to the long axis of the right atrium (Fig. 4.14).

Left Ventricular Wall Thickness

Assessing left ventricular wall thickness on ECG-gated cardiac CT requires measuring the maximal left ventricular wall thickness within each of the 17 left ventricular segments. The short-axis view of the left ventricle at end-diastole is used to obtain these measurements (Fig. 4.15). The radiologist must ensure that the short-axis view is truly orthogonal to the segment being evaluated (especially the basal cavity and apical segments); oblique angles will lead to a misrepresentation (overestimation) of wall thickness.

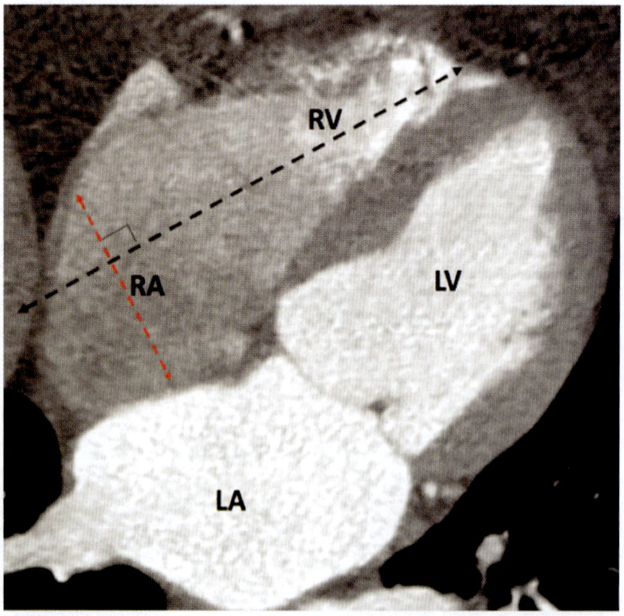

Figure 4.14 Quantification of right atrium *(RA)* chamber size. Quantitative assessment of RA chamber size requires obtaining the RA minor axis dimension from the four-chamber view at end-systole. The RA minor axis is defined as a dimension extending from the lateral border of the RA to the interatrial septum *(dashed red line with arrowheads)*, perpendicular to the long axis of the RA *(dashed black line)*. *LA*, Left atrium; *LV*, left ventricle; *RV*, right ventricle.

Evaluation of Global Left Ventricular Function and Regional Left Ventricular Wall Motion or Wall Thickening

Global left ventricular function and regional left ventricular wall motion or wall thickening on ECG-gated cardiac CT are usually assessed qualitatively (visual estimate on cine CT) and require dynamic assessment of the cardiac cycle. Generally, global left ventricular function on ECG-gated cardiac CT is quantitatively assessed with postprocessing software, which requires retrospective ECG gating acquisition. Regionally, each of the 17 left ventricular segments is subjectively evaluated for wall motion and systolic wall thickening during the cardiac cycle, usually in the short-axis view of the left ventricle. Normal regional left ventricular thickening is considered an increase of at least 40%, with hypokinesis noted with lesser degrees of thickening. Akinetic left ventricular wall motion is defined as a negligible increase in systolic wall thickness; dyskinetic left ventricular wall motion is defined as an outward movement of the wall during systole with associated systolic wall thinning.

Reference Values for the Cardiac Chambers on CT

Normal reference values for cardiac chamber quantification differ, depending on the imaging modality used (e.g., echocardiography, CT, MRI). Previously, cardiac

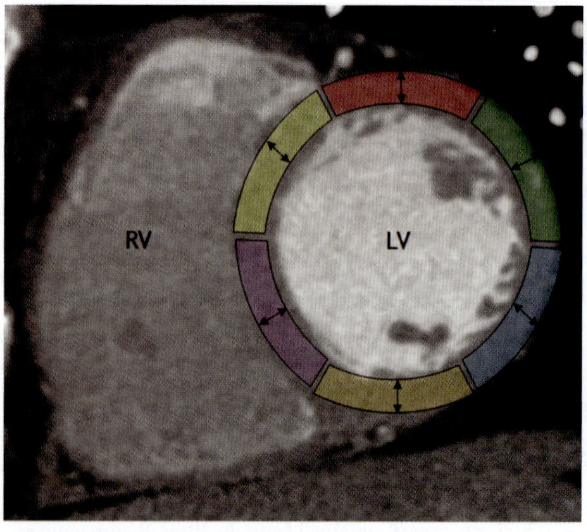

Figure 4.15 Short-axis view of the left ventricle *(LV)* midcavity segment. Assessment of LV wall thickness requires measuring the thickest LV myocardial wall thickness within each of the 17 LV segments. *RV*, Right ventricle.

TABLE 4.1 Cardiac Chamber Reference Values by Echocardiography

PARAMETER	WOMEN	MEN
LV end-diastolic diameter	3.9–5.3 cm	4.2–5.9 cm
LV end-diastolic diameter/ BSA	2.4–3.2 cm/m^2	2.2–3.1 cm/m^2
RV dimensions		
Basal RV diameter	2.0–2.8 cm	2.0–2.8 cm
Mid-RV diameter	2.7–3.3 cm	2.7–3.3 cm
Base-to-apex length	7.1–7.9 cm	7.1–7.9 cm
LA end-systolic diameter	2.7–3.8 cm	3.0–4.0 cm
LA end-systolic diameter/ BSA	1.5–2.3 cm/m^2	1.5–2.3 cm/m^2
LA area	≤20 cm^3	≤20 cm^3
RA minor axis dimension	2.9–4.5 cm	2.9–4.5 cm
RA minor axis dimension/ BSA	1.7–2.5 cm/m^2	2.9–4.5 cm/m^2

BSA, Body surface area; *LA*, left atrial; *LV*, left ventricular; *RA*, right atrial; *RV*, right ventricular.
From Lang RM, Bierig M, Devereux RB, et al; Chamber Quantification Writing Group; American Society of Echocardiography's Guidelines and Standards Committee; European Association of Echocardiography. Recommendations for chamber quantification: a report from the American Society of Echocardiography's Guidelines and Standards Committee and the Chamber Quantification Writing Group, developed in conjunction with the European Association of Echocardiography, a branch of the European Society of Cardiology. *J Am Soc Echocardiogr.* 2005;18(12):1440–1463.

chamber quantification on CT relied on echocardiographic reference values (Table 4.1); however, gender- and age-specific normalized reference values for the cardiac chambers on CT are now slowly being amassed.

■ Conclusion

Standardized imaging planes of the cardiac chambers can be derived from an axial dataset using a basic algorithm at the workstation during ECG-gated and non–ECG-gated CT of the thorax. These imaging planes, in combination with knowledge of cardiac chamber anatomy, are essential for clinically relevant and reproducible evaluation of cardiac morphology, size, and function.

Bibliography

Alfakih K, Thiele H, Plein S, Bainbridge GJ, Ridgway JP, Sivananthan MU. Comparison of right ventricular volume measurement between segmented k-space gradient-echo and steady-state free precession magnetic resonance imaging. *J Magn Reson Imaging.* 2002;16(3):253–258.

Cerqueira MD, Weissman NJ, Dilsizian V, et al. American Heart Association Writing Group on Myocardial Segmentation and Registration for Cardiac Imaging. Standardized myocardial segmentation and nomenclature for tomographic imaging of the heart: a statement for healthcare professionals from the Cardiac Imaging Committee of the Council on Clinical Cardiology of the American Heart Association. *Circulation.* 2002;105(4):539–542.

Ho SY. Cardiac morphology and nomenclature. In: Gatzoulis MA, Webb GD, Daubeney PEF, eds. *Diagnosis and Management of Adult Congenital Heart Disease.* New York: Elsevier; 2003:9–10.

Lang RM, Bierig M, Devereux RB, et al Chamber Quantification Writing Group; American Society of Echocardiography's Guidelines and Standards Committee; European Association of Echocardiography. Recommendations for chamber quantification: a report from the American Society of Echocardiography's Guidelines and Standards Committee and the Chamber Quantification Writing Group, developed in conjunction with the European Association of Echocardiography, a branch of the European Society of Cardiology. *J Am Soc Echocardiogr.* 2005;18(12):1440–1463.

Lee VL, Cardiovascular MRI. Physical principles to practical protocols. In: Lee VS, eds. *Cardiac Imaging Planes.* Philadelphia: Lippincott Williams & Wilkins; 2006:268.

Mahabadi AA, Truong QA, Schlett CL, et al. Axial area and anteroposterior diameter as estimates of left atrial size using computed tomography of the chest: comparison with 3-dimensional volume. *J Cardiovasc Comput Tomogr.* 2010;4(1):49–54.

Nevsky G, Jacobs JE, Lim RP, Donnino R, Babb JS, Srichai MB. Sex-specific normalized reference values of heart and great vessel dimensions in cardiac CT angiography. *AJR Am J Roentgenol.* 2011;196(4):788–794.

Schallert EK, Danton GH, Kardon R, Young DA. Describing congenital heart disease by using three-part segmental notation. *Radiographics.* 2013;33(2): E33–E46.

Shinebourne EA, Macartney FJ, Anderson RH. Sequential chamber localization: logical approach to diagnosis in congenital heart disease. *Br Heart J.* 1976;38(4):327–340.

Standardization of cardiac tomographic imaging. From the Committee on Advanced Cardiac Imaging and Technology, Council on Clinical Cardiology, American Heart Association; Cardiovascular Imaging Committee, American College of Cardiology; and Board of Directors, Cardiovascular Council, Society of Nuclear Medicine. *Circulation.* 1992;86:338–339.

Stojanovska J, Cronin P, Patel S, et al. Reference normal absolute and indexed values from ECG-gated MDCT: left atrial volume, function, and diameter. *AJR Am J Roentgenol.* 2011;197(3):631–637.

Wilkinson JL, Acerete F. Terminological pitfalls in congenital heart disease: reappraisal of some confusing terms, with an account of a simplified system of basic nomenclature. *Br Heart J.* 1973;35(11):1166–1177.

SECTION 2

Imaging Techniques

WHAT ARE THE ADVANTAGES OF HIGH-KILOVOLTAGE TECHNIQUES?

1. There is less obscuration of lung parenchyma by bony structures because the differences in coefficients of x-ray absorption of bones and soft tissues are minimized.
2. There is better penetration of the mediastinum, improving the visualization of airways.
3. Exposure time decreases, reducing motion artifact.

WHAT ARE THE ADVANTAGES OF LOW-KILOVOLTAGE TECHNIQUES?

1. Increased contrast between aerated lung and blood filled vessels gives better detail of the lung parenchyma—part of the lung parenchyma is not obscured by overlying bones.
2. Some lesions are better seen on low kilovoltage, such as calcification (e.g., pleural plaques) and lung nodules.

WHAT ARE THE FILM-SCREEN COMBINATIONS PRESENTLY USED?

Rare earth phosphor screens are preferred over calcium tungstate crystal screens because the improved light emission capability of rare earth phosphor screens reduces exposure time and gives sharper images.

Wide-latitude, low-contrast films are preferred in chest radiography because of the highly attenuated mediastinum and highly transmissive lung fields. Otherwise the cardiac outline would be too white and the lung parenchyma would be too dark on a processed film. Studies have shown that using a twin screen-film cassette gives a wide latitude, which helps with the proper visualization of the mediastinal soft tissues and air-filled lung.

WHAT IS SCANNING EQUALIZATION RADIOGRAPHY?

There is a significant difference in x-ray attenuation between the air-filled lung and soft tissues such as the mediastinum and diaphragm, precluding uniform exposure and increasing the scatter. One way to obtain a uniform exposure is the use of scanning equalization radiography (SER). This is a computer-assisted, electronically enhanced radiography technique in which a narrow x-ray beam is scanned over the patient, and its attenuation is measured. The beam intensity is then modulated, depending on this information to equalize the regional x-ray film exposure. An artificial dark band is created at the interfaces of high contrast, such as the diaphragm-lung interface.

WHAT IS AMBER?

AMBER stands for ***a**dvanced **m**ultiple-**b**eam **e**qualization **r**adiography*, one of the most widely used SER technologies. A horizontally oriented slit beam is used with this unit to scan the chest. The detectors are electronically connected to receive feedback information for changing exposure variables for different thickness of tissues.

WHY USE OTHER VIEWS IF PA AND LATERAL VIEWS ARE THE BEST?

It is not always possible to obtain a PA view (e.g., in an intensive care unit [ICU] setting); sometimes one can use an additional view to answer a specific clinical question. However, many views that were formerly used are no longer performed due to the easy availability of CT, which gives a more definite answer. Note that the cost of an additional radiographic view is still significantly less than a CT scan, and an additional view may solve a particular clinical question quickly and economically.

Standard Views

WHAT OTHER VIEWS ARE STILL CURRENTLY PERFORMED, AND WHY?

Anteroposterior View

Most portable radiographs (e.g., in an ICU setting) are performed in the anteroposterior (AP) projection. The main advantage of this position is that it can be done without changing the patient's position.

WHY NOT USE AP VIEWS IN ALL PATIENTS?

1. There is more magnification in an AP radiograph as compared to a PA radiograph due to a shorter focus-film distance. The heart is an anterior structure and is therefore magnified, suggesting apparent cardiomegaly (see Fig. 5.3). The apparent cardiac diameter may increase by 15% to 20% in the AP position.
2. One cannot use high-kilovoltage techniques for portable x-rays because portable machines have a limited kilovoltage setting. Similarly, maximum milliamperage is also limited as compared to stationary machines.
3. Grids to decrease scatter are not as effective.
4. Due to limited maximal kilovoltage capability, portable machines require longer exposures to have a proper penetration, resulting in increased motion-related artifacts.
5. Images are often rotated because critically ill patients are difficult to position.
6. Supine positioning elevates the diaphragm and compresses the lower lobes, thereby reducing lung volumes.
7. Because there is even a gravitational effect in the upper and lower lung zones, evaluation of pulmonary vascular congestion is often difficult on supine images.
8. The upper mediastinum is widened due to magnification and an increase in systemic venous return in the supine position.
9. Small effusions may be missed due to a layering effect in a supine patient.
10. A small pneumothorax may be missed because free air tends to move to an anteromedial or inferior location in a supine patient.

WHERE DO WE FREQUENTLY USE AP RADIOGRAPHY?

It is commonly used to evaluate cardiopulmonary status and various monitoring devices in an inpatient, particularly in the ICU setting. A sharper reconstruction algorithm is often used to evaluate positioning of support lines on a radiograph (Fig. 5.4).

Lateral Decubitus View

In this view side (not called a lateral view, because the name might be confusing), the patient is lying on the side, and a frontal x-ray is taken using a horizontal beam. One can use this view to demonstrate pleural fluid layering (and to differentiate loculated fluid or other causes of opacity) to the dependent position between the lung and chest wall (Fig. 5.5). This view has also been used to document a small pneumothorax in the nondependent lung (Fig. 5.6). According to the literature, as little as 5 mL of fluid or 15 mL of air can be visualized using lateral decubitus radiography.

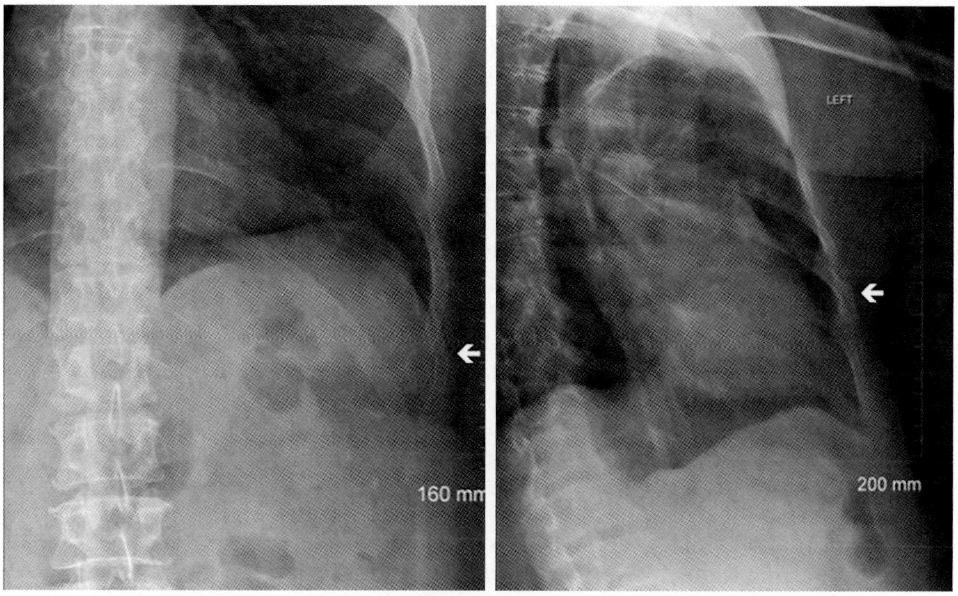

Figure 5.8 Dedicated rib radiographs on this patient with known trauma and localized chest pain showing mildly displaced left-sided rib fracture *(arrows)* not visualized on a frontal radiograph (not shown).

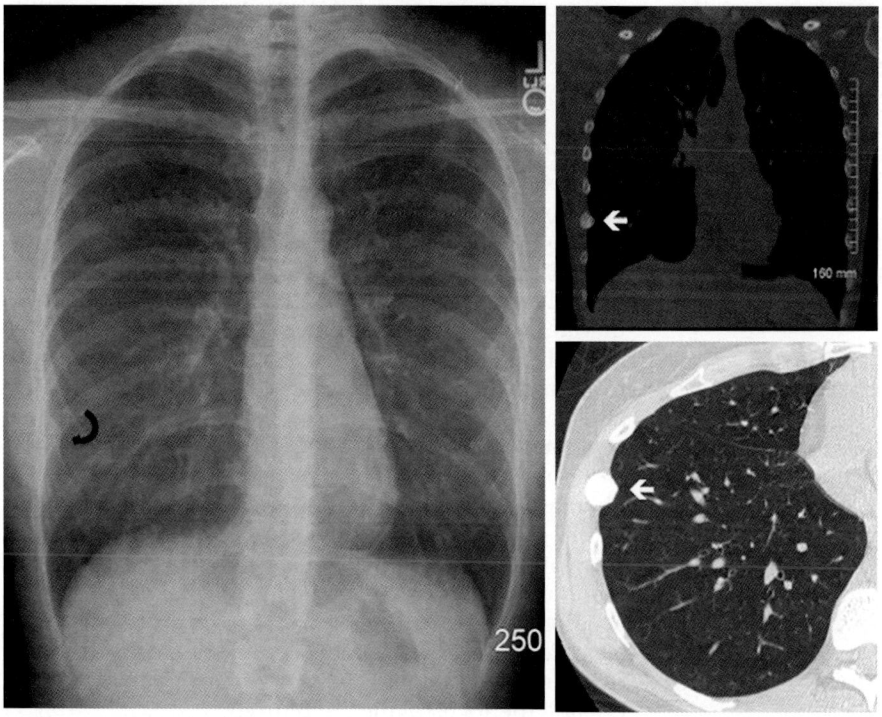

Figure 5.9 A nodule is noted in the right lateral hemithorax projecting over the sixth rib *(curved arrow)*. CT scan showing a healed right seventh rib fracture with callus formation *(straight arrows)*.

3. The screen fluoresces, depending on local energy deposition by x-rays.
4. This released light is used to form images using a computerized system.

Flat Panel Detector Technology

FPD technology is based on amorphous silicon thin-film transistors (TFTs) combined with an x-ray absorptive layer. This technology can be divided into direct or indirect FPD.

A phosphor screen is used to convert x-ray energy to light photons in indirect FPD. These light photons are detected by the photodiode array in the TFT layer. Each TFT has a capacitor and detects the charge created by the light energy.

Instead of a phosphor screen, a photoconductor layer is used in a direct FPD system. This photoconductor layer converts the energy liberated by the x-rays into a charge and, with the help of a strong magnetic field, this charge is directed to a TFT-capacitor combination. The charges in the TFT-capacitor array form a raw digital image data, which is used for processing and display.

Other ways of acquiring a digital chest radiograph include using a charge-coupled device (CCD) and complementary metal oxide semiconductor (CMOS) cameras. A phosphor layer is used to convert x-ray energy to light, and this light is used to create an image (a radiograph) by CCD or CMOS cameras. The main limitations of CCD and CMOS detectors are their smaller size and the need to minify the phosphor screen light image. A lens system or fiberoptic coupler is used to minify the light image, but this minification process decreases efficiency.

Processing of Digital Data

The images acquired in a digital system are usually processed before sending them to a display system.

WHAT ARE THE PROCESSING STEPS?

1. Correction of detector nonuniformity in raw data
2. Conversion of the dynamic range of raw data to the range of perception capability of the human eye
3. Postprocessing:
   a. Grayscale processing—converts detector signal information to grayscale values. This is mostly done by windowing and leveling.
   b. Edge enhancement—used to enhance fine details of an image. There are different unsharp masking techniques; the general rule is to create a blurred version of the image and subtract a part of the blurred version from the original.
   c. Multifrequency processing—this helps manipulate multiple portions of the frequency spectrum.

Displaying Digital Images

Digital radiography images are usually viewed on a computer screen in a soft copy format.

WHAT ARE THE DIFFERENT TYPES OF SOFT COPY DISPLAY?

1. Cathode ray tube displays
2. Active matrix liquid crystal displays (LCDs)

The advantages of cathode ray tube displays over LCDs are a wide viewing angle and less structured noise. However, an LCD display provides better resolution, less reflection, increased range of luminescence, decreased weight, and better bit depth.

HOW CAN COLOR MONITORS BE USEFUL?

Color monitors may not be useful for viewing a grayscale image. However, color monitors help in the use of different applications, which aids workflow.

WHAT ARE THE BENEFITS OF DIGITAL CHEST RADIOGRAPHY?

1. It improves the detection of subtle lesions missed on a conventional radiograph.
2. We can change an algorithm while viewing the images—similar to changing parameters such as peak kilovoltage and milliampere-second (mAs) on a conventional chest radiograph—and also increases lesion conspicuity (visibility).
3. A dual-energy imaging technique with digital imaging helps generate subtraction images.
4. A digital technique is used for temporal subtraction and digital tomosynthesis.

WHAT IS DUAL-ENERGY SUBTRACTION?

This technique uses low- and high-energy photons (usually 60 and 120 keV, respectively) to obtain different sets of images and mainly produces radiographs of two different tissue types. In chest imaging, we are mostly concerned about bone and soft tissues. This technique uses differences of the x-ray attenuation properties of bone and soft tissues and generates images of only bones or only soft tissues (Fig. 5.10).

HOW IS DUAL-ENERGY SUBTRACTION USED CLINICALLY?

1. Studies have shown that the ability to detect lung nodules can be improved by using dual-energy subtraction radiography, eliminating overlying bony structures.
2. This technique can also document calcification in a lung lesion.
3. Other uses include the detection of chest wall pleural lesions, lines, and tubes.

WHAT IS TEMPORAL SUBTRACTION?

This technique is used to subtract a previous radiograph of the same patient from the present radiograph to identify new findings. There are different registration techniques to reduce artifactual abnormalities related to differences in patient positioning at two different times.

HOW DOES TEMPORAL SUBTRACTION HELP IN DAILY PRACTICE?

1. Enhances detection of subtle changes
2. Reduces reading time

WHAT IS DIGITAL TOMOSYNTHESIS?

Digital tomosynthesis (DT) is a technique to generate three-dimensional (3D) images by using multiple x-rays of one object taken from a discrete number of angles.

HOW DOES DT COMPARE TO CT?

The main difference of tomosynthesis is that the range of angles used in DT is limited (usually from 15–60 degrees). At least a 180-degree rotation of the tube or detector is necessary in CT.

HOW DOES DT DIFFER FROM CT?

In DT, data obtained from multiple projections is digitally processed to obtain multiple thin images in one plane. Because the image processing is done digitally, we can change the slice thickness and depth from a single set of acquisition images. This saves time and reduces radiation as compared to conventional tomography.

HOW DOES DT WORK?

The basic principle of tomosynthesis is acquiring a set of images by moving the source and/or detector in a known fashion around the object being imaged and then mathematically reconstructing a 3D image. The images acquired during movement of the x-ray tube are called *projection images.* Different depths of acquisition are obtained by changing the amount of shift. Structures outside the focus plane are blurred.

Computer-Aided Detection

Computer-aided detection (CAD) is a technology in digital imaging in which artificial intelligence of the computer is used to decrease observational oversights, reducing false-negative rates. This technique is used commonly in digital mammography, and many prospective studies have shown an increase in breast cancer detection with the help of CAD. When the computer is used to give a diagnosis or differential diagnosis based on the detected abnormality, it is called *computer-aided diagnosis* (CADx). It has been reported that CAD be used for the detection of lung nodules; however, this area needs further validation and regulatory approval.

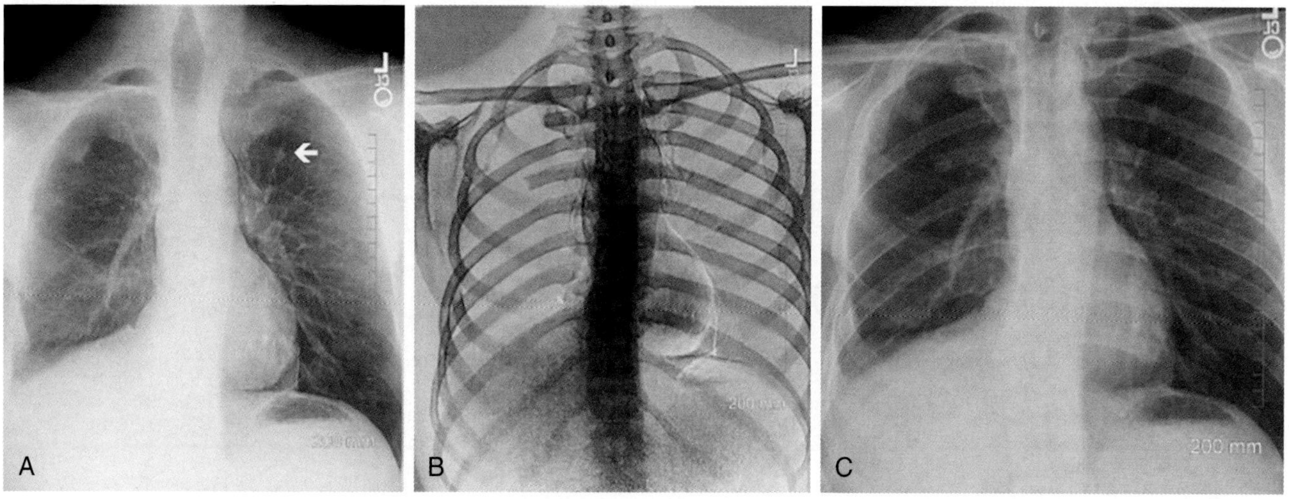

Figure 5.10 Dual-energy subtraction radiographs generating images of only soft tissues (A) and only bones (B) on this patient with a prior thoracotomy. A noncalcific nodule is only seen *(arrow in A)* in the soft tissue radiograph. (C) This nodule is difficult to differentiate from a bony lesion on a routine nonsubtracted radiograph.

Most CAD applications involve the detection of pulmonary nodules. Typically, morphology-based image processing is applied to detect nodular-appearing structures; more detailed morphologic and texture analyses can eliminate false-positive, nodule-like structures. Other potential areas of CAD and CADx use described in the literature have included assessing the malignant nature of lung nodules, differentiating interstitial lung diseases, and detecting pleural pathology such as pneumothorax, cardiac silhouette, and infectious diseases such as tuberculosis.

Bibliography

Abe K, Doi K, MacMahon H, et al. Computer-aided diagnosis in chest radiography. Preliminary experience. *Invest Radiol.* 1993;28:987–993.

Abe H, MacMahon H, Engelmann R, et al. Computer-aided diagnosis in chest radiography: results of large-scale observer tests at the 1996-2001 RSNA scientific assemblies. *Radiographics.* 2003;23:255–265.

Balassy C, Prokop M, Weber M, Sailer J, Herold CJ, Schaefer-Prokop C. Flat-panel display (LCD) versus high-resolution gray-scale display (CRT) for chest radiography: an observer preference study. *AJR Am J Roentgenol.* 2005;184: 752–756.

Bontrager KW, Lampignano JP. *Textbook of Radiographic Positioning and Related Anatomy.* 6th ed. St. Louis: Mosby; 2005:75–107.

Carlton RR, McKenna A. *Principles of Radiographic Imaging: An Art and a Science.* 5th ed. Boston: Cengage Learning; 2012.

Carmody DP, Nodine CF, Kundel HL. An analysis of perceptual and cognitive factors in radiographic interpretation. *Perception.* 1980;9:339–344.

Chotas HG, Floyd CE, Dobbins JT, Lo JY, Ravin CE. Scatter fractions in AMBER imaging. *Radiology.* 1990;177:879–880.

Dobbins JT, McAdams HP, Godfrey DJ, Li CM. Digital tomosynthesis of the chest. *J Thorac Imaging.* 2008;23:86–92.

Heelan RT, Rothenberg LN, Caravelli JF, Fleischman RC, Castellino RA. Low-density supradiaphragmatic band artifact on advanced multiple-beam equalization radiography of the chest. *Invest Radiol.* 1994;29:777–780.

Ishida T, Ashizawa K, Engelmann R, Katsuragawa S, MacMahon H, Doi K. Application of temporal subtraction for detection of interval changes on chest radiographs: improvement of subtraction images using automated initial image matching. *J Digit Imaging.* 1999;12:77–86.

Kakeda S, Nakamura K, Kamada K, et al. Improved detection of lung nodules by using a temporal subtraction technique. *Radiology.* 2002;224:145–151.

Kano A, Doi K, MacMahon H, Hassell DD, Giger ML. Digital image subtraction of temporally sequential chest images for detection of interval change. *Med Phys.* 1994;21:453–461.

Kelcz F, Zink FE, Peppler WW, Kruger DG, Ergun DL, Mistretta CA. Conventional chest radiography vs dual-energy computed radiography in the detection and characterization of pulmonary nodules. *AJR Am J Roentgenol.* 1994; 162:271–278.

Kelsey CA, Moseley RD, Mettler FA, Garcia JF, Parker TW, Briscoe DE. Comparison of nodule detection with 70-kvp and 120-kvp chest radiographs. *Radiology.* 1982;143:609–611.

Khan AN, Al-Jahdali H, Al-Ghanem S, Gouda A. Reading chest radiographs in the critically ill (part I): normal chest radiographic appearance, instrumentation and complications from instrumentation. *Ann Thorac Med.* 2009;4:75–87.

Kido S, Ikezoe J, Naito H, et al. Clinical evaluation of pulmonary nodules with single-exposure dual-energy subtraction chest radiography with an iterative noise-reduction algorithm. *Radiology.* 1995;194:407–412.

Marten K, Seyfarth T, Auer F, et al. Computer-assisted detection of pulmonary nodules: performance evaluation of an expert knowledge-based detection system in consensus reading with experienced and inexperienced chest radiologists. *Eur Radiol.* 2004;14:1930–1938.

McAdams HP, Samei E, Dobbins J, Tourassi GD, Ravin CE. Recent advances in chest radiography. *Radiology.* 2006;241:663–683.

McLean D, Gray JE, Swensen SJ, Vrieze TJ. Technical aspects of twin screen-film chest radiography: cost effective lung and mediastinal imaging. *Eur J Radiol.* 1998;27:53–60.

Monnier-Cholley L, MacMahon H, Katsuragawa S, Morishita J, Ishida T, Doi K. Computer-aided diagnosis for detection of interstitial opacities on chest radiographs. *AJR Am J Roentgenol.* 1998;171:1651–1656.

Morgan RA, Owens CM, Collins CD, Evans TW, Hansell DM. Detection of pneumothorax with lateral shoot-through digital radiography. *Clin Radiol.* 1993;48:249–252.

Oestmann JW, Greene R, Rhea JT, et al. "Single-exposure" dual energy digital radiography in the detection of pulmonary nodules and calcifications. *Invest Radiol.* 1989;24:517–521.

Oschatz E, Prokop M, Scharitzer M, Weber M, Balassy C, Schaefer-Prokop C. Comparison of liquid crystal versus cathode ray tube display for the detection of simulated chest lesions. *Eur Radiol.* 2005;15:1472–1476.

Parry RA, Glaze SA, Archer BR. The AAPM/RSNA physics tutorial for residents. Typical patient radiation doses in diagnostic radiology. *Radiographics.* 1999; 19:1289–1302.

Plewes DB, Wandtke JC. A scanning equalization system for improved chest radiography. *Radiology.* 1982;142:765–768.

Revesz G, Shea FJ, Kundel HL. The effects of kilovoltage on diagnostic accuracy in chest radiography. *Radiology.* 1982;142:615–618.

Samei E, Flynn MJ. An experimental comparison of detector performance for direct and indirect digital radiography systems. *Med Phys.* 2003;30:608–622.

Samei E, Flynn MJ, Eyler WR. Detection of subtle lung nodules: relative influence of quantum and anatomic noise on chest radiographs. *Radiology.* 1999;213: 727–734.

Shiraishi J, Abe H, Engelmann R, Aoyama M, MacMahon H, Doi K. Computer-aided diagnosis to distinguish benign from malignant solitary pulmonary nodules on radiographs: ROC analysis of radiologists' performance—initial experience. *Radiology.* 2003;227:469–474.

Trout ED, Kelley JP, Larson VL. A comparison of an air gap and a grid in roentgenography of the chest. *Am J Roentgenol Radium Ther Nucl Med.* 1975;124: 404–411.

Vlasbloem H, Kool LJ. AMBER: a scanning multiple-beam equalization system for chest radiography. *Radiology.* 1988;169:29–34.

CHAPTER 6

Pulmonary CT: The Scanner, the Protocol, and the Dose

Venkatesh Arumugam Murugan, Atul Padole, Azadeh Tabari, and Mannudeep K. Kalra

CHAPTER OUTLINE

Introduction

CT has become an indispensable part of diagnostic imaging in recent times. With the help of the money that the Beatles' records made for Electrical and Music Industries (EMI), Nobel Laureate Sir Godfrey Hounsfield invented CT in 1972, a technology that has evolved at a rapid pace since its introduction. The first CT scanner was an axial CT scanner, which took around 5 minutes for the acquisition of each image. Subsequent research in the early to mid-1970s led to the development of four generations of step-and-shoot CT scanners. The third generation of CT scanners, which used a cone-shaped x-ray beam and a rotating x-ray tube–detector assembly, has come to be the most widely used CT scanner design as of now. The major limitation of these axial CT scanners was their lack of temporal resolution and inability to generate volume images. The second phase of technologic overhaul for CT happened in 1989, with the introduction of slip ring technology, which enabled a continuous helical mode of volumetric CT data acquisition without the need for stopping the scan acquisition to uncoil the detector array or the x-ray tube. The introduction of single-detector row helical CT (SDCT) scanners virtually led to a revival of interest in CT in the 1990s.

The most recent wave of revolutionary change in CT technology started in the late 1990s with the introduction of multidetector-row CT (MDCT), which expanded the z-coverage and immensely enhanced the speed and z-resolution (ability to acquire thin-section images over the entire scan range). With multiple additions of detector rows to the MDCT, it is now possible to image long body regions in a matter of a few seconds. Modern MDCT scanners can allow up to 16-cm detector coverage in one x-ray tube rotation around the patient in under 0.4 second. Amid the rush to add rows to the detector array systems, some vendors also have added an additional x-ray tube and detector array panel, which led to the rise of dual-source MDCT technology; the impact on temporal resolution and dual-kilovoltage (kV) scanning has been revolutionary. Growth in CT technology has outpaced all other medical technologies in recent years.

With the increasing use of CT, the radiation dose from CT examinations has become a cause for concern. In 2006, there were an estimated 67 million CT examinations performed in the United States alone. Although CT contributed to only 17% of all radiologic and nuclear medicine procedures, it contributed to around 49% of the collective radiation dose. The National Council for Radiation Protection (NCRP) report 160 stated that the use of CT has increased at a rate of 8% to 15% per year, and there was an increase in effective dose per individual in the United States from 3.6 mSv in the early 1980s to 6.2 mSv in 2006, largely attributable to the increased utilization of radiation-based diagnostic imaging. The radiation doses associated with the same as well as different CT protocols vary widely. For example, the median CT dose index volume (CTDIvol) for pulmonary CT procedures in the United States ranges from 11 mGy for chest CT without intravenous contrast to 26 mGy for CT- guided lung biopsy. On the one hand, modern MDCT scanners enable the evaluation of a larger number of clinical applications at lower radiation doses, which was not possible with older CT systems but, on the other hand, spectacular imaging details and high-power x-ray tubes on modern scanners present the unique risk of overuse and misuse. This suggests the need for tailoring radiation dose protocols to individual patients and indications. In this chapter, we discuss the various options available while designing and tailoring CT protocols in terms of radiation dose.

CT Technology

Key Differences Between Multidetector-Row CT and Single-Detector Row CT Scanners for Chest Imaging

The introduction of multirow detectors has revolutionized CT imaging in many ways. The main advantages of MDCT over SDCT are as follows: (1) higher spatial resolution; (2) faster scanning; (3) ability to scan large volumes; (4) ability to generate superior three-dimensional (3D) reformations; (5) dual-kV scanning modes; and (6) radiation dose efficiency. Spatial resolution is the ability to differentiate between two adjacent points in an image and is measured in pixels. Modern MDCT scanners provide a resolution of up to 1024 × 1024 pixels in contrast to the first scanner designed by Sir Hounsfield, which generated images at a resolution of 80 × 80 pixels. MDCT scanners allow x-ray rotation times as low as 0.25 second, which, coupled with half-rotation reconstruction, enhances the temporal resolution to 0.125 second. With dual-source CT, a quarter-rotation is all that is needed from each x-ray source to generate CT images at a temporal resolution of about 0.063 second.

Acquisition of isotropic image resolution with MDCT allows for the creation of image postprocessing, such as multiplanar reformation (MPR), minimum intensity projection (MinIP), maximum intensity projection (MIP), and volume rendering techniques (VRTs), with exquisite details and without previously noted stairstep artifacts seen with SDCT scanners. These reformats are extremely useful, especially in the study of vascular and complex 3D anatomy.

MDCT also allows for more efficient use of intravenous contrast agents when compared to SDCT. These improvements mean that a chest CT can be completed in less than 1 second on state-of-the-art modern MDCT scanners versus the 15 to 30 seconds needed for SDCT. Such ultrafast scanning abilities at submillimeter resolution along the direction of scanning now allow for the routine generation of excellent 3D images in off-transverse planes. Different MDCT technologies are available to image patients simultaneously at two different levels of kV and generate virtual monoenergetic and material decomposition images while reducing some metal-related artifacts. Fortunately, heightened concerns over radiation dose have also led to significant improvements in radiation dose efficiency for MDCT as compared to SDCT. Modern MDCT scanners come equipped with several hardware and software technologies to enable radiation dose reduction while providing diagnostic image quality.

With the introduction of MDCT, each of the three basic hardware components of CT has advanced considerably. These include the x-ray tube, detector assembly, and data acquisition and processing hardware.

Demands for faster scanning over longer areas of the body with isotropic resolution have been responsible for driving the x-ray tube technology. Modern x-ray tubes now have higher power (100–120 kW) and smaller size. Some of these x-ray tubes can enable the use of 70 to 150 kV, with a maximum tube current of 1300 mA, to enable routine CT scanning at a low kV; this is closer to the k-edge of the iodine and provides better contrast enhancement, with a lower volume of required contrast media. Rapid kV switching on some scanners now allows dual-energy CT (DECT) data acquisition during the same x-ray tube rotation. The use of x-ray beam shaping filters helps carve out the shape of the x-ray beam according to patient size, enabling uniform noise distribution in the image and reducing radiation dose to the thinner peripheral portions of the patient.

Special x-ray beam filters (e.g., tin filter in dual-source CT) at the x-ray source provide better energy separation for DECT on dual-source CT scanners. Selective x-ray beam filtering for a 100-kV x-ray beam using a special tin filter allows for the delivery of a radiation dose as low as 0.1 mSv for lung nodule follow-up CT.

The photon output from an x-ray tube is a continuous spectrum. Although the low-energy photons contribute to the SDCT radiation dose to the patients, they do not contribute to projection generation. The x-ray photons in the scanning plane typically cross an ovoid path. Subsequently, the attenuation around the edges is minimal, and the attenuation is maximal at the center. This leads to an unnecessary radiation dose, as well as artifacts (e.g., beam-hardening artifacts). To minimize the absorption of low-energy photons and beam-hardening artifacts, metal filters (beam-shaping or bowtie shape) are used to shape the x-ray output from the x-ray tube. Bowtie filters are thicker at the periphery than at the center, so that the high-energy photons are filtered out from the periphery, thereby enabling homogeneous image quality as well as minimizing radiation dose. One disadvantage of using filters is that there is some loss of medium-energy photons, which might actually contribute to projection generation. Users must remember that appropriate functioning of these bowtie filters requires good patient centering. Some vendors now provide selectable filtration levels, whereby users can choose the degree of filtration as dictated by clinical needs. Bowtie filters are integral parts of most modern CT scanners.

Key Features of Current State-of-the-Art Modern Multidetector CT Scanners

CT technology has been evolving at an extremely rapid pace. Any discussion about state-of-the-art CT scanners now only holds true for an extremely short time because CT vendors are frequently introducing newer and better technologies.

At the time of this writing, the most modern dual-source CT scanner (Siemens SOMATOM Force) allows a tube current of 1300 mA, with an x-ray tube power of 120 kW for each x-ray tube. Such high milliamperage can now enable the routine use of lower kV (70–100 kV) to improve contrast resolution and reduce radiation dose and contrast volume requirements. Most contrast chest CTs can be performed at 70–80 kV on these scanners. In addition, a wider detector configuration and two sets of x-ray tubes and detector arrays enable the use of a high nonoverlapping pitch (1.6–3.4 : 1); this enables an ultrafast scanning mode in which the entire chest can be scanned in a fraction of a second.

Some other vendors have developed wide-area detectors (e.g., GE Revolution, Toshiba Aquilion One), with 256 to 320 detector rows along the scanning direction. These scanners allow 16-cm coverage in one gantry rotation. Most CT equipment now allows a gantry speed of well under 0.4 second, further shortening scan duration. Faster data acquisition systems with enhanced temporal resolution allow for near–real-time imaging (four-dimensional [4D] imaging).

To reduce radiation dose, most MDCT scanners now come equipped with x-ray beam collimation to improve radiation dose efficiency, which is the ratio of used x-rays falling on the detectors to the x-rays falling beyond the detectors. Postpatient 3D scatter grids help prevent scattered x-ray photons from reaching the detectors and thus help reduce the image noise, which also allows users to reduce the radiation dose. Furthermore, most vendors have introduced competitive iterative reconstruction (IR) techniques for low radiation dose scanning and have replaced traditionally used filtered backprojection (FBP) methods of image reconstruction.

Another vendor (Philips Healthcare) has introduced a multilayered detector to acquire spectral CT data from single-kV datasets. The advantages of such a system are manifold—improved radiation dose efficiency by eliminating the need to acquire simultaneous low- and high-energy acquisitions, ability to achieve a full field of view (FOV) (no disparity in the FOV between the tube-detector assemblies), and elimination of the cross scatter of photons from different tubes.

Modern CT technology is constantly evolving. Discussed in the next sections are a few important hardware features of modern MDCT scanners.

Better Detector Elements

No other component of CT has undergone as many changes in the past decade as the detector elements of CT equipment. With the increasing longitudinal width of detector arrays, coverage per rotation has improved tremendously, as has radiation dose efficiency. Wide-area detector MDCT (≥64 rows) has near-perfect dose efficiency, compared to older four- to eight-detector-row MDCT scanners. Modern MDCT scanners can have up to 256 to 320 detector rows, two detector array panels in a CT gantry (dual-source CT), or two layered detector assemblies (sandwich detector CT). A typical MDCT detector array, which is usually a solid state array, in contrast to the gas-filled detectors used in SDCT, consists of a scintillator, which converts incident x-ray photon flux into light. The latter is converted into an electrical potential by an adjacent layer of photo diode. The electric potential thus generated is amplified and used to generate CT projections using complex mathematical algorithms. Hence, the decay times, as well as the after-glow times of the detector elements, are major determinants of the temporal resolution of a CT scanner. The detector element most commonly used in modern MDCT scanners uses gadolinium oxide, with a ceramic material. This assembly has after-glow and decay times in the range of a few microseconds, which allow for faster acquisition of projection data and, in dual-energy scanners, rapid kV switching.

Prepatient Dose Efficiency

There are two factors that could affect CT radiation dose efficiency (see earlier). Overbeaming refers to the part of the x-ray beam that falls beyond the detector rows and cannot be used for image reconstruction. Modern MDCT scanners use real-time collimator cams to focus the x-ray beam on the detectors and reduce the extent of overbeaming.

Overranging refers to the portion of x-ray beam at the start and end locations of helical CT acquisition. Many contemporary MDCT scanners have prepatient adaptive shield collimators to reduce the extent of overranging at the start and end of a helical acquisition.

Scan Factors

Factors That Affect In-Plane Spatial Resolution in CT Imaging

The factors that affect in-plane spatial resolution in CT scanning can be classified as those acting during image acquisition and those acting during image processing. Configurations of the focal spot, detectors, scan FOV, and section thickness are a few image acquisition parameters that affect the resolution. Because CT images are generated by complex mathematical interpolation and calculation techniques, the algorithms used to generate images significantly affect image resolution. The pixel size of an image, which is determined by the scan FOV and matrix size, is given by this formula:

$$\text{Pixel size} = \text{Scan FOV}/(\text{Matrix size})$$

In general, a smaller FOV provides better spatial resolution but may not provide skin-to-skin coverage in larger patients. Thus routine chest CT may be limited to FOV spanning from skin to skin as much as possible. However, for specific protocols, such as workup of the aorta or diffuse lung disease, spatial resolution of images should be enhanced with the use of a smaller FOV. For example, rib-to-rib coverage with a smaller FOV is sufficient for a diffuse lung disease protocol and helps improve the in-plane spatial resolution.

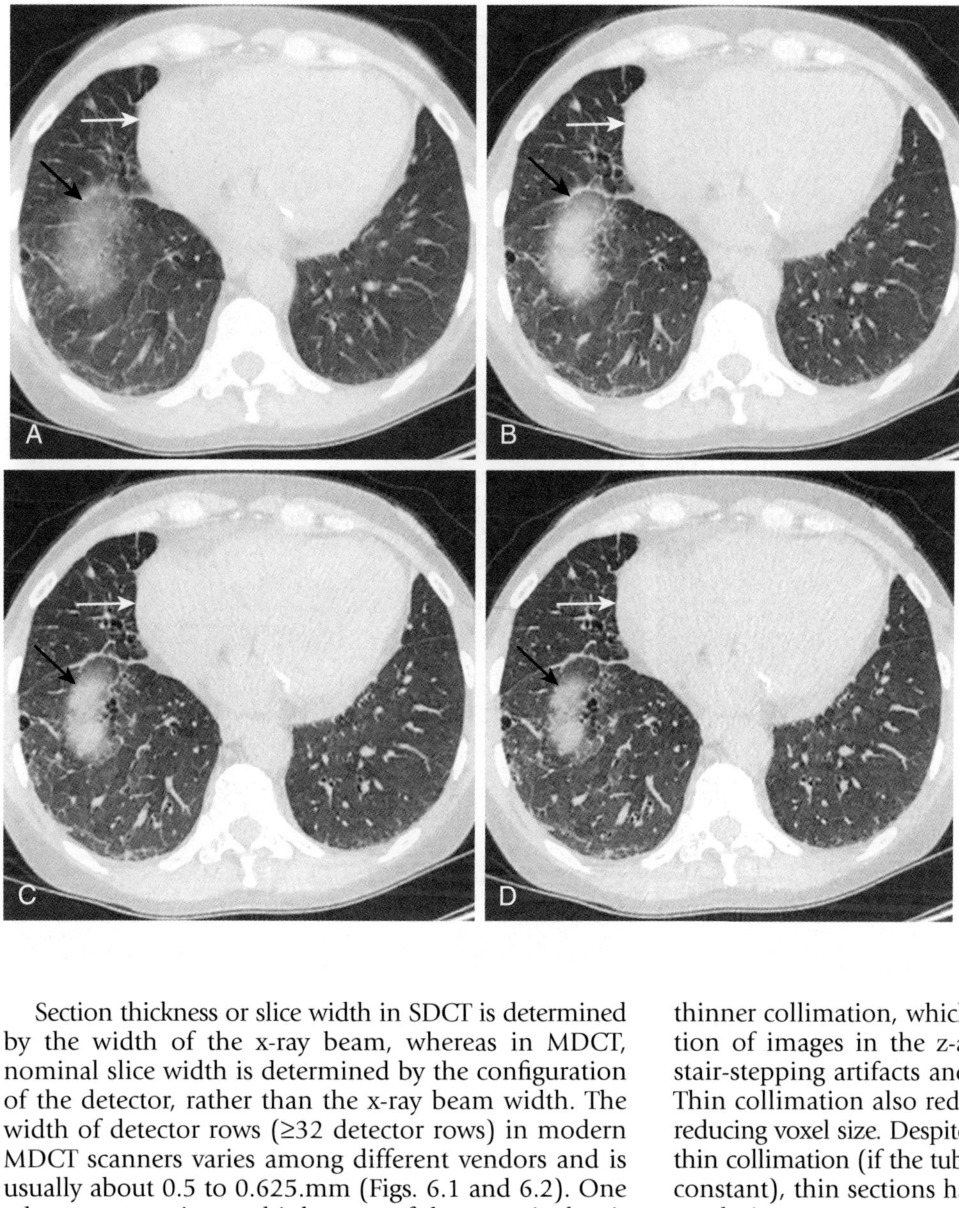

Figure 6.1 Reduced dose chest CT scan of a 61-year-old female patient (64 kg) on a 64-row multidetector CT scanner reconstructed with a slice thickness of 5 mm (A), 2.5 mm (B), 1.3 mm (C), and 0.6 mm (D; 120 kV; fixed mAs; CTDIvol, 2 mGy; dose length product, 68 mGy-cm). Transverse CT images demonstrate a right middle lobe peripheral nodule *(black arrows)* and bronchiectasis *(white arrows)*. The lung lesions and structures are better visualized and easier to find on thinner slices (0.6 mm, D) due to less partial volume average.

Section thickness or slice width in SDCT is determined by the width of the x-ray beam, whereas in MDCT, nominal slice width is determined by the configuration of the detector, rather than the x-ray beam width. The width of detector rows (≥32 detector rows) in modern MDCT scanners varies among different vendors and is usually about 0.5 to 0.625.mm (Figs. 6.1 and 6.2). One advantage to using multiple rows of detectors is that it allows the user to choose the nominal slice width. For example, let us assume that an MDCT scanner has an effective detector row width of 0.625 mm and a total of 40 detector rows. These rows could be adapted to attain a nominal slice width of 0.625, 1.25, 3.75, or 5 mm, depending on user preference and clinical indications. An important caveat to this is in the older generation of MDCT scanners (≤16 years), where variable thickness detector rows necessitate a priori specification of the required slice width. For example, on a 16-MDCT scanner, if a detector configuration of 16 × 1.25 mm is chosen for scanning, only 1.25-mm and wider slices can be generated, and 0.625-mm sections cannot be generated (will require use of a 16 × 0.625 mm configuration). For diffuse lung disease, it is desirable to obtain a section thickness of 1 mm or less, whereas most other chest indications can be imaged at a 1.25-mm slice width or more. Attaining isotropic resolution was a challenge in SDCT scanners. However, the detector configuration in modern MDCT scanners allows for thinner collimation, which in turn enhances the resolution of images in the z-axis. This has led to reduced stair-stepping artifacts and enhanced image resolution. Thin collimation also reduces partial volume effects by reducing voxel size. Despite increases in image noise with thin collimation (if the tube current–time product is held constant), thin sections have better contrast and spatial resolution.

Factors Affecting Scan Time

Wider x-ray beam or detector configuration is typically more dose-efficient compared to smaller detector configuration for covering longer scan volumes, such as the entire chest. If all scanning parameters are held constant, then wider detector configuration will enable quicker scanning across patient length. Thus, a 64- × 0.625-mm detector configuration will enable faster scanning as compared to 32 × 0.625 mm. For regions such as the thorax, where motion artifacts are not uncommon and can negatively affect assessment of the findings, a faster scanning mode is advantageous.

In addition to the detector configuration, beam pitch (ratio of table feed per rotation to the detector configuration) also affects the scan time. A higher nonoverlapping pitch ratio (>1 : 1) allows faster scanning as compared to smaller, overlapping pitch values (<1 : 1) if all other

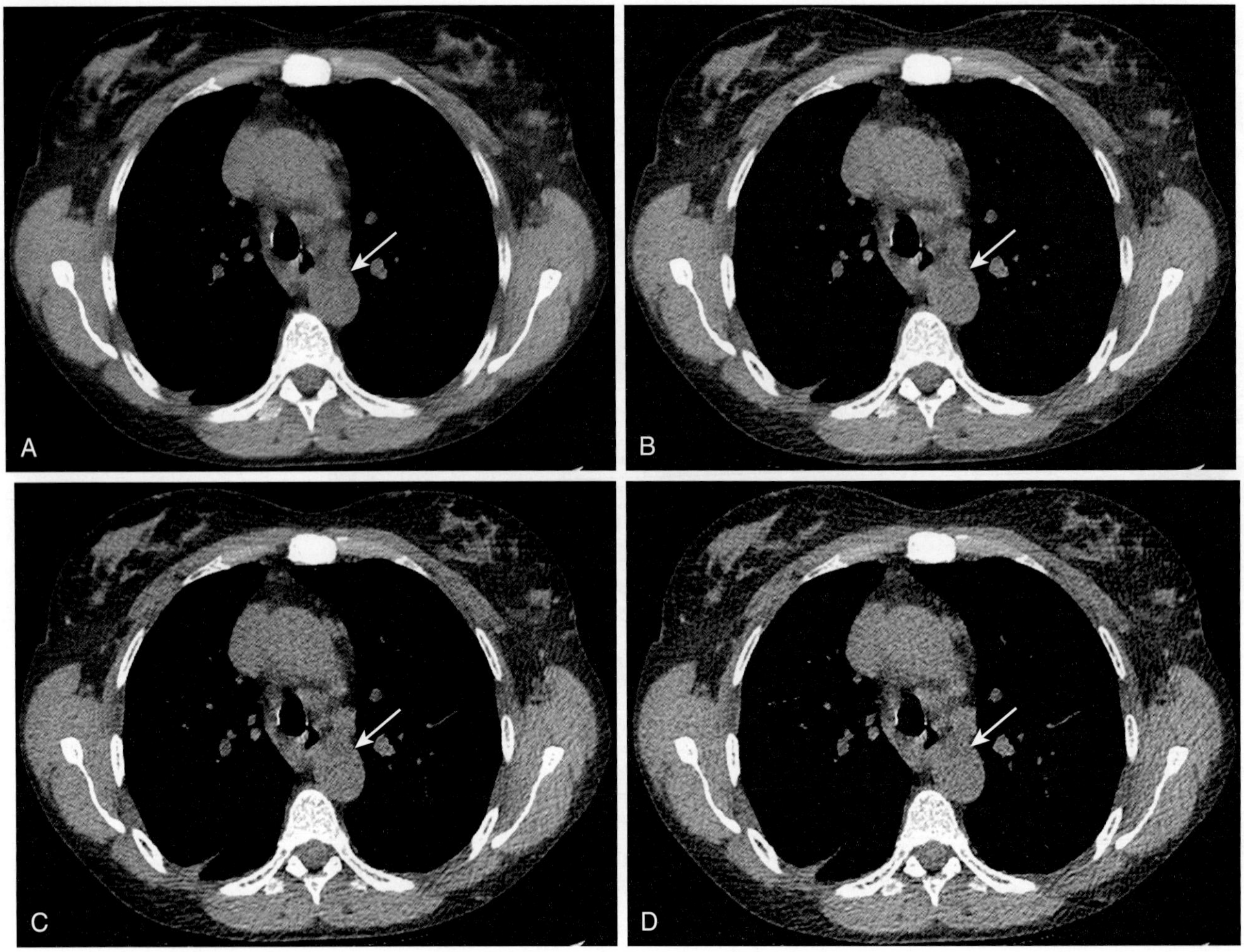

Figure 6.2 Reduced dose chest CT in a 61-year-old female patient (64 kg) on a 64-row multidetector CT scanner reconstructed with slice thickness of 5 mm (A), 2.5 mm (B), 1.3 mm (C), and 0.6 mm (D; 120 kV; fixed mAs; CTDIvol, 2 mGy; dose length product, 68 mGy-cm). Transverse CT images demonstrate a lymph node *(arrows)*. In the mediastinum, highest image noise is seen with thinner slices (0.6 mm, D).

scan parameters such as detector configuration and rotation time are kept constant. For most chest CT examinations, it is preferable to use a pitch ratio of 1 : 1 or higher to enable quicker scanning. On some scanners, use of a lower pitch is associated with a higher radiation dose, whereas on others there is no dose penalty with a change in pitch value. Another caveat is that on some MDCT scanners, the effective slice width is wider than the selected slice width at pitch values greater than 1 : 1. This should be considered specifically when developing a protocol for diffuse lung disease evaluation on these scanners. On some dual-source CT scanners, a very high nonoverlapping pitch ratio (>1.5 : 1) can enable scanning of the entire chest in about 0.5 second. In patients who are unable to hold their breath, such fast scanning mode can be used without breath-holding.

The scan time is also affected by the gantry rotation times. Most modern MDCT scanners allow at least a 0.5-second rotation time. For most chest CT examinations, a shorter scan time is preferred. For very large patients (weight ≥125 kg) on CT scanners with limited mA (especially on some scanners, with ≤16 detector rows), a slower gantry speed (>0.5 second) may be needed to obtain acceptable image quality. CT scanners (generally with ≥16 detector rows) with sufficiently higher tube current abilities usually will not require a slower gantry speed, even in larger patients undergoing chest CT. Some scanners (e.g., Siemens Definition Force) allow half-segment reconstruction at a gantry rotation time of 0.25 second to scan patients who cannot hold their breath.

In summary, pulmonary CT examinations on modern MDCT scanners should be performed in a single breath-hold, with the shortest scan duration, to minimize motion artifacts.

Dual-Energy CT

Introduction

Different tissues may have similar x-ray attenuation characteristics at certain x-ray photon energies. X-ray photons interact with tissues in two different ways: Compton scattering and a photoelectric effect. Intravenous contrast agents are best seen with a photoelectric effect.

Photoelectric effect refers to displacement of electrons from the innermost shell of an atom on interaction with x-ray photons of sufficient energy. The displaced electrons are then replaced by electrons from the outer shells, resulting in the production of characteristic radiation. Each element has a particular value of energy (k-edge), which an incident photon must possess to displace the innermost shell electrons. This value (k-edge) depends on the atomic number of the element. X-ray photons interacting with an atom are attenuated maximally if their energy is similar to the k-edge of the atom. X-ray photons produced at 80 kV have energy values close to the k-edge of iodine. Hence, attenuation of photons with iodinated contrast is maximal at 80 kV, which is the lowest allowed value on most CT scanners. However, such a low kV is practical in relatively few patients, given the limitations of maximal tube current constraints in most MDCT scanners. Although low kV imaging may be acceptable in relatively small patients, in larger patients such low-kV scanning will be associated with higher image noise and potential artifacts. These latter constrains often require an increase in tube current, with decreased kV, which may not be feasible or practical with most MDCT scanners.

The use of a dual-energy or dual-kV scanning mode enables near-simultaneous acquisition of a lower and higher kV datasets, which combine high-contrast, high-noise, low-kV information with lower noise and lower artifact information from high-kV scanning. In addition, DECT helps identify subtle differences in attenuation characteristics of tissues at different energy levels of photons. Although the term *dual-energy CT* indicates that x-rays of only two energy levels are used, in reality the output of x-ray photons from an x-ray tube is a continuous polychromatic spectrum. The tube voltage represents the maximum energy of the photons (kVp = peak voltage), but the mean energy of the photons in the spectrum is usually significantly lower than the peak energy. Subsequently, when two different values of tube voltage are used, the resulting photons have a significant overlap in their spectrum. Most scanners use tube voltages of 80 and 140 kV, although some newer scanners allow the use of 80/90/100 kV with 150 kV. Tin filters of varying thickness have been used to filter out low-energy x-ray output from the higher tube voltage spectrum to reduce the spectral overlap and enhance image contrast. There are a few ways in which DECT data can be acquired; the most commonly used methods are listed in Table 6.1.

TABLE 6.1 Commonly Used Methods for Acquiring Dual-Energy CT Images

TECHNIQUE	VENDOR
Rapid switching of tube voltage	GE Healthcare
Dual-source CT	Siemens Healthcare
Sequential acquisition	Toshiba Healthcare
Layer detector (sandwich detectors)	Philips Healthcare
Quantum counting detector	Work in progress with multiple vendors

Role of CT in Pulmonary Imaging

Studies have demonstrated the use of DECT for the delineation of several thoracic abnormalities. Usually, DECT is used for imaging patients with a known or suspected pulmonary embolism. Other reported applications of DECT of the thorax include pulmonary hypertension, pulmonary nodule characterization, and emphysema quantification. Initial studies with small sample sizes have shown promising results for differentiating benign and malignant mediastinal neoplasms with DECT, particularly with delayed contrast washout on DECT in malignant lesions as compared to benign lesions. However, these applications of DECT need further validation with larger sample sizes. Although the characterization of pulmonary nodules with dual energy was extensively evaluated in the 1990s using two separate acquisitions at different kV settings, the practice fell out of favor following statements from the Fleischner Society about the lack of accuracy. With the development of simultaneous DECT capabilities, interest in nodule characterization has been rekindled. A recent study has shown that DECT at 180 seconds following the administration of a contrast agent can help differentiate benign from malignant nodules with 90% accuracy. Another study has recently reported the ability of DECT to assess an early response to antiangiogenesis treatment in patients with lung cancer. These studies point to a potential future role for DECT in tissue characterization. Fig. 6.3 shows DECT images acquired using a CT pulmonary angiography (CTPA) protocol for the detection of pulmonary embolism.

Scan Protocols

Key Scan Parameters of CT Protocols

The key parameters while designing CT imaging protocols are tube current, tube voltage, pitch, detector collimation, scan region, gantry rotation speed, gantry tilt (if necessary), contrast considerations (e.g., type, mode of delivery, volume, rate, timing, saline flush volume and rate, site of injection), reconstruction algorithm (FBP vs. IR), reconstructed slice specification (width and reconstruction intervals), and reformats (e.g., type of reformats, slice thickness and intervals).

Stratifying Chest CT Protocols

Indications for chest CT must be the basis for stratifying chest protocols. Indication-based CT protocols ensure that reconstruction settings, image quality, and radiation dose are appropriate for desired radiologic information. Table 6.2 gives a lists of commonly used pulmonary CT protocols and their clinical indications. Figs. 6.4 to 6.6 are examples of images obtained by commonly used CT scanning protocols.

Contrast Considerations When Designing Chest CT Protocols

The factors that affect contrast medium enhancement in CT imaging can be divided into two main categories: patient factors and contrast factors.

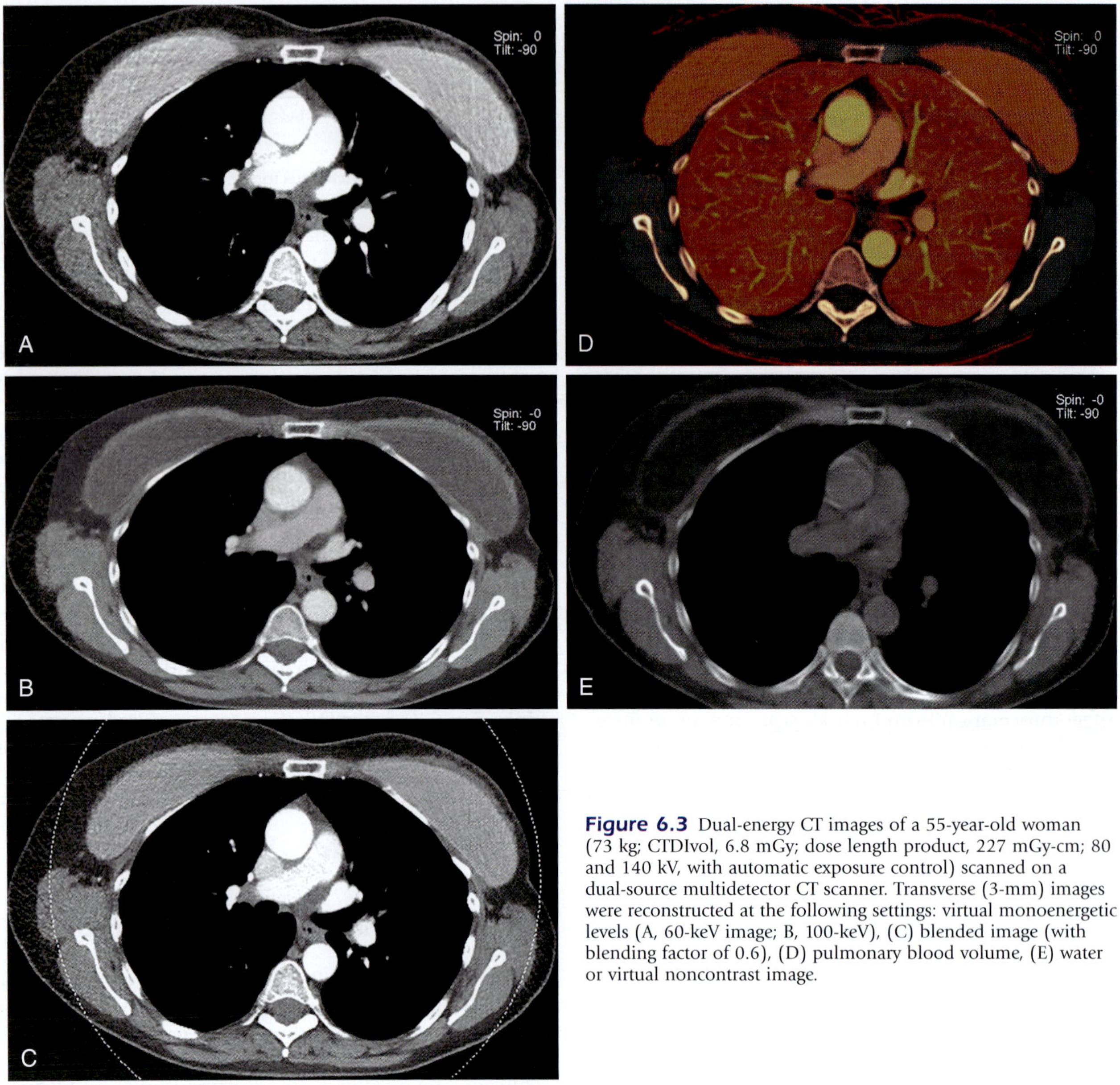

Figure 6.3 Dual-energy CT images of a 55-year-old woman (73 kg; CTDIvol, 6.8 mGy; dose length product, 227 mGy-cm; 80 and 140 kV, with automatic exposure control) scanned on a dual-source multidetector CT scanner. Transverse (3-mm) images were reconstructed at the following settings: virtual monoenergetic levels (A, 60-keV image; B, 100-keV), (C) blended image (with blending factor of 0.6), (D) pulmonary blood volume, (E) water or virtual noncontrast image.

PATIENT FACTORS

WEIGHT. Because larger patients have relatively large blood volumes, injected intravenous contrast agents tend to become more diluted. Subsequently larger volumes of contrast agent are required to achieve the same degree of contrast enhancement when compared to smaller patients. At a constant contrast volume and rate of delivery, the magnitude of contrast enhancement is inversely related to the weight of the patient.

Obese patients, however, have a larger percentage of body fat and a relatively smaller blood volume. In these patients, the use of body weight for calculating intravenous contrast volume may lead to an overestimation. Several studies have reported the use of body surface area and lean body mass as more accurate metrics to calculate the contrast agent requirement in patients. Although body weight plays an important role in determining the degree of contrast enhancement, it does not affect the timing of enhancement. This is because timing of contrast enhancement is largely dependent on the cardiac output and blood volume of the patient, and both tend to increase with increasing patient size.

Typically, contrast-enhanced CT can be performed at a much lower volume compared to abdominal CT. Another important determinant of contrast administration is the clinical indication for scanning—generally, most contrast-enhanced chest CT can be performed with 50 to 80 mL of contrast agent with a concentration of 300 to 370 mg%.

In patients with compromised renal function, some advanced CT scanners can allow low-kV or dual-energy scanning with a requirement of 20 to 30 mL of contrast, even for pulmonary embolism evaluation.

CARDIAC OUTPUT. Cardiac output is the most important patient factor that affects the timing and duration of contrast enhancement. In low cardiac output states, contrast material arrives slowly and clears slowly, resulting in delayed and prolonged peak contrast enhancement. Two approaches to individualize the scan delay are test bolus method and bolus tracking; bolus tracking is more widely used.

TABLE 6.2 Commonly Used Pulmonary CT Protocols and Their Indications

PROTOCOL	INDICATIONS
Routine chest	Pneumonia, diagnosis, and staging of suspected lung cancer, evaluation of mediastinal pathology, pulmonary nodule detection and characterization, pyrexia of unknown origin, pleural effusion, empyema, malignancy, air space disease
Pulmonary nodule follow-up	Follow-up of incidental pulmonary nodules
Pulmonary angiography	Pulmonary embolism and vascular malformation
Diffuse lung disease	Evaluation of unexplained chronic dyspnea, idiopathic interstitial pneumonia
Lung cancer screening	Screening for lung cancer in high-risk populations
Lung cancer follow-up	Long-term follow-up of lung cancer (see Fig. 6.13)
Tracheal	Tracheal stenosis, bronchial stenosis, tracheomalacia, tracheobronchomalacia, tracheoesophageal fistula, suspected tracheal or bronchial injury
Thoracic chest wall	Chest wall trauma, deformity, malignancy

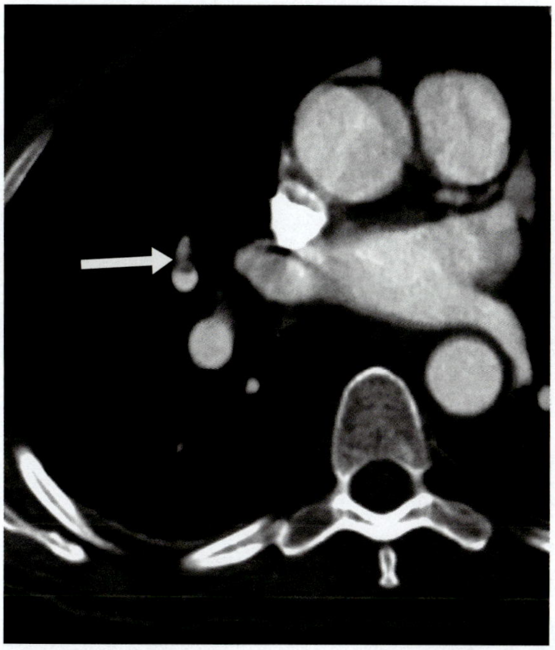

Figure 6.4 CT pulmonary angiography in a 69-year-old female patient (52 kg; 80 kV, with automatic exposure control; CTDIvol, 3.2 mGy; dose length product, 106 mGy-cm) was performed on a 128-row multidetector CT scanner. The transverse CT image depicts a pulmonary embolus in the right middle lobe pulmonary artery *(arrow)*.

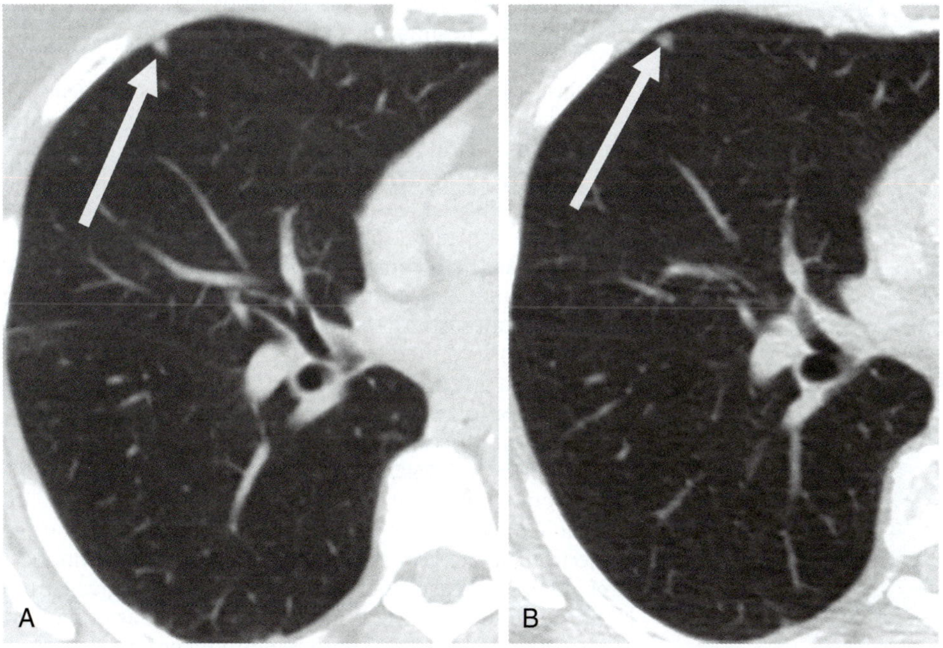

Figure 6.5 (A) Routine chest protocol images of a 66-year-old female patient. The initial routine chest CT image acquired (71 kg; 120 kV, with automatic exposure control; CTDIvol, 9 mGy; dose length product [DLP], 354 mGy-cm) on a 64-row multidetector CT scanner demonstrated a 3-mm nodule in the right middle lobe *(arrow)*. (B) Follow-up chest CT for evaluation of the lung nodule was performed at a low radiation dose (120 kV; 60 mAs; CTDIvol, 3.8 mGy; DLP, 140 mGy-cm). The right middle lobe nodule is seen equally well on a low–radiation dose CT scan.

AGE AND GENDER. Females tend to have lower blood volumes than males, which may account for the quicker peak contrast enhancement and higher magnitude of contrast enhancement in female patients. Because cardiac output is generally reduced in older people, the time to peak contrast enhancement is delayed.

SITE OF INJECTION. The antecubital veins are the most common sites for the injection of intravenous contrast agents. However, because of their small caliber, they are not suited for injection of contrast agents with a high iodine concentration or at faster rates. Studies have demonstrated that the use of central veins for injection of intravenous contrast agents is associated with distinct advantages, such as more predictable and early contrast enhancement. Forearm veins have also been used occasionally for injection of intravenous contrast agents.

HEPATIC AND RENAL DISORDERS. Hepatic cirrhosis may result in delayed and reduced contrast enhancement in the portal phase of hepatic imaging, while the arterial phase remains largely unaffected. This is because the

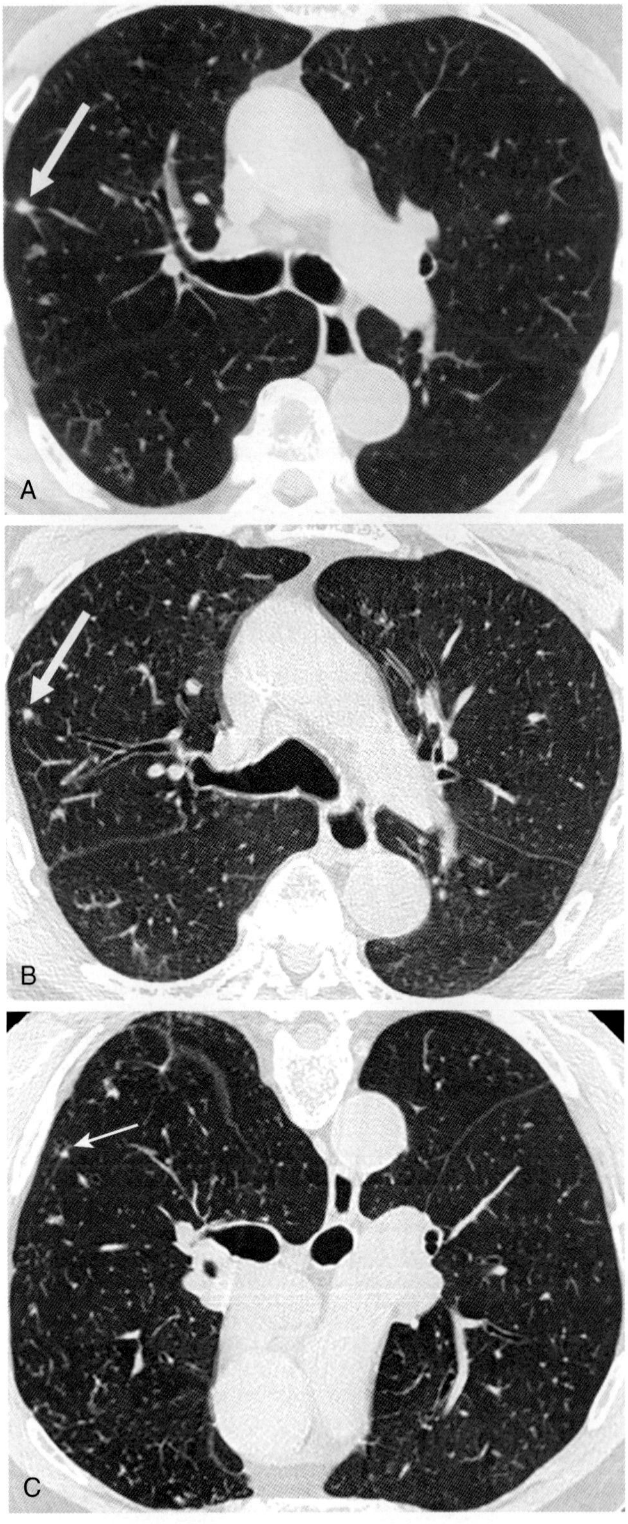

Figure 6.6 Diffuse lung disease protocol CT in an 80-year-old male patient (79 kg) on a 64-row multidetector CT scanner demonstrated no evidence of interstitial lung disease. There is a 4-mm noncalcified nodule in the right upper lobe on the inspiratory and expiratory images *(arrows)*. (A) Inspiratory images (120 kV, automatic exposure control; CTDIvol, 15 mGy; dose length product [DLP], 567 mGy-cm) were acquired in volumetric mode with helical mode. (B) Expiratory images (120 kV; 200 mAs; CTDIvol, 2.3 mGy; DLP, 66 mGy-cm) were acquired with a sequential scanning mode at 10-mm intervals. (C) Prone images (120 kV; 200 mAs; CTDIvol, 2.3 mGy; DLP, 61 mGy-cm) were acquired with a sequential scanning mode at 10-mm intervals.

liver is fibrotic and less vascular in cirrhosis. Iodinated contrast agents carry a risk of causing contrast-induced nephropathy. Although there is no safe threshold for the use of iodine in intravenous contrast agents, the Contrast-Induced Nephropathy Consensus Working Panel has recommended that a contrast material volume less than 100 mL is preferable in patients with an estimated glomerular filtration rate less than 60 mL/min per 1.73 m^2.

CONTRAST FACTORS

INJECTION DURATION. Injection duration is the duration of time from the start of the injection to the end of the injection. The selection of an appropriate injection duration is influenced by the clinical indications, as well as the scanning conditions. The main clinical factors that affect the injection duration include body size, the vessel or organ of interest, and the desired level of enhancement. At a constant contrast volume, longer injection durations are associated with delayed peak enhancement, and shorter injection durations are associated with a correspondingly reduced time for peak enhancement. In patients with normal cardiac output, peak contrast enhancement occurs shortly after termination of the injection. Hence, it is very important to design scan delays based on the injection duration. Injection duration thus plays a very important role in determining the scan delay. For example, a scan with a long injection duration is associated with delayed peak contrast enhancement, and hence the associated scan delay is also increased. Although shorter durations and rapid injection rates may be desirable for arterial enhancement, they are relatively less important for the venous and parenchymal enhancement phases. For vascular studies such as CT angiography, injection duration should be at least equal to or slightly longer than the scan duration.

INJECTION RATE. The magnitude of peak arterial enhancement increases with an increase in injection rate if the contrast concentration, volume, and injection duration are held constant. The magnitude of peak aortic enhancement has a linear relationship with increasing injection rates up to 10 mL/s. Generally, faster injection rates are more suited for shorter scan durations, and vice versa. For a given volume of contrast agent, increasing the rate of injection increases the magnitude of peak enhancement and reduces the duration of peak enhancement.

CONTRAST CONCENTRATION. The concentrations of intravenous contrast agents available commercially are variable. When the volume, injection duration, and rate of injection are held constant, a higher contrast concentration results in increased delivery of contrast at a given time and hence in increased magnitude, as well as enhanced temporal separation of contrast enhancement. The time to peak enhancement is unchanged, however, because the rate and duration of injection remain the same.

SALINE FLUSH. A saline flush of about 15 to 20 mL is routinely used after injection of intravenous contrast agents. The rationale behind the use of a saline flush is that after administration of an intravenous contrast agent, a small amount of contrast remains unused as it settles in the tubing and peripheral veins. The other advantages of using a saline flush is that it enhances bolus geometry by reducing dispersion, reduces streak artifacts caused by dense contrast material in the superior vena cava (SVC) and brachiocephalic vein, and reduces contrast requirement (variably reported in different studies), which may be helpful for patients in whom large contrast volumes are contraindicated. The volume of saline flush needed depends on the volume of the tubing and of the peripheral veins, the so-called dead space.

SCAN DIRECTION AND DURATION. Scan direction and duration play a major role in determining injection duration, rate, and volume. With modern MDCT scanners, most chest CT scans are completed in less than 5 to 10 seconds. In CTPA, the scanning proceeds in the caudocranial direction. This is because most of the pulmonary emboli tend to be in the lower lobes of the lungs, and the respiratory excursion in the lower lobes is more marked compared to that in the upper lobes. Another advantage to caudocranial scanning in CTPA is that it avoids the streak artifacts caused by dense contrast material in the SVC and right atrium.

Determination of contrast material arrival time is very important to determine scan start times. Two methods have been used. In the test bolus method, a small volume of contrast material is injected at the same rate as the contrast bolus to determine the duration to peak enhancement in a region of interest placed over an anatomic structure (usually the aorta). This time to peak enhancement is used to calculate the scan delay for the actual bolus. In the bolus tracking method, sequential low-dose acquisitions in a region of interest are carried out and, once the peak enhancement is reached, a trigger is set off, and the scanning starts after a predetermined delay (posttrigger delay).

Radiation Dose

Radiation Safety With CT

The first step toward ensuring radiation safety is appropriate justification of diagnostic procedures. This would prevent unnecessary radiation exposure. CT imaging has been widely used in thoracic imaging. Box 6.1 summarizes the most common clinical indications for pulmonary CT imaging.

BOX 6.1 Common Clinical Indications for Pulmonary CT Imaging

- Abnormal chest radiograph
- Cancer staging
- Pulmonary nodule detection and follow-up
- Interstitial lung disease
- Diffuse lung disease
- Large and small airway disease
- Myasthenia gravis (thymus)
- Hemoptysis evaluation
- Pulmonary vascular lesions (e.g., pulmonary embolism, arteriovenous malformations)
- Unknown source of infection in an immunocompromised host
- Mediastinal lesions (e.g., mass, widening)
- Pleural lesions (e.g., effusion, calcification)
- Chest wall lesions (e.g., tumors, trauma, deformities)
- Lung cancer screening

Parameters That Affect Radiation Dose in Chest CT

Scanning parameters that affect CT radiation doses are summarized in Table 6.3.

Setting the Tube Current

Tube current is perhaps the most important scan parameter from both the image quality and radiation dose perspectives. Most chest CT must be performed with automatic exposure control (AEC) techniques. In general, the image quality depends on the applied radiation dose, regional dimension, and tissue attenuation. The body dimension and tissue attenuation provide an estimate of patient size to be used with AEC techniques. If the radiation dose is held constant, a chest with low-attenuation organs will have better image quality compared to the abdomen and pelvis, which have higher attenuation organs. Thus chest CT can be performed at a much lower dose compared to abdominal CT. AEC technology estimates regional body attenuation from the planning x-ray and adapts the tube current according to varying body attenuation. Thus for chest CT, a higher tube current will be selected for the shoulder (higher attenuation due to bones) as compared to the other regions of the chest (lower attenuation due to lungs; Figs. 6.7 and 6.8).

There are three types of AEC techniques. The angular modulation technique adapts the tube current according to the geometric cross-sectional asymmetry of the body. If the radiation dose is kept constant, the image quality varies according to the length (thickness) of the body part through which the x-rays travel. Thus thinner portions of the cross sections (anteroposterior or posteroanterior) are scanned at a lower tube current as compared to thicker portions (lateral) of the body, with angular modulation.

The longitudinal AEC technique tailors the tube current along the patient's length from one section (portion) to the next. This technique enables automatic modulation of the tube current based on changes in tissue attenuation along the patient's length, as described above. The combined modulation techniques both angular and longitudinal AEC techniques.

Most AEC techniques require users to specify an image quality metric (e.g., noise index [GE Healthcare], quality mAs [Siemens Healthcare], standard deviation [Toshiba], mA and slice [Philips Healthcare]). All AEC techniques automatically adapt tube current according to patient size (tissue attenuation and regional dimension). Thus AEC techniques will apply a lower tube current and radiation dose for smaller patients and a higher tube current and radiation dose for larger patients, if all other parameters are held constant. Image quality requirements can be set for AEC techniques for patients of different sizes; however, there are considerable variations for patients at extreme ends of the body habitus.

TABLE 6.3 Scanning Parameters That Affect the CT Radiation Dose

SCAN PARAMETER	EFFECT ON RADIATION DOSE
Tube current (mA)	Linear, direct relationship; 50% reduction in tube current = 50% reduction in radiation dose; most commonly used parameter for managing radiation dose; lower mA = lower radiation dose = higher image noise (and no change in image contrast; see Figs. 6.7 and 6.8)
Tube potential (kV)	Directly related to radiation dose; change in radiation dose = (change in kV)^2; lower kV = lower radiation = higher image noise = higher image contrast (especially for contrast enhanced CT)
Pitch	Pitch is defined as the ratio of the nominal beam width to the tube feed per gantry rotation. For some CT vendors, radiation dose is independent of pitch because mA changes with pitch automatically to maintain a constant dose. For other CT vendors, higher pitch implies lower dose, and vice versa. Pitch values >1 : 1 are generally preferred for chest CT to ensure faster coverage and less motion artifacts.
Detector collimation	Refers to the combination of detector element width and number of detector rows along the patient length; wider detector configuration = faster scanning if all other parameters are constant; for most (≥64-slice MDCT), wider detector collimation is preferable
Gantry rotation time (seconds)	If all scan parameters are constant, faster rotation time = faster scan time = less motion artifacts = lower radiation dose; <0.5-second rotation time preferred in chest CT
Scan length	Longer scan length = more body region irradiated = higher dose. For lung nodule follow-up, lung cancer screening, and pulmonary embolism CT, cover up to lung bases only. For cancer staging and other indications, coverage generally extends up to the adrenals.
Scan overlap	Greater scan overlap = greater radiation dose; when scanning multiple body regions, limit the extent of overlapping in different scan series.
Scan phases	Most chest CT should be noncontrast or postcontrast only. For multiphase chest CT: radiation dose for expiratory and/or prone images should be substantially lower than the inspiratory images.
Number of CT examinations	Follow-up chest CT must be performed according to established guidelines. Unnecessary follow-up chest CT should be avoided.
Breathing instruction and contrast injection	Inappropriate breath-hold and contrast injection may result in repeat CT image acquisition and thus increase the radiation dose.
Arm positioning	When possible, arms must be kept overhead to avoid artifacts and an increase in radiation dose with automatic exposure control techniques.
Reconstruction settings	These do not have any direct effect on radiation. However, based on reconstruction parameters, image quality can vary substantially. Higher kernels give better image sharpness and can allow dose reduction.

In general, chest CT can be performed with at least a 30% to 50% lower dose as compared to routine abdominal CT. The image quality metric for chest CT must therefore be lower than for routine abdominal CT. Similarly, lung nodule follow-up and lung cancer screening CT can be performed at a fraction of the image quality and radiation dose requirement compared to routine chest CT protocol.

In addition to patient size and clinical indication, AEC techniques should also be adjusted to obtain the desired radiation dose reduction for IR techniques. A good starting point for a new application of IR techniques can involve about a 25% to 30% reduction in radiation dose compared to FBP. This reduction in radiation dose can be achieved with a suitable modification in AEC techniques or tube voltage reduction. Iterative reconstruction techniques (such as adaptive statistical iterative reconstruction [GE healthcare]) can reduce radiation dose by up to 65%.

When setting image quality requirements for AEC techniques, it is important to keep target or desired CTDIvol in mind. For example, most lung nodule follow-up CTs can be performed with a CTDIvol of 1 to 3 mGy. The target CTDIvol can then help users set a correct image quality requirement from AEC techniques.

Selecting the Best Tube Voltage

The importance of appropriate kV selection cannot be overemphasized for chest CT, particularly with the availability of x-ray tubes with higher power (ability to go up to high values of tube current at low kV) and IR techniques. Tube potential has a profound effect on radiation dose, as well as image contrast, particularly for contrast-enhanced chest CT. For contrast-enhanced chest CT, including CTPA, a lower tube potential (<120 kV) should be applied in most average or smaller patients to reduce radiation dose and enhance image contrast. Most chest CT can be performed at 80 to 100 kV, except in morbidly obese patients. In the latter, 120 kV may be required for chest CT. Use of a lower tube potential for CTPA can not only enable better contrast, but also aid in the diagnosis of smaller, subsegmental pulmonary emboli.

For noncontrast-enhanced chest CT, with the availability of IR techniques, it should be possible to use 80 to 100 kV to reduce radiation dose. A recently introduced CT scanner (Definition Force, Siemens Healthcare) enables 100-kV acquisition with a tin filter to reduce the radiation dose to well under 1 mSv, in combination with an IR technique.

A few CT scanners allow automatic kV selection technique. These automatic kV selection techniques enable users to specify the examination type (e.g., noncontrast CT, postcontrast CT, CTPA). It then selects the most appropriate kV to maintain a constant contrast-to-noise ratio at a similar or lower radiation dose. Users can control the range of kV adjustments for different indications and body regions. These techniques work synchronously with

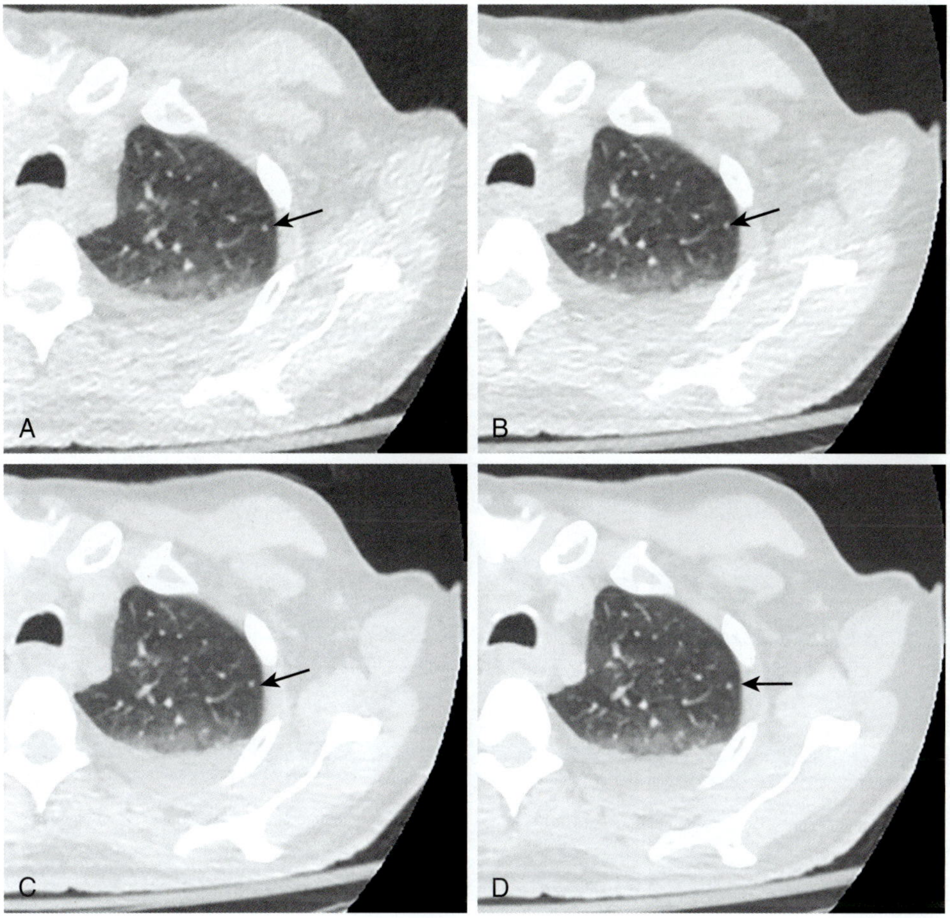

Figure 6.7 Transverse postmortem chest CT images of a 67-year-old male cadaver (79 kg) acquired on a 64-row multidetector CT scanner (GE Discovery CT750 HD) at four different dose levels at 120 kV with automatic exposure control and reconstructed with adaptive statistical iterative reconstruction 50%. (A) 36 mA, CTDIvol, 1.4 mGy; dose length product (DLP), 62 mGy-cm. (B) 68 mA, CTDIvol, 2.6 mGy, DLP, 114 mGy-cm. (C) 207 mA, CTDIvol, 6 mGy, DLP, 267 mGy-cm. (D) 351 mA, CTDIvol, 14 mGy, DLP, 606 mGy-cm. The left upper lobe lung nodule *(black arrows)* is seen well at all four dose levels.

AEC techniques to adjust the tube current automatically with changes in kV.

An additional benefit of kV reduction includes the potential for reducing the amount of contrast medium required for a chest CT examination. In general, the required contrast volume can be reduced by 25% to 50% at a lower kV as compared to higher kV scanning.

Role of Iterative Reconstruction in Chest CT

IR algorithms are replacing conventional FBP algorithms in modern MDCT scanners. In IR, the measured projection raw data are compared with the estimated raw dataset in sequential steps leading to the generation of CT images. The first CT scanner, developed by Sir Hounsfield, used IR techniques for image reconstruction. However, the progressively increasing matrix configurations in modern CT scanners demand faster computational abilities. Hence, FBP techniques gained prominence because they were relatively less demanding in terms of computational ability. The recent development of faster data processors has revived interest in IR techniques. Most major CT vendors now offer IR algorithms; IR techniques have been demonstrated to reduce radiation dose and improve image quality for varied clinical indications and age groups.

In simpler terms, IR techniques reduce image noise and artifacts in CT examinations performed at a lower radiation dose compared to FBP techniques. Thus users need to reduce the radiation dose appropriately for deriving the desired benefit of IR techniques. Most IR techniques take almost the same time for reconstruction as conventional FBP techniques. A notable exception is model-based iterative reconstruction (MBIR; GE Healthcare), which can take 30 to 60 minutes to reconstruct single-image series. The radiation dose can be reduced by adjusting the tube current or tube potential, as described earlier. Depending on the extent of radiation dose reduction, patient size, and radiologist preference, different strengths of IR techniques can be applied. In general, higher strengths of IR have lesser noise but can have a distinctive image appearance, which may not be acceptable to all interpreting physicians.

When applying IR techniques for the first time, it is prudent to target about a 25% to 30% reduction in radiation dose at lower IR strengths. With experience and confidence, the radiologist can step up the strength of IR and further reduce radiation dose to a desired level. In addition to reducing image noise in LDCT, the IR techniques can help in increased usage of lower kV to improve image contrast while reducing radiation dose. Figs. 6.9 to 6.13 show the effect of IR techniques on image quality and radiation dose; these chest CT images with FBP and IR techniques were obtained from different CT vendors.

■ Conclusion

Developments in CT technology have enabled faster, often non–breath-hold, low-radiation dose CT examinations,

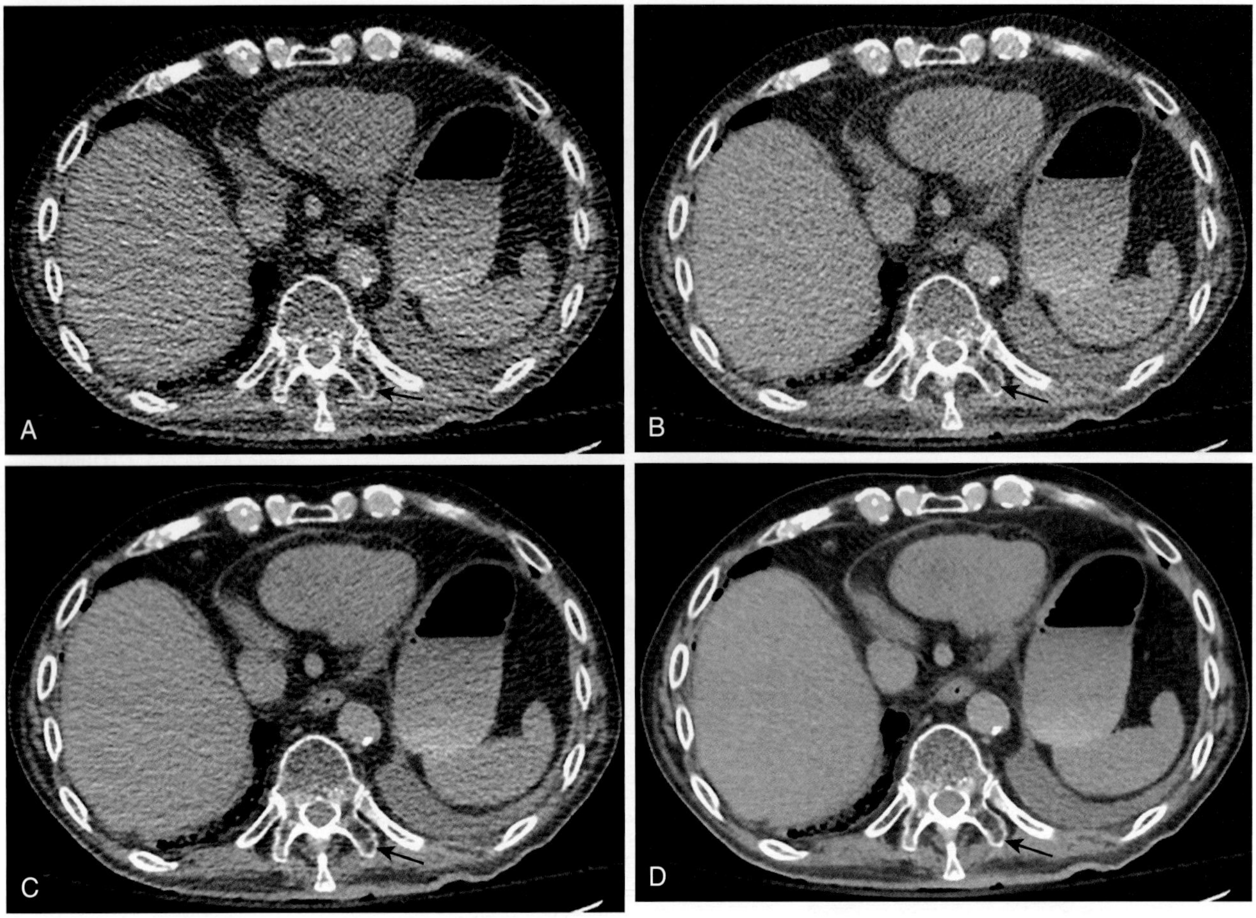

Figure 6.8 Transverse postmortem chest CT images of a 82-year-old male cadaver (57 kg) acquired on a 64-row multidetector CT scanner (GE Discovery CT750 HD) at four different dose levels at 120 kV with automatic exposure control and reconstructed with adaptive statistical iterative reconstruction 50%. (A) 21 mA; CTDIvol, 0.8 mGy; dose length product (DLP), 38 mGy-cm. (B) 37 mA; CTDIvol, 1.5 mGy; DLP, 68 mGy-cm. (C) 85 mA; CTDIvol, 3.4 mGy; DLP, 156 mGy-cm. (D) 341 mA; CTDIvol, 13 mGy; DLP, 608 mGy-cm. The left pleural effusion *(arrows)* is not seen well at CTDIvol of 0.8 mGy (21 mA, A). Image noise increases with a decrease in tube current, which also affects the conspicuity of mediastinal lesions.

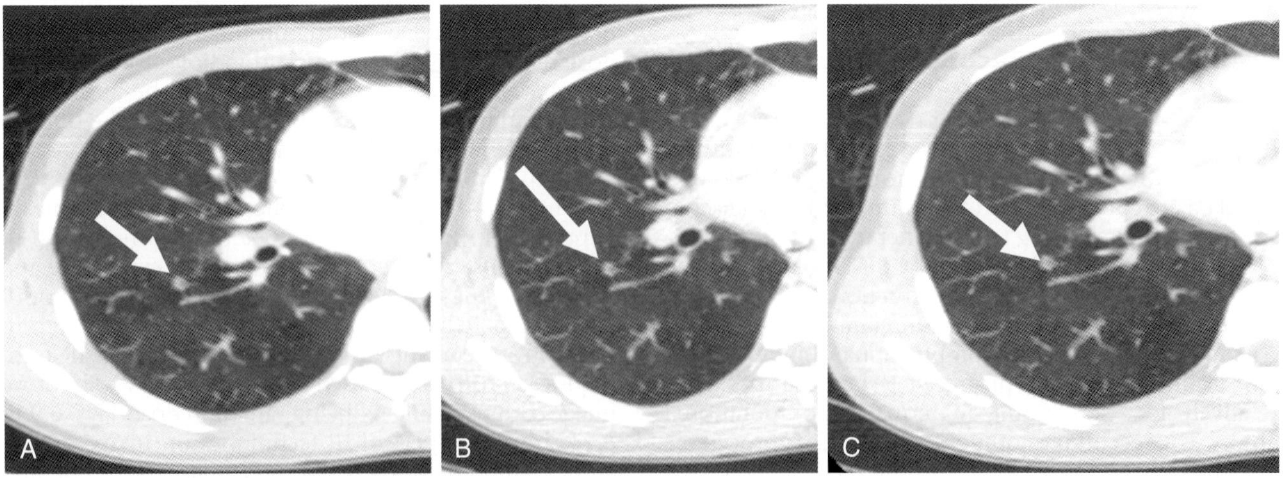

Figure 6.9 Routine chest CT scan of a 26-year-old male patient (57 kg) on 64-row multidetector CT scanner (GE Discovery CT750 HD) at a standard of care radiation dose with filtered backprojection (FBP)–based reconstruction (A; 120 kV; automatic exposure control; CTDIvol, 5 mGy; dose length product [DLP], 191 mGy-cm) and low radiation dose (20 mA; 120 kV; CTDIvol, 0.8 mGy; DLP, 30 mGy-cm) with FBP (B) and adaptive statistical iterative reconstruction at a 70% blending level (C). Both the standard and low–radiation dose chest CT images demonstrate a 6- to 7-mm nodule in the superior segment of the right lower lobe *(white arrows)*.

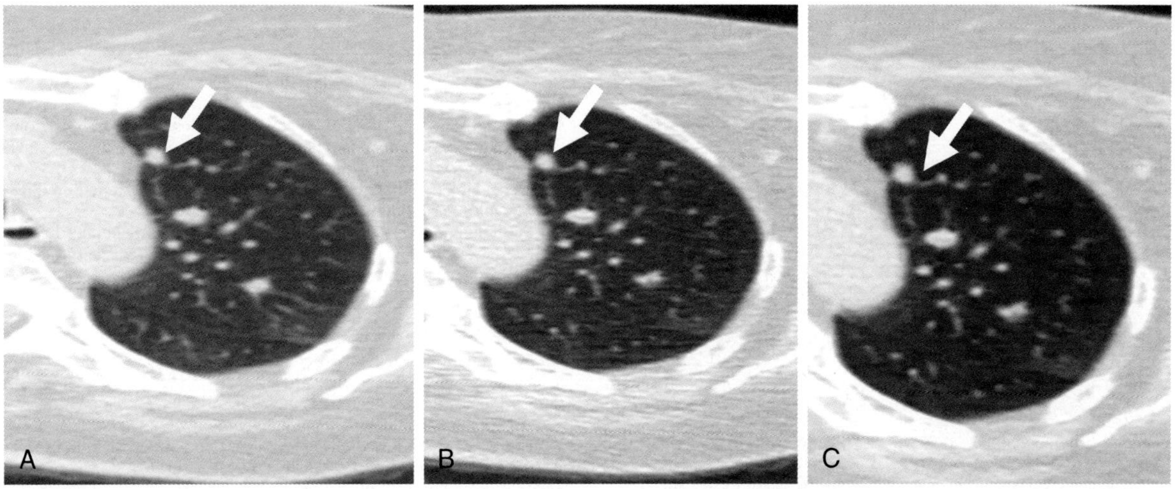

Figure 6.10 Routine chest CT scan of a 66-year-old female patient (57 kg) on a 128-row multidetector CT scanner (Philips iCT) at a standard of care radiation dose with filtered backprojection (FBP)–based reconstruction (A; 120 kV; automatic exposure control; CTDIvol, 5.0 mGy; dose length product [DLP], 171 mGy-cm) and low radiation dose (120 kV; 55 mA; CTDIvol, 0.7 mGy; DLP, 28 mGy-cm) with FBP (B) and iDose (C). Both the standard and low–radiation dose chest CT images demonstrate an 8-mm nodule in the left upper lobe *(arrows)*.

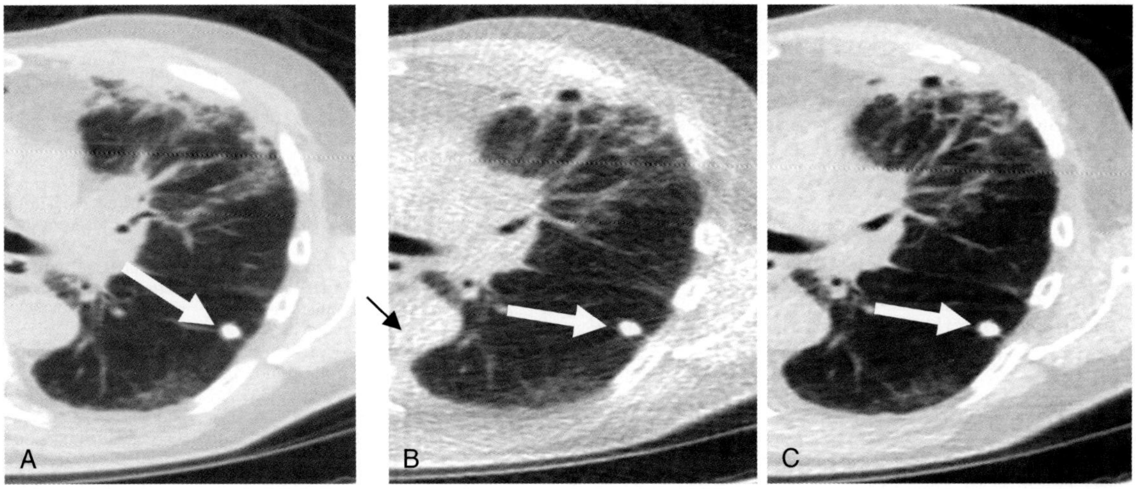

Figure 6.11 Routine chest CT scan of a 67-year-old male patient (60 kg) on a 64-row multidetector CT scanner (Siemens Definition Flash) at standard of care radiation dose with filtered backprojection (FBP)–based reconstruction (A; 120 kV; automatic exposure control; CTDIvol, 8.6 mGy; dose length product [DLP], 267 mGy cm) and low radiation dose (36 mA; 120 kV; CTDIvol, 1.1 mGy; DLP, 35 mGy-cm) with FBP (B) and SAFIRE (Siemens Healthineers; C). Both the standard- and low-dose images demonstrate an 8-mm calcified nodule in the left lower lobe.

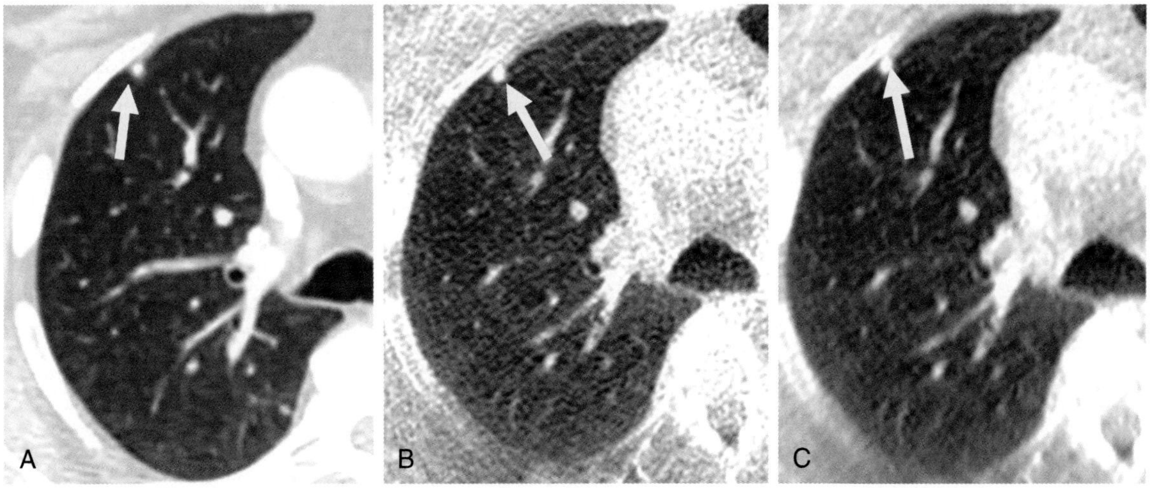

Figure 6.12 Routine chest CT scan of a 78-year-old male patient (82 kg) on a 320-row multidetector CT (Toshiba Aquilion One) at a standard of care radiation dose with filtered backprojection (FBP)–based reconstruction (A; 120 kV; automatic exposure control; CTDIvol, 22.2 mGy; dose length product [DLP], 774 mGy-cm) and low radiation dose (135 kV; 10 mA fixed; CTDIvol, 0.3 mGy; DLP, 11 mGy-cm) with FBP (B) and AIDR3D (Canon Medical Systems; C). Both the standard- and low-dose images demonstrate a 4-mm nodule in the right upper lobe *(arrows)*.

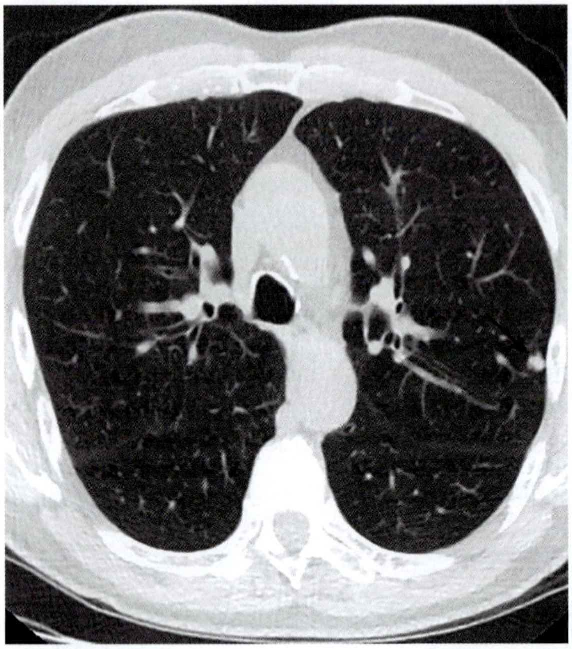

Figure 6.13 Lung cancer screening—CT examination of a 73-year-old male patient (69 kg; 120 kV, with fixed mAs; CTDIvol, 1.3 mGy; dose-length product, 56 mGy-cm) performed on a 64-slice multidetector CT scanner. The transverse CT image demonstrates a solid pulmonary nodule in the left upper lobe *(arrow)*.

particularly in the thorax. Modern MDCT scanners have a plethora of techniques to enhance image quality and drastically reduce the radiation dose to heretofore unprecedented levels.

Bibliography

American Cancer Society. *Cancer Facts & Figures*. Atlanta: American Cancer Society; 2013:2013.

Bae KT, Heiken JP. Scan and contrast administration principles of MDCT. *Eur Radiol*. 2005;15:e46–e59.

Bae KT, Tao C, Gurel S, et al. Effect of patient weight and scanning duration on contrast enhancement during pulmonary multidetector CT angiography. *Radiology*. 2007;242:582–589.

Bae KT. Intravenous contrast medium administration and scan timing at CT: consideration and approaches. *Radiology*. 2010;256:32–61.

Braun FM, Johnson TRC, Sommer WH, et al. Chest CT using spectral filtration: radiation dose, image quality and spectrum of clinical utility. *Eur Radiol*. 2015;25:1598–1606.

Eller A, Wuest W, Scharf M, et al. Attenuation-based automatic kilovolt (kV)-selection in computed tomography of the chest: effects on radiation exposure and image quality. *Eur J Radiol*. 2013;82:2386–2391.

GE Healthcare. Revolution CT. http://www3.gehealthcare.com/en/Products/Categories/Computed_Tomography/Revolution_CT#tabs/tab8CB733F2821249EDA32FB25F78A47A70. Accessed January 28, 2015.

Goldman LW. Principles of CT: radiation dose and image quality. *J Nucl Med Technol*. 2007;35:213–225.

Gordic S, Morsbach F, Schmidt B, et al. Ultralow-dose chest computed tomography for pulmonary nodule detection: first performance evaluation of single energy scanning with spectral shaping. *Invest Radiol*. 2014;49:465–473.

Henzler T, Fink C, Schoenberg SO, et al. Dual energy CT: radiation dose aspects. *AJR Am J Roentgenol*. 2012;199:s16–s25.

Hu XH, Ding XF, Wu RZ, et al. Radiation dose of non-enhanced chest CT can be reduced 40% by using iterative reconstruction in image space. *Clin Radiol*. 2011;66:1023–1029.

Ichikawa Y, Kitagawa K, Nagasawa N, et al. CT of the chest with model-based, fully iterative reconstruction: comparison with adaptive statistical iterative reconstruction. *BMC Med Imaging*. 2013;13:27.

Jan SC, Weiland S, Klement N, et al. Dual energy CT of the chest: how about the dose? *Invest Radiol*. 2010;45:347–353.

Johnson TRC. Dual-energy CT: general principles. *AJR Am J Roentgenol*. 2012;199:s3–s8.

Johnson TRC, Kraub B, Sedlmair M, et al. Material differentiation by dual energy CT: initial experience. *Eur Radiol*. 2007;17:1510–1517.

Kalender W. X-ray computed tomography. *Phys Med Biol*. 2006;51:R29–R43.

Kalra MK, Maher MM, Toth TL, et al. Techniques and applications of automatic tube current modulation for CT. *Radiology*. 2004;233:649–657.

Kalra MK, Maher MM, Toth TL, et al. Strategies for CT radiation dose optimization. *Radiology*. 2004;230:619–628.

Kalra MK, Rizzo S, Maher MM, et al. Chest CT performed with z-axis modulation: scanning protocol and radiation dose. *Radiology*. 2005;237:303–308.

Kubo T, Lin PJP, Stiller W, et al. Radiation dose reduction in chest CT: a review. *AJR Am J Roentgenol*. 2008;190:335–343.

Leipsic J, Nguyen G, Brown J, et al. A prospective evaluation of dose reduction and image quality in chest CT using adaptive statistical iterative reconstruction. *AJR Am J Roentgenol*. 2010;195:1095–1099.

Lu GM, Zhao Y, Zhang LJ, et al. Dual energy CT of the lung. *AJR Am J Roentgenol*. 2012;199:s0–s53.

Mayer C, Meyer M, Fink C, et al. Potential for radiation dose savings in abdominal and chest CT using automatic tube voltage selection in combination with automatic tube current modulation. *AJR Am J Roentgenol*. 2014;203:292–299.

McCollough CH, Bruesewitz MR, Kofler JM. CT dose reduction and dose management tools: overview of available options. *Radiographics*. 2006;26:503–512.

Mettler FA, Bhargavan M, Faulkner K, et al. Radiologic and nuclear medicine studies in the United States and worldwide: frequency, radiation dose, and comparison with other radiation sources—1950-2007. *Radiology*. 2009;253:520–531.

Mulkens TH, Bellinck P, Baeyaert M, et al. Use of an automatic exposure control mechanism for dose optimization in multi-detector row CT examinations: clinical evaluation. *Radiology*. 2005;237:213–223.

National Cancer Institute. *Cancer of the Lung and Bronchus: SEER Stat Fact Sheets* [database online]. Bethesda, MD: National Cancer institute; 2014.

Pan X, Siewerdsen J, La Riviere P, et al. Development of x-ray computed tomography: the role of *Medical Physics* and *AAPM* from the 1970s to present. *Med Phys*. 2008;35:3728–3739.

Pontana F, Pagniez J, Duhamel A, et al. Reduced-dose low-voltage chest CT angiography with sinogram-affirmed iterative reconstruction versus standard-dose filtered back projection. *Radiology*. 2013;267:609–618.

Siemens. SOMATOM Force. http://www.healthcare.siemens.com/computed-tomography/dual-source-ct/somatom-force/technical-specifications. Accessed January 28, 2015.

Singh S, Kalra MK, Gilman MD, et al. Adaptive statistical iterative reconstruction technique for radiation dose reduction in chest CT: a pilot study. *Radiology*. 2011;259:565–573.

Singh S, Kalra MK, Khawaja RD, et al. Radiation dose optimization and thoracic computed tomography. *Radiol Clin North Am*. 2014;52:1–15.

Singh S, Kalra MK, Shenoy-Bhangle AS, et al. Radiation dose reduction with hybrid iterative reconstruction for pediatric CT. *Radiology*. 2012;263:537–546.

Yu L, Li H, Fletcher JG, et al. Automatic selection of tube potential for radiation dose reduction in CT: a general strategy. *Med Phys*. 2010;37:234–243.

CHAPTER 7
Cardiovascular CT

Rachel Edwards, Gregory A. Kicska, and Guatham P. Reddy

CHAPTER OUTLINE

■ Introduction

CT imaging of the heart plays an important role in anatomic and sometimes functional evaluation of the heart and coronary arteries. Coronary artery cardiac CT angiography (CTA) has substantially gained popularity, specifically for imaging acute chest pain in urgent care settings, allowing for a more rapid rule-out of acute coronary syndrome (ACS) and for imaging patients before and after coronary artery bypass graft (CABG) surgery. Before the imaging specialist interprets the images from a cardiac CT examination, it is important to understand the basics of image acquisition.

■ Basics of Cardiac CT

Electrocardiogram Gating

Electrocardiogram (ECG) gating allows for image acquisition during certain time points in the cardiac cycle. Usually, images are acquired during the later third of the R-R interval, which corresponds to cardiac diastole when the images will be subject to less motion artifact. There are three main types of ECG synchronization: (1) prospective triggering (axial, sequential); (2) retrospective gating (spiral, helical); and (3) retrospective gating with tube modulation (Fig. 7.1). A newer type is a high-pitch spiral prospectively triggered acquisition, which requires a dual-source scanner.

In prospective triggering, images are acquired in a step-and-shoot fashion. The tube current is only applied for a specific percentage of the R-R interval, usually end-diastole. The minimum amount of time that the patient can be irradiated during the cardiac cycle is determined by the gantry rotation time. On single-source scanners, this is typically between 135 and 210 ms, and on dual source scanners this may less than 70 ms, depending on exact scanner type. When the minimum time for image acquisition is used, this results in a solitary image (frame) from a single time point during the cardiac cycle. If this image is blurred by motion artifact, images from other points in the cardiac cycle cannot be reconstructed. The amount of time a patient can be irradiated during the cardiac cycle can be increased so that additional images or frames can be reconstructed, but this increases radiation dose.

Therefore, prospective gating is ideally performed in patients with low, regular heart rates, ideally less than 60 beats/min, although some sites use this mode when the heart rate is less than 65 beats/min.

When prospective triggering is performed, the patient may be imaged every other heartbeat, as opposed to retrospective gating, which images each heartbeat. Between heartbeats, the table moves within the CT gantry to the

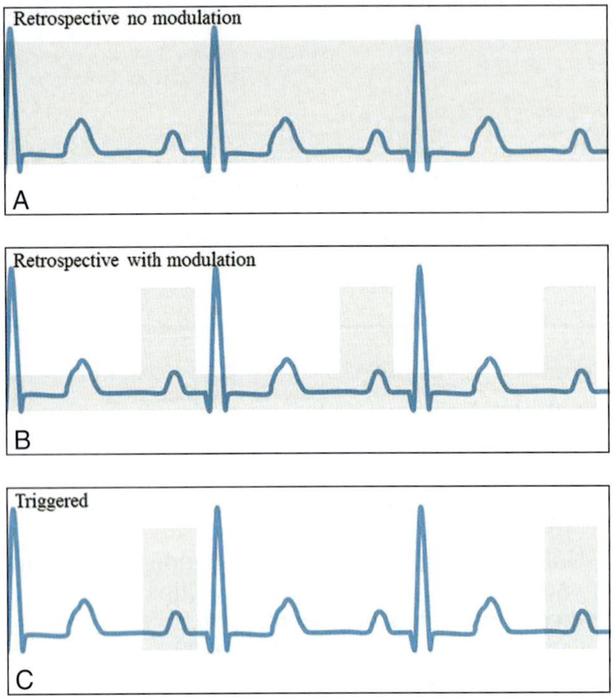

Figure 7.1 Three most commonly used gating and triggering techniques. Gray areas indicate the amount of tube current being applied during the cardiac cycle. (A) In retrospective gating without modulation, data are acquired continuously, with the tube current set to the same value throughout the cardiac cycle. (B) In retrospective gating with tube current modulation, the tube current is decreased during suboptimal phases of the cardiac cycle, which is usually systole and early diastole. (C) In prospective triggering, data are acquired discontinuously, every other heartbeat, with the tube current only being applied during the optimal cardiac phase, which is usually diastole.

next location of image acquisition. Therefore, prospective examinations usually take longer, resulting in a slightly longer breath-hold and the need for more IV contrast.

In retrospective gating, images are acquired throughout the cardiac cycle using a helical acquisition, producing a cine clip of heart motion. Images acquired during numerous points in the cardiac cycle can be used to measure function. In addition, images from various stages in the cardiac cycle can serve to display anatomy that may be blurred by motion artifact on some cardiac phases.

A variation of retrospective gating called *retrospective gating with modulation* also acquires images throughout the cardiac cycle, but the tube current is varied based on the cardiac cycle. This is typically used to produce low-noise images during diastole, allowing for visualization of the coronary arteries and higher noise, and lower dose images during the remainder of the cardiac cycle. This approach minimizes radiation dose, yet allows cardiac function to be evaluated.

Image Reconstruction and Analysis

Imaging reconstruction depends on whether prospective or retrospective gating is used. For example, for examinations using a CT scanner with a minimum slice thickness of 0.625 mm, prospective triggering may be reconstructed at a 0.625-mm slice thickness, with a 0.625-mm interval. When using retrospective gating, slices may be reconstructed at a 0.625-mm thickness but with a 0.3125-mm interval. In both cases, the field of view should be confined to the anatomy of interest, but there is little benefit in a field of view less than 15 cm. Images should be reconstructed using an appropriately smooth kernel, which will have a different name based on the CT vendor.

Reconstructed images can be reformatted in real time using a three-dimensional workstation. Coronary artery stenosis is best diagnosed using multiplanar reconstruction (MPR) images when the reformatted plane shows the vessel through-plane. Axial images are nearly as effective as MPR images for diagnosing coronary stenosis. Maximum intensity projection images should be used with caution when diagnosing coronary stenosis (Fig. 7.2).

Common Indications for Imaging

Chest Pain

Chest pain is one of the most common indications for cardiac CT. Recently, multiple randomized trials have demonstrated that cardiac CTA has an excellent negative predictive value for excluding coronary artery disease for emergency department patients with chest pain. In low- to intermediate-risk patients, ACS can be safely excluded if there is no coronary artery stenosis greater than 50% (Fig. 7.3).

Additionally, in the setting of a nondiagnostic cardiac stress test, cardiac CTA can provide information that may obviate the need for an unnecessary conventional coronary angiogram. If the cardiac CTA is normal in the setting of a nondiagnostic stress test, the patient often does not need to undergo conventional coronary angiography.

Sudden Cardiac Death

Sudden cardiac death (SCD) is defined as unexpected death occurring within a short time period from symptom onset. In patients for whom SCD has been successfully aborted, cardiac CTA can be used to diagnose structural heart disease–related causes. SCD in patients older than 35 years is usually due to coronary atherosclerosis and myocardial ischemia. In patients younger than 35 years, an anomalous coronary artery or a cardiomyopathy, such as arrhythmogenic right ventricular cardiomyopathy (ARVC), arrhythmogenic right ventricular dysplasia (ARVD), or hypertrophic cardiomyopathy, becomes more common. In the approximately 20% of SCD patients who have no structural heart disease, mostly represented by channelopathic disorders, cardiac CT does not yield a diagnosis.

Coronary Artery Disease Risk Stratification

Obtaining the coronary artery calcium score (CACS) using noncontrast cardiac CT has been shown to assist in the risk stratification of patients with atypical chest pain and asymptomatic patients with cardiovascular disease risk factors. CACS has been shown to correlate strongly with the risk of future adverse cardiac events and mortality.

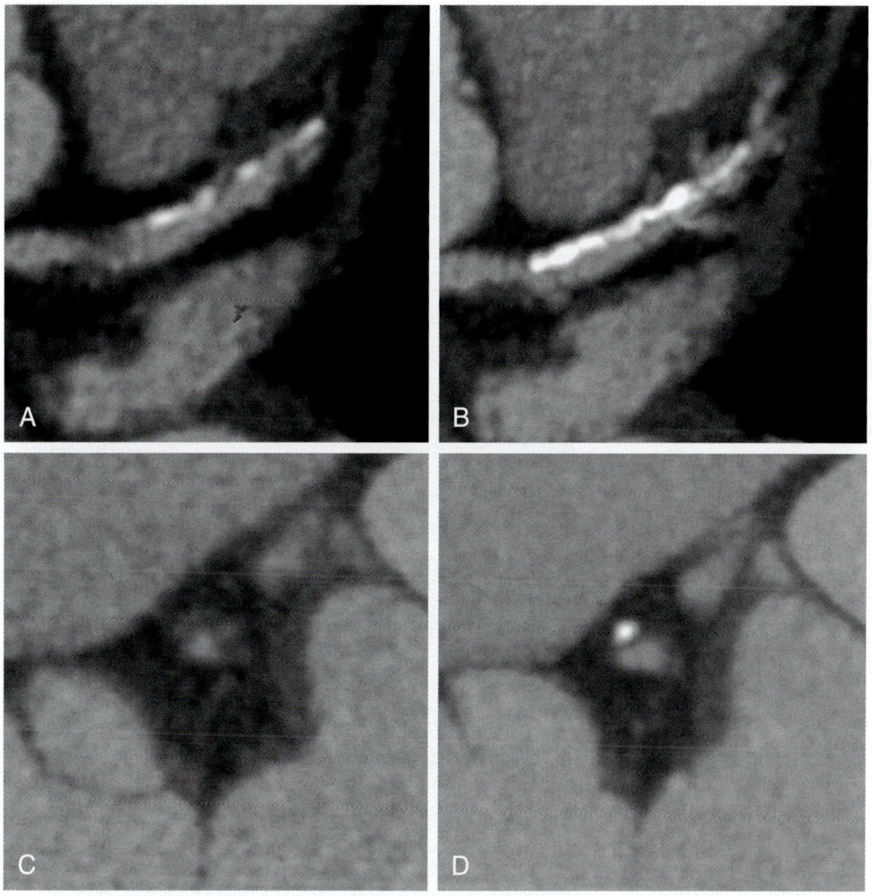

Figure 7.2 Diagnostic pitfall of evaluating coronary stenosis using reformatted maximum intensity projection (MIP) compared to multiplanar reconstruction (MPR) images. Proximal coronary atherosclerosis is shown in-plane on (A), 0.6-mm MPR, and (B), 1.5-mm MIP images. (B) The amount of stenosis is overestimated in the MIP image. Image of the same stenosis is shown through-plane on (C), 0.6-mm MPR, and (D), 1.5-mm MIP images. (D) Using the through-plane images, the stenosis is underestimated on the MIP images.

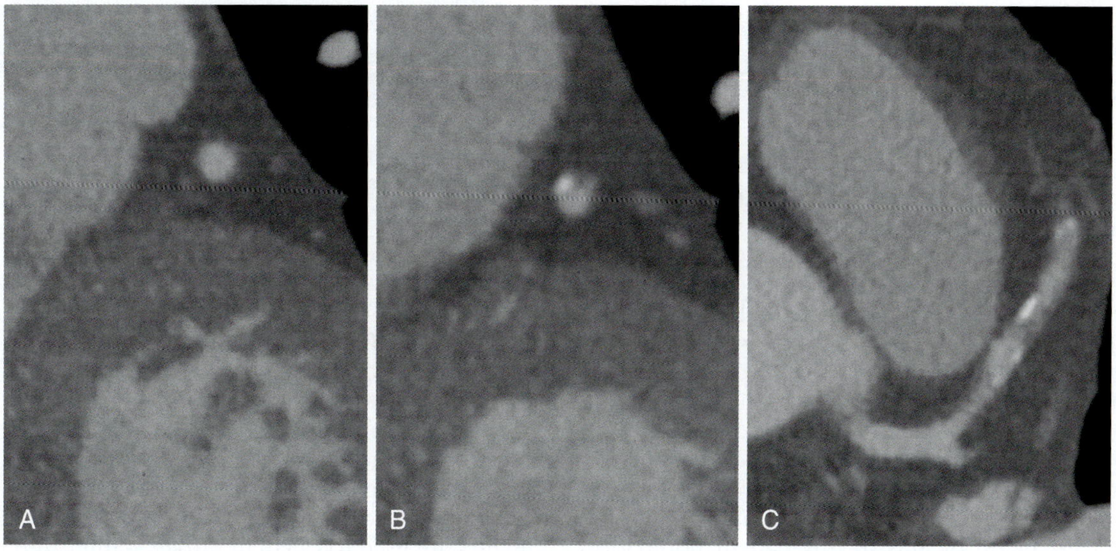

Figure 7.3 (A, B) Through-plane and in-plane (C) images representing less than 50% luminal narrowing of the left anterior descending. The image in (A) demonstrates the normal luminal diameter for comparison. Image (B) is at the level of the lesion resulting in less than 50% luminal stenosis.

The CACS inversely correlates with cardiac CTA performance for diagnosing coronary stenosis. In some cases, if a patient being evaluated for ACS has a calcium score >1000 Agatston units, cardiac CTA may be unreliable, and the patient will undergo conventional coronary angiography, regardless of the cardiac CTA findings.

Contraindications to Cardiac Catheterization

Cardiac CTA can be performed safely in patients who have a contraindication to cardiac catheterization. There are few contraindications to cardiac catheterization, but they include coagulopathy (both iatrogenic and intrinsic), uncontrolled systemic hypertension, unexplained fever, and/or untreated infection.

Coronary Artery Bypass Patency

Cardiac CTA is a noninvasive method for determining the patency of CABG surgery and for detecting complications following CABG, such as an aneurysm of the graft vessel. Using multidetector CT (MDCT), cardiac CTA has an excellent sensitivity (97%–100%) and specificity (98%) in determining if there is a stenosis in the bypass graft or the distal runoff vessel. Evaluation of the native vessels is more difficult due to the high prevalence of calcium and, often, stents.

Presurgical Planning

Cardiac CTA is often performed prior to initial cardiothoracic surgical intervention and in cases of reoperation. In cases prior to initial surgical intervention, cardiac CTA provides anatomic information that allows the surgeon to determine the best surgical approach for the desired sites of intervention. In patients undergoing reoperation, preoperative cardiac CTA provides information confirming the prior surgical interventions, as well as information used to decrease the risk of intraoperative and postoperative complications associated with the positioning of prior grafts within the thorax and their proximity to the expected access site (usually sternotomy or thoracotomy).

■ Problem-Solving Issues

Causes of Acute Chest Pain

Determining if Coronary Atherosclerosis Is Present

Cardiac CTA, specifically coronary CTA, can be used in the emergency department setting in patients with acute chest pain who are predetermined to have a low to intermediate risk for ACS. The risk for ACS is often calculated using the Thrombolysis In Myocardial Infarction (TIMI) score. A TIMI score of less than or equal to 4 is considered low to intermediate risk. The negative predictive value of a coronary CTA that does not demonstrate significant coronary artery stenosis, defined as less than 50% luminal stenosis, is 99%, allowing for the confident exclusion of ACS in this patient population (see Fig. 7.3). If a significant coronary artery stenosis greater than 50% is identified by coronary CTA, then the likelihood of ACS increases, and the patient should undergo an immediate workup for ischemic cardiac chest pain, such as cardiac catheterization (Fig. 7.4). In all cases, the region of suspected stenosis should be measured by comparing it to an adjacent normal segment (Fig. 7.5). Cardiac CTA can also be used to identify the sequelae of ischemia, such as true and false cardiac aneurysms (Fig. 7.6).

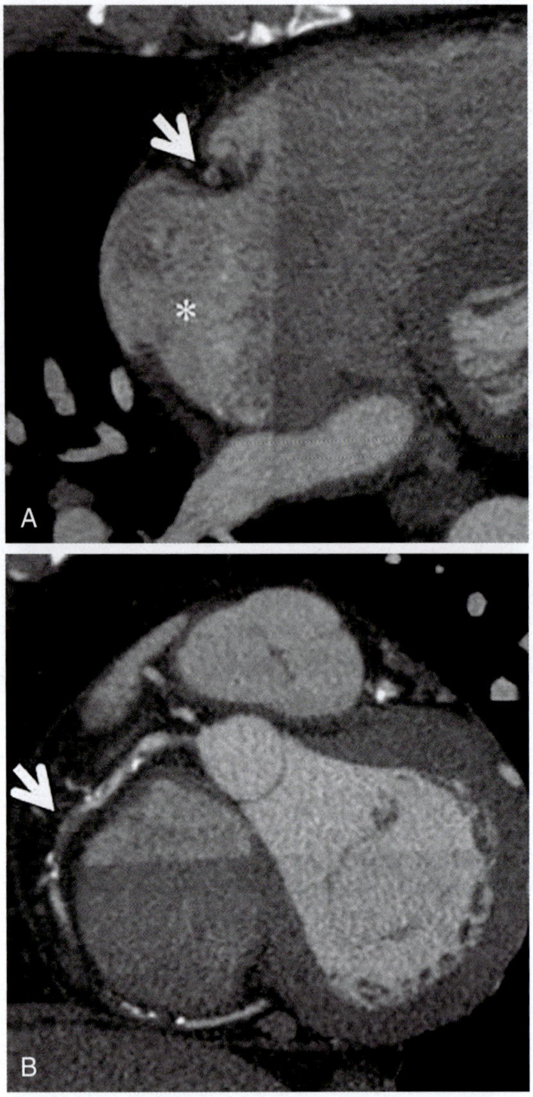

Figure 7.4 (A) In plane and (B) through-plane multiplanar reconstruction images showing an occluded right coronary artery (RCA; *arrows*). Abnormal enhancement of the RCA in (A) can be determined by comparing to enhancement of the right atrium *(asterisk)*. Note that contrast enhancement is present in the distal RCA, which is due to collateral flow.

Evaluation of Cardiac Function

Cardiac function can be evaluated when cardiac CTA is performed with retrospective ECG gating, producing multiple snapshots of cardiac anatomy at evenly spaced time points throughout the cardiac cycle. This allows for the measurement of overall ventricular function, as well as focal ventricular wall motion. Systolic and diastolic images are used to calculate stroke volume and ejection fraction. In the setting of acute chest pain, a focal wall motion abnormality that corresponds to a coronary artery territory may indicate acute myocardial ischemia. Wall motion can be described as normal, hypokinetic (decreased thickening during systole), akinetic (no systolic thickening), or dyskinetic (outward motion of myocardium during systole).

Cardiac valves can be evaluated for vegetations, masses, or stenosis. The aortic valve can be assessed for regurgitation. Incomplete coaptation of the aortic

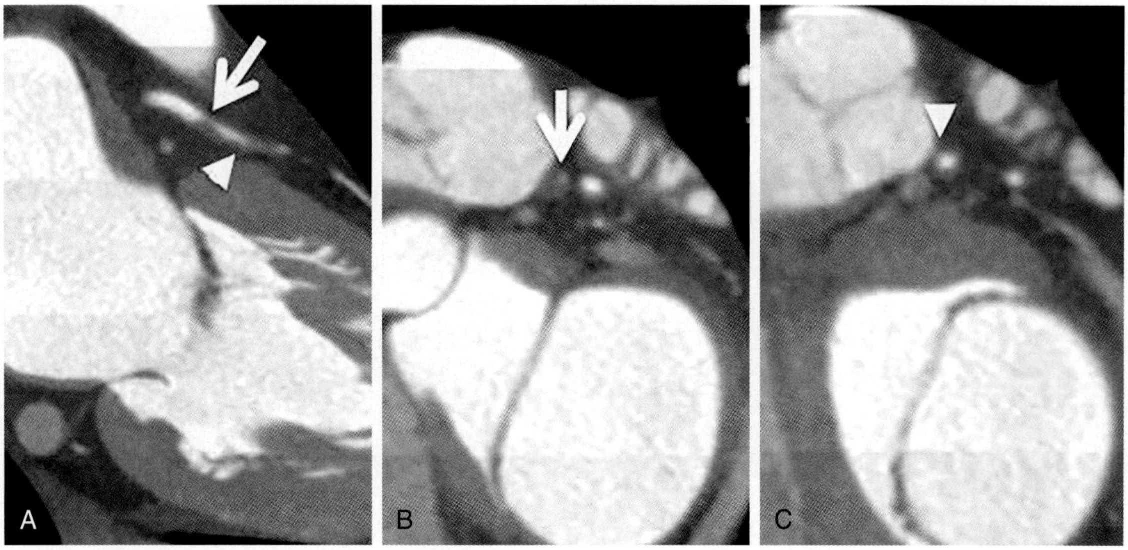

Figure 7.5 Coronary stenosis of the proximal left anterior descending artery (LAD; *arrows*) due to noncalcified plaque is shown (A) in-plane and (B) through-plane. The amount of stenosis is determined by comparing the lumen to the closest segment of the LAD that is disease-free *(arrowheads)*.

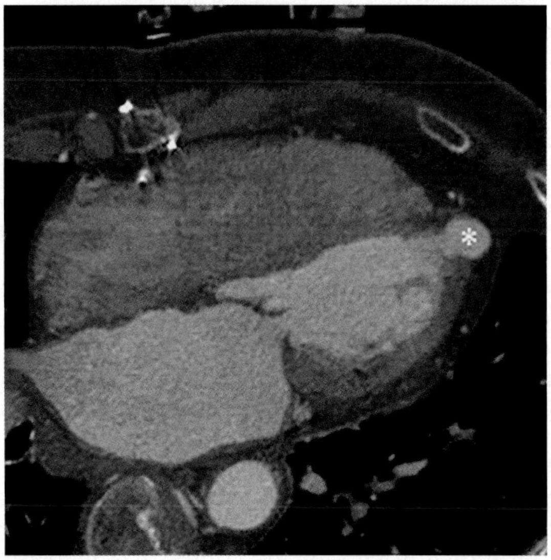

Figure 7.6 Four-chamber view in a patient with a rare left ventricular apical pseudoaneurysm *(asterisk)*. Note that the maximum internal diameter of the aneurysm is greater than the diameter of the neck. Pseudoaneurysms are more commonly found at the posterolateral base of the heart.

valve cusps, seen as a central dot sign, indicates aortic regurgitation, although the amount of regurgitation cannot be determined.

Sudden Cardiac Death

Coronary Artery Anomaly

Conventional coronary artery anatomy is described as the left coronary artery arising from the left coronary sinus and the right coronary artery arising from the right coronary cusp. There are numerous variations on this conventional anatomy. These anatomic variations can be classified into two main groups: (1) anomalous coronary artery arising from the opposite coronary cusp; and (2) anomalous coronary artery arising from the pulmonary artery. The risk of SCD is related to the course of the coronary artery and the coronary artery origin. Therefore, a decision to correct any coronary anomaly surgically incorporates both the arterial course and origin morphology.

The most commonly encountered anomaly associated with SCD or cardiac symptoms is an anomalous origin of the left coronary artery from the right coronary cusp with an interarterial course, otherwise known as a *malignant course* (Fig. 7.7).

The coronary artery origin is also related to the risk of SCD. If a coronary origin has an acute angle or travels within the aortic wall, it is considered to have a higher associated risk of SCD.

Hypertrophic Cardiomyopathy

Hypertrophic cardiomyopathy is an autosomal dominant disease characterized by an abnormally thick, often hyperdynamic, myocardium (Fig. 7.8). Cardiac CTA can be used to diagnose hypertrophic cardiomyopathy by measuring left ventricular wall thickness on the end-diastolic phase image. Hypertrophy can be diffuse or segmentally distributed. A wall thickness of 12 mm or greater is considered abnormal, and greater than 15 mm is suspicious for hypertrophic cardiomyopathy. A thickness greater than 30 mm is considered a risk factor for SCD.

There are various described phenotypic distributions of hypertrophy. In the asymmetric septal phenotype, the most common form, hypertrophy is confined to the basal septum. It is important to identify patients for whom this hypertrophy leads to subaortic stenosis during systole. Subaortic stenosis can result in the anterior leaflet of the mitral valve being pulled toward the left ventricular septum during systole (systolic anterior motion of the mitral valve), causing further outflow obstruction and mitral regurgitation.

Symmetric or concentric phenotypic distribution of hypertrophy is less common and can be confused with other diseases, such as hypertension, aortic stenosis, and

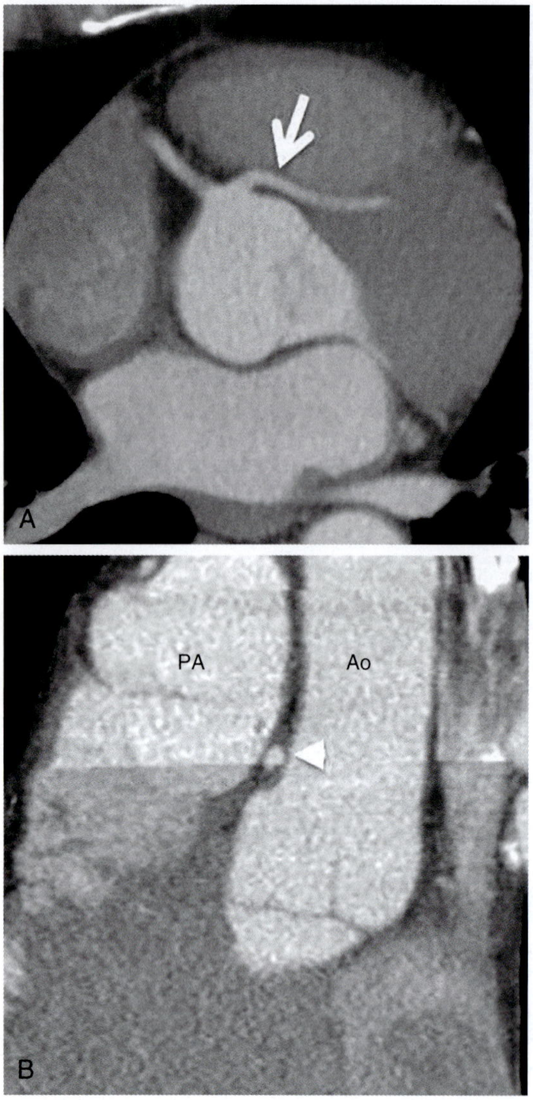

Figure 7.7 Anomalous left coronary artery originating from the right coronary cusp *(arrow)* shown (A) in-plane and (B) in a double-oblique multiplanar reconstruction image that illustrates the interarterial course *(arrowhead)*. *Ao*, Aorta; *PA*, pulmonary artery.

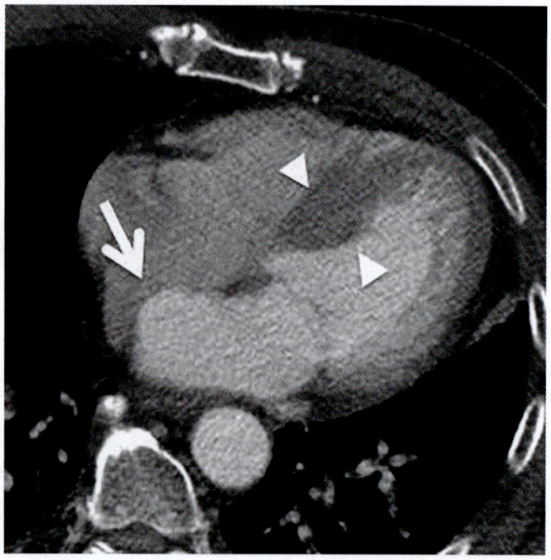

Figure 7.8 End-diastolic image, four-chamber CT scan in a patient with asymmetric septal hypertrophic cardiomyopathy. The basal septum thickness exceeds 15 mm *(arrowheads)*. This patient could be imaged with retrospectively gated CT to look for systolic anterior motion of the mitral valve, which is best performed on the three-chamber view (not shown). There is an incident interatrial septal aneurysm *(arrow)*.

amyloidosis. Athlete's heart can also be confused with symmetric hypertrophic cardiomyopathy. In these cases, the patient must have a history of engaging in sustained cardiovascular activity, usually basketball players, cyclists, and long-distance athletes. The diagnosis of athlete's heart can be made by having the patient cease all exercise and return for imaging in 3 to 6 months. At follow-up, the diastolic volume will then be seen to have returned to normal limits.

Alternative diagnoses should be excluded because patients with these diagnoses are managed differently compared to those with hypertrophic cardiomyopathy.

Coronary Artery Bypass Grafts and Stents

Patency of a Bypass Graft

Cardiac CTA is a noninvasive method for determining the patency of CABGs. Ideally, prior to performing a cardiac CTA for graft patency, the imaging specialist should determine the surgical history of the patient. Craniocaudal coverage of the examination must include the origin and touchdown site of the graft in question. If patients have an internal mammary artery graft, CT should begin above the subclavian arteries. If the patient has vein bypass grafts, CT should begin above any bypass graft markers seen along the ascending aorta. If bypass graft markers are not observed on the CT topogram, scanning should include the entire aortic arch.

Internal mammary grafts can become stenotic or occlude anywhere along their course, although they usually become stenotic at the touchdown site. Occasionally, there is a surgical clip adjacent to the graft at the touchdown site, which can result in a streak artifact that limits evaluation of this area (Fig. 7.9). In these cases, opacification throughout the course of a graft can be used to suggest patency, even though the touchdown site cannot be inspected due to streak artifacts, and a focal stenosis there may not be excluded.

A bypass graft created from a reversed segment of saphenous vein typically originates from the anterior surface ascending aorta. The use of CTA in the assessment of bypass graft patency has been shown to be 100% accurate in cases of saphenous vein grafts. However, the native vessel assessment is more difficult and has lower accuracy values.

In addition to patency, postoperative complications can be detected, including bypass graft aneurysms. Bypass graft aneurysms are usually described in saphenous vein grafts; they are most commonly asymptomatic and are detected years after initial CABG surgery (Fig. 7.10).

Patency of a Coronary Artery Stent

It is more difficult to interpret coronary artery stent patency compared to bypass graft patency due to increased motion artifacts and the blooming and streak artifacts generated by the metal stent. Conventional coronary

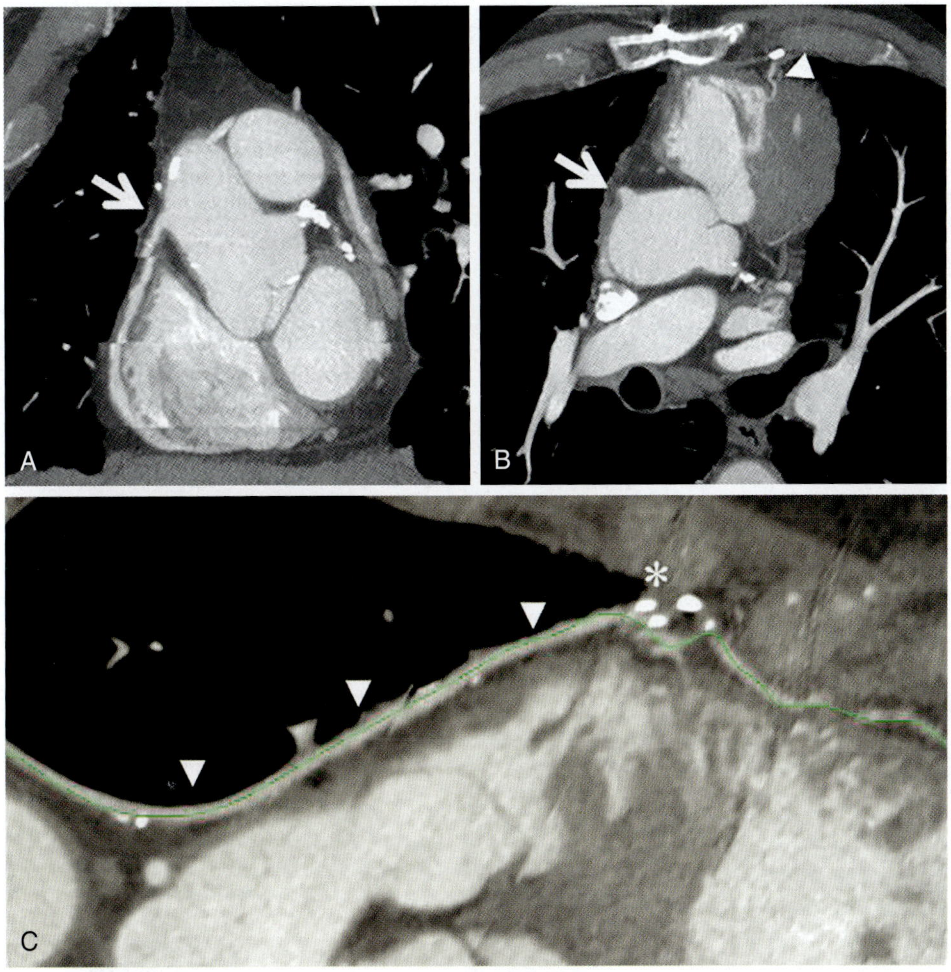

Figure 7.9 CT examination of bypass grafts in a patient with both a saphenous vein bypass *(arrows)* and a left internal mammary artery (LIMA) bypass *(arrowheads)*. (A, B) Double-oblique multiplanar reconstruction image shows the origin of the saphenous vein graft *(arrow)*. Surgical clips in the anterior chest wall indicate that a LIMA graft is also present *(arrowhead)*. (C) Curved planar reformatted image shows the course of the LIMA *(arrowheads)*. The final surgical clips seen in the course of the artery *(asterisk)* indicate the touchdown site on the left anterior descending artery.

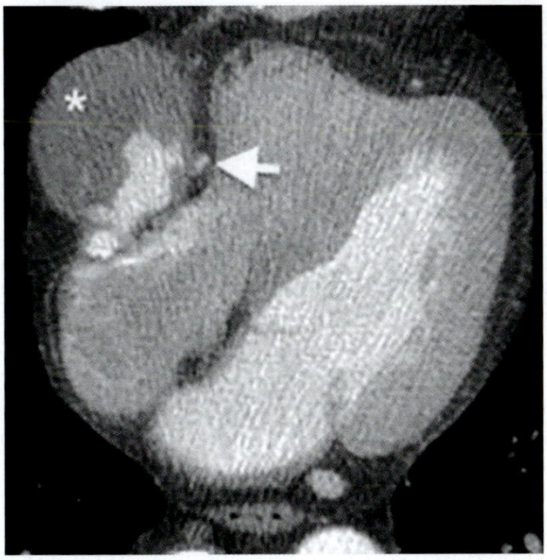

Figure 7.10 Bypass graft aneurysm. This CT examination demonstrated a pseudoaneurysm *(asterisk)* of the bypass graft to the posterior descending artery located adjacent to the right coronary artery *(arrow)*.

angiography is traditionally used for the evaluation of stenosis or thrombosis within a coronary artery stent, although this is an invasive procedure.

Stents within a luminal diameter less than 3 mm are not well evaluated by CTA. However, CTA can diagnose stenosis in stents 3 mm or greater. Contrast opacification of the stent lumen may be directly measured to diagnose stent patency confidently. Contrast opacification of the coronary artery segments proximal and distal to the stent cannot be used to determine stent patency because the distal coronary artery may be opacified through collateral vessels.

Conventional coronary angiography can be used to evaluate stent patency in cases in which CTA is insufficient.

Presurgical Planning

Determining the Best Site for Revascularization

Patients undergoing reoperative cardiac surgery following a prior sternotomy, specifically for CABG, often undergo preoperative imaging, which may include cardiac CTA. Reoperative cardiac surgery is associated with a potential risk for injury to CABGs, aorta, and right ventricle that are located deep to the expected site of the re-do sternotomy (Fig. 7.11).

Preoperative CTA allows for the visualization of the CABGs and their approximate distance from the expected surgical access site, which can affect surgical planning and may influence the surgeon to change from a sternotomy approach to a thoracotomy. Also, the distance between the sternum and aorta and right ventricle can be measured, aiding in the determination of risk for injury if a repeat sternotomy is performed.

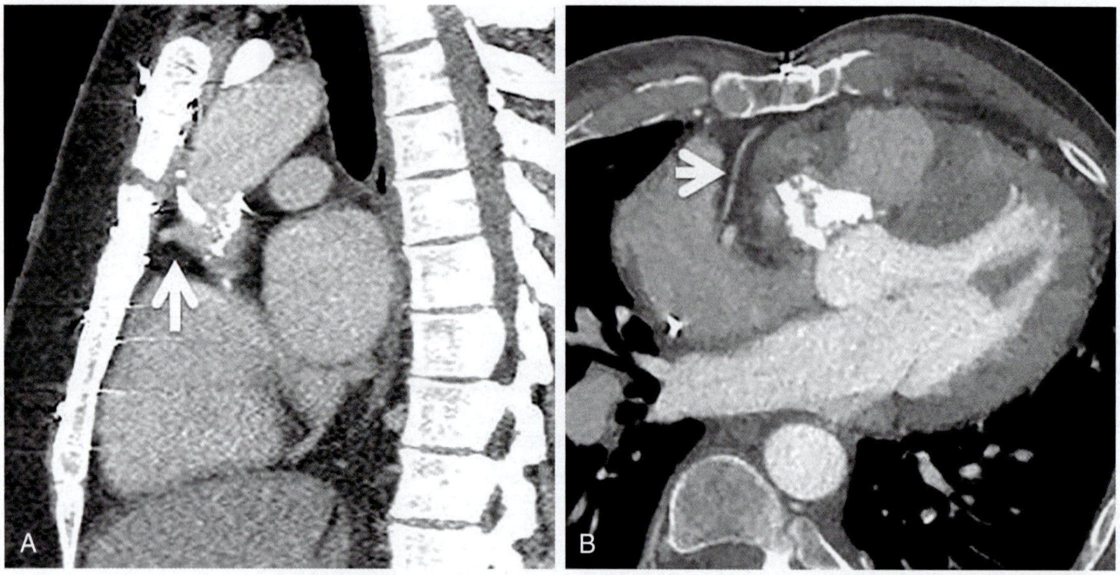

Figure 7.11 CT images in two different patients who were planned for a repeat sternotomy. (A) The right coronary artery (RCA) originates immediately behind the sternum *(arrow)*, placing it at risk of injury during sternotomy. (B) An acute marginal branch of the RCA *(arrow)* passes immediately behind the sternum.

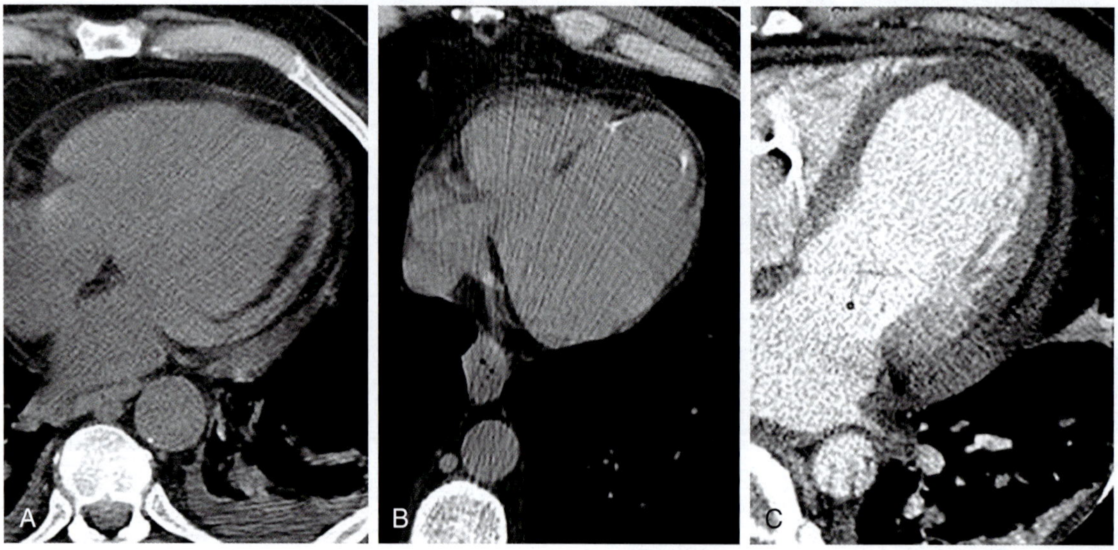

Figure 7.12 CT images in different patients showing the sequelae of myocardial ischemia and infarction. (A) Unenhanced axial image shows subendocardial fat compatible with fatty metaplasia from a prior infarct in a left circumflex coronary distribution (lateral wall). (B) Unenhanced axial image shows apical wall thinning with subendocardial fat and calcium due to a prior left anterior descending artery territory infarct. (C) Enhanced axial image in another patient with apical infarct shows an apical thrombus.

Pitfalls

Differentiating Ischemic From Nonischemic Myocardial Fat

Ischemic left ventricular fat is almost always located in the subendocardium and is linear and confined to a coronary artery distribution (Fig. 7.12). This fat may also be associated with linear calcification, wall thinning, or motion abnormalities. Coronary artery calcium or stenosis further increases confidence that the fat is due to a prior infarct.

Nonischemic left ventricular myocardial fat can also be located in the subendocardium but is usually associated with a normally functioning left ventricle, with normal myocardial thickness. This nonischemic fat is commonly located in the inferoseptal segments of the base through the apex, as well as the apical segment of the left ventricle. It is associated with obesity, steroid use, and older age.

Right ventricular myocardial fat is usually nonischemic. It can be observed in the moderator band or, less commonly, in other trabeculations of the right ventricle. In some cases, there can be diffuse fatty infiltration of the anterior free wall of the right ventricle, a condition referred to as *adipositas cordis*.

Less commonly, myocardial fat is seen in other nonischemic diseases. ARVD or ARVC may demonstrate myocardial fat in the free wall of the right ventricle, right ventricular outflow tract, moderator band, trabeculae in the right ventricle, or left ventricular free wall and is typically located in the subepicardium. However, it is important to note that the presence of myocardial fat is not a criterion for the diagnosis of ARVD. ARVC is diagnosed based on right ventricular diastolic volume and ejection fraction, along with focal wall motion abnormalities.

Misinterpreting Stair Step Artifact as Coronary Artery Stenosis

A CT stair step artifact occurs when a patient's R-R interval varies during scanning. It appears when different phases of the cardiac cycle are present on adjacent axial images. The resulting coronary motion can be misinterpreted as stenosis or occlusion (see Fig. 7.9). This pitfall can be avoided by examining the coronary artery in multiple planes, which can confirm the presence of a stair step artifact if all the anatomy demonstrates a shift between the two axial acquisitions. The coronal and sagittal planes are particularly useful in identifying the levels were the artifact is present.

Understanding Limits of Interpretation in Anatomy Adjacent to Calcium or Surgical Clips

Evaluation of cardiac structures, specifically blood vessels, adjacent to calcium or metallic surgical clips is limited due to blooming artifacts from beam hardening (Fig. 7.13). The visualization of blood vessels such as coronary arteries can be improved with use of the edge-enhancing convolution kernel, although evaluation remains somewhat limited. This blooming artifact can result in an artifactual appearance of stenosis at the proximal and distal ends of the coronary artery stent, where the metallic struts are located, or poor visualization of CABGs adjacent to the metallic surgical clips used for marking the surgical anastomoses on subsequent, conventional, coronary artery angiograms.

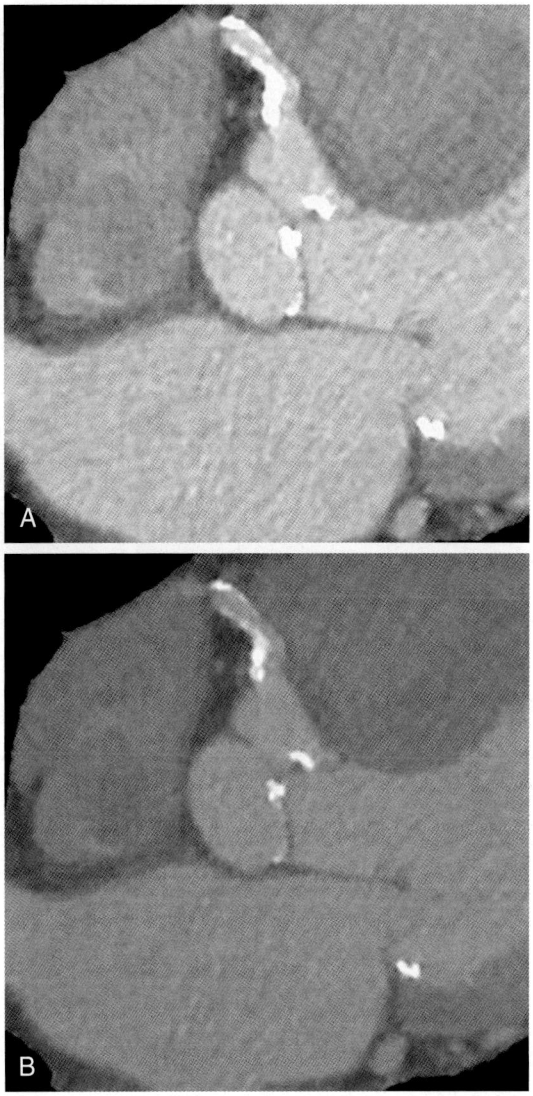

Figure 7.13 Blooming artifact from coronary calcium. Coronary CT angiography demonstrates dense atherosclerotic calcification of the proximal right coronary artery. Axial images are reconstructed in a soft tissue algorithm (A) and bone algorithm (B). Blooming artifact from calcification is more pronounced in the soft tissue algorithm images.

■ Overcoming Technical Obstacles

Patient Is Unable to Hold Breath

A patient's inability to hold the breath is less of a technical obstacle than in prior years as the acquisition times get shorter, with faster gantry rotation times, increasing number of detectors, and increasing table speeds. Modern 320-slice CT scanners or dual-source, high-pitch scanners have been reported to image patients during free breathing. If a patient is unable to hold his or her breath, retrospective gating can be used to decrease the breath-hold time compared to prospective triggering (see Fig. 7.1). Limiting z-axis coverage will also decrease the breath-hold time.

Patient Has Metal in Chest

Metal within the patient's chest (e.g., surgical clips, pacer leads, shrapnel) can result in a blooming artifact and limit the diagnostic quality of the CT examination. Surgical clips within the mediastinum placed during CABG surgery and intracardiac leads and pulse generators from defibrillators and pacers are some of the most commonly encountered metallic objects on cardiac CTA. If the surgical history is not known prior to the examination, these metallic objects can be identified on the topogram obtained for CT planning.

If the metal object is located next to a structure that is to be evaluated with CT, there are a few techniques that can improve image quality. Using an edge-enhancing convolution filter can decrease the blooming artifact encountered with metallic objects. Imaging at a higher kVp value will also reduce blooming artifacts. Dual-energy or spectral CT imaging can also be used to reduce metallic streak artifacts (Fig. 7.14). Generally, virtual monochromatic reconstructions at a higher keV level are most useful.

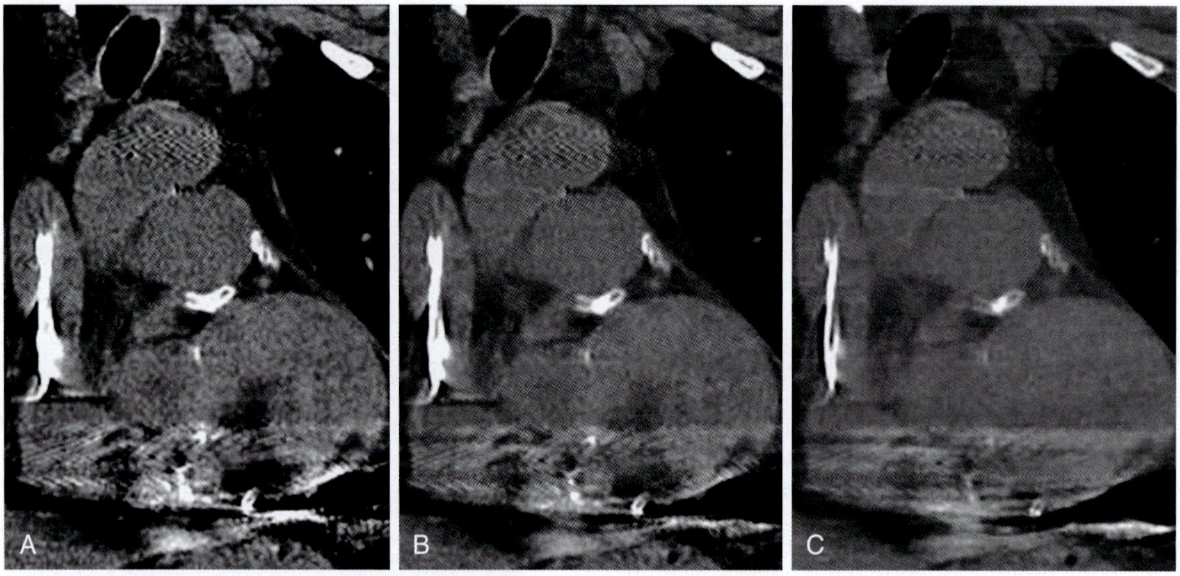

Figure 7.14 Dual-energy CT examination in a patient with an intracardiac pacer. Coronal reformats demonstrate the varying appearance of the pacer leads at 50 keV (A), 70 keV (B), and 140 keV (C). As the keV increases, less streak artifact is seen at the pacer leads.

TABLE 7.1 Heart Rate–Based Recommended Pulsing Width

HEART RATE (BEATS/MIN)	DUAL-SLICE CT PULSING WIDTH (% OF RR)	SINGLE-SLICE CT PULSING WIDTH (% OF RR)
<60	60–70	60–77
60–70	60–80	30–77
70–80	55–80	30–77
>80	30–46	30–46

RR, Interbeat interval.

Patient Has Poor Renal Function

Patients with acute or chronically impaired renal function may be at risk for developing contrast-induced nephropathy, although guidelines for iodinated contrast administered to these individuals vary, with no global consensus.

Patient Is Tachycardic

Prior to performing cardiac CT, the ECG rhythm should be interpreted. Ideally, the heart rate should be below 60 beats/min. If the rate is above 65 beats/min, a beta blocker can be administered to lower the heart rate. Metoprolol can be given intravenously or orally prior to cardiac CT to decrease the heart rate and help control cardiac rhythm. If the rate cannot be controlled, the pulsing width can be adjusted to increase the chance of visualizing all coronary segments (Table 7.1).

Patient Is Not in Sinus Rhythm

Prior to performing cardiac CT, the cardiac rhythm should be interpreted on the ECG. If the rhythm is irregular despite beta blockade, retrospective gating should be considered, because this will provide the ability to reconstruct the heart at multiple phases and recover blurred anatomy.

Bibliography

Agrawal H, Mery CM, Krishnamurthy R, Molossi S. Anatomic types of anomalous aortic origin of a coronary artery: a pictorial summary. *Congenit Heart Dis.* 2017;12(5):603–606.

Ashrafpoor G, Danchin N, Houyel L, Ramadan R, Belli E, Paul JF. Anatomical criteria of malignancy by computed tomography angiography in patients with anomalous coronary arteries with an interarterial course. *Eur Radiol.* 2015;25(3):760–766.

Beck KS, Kim JA, Choe YH, et al. 2017 multimodality appropriate use criteria for noninvasive cardiac imaging: expert consensus of the Asian Society of Cardiovascular Imaging. *Korean J Radiol.* 2017;18(6):871–880.

Chan M, Ridley L, Dunn DJ, et al. A systematic review and meta-analysis of multidetector computed tomography in the assessment of coronary artery bypass grafts. *Int J Cardiol.* 2016;221:898–905.

Chheda SV, Srichai MB, Donnino R, Kim DC, Lim RP, Jacobs JE. Evaluation of the mitral and aortic valves with cardiac CT angiography. *J Thorac Imaging.* 2010;25(1):76–85.

Cury RC, Budoff M, Taylor AJ. Coronary CT angiography versus standard of care for assessment of chest pain in the emergency department. *J Cardiovasc Comput Tomogr.* 2013;7(2):79–82.

Earls JP, Woodard PK, Abbara S, et al. ACR appropriateness criteria asymptomatic patient at risk for coronary artery disease. *J Am Coll Radiol.* 2014;11(1):12–19.

Gasparovic H, Rybicki FJ, Millstine J, et al. Three dimensional computed tomographic imaging in planning the surgical approach for redo cardiac surgery after coronary revascularization. *Eur J Cardiothorac Surg.* 2005;28(2):244–249.

Kalisz K, Buethe J, Saboo SS, Abbara S, Halliburton S, Rajiah P. Artifacts at cardiac CT: physics and solutions. *Radiographics.* 2016;36(7):2064–2083.

Kim SS, Ko SM, Choi SI, Choi BH, Stillman AE. Sudden cardiac death from structural heart diseases in adults: imaging findings with cardiovascular computed tomography and magnetic resonance. *Int J Cardiovasc Imaging.* 2016;32(suppl 1):21–43.

Nasis A, Meredith IT, Sud PS, Cameron JD, Troupis JM, Seneviratne SK. Long-term outcome after CT angiography in patients with possible acute coronary syndrome. *Radiology.* 2014;272(3):674–682.

Opolski MP. Cardiac computed tomography for planning revascularization procedures. *J Thorac Imaging.* 2018;33(1):35–54.

Roobottom C. Radical changes to the investigation of stable chest pain following the 2016 NICE update. *Br J Radiol.* 2018;91(1087):20170694.

Shambrook JS, Chowdhury R, Brown IW, Peebles CR, Harden SP. Cross-sectional imaging appearances of cardiac aneurysms. *Clin Radiol.* 2010;65(5):349–357.

Sun Z, Almutairi AM. Diagnostic accuracy of 64 multislice CT angiography in the assessment of coronary in-stent restenosis: a meta-analysis. *Eur J Radiol.* 2010;73(2):266–273.

Sundaram B, Patel S, Agarwal P, Kazerooni EA. Anatomy and terminology for the interpretation and reporting of cardiac MDCT: part 2, CT angiography, cardiac function assessment, and noncoronary and extracardiac findings. *AJR Am J Roentgenol.* 2009;192(3):584–598.

Winchester DE, Wymer DC, Shifrin RY, Kraft SM, Hill JA. Responsible use of computed tomography in the evaluation of coronary artery disease and chest pain. *Mayo Clin Proc.* 2010;85(4):358–364.

CHAPTER 8

Pulmonary, Mediastinal, Vascular, and Chest Wall MRI

Daniel Jeong, Scott K. Nagle, and Christopher J. François

CHAPTER OUTLINE

■ Introduction and Background: Considerations for Using MRI

Magnetic resonance imaging (MRI) is an important tool in imaging the mediastinum, chest wall, and chest vasculature, with a continuously expanding role. Excellent soft tissue contrast makes MRI a useful tool in the diagnosis, staging, surgical planning, and response to treatment evaluation in many cancers. MRI offers sensitivity to blood flow without ionizing radiation, which is particularly useful for multiphase vascular imaging. Multiplanar imaging capabilities allow the precise evaluation of complex thoracic lesion configuration and margins when chest wall, mediastinal, or spinal invasion is suspected.

Although computed tomography (CT) is often the primary means of imaging the chest, the role of MRI is increasing. The indications and application of thoracic MRI and magnetic resonance angiography (MRA) will be reviewed in this chapter while highlighting the MRI appearance of common thoracic pathology.

Recent Technologic Advances That Make Chest MRI More Feasible

Clinically available MRI sequences and those that are frequently used in lung MRI research are summarized in Table 8.1. Magnetic resonance has shown an increasing role in the imaging of chest disease due to faster sequences with shorter breath-hold times and more robust cardiac gating. The availability of multichannel phased array MRI coils and improvements in parallel imaging are partially responsible for the significant improvements in scan times. In addition, newer gadolinium contrast agents, such as the macrocyclic agents, have decreased the risk of nephrogenic systemic fibrosis.

Newer proton-based sequences, including ultrashort echo times (TEs) and pulmonary perfusion, are improving the ability of MRI in pulmonary parenchymal evaluation using commercial hardware. The use of hyperpolarized gases has also been increasing the capabilities of pulmonary MRI. With these applications, interstitial lung diseases

TABLE 8.1 Summary of Commonly Used Lung MRI Sequences

SEQUENCE	UTILITY	COMMENTS
Commercially Available		
T1	Mass evaluation	Pre- and postcontrast
T2	Mass evaluation, radiation fibrosis vs. recurrence	
DCE T1-weighted perfusion	Pulmonary hypertension, chronic obstructive disease, pulmonary embolism	3D full-chest coverage
ASL perfusion	Pulmonary hypertension, chronic obstructive disease	No IV contrast required; better absolute quantitation than DCE 2D evaluation of limited number of slices
Diffusion-weighted imaging	Nodule or mass evaluation	
Research Tools		
Hyperpolarized ^{3}He, ^{129}Xe	Ventilation defects in chronic obstructive disease, asthma, bronchospasm	Requires broadband-capable hardware, polarizer, and specialized physics support
Ultrashort TE	Lung cancer, diffuse lung disease, pulmonary edema, air trapping	Not yet available commercially

2D, Two-dimensional; *3D*, three dimensional; *ASL*, arterial spin labeling; *DCE*, dynamic contrast-enhanced; *IV*, intravenous; *TE*, echo time.

and chronic obstructive pulmonary disease (COPD) can be evaluated with MRI.

With faster imaging, MRA is now becoming more robust in the rapid evaluation of acute and chronic vascular disease, including pulmonary embolism (PE). Compared to computed tomography angiography (CTA), MRA has the benefit of not requiring the use of ionizing radiation and the ability to scan multiple postcontrast phases following a single contrast dose. In addition, noncontrast MRA sequences are improving and can offer diagnostic evaluation of vasculature when contrast is not used.

Lung MRI

Sequences Used to Evaluate the Lung Parenchyma and Lung Masses

T1 and T2 signal characterization of lung masses (Fig. 8.1) alone has not been shown to be a reliable means of distinguishing between benign and malignant processes. However, more recent studies have suggested restricted diffusion on diffusion-weighted imaging (Fig. 8.2) and offers promise in characterizing benign and malignant lesions.

Three-dimensional (3D) MRI with an ultrashort TE has allowed for high-resolution, whole-lung imaging. Shortening the TE in fast spin-echo sequences is crucial for maintaining image quality in the lungs and has demonstrated clinical utility in assessing non–small cell lung cancer, diffuse lung disease, and pulmonary edema.

Pulmonary imaging with hyperpolarized agents, such as helium-3 (^{3}He) and xenon-129 (^{129}Xe), has allowed functional pulmonary analysis on MRI, which has proven useful in asthma, COPD, and cystic fibrosis. Although the image quality with these agents is high, the need for specialized hardware, technical expertise, and expensive gas has limited the use of these techniques to a few academic centers.

A recent study has shown that 3-T MRI, including T2 half-Fourier acquisition single-shot turbo spin-echo (HASTE) and 3D gradient echo (GRE) sequences, offers sensitivity of 82% and a specificity of 79% in detecting pulmonary abnormalities compared to high-resolution CT (HRCT). MRI was sufficient for detecting infectious nodules and consolidations in neutropenic patients with acute myeloid leukemia; however, MRI failed to detect ground-glass opacities that were noted on HRCT.

The postcontrast enhancement pattern on MRI has proven more useful for evaluating benign and malignant lesions in the lungs, compared to precontrast T1- and T2-weighted imaging. Malignant pulmonary lesions demonstrate higher maximum enhancement values, with increased slope and earlier peak enhancement, than benign lesions (Fig. 8.3). Delayed enhancement is also higher in malignant compared to benign lesions.

MRI perfusion of the lungs correlates well with pulmonary function tests in COPD patients and can be used to distinguish mild from severe cases of COPD. Pulmonary perfusion data can be acquired using dynamic contrast-enhanced (DCE) or arterial spin labeling (ASL) techniques. With dynamic contrast injection, parenchymal enhancement can be measured precontrast and during multiple postcontrast acquisitions. Lung parenchymal signal intensity is higher with gadobenate dimeglumine (Multihance) compared to gadolinium dimeglumine (Magnevist). There is a nonlinear relationship between contrast agent concentration and MRI signal in the arterial input function, and therefore a nonlinear correction method is useful for perfusion quantification using DCE techniques. ASL is another established technique that can evaluate pulmonary parenchymal perfusion without

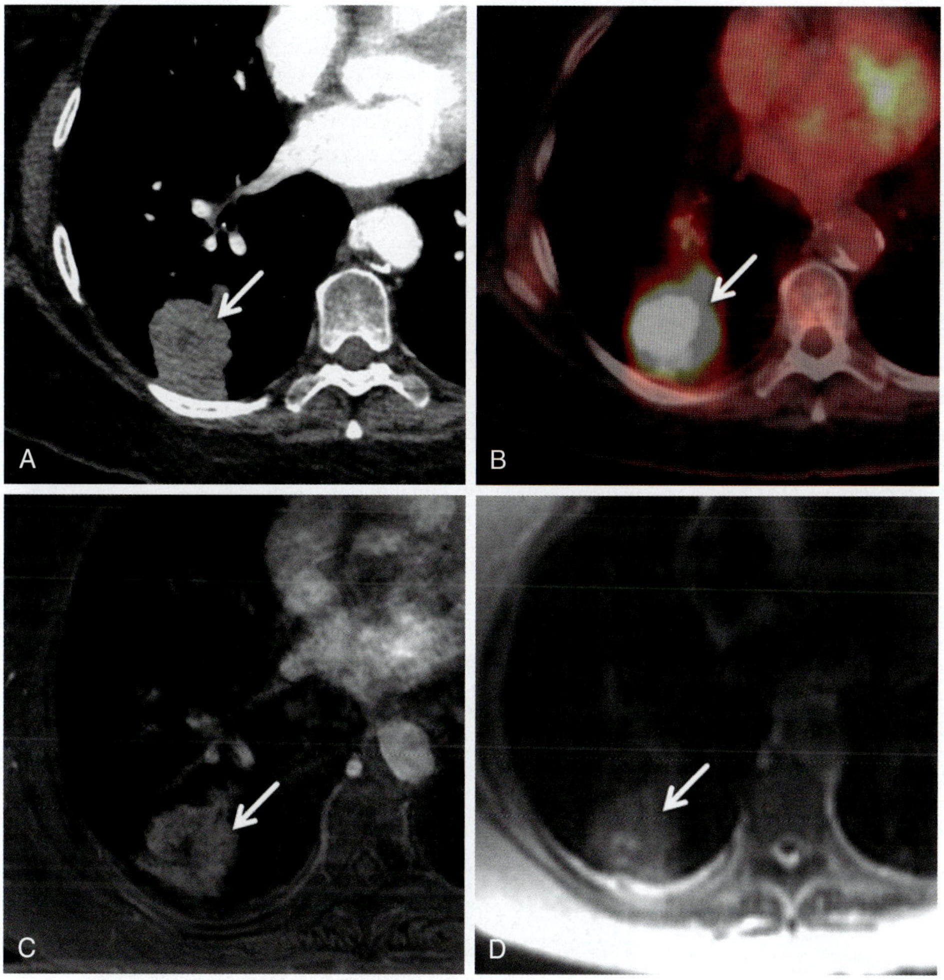

Figure 8.1 A 67-year-old woman with right lower lobe primary lung adenocarcinoma *(arrows)*. (A) Contrast-enhanced CT. (B) Fluorodeoxyglucose–positron emission tomography CT. (C) T1 with fat saturation after contrast administration. (D) T2 without fat saturation. The mass enhances heterogenously (C), with an area of hypoenhancement corresponding to an area of necrosis that is hyperintense on the T2-weighted image (D).

intravenous (IV) contrast. ASL involves cardiac-gated images obtained during a breath-hold, where the only differing factor between images is the radiofrequency (RF) tagging of the blood flowing into the image. Subtracted images can provide signal proportional to the arterial blood delivered to the lung during a cardiac cycle, which can be quantified. It is, however, more technically challenging than DCE to perform and usually results in only a small number of two-dimensional (2D) images.

When to Use MRI for Characterizing Lung Tumors

Traditionally, pulmonary imaging with MRI has been limited by a paucity of protons in the lung parenchyma, respiratory motion due to longer imaging times, and magnetic field inhomogeneities with air-tissue interfaces in the lungs. In most cases, CT offers better pulmonary imaging than MRI due to its higher spatial resolution and shorter scan times, reducing the possibility of motion artifact.

Solitary Pulmonary Nodules

Solitary pulmonary nodule imaging with MRI has been shown to differentiate lung cancers from tuberculomas and hamartomas reliably using DCE methods and washout ratios. Lung malignancies (see Fig. 8.3) have rapid enhancement with mild delayed washout at 8 minutes, whereas tuberculomas and hamartomas have slower steady enhancement over 8 minutes with a lower peak. However, dynamic MRI cannot reliably differentiate between lung cancers and focal organizing pneumonias because both display relatively rapid enhancement, with mild delayed washout. Additional signs that may help differentiate benign and malignant nodules include an enhancing rim at the periphery of a lesion (a thin rim enhancement pattern), which may be a sign of benignity. Similarly, a heterogeneous enhancement pattern with areas of irregular linear enhancement, so-called network enhancement, was more commonly seen in hamartomas than other solitary pulmonary nodules.

Assessing Extrapulmonary Invasion

MRI is the primary imaging modality for the local staging of superior sulcus (Pancoast) tumors (Fig. 8.4) due to excellent soft tissue contrast. In addition, MRI can offer definitive evaluation of tumor extension into the great vessels, mediastinum, pericardium, chest wall (Fig. 8.5), and spine in cases where CT is equivocal. MRI is also appropriate for evaluating the pleural involvement of tumors or differentiating pleural metastases from primary

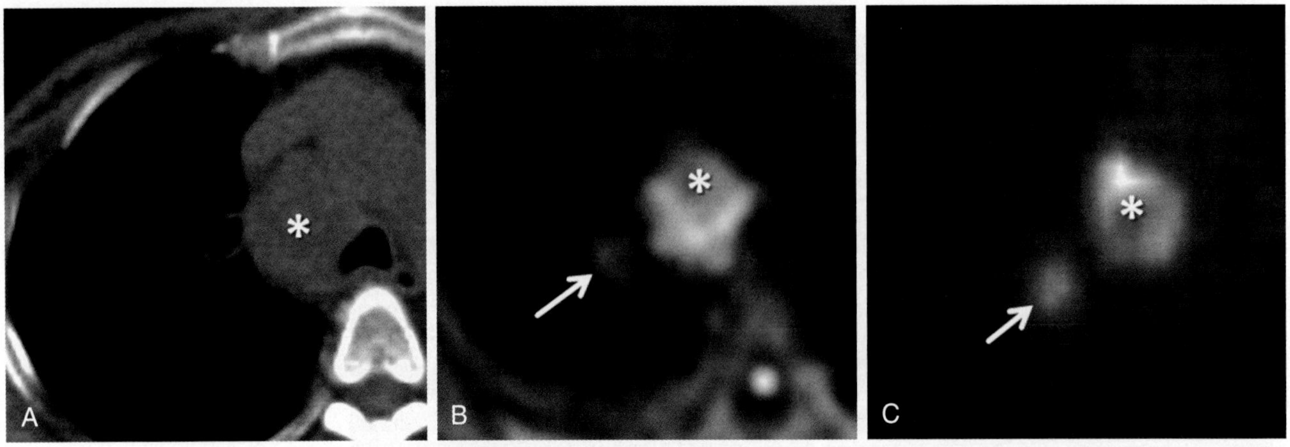

Figure 8.2 A 48-year-old woman with poorly differentiated adenocarcinoma of the lung with paratracheal lymph node metastasis *(asterisks)*. (A) CT chest scan without contrast. (B) MRI diffusion-weighted image (DWI; *arrow*). (C) Fluorodeoxyglucose (FDG)–positron emission tomography (PET; *arrow*). The lymph node metastasis is restrictive on the DWI and is hypermetabolic on FDG-PET. The edge of the primary tumor in the right upper lobe *(arrows)* has similar imaging characteristics.

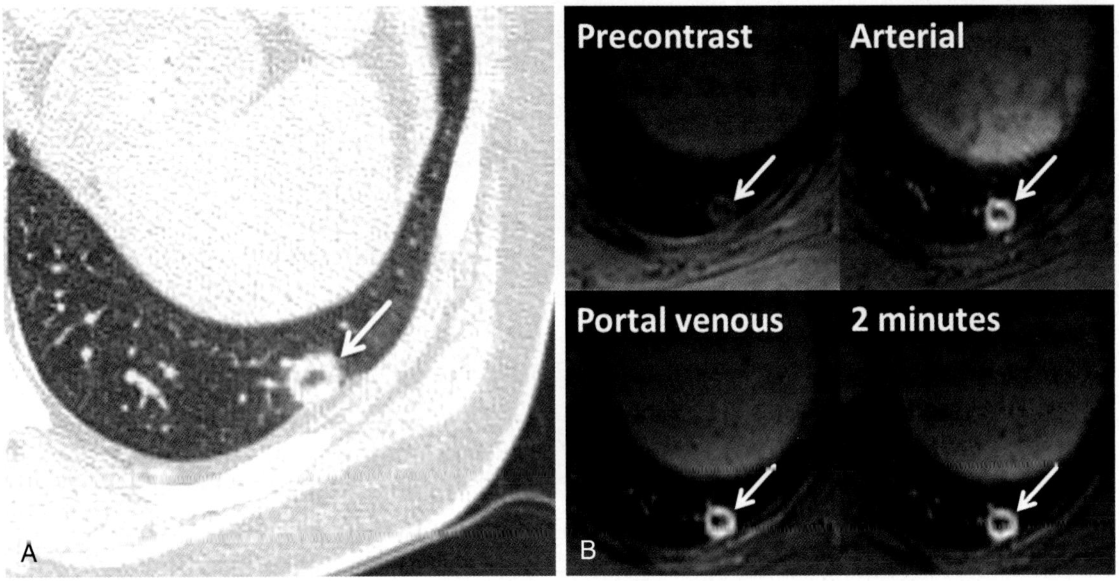

Figure 8.3 A 61-year-old man with hepatocellular metastasis to the left lower lobe *(arrows)*. (A) CT chest scan reveals a subpleural nodule with irregular margins and central area of ground-glass attenuation. (B) Precontrast, arterial phase, portal venous phase, and 2-minute delay T1-weighted gradient echo images reveal dynamic enhancement of the left lower lobe nodule. The nodule had rapid enhancement, with only mild delayed washout.

tumors of the pleura, such as a solitary fibrous tumor of the pleura (Fig. 8.6). Patients who cannot receive iodinated contrast can undergo MRI, in addition to noncontrast CT, for the evaluation of hilar and mediastinal involvement and lymph node metastases.

Brachial plexus invasion is well evaluated with MRI. Thin-section (3–4 mm), axial, coronal, and oblique sagittal plane T1 and T2 fat-saturated imaging is a suitable protocol. Some authors have recommended the use of short tau inversion recovery (STIR) methods for T2 imaging to increase the conspicuity of abnormal signal from adjacent fat; however, STIR has a relatively low signal-to-noise ratio with low tissue contrast and is more susceptible to flow artifacts than other methods. With MRI, normal brachial plexus components demonstrate an intermediate to low signal on all sequences and are surrounded by fat. Abnormal nerves typically appear focally or diffusely enlarged, with deviation or discontinuity. These abnormal nerves demonstrate high T2 signal, and there is associated effacement of perineural fat planes. Postcontrast T1 imaging demonstrates segmental or confluent enhancement in the setting of tumor or infection.

Assessing Metastases

Lung cancer has been reported to be the most common malignancy causing cardiac metastasis. Cardiac and

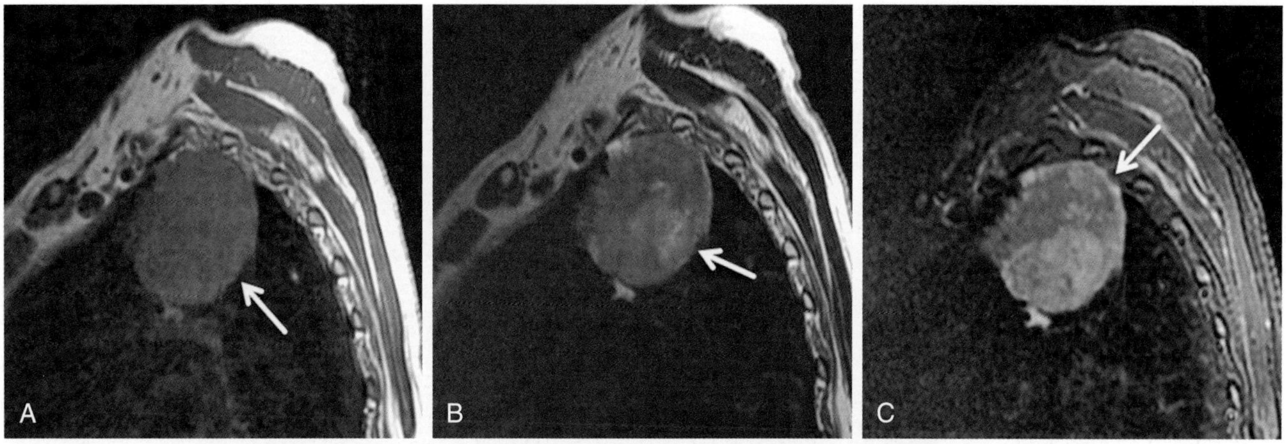

Figure 8.4 A 50-year-old woman with large left apical primary lung adenocarcinoma *(arrows)*. (A) T1 spin echo without fat saturation. (B) T1 spin echo without fat saturation after contrast administration, (C) T2-weighted short tau inversion recovery images reveal a mass that is isointense to skeletal muscle on T1-weighted images precontrast, enhances heterogeneously, and is heterogeneously hyperintense to skeletal muscle on T2-weighted images. Furthermore, MRI confirms the absence of chest wall extension of the tumor.

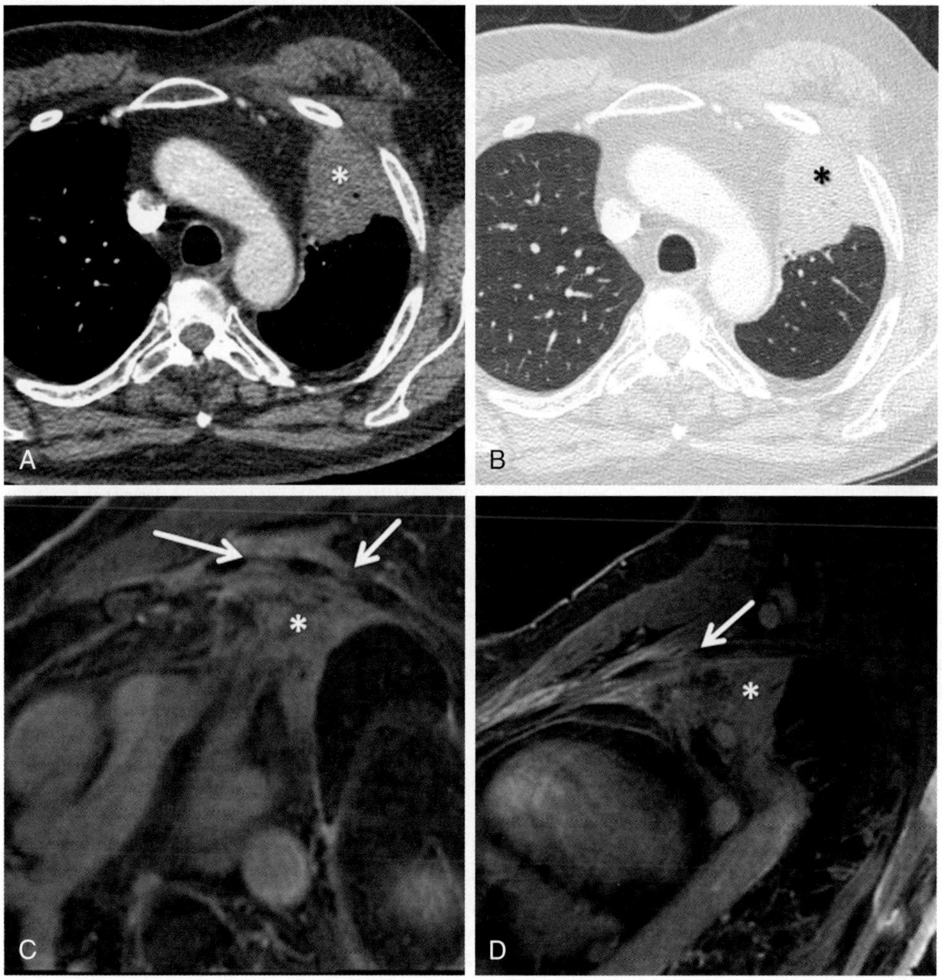

Figure 8.5 A 63-year-old man with a left upper lobe primary lung adenocarcinoma *(asterisks)*. Contrast-enhanced CT with (A) soft tissue and (B) lung tissue windows and levels. (C) Axial and sagittal oblique (D) postcontrast T1-weighted, gradient echo imaging with fat saturation. The mass enhances heterogeneously (C and D) and extends into the chest wall between the adjacent ribs *(arrows)*.

pericardial involvement is found in 17%–31% of patients with bronchogenic carcinoma. Cardiac metastases have been associated with life-threatening complications, including conduction disruptions such as complete atrioventricular block or ventricular fibrillation. Therefore, detection of cardiac metastases can be very important in a patient's clinical management.

On MRI, cardiac metastases typically demonstrate low T1 (Fig. 8.7) and high T2 signals with gadolinium enhancement. Postcontrast enhancement is necessary to

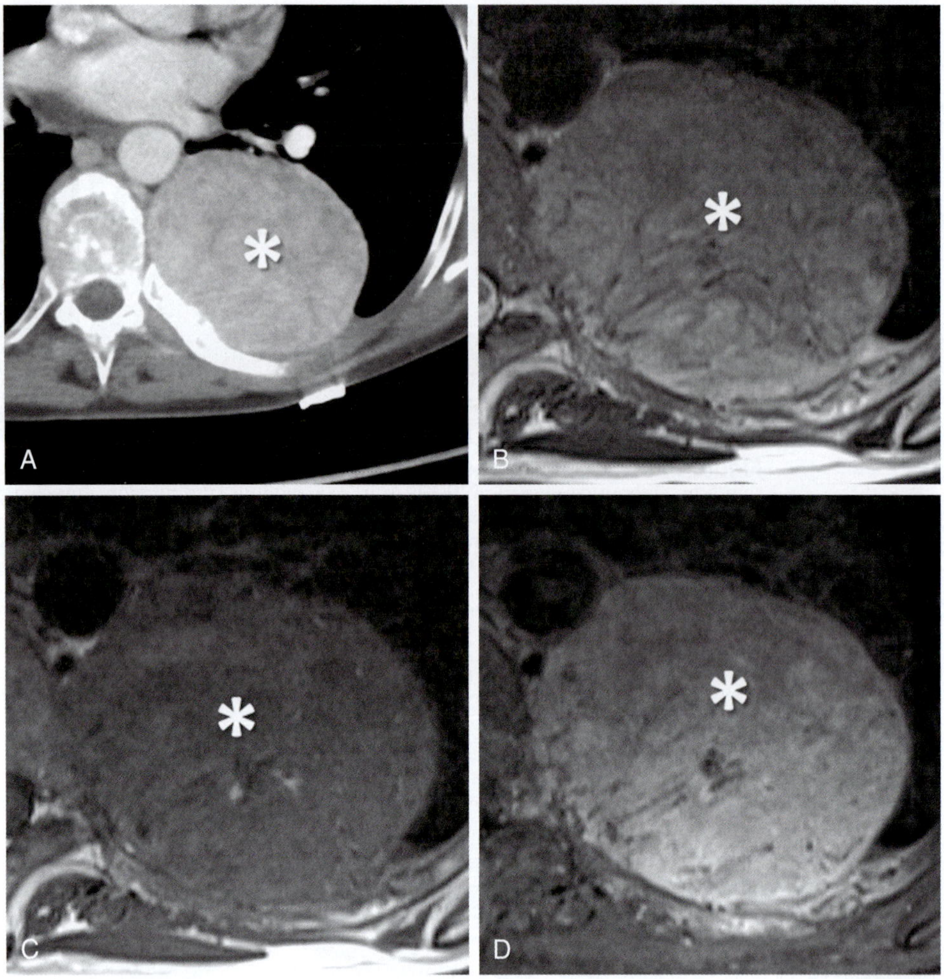

Figure 8.6 A 47-year-old woman with solitary fibrous tumor of the pleura *(asterisks)*. (A) Contrast-enhanced CT, (B) T2-weighted. (C) T1-weighted precontrast. (D) T1-weighted postcontrast. These images reveal a large heterogeneous mass that is intermediate intensity on T2-weighted imaging, hypointense on T1 precontrast, and diffusely enhancing on T1 postcontrast images.

differentiate true tumor from thrombus because chronic thrombus can appear to enhance peripherally. An inversion recovery delayed enhancement sequence with very long inversion time (TI = 600 ms) has been suggested as the best technique to demonstrate true enhancement of tumor, apart from thrombus. Metastatic tumor that has invaded a cardiac chamber will demonstrate a hyperintense filling defect on black blood imaging. In addition, secondary hemodynamic consequences of the mass may be present, including inflow or outflow obstruction of cardiac chambers or valves. Valvular regurgitation in the presence of tumor infiltration could also be identified as flow jets on cine imaging or by using phase contrast techniques.

Some studies have suggested that tumor recurrence can be distinguished from radiation fibrosis using T2 imaging. Chronic fibrosis demonstrates a low T2 signal, whereas tumor tissue tends to demonstrate a higher T2 signal. However, a low signal within a lesion does not preclude residual tumor. In addition, a high signal can also be seen with postradiation therapy, early fibrosis, and acute inflammation.

Tumor can be distinguished from atelectasis with postcontrast MRI. Atelectasis usually demonstrates greater signal intensity than tumor due to its better blood supply. Additionally, the peak signal intensity of atelectasis is seen earlier than with tumors. This relationship can change if vascular obstruction is present.

MRI also offers value in characterizing adrenal lesions in patients with lung cancer. Adrenal lesions are detected in up to 21% of lung cancer staging CT examinations, and a high percentage represents benign adenomas. When MRI demonstrates signal loss within the lesion on out-of-phase imaging or fat-saturated sequences, a confident diagnosis of adenoma can be made.

Emerging Roles for Lung MRI in Diffuse Lung Diseases

When conventional MRI sequences are applied to the lungs, there is a rapid decay of signal before it can be observed due to the short T2* of the lungs (~1.5 ms). However, new techniques allow adequate signal acquisition from the lungs by shortening the effective TE. It is possible to image the entire lung parenchyma in vivo during a single breath-hold using a multislice, interleaved, submillisecond TE GRE sequence. The technique involves fractional echo sampling, high bandwidth, and a shortened RF pulse to minimize TE. In addition, using a 3D radial ultrashort TE sequence with TE less than 100 μs enables significantly improved

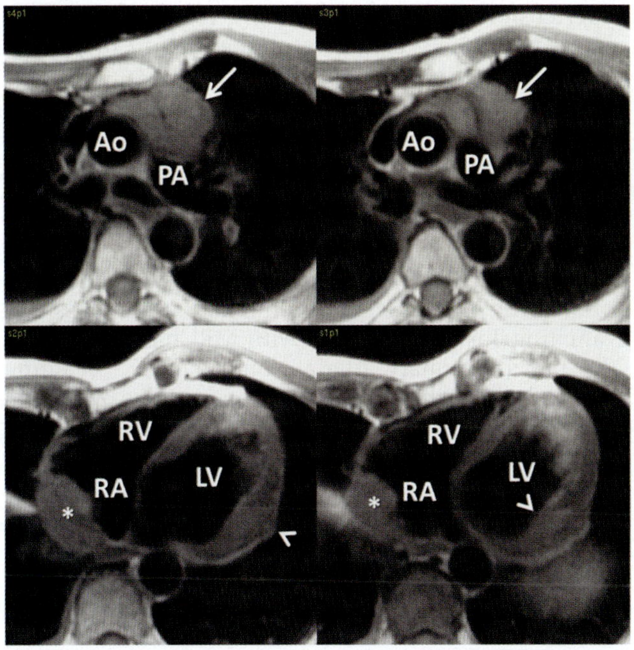

Figure 8.7 A 63-year-old man with metastatic adenocarcinoma to the mediastinum and heart. Axial black blood double-inversion recovery images through the mediastinum *(top row)* and heart *(bottom row)* reveal large, lobular masses in the anterior mediastinum abutting the great vessels *(arrows)* and within the wall of the right atrium *(RA; asterisks)* and left ventricle *(LV; arrowheads)*. *Ao,* Aorta; *PA,* main pulmonary artery; *RV,* right ventricle.

visualization of lung parenchyma. Variations on this 3D radial technique can be used to image lung parenchyma and postcontrast perfusion simultaneously during a single breath-hold.

MRI pulmonary perfusion imaging has correlated to pulmonary function tests in COPD patients. MRI perfusion data, including the pulmonary signal intensity and signal ratio of diseased lung to normal lung, have shown correlation with pulmonary function tests. In addition, significant differences were seen in signal intensity between mild and very severe COPD patients.

The use of hyperpolarized gases, including ^{3}He and ^{129}Xe, has improved MRI evaluation of lung ventilation. The use of hyperpolarized ^{3}He allows for the detection of focal ventilation defects during the approximate 8.16-second breath-hold. Initial studies using hyperpolarized ^{3}He have shown promise in imaging ventilation defects in patients with exercise-induced bronchospasm. Ventilation defects are also observed in those with asthma and COPD. In asthma, heterogeneous defects have been noted involving the central airways, even in asymptomatic patients.

Unfortunately, hyperpolarized ^{3}He is expensive, and the supply is limited, given that it is not naturally occurring and is obtained from the decay of tritium. Costs are estimated at $800 to $2000/L of the ^{3}He gas, depending on the use, which can be prohibitive. The need for a technically complex polarizer and specialized MRI coils and broadband transmit-receive capability has limited the availability of hyperpolarized gas imaging to a few academic centers.

Pulmonary MRA

Sequences Used to Evaluate the Pulmonary Arteries

MRI protocols used for the diagnosis of PE include a combination of noncontrast and contrast-enhanced MRA sequences, DCE perfusion sequences, and steady-state GRE sequences. With respect to maximizing spatial resolution and minimizing acquisition time, 3D contrast-enhanced MRA using parallel imaging and bolus tracking has proven to be the most promising approach and has been reported most extensively in the literature. Using current acceleration methods, it is now possible to carry out whole-chest MRA with 1.0 to 1.5 mm^3 isotropic spatial resolution in approximately 15 to 18 seconds. At our institutions, 0.1 mmol/kg of gadobenate dimeglumine is used, diluted to 30 mL with normal saline, injected at a rate of 1.5 mL/s. This ensures that the contrast bolus remains in the pulmonary arteries throughout the duration of the scan, minimizing the risk of artifact (particularly blurring when using an elliptic, centric, k-space encoding order).

With MRA, it is possible to repeat the acquisition without any concern for ionizing radiation; therefore the 3D MRA sequence is typically repeated two or three times after the injection of IV contrast (Fig. 8.8) to obtain additional steady-state images. These can be acquired using the same parameters as the first-pass acquisition or with parameters adjusted to optimize blood pool to soft tissue contrast. In addition to standard GRE 3D MRA sequences, fat-suppressed T1 GRE acquisitions can be helpful for imaging nonvascular structures. If prescribed breath-holding times are too long for a particular patient, several options are available, including the following: slice thickness can be increased, phase field of view can be decreased, matrix size can be decreased, bandwidth can be increased, and the number of signal averages can be decreased. Cardiac gating is not necessary to achieve high-quality imaging of the pulmonary arteries. The appearance of pulmonary emboli on MRA is similar to CTA, typically appearing as central, low signal intensity filling defects within the center of the pulmonary arteries (Fig. 8.9).

When to Use MRA for the Evaluation of Pulmonary Embolism and Other Pulmonary Vascular Abnormalities

MRA for Pulmonary Embolism

Up to 24% of patients had a contraindication to CTA in the Prospective Investigation of Pulmonary Embolism Diagnosis (PIOPED) II study. In patients with clinically suspected PE and a contraindication to CTA, both ventilation-perfusion scintigraphy and MRA serve as alternative imaging modalities to diagnose PE. MRA offers the benefit that it can be repeated without or with a second IV contrast injection, without radiation exposure or contrast-induced nephropathy risks. In addition, MRA of the lower extremities can evaluate for deep venous thrombosis without additional IV contrast.

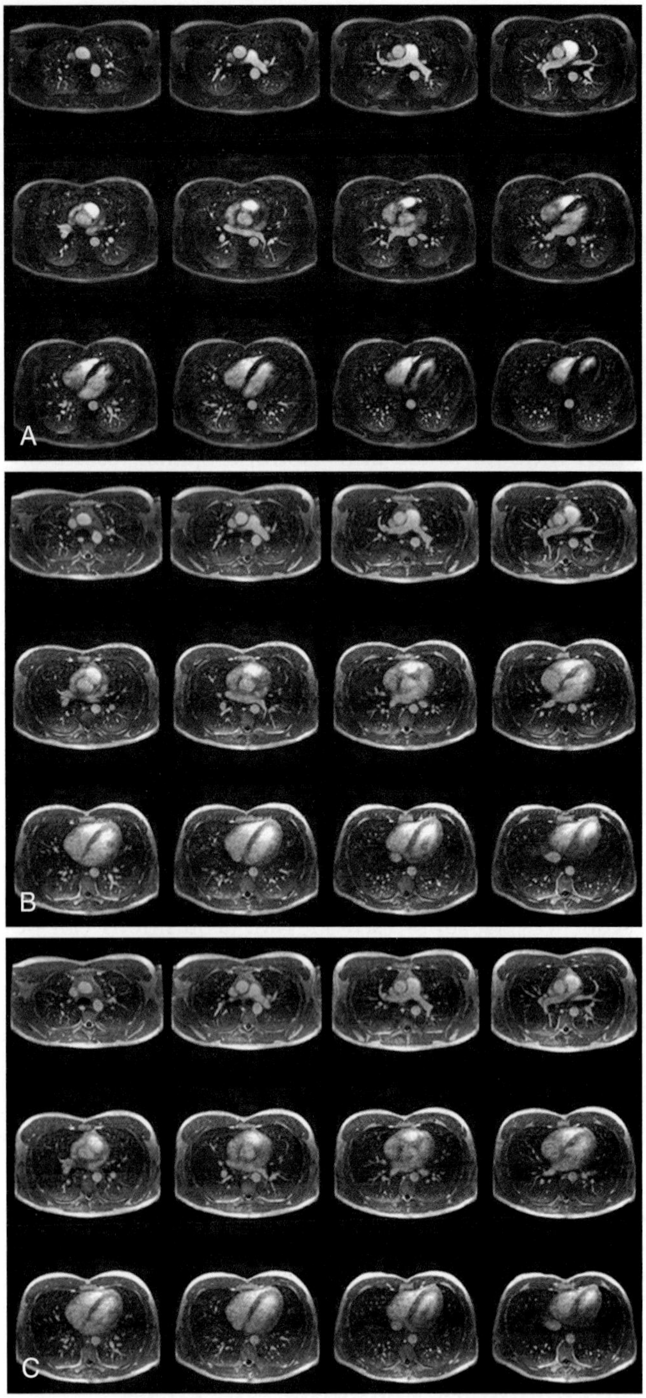

Figure 8.8 A 28-year-old woman with normal pulmonary MRA. Contrast-enhanced pulmonary MRA consisting of (A) arterial, (B) early delayed, and (C) later delayed phase acquisitions. The later delayed phase acquisition uses a lower flip angle to increase contrast between the blood pool and surrounding soft tissues.

MRA for Pulmonary Hypertension

Pulmonary hypertension can arise from a variety of causes and is often evidenced on cross-sectional imaging by a dilated main pulmonary artery (>29 mm). Early investigation of the role of MRI in assessing pulmonary hypertension revealed an increased cine GRE signal in the pulmonary arteries of patients with pulmonary hypertension compared to healthy volunteers. Dilated central pulmonary arteries and attenuation of peripheral branches are also seen (Fig. 8.10). There is loss of systolic normal distention and diastolic collapse in the right pulmonary artery, suggesting decreased pulmonary arterial compliance.

MRA for Vasculitis

MRA can be useful in the evaluation of vasculitis involving the pulmonary arteries. Takayasu arteritis can affect the aorta, aortic branches, and pulmonary arteries. A study evaluating Takayasu arteritis with MRI has shown that 70% had pulmonary arterial abnormalities, including dilation in 17%, thrombus in 3%, and treelike peripheral branching suggesting peripheral occlusive disease in 66%. Behçet disease is caused by an autoimmune vasculitis associated with recurrent oral and genital ulcers, with relapsing uveitis. Vasculitis of the pulmonary arteries is rare but has been seen in 5% of Behçet patients. On MRI, associated pulmonary vasculitis can manifest as thrombosis, pulmonary artery aneurysms, and rupture of aneurysms. T2 fat-saturated imaging is necessary for the evaluation of vasculitis. A high T2 signal in the wall of the vessel suggests edema and active vasculitis.

MRA for Congenital Abnormalities

MRA can also be used to evaluate congenital cardiopulmonary abnormalities (Fig. 8.11), both for diagnosis, preoperative planning, and postoperative follow-up. Although standard dynamic postcontrast MRA will offer overall anatomic evaluation, time-resolved 3D MRA can offer more sensitive evaluation of vascular anomalies and flow patterns. Evaluation of total and partial anomalous pulmonary venous connections also benefits from time-resolved 3D MRA through its ability to show the sequence of vessel filling and directionality of flow.

Tetralogy of Fallot (TOF) patients routinely undergo surgical correction early in life, relief of right ventricular (RV) outflow tract obstruction, ventricular septal defect closure, pulmonary valve repair, and RV outflow patch. Monitoring of these repaired TOF patients relies heavily on ventricular volumetrics. Flow quantification using phase contrast MRI allows shunt fraction calculation, in which pulmonary flow in the main pulmonary artery is divided by systemic flow in the aortic root (Qp:Qs). Pulmonic regurgitant fraction can also be calculated from phase contrast data. In addition, newer four-dimensional (4D) flow techniques are available, in which a time-resolved 3D volume of phase contrast data is acquired over the cardiac cycle, allowing flow through any arbitrary plane to be measured retrospectively.

Evidence Supporting the Use of MRA in These Indications

A 2006 study by Kluge et al. with 62 subjects compared three MRI sequences (real-time balanced steady-state free precession [bSSFP], contrast-enhanced MRA, and MRI perfusion) with CTA for the detection of PE. They found that per patient sensitivities were 77%–100% and specificities were 91%–100% for PE evaluation, depending on

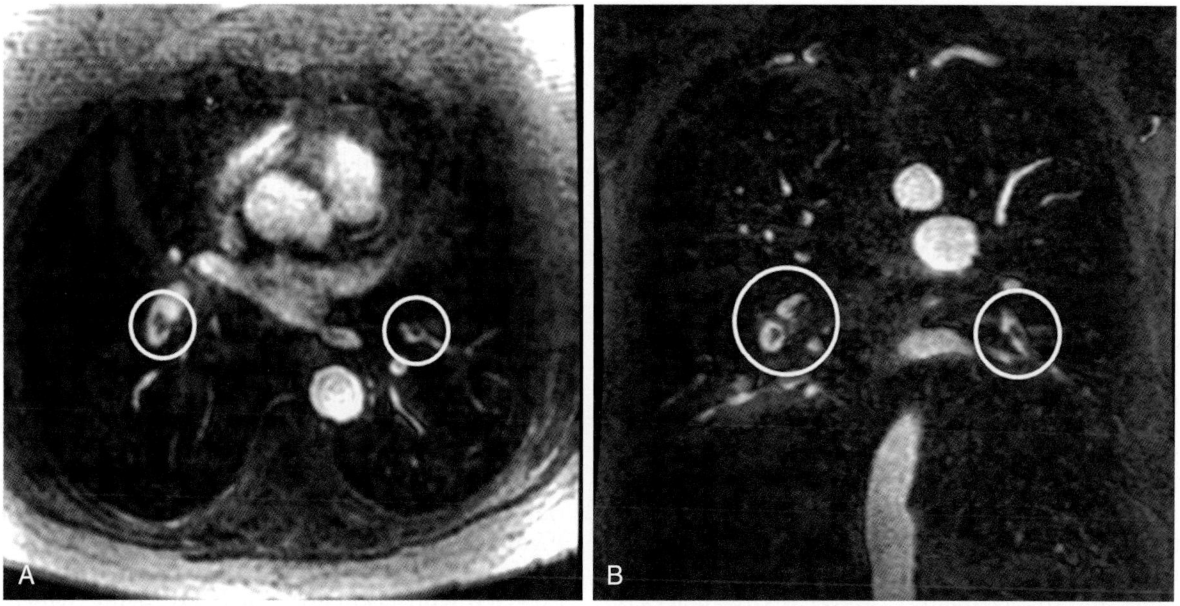

Figure 8.9 A 67-year-old woman with bilateral lower lobe segmental pulmonary emboli *(circles)*. (A) Axial and (B) coronal reformatted images from contrast-enhanced MRA.

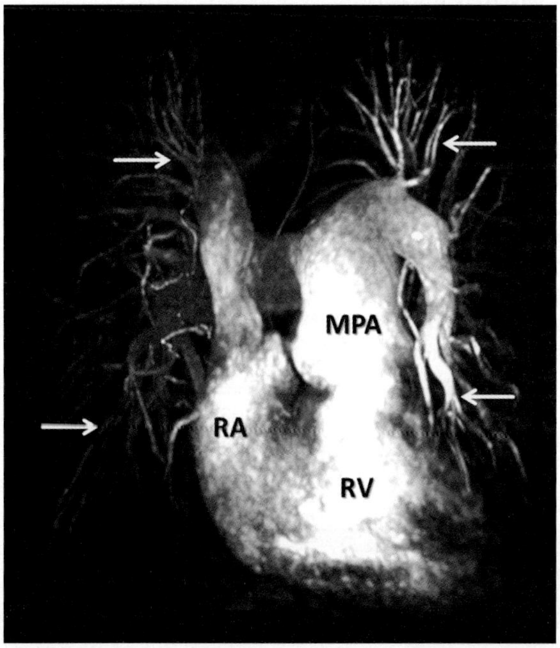

Figure 8.10 A 32-year-old woman with pulmonary arterial hypertension. Maximum intensity projection image from MRA shows typical features of pulmonary arterial hypertension, included a dilated main pulmonary artery *(MPA)*, with pruning of the branch pulmonary arteries *(arrows)*. *RA*, Right atrium; *RV*, right ventricle.

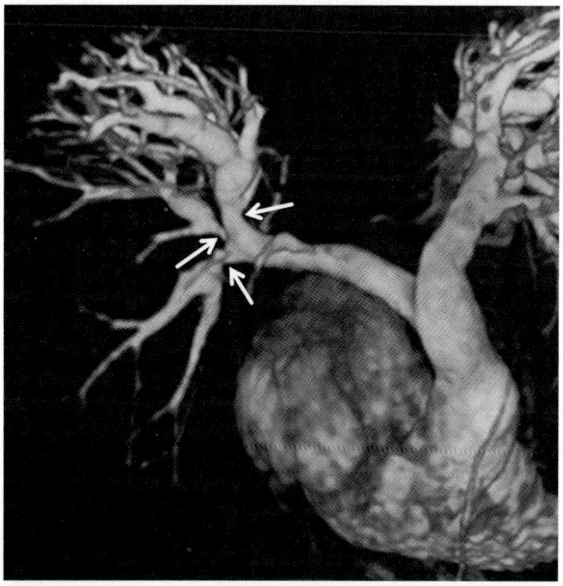

Figure 8.11 A 28-year-old man with Alagille syndrome. MRA of the pulmonary arteries reveals multiple branch pulmonary artery stenoses *(arrows)*.

the sequence. A 2012 study from Kalb et al. has reported that combining respiratory-triggered bSSFP, contrast-enhanced MRA, and steady-state GRE imaging offers the greatest sensitivity for PE evaluation. Ohno et al. have suggested that dynamic MRI perfusion has a higher accuracy in assessing disease severity and predicting clinical outcomes than either MRA or CTA.

PIOPED II reported the sensitivity and specificity of contrast-enhanced MRA in the detection of PE as 78% and 99%, respectively. When combined with lower extremity MRI venography, sensitivity was increased to 92%. It was reported that 25% of the MRA examinations were considered technically inadequate. Based on this, the authors recommended that pulmonary MRA should be considered only at institutions that can perform the examination well and when CTA is contraindicated.

Schiebler et al. have retrospectively evaluated the 1-year incidence of thromboembolism following contrast-enhanced MRA for PE evaluation in 190 patients. They reported a negative predictive value of MRA for PE of 97% at 3 months and 96% at 1-year follow-up.

Mediastinal MRI

When to Use MRI for the Evaluation of Mediastinal Lesions

MRI demonstrates excellent soft tissue contrast when compared to CT, despite the higher spatial resolution of CT. The margins of a lesion can be confidently identified with MRI (Figs. 8.12 and 8.13), which can affect resectability and surgical planning. MRI is particularly useful in depicting the amount of intraspinal extension of a lesion. MRI offers excellent identification of pericardial masses and can distinguish potential pericardial fluid and soft tissue boundaries better than CT. MRI can confirm the cystic nature of lesions that have a solid appearance on CT. MRI also allows evaluation of vessels and vascular invasion in patients who cannot receive iodinated contrast. In addition, double- and triple-inversion recovery techniques can be used to evaluate the epicardial and pericardial fat planes and involvement. However, disadvantages of MRI compared to CT include the decreased ability to demonstrate calcification and the relatively decreased spatial resolution.

MRI is effective in evaluating anterior mediastinal lesions, including thymic cysts (Figs. 8.14 and 8.15) and neoplasms (Figs. 8.16 and 8.17). Although CT is the primary modality for the evaluation of anterior mediastinal lesions, MRI offers specific benefits in thymic evaluation. MRI is superior in differentiating cystic and solid lesions (see Figs. 8.14 to 8.17) compared to CT, and MRI offers chemical shift imaging to detect interspersed fat that is found in the normal thymus. The normal thymus achieves its maximal mass between 12 and 19 years. After this, it slowly involutes until it is mostly fatty by age 40 and completely fatty by age 60 years. Early in life, the thymus appears as a soft tissue mass with convex contours. These contours straighten throughout puberty and eventually become concave before involuting completely later in life. The MR signal of normal thymus reflects this slow fatty replacement process with gradually increasing T1 and T2 signals toward that of fat throughout life. During the involution process, reticulonodular strands or small rounded islands (≤7 mm) of residual thymic tissue are considered normal. Thymic hyperplasia should have signal characteristics of normal thymic tissue but may differ in thymic configuration. For example, soft tissue lobulations, convex contour after age 19 years, excessive thickness more than 1.3 cm after age 20 years, or rounded nodules more than 7 mm all suggest hyperplasia. In addition, certain diagnoses are associated with thymic hyperplasia, including hyperthyroidism, Graves disease (Fig. 8.18), acromegaly, Addison disease, and thyroid malignancies. Recent chemotherapy, steroids, or surgery can be a cause for rebound thymic hyperplasia.

Inaoka et al. (2007) have suggested that in-phase and out-of-phase GRE imaging can differentiate normal thymus and thymic hyperplasia from thymic neoplasms. Uniform signal suppression on out-of-phase imaging is expected with normal thymus and thymic hyperplasia due to interspersed fat, whereas thymic neoplasms do not contain fat and therefore do not suppress. Inversion recovery (black blood) imaging can be helpful in evaluating vascular invasion.

Thymomas demonstrate low to intermediate T1 and high T2 signals and demonstrate homogenous enhancement. Fat-saturated T2 sequences can differentiate a thymoma from adjacent mediastinal fat. Hemorrhage within the lesion may also focally alter T1 and T2 signals based on chronicity. Thymomas can have internal cystic changes with necrosis, fibrous septa, and nodularity. Sadohara et al. (2006) have shown that lower risk thymomas tend to have a complete capsule and septum with homogenous postcontrast enhancement, whereas higher risk thymic carcinomas present with necrosis, cystic components, irregular margins, and heterogeneous enhancement.

MRI provides a comprehensive evaluation of the pericardium and pericardial lesions. With the combination

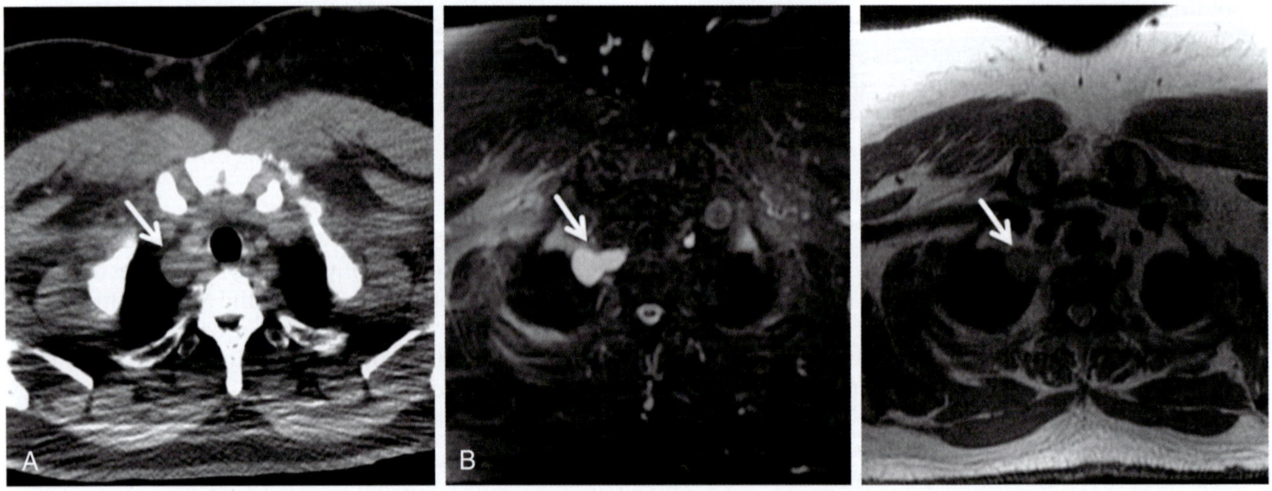

Figure 8.12 A 43-year-old man with duplication cyst in upper mediastinum. (A) CT. (B) T2 with fat saturation. (C) T1 without fat saturation. Shown is a well-circumscribed hyperintense T2 and intermediate-intensity T1 lesion in the anterior mediastinum *(arrows)*.

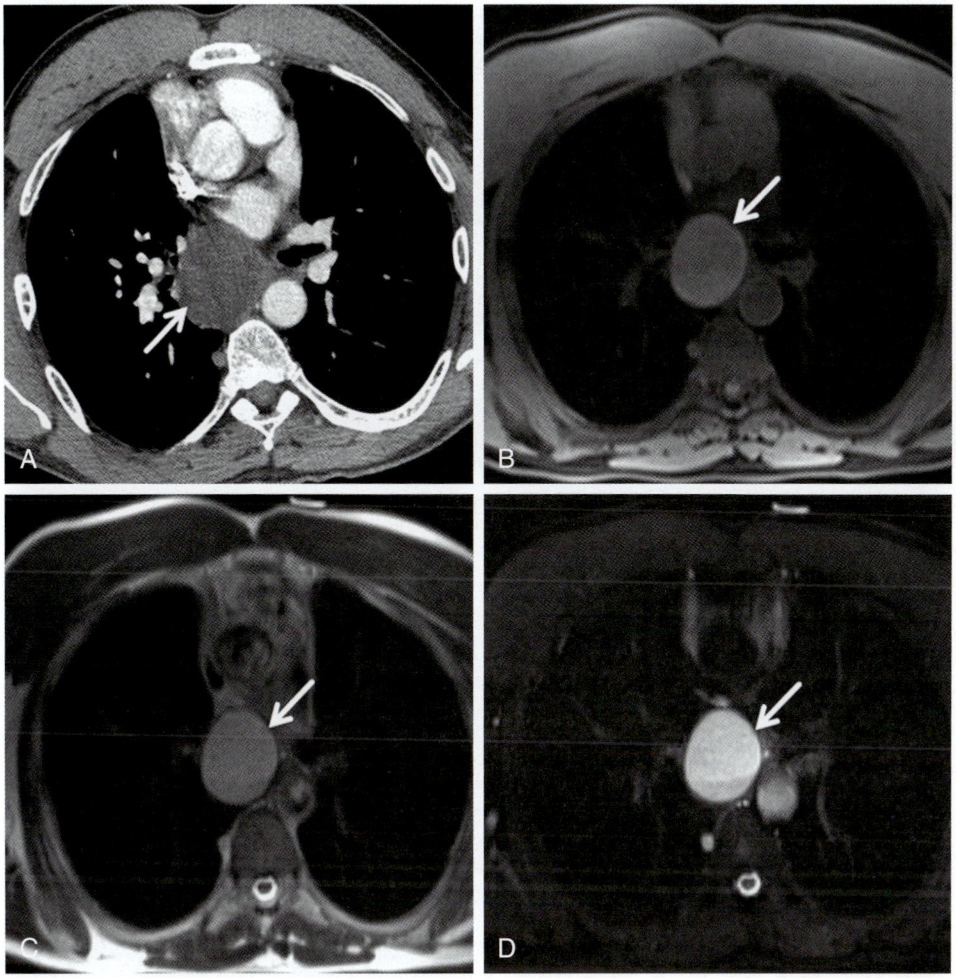

Figure 8.13 A 57-year-old man with enteric duplication cyst. (A) Contrast-enhanced CT. (B) T1 with fat saturation. (C) T2 without fat saturation. (D) T2 with fat saturation. Shown is a well-circumscribed hyperintense T2 and intermediate-intensity T1 lesion in the anterior mediastinum *(arrows)*.

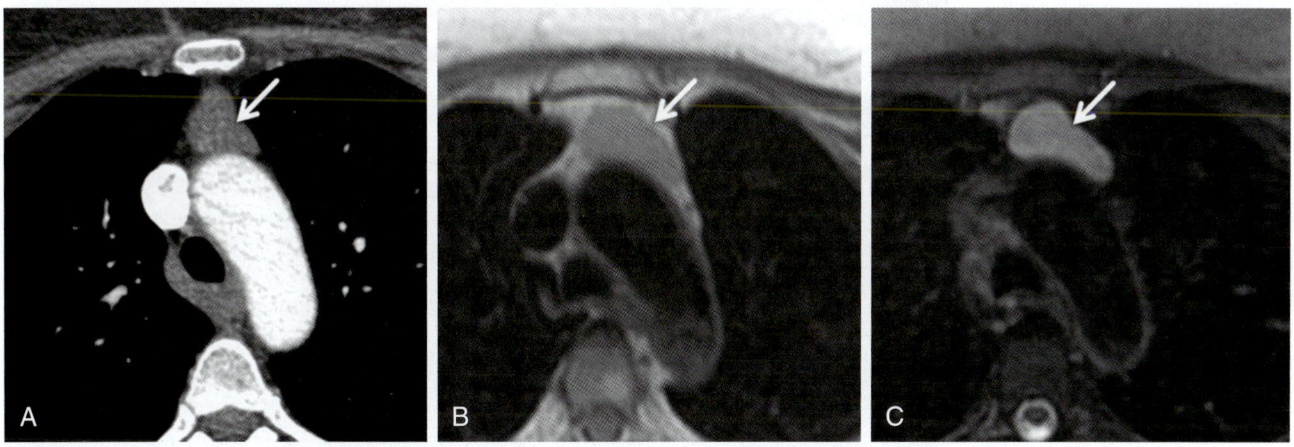

Figure 8.14 A 63-year-old man with a thymic cyst. (A) Contrast-enhanced CT. (B) T1 without fat saturation. (C) T1 with fat saturation. Shown is a well-circumscribed hyperintense T2 and intermediate-intensity T1 lesion in anterior mediastinum *(arrows)*.

of T1, T2, and cine GRE sequences, MRI demonstrates superior characterization of pericardial effusion and masses. Normal pericardium appears as a thin intermediate T1 and low T2 structure that is easily identified over the right atrium and ventricle in most individuals. The pericardium often is not visible over the lateral and posterior walls of the left ventricle, and the left atrium is only partially covered by pericardium. The pericardium is more easily distinguished during end-systole on cine imaging. In the setting of acute inflammation, the

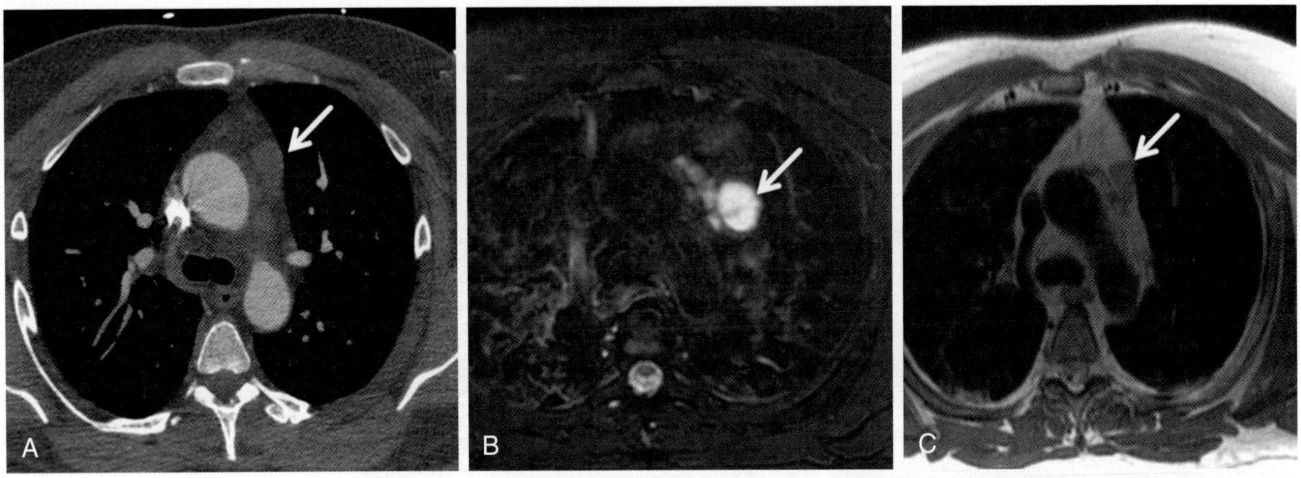

Figure 8.15 A 44-year-old man with a thymic cyst. (A) Contrast-enhanced CT. (B) T2 with fat saturation. (C) T1 without fat saturation. Shown is a well-circumscribed hyperintense T2 and intermediate intensity T1 lesion in anterior mediastinum *(arrows)*.

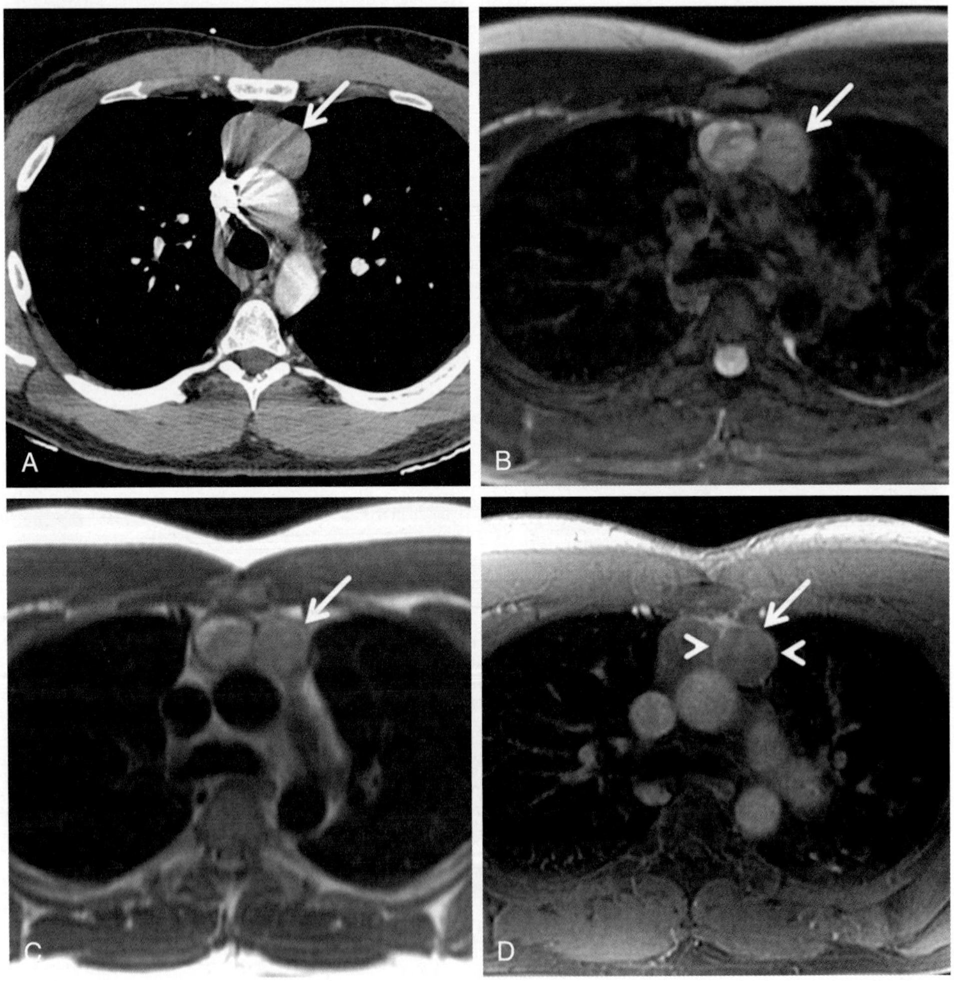

Figure 8.16 A 26-year-old man with thymoma *(arrows)*. (A) Axial CT. (B) Axial T2 with fat saturation. (C) Axial T1 without fat saturation. (D) Axial T1 with fat saturation after intravenous contrast administration. The thymoma is very hyperintense on T2 and mildly hyperintense on T1 and has enhancing septations and walls after the administration of contrast *(arrowheads)*.

pericardium demonstrates thickening of both pericardial layers, with high T2 signal and postcontrast enhancement. The pericardium can also become obscured by chemical shift and cancellation artifacts.

MRI is appropriate when echocardiography is indeterminate or in the setting of pericardial masses, complex pericardial effusion, or pericardial thickening. Congenital pericardial cysts typically have smooth walls without internal septa and will demonstrate homogenous low to intermediate T1 and high T2 signals without enhancement. Pericardial hematomas demonstrate signal related to the chronicity of blood. Primary pericardial neoplasms are

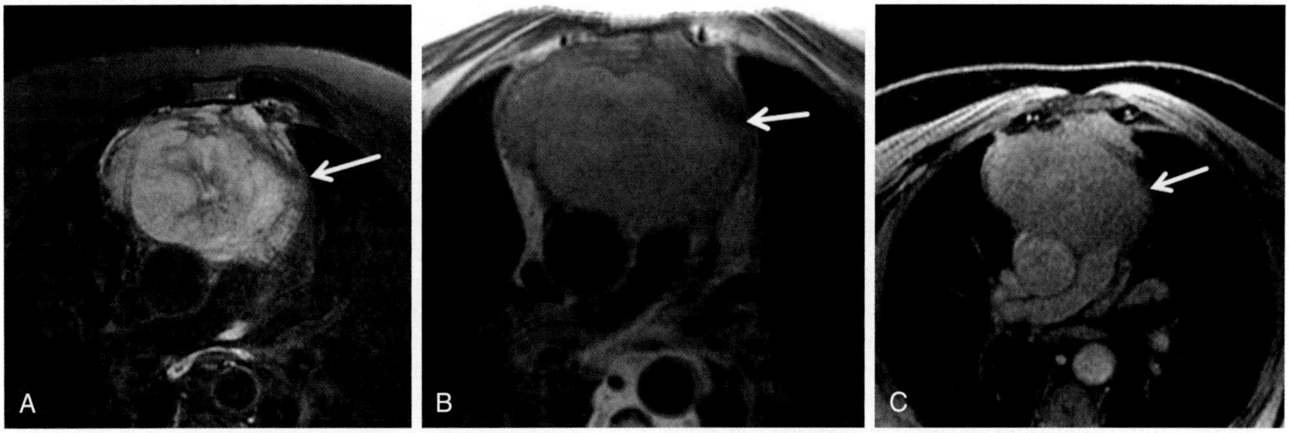

Figure 8.17 A 68-year-old man with thymic carcinoid *(arrows)*. (A) Axial T2 with fat saturation. (B) Axial T1 without fat saturation. (C) Axial T1 with fat saturation after intravenous contrast administration images reveal an anterior mediastinal mass that is heterogeneously hyperintense on T2, mildly hyperintense on T1, and diffusely enhancing *(arrows)*.

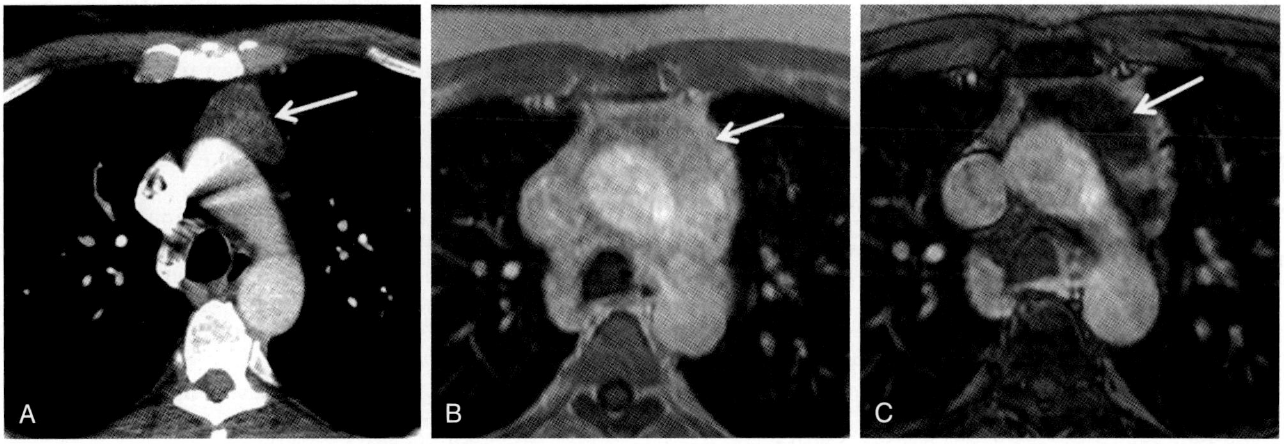

Figure 8.18 A 51-year-old woman with Graves disease and thymic hyperplasia. (A) CT chest scan with IV contrast. (B) Axial in-phase image. (C) Axial out-of-phase images. These reveal a well-circumscribed anterior mediastinal mass *(arrows)* that has abundant macroscopic fat evident on the out-of-phase images (C).

rarer but include both benign and malignant entities. Relatively common benign masses include lipoma, teratoma, fibroma, and hemangioma; malignant masses include mesothelioma, lymphoma, sarcoma, and liposarcomas.

In the acute setting, pericardial effusions are often evaluated with echocardiography; however, MRI can provide more advanced characterization. When a pericardial effusion is secondary to malignancy, irregular thickening of the pericardium with pericardial nodularity can be expected. Metastases tend to have low T1 and high T2 signals with enhancement, except in the setting of melanoma, where hyperintense T1 signal would be expected due to melanin. Cardiac tamponade can result from a large pericardial effusion and is characterized by early diastolic collapse of the right ventricular free wall, late diastolic right atrial inversion, swinging heart, abnormal ventricular septal motion, and respiratory variation in chamber size.

Imaging of the mediastinum, especially between the carina and diaphragm, relies heavily on cardiac gating to image around the beating heart and minimize cardiac motion artifacts; thus arrhythmias may cause significant artifacts. In addition, cardiac involvement of a mediastinal mass can be demonstrated using cine tagged images. Cine tagged images are obtained using RF prepulses that selectively null signal in a specified pattern (parallel lines or grid). During motion, the tissues move, and nulled lines deform following the motion of the tissue. The lack of shearing at the interfaces implies adherence or invasion. At the normal mediastinal pericardial interface, clean shearing of tag lines would be expected, and this finding would rule out invasion in the setting of a mediastinal mass abutting the pericardium.

Finally, MRI does not require ionization radiation, unlike CT. This is of particular importance for pediatric patients. Noncardiovascular mediastinal MRI in pediatric populations is primarily focused on anterior mediastinal mass imaging, congenital malformations, and posterior mediastinal lesions.

Sequences Used to Evaluate the Mediastinum

Multiplanar T1 and T2 fat-suppressed, spin-echo imaging allows for the basic assessment of soft tissue abnormalities in the mediastinum. However, these sequences can be limited in the lower mediastinum and perivascular regions due to cardiac and vascular pulsation artifacts; these can be reduced by applying cardiac gating. Respiratory triggering applied to the longer T2 sequences also reduces motion artifact. Inversion recovery sequences with cardiac gating offer excellent soft tissue contrast, with suppression of signal from the blood pool (double inversion) and epicardial and mediastinal fat (triple inversion). Depending on the clinical imaging question, additional sequences can be added, such as MRA or phase contrast imaging for vascular abnormalities. In-phase and out-of-phase GRE imaging can be helpful in thymic evaluation to assess for interspersed fat in the normal or hyperplastic thymus. IV gadolinium contrast may also be used to characterize mediastinal lesions further. In addition, if there is concern that a mass invades the pericardium, cine tagged imaging can be applied to assess for invasion or adhesions.

■ Chest Wall MRI

Sequences Used to Evaluate Chest Wall Lesions

MRI evaluation of the chest wall (Fig. 8.19) includes multiplanar T1 and T2 fat saturation with respiratory triggering and T1 fat-saturated pre- and postcontrast evaluation. T1 sequences demonstrate bright blood signal and allow for excellent evaluation of vascular encasement or vascular invasion. T2 sequences are suited for characterizing specific lesions and areas of cystic degeneration, inflammation, and edema. STIR imaging may be useful if an osseous lesion or osseous involvement is suspected, in which mild marrow edema may become more evident. Fat suppression preparation pulses are useful to confirm the presence of fat within lesions (Fig. 8.20).

Diffusion-weighted imaging may be added to the examination if primary lesion characterization is needed (e.g., chest wall metastasis vs. benign nodule). In addition, if there is a question of mediastinal adherence or extension of a chest wall mass, cine tagging can also be applied.

The multiplanar nature of MRI allows imaging in arbitrary user-defined planes, which provides an advantage over CT in the assessment of complex regions such as the lung apices, diaphragms, and spinal column.

When to Use MRI for the Evaluation of Chest Wall Pathology

MRI is the imaging modality of choice to demonstrate the extent of chest wall invasion by primary lung cancer or similar invasion of the chest wall by infection (Fig. 8.21), including actinomycosis. In addition, the extent of thoracic invasion of primary chest wall masses, such as the neuroectodermal Askin tumor, are well visualized on MR. A T1 postcontrast sequence delineates tumor margins and is helpful in planning for biopsy or mass resection.

MRI excels in the imaging of paraspinal lesions. The craniocaudal extent of disease can be made clearly evident using multiplanar imaging, and extension into the spinal canal can be delineated on T1 and T2 sequences. Although CT offers better visualization of cortical bone destruction, bone marrow involvement by tumor is more sensitively characterized by MR. The extent of vertebral body invasion is well defined by edema-like marrow signal changes, whereas on CT poorly defined cortical destruction may be the only evidence of a vertebral lesion. CT may also suffer from beam-hardening artifact produced by the high-attenuation spinal column, which is not present

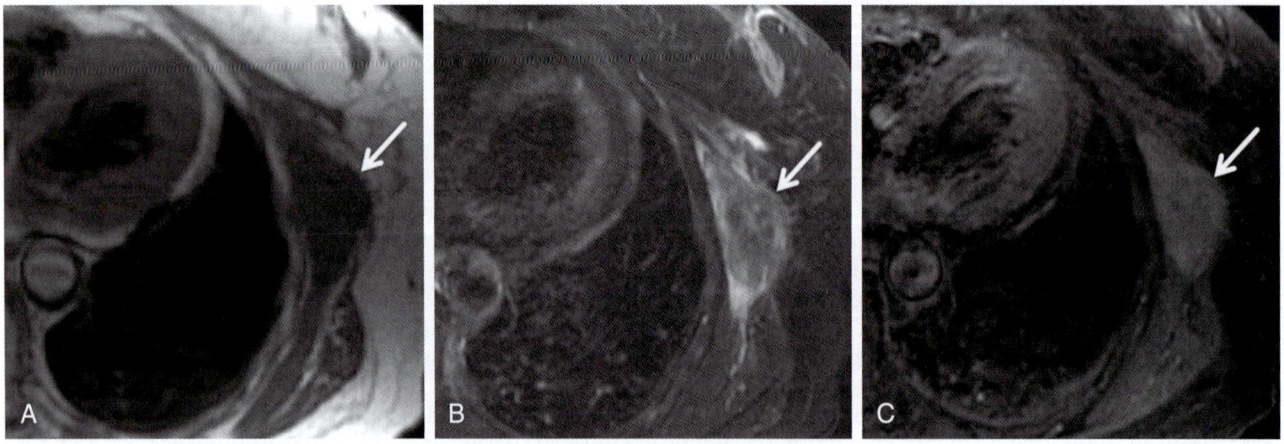

Figure 8.19 A 71-year-old woman with undifferentiated pleomorphic sarcoma of the left chest wall *(arrows)*. (A) T1 fast spin echo without fat saturation. (B) T1 fast spin echo with fat saturation after contrast administration. (C) T2 fast spin echo with fat saturation. The mass is isointense to skeletal muscle on T1-weighted images precontrast, enhances heterogeneously, and is heterogeneously hyperintense to skeletal muscle on T2-weighted images.

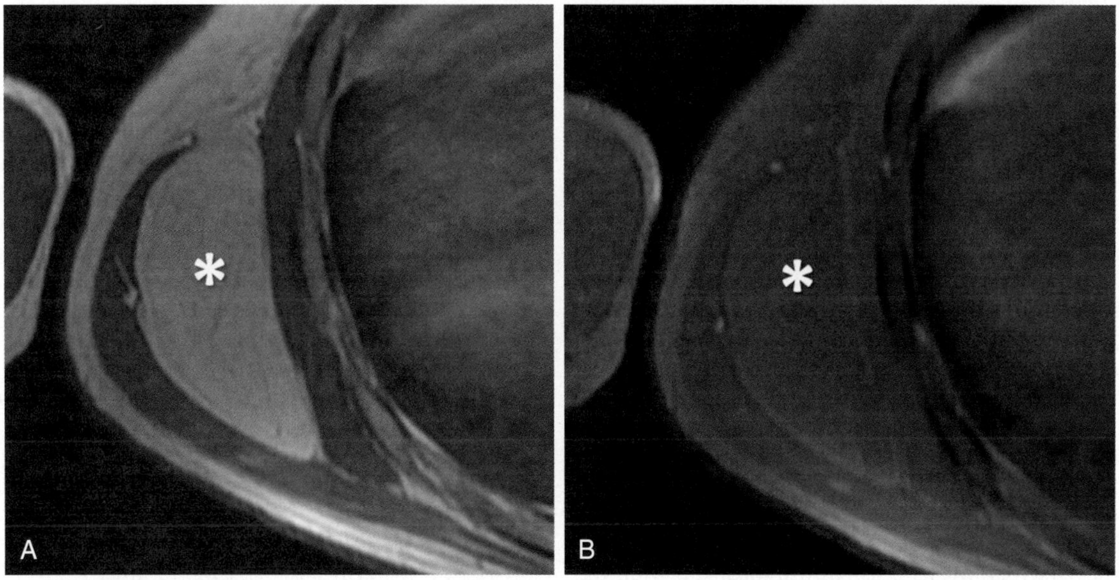

Figure 8.20 A 56-year-old woman with simple lipoma in the right latissimus dorsi muscle. (A) T1 without fat saturation. (B) T1 with fat saturation. These images reveal a well-circumscribed, homogenous mass *(asterisks)* that is isointense to fat signal.

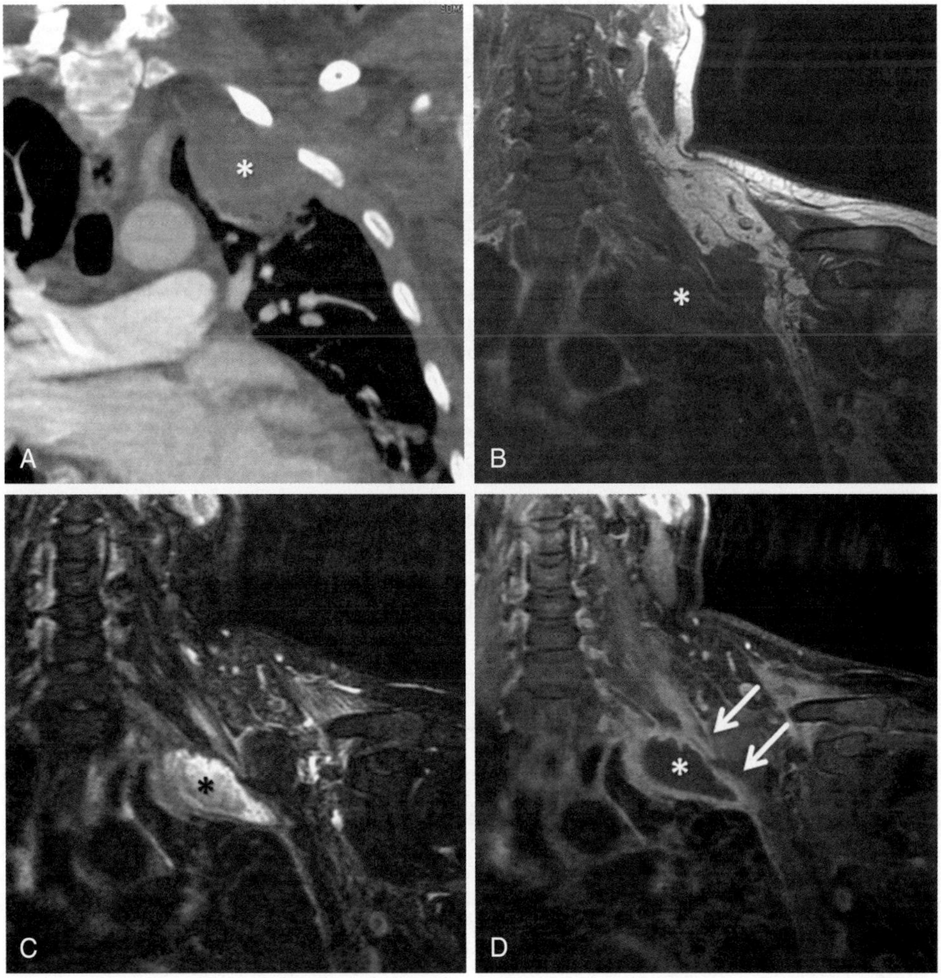

Figure 8.21 A 40-year-old man with lung abscess *(asterisks)* and chest wall invasion. (A) Contrast-enhanced CT. (B) T1 without fat saturation. (C) T2 with fat saturation. (D) T1 with fat saturation postcontrast administration. The abscess is hyperintense on T2-weighted imaging and hypointense on T1-weighted imaging. Postcontrast T1-weighted images reveal extension of the abscess into the chest wall, in between the ribs *(arrows)* and along the brachial plexus.

in MRI. Similar benefits are seen in the imaging of rib lesions. Rib lesions on CT may only be evident by subtle cortical destruction, whereas the edema pattern on MRI is often much more obvious. Some of the pathologic conditions for which MRI is useful are highlighted below.

Benign Chest Wall Disease

Lipomas are the most common benign soft tissue lesion involving the chest wall (see Fig. 8.20). On MRI, lipomas will demonstrate homogenous high T1 and T2 signals and may contain several hypointense internal fibrous septations. A markedly heterogenous fat signal or regions of enhancing soft tissue within the fatty mass should raise suspicion for liposarcoma. MRI can assist with surgical planning for symptomatic lipomas that infiltrate the chest wall or have proximity to neurovascular structures.

Costochondritis (Tietze syndrome) is a benign inflammatory process involving one or more of the costochondral cartilages which presents as painful localized swelling of the costochondral, costosternal, and/or sternoclavicular joints. On MRI, there is no discrete mass at the site of the complaint but there is enlargement and thickening of hyaline cartilage presenting as avidly enhancing thickened low T1 and increased T2 signals. Underlying bone marrow edema can be seen in the subchondral bone of the involved cartilage. In most cases, a single level of costal cartilage is involved, most commonly the second or third rib level.

Malignant Chest Wall Masses

Lung cancer spread to the chest wall can be well evaluated on MRI (see Figs. 8.4 and 8.5). MRI demonstrates tumor infiltration of extrapleural fat and chest wall muscles better than CT. In chest wall invasion, MRI shows loss of the normal T1 hyperintense extrapleural fat with disruption of soft tissue planes and T2 hyperintensity replacing the normal muscle signal. However, T2 hyperintensity can also be seen with inflammation or edema. Breast carcinomas may be seen on chest MRI but would warrant dedicated breast imaging evaluation and possibly breast protocol MRI. Desmoid tumors, classified as low-grade fibrosarcomas, can have locally aggressive behavior. On MRI, desmoid tumors show isointense to a muscle T1 signal and variable T2 signal and variable enhancement.

Masses arising from osseous structures of the chest can also invade the chest wall. Metastasis and multiple myeloma account for the most common causes of chest wall masses with an associated destructive rib lesion. Primary chest wall neoplasms include osteosarcoma, fibrosarcoma, chondrosarcoma, and osteochondroma (see Fig. 8.19). Askin's tumor and Ewing's sarcoma are uncommon masses but can also present in the chest with bony destruction.

Askin's tumor is a neuroectodermal neoplasm that presents as a chest wall or paravertebral lesion in young adults. On MRI, a soft tissue mass is present with associated bony erosions. T1 hyperintensity to skeletal muscle and T2 hyperintensity are common, with heterogeneity of signal due to hemorrhage and necrosis.

Ewing's sarcoma is most common in adolescent boys and presents as a rapidly enlarging and painful mass. Although it usually arises in the diaphysis or metadiaphysis of long bones in the younger age group (first and early second decades), Ewing's sarcoma can also arise in the scapula and chest wall bones, usually in an older age group (late second and third decades). On MRI, Ewing's sarcoma presents with a mass arising from bone, with a T1 signal hypoisointense to muscle, heterogenous hyperintensity on fluid-sensitive sequences, and heterogenous enhancement. Permeative osseous destruction and marrow edema are also expected.

Chest Wall Infections

Patients with diabetes mellitus, history of surgery or trauma, and immunocompromised status are at increased risk for chest wall infections, which are rare but can have high morbidity and potential mortality. With the benefit of coronal and sagittal imaging, MRI can delineate the extent of soft tissue infection, even without IV contrast. However, IV contrast will increase diagnostic specificity. Abscesses will present as low T1 and high T2 signal collections with peripheral enhancement. However, CT offers more sensitive detection of gas in these collections. Osteomyelitis of bony structures of the chest is best imaged with MRI. MRI will demonstrate a low T1 and high T2 or STIR marrow edema pattern with focal enhancement.

MRI can be complementary to CT in evaluating pleural disease. Pleural lipomas are typically located in the lateral pleura and will show signal-matching subcutaneous fat on all sequences. Fibrous tumors of the pleura occur later in life and demonstrate T1 signal that is isointense to muscle and high T2 signal with postcontrast enhancement (see Fig. 8.6). Mesothelioma often presents with unilateral nodular pleural thickening, with an associated pleural effusion. The tumor can be diffuse and encase the lung, with extent into fissures. On MRI, there is mildly increased T1 and moderately increased T2 signals. Metastases are the most common tumor involving the pleura, and lung, breast, gastric, and ovarian carcinomas are the common primary sites of primary disease.

Evidence Supporting the Use of MRI in These Indications

Many studies have shown the utility of diffusion-weighted imaging in characterizing lesions and lymph nodes. The mean apparent diffusion coefficient (ADC) has been shown to be lower in malignant tumors than in benign masses. In addition, malignant lymph nodes demonstrate lower ADC values than benign lymph nodes; however, tuberculous lymphadenopathy has also been also shown to demonstrate low ADC values.

Bibliography

LUNG MRI

Attenberger UI, Morelli JN, Henzler T, et al. 3 tesla proton MRI for the diagnosis of pneumonia/lung infiltrates in neutropenic patients with acute myeloid leukemia: initial results in comparison to HRCT. *Eur J Radiol*. 2014;83(1):e61–e66.

Bell LC, Johnson KM, Fain SB, et al. Simultaneous MRI of lung structure and perfusion in a single breathhold. *J Magn Reson Imaging*. 2015;41(1):52–59.
Bell LC, Wang K, Munoz Del Rio A, Grist TM, Fain SB, Nagle SK. Comparison of models and contrast agents for improved signal and signal linearity in dynamic contrast-enhanced pulmonary magnetic resonance imaging. *Invest Radiol*. 2015;50(3):174–178.
Fain SB. Functional lung imaging using hyperpolarized gas MRI. *J Magn Reson Imaging*. 2007;25:910–923.
Fain S, Schiebler ML, McCormack DG, Parraga G. Imaging of lung function using hyperpolarized helium-3 magnetic resonance imaging: review of current and emerging translational methods and applications. *J Magn Reson Imaging*. 2010;32(6):1389–1408.
Fujimoto K. Usefulness of contrast-enhanced magnetic resonance imaging for evaluating solitary pulmonary nodules. *Cancer Imaging*. 2008;8:36–44.
Hatabu H, Stock KW, Sher S, et al. Magnetic resonance imaging of the thorax. *Clin Chest Med*. 1999;4:775–803.
Koenigkam-Santos M, Optazaite E, Sommer G, et al. Contrast-enhanced magnetic resonance imaging of pulmonary lesions: description of a technique aiming clinical practice. *Eur J Radiol*. 2015;84(1):185–192.
Li B, Li Q, Chen C, et al. A systematic review and meta-analysis of the accuracy of diffusion-weighted MRI in the detection of malignant pulmonary nodules and masses. *Acad Radiol*. 2014;21(1):21–29.
Lilburn DM, Pavlovskaya GE, Meersmann T. Perspectives of hyperpolarized noble gas MRI beyond 3He. *J Magn Reson*. 2013;229:173–186.
Webb WR, Gatsonis C, Zerhouni EA, et al. CT and MRI imaging of staging non-small cell bronchogenic carcinoma: report of the radiologicl diagnostic oncology group. *Radiology*. 1991;178:705.
Xia Y, Guan Y, Fan L, et al. Dynamic contrast enhanced magnetic resonance perfusion imaging in high-risk smokers and smoking-related COPD: correlations with pulmonary function tests and quantitative computed tomography. *COPD*. 2014;11:510–520.

PULMONARY MRA

Bannas P, Schiebler ML, Motosugi U, et al. Differentiation of pulmonary embolism from truncation artefact. *Eur Radiol*. 2014;24(8):1942–1949.
Kalb B, Sharma P, Tigges S, et al. MRI imaging of pulmonary embolism: diagnostic accuracy of contrast-enhanced 3D MRI pulmonary angiography, contrast-enhanced low-flip angle 3D GRE, and nonenhanced free-induction FISP sequences. *Radiology*. 2012;263(1):271–278.
Kluge A, Mueller C, Strunk J, et al. Experience in 207 combined MRI examinations for acute pulmonary embolism and deep vein thrombosis. *Am J Roentgenol*. 2006;186(6):1686–1696.
Ohno Y, Koyama H, Matsumoto K, et al. Dynamic MRI perfusion imaging: capability for quantitative assessment of disease extent and prediction of outcome for patients with acute pulmonary thromboembolism. *J Magn Reson Imaging*. 2010;31(5):1081–1090.
Schiebler ML, Nagle SK, Francois CJ, et al. Effectiveness of MR angiography for the primary diagnosis of acute pulmonary embolism: clinical outcomes at 3 months and 1 year. *J Magn Reson Imaging*. 2013;38(4):914–925.
Stein PD, Chenevert TL, Fowler SE, et al. Gadolinium enhanced magnetic resonance angiography for pulmonary embolism. *Ann Intern Med*. 2010;152:434–443.
Yamada I, Numano F, Suzuki S. Takayasu arteritis: evaluation with MR imaging. *Radiology*. 1993;188:89.

MEDIASTINAL MRI

Ackerman JB, Wu CC. MRI of the thymus. *AJR Am J Roentgenol*. 2011;197:W15–W20.
Inaoka T, Takahashi K, Mineta M, et al. Thymic hyperplasia and thymus gland tumors: differentiation with chemical shift MR imaging. *Radiology*. 2007;243: 869–876.
Sadohara J, Fujimoto K, Muller NL, et al. Thymic epithelial tumors: comparison of CT and MR imaging findings of low-risk thymomas, high-risk thymomas, and thymic carcinomas. *Eur J Radiol*. 2006;60:70–79.
Tamura A, Matsubara O, Yoshimura N, Kasuga T, Akagawa S, Aoki N. Cardiac metastasis of lung cancer: a study of metastatic pathways and clinical manifestations. *Cancer*. 1992;70:437–442.
Wang ZJ, Reddy GP, Gotway MB, et al. CT and MRI imaging of pericardial disease. *Radiographics*. 2003;23:S168–S180.

CHEST WALL MRI

El-Badrary A, Elzaafarany M, Youssef TF, et al. Role of diffusion-weighted MRI imaging in chest wall masses. *Egyptian J Radiol Nuclear Med*. 2011;42:147–151.
Padovani B, Mouroux J, Seksik L, et al. Chest wall invasion by bronchogenic carcinoma: evaluation with MRI imaging. *Radiology*. 1993;187:33.

CHAPTER 9
Cardiac MRI

Rachel Edwards, Gregory A. Kicska, and Guatham P. Reddy

CHAPTER OUTLINE

■ Introduction

Cardiac MRI is a study often used for the evaluation and diagnosis of a wide range of acquired and congenital cardiac abnormalities. Cardiac MRI offers excellent soft tissue contrast that is useful in evaluating cardiac masses and infiltrative diseases of the myocardium. Both ECG and respiratory gating improve temporal resolution, allowing for the detection of cardiac motion abnormalities and evaluation of small structures adjacent to the contracting myocardium, such as the coronary arteries. In addition to the anatomic information provided by cardiac MRI, ventricular function and blood flow can be calculated using cine sequences and velocity-encoded cine (VEC) phase contrast imaging.

■ Basic Cardiac MRI

MRI Pulse Sequences

There are two broad categories of MRI sequences used in cardiac MRI: black blood imaging and bright blood imaging. Black (dark) blood imaging is predominantly used to evaluate anatomy and characterize the T1 and T2 properties of tissue. The sequence is referred to as black blood because double-inversion pulse, fast-flowing blood in the imaged slice appears black. Black blood images can be obtained with spin-echo (SE), turbo spin-echo (TSE), or fast spin-echo (FSE) pulse sequences, with echo and repetition times chosen to create a T1- or T2-weighted image.

Bright blood imaging can be used to evaluate both anatomy and motion, usually myocardial contraction, cardiac valve function, and visualization of stenotic or regurgitant flow jets. The sequence is referred to as bright blood because, in contrast to black blood images, the blood pool is brighter than the myocardium. Bright blood images are usually obtained with balanced steady-state free precession (bSSFP) but can also be obtained with spoiled steady-state free precession (sSSFP).

VEC phase contrast imaging is used to measure the velocity of blood throughout the cardiac cycle. This is usually applied to the aorta and pulmonary arteries, where velocity measurements can be used to calculate net forward flow, regurgitant fraction, peak velocity, and pressure gradient. The pulmonary to systemic blood flow ratio (Qp:Qs) can be calculated using VEC MRI to look for evidence of shunts.

Delayed contrast enhancement (DCE) imaging is used to detect any cause of an expanded extravascular space,

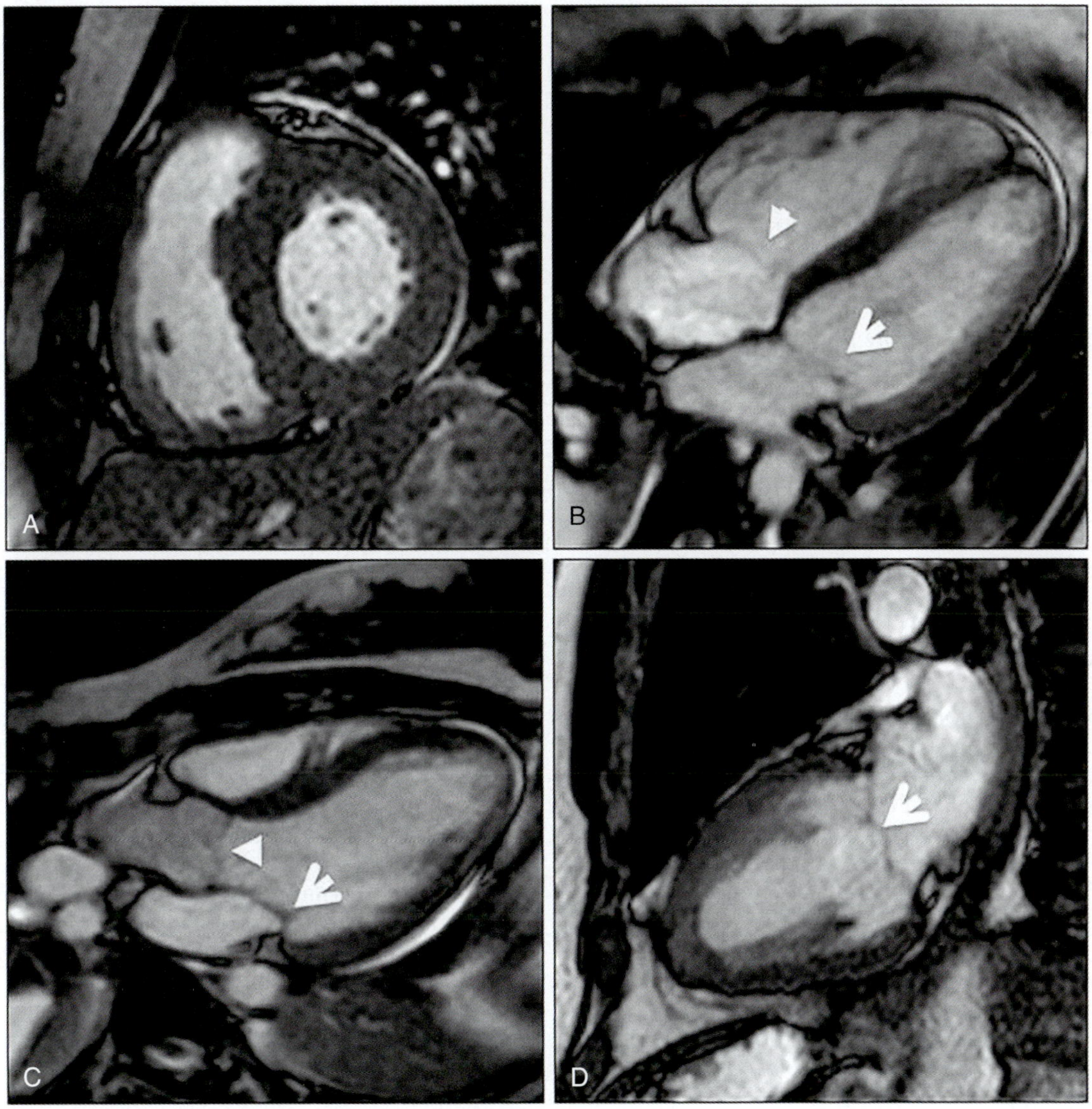

Figure 9.1 Most commonly used planes in cardiac MRI. (A) The short-axis view is primarily used to assess the left ventricle for wall motion abnormalities and calculate function. (B) The four-chamber view is used to assess function of the mitral *(arrow)* and tricuspid *(arrowhead)* valves. (C) The left ventricular outflow tract view is used to assess the aortic *(arrowhead)* and mitral *(arrow)* valves. (D) The vertical long-axis view is used to assess the mitral valve *(arrow)* and left ventricular contraction.

such as myocardial fibrosis in the setting of ischemia and cardiomyopathy or myocyte injury in myocarditis. DCE can also be used to determine if a myocardial mass has a blood supply, which can differentiate thrombus from tumor.

Imaging Planes

The standard cardiac planes are short-axis, four-chamber (horizontal long axis), and vertical long-axis (two-chamber) views. Additional commonly used cardiac planes include the right ventricular outflow tract, left ventricular outflow tract, right horizontal long axis, and an oblique sagittal used for the evaluation of the aortic arch and descending aorta. These planes are illustrated in Fig. 9.1. In respiratory gating, imaging is only performed when the diaphragm is in an acceptable position and the heart is in diastole (Fig. 9.2). In this example, imaging was only possible during the first diastole (gray box), ECG signal (blue line), diaphragm displacement (red line), and acceptable diaphragm position (dotted lines).

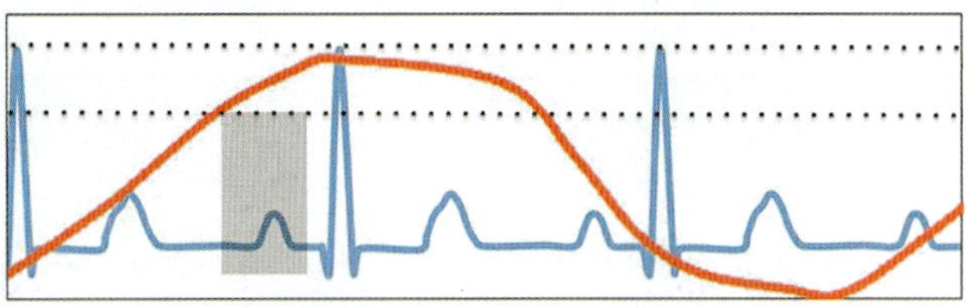

Figure 9.2 In respiratory gating, imaging is only performed when the diaphragm is in an acceptable position, and the heart is in diastole. In this example, imaging was only possible during the first diastole *(gray box)*, ECG signal *(blue line)*, diaphragm displacement *(red line)*, and acceptable diaphragm position *(dotted lines)*.

ECG and Respiratory Gating

ECG gating makes it possible to create cine video clips of cardiac motion throughout the entire cardiac cycle. Alternatively, images can be obtained during preselected segments of the cardiac cycle, most commonly during the R-R interval corresponding to late diastole, when the least amount of cardiac motion is present. Usually, patients are required to hold their breath during the scan.

Respiratory gating is used to compensate for respiratory motion when the patient is breathing freely (see Fig. 9.2). The scanner can use the MR signal to monitor the position of the diaphragm and image only when the diaphragm is in an acceptable location. An alternative approach to respiratory gating uses respiratory bellows, which are devices encircling the abdomen and chest that correlate body wall motion with the phase of respiration.

Common Indications for Cardiac MRI

Ischemic Heart Disease

Cardiac MRI plays an important role in evaluating both acute and chronic myocardial ischemia. Cardiac MRI can be used to evaluate for myocardial edema, myocardial infarction (MI), and wall motion abnormalities. An important characteristic of ischemia is the distribution of the abnormal findings, which should conform to the coronary artery vascular distributions and, in the case of fibrosis, should be subendocardial.

Myocardial edema appears as high signal on T2-weighted black blood sequences. An abnormally high T2 signal can be difficult to perceive; it has been defined as signal that is two standard deviations (SDs) higher than in remote, presumably normal, myocardium. Alternatively, an abnormal T2 signal is defined as two SDs greater than signal in skeletal muscle on the same slice. In the setting of acute MI, the myocardium that has a high T2 signal but no late gadolinium enhancement (LGE) is at risk for future infarction if the blood flow is not restored.

An MI begins in the endocardium and progressively extends outward, toward the epicardium. The pattern of LGE reflects this physiology, with enhancement beginning in the subendocardium and progressing toward the epicardium. As ischemia persists, there is eventual transmural enhancement. The larger the percentage of myocardial wall thickness demonstrating LGE, the less likely that function will be recovered if the patient is revascularized. It is commonly accepted that the myocardium will be unlikely to recover function if more than 50% of its wall thickness shows LGE.

Another imaging feature associated with nonviable myocardium is microvascular obstruction. This occurs in cases of severe MI, in which myocardial capillaries are obstructed due to cellular debris from myocardial necrosis and vessel damage. Because of the microvascular obstruction, gadolinium (Gd) contrast agent cannot penetrate these areas, and they appear dark on LGE images. The imaging hallmark is a dark endocardial region, commonly referred to as a no-reflow zone, surrounded by bright myocardium, which is infarcted (Fig. 9.3).

Wall motion abnormalities are associated with MI and, when they are present in the absence of LGE, they may reflect hibernating myocardium that will recover function following revascularization. Wall motion is reported as normal, hyperkinetic, akinetic, or dyskinetic. Location of the abnormality is commonly reported using the 17-segment heart model nomenclature. Wall motion is best assessed with bright blood cine imaging

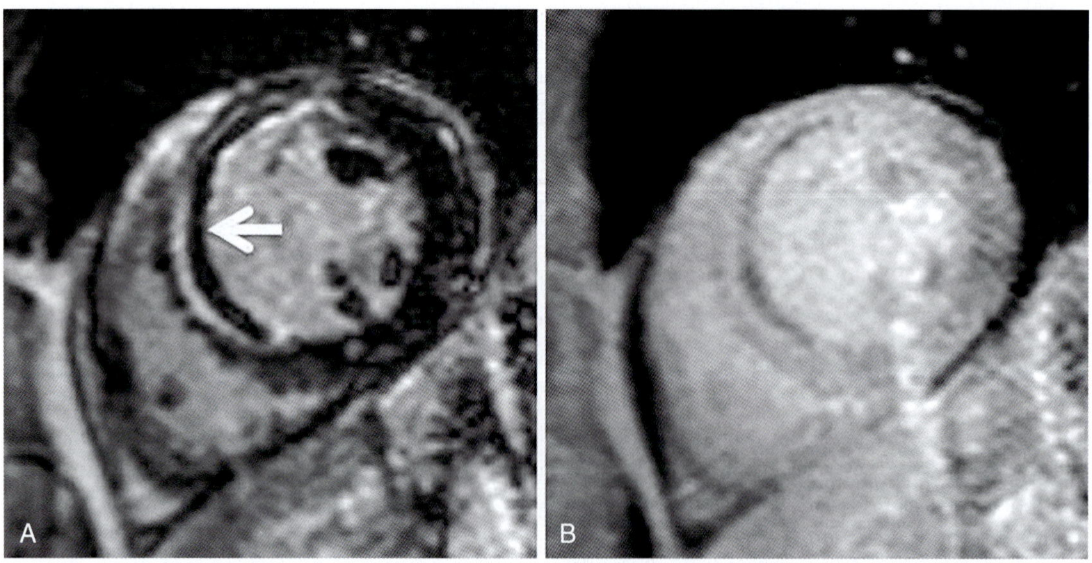

Figure 9.3 Midchamber short-axis magnitude (A) and phase-preserved (B) late gadolinium enhancement images in a patient with a left anterior descending artery distribution infarct. In (A), there is a subendocardial rim of low signal *(arrow)* that indicates a region of microvascular obstruction. The phase-preserved images (B) can be used to increase confidence of this finding, showing that this region has lower signal intensity (longer T1) compared to normal myocardium.

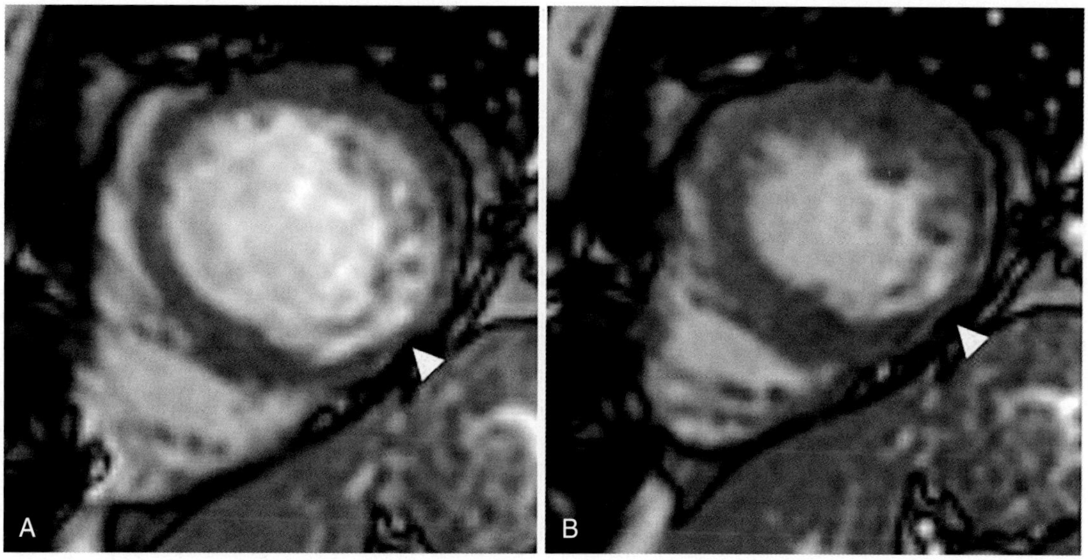

Figure 9.4 Short-axis bright blood cine images during (A) diastole and (B) systole show an akinetic midchamber inferior wall *(arrowheads)*. Note how other portions of the left ventricle increase in thickness from diastole to systole.

(Fig. 9.4). A stack of short-axis images can be inspected for both wall motion and, more importantly, at least 50% wall thickening from diastole to systole. Some centers will routinely apply grid tags as a prepulse sequence so that strain can be measured. More recently, strain has been measured using feature tracking, without the need for tagging.

Cardiac MRI also plays a role in imaging chronic myocardial ischemia. In addition to the findings of myocardial ischemia described above, the presence of myocardial thinning suggests that the ischemia is long-standing. Patients with a hibernating myocardium can be identified as having a wall motion abnormality, with no LGE. These patients are likely to recover function if they are revascularized.

Cardiomyopathy

Cardiac MRI is used to diagnose and evaluate the functional impact of cardiomyopathy (e.g., hypertrophic, arrhythmogenic right ventricular dysplasia [ARVD]). A wide variety of conditions fall into the category of what is referred to as cardiomyopathy, which is a diagnosis of myocardial disease with associated cardiac dysfunction. The types of cardiomyopathy most often imaged and those with characteristic cardiac MRI findings include (1) hypertrophic cardiomyopathy (HCM); (2) ARVD; (3) dilated cardiomyopathy; (4) sarcoidosis; and (5) amyloidosis.

HCM is an autosomal dominant disease of incomplete penetrance. The imaging diagnosis is based predominantly on a left ventricular (LV) wall thickness, 15 mm or more, measured at end-diastole. A septal-to-lateral wall ratio greater than 1.3 is an often-discussed criterion for diagnosis but is not as widely accepted.

Cardiac MRI also provides additional information to assist in risk stratification and determine the treatment plan. HCM patients have an increased risk of arrhythmia if there is LGE in areas of thickened myocardium. A myocardial thickness greater than 30 mm is associated with an increased risk of sudden cardiac death. An LV mass can be calculated using cardiac MRI and is associated with overall risk. HCM has several morphologic subtypes described by the distribution of hypertrophy, including septal, midventricular, apical, and symmetric. Cardiac MRI provides an excellent delineation of myocardial hypertrophy distribution when compared to echocardiography. The septal distribution of HCM can often cause a subaortic stenosis that results in systolic anterior motion (SAM) of the mitral valve leaflet. This effect can be exacerbated by exercise.

ARVD is a progressive disease in which the myocardium is replaced by fibrofatty tissue over time. ARVD is associated with ventricular arrhythmias and sudden cardiac death. Patients are typically diagnosed in adulthood based on a combination of major and minor criteria encompassing imaging characteristics, ECG findings, histopathology, and family history. Cardiac MRI findings are included as major and minor criteria in the diagnostic criteria for ARVD. A regional right ventricular (RV) wall motion abnormality, in combination with a decreased RV ejection fraction or abnormal ratio of RV end-diastolic volume relative to body surface area, can fulfill major or minor criteria, depending on the severity of the abnormality. Although detection of fat within the myocardium using cardiac MRI is often discussed, this is no longer a criterion for diagnosis. More commonly seen is RV dilation with regional wall motion abnormalities. Additionally, aneurysms of the RV wall can be seen in ARVD. Abnormal fibrofatty tissue may also be present in the LV myocardium, not only the RV wall.

Dilated cardiomyopathy is often described as ischemic or nonischemic in regard to cause. As described above, ischemic cardiomyopathy is due to coronary artery disease and myocardial ischemia, resulting in thinning and poor contractility of the myocardium. Nonischemic cardiomyopathy has a number of causes, including familial forms of cardiomyopathy, myocarditis, alcoholism, toxins, and cardiomyopathy in pregnancy. Due to the dilation of the ventricular chambers and frequently poor contractility of the myocardium, dilated cardiomyopathy is typically associated with impaired systolic function. Calculation of end-diastolic and end-systolic ventricular volumes is of paramount importance in these patients, who often undergo serial evaluations to monitor ventricular dilation and ejection fraction. It is especially important in these patients to maintain a consistent method of calculating cardiac function.

Cardiac amyloidosis is characterized by the extracellular deposition of glycoproteins (amyloid) within the myocardium. On cardiac MRI, the myocardium is diffusely thickened and hypokinetic. Typically, amyloid deposition in the myocardium delays clearance of Gd, which leads to globally increased T1 relaxation. Therefore, the LV MR signal nulls at the same rate as the blood pool. Another pattern seen with LGE is circumferential subendocardial enhancement. Amyloid can present with patchy LGE that is neither confined to a coronary artery distribution nor exclusively subendocardial (Fig. 9.5).

Congenital Heart Disease

Congenital heart disease (CHD) encompasses a broad spectrum of abnormalities. CHD is most often seen in the pediatric population but, with the advent of new surgical procedures and interventions that prolong life, the imaging specialist encounters more adults with CHD. Imaging plays an integral role in the diagnosis and management of these patients. Echocardiography is generally used when imaging the fetus and neonate. Cardiac MRI has been gaining popularity as a noninvasive method of imaging that does not use ionizing radiation. Cardiac MRI can provide anatomic and functional information about these complex lesions, thereby assisting in medical management and surgical planning.

Cardiac Mass

Cardiac MRI has unique capabilities for the evaluation of a cardiac mass that is not matched by other modalities. One of the most commonly encountered problems in cardiac imaging is differentiating a cardiac tumor from a thrombus. Thrombus, being devoid of a blood supply, has low signal compared to the myocardium on LGE imaging. In systems that only generate magnitude LGE images, low signal intensity in the thrombus should be confirmed by repeating the LGE sequence with a long inversion time, usually 550 to 600 ms, which causes a thrombus to become even darker. On nonenhanced images, thrombus will generally be hyperintense or isointense, depending on the age of the thrombus.

Cardiac MRI is also useful for the characterization of cardiac tumors, allowing determination of myocardial invasion and vascular invasion that may not be evident on echocardiography or CT. Most cardiac tumors are metastases, and any mass in the heart should be correlated with a clinical history of cancer. Primary cardiac tumors are rare. Benign cardiac tumors are more common than malignant cardiac tumors. Cardiac myxomas are the most common benign tumor in the adult population, and rhabdomyomas are the most common benign tumor in the pediatric population. Sarcomas account for the vast majority of malignant primary cardiac tumors.

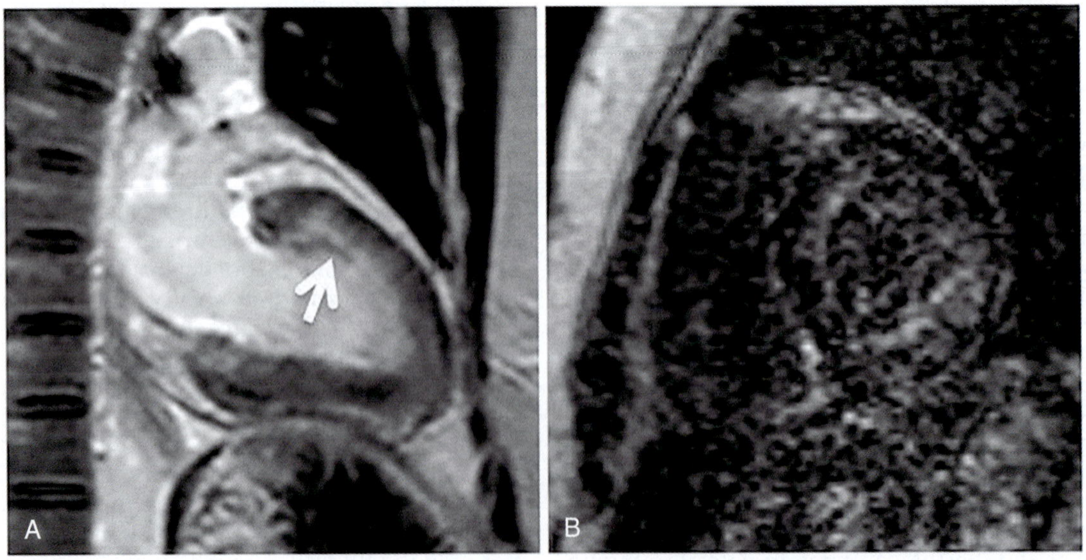

Figure 9.5 Cardiac amyloid in two different patients. (A) Vertical long-axis late gadolinium enhancement (LGE) image shows diffuse subendocardial enhancement *(arrow)*, a pattern characteristic of amyloid. (B) The midchamber of a short-axis LGE image in a different patient shows equal signal intensity in ventricular myocardium and blood pool, which is caused by diffuse retention of gadolinium contrast throughout the myocardium.

Problem-Solving Issues

Ischemic Heart Disease

Evaluating Viability of Myocardial Segments

Cardiac MRI is increasingly being used in the evaluation of myocardial tissue viability prior to and after revascularization procedures. Cardiac MR LGE is used to detect infarcted or fibrotic myocardium. Gd chelate MR contrast agents are called *extracellular contrast agents* because the Gd chelate exits the vessel, accumulating in the extracellular space, with normal cells excluding the Gd chelate. The injured myocytes in myocardial infarct cannot exclude the Gd chelate and demonstrate LGE in comparison to the adjacent normal myocardium, with intact myocytes.

The extent of the infarct can be evaluated in two ways—in determining which coronary artery territories are involved and the thickness of the myocardium demonstrating LGE. Coronary artery territories are described using the American Heart Association's 17-segment model.

LGE extending through 100% of the myocardial thickness (transmural) is considered nonviable and has a very low likelihood of improvement in contractility following revascularization. If the extent of LGE involves a 51%–75% thickness of the myocardium, it has been shown that approximately 90% of these infarcts do not recover function following revascularization. Based on these results, a more than 50% thickness myocardial LGE is considered to have a low likelihood of treatment response; often, intervention is not pursued, and patients are treated medically. Alternatively, if LGE is not present in at-risk myocardium, this tissue has a high likelihood of recovering function following revascularization, even in the presence of wall motion abnormality.

Evaluating How Well the Heart Is Functioning

Cine SSFP sequences are used to assess for wall motion abnormalities that conform to a coronary artery territory. Segmental motion abnormalities can be present in both acute and chronic myocardial ischemia. Wall motion is described as normokinetic, hypokinetic, akinetic, or dyskinetic (see Fig. 9.4). Abnormal myocardial contractility can also contribute to poor cardiac function and can be quantitatively assessed using cardiac MRI by calculating the ejection fraction using end-diastolic and end-systolic volumes.

Additionally, LGE imaging combined with cine SSFP sequences can detect stunned myocardium in the acute MI setting and hibernating myocardium in chronic ischemia. Stunned myocardium is dysfunctional but viable and demonstrates normal contrast kinetics without LGE, although segmental wall motion abnormalities may be present.

Hibernating myocardium is due to chronic reduced coronary blood flow resulting in impaired myocardium, which can be restored to normal or near-normal function if myocardial perfusion is improved (Fig. 9.6). Because hibernating myocardium occurs in the setting of chronic ischemia, LGE may be present related to a prior infarct, although there should be less than 50% thickness if a combination of infarct and hibernating myocardium is considered.

Cardiomyopathy

Evaluating a Patient for Suspected Hypertrophic Cardiomyopathy

When evaluating a patient for suspected HCM with cardiac MRI, the LV wall thickness should be evaluated in all LV segments during diastole (Fig. 9.7). There are two imaging criteria used in the diagnosis of HCM: (1) LV

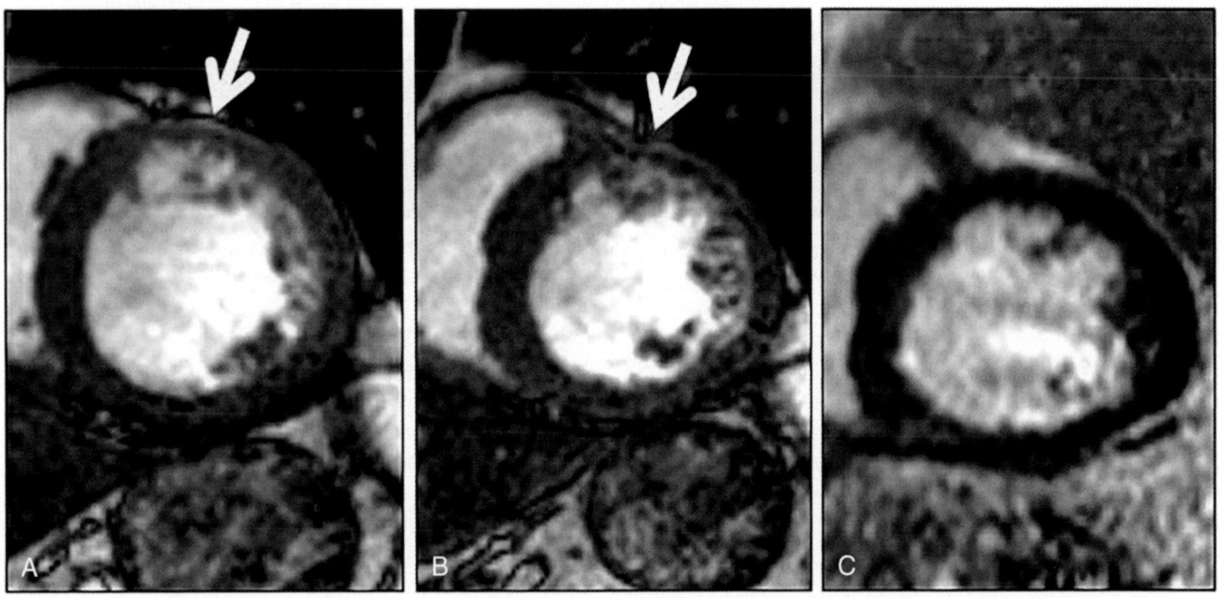

Figure 9.6 Hibernating myocardium. Short-axis bright blood images during diastole (A) and systole (B) show an akinetic anterior wall *(arrows)*. (C) The corresponding location on the late gadolinium enhancement image shows no enhancement. This finding is compatible with hibernating myocardium and suggests that function will return if perfusion is restored.

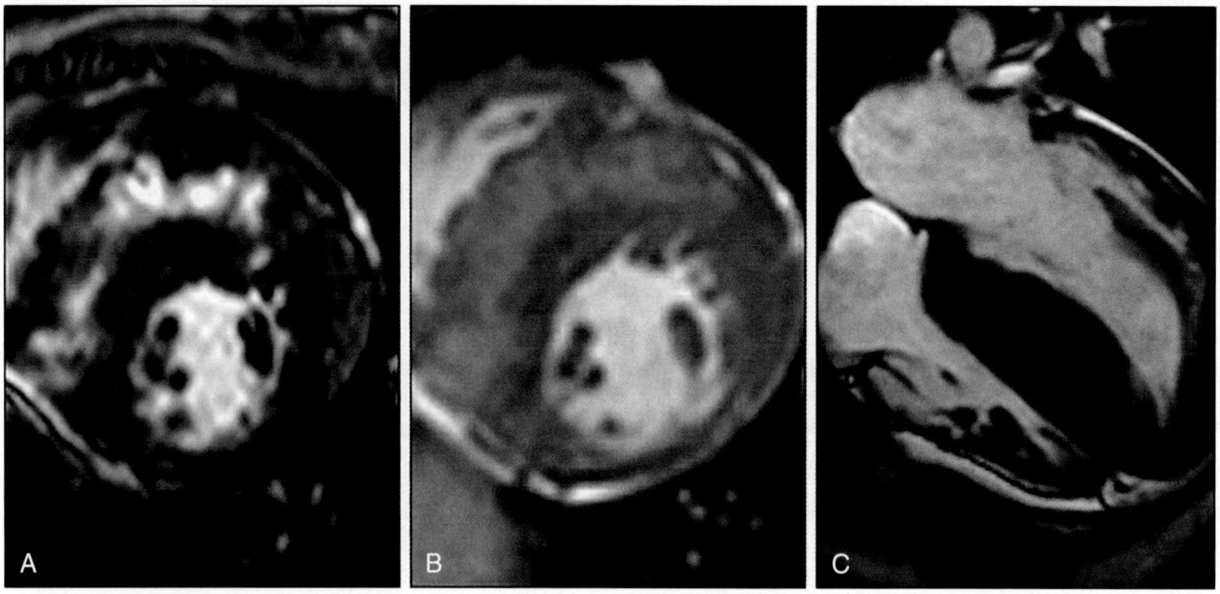

Figure 9.7 Asymmetric septal hypertrophic cardiomyopathy. (A) The late gadolinium enhancement sequence shows patchy midmyocardial enhancement in areas of hypertrophy myocardium, but no enhancement in normal-thickness myocardium. Asymmetric thickening of the myocardium is seen on the short-axis (B) and four-chamber (C) bright blood images.

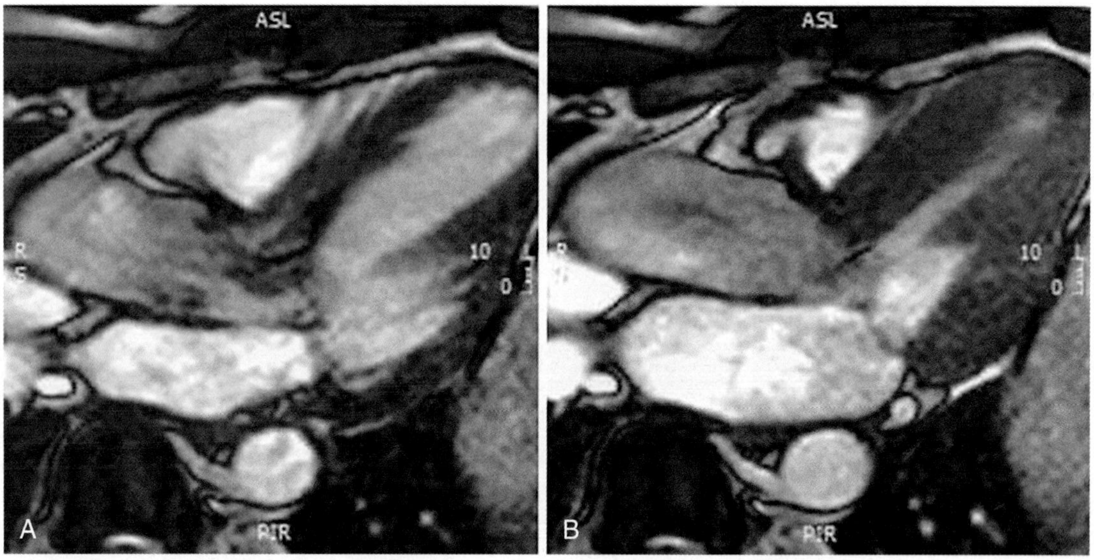

Figure 9.8 Left ventricular outflow tract views during diastole (A) and systole (B) in a patient with hypertrophic obstructive cardiomyopathy and systolic anterior motion of the mitral valve leaflet.

wall thickness 15 mm or more at end-diastole, and (2) a ratio of the septal to lateral LV wall more than 1.3, with no other diagnosis to alter the myocardial thickness, such as dilated cardiomyopathy. The ratio of the septal to lateral LV wall is a less commonly used measurement and not as widely accepted.

Additionally, the LV myocardial mass should also be calculated using cardiac MRI. An increased LV mass is associated with a poorer outcome in patients with HCM.

These imaging criteria are not used in isolation. They are combined with genetic profiles, family history, and clinical history when making a diagnosis of HCM.

Determining the Presence of Systolic Anterior Motion of the Mitral Valve Leaflet

SAM of the mitral valve leaflet is diagnosed on cine SSFP cardiac MRI when the mitral valve leaflet, usually the anterior leaflet, paradoxically moves anteriorly toward the ventricular septum during systole (Fig. 9.8). SAM of the mitral valve can result in left ventricular outflow tract, which may occur at rest or during stress alone. A pressure gradient across the left ventricular outflow tract of 30 mm Hg or higher is considered significant and can be calculated with VEC phase contrast MRI.

Determining the Presence of Delayed Enhancement

One of the benefits of cardiac MRI relative to echocardiography is the ability to assess for LGE in patients with HCM. The cause of myocardial fibrosis in HCM is unknown at this time, but the presence of LGE in a patient with known HCM is associated with sudden cardiac death and a poorer outcome relative to a patient without LGE. Patients with LGE and HCM often receive intracardiac defibrillators. LGE due to HCM is patchy, midmyocardial, and only occurs in abnormally thickened myocardium and right ventricular (RV) insertion sites. The latter pattern of LGE is characteristic of HCM, but not specific for it, and can be seen in RV hypertension. Additionally, the pattern of LGE is not confined to coronary artery territories (nonischemic pattern).

Congenital Heart Disease

Evaluating the Function of the Heart

Cine bright blood imaging is used to evaluate function by calculating end-diastolic and end-systolic volumes. In the setting of complex anatomy, such as a functional single ventricle, it can be helpful to use multiple imaging planes to verify that the placement of contours is correct.

Determining the Presence of a Shunt

VEC phase contrast imaging is used to detect a shunt by measuring flow volumes through the pulmonary artery (Qp) and aorta (Qs). The ratio of Qp:Qs designates the severity of the shunt. However, a 10% error is commonly accepted, suggesting that a patient with a Qp:Qs of 1.1 to 1 may, in fact, be normal. In surgically corrected CHD, phase contrast imaging may be performed through other vessels or conduits to measure blood flow.

Determining the Presence of Postsurgical Complications

CHD encompasses a large variety of cardiac anomalies, many of which are surgically repaired. Surgical repair often involves vascular anastomoses and the placement of a vascular conduit or other surgical device. The MR sequences used depend on the specific clinical question, but likely will use a combination of bright blood, VEC phase contrast, and three-dimensional (3D) postcontrast MRA imaging.

As an example, VEC phase contrast imaging can detect shunts, which may suggest postsurgical complications, such as anastomotic leaks or the formation of collateral vessels. Cine bright blood images can detect aneurysms, which may form at sites of a prior ventriculotomy or vascular anastomosis.

Cardiac Mass

Determining if the Mass Enhances

Intracardiac thrombus is the most common intracardiac mass, especially if there is no history of malignancy. Echocardiography often cannot differentiate between cardiac tumor and cardiac thrombus based on tissue properties, and these patients often undergo cardiac MRI to determine the composition of the mass.

A thrombus will not enhance or retain contrast. During injection of Gd MR contrast, the first-pass perfusion should be imaged, and the signal intensity of the mass should be measured on each frame. The MR sequence used for first-pass perfusion varies by MR manufacturer.

After first-pass perfusion, LGE should be measured. It is important to include the mass and the LV in the same image because enhancement should be evaluated relative to the myocardium. If phase-sensitive LGE images are not available, additional LGE images should be acquired at a longer inversion time, typically 550 to 600 ms (Fig. 9.9).

If the mass displays dynamic or delayed Gd uptake, then a thrombus is excluded.

Determining if the Mass Has a Characteristic T1 or T2 Signal Property

Certain cardiac masses have characteristic signal properties. Lipomas will be hyperintense on T1-weighted images and convert to hypointense when fat saturation is applied. Congenital cysts will be T2 hyperintense but do not demonstrate contrast uptake. Hemangiomas will be T2 hyperintense but will have contrast uptake (Fig. 9.10).

Determining if Malignant Imaging Features Are Present

Imaging features suggestive of malignancy include ill-defined borders with soft tissue invading adjacent structures. Additionally, the presence of a pericardial effusion raises the suspicion for malignancy. Calcifications can be seen in both benign and malignant masses but, if the calcification is large relative to the size of the mass cardiac osteosarcoma, although rare, it should be included in the differential diagnosis (Fig. 9.11).

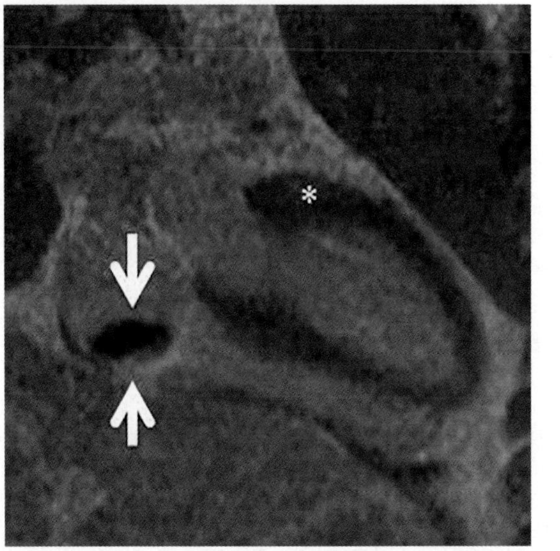

Figure 9.9 Double-oblique late gadolinium enhancement image in a patient with a right atrial thrombus *(arrows)*. The inversion time for the image was 550 ms, which is longer than the usual 320 ms. This resulted in a myocardium with intermediate signal intensity *(asterisk)*, but the thrombus remained low in signal intensity.

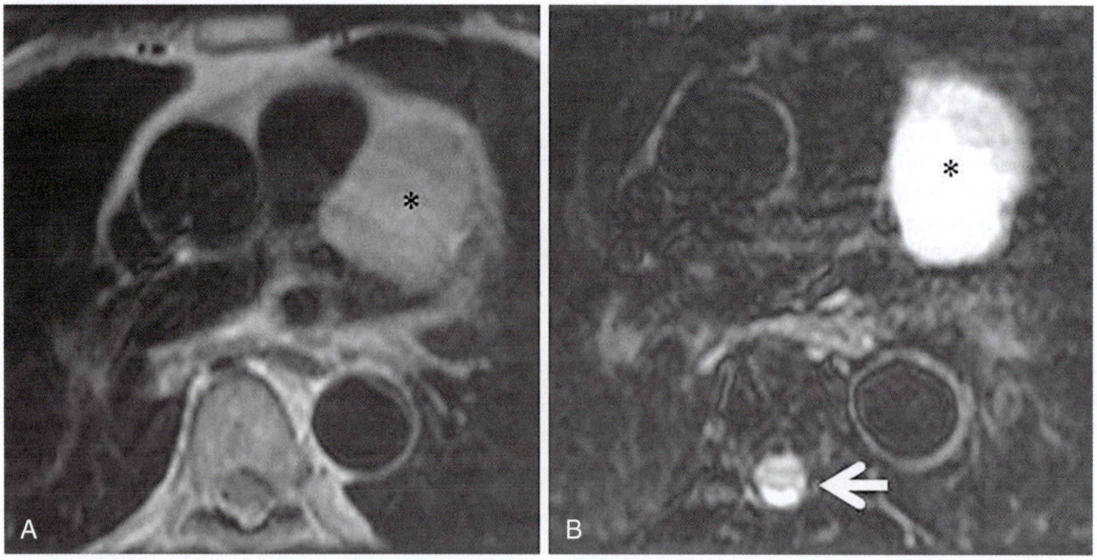

Figure 9.10 Axial T2-weighted black blood images without (A) and with (B) fat saturation at the level of the proximal pulmonary artery. (A) The mass *(asterisk)* is intermediate signal intensity similar to the fat. However, in (B), fat saturation decreases signal intensity of the fat but not the mass *(asterisk)*, which is now similar in signal intensity to cerebral spinal fluid *(arrow)*. Other sequences (not shown) demonstrated gadolinium enhancement of the mass. The final diagnosis was a hemangioma.

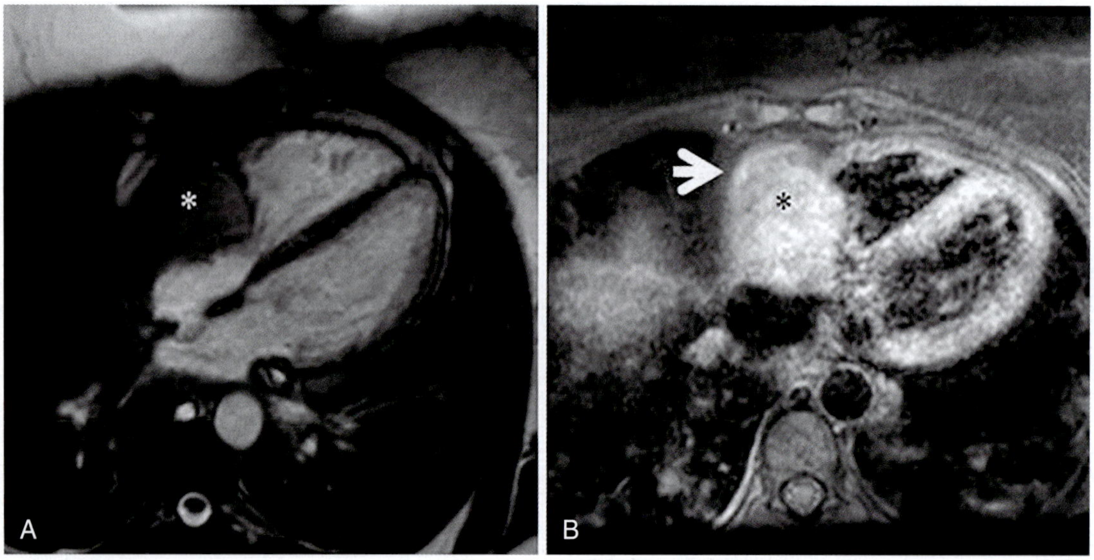

Figure 9.11 Four-chamber bright blood sequence (A) and axial T1-weighted fat saturation image shows an enhancing mass *(asterisk)* in the right atrium that extends beyond the atrial border into the epicardial fat and possibly pericardium *(arrow)*. This is compatible with a malignant neoplasm. The final diagnosis, based on pathology, was angiosarcoma.

Pitfalls

Differentiation of Late Gadolinium Enhancement From Blood Pool Signal

The signal of the blood pool following the administration of intravenous Gd may be difficult to distinguish from subendocardial LGE, given the similarly high signal. This pitfall can be avoided by correlating anatomy on the LGE images with bright blood images in the same plane (Fig. 9.12).

Misinterpreting Hypokinesis in Patients With Irregular Cardiac Rhythm

When interpreting imaging of patients with an irregular cardiac rhythm, the imaging specialist should be aware of the potential pitfall leading to a misdiagnosis of wall hypokinesis. Despite ECG gating, if a patient has an irregular rhythm, images may be composed of acquisitions at different time points in the cardiac cycle. When viewed as a cine loop, this may give the false appearance of a hypokinetic wall motion abnormality because one or more images are composed from different time points

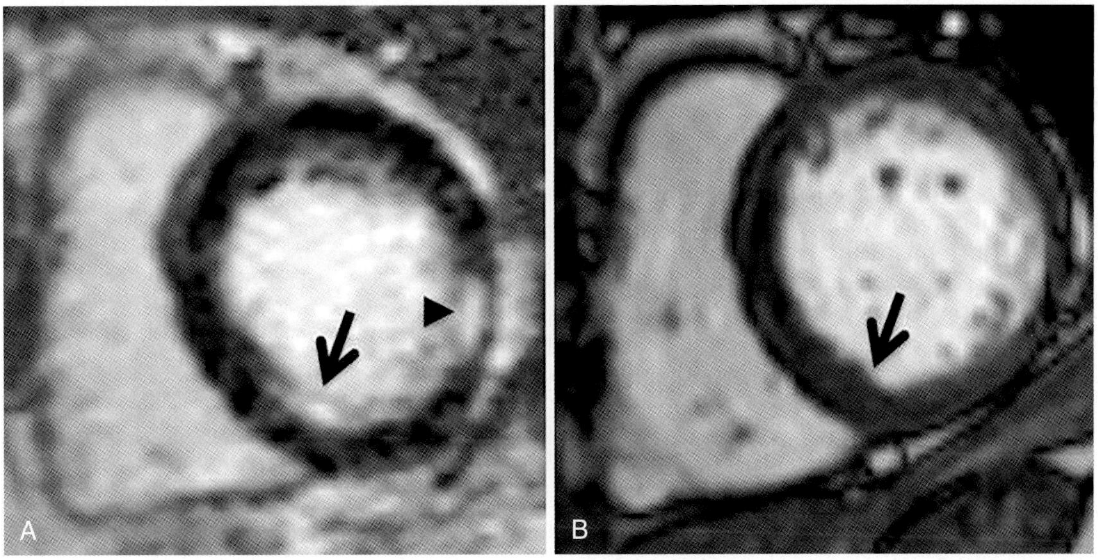

Figure 9.12 Avoiding a false-negative pitfall in diagnosing late gadolinium enhancement (LGE). (A) In the LGE sequence, an area of enhancement is present in the subendocardial inferoseptal wall *(arrow)*. Because the signal intensity of this region is similar to that of the blood pool, it can be missed. (B) However, if the image is correlated with the bright blood sequence, the diagnosis of LGE is more easily made. Note the additional area of LGE in the lateral wall *(arrowhead in A)*.

of cardiac contraction. The imaging specialist can be alerted to this pitfall by inspecting the patient's rhythm strip at the scanner console. Real-time imaging can be used to determine cardiac function in patients with high heart rate variability, although real-time images are more cumbersome to process.

Differentiation of Ischemic From Nonischemic Enhancement Patterns

As discussed in prior sections, when interpreting LGE imaging, the pattern of myocardial enhancement can suggest an ischemic versus nonischemic pattern of injury. Ischemic patterns of injury follow coronary artery territories and are typically subendocardial and extend outward (see Fig. 9.3). Nonischemic patterns of LGE are not confined to coronary artery territories and are usually midmyocardial and patchy in distribution.

Misinterpreting Subaortic Stenosis From Interventricular Thickening

A frequently encountered question when imaging patients with HCM is determining if SAM of the mitral valve leaflet is present and differentiating this diagnosis from subaortic stenosis due to interventricular thickening. To avoid this pitfall, the imaging specialist should view the SSFP cine images of the three-chamber view, which includes the ventricular septum, mitral valve, and left ventricular outflow tract. SAM is diagnosed when anterior motion of the mitral valve leaflet, often the anterior leaflet, toward the left ventricular outflow tract during systole is observed on the cine SSFP images; this often results in blood flow turbulence, resulting in a spin-dephasing artifact at the mitral valve leaflet. If only single still images are viewed, this may give the false impression of SAM when a subaortic stenosis is present due to hypertrophy of the interventricular septum, resulting in a spin-dephasing artifact from the subaortic stenosis.

Failure to Include Left Ventricle in Images When Evaluating a Cardiac Mass

Unlike CT, signal intensity in MRI is relative. When acquiring images in the setting of a cardiac mass, the image field of view should include the mass and LV myocardium as an internal reference. Without inclusion of the LV myocardium to function as a reference for the MRI signal, the composition of the cardiac mass is difficult to determine because intrinsic MRI signal characteristics, including inversion times for myocardial signal nulling and enhancement, cannot be interpreted accurately.

Choosing the Correct Inversion Time in Amyloidosis

Cardiac amyloidosis is a diagnosis associated with characteristic MRI findings, specifically when inversion time scouts are used to determine the optimal inversion time for myocardial signal nulling. The imaging specialist and technologist should be cognizant that the inversion time for myocardial nulling in the setting of cardiac amyloid deposition is often shorter than expected, because the myocardium with amyloid deposits nulls before the blood pool (see Fig. 9.5). Normally, the myocardium should null after the blood pool.

Overcoming Technical Obstacles

Patient Cannot Hold Breath

When imaging patients who are unable to hold their breath, respiratory gating can be performed to decrease motion artifact. Unfortunately, respiratory gating significantly increases scan time. If the patient is not able to tolerate the longer examination time, then real-time imaging can be performed.

Patient Is in Irregular Cardiac Rhythm

As discussed above, irregular cardiac rhythm can predispose to motion artifacts, which can lead to imaging misinterpretation. ECG gating may be suboptimally triggered in the setting of an irregular cardiac rhythm. The imaging specialist should always evaluate the ECG rhythm strip to detect abnormal cardiac rhythm and at which time points during the cardiac cycle imaging was obtained, because this may differ with poor ECG triggering. If artifact from the irregular rhythm limits the diagnostic quality of the ECG-gated MRI scans too greatly, images can be acquired in real time, without triggering. Real-time imaging, however, is associated with decreased temporal and spatial resolution.

Patient Has Poor Renal Function

The use of Gd-containing contrast agents in the setting of impaired renal function often varies by institution. However, if a patient has known end-stage renal disease (estimated glomerular filtration rate [GFR] <30 mL/min/1.73 m^2), the vast majority of practices do not administer Gd-containing contrast agent due to the risk of nephrogenic systemic fibrosis (NSF). Although the risk for NSF is small and not well studied in many of the newer Gd-containing contrast agents, the severe morbidity and mortality rates of NSF lead many institutions to advise against their use in patients with a GFR less than 30 mL/min/1.73 m^2.

Bibliography

Biglands JD, Radjenovic A, Ridgway JP. Cardiovascular magnetic resonance physics for clinicians: part II. *J Cardiovasc Magn Reson.* 2012;14:66.

Bogaert J, Francone M. Pericardial disease: value of CT and MR imaging. *Radiology.* 2013;267(2):339–355.

Hansen MW, Merchant N. MRI of hypertrophic cardiomyopathy: part I. MRI appearances. *AJR Am J Roentgenol.* 2007;189(6):1335–1343.

Hoey ETD, Mankad K, Puppala S, Gopalan D, Sivananthan MU. MRI and CT appearances of cardiac tumours in adults. *Clin Radiol.* 2009;64(12):1214–1230.

Indik JH, Gimbel JR, Abe H, et al. 2017 HRS expert consensus statement on magnetic resonance imaging and radiation exposure in patients with cardiovascular implantable electronic devices. *Heart Rhythm.* 2017;14(7):e97–e153.

Ishida M, Kato S, Sakuma H. Cardiac MRI in ischemic heart disease. *Circ J.* 2009;73(9):1577–1588.

Jackson E, Bellenger N, Seddon M, Harden S, Peebles C. Ischaemic and non-ischaemic cardiomyopathies—cardiac MRI appearances with delayed enhancement. *Clin Radiol.* 2007;62(5):395–403.

Jordan JH, Todd RM, Vasu S, Hundley WG. Cardiovascular magnetic resonance in the oncology patient. *JACC Cardiovasc Imaging.* 2018;11(8):1150–1172.

Maraj S, Pressman GS, Figueredo VM. Primary cardiac tumors. *Int J Cardiol.* 2009;133(2):152–156.

Messroghli DR, Moon JC, Ferreira VM, et al. Clinical recommendations for cardiovascular magnetic resonance mapping of T1, T2, T2* and extracellular volume: a consensus statement by the Society for Cardiovascular Magnetic Resonance (SCMR) endorsed by the European Association for Cardiovascular Imaging (EACVI). *J Cardiovasc Magn Reson.* 2017;19(1):75.

O'Donnell DH, Abbara S, Chaithiraphan V, et al. Cardiac tumors: optimal cardiac MR sequences and spectrum of imaging appearances. *AJR Am J Roentgenol.* 2009;193(2):377–387.

Rajiah P, Bolen MA. Cardiovascular MR imaging at 3 T: opportunities, challenges, and solutions. *Radiographics.* 2014;34(6):1612–1635.

Ridgway JP. Cardiovascular magnetic resonance physics for clinicians: part I. *J Cardiovasc Magn Reson.* 2010;12:71.

Schulz-Menger J, Bluemke DA, Bremerich J, et al. Standardized image interpretation and post processing in cardiovascular magnetic resonance: Society for Cardiovascular Magnetic Resonance (SCMR) board of trustees task force on standardized post processing. *J Cardiovasc Magn Reson.* 2013;15:35.

Shinbane JS, Colletti PM, Shellock FG. Magnetic resonance imaging in patients with cardiac pacemakers: era of "MR conditional" designs. *J Cardiovasc Magn Reson.* 2011;13:63.

Wieben O, Francois C, Reeder SB. Cardiac MRI of ischemic heart disease at 3 T: potential and challenges. *Eur J Radiol.* 2008;65(1):15–28.

CHAPTER 10
Angiography and Interventions

Anil K. Pillai, Jerry Kovoor, and Sanjeeva P. Kalva

CHAPTER OUTLINE

Introduction

The bony thoracic cage and crowded vital organs in the thorax make open surgical access difficult and challenging. For these same reasons, the thorax is ideal for image-guided interventions. In addition to procedural skills, a thorough knowledge of the anatomy, physiology, pathology, imaging findings, and preprocedure and postprocedure care is required for successful practice of various interventional procedures. Thoracic interventions can be broadly divided into vascular and nonvascular interventions. Nonvascular interventions include image-guided biopsy and drainage procedures, tumor ablation, lymphatic interventions, and esophageal and tracheobronchial interventions. Some of these procedures are covered elsewhere in this text. Vascular interventions involve the aorta and its branches, pulmonary arteries, and venous structures and include revascularization procedures (angioplasty, stent placement), vascular occlusion procedures (embolization and exclusion), and venous access procedures. This chapter provides a brief overview of some vascular and lymphatic interventions for a diagnostic radiologist.

Pulmonary Angiography

For several years, catheter-based pulmonary angiography was the standard imaging technique for the evaluation of the pulmonary arteries. Technical advances in cross-sectional imaging, especially with the introduction of multidetector computed tomography (MDCT), have had a significant impact on imaging of the pulmonary arteries. CT pulmonary angiography is now the first-line imaging technique to evaluate pulmonary arterial diseases, including acute pulmonary embolism (PE). Catheter-based pulmonary arteriography is now essentially used as a problem-solving tool or as an a priori imaging technique for endovascular interventions. The current indications for performing catheter-based pulmonary arteriography are as follows:

1. Clinically suspected acute PE when CT pulmonary angiography is nondiagnostic
2. Chronic PE, especially prior to surgical endarterectomy
3. Suspected pulmonary vascular abnormalities, such as vasculitis, congenital and acquired anomalies, and tumor encasement
4. As part of a pulmonary arterial intervention

Workup of a Patient for Pulmonary Angiography

Clinical history, laboratory values, and medications should be reviewed. A clinical history of left bundle branch block places the patient at risk of a complete heart block while catheterizing the pulmonary arteries. Temporary cardiac pacing prior to the procedure may be considered in elective cases to mitigate this risk. Moderate pulmonary hypertension is a relative contraindication for pulmonary angiography. Iodinated contrast materials are known to cause pulmonary vasoconstriction and pulmonary edema, leading to increased right heart strain. The use of low-osmolar contrast material and limiting the injection volume can mitigate this risk. Similar to any other vascular procedure involving the use of contrast material, renal function tests, coagulation parameters, and platelet counts should be checked.

Performing Pulmonary Arteriography

The procedure can be safely performed under local anesthesia. Moderate sedation is often administered to reduce anxiety. Patients who cannot lay flat or hold their breath for 10 seconds or have a poor airway are best intubated for pulmonary angiography. If a left bundle branch is known, a temporary pacer is placed. Jugular or femoral vein access is established after administering local anesthesia. The choice of venous access is dependent on the operator's preference and length of the catheter or devices anticipated for the procedure. Shorter catheters and devices will require a jugular access. Most of the catheters used for pulmonary angiography are between 6 and 8 Fr. Standard pulmonary flush catheters (Grollman, Van Aman, Berman) have a 90-degree curve to facilitate maneuverability through the right heart. A pigtail catheter and a tip-deflecting guidewire can also be used to catheterize the pulmonary artery.

Pulmonary arterial pressures are measured with the catheter positioned in the right or left main pulmonary artery. A nonselective pulmonary trunk arteriography is rarely performed. Selective arteriography with the catheter tip in the right and left pulmonary arteries in the frontal and lateral projections is typically performed. The contrast material is injected at a rate of 15 to 20 mL/s, for a total volume of 30 to 40 mL (Figs. 10.1 and 10.2). The images are acquired at a rate of six frames/s using digital subtraction angiography during a single breath-hold.

Complications of Pulmonary Arteriography

Minor complications, including access site complications, transient arrhythmias, and allergy to contrast materials occur in 5% of patients. Major complications include contrast-induced nephropathy, which occurs in 1%, and fatalities, which occur in 0.5%. With the advent of flexible catheters and nonionic contrast materials, the complication rates are even lower.

Pulmonary Arterial Interventions

Image-guided interventions of the pulmonary arterial circulation involve treatment of pulmonary arteriovenous malformations (PAVMs), pulmonary artery aneurysms and pseudoaneurysms, pulmonary arterial embolism, and pulmonary arterial stenosis.

Pulmonary Arteriovenous Malformations

PAVMs are rare vascular anomalies of the lungs, in which abnormal dilated vessels provide a direct high-flow, low-resistance, right-to-left shunt between the pulmonary artery and vein. PAVMs are usually part of hereditary hemorrhagic telangiectasia (HHT), although sporadic cases occur in 30% of patients. Conversely, one-third of patients with HHT harbor a PAVM. Uncommon causes of PAVMs include trauma, malignancy, and hepatopulmonary syndrome. Patients may be asymptomatic, especially with a small PAVM, but larger lesions may present with hypoxia or heart failure from a right-to-left shunt. Other presentations are usually secondary to systemic emboli; these include transient ischemic attacks (37%), stroke (18%), brain abscess (9%), and seizures (8%). Rupture leading to pulmonary hemorrhage or hemothorax is a rare but well-known and dreaded complication. Diagnosis is usually with CT pulmonary angiography and bubble echocardiography. Endovascular occlusion of the feeding artery with fibered coils or vascular plugs is the mainstay of treatment.

Indications for Treatment

PAVMs are classified into simple (single pulmonary artery directly communicating with a single pulmonary vein, with or without an aneurysm), complex (two or more segmental arteries feeding the PAVM), and a telangiectatic type. The latter does not need treatment. Treatment of nontelangiectatic PAVM is indicated in all patients who are symptomatic and when the feeding artery of the PAVM is 3 mm or more in diameter, irrespective of symptoms.

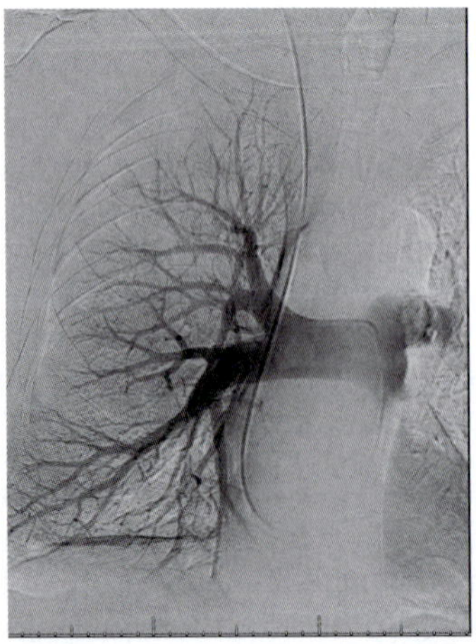

Figure 10.1 Frontal digital subtraction angiogram with a catheter in the right pulmonary artery demonstrating the normal branching anatomy of the pulmonary arteries.

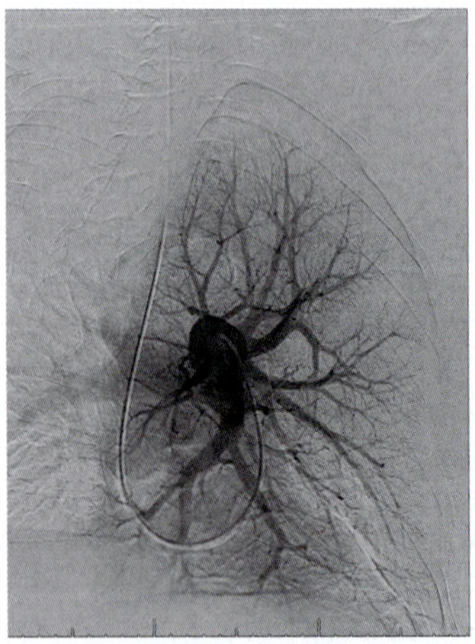

Figure 10.2 Digital subtraction angiogram, right anterior oblique projection, with the catheter tip in the right pulmonary artery demonstrating the normal anatomy.

Patients require lifelong antibiotic prophylaxis for dental or surgical procedures, despite therapy.

Performing Embolization

Based on the location of the PAVM on CT pulmonary angiography, selective pulmonary angiography of the lung is performed. The feeding pulmonary arteries are identified (Figs. 10.3 and 10.4). At our institution, the 7.0/5.0-Fr Lumax guiding catheter (Cook Medical, Bloomington, IN) is used to cannulate the feeding artery. Microcatheters are used if a more selective catheter position is desired. The feeding artery is occluded with fibered coils or vascular plugs (Fig. 10.5). Coils or vascular plugs are selected based on the size of the feeding artery, with the coil usually oversized by 2 mm or 20% and vascular plugs by 30% to 50%. Embolization of the aneurysmal segment is not indicated. In the presence of a high-flow PAVM, a technique known as the *anchor technique* is used to prevent paradoxic embolization of the coil. In this technique, the initial segment of a long coil is first deployed in a proximal branch vessel (to anchor it to the branch) and the rest of the coil is then prolapsed into the feeding artery supplying the PAVM. The embolization procedure is much simpler with the use of detachable vascular plugs, especially in PAVMs with large but short feeding arteries.

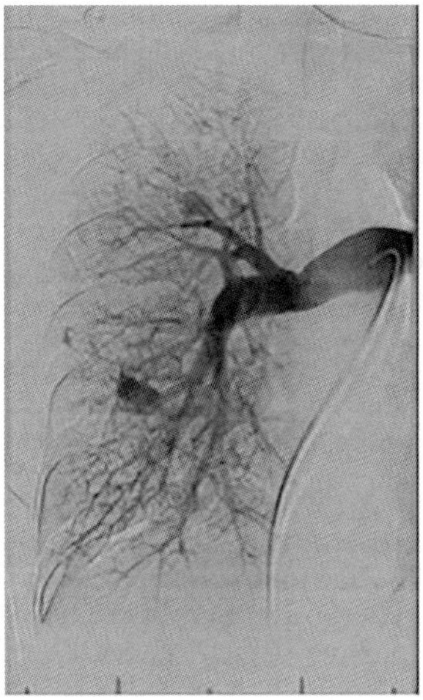

Figure 10.3 Arterial phase digital subtraction angiogram with the catheter in the right pulmonary artery demonstrates two pulmonary arteriovenous malformations.

Results of Embolization Therapy

Embolization procedures are highly successful (close to 100%), but recanalization is known to occur in 5% to 19% of cases. With the use of the vascular plugs, the recanalization rates are much lower. In addition, smaller PAVMs may grow with time and may require therapy during follow-up. Posttreatment, contrast-enhanced CT is performed within 6 to 12 months and then at least every 3 years to assess reperfusion or growth of the PAVM. Minor complications include chest pain and pleural reactions, which occur in 10% to 14% of patients. These are self-limiting and resolve within 1 week, with supportive care and antiinflammatories on an outpatient basis. Other complications include hemothorax, pulmonary infarct, coil migration and nontarget embolization, stroke, severe pulmonary hypertension, access site complications, and persistent cardiac arrhythmia.

Pulmonary Embolism

Systemic anticoagulation is the mainstay of therapy for acute PE. Systemic thrombolysis for massive and

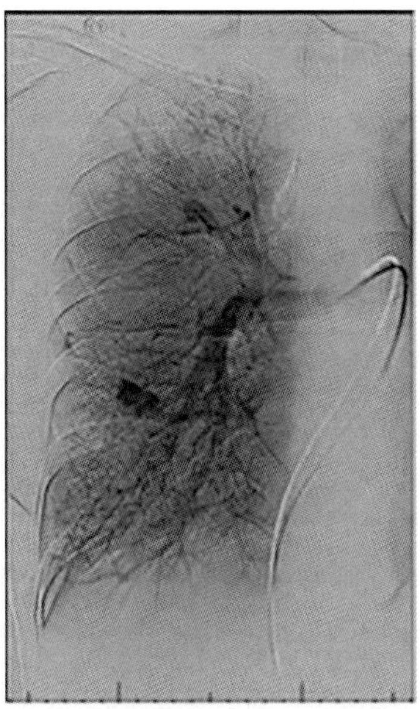

Figure 10.4 Venous phase digital subtraction angiography with the catheter in the right pulmonary artery demonstrates pulmonary arteriovenous malformations with the hypertrophied early draining veins.

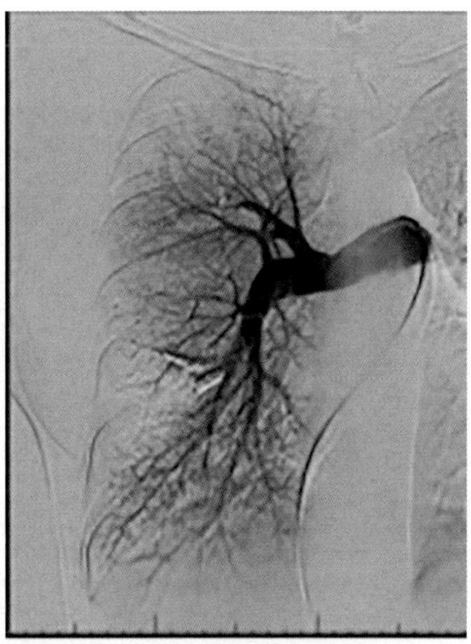

Figure 10.5 Arterial phase digital subtraction angiography with the catheter in the right pulmonary artery demonstrates complete occlusion of the pulmonary arteriovenous malformations after coil embolization.

submassive PE has been well established. Intravenous infusion of tissue plasminogen activator (tPA) along with systemic anticoagulation decreases the risk of death (41% risk reduction compared to anticoagulation alone) and recurrence. However, systemic thrombolysis is contraindicated in the presence of a recent stroke or intracranial injury, intracranial malignancy, bleeding from any source in the body, and recent surgery. Intracranial bleeding is the most devastating complication of systemic thrombolysis, occurring with a frequency of 2% to 5%. Major bleeding complications, including retroperitoneal and gastrointestinal bleeding, occur in 9%. Catheter-directed thrombolysis (CDT) has been gaining acceptance in the treatment protocol for massive and submassive PEs by limiting the systemic side effects of thrombolysis.

Indications for Catheter-Directed Thrombolysis for a Pulmonary Embolism

Aggressive therapy with the use of systemic or regional thrombolytic drugs or mechanical disruption of the thrombus is indicated for acute massive and submassive PEs (Fig. 10.6). A massive PE is defined as an acute PE causing systemic hypotension, with a systolic blood pressure less than 90 mm Hg for more than 15 minutes or circulatory collapse requiring ionotropic support, or a more than 40 mm Hg decrease in systolic blood pressure from baseline. A submassive PE is defined as an acute PE causing right ventricular dilation and hypokinesis on echocardiography, chest CT scan (RV/LV ratio ≥0.9), or both, elevated cardiac biomarkers (troponin and/or B-type natriuretic peptide [BNP]), without systemic hypotension.

Performing Percutaneous Pulmonary Embolectomy

There are two methods of performing a pulmonary embolectomy: pharmacomechanical and mechanical thrombolysis. The former is the most commonly used technique. Mechanical disruption is performed when there is a contraindication to using thrombolytic therapy. Pharmacomechanical thrombolysis involves mechanical disruption of the thrombus with sequential or simultaneous infusion of a thrombolytic drug into the thrombus. Mechanical disruption is achieved by using a variety of devices, including various suction devices (Greenfield embolectomy device, AngioVac, Penumbra Indigo), catheter or balloon fragmentation techniques, and other mechanical disruption maceration techniques (Trerotola device, Impella catheter, Amplatz aspiration thrombectomy device). Rheolytic thrombectomy catheters (AngioJet) are not commonly used due to severe bradycardia associated with their use in the pulmonary circulation. CDT has the advantage of decreased systemic complications while providing high thrombus resolution. This is achieved through placement of a multiside hole infusion catheter directly into the thrombus and infusion of a thrombolytic drug (recombinant tPA [rtPA], infused at 1 mg/h though a single catheter or a split dose of 0.5 mg/h each through two catheters, in the right and left pulmonary artery; Figs. 10.7 and 10.8). Some authors have reported the use of ultrasound-assisted infusion catheters, with good clinical outcomes. The major advantage of endovascular thrombectomy is rapid restoration of pulmonary arterial blood flow, with a significant reduction of pulmonary arterial pressures and right ventricular strain. Following local therapy, patients are managed with systemic anticoagulation.

Results of Catheter-Directed Thrombolysis for Pulmonary Embolism

A meta-analysis for catheter-directed therapy for the treatment of massive PE has reported a success rate of 86.5%, which is comparable to the historical survival rates of 77% after systemic thrombolysis. Major complications, including right ventricular damage and pulmonary hemorrhage, occur in 2.4% of cases, whereas minor complications, including self-limiting arrhythmias, distal embolism, and access site complications, occur in 8%.

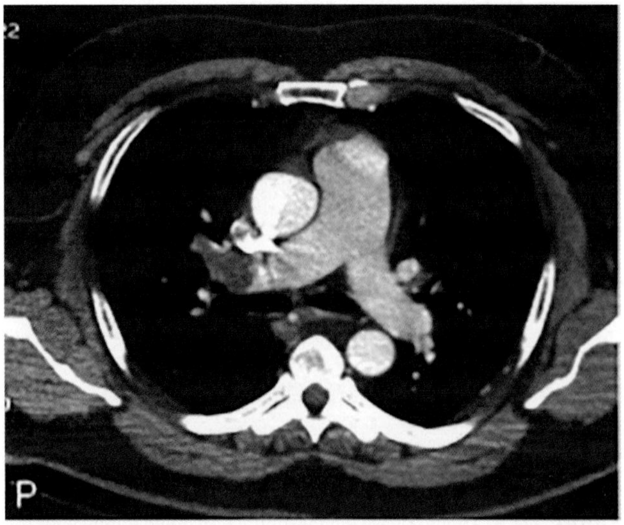

Figure 10.6 Axial contrast-enhanced CT scan at the level of the carina demonstrating a large pulmonary embolus involving the right main pulmonary artery.

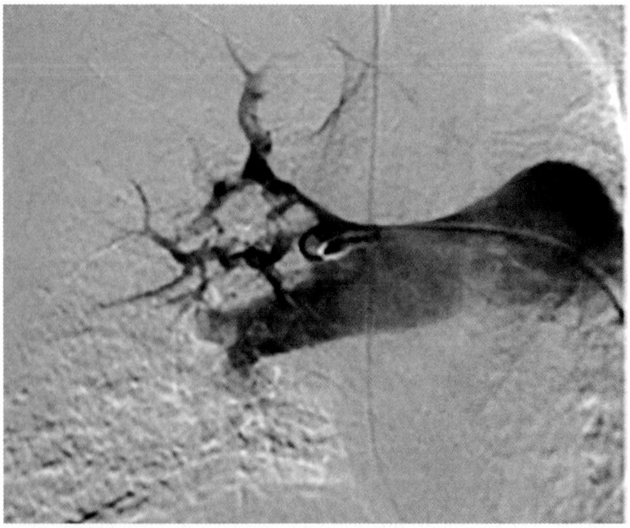

Figure 10.7 Selective right pulmonary digital subtraction angiogram demonstrating a large pulmonary embolus involving the right upper and midlobar pulmonary artery.

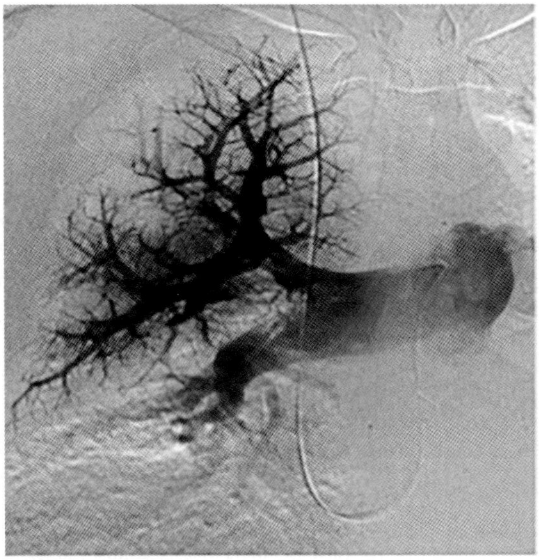

Figure 10.8 Selective right pulmonary digital subtraction angiogram demonstrating resolution of the thrombus after 24 hours of catheter-directed thrombolysis.

Pulmonary Artery Aneurysms and Pseudoaneurysms

Pulmonary artery aneurysms and pseudoaneurysms are rare and are usually secondary to iatrogenic trauma (e.g., from a Swan-Ganz catheter lung biopsy [Figs. 10.9 and 10.10]), penetrating injuries, septic emboli (e.g., tricuspid endocarditis), pulmonary infection (e.g., tuberculosis, mucormycosis, pyogenic infection), vasculitis (e.g., Behçet disease, Takayasu arteritis), pulmonary hypertension, connective tissue abnormalities, neoplasm, and, rarely, congenital. These are associated with high mortality if left untreated. Patients may present with hemoptysis, dyspnea, chest pain, hypoxia, and an enlarging aneurysm on imaging. Contrast material–enhanced CT is the imaging modality of choice for an accurate diagnosis. Treatment is indicated for all patients, irrespective of the size of the aneurysm, and involves embolization of the feeding artery and/or the aneurysm with fibered coils or vascular plugs (Figs. 10.11 to 10.13). Complications include intraprocedural rupture leading to hemoptysis, pleurisy from segmental infarction, and nontarget embolization.

■ Arterial Interventions

Bronchial Artery Embolization

Hemoptysis refers to the expectoration of blood that originates from the respiratory tract. Massive hemoptysis is a life-threatening condition, with a mortality rate of 50% to 100% with conservative management. The cause of death is usually asphyxiation, not exsanguination. The source of massive hemoptysis is bronchial circulation (90%) rather than the pulmonary circulation (5%). Bronchial artery embolization (BAE) is the mainstay of treatment of patients with massive hemoptysis. It provides a temporary measure before the patient can undergo a

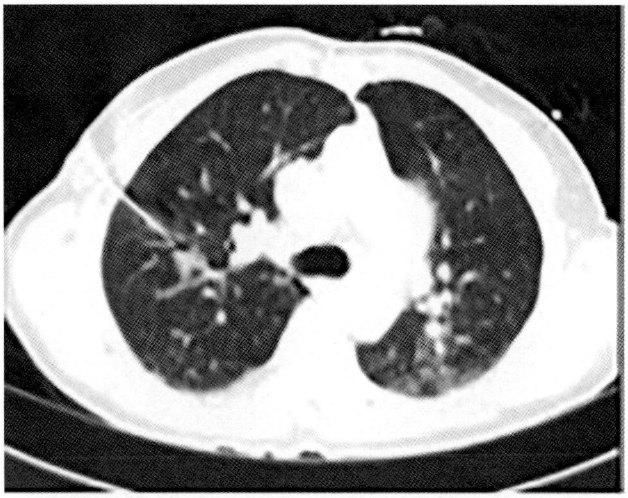

Figure 10.9 Axial CT scan of the thorax demonstrating a needle biopsy targeting a right upper lobe lung mass.

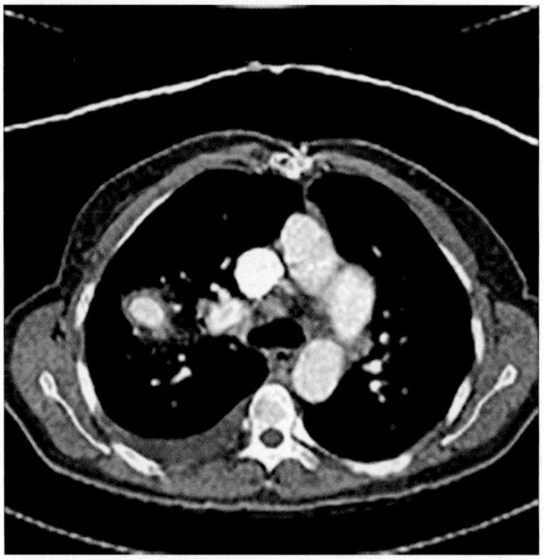

Figure 10.10 Contrast-enhanced axial CT scan of the same patient as in Fig. 10.9 performed for persistent hemoptysis 3 days after the biopsy demonstrating a large pseudoaneurysm near the previous biopsy site.

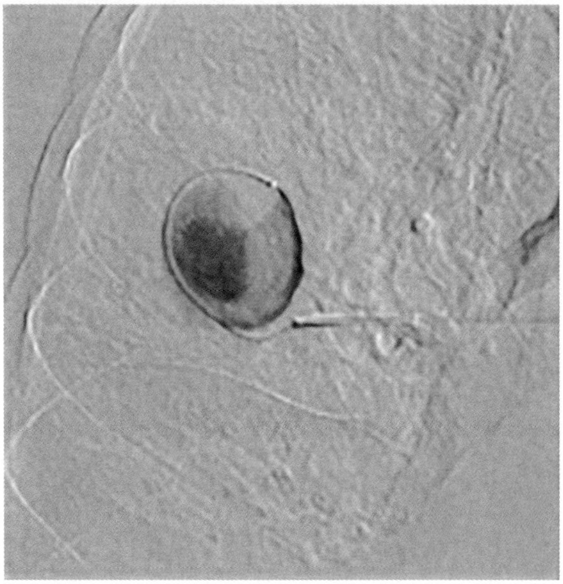

Figure 10.11 Digital subtraction angiogram through a microcatheter demonstrating a large pseudoaneurysm.

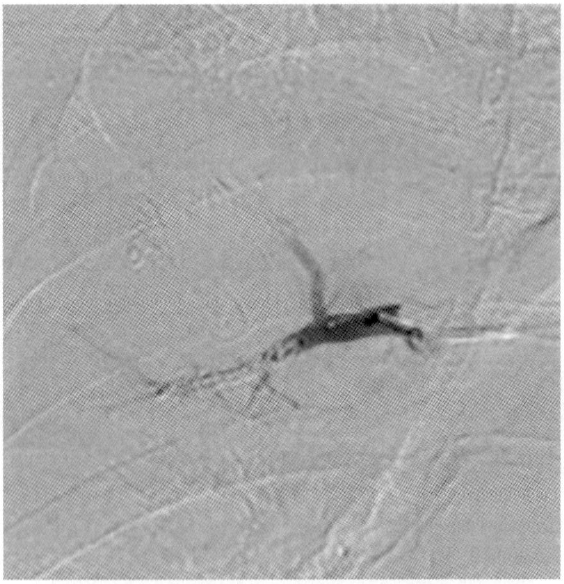

Figure 10.12 Digital subtraction angiogram through a microcatheter within the feeding artery after coil embolization demonstrating complete obliteration of the pseudoaneurysm.

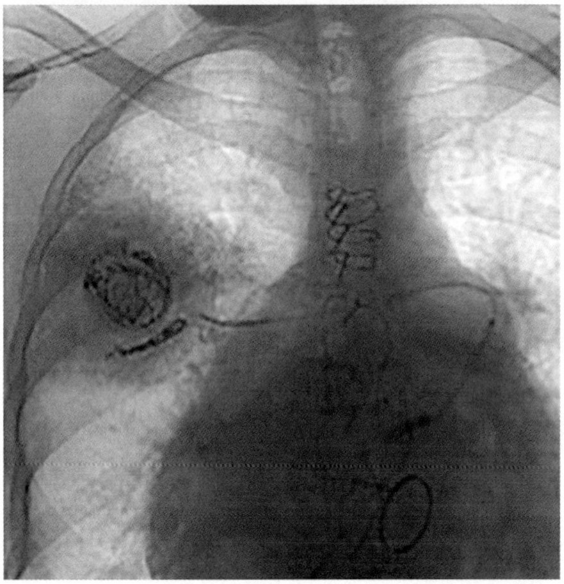

Figure 10.13 Chest radiograph at the end of the procedure demonstrating the coil pack within the aneurysm and in the feeding artery.

definitive treatment, such as surgical resection. In a palliative setting, BAE is performed to stop active expectoration of blood, which is disturbing to patients and their families. It is not a definitive therapy because the recurrence rate after BAE is around 10% to 52%.

Indications for Bronchial Artery Embolization

The main indication for BAE is massive hemoptysis. Massive hemoptysis is defined as blood loss totaling 300 to 600 mL over a 24-hour period or recurrent small amounts of hemoptysis causing blood loss exceeding more than 100 mL/day over 3 days in a week. BAE is also indicated in patients who develop clinically significant airway and/or ventilatory compromise, irrespective of the amount of blood loss or hemodynamic stability.

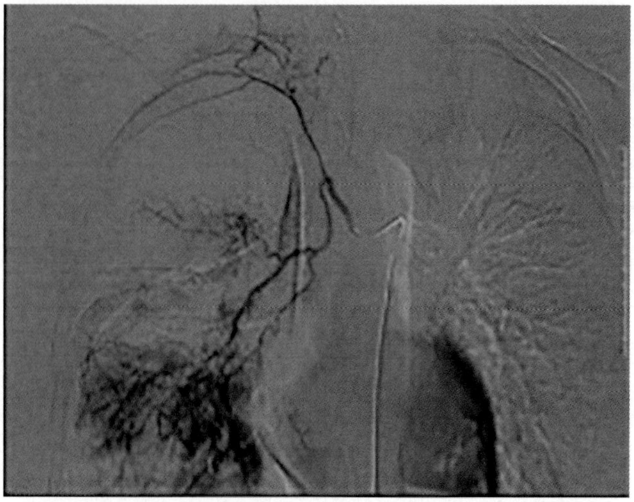

Figure 10.14 Digital subtraction angiogram after selective catheterization of the right inferior phrenic artery demonstrates intense tumor blush in a patient with metastatic lung disease.

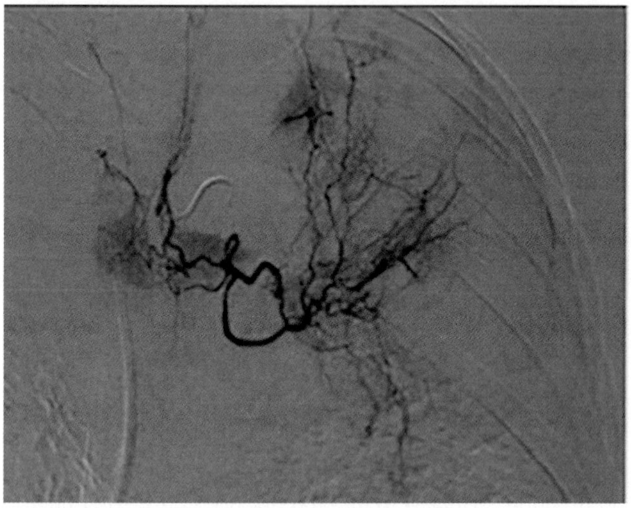

Figure 10.15 Digital subtraction angiogram after selective catheterization of the right intercostobronchial trunk demonstrates multiple tumor blushes in a patient with metastatic lung disease.

Performing Bronchial Artery Embolization

Arterial access is obtained through a femoral or brachial or radial artery approach. A thoracic aortogram with a flush catheter placed at the distal aortic arch is obtained to identify the origin, number, and course of the bronchial arteries and nonbronchial systemic arteries—thyrocervical trunk, internal mammary, intercostal, long thoracic, dorsal scapular, inferior phrenic arteries (Fig. 10.14). Normal bronchial arteries are less than 1.5 mm in diameter and may not be seen on the aortogram. Selective bronchial artery catheterization is performed using various catheter configurations, including Mikaelsson, Simmons, Cobra, or Yashiro catheter. The bronchial arteries arise at the level of T5 and T6, with the most common anatomy being two left bronchial arteries and single right intercostal bronchial trunk (Fig. 10.15). Less common variations include one left and one right, two left and two right, followed by one left and two right bronchial arteries (Fig. 10.16). Angiography findings that suggest bleeding

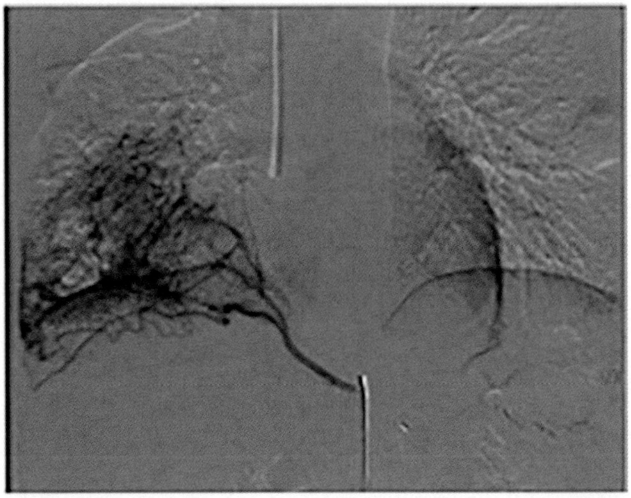

Figure 10.16 Digital subtraction angiogram after selective catheterization of the left bronchial artery demonstrates multiple tumor blushes in a patient with metastatic lung disease.

are active extravasation (3.6%–10.7%), pseudoaneurysm, bronchial artery to pulmonary artery vein shunting, hypertrophy and tortuosity of the bronchial arteries (most common), and neovascularity-hypervascularity of the lung parenchyma. After identifying the abnormal bronchial or nonbronchial systemic artery, a microcatheter is introduced coaxially through the selective catheter and advanced into a stable location. Bronchial and intercostal arteries often give a branch to the spinal cord, and this must be carefully excluded before embolization of the arteries. Embolization is performed with 300- to 500-μm microspheres or Gelfoam. Coils are avoided but can be used to divert the flow within the collaterals.

Results of Bronchial Artery Embolization

Technical success in embolizing the bronchial arteries and nonbronchial systemic arteries can be achieved in more than 90% of cases. Immediate clinical success in controlling bleeding is achieved in 75% to 90% of cases. Early recurrent hemoptysis occurs in less than 10% of patients following embolization and is usually due to incomplete embolization or an unidentified nonbronchial systemic artery supplying the lung. Late recurrences are due to disease progression and occur in up to 52% of cases. Minor complications, including chest pain (24%–71%), dysphagia (0.7%–18.2%), and fever, are transient and self-limiting. These are attributed to the ischemic phenomenon caused by the embolization. The most disastrous complication of BAE is spinal cord ischemia due to inadvertent occlusion of the spinal arteries. The reported incidence of spinal cord ischemia is between 1.4% and 6.5%. Other rare complications, including stroke and blindness, have been reported, resulting from bronchial pulmonary venous shunting.

Arterial Embolization of the Chest Wall

Bleeding into the chest wall is usually due to trauma, iatrogenic surgical procedures such as biopsy, thoracentesis, chest tube placement, and, rarely, neoplasms (Figs. 10.17 and 10.18). Rarely, embolization may be required preoperatively prior to tumor resection to decrease the intraoperative bleeding. It is also part of the treatment for arteriovenous malformations involving the chest wall. The arterial supply to the chest wall comes from the branches of the aorta and intercostal arteries, internal mammary arteries, and other branches of the subclavian and inferior phrenic arteries. Embolization is performed with particles of Gelfoam or coils, depending on the underlying arterial pathology and desired level of vascular occlusion (Figs. 10.19 and 10.20).

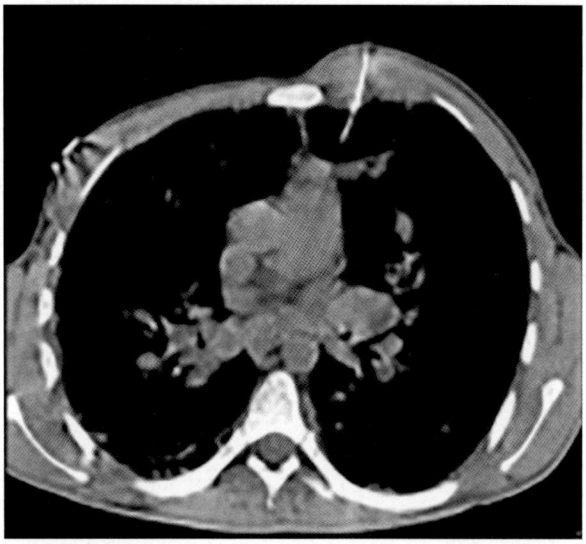

Figure 10.17 Axial CT scan demonstrating needle access into a pneumothorax in a patient with cystic fibrosis. Note the relation between the needle and the internal mammary artery.

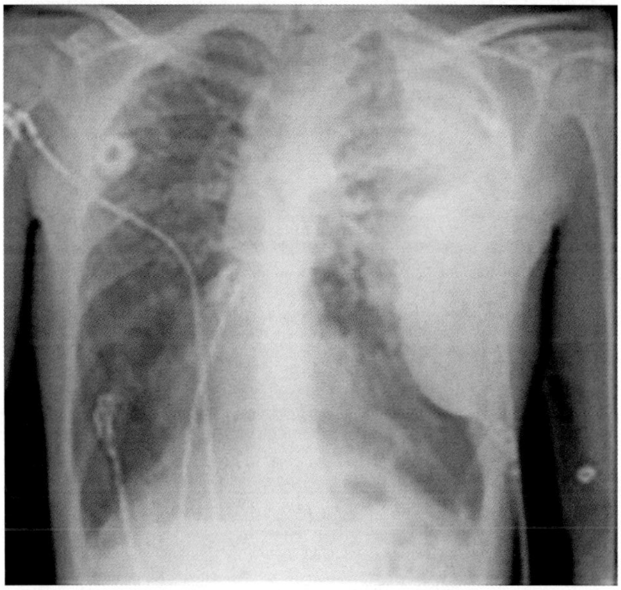

Figure 10.18 Frontal chest x-ray 2 hours after removal of a chest tube shows an opacity involving the left chest wall, indicative of a hematoma.

Thoracic Aortic Stent Grafts

Detailed descriptions of the technical aspects of thoracic aortic interventions are beyond the scope of this text.

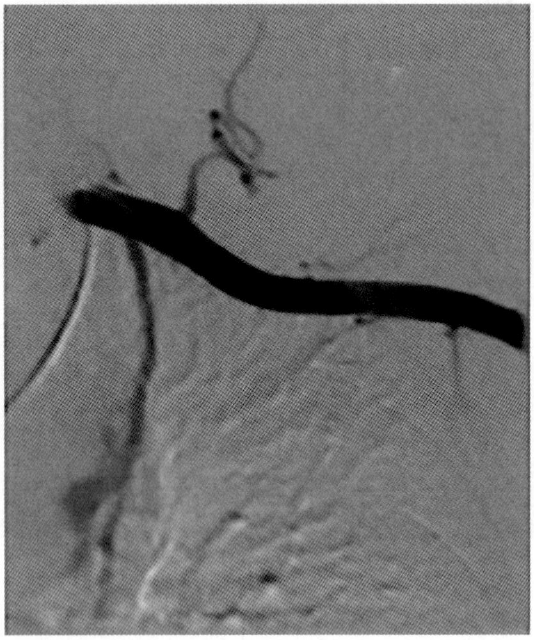

Figure 10.19 Digital subtraction angiogram after selective catheterization of the left subclavian artery demonstrates contrast extravasation from the internal mammary artery.

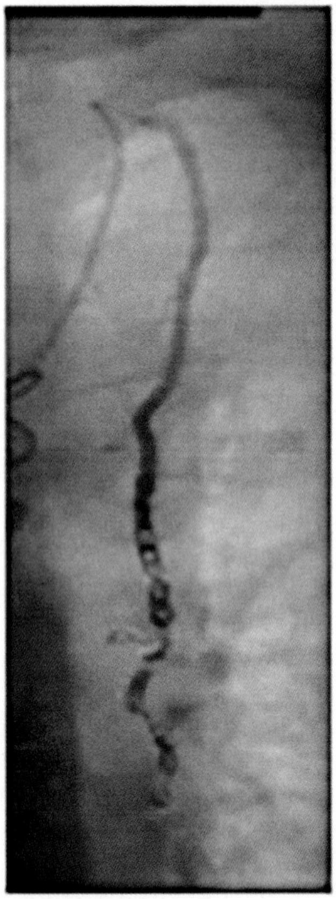

Figure 10.20 Digital angiogram after selective catheterization and coil embolization of the left internal mammary artery shows no further extravasation.

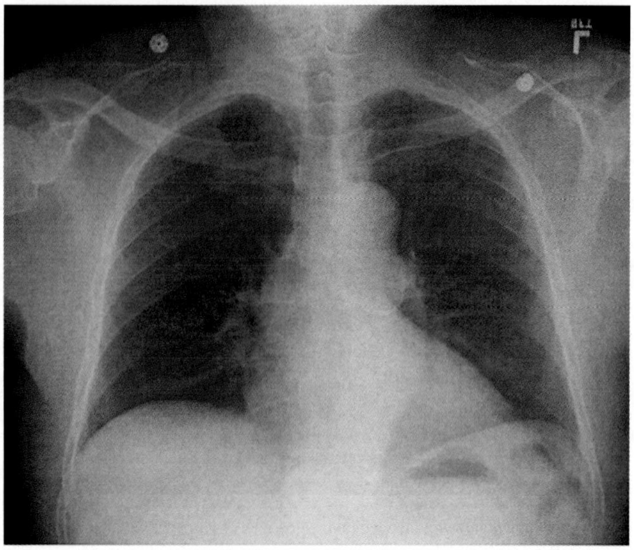

Figure 10.21 Frontal chest radiograph demonstrating a mass overlapping the left hilum, with curvilinear calcific borders.

With the advent of commercially available, dedicated, branched thoracic aortic stent grafts, hybrid reconstruction techniques, advancements in intraprocedural navigation tools, CT fluoroscopy overlay, and intravascular ultrasound imaging, thoracic aortic interventions have progressed immensely.

Indications for a Thoracic Aortic Stent Graft

The current indications for the use of thoracic aortic stent grafts include treatment of thoracic aortic aneurysms more than 5.5 to 6 cm in diameter, acute Stanford type B thoracic aortic dissection, penetrating aortic ulcer, aortic transection and pseudoaneurysms after trauma, aortic coarctation, and aortoesophageal–aortobronchial fistulae.

The success of stent grafting in the thoracic aorta is mainly dependent on the anatomic suitability of the aorta (Figs. 10.21 to 10.23). At least a 2-cm landing zone is required on either end for standard aortic stent grafts. This can be altered if hybrid reconstruction techniques are applied. Relative contraindications for thoracic aortic stent grafts include active infection or inflammation of the aorta, renal failure, and young age. Preoperative CT angiography is the main tool to plan for thoracic aortic stent grafting. The size of the aneurysm (diameter, length), landing zones, mural thrombus, location of entry and reentry tears in case of dissection, length of aortic injury, branch vessel location, origin from the aneurysm or dissection, and diameter of access arteries are assessed by preoperative CT angiography. For successful proximal deployment, aortic arch vessels may be intentionally occluded with the creation of a cervical carotid to carotid or carotid to subclavian bypass. In addition, the stent grafting may be combined with open surgical repair of the ascending aorta, especially with type A aortic dissection or if the aneurysm involves the proximal arch.

Complications of Thoracic Aortic Stent Grafting

Complications of the procedure include stent thrombosis, bleeding, rupture, endoleak, thromboembolism resulting

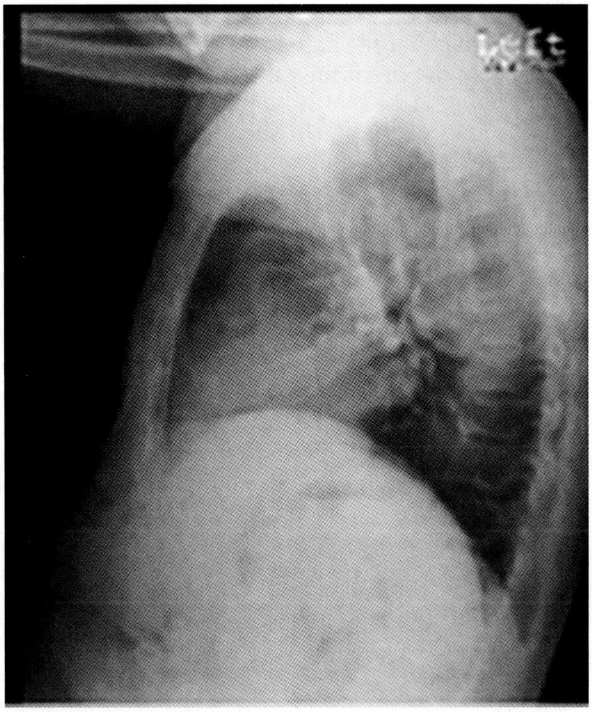

Figure 10.22 Lateral chest radiograph showing that the mass is contiguous with the inferior surface of the thoracic aorta.

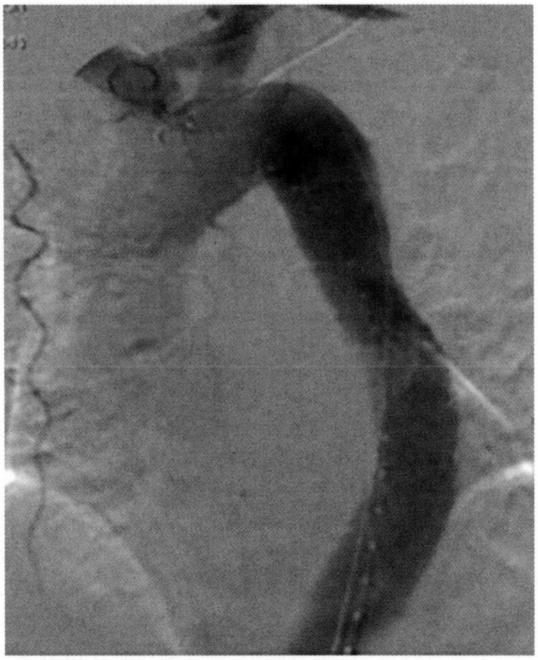

Figure 10.23 Digital subtraction angiogram after stent graft exclusion of the thoracic aortic aneurysm.

in stroke or transient ischemic attack, spinal cord ischemia resulting in paralysis, new aortic dissection, and injury to the esophagus and bronchi. Patients are regularly followed with CT angiography at 1, 3, 6, and 12 months and then annually to assess for stent graft integrity, endoleak, and branch vessel occlusion. The definition of endoleak differs depending on whether the stent graft is used for an aneurysm or for dissection. Persistent perfusion of the aneurysm sac defines endoleak in aneurysm repair and is classified depending on the site and cause of the leak, as follows:

Type 1: endoleak from the attachment sites of the graft
Type 2: endoleak due to retrograde perfusion of the sac from aortic branch vessels
Type 3: endoleak due to defects or separation of components of the stent graft
Type 4: endoleak from porosity of the graft
Type 5: continued sac enlargement despite the lack of a detectable sac perfusion on imaging (also known as *endotension*)

In the case of an aortic dissection, persistent perfusion of the false lumen is considered an endoleak.

Venous Interventions

The two most common venous interventional procedures performed in the thorax are placement of central venous access catheters, with or without an implantable port, and recanalization of occluded central veins.

Central Venous Catheters

Central venous catheters are placed for short-term or long-term venous access and include those that are temporary, nontunneled catheters or tunneled catheters, with or without an implantable port. The number of lumens vary from one to three and the size of the catheters ranges from 6 to 15 Fr. Small-bore catheters are routinely used for drug infusion (e.g., chemotherapy, antibiotics, vasoactive drugs) or total parenteral nutrition, and large-bore catheters are used for dialysis, plasmapheresis, and extracorporeal membrane oxygenation. Multilumen large-bore catheters may have a split end or staggered end to prevent recirculation of blood. An implantable subcutaneous port attached to the catheter allows for long-term accessibility while decreasing the risk of infection and is commonly used for chemotherapy. The catheters are radiopaque and can be easily visualized on plane radiographs. The implantable ports may be radiopaque with specific letters (CT with ports made by Bard [Tempe, AZ]) to denote their orientation and ability to accept high injection rates through the ports. The contraindications for tunneled and implantable catheters are the presence of active bloodstream infection, access site skin infection, and severe coagulopathy. An international normalized ratio less than 1.5 and platelet count of more than 50,000 mm^3 are recommended.

Considerations Before Placing a Central Venous Catheter

Venous access for central venous catheters is obtained via the internal jugular, external jugular, and subclavian veins (the preferred order). Right chest catheters are preferred due to the straight course of the right brachycephalic vein and superior vena cava. Left chest catheters are often associated with migration into the azygos vein and an increased incidence of complications. However, the presence of breast cancer, axillary lymph node dissection, chest wall wound or deformity, and venous occlusion (in the neck or chest) determine the choice of venous access and catheter placement. Subclavian venous access is rarely preferred because it is associated with a more than 50% incidence of venous thrombosis and high rate of catheter pinch-off syndrome, a condition in which the catheter is compressed between the first rib and clavicle, leading to the catheter breaking off at the site of the compression. The catheters are positioned at the cavoatrial junction under fluoroscopy; however, large-bore catheters are preferentially positioned in the proximal right atrium to obtain better flow during blood withdrawal for dialysis.

Complications

The main complications of the procedure are inadvertent arterial puncture, leading to hematoma, injury to the lung apex causing pneumothorax or hemothorax, infection, air embolism, and malposition of the catheter. Rare complications include cardiac or vena cava perforation leading to hemopericardium and extravascular migration of the catheter. Although an anteroposterior radiograph of the chest is often sufficient to visualize the catheter position, oblique views may be necessary to detect a kink in the catheter or malposition into the internal mammary vein, aorta, mediastinum, or esophagus. In difficult cases, CT imaging is helpful.

Late complications include catheter malposition due to migration, fibrin sheath formation around the catheter leading to nonfunctioning, central venous thrombosis, or chronic stenosis or occlusion. A fibrin sheath forms around the tip of the catheter and acts as one-way valve, preventing blood draw (Fig. 10.24). This can be diagnosed on fluoroscopy by injecting contrast material through the catheter or port. The contrast material often tracks along the length of the catheter and exits at a different location than the tip of the catheter. Treatment involves infusion of low dose tPA through the catheter, endovascular stripping of the fibrin sheath, or replacement of the catheter. Catheter pinch-off syndrome can be diagnosed on chest radiographs based on the characteristic compresssion or kink of the catheter between the first rib and clavicle. A detached catheter can easily be identified in the heart or pulmonary circulation and can present with arrhythmia (Figs. 10.25 to 10.27). Venous thrombosis associated with a central venous catheter occurs in 3% to 11% of cases and is more common with subclavian venous access. The position of the catheter tip in the cranial third of the superior vena cava or brachiocephalic veins is associated with a higher incidence of venous thrombosis (45% vs. 5.7% with placement in the middle

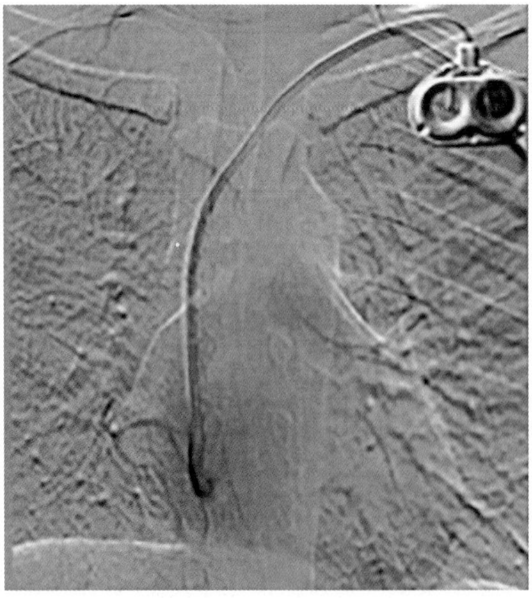

Figure 10.24 Digital subtraction angiogram after injecting contrast into one lumen of a dual-lumen mediport demonstrating contrast outlining the catheter tip, indicating the presence of a fibrin sheath around the catheter tip.

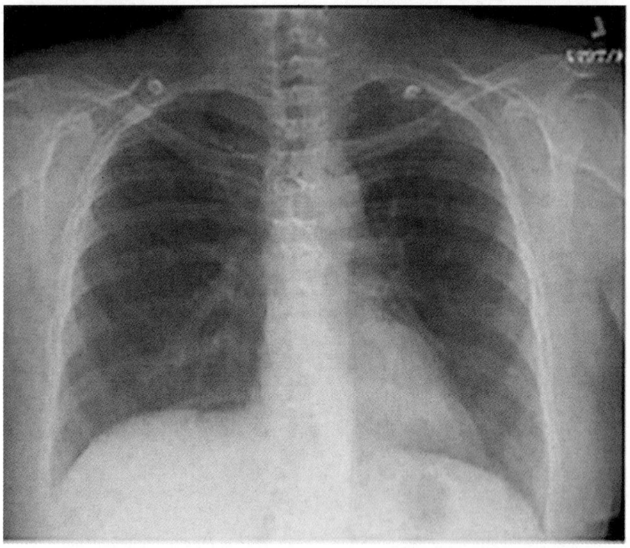

Figure 10.25 Frontal chest radiograph showing a dislodged catheter tip in the left pulmonary artery.

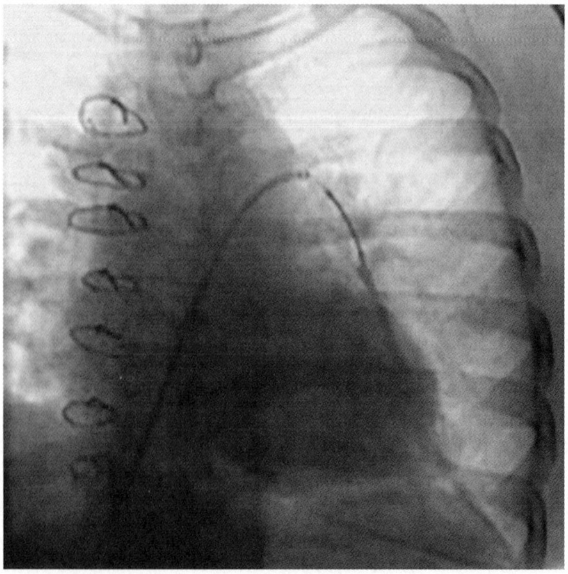

Figure 10.26 Digital fluoroscopic image demonstrating the engagement of the dislodged catheter using a loop snare.

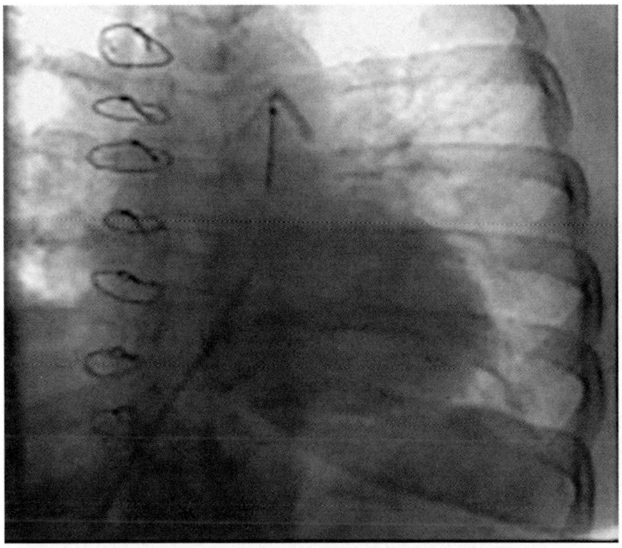

Figure 10.27 Digital fluoroscopic image showing the catheter being removed from the left pulmonary artery.

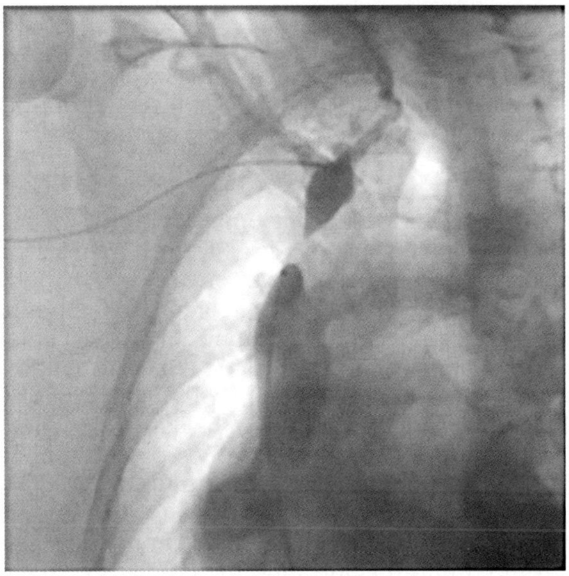

Figure 10.28 Digital fluoroscopic image showing a short-segment occlusion of the right brachiocephalic vein.

or distal third of the superior vena cava). Thrombosis of the jugular and subclavian veins is diagnosed with duplex ultrasound, but contrast-enhanced CT is used when brachiocephalic veins or the superior vena cava is affected. Treatment involves systemic anticoagulation and, in some cases, removal of the catheter. Chronic venous occlusion can result in enlarged collaterals in the neck and upper chest and may be symptomatic, with arm swelling, headache, and blurred vision (Fig. 10.28).

Venous Revascularization

Central venous occlusion may have benign causes, especially with the long-term use of central venous catheters, mediastinal fibrosis, postsurgical anastomotic strictures, infection, and radiotherapy or can occur with malignant tumor invasion or compression from lung cancer,

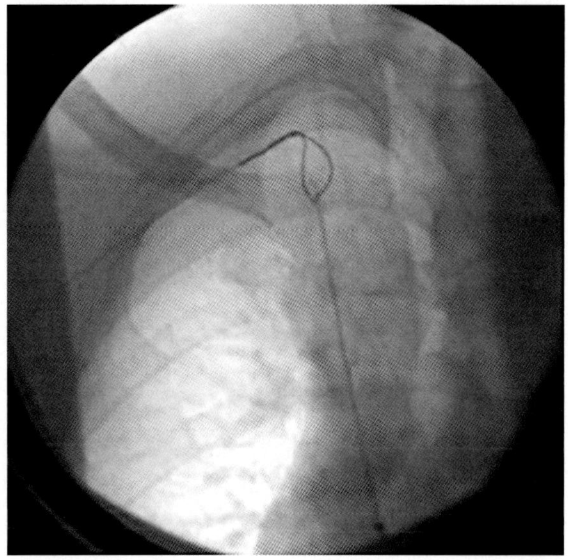

Figure 10.29 Digital fluoroscopic image demonstrating sharp recanalization of the occlusion using a long needle targeting an open snare.

lymphoma, or metastases. The most common cause of malignant superior vena cava occlusion is bronchogenic carcinoma. Patients may be asymptomatic or may present with arm or neck swelling, pain, blurred vision, or headache. In patients with a working dialysis circuit, increased bleeding following dialysis, incomplete urea clearance, high pressures during dialysis, and recurrent thrombosis of the dialysis access may occur. Treatment is indicated in the presence of symptoms or a failing dialysis circuit. Contrast-enhanced CT and conventional venography are the mainstays for planning therapy. Acute venous thrombosis is treated with local infusion of thrombolytics and mechanical thrombectomy. Benign stenoses are preferentially treated with angioplasty, and stents are used when angioplasty fails or when complicated by dissection or rupture (Figs. 10.29 to 10.31). Malignant strictures are preferentially treated with a stent or stent grafts. These therapies are effective in 70% to 90% of patients in relieving the symptoms. Complications include rupture, leading to hemopericardium or hemomediastinum, stent migration into the heart or the pulmonary vessels, PE, and infection. Patients are followed with CT for recurrent venous occlusion or stent thrombosis. Recurrent stenoses are treated with repeat angioplasty, without additional stent placement.

■ Lymphatic Interventions

Thoracic Duct Embolization

The thoracic duct is the central drainage pathway for the lymphatic system of the abdomen and lower extremities. It commences as the cranial continuation of the cisterna chyli, courses posterior to the esophagus in the posterior mediastinum, and terminates at the junction of the left subclavian vein and left internal jugular vein. It is usually

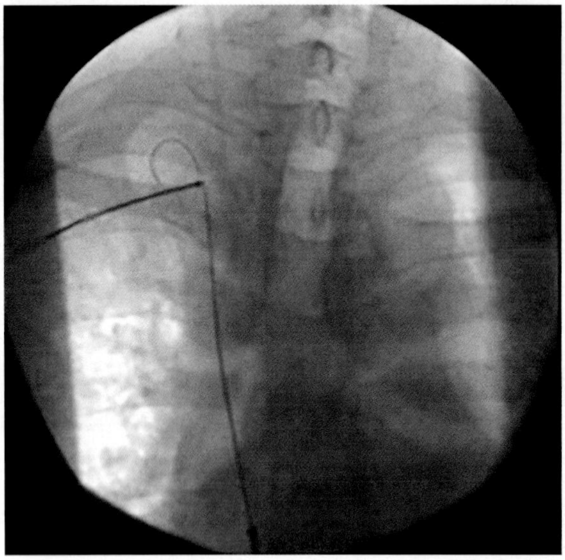

Figure 10.30 Digital fluoroscopic image showing the snare being closed around a wire fed through the hollow needle to obtain through and through access.

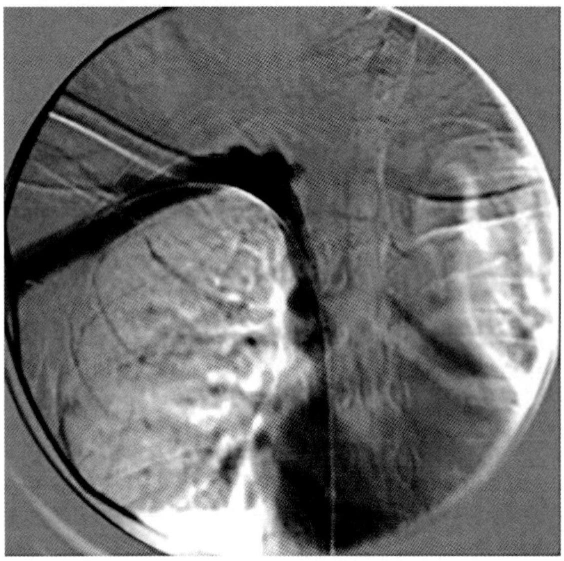

Figure 10.31 Digital subtraction angiogram after stent placement demonstrating a successful recanalization.

a single channel, but duplication and multichannel structure occur in 10% of cases.

Interventions on the thoracic duct aim at occlusion of the duct in the presence of thoracic duct injury resulting in clinically significant chylothorax. Thoracic duct injury is most common with esophageal and other mediastinal surgeries and occurs at a frequency of 0.5% to 2%. Malignant occlusion of the thoracic duct from mediastinal tumors can also result in its rupture and in chylothorax.

Indications for Thoracic Duct Embolization

Conservative therapy with fat restriction results in spontaneous resolution of iatrogenic chylothorax in 28% of patients. Thoracic duct embolization is recommended

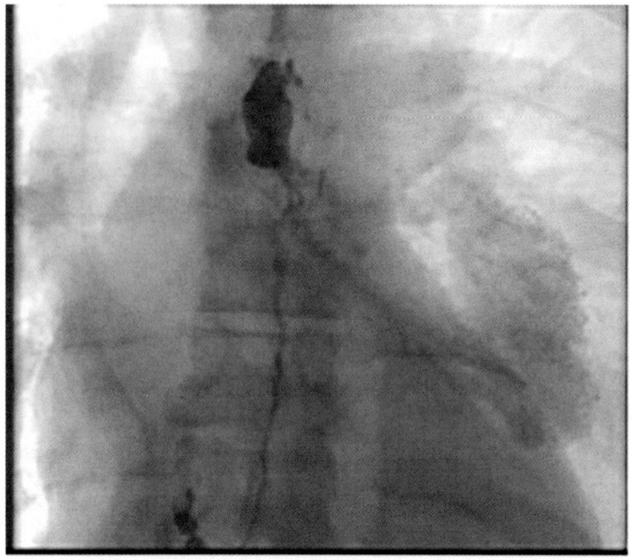

Figure 10.32 Intranodal lymphangiogram demonstrates the thoracic duct, which is disrupted in the upper thorax with extravasation of ethiodized oil (Lipiodol or Ethiodol) into the right pleural space.

for persistent chylothorax after 2 weeks of conservative therapy, high-output (>1000 mL/day) chylothorax, and progressively worsening chylothorax on conservative therapy.

Performing Thoracic Duct Embolization

Initially, lymphangiography is performed to opacify the thoracic duct. This is achieved through a pedal lymphangiography or nodal lymphangiography. We routinely practice nodal lymphangiography. In this technique, 5 mL of ethiodized oil (Lipiodol or Ethiodol) is injected into the lymph nodes at either groin under ultrasound guidance. Within a few minutes, the iliac lymphatics are opacified and can be seen on fluoroscopy. The thoracic duct is visualized in 30 to 60 minutes. The duct is accessed percutaneously from the epigastric region using a 22-gauge long Chiba needle under fluoroscopy. A wire is advanced into the duct, and the needle is exchanged for a 3-Fr microcatheter. A contrast material injection under fluoroscopy confirms the injury and extravasation of contrast material into either thoracic cavity (Fig. 10.32). Embolization is performed across the injured segment using coils and/or *n*-butyl cyanoacrylate glue (Fig. 10.33). Other approaches to access the thoracic duct from the neck and subclavian vein are also described. If thoracic duct cannulation is not feasible, the cisterna chyli and adjacent lymphatics are disrupted with serial needle passes to decompress the thoracic duct into the retroperitoneal spaces.

Results of Thoracic Duct Embolization

Thoracic duct embolization is effective in 50% to 70% of patients. One study reported a complete response in 61%, partial response in 23% and clinical failure in 15%. Disruption of the cisterna chyli is less effective, with 56% failure rates.

The main complications include chemical pneumonitis, infection, and nontarget embolization. Chemical

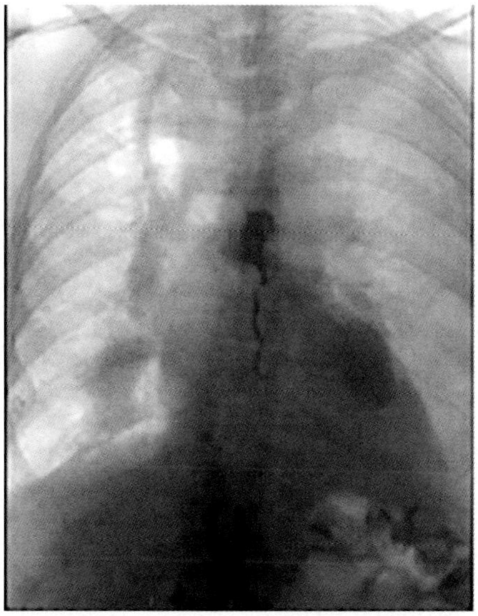

Figure 10.33 Chest x-ray demonstrating occlusion of the thoracic duct with a combination of coils and *n*-butyl cyanoacrylate glue.

pneumonitis is managed conservatively; infection after embolization will require antibiotic treatment. Nontarget embolization is managed according to the site of affliction.

Conclusion

Vascular and lymphatic interventions in the thorax are highly effective and very important in patient management. The practice and patient care are highly dependent on preoperative and postoperative imaging with CT angiography. The success of these procedures requires dedication and commitment from the physician for continued long-term success.

Bibliography

Bashir MR, Ferral H, Jacobs C, McCarthy W, Goldin M. Endoleaks after endovascular abdominal aortic aneurysm repair: management strategies according to CT findings. *AJR Am J Roentgenol*. 2009;192:W178–W186.

Burrel M, Real MI, Barrufet M, et al. Pulmonary artery pseudoaneurysm after Swan-Ganz catheter placement: embolization with vascular plugs. *J Vasc Interv Radiol*. 2010;21:577–581.

Cartin-Ceba R, Swanson KL, Krowka MJ. Pulmonary arteriovenous malformations. *Chest*. 2013;144:1033–1044.

Cody O'Dell M, Gill AE, Hawkins CM. Bronchial artery embolization for the treatment of acute hemoptysis. *Tech Vasc Interv Radiol*. 2017;20(4): 263–265.

Colotto M, Da Ros S, Barbarossa G, et al. Atrial fibrillation and right bundle branch block complicating coil embolization of a huge pulmonary arterio-venous malformation. *Intern Med*. 2011;50:2983–2986.

Dariushnia SR, Gill AE, Martin LG, et al. Quality improvement guidelines for diagnostic arteriography. *J Vasc Interv Radiol*. 2014;25:1873–1881.

Davies MG, El-Sayed HF. Current status of clot removal for acute pulmonary embolism. *Ann Vasc Surg*. 2016;31:211–220.

Faughnan ME, Palda VA, Garcia-Tsao G, et al. International guidelines for the diagnosis and management of hereditary haemorrhagic telangiectasia. *J Med Genet*. 2011;48:73–87.

Hao Q, Dong BR, Yue J, Wu T, Liu GJ. Thrombolytic therapy for pulmonary embolism. *Cochrane Database Syst Rev*. 2015;(9):CD004437.

Itkin M, Kucharczuk JC, Kwak A, Trerotola SO, Kaiser LR. Nonoperative thoracic duct embolization for traumatic thoracic duct leak: experience in 109 patients. *J Thorac Cardiovasc Surg*. 2010;139:584–589. discussion 589-590.

Jaff MR, McMurtry MS, Archer SL, et al. Management of massive and submassive pulmonary embolism, iliofemoral deep vein thrombosis, and chronic thromboembolic pulmonary hypertension: a scientific statement from the American heart association. *Circulation*. 2011;123:1788–1830.

Kalva SP. Bronchial artery embolization. *Tech Vasc Interv Radiol*. 2009;12:130–138.

Kische S, Akin I, Ince H, et al. Stent-graft repair in acute and chronic diseases of the thoracic aorta. *Rev Esp Cardiol*. 2008;61:1070–1086.

Kucukay F, Ozdemir M, Senol E, Okten S, Ereren M, Karan A. Large pulmonary arteriovenous malformations: long-term results of embolization with AMPLATZER vascular plugs. *J Vasc Interv Radiol*. 2014;25:1327–1332.

Kuhajda I, Milosevic M, Ilincic D, et al. Pulmonary arteriovenous malformation-etiology, clinical four case presentations and review of the literature. *Ann Transl Med*. 2015;3:171.

Kuo WT, Banerjee A, Kim PS, et al. Pulmonary embolism response to fragmentation, embolectomy, and catheter thrombolysis (PERFECT): initial results from a prospective multicenter registry. *Chest*. 2015;148:667–673.

Kuo WT, Gould MK, Louie JD, Rosenberg JK, Sze DY, Hofmann LV. Catheter-directed therapy for the treatment of massive pulmonary embolism: systematic review and meta-analysis of modern techniques. *J Vasc Interv Radiol*. 2009;20: 1431–1440.

Nadolski G, Itkin M. Thoracic duct embolization for the management of chylothoraces. *Curr Opin Pulm Med*. 2013;19:380–386.

Najarian KE, Morris CS. Arterial embolization in the chest. *J Thorac Imaging*. 1998;13:93–104.

Nguyen ET, Silva CI, Seely JM, Chong S, Lee KS, Muller NL. Pulmonary artery aneurysms and pseudoaneurysms in adults: findings at CT and radiography. *AJR Am J Roentgenol*. 2007;188:W126–W134.

Pamarthi V, Stecker MS, Schenker MP, et al. Thoracic duct embolization and disruption for treatment of chylous effusions: experience with 105 patients. *J Vasc Interv Radiol*. 2014;25:1398–1404.

Patel N, Patel NJ, Agnihotri K, et al. Utilization of catheter-directed thrombolysis in pulmonary embolism and outcome difference between systemic thrombolysis and catheter-directed thrombolysis. *Catheter Cardiovasc Interv*. 2015;86:1219–1227.

Piazza G, Hohlfelder B, Jaff MR, et al. A prospective, single-arm, multicenter trial of ultrasound-facilitated, catheter-directed, low-dose fibrinolysis for acute massive and submassive pulmonary embolism: the SEATTLE II study. *JACC Cardiovasc Interv*. 2015;8:1382–1392.

Pollak JS, Saluja S, Thabet A, Henderson KJ, Denbow N, White RI Jr. Clinical and anatomic outcomes after embolotherapy of pulmonary arteriovenous malformations. *J Vasc Interv Radiol*. 2006;17:35–44. quiz 5.

Schoepf UJ. Pulmonary artery CTA. *Tech Vasc Interv Radiol*. 2006;9:180–191.

Schoepf UJ, Savino G, Lake DR, Ravenel JG, Costello P. The age of CT pulmonary angiography. *J Thorac Imaging*. 2005;20:273–279.

Stein PD, Athanasoulis C, Alavi A, et al. Complications and validity of pulmonary angiography in acute pulmonary embolism. *Circulation*. 1992;85: 462–468.

White RI Jr. Pulmonary arteriovenous malformations: how do I embolize? *Tech Vasc Interv Radiol*. 2007;10:283–290.

White RI Jr, Pollak JS, Wirth JA. Pulmonary arteriovenous malformations: diagnosis and transcatheter embolotherapy. *J Vasc Interv Radiol*. 1996;7:787–804.

Yoon W, Kim JK, Kim YH, Chung TW, Kang HK. Bronchial and nonbronchial systemic artery embolization for life-threatening hemoptysis: a comprehensive review. *Radiographics*. 2002;22:1395–1409.

Zuckerman DA, Sterling KM, Oser RF. Safety of pulmonary angiography in the 1990s. *J Vasc Interv Radiol*. 1996;7:199–205.

CHAPTER 11

Problem-Oriented Radionuclide Myocardial Perfusion Imaging

Vikas Veeranna and Sharmila Dorbala

CHAPTER OUTLINE

Introduction

Radionuclide myocardial perfusion imaging (MPI) plays a key role in the diagnosis and management of individuals with known or suspected coronary artery disease (CAD). Recent breakthroughs in single-photon emission computed tomography (SPECT) technology and software, along with the increasing availability of positron emission tomography (PET) scanners, are rapidly changing the existing paradigm of MPI. Cardiac SPECT MPI is a versatile tool to diagnose obstructive CAD noninvasively; it has a sensitivity of 82% to 88% for exercise and 88% to 91% for pharmacologic stress and a specificity of 70% to 88% for exercise and 75% to 90% for pharmacologic stress. Perfusion defect size, severity, location, and reversibility are powerful markers, not only to identify the extent and severity of CAD, but also to estimate the risk of future myocardial infarction and cardiac death. The left ventricular ejection fraction (LVEF) and volumes are critical to guide patient management. Cardiac PET MPI is more accurate than SPECT MPI to diagnose obstructive CAD. Peak stress ejection fraction (EF) by PET provides significant incremental value over perfusion imaging to identify obstructive multivessel CAD. Quantitative PET with myocardial blood flow and coronary flow reserve (CFR) are powerful tools to stratify risk, exclude multivessel CAD, and identify coronary microvascular dysfunction. Hybrid PET-CT imaging with calcium scores and CT coronary angiography can significantly enhance the diagnostic value of quantitative MPI. Multiple factors, however, can compromise the quality of study, affect the eventual scan interpretation, and thereby affect patient management and outcomes. In this chapter, we will address the challenges of stress MPI before and during the test and during reporting, along with solutions to optimize radionuclide MPI.

Before the Test: Appropriate Patient Selection

Rest myocardial blood flow may remain normal, even with severe underlying coronary stenosis, due to compensatory coronary microvascular vasodilation. Therefore detection of inducible ischemia with exercise or pharmacologic stress remains the cornerstone in the diagnosis of CAD. Whereas exercise and dobutamine stress increase myocardial oxygen demand, vasodilator stress agents produce differential hyperemia between the diseased and nondiseased territories. All forms of stress testing have inherent risks, which can be minimized by appropriate selection of patients and stress tests.

Challenge: Patient Selection

Appropriate patient selection is critical to ensure the optimal risk versus benefit of MPI, including the type of stress test. As radionuclide MPI is rapidly expanding with conventional SPECT, novel semiconductor detector SPECT, and PET MPI, referring physicians may find it challenging to identify the right test for a given clinical question.

Radionuclide MPI and the more recent, multisocietal, appropriate use criteria (AUC) documents provide valuable information regarding the clinical use of radionuclide imaging—SPECT and PET are used interchangeably in the AUC document. The RAND Corporation has defined appropriate use as one wherein the expected clinical benefit of the test outweighs the risks of the procedure, including the radiation risk. The radionuclide AUC were developed based on expert opinion, with the test indications categorized as appropriate, may be appropriate (previous term *uncertain*), and rarely appropriate (previous term *inappropriate*) by an expert panel. Several clinical studies have confirmed that although most MPI studies (70%–85%) are performed for appropriate indications, a smaller but significant proportion of tests is performed for may be appropriate or rarely appropriate indications. To reduce the use of stress testing in the latter two categories, the Choosing Wisely initiative of the American Board of Internal Medicine (ABIM), in conjunction with *Consumer Reports*, has listed specific recommendations for physicians and patients to be aware of prior to performing a study; it is summarized as follows:

1. Don't perform stress cardiac imaging or coronary angiography in patients without cardiac symptoms unless high-risk markers are present.
2. Don't perform cardiac imaging for patients who are at low risk.
3. Don't perform radionuclide imaging as part of routine follow-up in asymptomatic patients.
4. Don't perform cardiac imaging as a preoperative assessment in patients scheduled to undergo low- or intermediate-risk noncardiac surgery.
5. Use methods to reduce radiation exposure in cardiac imaging, whenever possible, including not performing such tests when limited benefits are likely.

Potential Solutions

A careful review of the reason for the study will ensure appropriate patient selection. This may sometimes involve a discussion with the referring physician to clarify that the clinical question can be appropriately answered by radionuclide MPI or any alternative tests.

An online app (radionuclide appropriateness use criteria) is helpful to evaluate the AUC for any given indication. As of January 2017, Medicare payments have been linked to documentation of AUC in the study report. Several decision support systems now incorporate professional societal AUC criteria into physician order entry systems.

Stress Test: Exercise and Pharmacologic Stress

Exercise is physiologic and preferred in patients able to perform routine daily activities. Exercise stress also provides information on functional capacity and symptoms, and is a powerful prognostic marker. Treadmill exercise with a Bruce or modified Bruce protocol is the most common type of stress test in the United States; bicycle stress tests are more commonly used in Europe. Although functional testing has good diagnostic accuracy, nonobstructive disease may not be detected, especially if the test is submaximal. Exercise stress alone, without imaging, is appropriate in low- or intermediate-risk patients with an interpretable electrocardiogram (ECG). Even in patients who need imaging, those with moderate physical functioning should undergo a symptom-limited exercise stress test. Pharmacologic stress testing is an excellent alternative in patients who are unable to exercise, have contraindications to exercise stress, or achieve a submaximal target heart rate during exercise.

Imaging in these patients is driven by other patient characteristics, such as intermediate to high risk for CAD, known CAD, or a baseline ECG that makes ischemic changes uninterpretable. Incremental diagnostic and prognostic information is obtained from the exercise from parameters such as the Duke treadmill score and heart rate recovery. For a standard Bruce protocol, the Duke treadmill score is calculated as exercise duration in minutes minus five times the maximal ST segment depression (in millimeters), minus four times the chest pain score (0 = no angina, 1 = nonlimiting angina, and 2 = exercise-limiting angina), and heart rate recovery as heart rate at peak exercise minus heart rate at 1 minute into recovery (normal >12 beats/min). A mildly abnormal SPECT MPI portends a higher risk in patients with an intermediate or high Duke treadmill score than in patients with a low Duke treadmill score.

Challenge: Rest Chest Pain

Occasionally, patients referred for a stress test may experience rest chest pain at the time of the test.

Potential Solutions

Examine the patient clinically, ensure hemodynamic stability, and obtain a rest ECG. If clinically unstable, refer the patient to the emergency room for further evaluation.

If the patient has ongoing chest pain but is stable hemodynamically, consider injection of a perfusion tracer (SPECT or PET) during chest pain and rest imaging. In a randomized clinical trial of patients presenting with chest pain to the emergency room, rest MPI, with radionuclide injected during ongoing chest pain or within 3 hours of pain resolution, significantly reduced unnecessary hospitalizations without differences in clinical outcomes. The extent of perfusion abnormality correlated well with the anatomic extent of myocardial ischemia. The sensitivity and specificity of rest MPI performed at <6 hours of the onset of symptoms are >90% and 80%, respectively. However, the reduced specificity is due to lack of differentiation between acute reduction in blood flow versus hibernation or a chronic infarct. The negative predictive value of a completely negative rest MPI in patients with acute chest pain is >99%. Furthermore, resting MPI in these patients has prognostic clinical implications. A positive resting MPI has up to a 30% short-term event rate as opposed to a <1% 30-day event rate for a normal MPI.

If the patient is clinically stable and the rest MPI (during chest pain) is normal, the next step is to proceed with the stress test and imaging. If the rest MPI is abnormal and the patient is clinically unstable, referral to coronary angiography may be warranted. If the patient is clinically

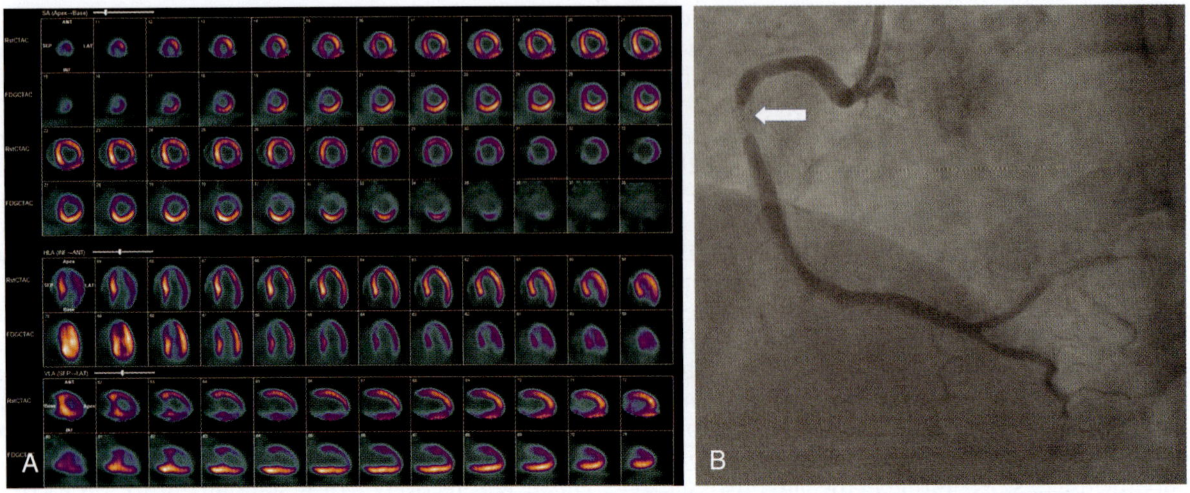

Figure 11.1 A 55-year-old woman with known coronary artery disease referred for evaluation of ischemia. (A) At the time of rest image acquisition, the patient complained of typical chest pain, with no electrocardiographic changes. ^{13}N-Ammonia resting perfusion images show a large perfusion defect in the entire inferior and inferolateral walls, with significant mismatch pattern on ^{18}F-fluorodeoxyglucose images, suggestive of rest myocardial ischemia. (B) Subsequent invasive coronary angiogram demonstrates a severe proximal right coronary artery in-stent restenosis *(arrow)*.

stable and has no active chest pain, ^{18}F-fluorodeoxyglucose (FDG) PET can be performed. A mismatch between rest myocardial perfusion and FDG metabolic imaging suggests hibernating myocardium as a potential cause for the rest angina (Fig. 11.1).

Exercise Stress Testing

A Bruce or modified Bruce protocol with 3-minute stages is the most commonly used exercise treadmill protocol. During the treadmill test, the ECG is monitored, blood pressure is obtained at regular intervals, and symptoms are assessed. The physician performing the test should be aware of the indications for early termination of the exercise stress. Unlike stress echocardiography (echo), where the exercise is terminated at maximal exercise, the exercise during MPI should be continued for at least 1 minute after injection of the radiotracer to ensure adequate radiotracer circulation and myocardial uptake.

Challenges During Exercise Stress Testing

During the stress test, patients can experience chest pain, hypotension, ischemic ST segment changes, tachyarrhythmias or bradyarrhythmias, syncope, falls, or other complications.

Potential Solutions

Objective evidence of significant ischemia on the ECG, horizontal or downsloping ST depression (>2 mm), and significant ST elevation (>1 mm; Fig. 11.2) are reasons to inject the radiotracer (if feasible) and terminate the exercise, even if the patient is asymptomatic and the age-predicted maximal heart rate (85% of 220 minus age in years) has not been achieved. When significant ST segment elevation is noted during exercise, it localizes the ischemia to a coronary territory. Therefore radiotracer injection and imaging are typically avoided and the patient scheduled for emergent coronary angiography—unless the patient is stable and there is a delay for coronary angiography.

Subjective complaints of moderate to severe chest pain during exercise may be reasons to terminate exercise. In a patient experiencing exercise-limiting chest pain, if the heart rate is submaximal, the exercise test is terminated, without radiotracer injection. A vasodilator study is performed after the chest pain resolves. Reproducible angina during stress, even in the absence of ECG changes, may warrant additional workup. In hemodynamically stable patients, sublingual nitroglycerin can be administered for moderate to severe chest pain. Persistent or worsening chest pain, even after three doses of sublingual nitroglycerin (0.4 mg) at 5-minute intervals, or hemodynamic instability may be a reason for referral to urgent coronary angiography.

Hypotension, a decrease in systolic blood pressure below the preexercise standing blood pressure, especially when accompanied by other ischemic signs or symptoms, is a marker of underlying significant CAD and death. Exercise-induced hypotension is typically managed by IV fluids and, if necessary, referral to coronary angiography. Nitroglycerin and beta blockers are contraindicated in patients with exercise-induced hypotension.

Symptomatic arrhythmias are managed as per the American Heart Association's advanced cardiac life support algorithms. Falls or syncope should be addressed immediately with evaluation of hemodynamic status, arrhythmias, and orthopedic limitations and assessment of injuries.

Submaximal Heart Rate Response

Chronotropic incompetence is defined as the inability to attain 85% of the age-predicted maximal heart rate during exercise. It may be related to cardiac disease, medication use (e.g., beta blockers, calcium channel blockers), or orthopedic limitations. The diagnostic accuracy of MPI to identify significant obstructive CAD is limited in patients with a submaximal heart rate response. Therefore if the reason for the MPI is to assess response to medical therapy

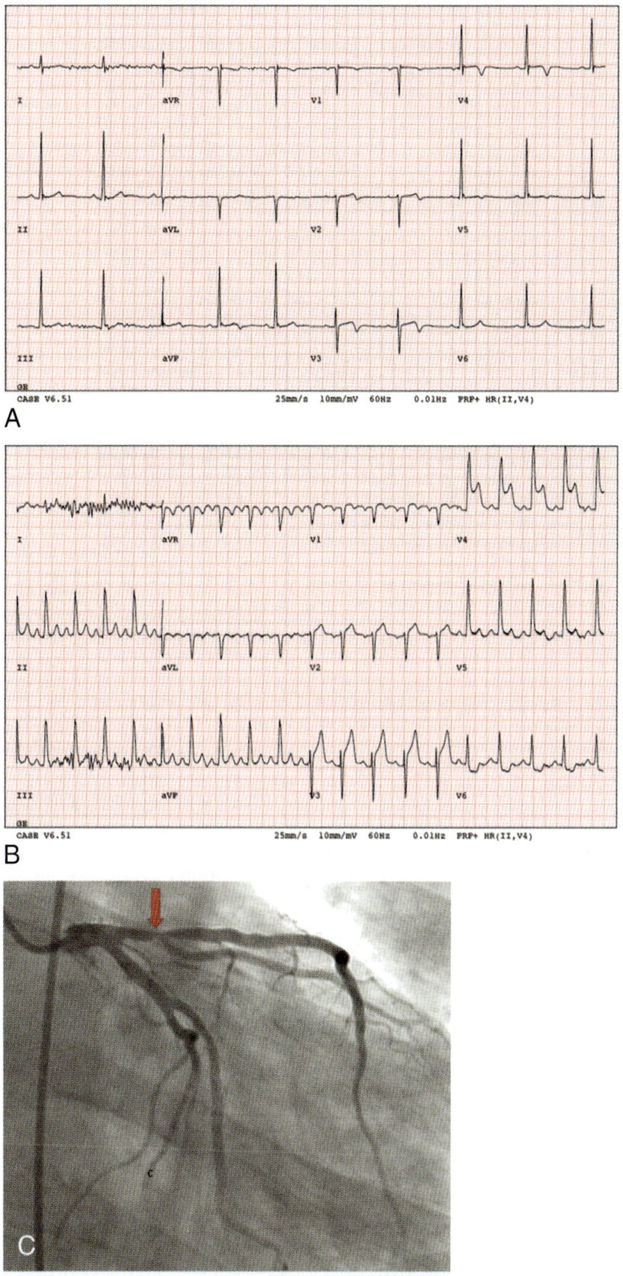

Figure 11.2 Resting (A) and peak (B) exercise electrocardiograms (ECGs). The peak exercise ECG demonstrates ST segment elevation of >1 mm in leads V3 and V4. (C) Corresponding invasive coronary angiogram image demonstrates a severe (>70%) stenosis of the proximal left anterior descending coronary artery *(arrow)*.

(as in medically managed patients with CAD), radiotracer may be injected at the heart rate achieved despite submaximal heart rate, especially if a workload of 5 METs (metabolic equivalent of task [or just metabolic equivalent]) is achieved. However, if the reason for the study is to identify ischemia or understand the hemodynamic significance of stenoses of indeterminate significance or preoperative evaluation, a maximal heart rate response is preferred for administration of the radiotracer. Whatever the reason, chronotropic incompetence is a marker of high 2-year mortality, particularly when associated with perfusion defects on MPI. The reasons for high mortality with chronotropic incompetence are not known but may reflect cardiac autonomic function, which may be evident in individuals with advanced heart disease.

Potential Solutions

In patients with submaximal heart rate response to exercise, pharmacologic stress testing (with a vasodilator or dobutamine) is an excellent alternative. Adenosine and dobutamine infusions are typically administered after the treadmill test is terminated. Regadenoson, a novel A2A receptor agonist, is supplied as a prefilled syringe and is not weight-based but can be administered during standard Bruce treadmill protocol when the heart rate is noted to be submaximal, followed by radiotracer injection. When used appropriately, regadenoson with treadmill exercise is safe and yields a result similar to that with vasodilator stress without exercise.

Pharmacologic Stress Testing: Vasodilators and Dobutamine

Adenosine, dipyridamole, and regadenoson are the most commonly used vasodilators for stress MPI. Adenosine and dipyridamole are nonselective adenosine receptor agonists (bind to adenosine A1, A2A, A2B, and A3 receptors), whereas regadenoson is a selective adenosine A2A receptor agonist. In addition to general contraindications for stress testing, vasodilators are contraindicated in patients with sinus node dysfunction or high-degree atrioventricular (AV) block without a functioning pacemaker, active wheezing, oxygen-dependent chronic obstructive lung disease, recent use of methylxanthines (within 12 hours) or oral dipyridamole (48 hours), and systolic blood pressure <90 mm Hg. Administration of IV adenosine to individuals who are on oral dipyridamole (sometimes used in patients with transient ischemic attacks) can result in prolonged heart block and hemodynamic collapse. Dobutamine infusion is an alternative for patients with contraindications to vasodilator stress and patients with caffeine or oral dipyridamole intake. Dobutamine is preferred mainly in patients with active reactive airway disease and is avoided in patients with acute myocardial infarction, uncontrolled atrial or ventricular tachyarrhythmias, uncontrolled hypertension, aortic dissection, or a large aortic aneurysm (>6 cm).

Challenges During Pharmacologic Stress Testing

In carefully screened and selected individuals, adverse effects during pharmacologic stress testing are uncommon. Severe chest pain, ischemic ECG changes (ST elevation >1 mm in non–Q wave leads or >2-mm ST depression in three consecutive beats), hemodynamic instability (decrease in systolic blood pressure <90 mm Hg), signs of poor perfusion (e.g., pallor, cool extremities), high-degree AV block (Fig. 11.3), wheezing, atrial or ventricular tachyarrhythmias or bradyarrhythmias, or intolerance to the infusion have been reported. Low-grade exercise with vasodilator infusion can attenuate side effects and improve image quality by reducing the subdiaphragmatic uptake of the tracer.

Potential Solutions

Mild side effects are common and usually well tolerated. Moderate to severe adverse effects during adenosine or

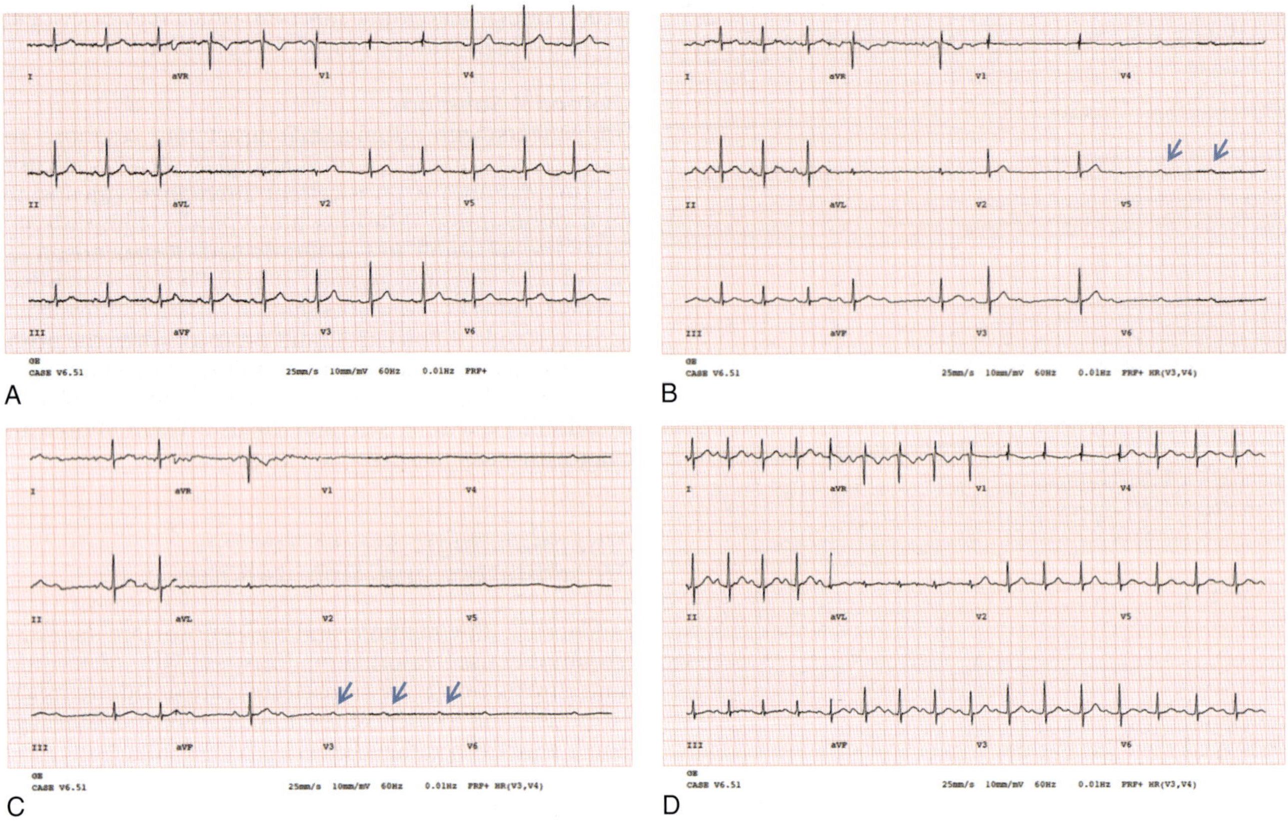

Figure 11.3 (A) Normal sinus rhythm at baseline. (B and C) Complete atrioventricular node block seen during adenosine infusion (p waves *[blue arrows]*, followed by no QRS complexes), with resolution of the block after discontinuation of the infusion (D).

dobutamine infusions may necessitate premature termination of the infusion.

Infusion of regadenoson (administered as a bolus over 10 seconds) or dipyridamole (administered over 4 minutes but with symptoms occurring at 7 minutes) typically is not terminated, but the hyperemia is counteracted by IV aminophylline.

Aminophylline (50–150 mg slow IV push, 1–1.5 mg/kg) given as a slow IV bolus over 60 to 90 seconds can be used to reverse the hyperemic effects of vasodilator agents. Due to the short half-life of adenosine, aminophylline is not typically needed unless the patient has wheezing or prolonged heart block, despite termination of the adenosine infusion.

For hypotension, IV fluids may be administered (100–150 mL of normal saline IV as a rapid bolus), followed by IV aminophylline, as described above.

Chest pain typically resolves with termination of the infusion agent and after IV aminophylline. If chest pain persists, especially with ST depression, sublingual nitroglycerin, 0.4 mg, can be administered, provided that the systolic blood pressure is >90 mm Hg and there is no recent history of the use of sildenafil or other phosphodiesterase inhibitors. IV beta blockers (5 mg IV metoprolol [Lopressor] over 30 seconds) can be administered for chest pain, especially during dobutamine infusion.

Wheezing is managed with inhaled albuterol via a nebulizer every 10 minutes, as needed. If wheezing does not improve after two units of nebulizer therapy with albuterol have been administered, consider referral to the emergency room.

High-grade AV block, usually transient, is common with IV adenosine infusion, especially following radiotracer injection at 2 minutes into the infusion. Exercise, hand grip, or supine leg exercise typically improves the heart block. In patients with persistent or symptomatic high-grade AV block, adenosine infusion may be prematurely terminated. Persistent or symptomatic heart block, although less frequent after termination of the adenosine infusion or with dipyridamole or regadenoson, is managed with IV aminophylline.

In cases of hemodynamic instability, signs of hypoperfusion, or sustained ventricular arrhythmias, advanced cardiac life support measures are instituted.

Imaging

Attenuation Artifacts

Artifacts can arise during each step of the scan from patient-related factors or from errors during image acquisition, reconstruction, or processing.

The Challenge

Attenuation of the photons from the patient's body, typically because of a large body habitus, breast tissue in females, and muscular diaphragm in males, or from arms-down imaging, is a major source of artifact with radionuclide MPI (Figs. 11.4–11.6). Breast tissue typically reduces counts in the anterior or lateral wall of the left ventricle, depending on the size and position of the breasts. Although more often these so-called defects appear fixed, a shift in breast tissue position (especially the left) between the rest and stress scans can produce an apparently reversible perfusion defect (see Fig. 11.4). Inferior wall attenuation is seen more commonly in men due to attenuation from a muscular diaphragm (see Fig. 11.5).

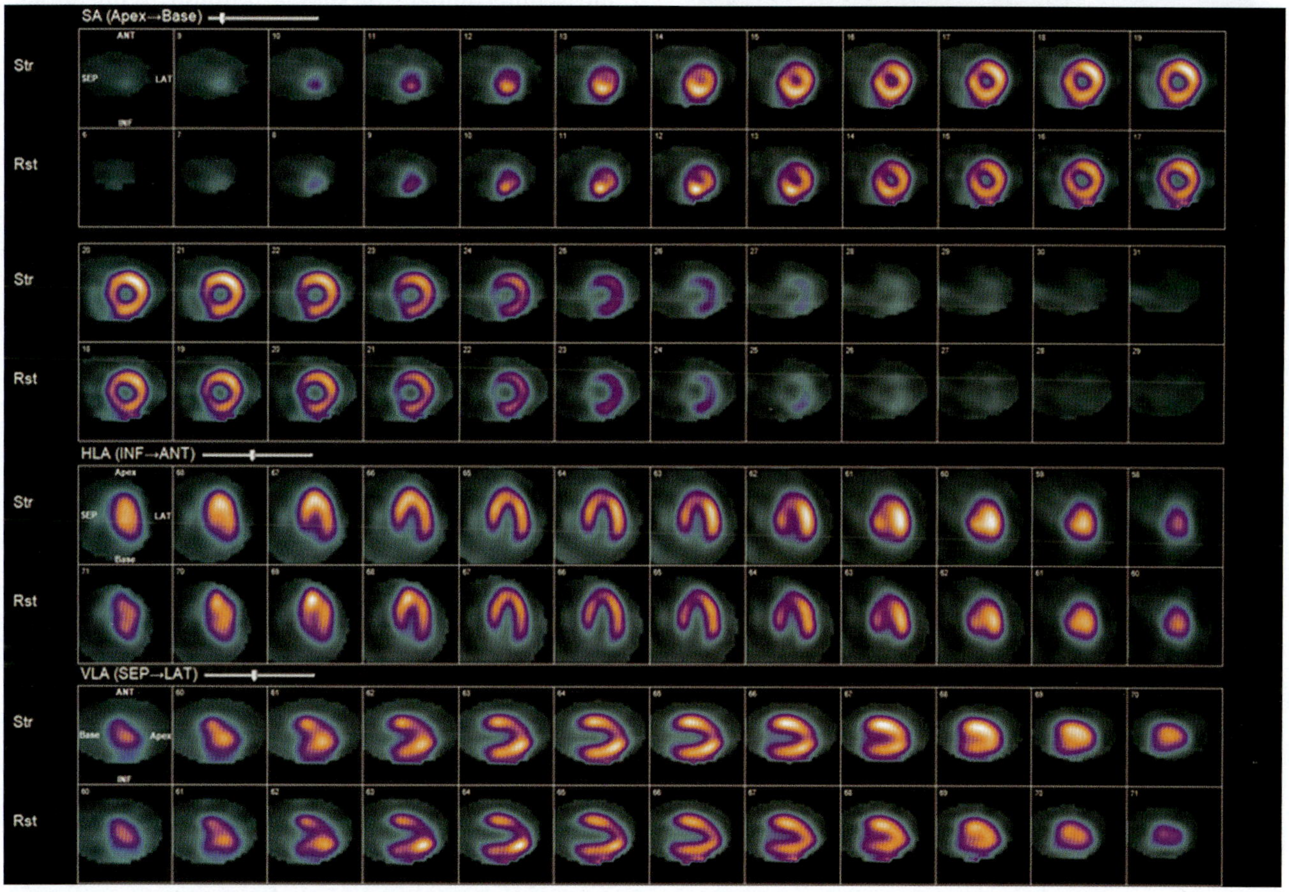

Figure 11.4 Rest and stress ^{99m}Tc- SPECT perfusion images of a 70-year-old woman for evaluation of atypical chest pain. There is a small, mild-intensity, fixed perfusion abnormality in the mid- to apical anterior-anteroseptal wall. Gated images (not shown) showed normal wall motion and thickening, consistent with a breast attenuation artifact.

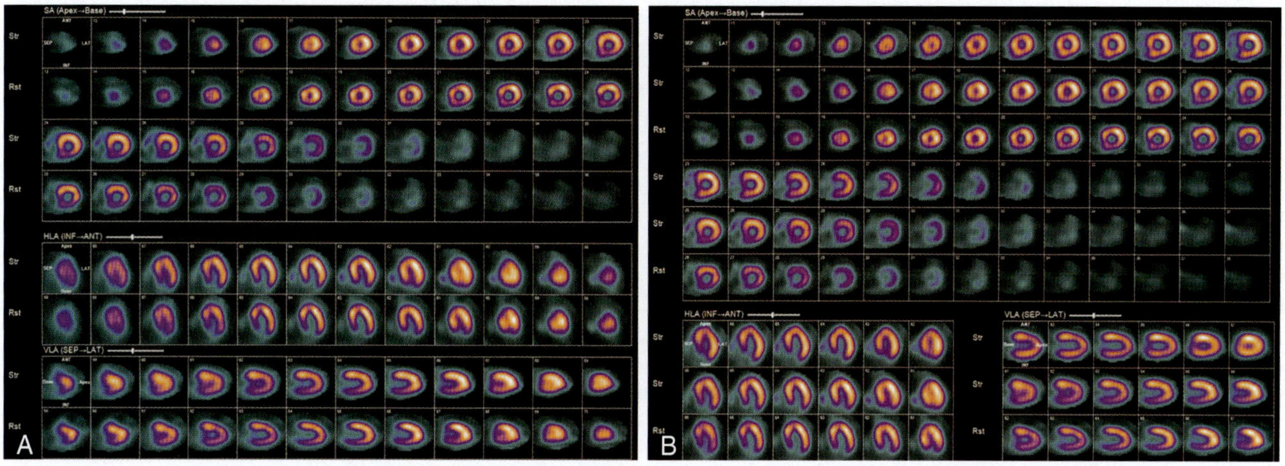

Figure 11.5 Rest (A) and stress (B) supine images in a 56-year-old man show reduced counts in the inferior wall. Gated images (not shown) showed normal wall motion and thickening. With prone imaging (top row in B), an increase in the inferior wall counts is seen, confirming the diaphragmatic attenuation.

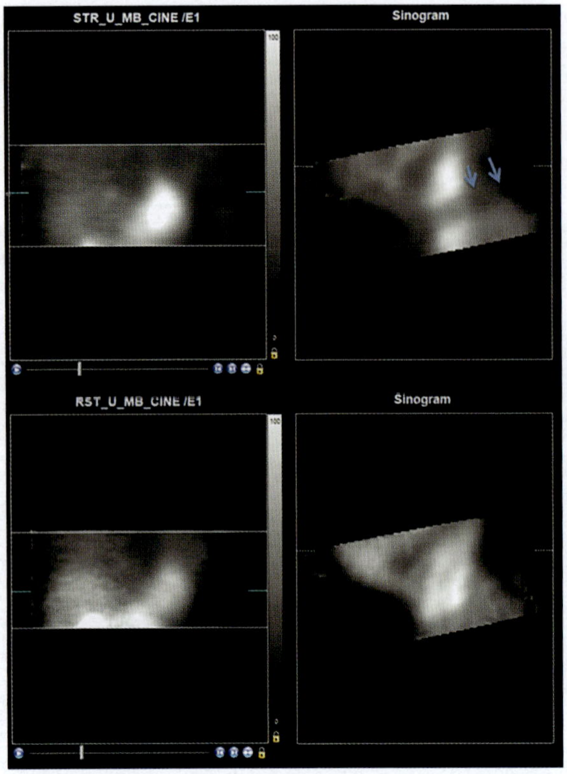

Figure 11.6 Arms down during stress images as seen on rotating projection images, leading to attenuation and reduced counts on the sinogram *(arrows)*.

Identifying the Artifact

A careful review of the raw rotating planar and projection images will help identify attenuation from breast tissue or from the diaphragm. It is also important to identify breast tissue on the stress and rest images to ensure that they are in a similar position.

Potential Solutions

If breast tissue attenuation is the suspected cause of a fixed perfusion defect, gated SPECT, repeat imaging, and attenuation correction can be considered.

GATED SPECT

The advent of technetium-99m (^{99m}Tc) perfusion tracers and gated SPECT was a major breakthrough for the differentiation of breast tissue attenuation artifacts from a myocardial scar. Normal regional wall thickening and wall motion confirm the fixed defect as an attenuation artifact, whereas abnormal wall motion confirms a real perfusion defect (hibernation or scar).

REPEAT IMAGING

If the breast position is different on the rest of the stress images, image acquisition may be repeated with the hope of mitigating the problem. Breast binders are not recommended because they may increase the chance of variable breast tissue attenuation. Imaging in a prone position is helpful for the correction of artifacts related to the diaphragm but can worsen anterior wall attenuation and thus is not recommended.

HIGHER RADIOTRACER DOSE IMAGING

A generalized reduction in the counts resulting from a large body habitus can be mitigated by using a higher radiotracer dose to increase image counts or using 2-day imaging protocols.

With some of the dedicated cardiac SPECT scanners, imaging is performed with the patient in the upright and semirecumbent or supine position. With upright imaging, a breast attenuation artifact results in an inferoapical defect rather than the usual anterior wall perfusion defect. Acquiring stress images with the patient in a supine position, in addition to upright imaging, may help differentiate an artifact from a real defect (seen in both and supine images).

SOFTWARE

Most commercially available semiquantitative programs compare the perfusion data with gender-specific, normal limits databases and delineate attenuation artifacts. The most specific solution for attenuation artifacts, however, is to measure attenuation and correct for it.

ATTENUATION CORRECTION

Attenuation correction (AC) is the most direct solution for attenuation artifacts. Soft tissue attenuation can be accurately measured and corrected using a transmission map derived from a radioactive line source, commonly gadolinium-135 (^{135}Gd), with conventional scanners, or using a CT-derived transmission map with hybrid scanners (SPECT CT or PET CT). Currently, the transmission scans are typically sequential to the emission scans (either before or after). Therefore appropriate coregistration between the emission and transmission scans is important. If misregistration is observed, special software is used to realign the images, develop a new attenuation map, and derive a new reconstruction of the emission images, using the revised attenuation map. In cases in which significant attenuation is anticipated, as in patients with a large body habitus or left arm–down imaging, PET MPI may be a preferred alternate study. PET imaging is based on coincidence detection of photons and provides improved spatial and temporal resolution when compared to SPECT. Due to the coincidental detection of photons with PET, attenuated photons are not counted as true counts and may be discarded by the scanners. Hence, attenuation is paradoxically higher, and AC is always used. Compared to SPECT, AC with PET is depth-independent and more robust.

Patient Motion

The Challenge

Patient motion during MPI is an important and common source for artifacts with both SPECT and PET MPI. Motion can be vertical, horizontal (side to side), or complex. Motion may also be gradual or abrupt. A 0.5-pixel movement does not cause a detectable defect, whereas a 1- pixel movement could cause a defect that is detectable but may not be clinically significant; motion of 2 pixels or more causes a clinically significant artifact. With the newer cardiocentric scanners, the acquisition is quick and, due to the reduced scan time and more comfortable position, the frequency of patient motion may be reduced. Patient motion during the transmission scan may also be a significant source of artifacts.

Identifying Patient Motion

TRADITIONAL ANGER SPECT SCANNERS

With traditional SPECT, images are acquired in a temporal sequence using a multiframe acquisition (step and shoot or continuous), with a series of 32 to 34 image frames acquired by each scanner detector, for a total of 60 to 64 frames. A review of rotating projection images can identify patient motion, especially vertical or complex motion. The sinogram may be better at identifying horizontal motion, and a linogram can further provide information about motion (Fig. 11.7).

CARDIOCENTRIC SPECT SCANNERS AND PET

Identification of patient motion during the scan is challenging with the newer cardiocentric SPECT scanners (e.g., D-SPECT, GE Alcyone), as well as with PET scanners, in which the imaging mode is continuous, and counts are acquired simultaneously in a tomographic mode (not as multiple projection images). Because the images are not acquired in a multiframe format, the rotating projection images cannot be used to identify patient motion. For the same reason, identification of patient motion is challenging with PET MPI unless images are acquired in a dynamic or list mode. With dynamic imaging, motion can be identified by playing the multiple frames of the dynamic images in a cine loop format. A review of the sinogram or pannogram (D-SPECT) may provide clues about patient motion.

TRANSMISSION SCANS

Motion during the transmission scan can be detected by a careful review of the transmission images. CT-based transmission scans are quick and typically not associated with motion (unless the patient has unexpected movement, such as sneezing or coughing). Radionuclide transmission scans are more prone to motion, but motion during a transmission scan is very challenging to detect.

Potential Solutions

Prevention of motion by careful patient instruction is important. If the patient moves despite instructions, the scan acquisition can ideally be repeated with SPECT.

If that is not feasible, automatic and semiautomatic software-based motion correction techniques are now available that can mitigate motion artifacts, but are not optimal. These programs work best for motion in vertical direction. Side-to-side motion results in more complex artifacts, which may remain uncorrected.

Imaging in the prone position can help minimize patient motion. With PET, careful attention should be paid during image acquisition to minimize motion and prevent motion. Novel motion correction software is available to correct for patient motion identified on dynamic PET images.

Patient motion during the transmission scan cannot be corrected by software, however, and may necessitate a repeat study.

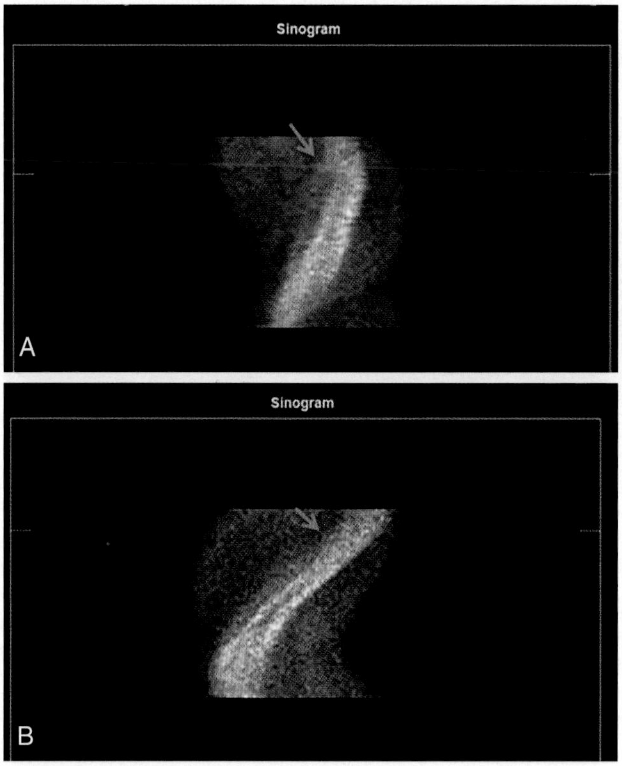

Figure 11.7 (A) Sinogram showing motion on supine imaging *(arrow)*. On prone imaging (B), there is a reduction in patient motion.

Transmission and Emission Misregistration Artifacts

Although radionuclide- or CT-based AC with SPECT or PET MPI significantly improves soft tissue attenuation and diagnostic accuracy, the use of AC itself is not free from artifacts. Due to the nature of sequential transmission and emission imaging and the inherent differences in image resolution between radionuclide and CT images, misregistration of transmission and emission images is more common with hybrid-based (40%) than with radionuclide-based (21.4%) AC imaging.

Identification of the Artifact

Registration between the transmission and emission scans is checked manually or by the use of software. This review must be performed in the transaxial, sagittal, and coronal planes because axial and vertical displacement of the heart may occur from changes in breathing pattern during hyperemia from stress testing. Due to the significantly different attenuation coefficients of soft tissue and air in the lungs, if the myocardium on the emission images overlies the lung tissue on the transmission images, significant perfusion defects may result (Fig. 11.8). These defects are typically seen in the anterolateral wall. Overcorrection artifacts are more frequent with high-density objects such as a pacemaker or automated implantable cardioverter-defibrillator leads and typically a pose

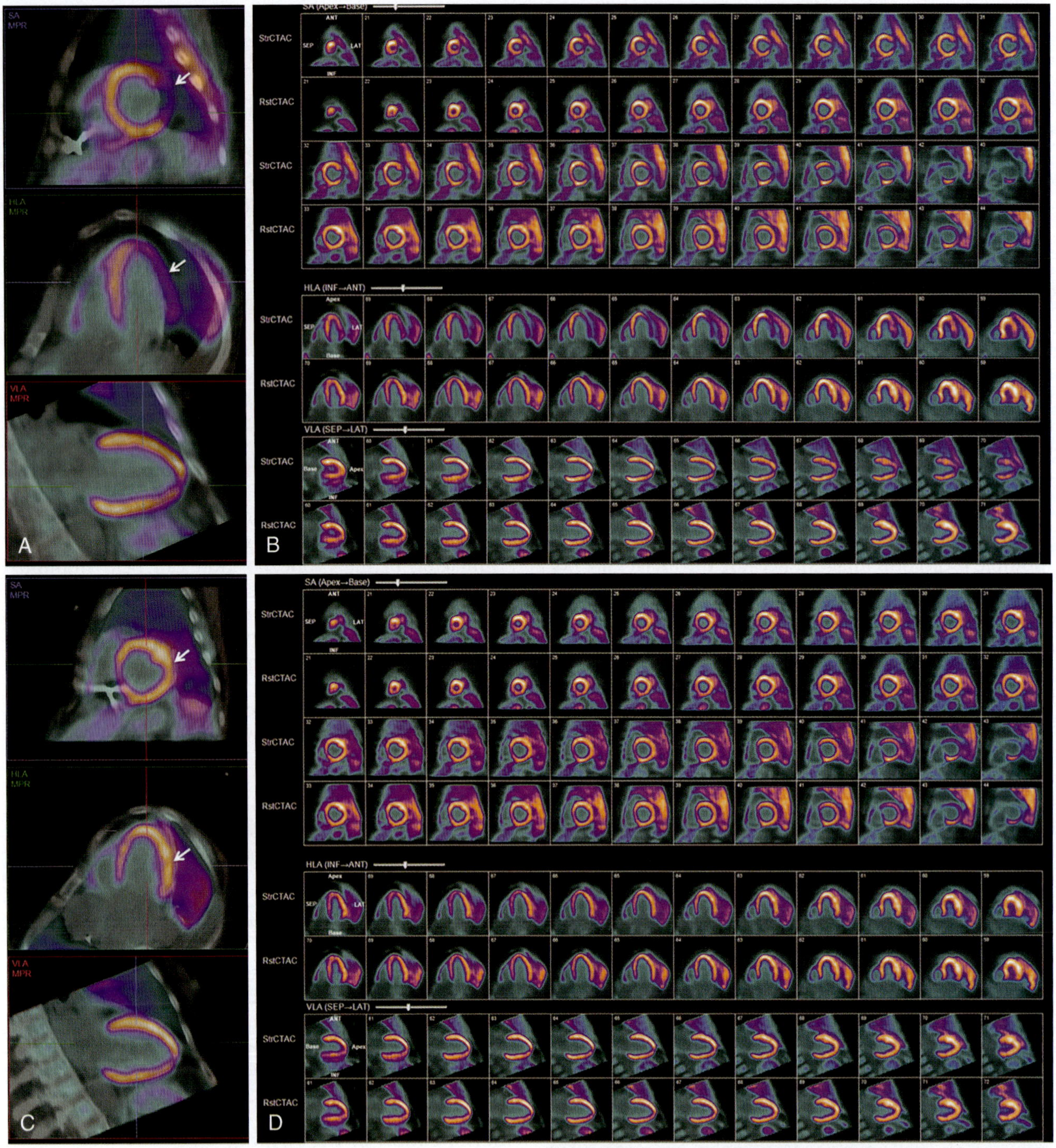

Figure 11.8 (A) Misregistration of the CT transmission and ^{13}N-ammonia emission maps *(arrows)* creating a perfusion defect in the lateral wall on the stress images (B). (C) Realignment of the transmission and emission images and a new image reconstruction resolves the artifact (D). Note intensely increased ^{13}N-ammonia uptake in the lungs in this patient with left ventricular dysfunction and an ejection fraction of 35%.

problem with hot spot imaging studies, such as cardiac sarcoid imaging. Metallic heart valves typically do not pose a problem because they are too basal and typically do not overlie myocardial tissue.

Potential Solutions

Investigators have attempted to minimize misregistration artifacts by using slow CT scans, end-expiratory CT scans, or even high-pitch CT scans, with variable results. The current recommendation is to use a free tidal breathing transmission scan.

Several software solutions are available for correcting misregistration artifacts. Typically, the steps for correction of misregistration include identification, realignment of the transmission and emission images, development of a new attenuation map, and application of the new attenuation map to reconstruct new emission images.

Subdiaphragmatic Activity

Radiopharmaceuticals used for SPECT and PET MPI have hepatobiliary excretion, resulting in activity in the liver and intestines that may overlap the cardiac activity and increase Compton scatter or cause a ramp filter artifact. Compton scatter from intense subdiaphragmatic activity may mask true inferior wall perfusion defects (Fig. 11.9), whereas the use of filtered backprojection for image reconstruction may create an inferior wall perfusion defect and a ramp filter artifact.

Identifying the Artifact

A review of the reconstructed static images, as well as the rotating projection images, can identify excessive subdiaphragmatic activity.

Potential Solutions

With SPECT tracers, images are acquired about 45 to 60 minutes after the injection of radiotracer to minimize interference from gut activity. Other options to minimize gut activity include a drink of water or milk, addition of low-level exercise with vasodilator stress, or imaging in the prone position. If excessive subdiaphragmatic activity causes a fixed perfusion defect, gated imaging may help differentiate an artifact from a scar.

Iterative reconstruction protocols improve image quality by removing the ramp filter artifact. Prone imaging or repeat imaging after a delay may also reduce the artifact (see Fig. 11.9). If all measures fail, a repeat study using thallium-201 (^{201}Tl), instead of ^{99m}Tc radiotracers, can help improve subdiaphragmatic activity.

Image Acquisition and Reconstruction Artifacts

Artifacts may occur due to errors during image acquisition, reconstruction, or display. Fig. 11.10 shows an artifact resulting from acquiring ^{99m}Tc sestamibi images using a ^{201}Tl window. Also important is aligning the long axes of the images similarly at rest and stress because small differences can introduce artifactual, reversible, perfusion defects. The same principles are applied to quantitative parameters, including polar plots, gated SPECT for the accurate estimation of LVEF, and the transient ischemic dilation (TID) ratio.

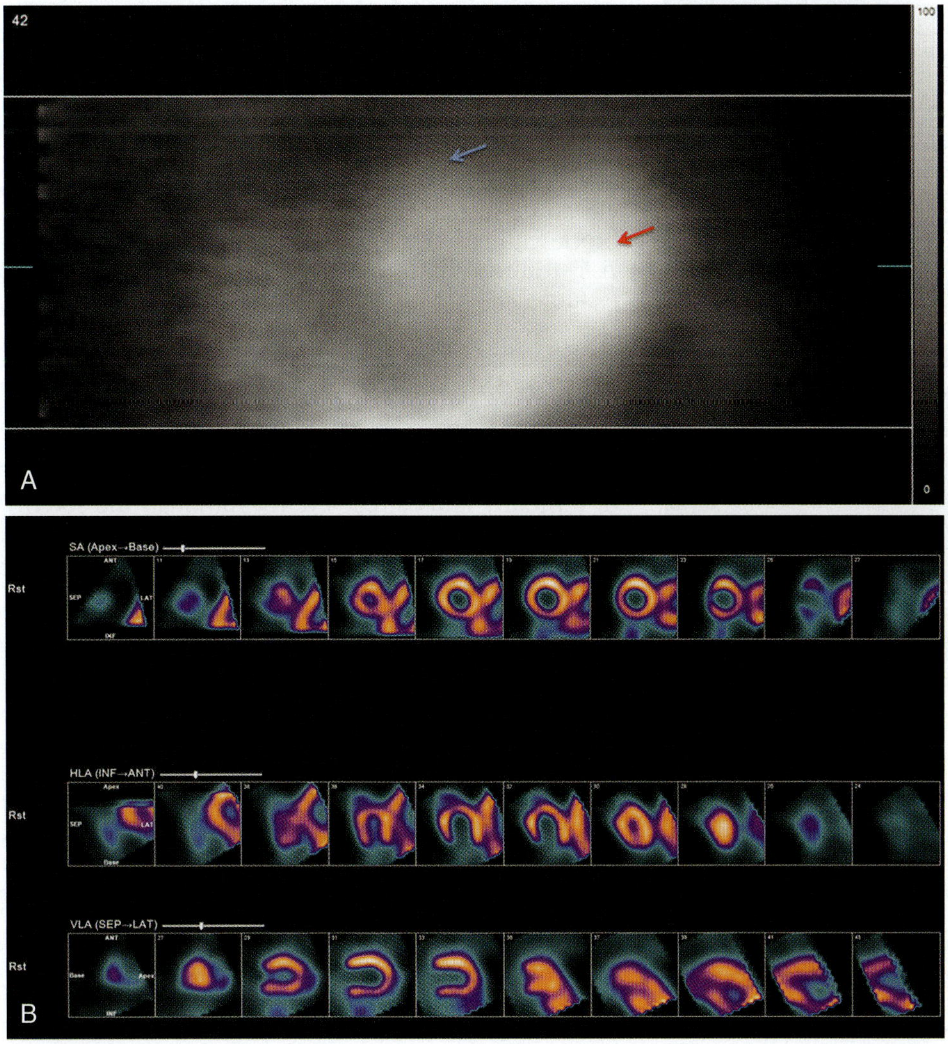

Figure 11.9 (A) Rotating projection image demonstrating loop of bowel *(red arrow)* in the cardiac field of view *(blue arrow)*, with corresponding perfusion images (B) demonstrating the overlapping bowel loop along the inferolateral wall.

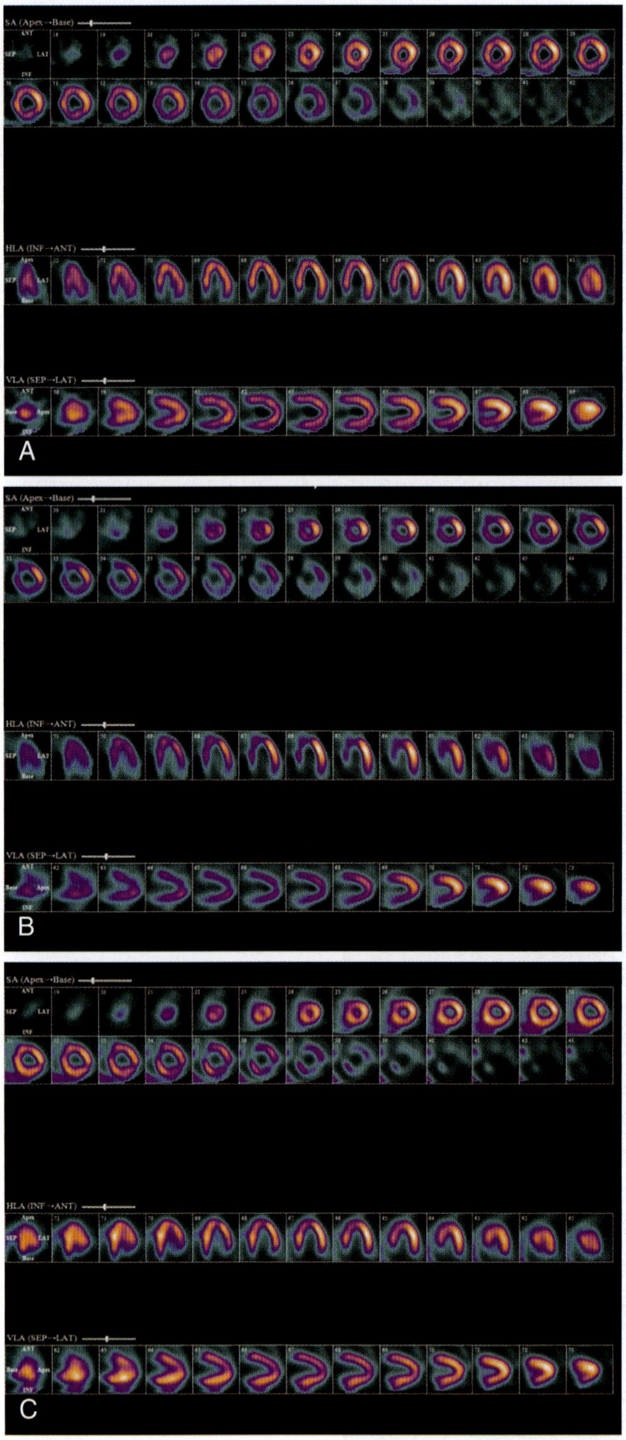

Figure 11.10 Rest ^{99m}Tc sestamibi images (A) and ^{99m}Tc sestamibi stress images obtained using a ^{201}Tl energy window (B). (C) Repeat stress images obtained with the correct energy window show resolution of the artifact.

Potential Solutions

In cases of image acquisition artifacts, repeat imaging may be needed. For proper evaluation of the polar plots, myocardial limits are set carefully to exclude any extracardiac activity. Careful selection of the basal and apical slices during image display is critical for calculation of the TID ratio. Usually the software-generated TID ratio is not reported alone because it is also appreciated visually.

Other Artifacts

Review of the rotating projection images may identify artifacts generated from extracardiac hardware such as implantable cardioverter-defibrillator generators, arrhythmias, scanner quality control, and detector malfunction (Fig. 11.11). Artifacts in images such as septal defects secondary to left bundle branch block should be recognized, especially when stress testing has been performed with exercise.

High-Risk Features

The scans are closely scrutinized for high-risk features during stress testing, MPI, or CT scanning of hybrid studies. All stress and MPI studies must be quickly reviewed for high-risk features before discharging the patient from the laboratory. Due to important clinical implications, high-risk features should be incorporated into the final MPI report and appropriately communicated to the referring physician.

Exercise Findings

Low exercise capacity, exercise-induced hypotension, angina at a low workload, ischemic ST depression at a low workload, >2-mm ST depression or ST segment elevation, sustained ventricular tachyarrhythmias, heart block with exercise, and syncope are some of the high-risk features that can occur during exercise stress testing.

Myocardial Perfusion Imaging Findings

Perfusion Defects

Large and severe perfusion defects indicate a high risk of mortality and cardiac events. Although the severity of perfusion defects is an indicator of the severity of underlying CAD, the extent of perfusion defects correlates with the extent of CAD. With increasing extent and severity of perfusion defects, the risk of cardiac events increases exponentially. A perfusion defect involving >10% of the left ventricle is associated with a high risk of adverse cardiac events.

Increased Lung Uptake

Increased lung uptake of myocardial perfusion tracers often indicates high left ventricular (LV) end-diastolic pressures or high wedge pressures and is a poor prognostic indicator. Increased lung uptake (Fig. 11.12), when seen only on the stress images (exercise or pharmacologic), is typically a marker of severe and multivessel obstructive CAD; this sign may also be evident postexercise in patients with significant mitral valve stenosis or poor pulmonary reserve. With ^{13}N-ammonia, however, increased

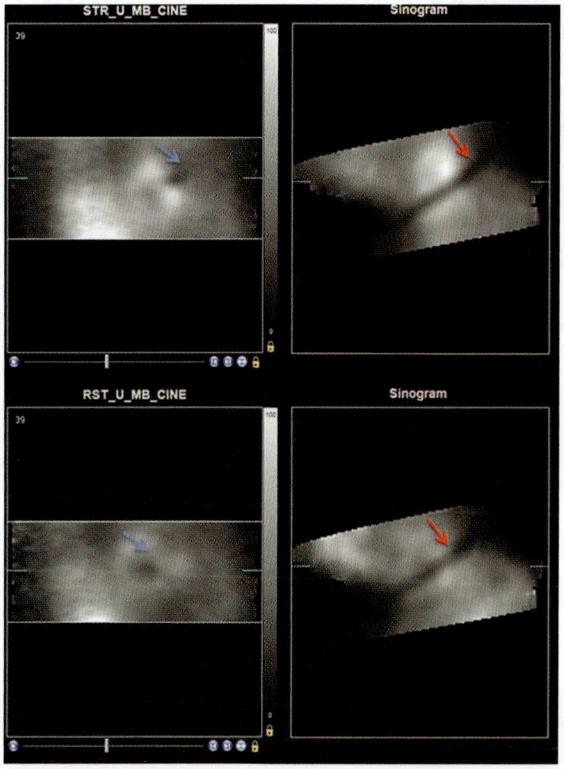

Figure 11.11 Rotating projection images showing an implantable cardioverter-defibrillator in the cardiac field of view on both stress and rest images *(blue arrows)*, with corresponding sinogram images showing an absence of counts *(red arrows)*.

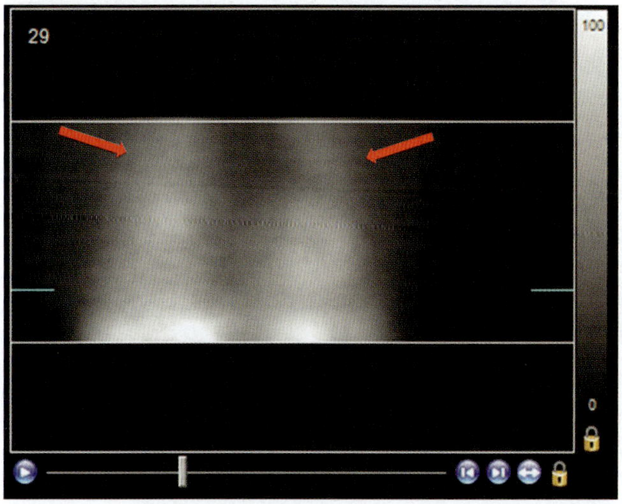

Figure 11.12 Rotating projection image showing increased lung uptake of the ^{99m}Tc sestamibi *(red arrows)*.

lung uptake may be noted in smokers, for unclear reasons.

Increased Right Ventricular Tracer Uptake

Normally right ventricular (RV) tracer uptake is barely noticeable on rest and stress MPI. Increased RV tracer uptake can be seen with right heart or pulmonary disease (e.g., RV hypertrophy, pulmonary hypertension) or it can be a marker of global LV ischemia, with a relative increase in RV tracer uptake. Regional defects in RV uptake may suggest right coronary artery ischemia and/or infarct. Increased RV tracer uptake is commonly seen in patients with complex congenital heart disease and in those with systemic right ventricles. Transiently increased RV tracer uptake (20% increased RV/LV ratio at stress compared to rest) is a specific marker for left main CAD (93% specificity), in which the ostial left main disease is more severe than the proximal right coronary disease.

Transient Ischemic Dilation Ratio of the Left Ventricle

An increase in the LV cavity size during stress compared to rest (TID ratio of the left ventricle) is a marker of severe and extensive obstructive CAD (Fig. 11.13). The normal limits of the TID ratio vary based on the radiotracer used (higher with dual-isotope protocols using ^{201}Tl) and the protocol used (higher with single-day protocols compared to 2-day equal dose protocols). With SPECT radionuclide MPI, the TID ratio most likely represents diffuse subendocardial ischemia, whereas with PET it may also represent true ischemic LV dilation (see Fig. 11.13). Patients with coronary microvascular disease, diabetes, or LV hypertrophy may manifest a TID ratio in the absence of CAD, reducing its specificity in these patients.

Left and Right Ventricular Ejection Fraction

Gated SPECT and PET MPI provide information regarding LV volumes, regional wall motion, and EF. A decline in LVEF from rest to stress (≥5%), LVEF ≤45%, and regional wall motion abnormalities predict a high risk of cardiac death. Transient regional wall motion abnormalities (noted only on the stress images) on ^{99m}Tc SPECT are highly specific for underlying severe obstructive CAD. Among patients with mild to moderate or severe ischemia, those with a lower LVEF (30%–50%) have a higher rate of cardiac death compared to patients with a higher LVEF (>50%). A decline in LVEF, particularly with rubidium-82 (^{82}Rb) PET, is a marker of underlying left main or multivessel severe CAD and predicts a significantly worse survival free of cardiac death or myocardial infarction.

High-Risk Markers on PET Myocardial Perfusion Imaging

Persistent blood pool activity and reduced CFR on PET MPI are powerful prognostic markers for cardiac death and myocardial infarction. Persistent blood pool activity on ^{82}Rb MPI is seen in patients with a low LVEF, with a concomitant high risk. CFR is the ratio of hyperemic myocardial blood flow to myocardial blood flow at rest. Although normal values may vary, a CFR >1.9 is considered normal. A reduced vasodilator CFR signifies coronary microvascular dysfunction, with or without epicardial CAD (Fig. 11.14). Multiple studies have confirmed the powerful prognostic value of reduced CFR in individuals with ischemic heart disease, as well as in those with nonischemic cardiomyopathies. Defining patient management based on an abnormal CFR, reflecting integrated epicardial and microvascular dysfunction, is complex; it requires the integration of patient symptoms with findings from MPI and coronary angiography. The most important clinical application of CFR in clinical

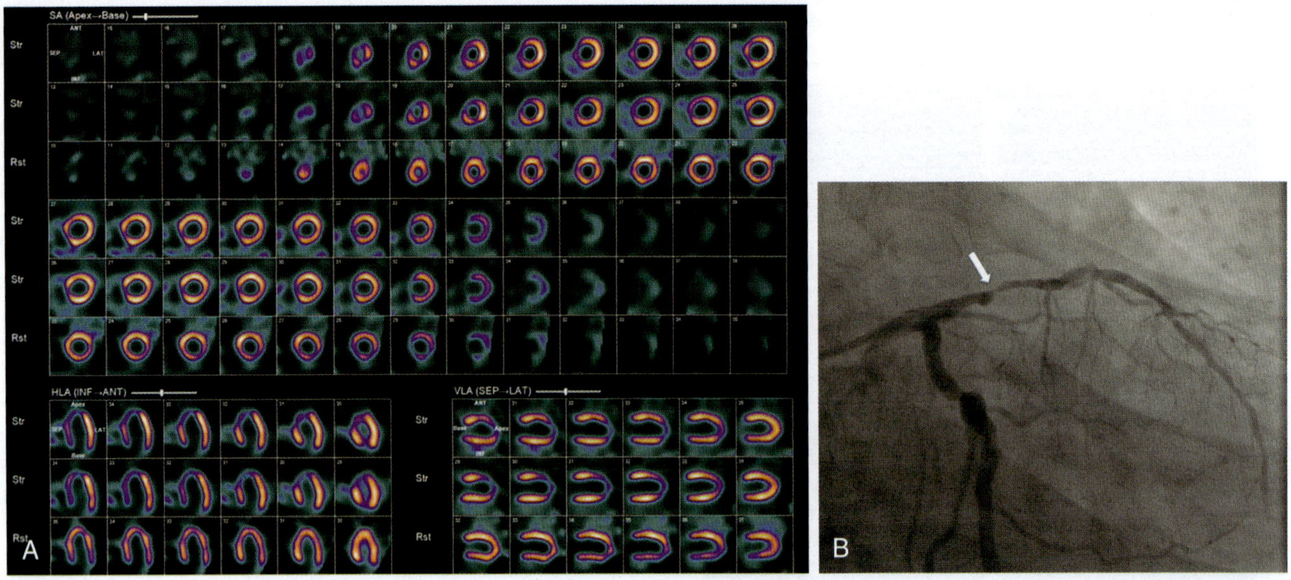

Figure 11.13 (A) Stress and rest images of a 56-year-old man for evaluation of chest pain showing a large and severe perfusion defect in the distribution of the left anterior descending coronary artery (LAD), which is reversible (24% myocardium involved). Transient ischemic dilation (TID) of the left ventricle was noted (TID ratio, 1.45). Another high-risk feature was a drop in left ventricular ejection fraction, 70% at rest to 54% on post–stress-gated images, suggesting a postischemic stunning (not shown). (B) Invasive coronary angiogram of the same patient shows a proximal 90% stenosis of the LAD *(arrow)*.

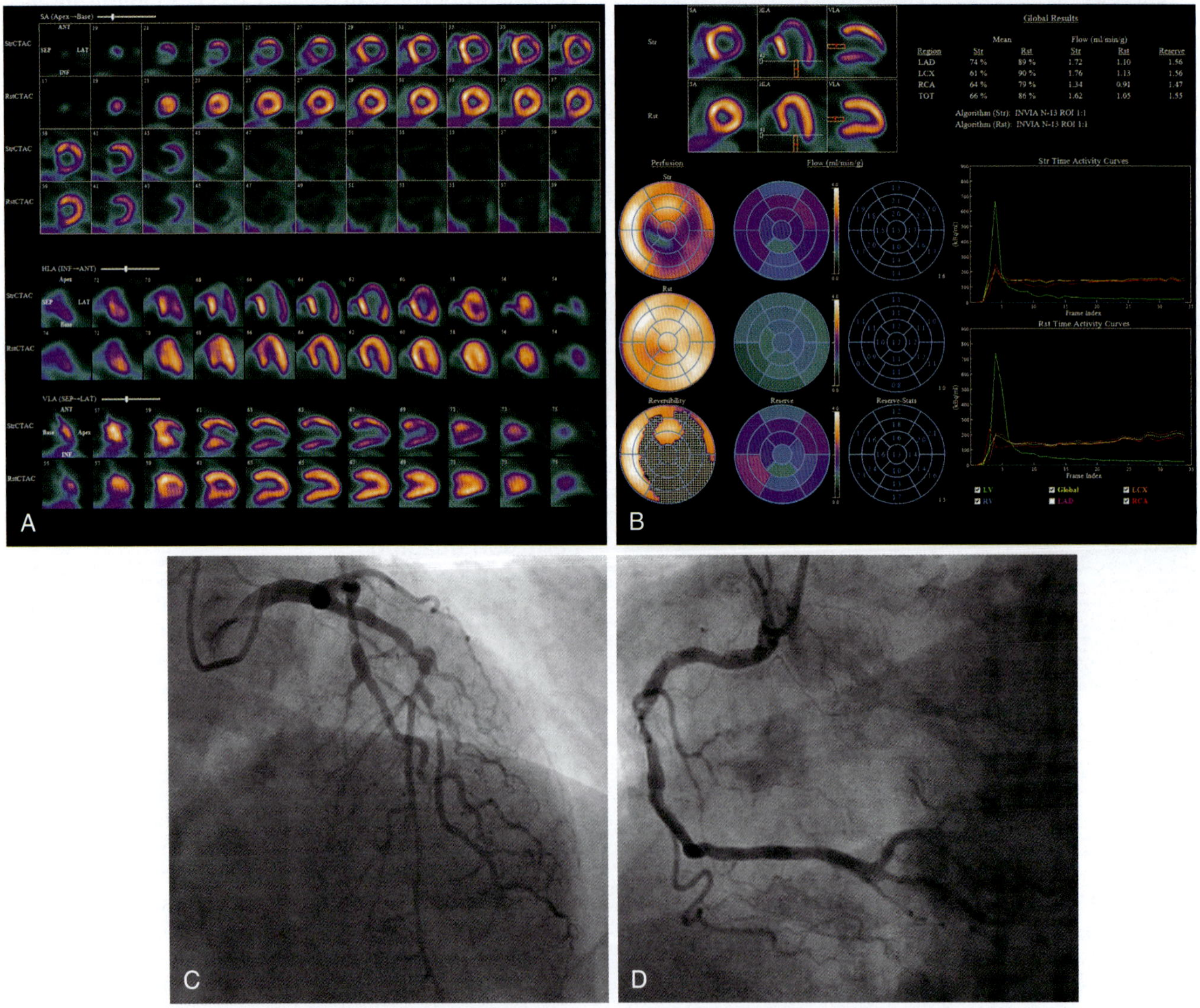

Figure 11.14 A 71-year-old woman with cardiac risk factors referred for evaluation of dyspnea on exertion. This ^{13}N-ammonia PET regadenoson study demonstrated a large reversible perfusion abnormality in the midanterior, anteroseptal walls, apical segments, and apex, as well as a large reversible perfusion abnormality in the entire lateral and inferior walls (A), with a diminished coronary flow reserve (B). An invasive coronary angiogram demonstrates severe lesions in the proximal left anterior descending, diagonal, left circumflex (C), and right coronary (D) arteries.

practice, however, may be when it is normal. Normal global and regional CFR values identify the adequacy of the hyperemic response and excludes balanced ischemia, obviating the need for further testing. With a revolutionary shift under way—PET scanners to acquire dynamic images for flow quantitation, commercial software to measure myocardial blood flow, and a clinical evidence base—CFR has entered mainstream clinical practice.

High-Risk CT Findings

Extensive studies have supported the diagnostic and adverse prognostic impact of calcified and noncalcified coronary atherosclerosis. MPI with hybrid scanners can provide valuable information about the coronary artery calcium score based on the CT-based transmission scan or based on a dedicated, gated calcium score protocol CT scan. The calcium score combined with perfusion imaging may be most valuable for the management of individuals with normal MPI. A normal MPI portends an excellent short-term risk, but a high calcium score indicates an intermediate-risk, long-term prognosis; these patients may thus warrant a more aggressive risk factor modification. CT coronary angiography is typically not combined with MPI unless specifically indicated to answer a clinical question. When the coronary arteries are extensively calcified (due to concern of overestimation of stenosis) or equivocally narrowed on CT coronary angiography, stress MPI may be considered to assess the hemodynamic significance of the stenosis.

Balanced Ischemia

Because relative perfusion imaging relies on uptake of the radiotracer in one distribution compared to another, a diffuse reduction in blood flow may be underrecognized. The most common form of balanced ischemia is one in which MPI is abnormal but underestimates the extent of underlying CAD in the other two territories. The presence of a high-risk clinical stress test or CT markers or low functional capacity with ischemic ECG changes should raise the suspicion of multivessel CAD, even when MPI is normal. With normal PET MPI, CFR is a useful tool to exclude balanced ischemia effectively. Fortunately, true balanced ischemia with a completely normal SPECT MPI and no high-risk features is rare.

Abnormal ECG With Normal Perfusion

An abnormal ECG with normal MPI is not infrequent. Usually, with ischemic ECG changes, a normal MPI is of relatively low risk and is reassuring. However, in patients with certain high-risk ECG features, such as ST segment elevation (>1 mm) or a high Duke treadmill score (≤–11, associated with an annual cardiac mortality rate of >5%), coronary angiography is recommended, irrespective of MPI results (Fig. 11.15). Exercise-induced

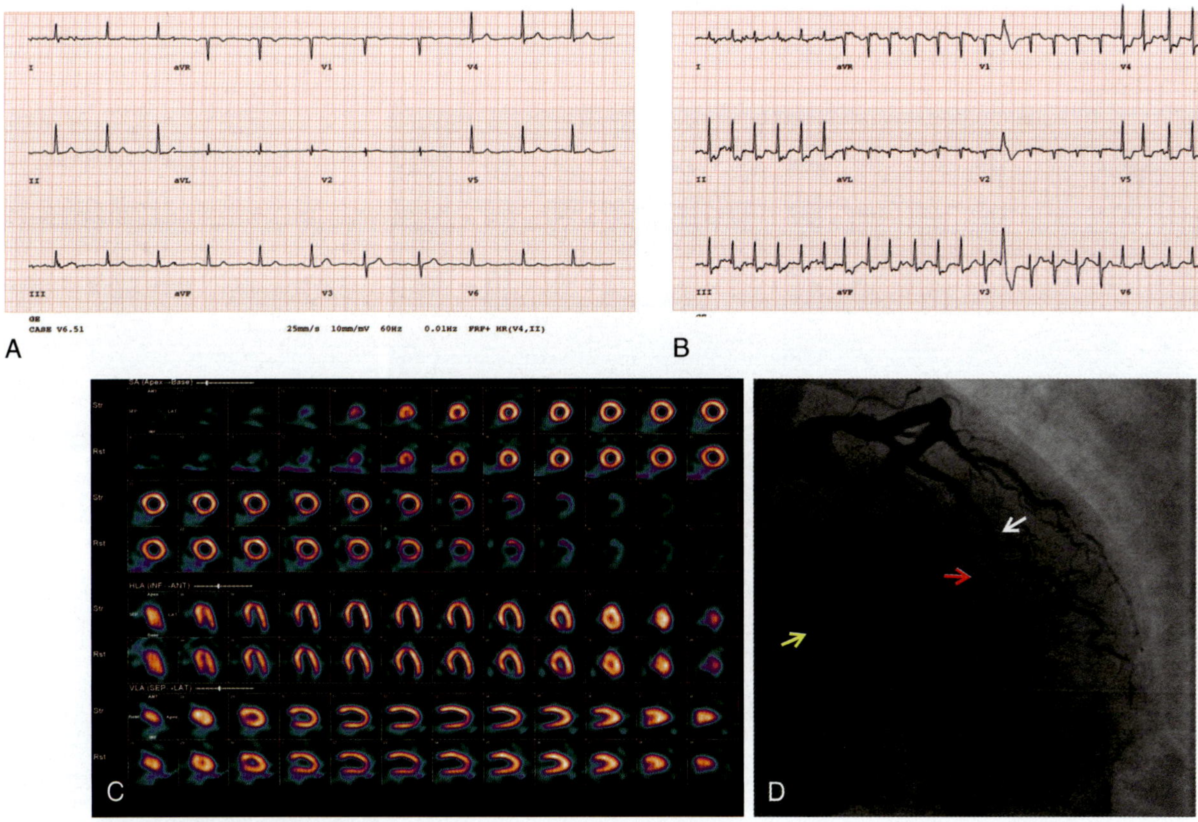

Figure 11.15 A 73-year-old man with cardiac risk factors for evaluation of typical chest pain. Exercise was terminated due to a >2-mm ST segment depression in leads II, III, aVF, V4–6 with reciprocal ST elevations in aVR and V1 (B) at 3 minutes. (C) Perfusion images demonstrate no evidence of ischemia or infarction. (D) Invasive coronary angiogram demonstrating mid–left anterior descending coronary artery stenosis of 80% *(red arrow)*, proximal first diagonal has 80% stenosis *(white arrow)*, and proximal left posterior descending coronary artery stenosis of 90% *(yellow arrow)*.

hypotension, ischemic ECG changes at a low workload or with vasodilator stress (Fig. 11.16), and sustained ventricular arrhythmias can be markers of more extensive CAD, even in the absence of any perfusion abnormalities. Reproducible typical anginal symptoms without ECG changes or perfusion abnormalities can also suggest underlying disease. A further invasive or noninvasive workup may be considered in each of these scenarios.

Reporting Stress Test and Myocardial Perfusion Imaging Results: Appropriate Communication and Follow-Up

An accurate assessment of the entire test, including the study protocol, stress parameters, reporting, and communication of results, has important implications for patient management. For example, in patients who are low or intermediate risk, a stress scan can be performed first, with rest images performed only if stress images are abnormal, with resultant time, cost, and radiation dose savings. Furthermore, a normal stress-only MPI is associated with an excellent prognosis, equivalent to that of a stress and rest MPI.

The American Society of Nuclear Cardiology has published guidelines for standardized reporting of MPI stress testing to provide high-quality reports. The elements of an MPI report include patient demographics, reason for the test, clinical information, including coronary risk factors, prior cardiac history and procedures, medications, rest and stress ECG data, data from stress testing, imaging parameters, including radionuclide dose, a qualitative,

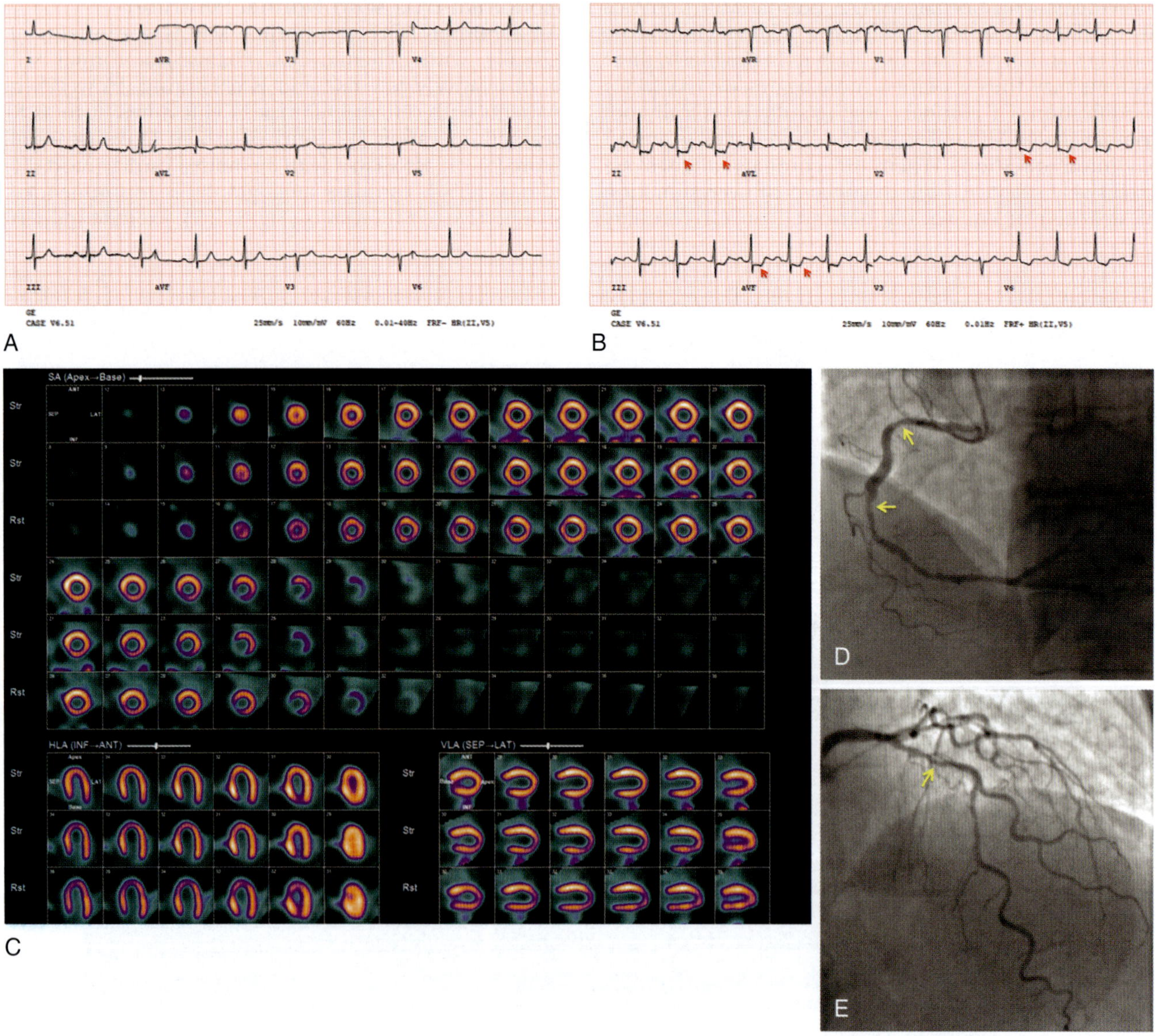

Figure 11.16 An 84-year-old woman presented for evaluation of typical chest pain. (A, B) ST segment depressions seen in leads II, III, aVF, and V4–6 *(red arrows)* during adenosine infusion. (C) Perfusion images demonstrate no ischemia or infarction. (D) Invasive coronary angiogram demonstrates significant proximal and mid-right coronary artery stenosis *(yellow arrows)* and moderate mid-left anterior descending coronary artery stenosis (E; *yellow arrow*).

semiquantitative, and quantitative assessment of perfusion images, LV and RV function assessments, and any extra cardiac findings and comparison to prior studies. High-risk features should be communicated in a timely manner—preferably prior to discharging the patient home from the laboratory—so that appropriate management may be instituted.

Appropriate and timely communication with the referring physician is essential to minimize layered testing and reduce radiation doses and costs of testing. Follow-up on a downstream workup of patients with MPI, such as cardiac catheterization or CT angiography results, is invaluable to improve scan interpretation.

Summary

Radionuclide MPI has transformed the management of individuals with known or suspected CAD. The wealth of diagnostic and prognostic information from MPI is indispensable in the care for these individuals. Yet, as discussed in this chapter, performing, interpreting, and reporting of radionuclide MPI comprise an intricate process that involves careful consideration of several clinical, stress, and imaging parameters. The optimal performance of rest and stress MPI begins with appropriate selection of patients and mode of stress to minimize complications and maximize the yield of stress testing. A problem-oriented approach to image interpretation with the application of effective solutions to imaging challenges will maximize the value of radionuclide MPI. Timely and comprehensive reporting of MPI findings will ultimately affect management and improve patient outcomes.

Bibliography

Abbott BG. The vasodilator stress ECG: should depression cause anxiety? *J Nucl Cardiol*. 2012;19:13–15.

Abidov A, Bax JJ, Hayes SW, et al. Transient ischemic dilation ratio of the left ventricle is a significant predictor of future cardiac events in patients with otherwise normal myocardial perfusion SPECT. *J Am Coll Cardiol*. 2003;42:1818–1825.

Al Jaroudi W, Iskandrian AE. Regadenoson: a new myocardial stress agent. *J Am Coll Cardiol*. 2009;54:1123–1130.

American Society of Nuclear Cardiology. Five things physicians and patients should question. *J Okla State Med Assoc*. 2013;106:150–151.

Berman DS, Kang X, Slomka PJ, et al. Underestimation of extent of ischemia by gated SPECT myocardial perfusion imaging in patients with left main coronary artery disease. *J Nucl Cardiol*. 2007;14:521–528.

Burmahl B. New law mandates use of imaging appropriateness criteria; June 1, 2014. http://www.rsna.org/NewsDetail.aspx?id=12360. Accessed August 15, 2018.

Burrell S, MacDonald A. Artifacts and pitfalls in myocardial perfusion imaging. *J Nucl Med Technol*. 2006;34:193–211, quiz 212–214.

Camici PG, Crea F. Coronary microvascular dysfunction. *N Engl J Med*. 2007;356:830–840.

Cecchi F, Olivotto I, Gistri R, Lorenzoni R, Chiriatti G, Camici PG. Coronary microvascular dysfunction and prognosis in hypertrophic cardiomyopathy. *N Engl J Med*. 2003;349:1027–1035.

Chang SM, Nabi F, Xu J, et al. The coronary artery calcium score and stress myocardial perfusion imaging provide independent and complementary prediction of cardiac risk. *J Am Coll Cardiol*. 2009;54:1872–1882.

Chang SM, Nabi F, Xu J, et al. Value of CACS compared with ETT and myocardial perfusion imaging for predicting long-term cardiac outcome in asymptomatic and symptomatic patients at low risk for coronary disease: clinical implications in a multimodality imaging world. *JACC Cardiovasc Imaging*. 2015;8:134–144.

Chang SM, Nabi F, Xu J, Raza U, Mahmarian JJ. Normal stress-only versus standard stress/rest myocardial perfusion imaging: similar patient mortality with reduced radiation exposure. *J Am Coll Cardiol*. 2010;55:221–230.

Christman MP, Bittencourt MS, Hulten E, et al. Yield of downstream tests after exercise treadmill testing: a prospective cohort study. *J Am Coll Cardiol*. 2014;63:1264–1274.

Cole CR, Blackstone EH, Pashkow FJ, Snader CE, Lauer MS. Heart-rate recovery immediately after exercise as a predictor of mortality. *N Engl J Med*. 1999;341:1351–1357.

Congress passes legislation linking physician payments to appropriate use criteria; March 31, 2014. http://www.snmmi.org/NewsPublications/NewsDetail.aspx?ItemNumber=11205. Accessed August 15, 2018.

Dilsizian V. 18F-FDG uptake as a surrogate marker for antecedent ischemia. *J Nucl Med*. 2008;49:1909–1911.

Dilsizian V, Bacharach SL, Beanlands RS, et al. ASNC imaging guidelines/SNMMI procedure standard for positron emission tomography (PET) nuclear cardiology procedures. *J Nucl Cardiol*. 2016;23:1187–1226.

Dorbala S, Blankstein R, Skali H, et al. Approaches to reducing radiation dose from radionuclide myocardial perfusion imaging. *J Nucl Med*. 2015;56:592–599.

Dorbala S, Di Carli MF. Cardiac PET perfusion: prognosis, risk stratification, and clinical management. *Semin Nucl Med*. 2014;44:344–357.

Dorbala S, Di Carli MF, Delbeke D, et al. SNMMI/ASNC/SCCT guideline for cardiac SPECT/CT and PET/CT 1.0. *J Nucl Med*. 2013;54:1485–1507.

Dorbala S, Hachamovitch R, Curillova Z, et al. Incremental prognostic value of gated Rb-82 positron emission tomography myocardial perfusion imaging over clinical variables and rest LVEF. *JACC Cardiovasc Imaging*. 2009;2:846–854.

Dorbala S, Vangala D, Sampson U, Limaye A, Kwong R, Di Carli MF. Value of vasodilator left ventricular ejection fraction reserve in evaluating the magnitude of myocardium at risk and the extent of angiographic coronary artery disease: a 82Rb PET/CT study. *J Nucl Med*. 2007;48:349–358.

Dubach P, Froelicher VF, Klein J, Oakes D, Grover-McKay M, Friis R. Exercise-induced hypotension in a male population. Criteria, causes, and prognosis. *Circulation*. 1988;78:1380–1387.

Emmett L, Iwanochko RM, Freeman MR, Barolet A, Lee DS, Husain M. Reversible regional wall motion abnormalities on exercise technetium-99m-gated cardiac single photon emission computed tomography predict high-grade angiographic stenoses. *J Am Coll Cardiol*. 2002;39:991–998.

Emmett L, Magee M, Freedman SB, et al. The role of left ventricular hypertrophy and diabetes in the presence of transient ischemic dilation of the left ventricle on myocardial perfusion SPECT images. *J Nucl Med*. 2005;46:1596–1601.

Fihn SD, Blankenship JC, Alexander KP, et al. 2014 ACC/AHA/AATS/PCNA/SCAI/STS focused update of the guideline for the diagnosis and management of patients with stable ischemic heart disease: a report of the American College of Cardiology/American Heart Association task force on practice guidelines, and the American Association for Thoracic Surgery, Preventive Cardiovascular Nurses Association, Society for Cardiovascular Angiography and Interventions, and Society of Thoracic Surgeons. *J Am Coll Cardiol*. 2014;64:1929–1949.

Fukushima K, Javadi MS, Higuchi T, et al. Prediction of short-term cardiovascular events using quantification of global myocardial flow reserve in patients referred for clinical 82Rb PET perfusion imaging. *J Nucl Med*. 2011;52:726–732.

Garcia EV. SPECT attenuation correction: an essential tool to realize nuclear cardiology's manifest destiny. *J Nucl Cardiol*. 2007;14:16–24.

Garcia EV, Faber TL, Esteves FP. Cardiac dedicated ultrafast SPECT cameras: new designs and clinical implications. *J Nucl Med*. 2011;52:210–217.

Germano G, Slomka PJ, Berman DS. Attenuation correction in cardiac SPECT: the boy who cried wolf? *J Nucl Cardiol*. 2007;14:25–35.

Gibbons RJ, Balady GJ, Bricker JT, et al. ACC/AHA 2002 guideline update for exercise testing: summary article: a report of the American College of Cardiology/American Heart Association task force on practice guidelines (committee to update the 1997 exercise testing guidelines). *Circulation*. 2002;106:1883–1892.

Gould KL, Lipscomb K, Hamilton GW. Physiologic basis for assessing critical coronary stenosis. Instantaneous flow response and regional distribution during coronary hyperemia as measures of coronary flow reserve. *Am J Cardiol*. 1974;33:87–94.

Gould KL, Pan T, Loghin C, Johnson NP, Guha A, Sdringola S. Frequent diagnostic errors in cardiac PET/CT due to misregistration of CT attenuation and emission PET images: a definitive analysis of causes, consequences, and corrections. *J Nucl Med*. 2007;48:1112–1121.

Hachamovitch R, Berman DS, Kiat H, et al. Exercise myocardial perfusion SPECT in patients without known coronary artery disease: incremental prognostic value and use in risk stratification. *Circulation*. 1996;93:905–914.

Hachamovitch R, Hayes SW, Friedman JD, Cohen I, Berman DS. Comparison of the short-term survival benefit associated with revascularization compared with medical therapy in patients with no prior coronary artery disease undergoing stress myocardial perfusion single photon emission computed tomography. *Circulation*. 2003;107:2900–2907.

Halligan WT, Morris PB, Schoepf UJ, et al. Transient ischemic dilation of the left ventricle on SPECT: correlation with findings at coronary CT angiography. *J Nucl Med*. 2014;55:917–922.

He ZX, Shi RF, Wu YJ, et al. Direct imaging of exercise-induced myocardial ischemia with fluorine-18-labeled deoxyglucose and Tc-99m-sestamibi in coronary artery disease. *Circulation*. 2003;108:1208–1213.

Heller GV, Stowers SA, Hendel RC, et al. Clinical value of acute rest technetium-99m tetrofosmin tomographic myocardial perfusion imaging in patients with acute chest pain and nondiagnostic electrocardiograms. *J Am Coll Cardiol*. 1998;31:1011–1017.

Hendel RC, Thomas GS. The time and place for appropriate radionuclide imaging: now and everywhere. *J Nucl Cardiol.* 2011;18:997–999.

Hendel RC, Berman DS, Di Carli MF, et al. ACCF/ASNC/ACR/AHA/ASE/SCCT/SCMR/SNM 2009 appropriate use criteria for cardiac radionuclide imaging: a report of the American College of Cardiology Foundation Appropriate Use Criteria Task Force, the American Society of Nuclear Cardiology, the American College of Radiology, the American Heart Association, the American Society of Echocardiography, the Society of Cardiovascular Computed Tomography, the Society for Cardiovascular Magnetic Resonance, and the Society of Nuclear Medicine. *J Am Coll Cardiol.* 2009;53:2201–2229.

Hendel RC, Cerqueira M, Douglas PS, et al. A multicenter assessment of the use of single-photon emission computed tomography myocardial perfusion imaging with appropriateness criteria. *J Am Coll Cardiol.* 2010;55:156–162.

Henzlova MJ, Cerqueira MD, Mahmarian JJ, Yao SS. Stress protocols and tracers. *J Nucl Cardiol.* 2006;13:e80–e90.

Holly TA, Abbott BG, Al-Mallah M, et al. Single photon-emission computed tomography. *J Nucl Cardiol.* 2010;17:941–973.

Iskandrian AS. Adenosine myocardial perfusion imaging. *J Nucl Med.* 1994;35:734–736.

Klocke FJ, Baird MG, Lorell BH, et al. ACC/AHA/ASNC guidelines for the clinical use of cardiac radionuclide imaging—executive summary: a report of the American College of Cardiology/American Heart Association task force on practice guidelines (ACC/AHA/ASNC committee to revise the 1995 guidelines for the clinical use of cardiac radionuclide imaging). *Circulation.* 2003;108:1404–1418.

Lauer MS, Francis GS, Okin PM, Pashkow FJ, Snader CE, Marwick TH. Impaired chronotropic response to exercise stress testing as a predictor of mortality. *JAMA.* 1999;281:524–529.

Loghin C, Sdringola S, Gould KL. Common artifacts in PET myocardial perfusion images due to attenuation-emission misregistration: clinical significance, causes, and solutions. *J Nucl Med.* 2004;45:1029–1039.

Madsen MT. Recent advances in SPECT imaging. *J Nucl Med.* 2007;48:661–673.

Mandour Ali MA, Bourque JM, Allam AH, Beller GA, Watson DD. The prevalence and predictive accuracy of quantitatively defined transient ischemic dilation of the left ventricle on otherwise normal SPECT myocardial perfusion imaging studies. *J Nucl Cardiol.* 2011;18:1036–1043.

Mc Ardle BA, Dowsley TF, deKemp RA, Wells GA, Beanlands RS. Does rubidium-82 PET have superior accuracy to SPECT perfusion imaging for the diagnosis of obstructive coronary disease? A systematic review and meta-analysis. *J Am Coll Cardiol.* 2012;60:1828–1837.

McLaughlin MG, Danias PG. Transient ischemic dilation: a powerful diagnostic and prognostic finding of stress myocardial perfusion imaging. *J Nucl Cardiol.* 2002;9:663–667.

Murthy VL, Naya M, Foster CR, et al. Improved cardiac risk assessment with noninvasive measures of coronary flow reserve. *Circulation.* 2011;124:2215–2224.

Murthy VL, Naya M, Taqueti VR, et al. Effects of sex on coronary microvascular dysfunction and cardiac outcomes. *Circulation.* 2014;129:2518–2527.

Naya M, Murthy VL, Taqueti VR, et al. Preserved coronary flow reserve effectively excludes high-risk coronary artery disease on angiography. *J Nucl Med.* 2014;55:248–255.

Neumar RW, Otto CW, Link MS, et al. Part 8: adult advanced cardiovascular life support: 2010 American Heart Association guidelines for cardiopulmonary resuscitation and emergency cardiovascular care. *Circulation.* 2010;122:S729–S767.

Parker MW, Iskandar A, Limone B, et al. Diagnostic accuracy of cardiac positron emission tomography versus single photon emission computed tomography for coronary artery disease: a bivariate meta-analysis. *Circ Cardiovasc Imaging.* 2012;5:700–707.

Partington SL, Lanka V, Hainer J, et al. Safety and feasibility of regadenoson use for suboptimal heart rate response during symptom-limited standard bruce exercise stress test. *J Nucl Cardiol.* 2012;19:970–978.

Rischpler C, Higuchi T, Fukushima K, et al. Transient ischemic dilation ratio in 82Rb PET myocardial perfusion imaging: normal values and significance as a diagnostic and prognostic marker. *J Nucl Med.* 2012;53:723–730.

Ross MI, Wu E, Wilkins JT, et al. Safety and feasibility of adjunctive regadenoson injection at peak exercise during exercise myocardial perfusion imaging: the both exercise and regadenoson stress test (BERST) trial. *J Nucl Cardiol.* 2013;20:197–204.

Rozanski A, Gransar H, Shaw LJ, et al. Impact of coronary artery calcium scanning on coronary risk factors and downstream testing the EISNER (early identification of subclinical atherosclerosis by noninvasive imaging research) prospective randomized trial. *J Am Coll Cardiol.* 2011;57:1622–1632.

Rozanski A, Gransar H, Wong ND, et al. Clinical outcomes after both coronary calcium scanning and exercise myocardial perfusion scintigraphy. *J Am Coll Cardiol.* 2007;49:1352–1361.

Saifi S, Taylor AJ, Allen J, Hendel R. The use of a learning community and online evaluation of utilization for SPECT myocardial perfusion imaging. *JACC Cardiovasc Imaging.* 2013;6:823–829.

Sechtem U, Achenbach S, Friedrich M, Wackers F, Zamorano JL. Non-invasive imaging in acute chest pain syndromes. *Eur Heart J Cardiovasc Imaging.* 2012;13:69–78.

Sharir T, Berman DS, Lewin HC, et al. Incremental prognostic value of rest-redistribution (201)Tl single-photon emission computed tomography. *Circulation.* 1999;100:1964–1970.

Sharir T, Germano G, Kang X, et al. Prediction of myocardial infarction versus cardiac death by gated myocardial perfusion SPECT: risk stratification by the amount of stress-induced ischemia and the poststress ejection fraction. *J Nucl Med.* 2001;42:831–837.

Shaw LJ, Hage FG, Berman DS, Hachamovitch R, Iskandrian A. Prognosis in the era of comparative effectiveness research: where is nuclear cardiology now and where should it be? *J Nucl Cardiol.* 2012;19:1026–1043.

Shaw LJ, Mieres JH, Hendel RH, et al. Comparative effectiveness of exercise electrocardiography with or without myocardial perfusion single photon emission computed tomography in women with suspected coronary artery disease: results from the what is the optimal method for ischemia evaluation in women (WOMEN) trial. *Circulation.* 2011;124:1239–1249.

Slomka PJ, Berman DS, Germano G. New cardiac cameras: single-photon emission CT and PET. *Semin Nucl Med.* 2014;44:232–251.

Taillefer R, Ahlberg AW, Masood Y, et al. Acute beta-blockade reduces the extent and severity of myocardial perfusion defects with dipyridamole Tc-99m sestamibi SPECT imaging. *J Am Coll Cardiol.* 2003;42:1475–1483.

Takx RA, Blomberg BA, El Aidi H, et al. Diagnostic accuracy of stress myocardial perfusion imaging compared to invasive coronary angiography with fractional flow reserve meta-analysis. *Circ Cardiovasc Imaging.* 2015;8.

Taylor AJ, Cerqueira M, Hodgson JM, et al. ACCF/SCCT/ACR/AHA/ASE/ASNC/NASCI/SCAI/SCMR 2010 appropriate use criteria for cardiac computed tomography. A report of the American College of Cardiology Foundation Appropriate Use Criteria Task Force, the Society of Cardiovascular Computed Tomography, the American College of Radiology, the American Heart Association, the American Society of Echocardiography, the American Society of Nuclear Cardiology, the North American Society for Cardiovascular Imaging, the Society for Cardiovascular Angiography and Interventions, and the Society for Cardiovascular Magnetic Resonance. *J Am Coll Cardiol.* 2010;56:1864–1894.

Tilkemeier PL, Cooke CD, Ficaro EP, Glover DK, Hansen CL, McCallister BD Jr. American Society of Nuclear Cardiology information statement: standardized reporting matrix for radionuclide myocardial perfusion imaging. *J Nucl Cardiol.* 2006;13:e157–e171.

Udelson JE, Beshansky JR, Ballin DS, et al. Myocardial perfusion imaging for evaluation and triage of patients with suspected acute cardiac ischemia: a randomized controlled trial. *JAMA.* 2002;288:2693–2700.

Weiss AT, Berman DS, Lew AS, et al. Transient ischemic dilation of the left ventricle on stress thallium-201 scintigraphy: a marker of severe and extensive coronary artery disease. *J Am Coll Cardiol.* 1987;9:752–759.

Williams KA, Schneider CM. Increased stress right ventricular activity on dual isotope perfusion SPECT: a sign of multivessel and/or left main coronary artery disease. *J Am Coll Cardiol.* 1999;34:420–427.

Wolk MJ, Bailey SR, Doherty JU, et al. ACCF/AHA/ASE/ASNC/HFSA/HRS/SCAI/SCCT/SCMR/STS 2013 multimodality appropriate use criteria for the detection and risk assessment of stable ischemic heart disease: a report of the American College of Cardiology Foundation Appropriate Use Criteria Task Force, American Heart Association, American Society of Echocardiography, American Society of Nuclear Cardiology, Heart Failure Society of America, Heart Rhythm Society, Society for Cardiovascular Angiography and Interventions, Society of Cardiovascular Computed Tomography, Society for Cardiovascular Magnetic Resonance, and Society of Thoracic Surgeons. *J Am Coll Cardiol.* 2014;63:380–406.

Ziadi MC, Dekemp RA, Williams KA, et al. Impaired myocardial flow reserve on rubidium-82 positron emission tomography imaging predicts adverse outcomes in patients assessed for myocardial ischemia. *J Am Coll Cardiol.* 2011;58:740–748.

CHAPTER 12
Thoracic Nuclear Imaging

Yingbing Wang

CHAPTER OUTLINE

Introduction

Historically, radionuclide lung imaging was used mainly for the diagnosis of pulmonary embolism (PE) and lung function. The advent of fluorodeoxyglucose (FDG) positron emission tomography (PET) computed tomography (CT) scanning, with its integration of both functional and anatomic information into coregistered datasets, has heralded a new age of radionuclide imaging for lung cancer evaluation and staging. Expanded applications of FDG PET/CT now also include non-neoplasm imaging. Although the interpretation of nuclear studies remains primarily qualitative, an important advantage of modern nuclear medicine instrumentation and computing power is the availability of quantitative imaging analysis, which can supplement and support qualitative observations.

Part I: Principles of Pulmonary Scintigraphy

Pulmonary scintigraphy—or V/Q scanning—allows for the noninvasive interrogation of two key aspects of lung function: bronchopulmonary ventilation and pulmonary vasculature perfusion. The underlying principle is that inhaled radioactive gases or radioaerosols and intravenous radiolabeled small particles will distribute according to air and blood flow, respectively. Radiotracer distribution creates a physiologic map of ventilation and perfusion; areas of low radiotracer distribution suggest an obstructed flow, shunting, or surgical defect.

Historically, pulmonary scintigraphy has been the most important diagnostic tool for evaluating PE. In the modern era, CT has become the first-line imaging modality for detecting and monitoring most thoracic pathology; however, pulmonary scintigraphy continues to provide unique physiologic information and remains an indispensable adjunct to anatomic imaging.

Radiopharmaceuticals

Ventilation

Ventilation imaging can be performed with radioactive gases or radioaerosols. Only xenon-133 (^{133}Xe), a radioactive gas, and technetium-99m (^{99m}Tc) diethylenetriamine pentaacetic acid (^{99m}Tc-DTPA), a radioaerosol, are currently available in the United States. Comparative studies between ^{133}Xe and ^{99m}Tc-DTPA have not shown significant differences in overall accuracy. The choice of agent varies by institution and depends largely on available equipment and physician preference.

XENON-133

^{133}Xe is a noble gas produced by fission of uranium-235 (^{235}U) in a nuclear reactor. ^{133}Xe has a half-life of 5.3 days. The principle photon energy is 81 keV. Although ^{133}Xe is partially soluble in blood, it clears rapidly from the blood as it is exhaled, resulting in a biologic half-life of 30 seconds by current imaging standards. A typical adult dose of ^{133}Xe for a ventilation scan is 10 to 30 mCi.

TECHNETIUM-99m DTPA

^{99m}Tc-DTPA is produced by nebulizing its liquid form into a fine mist that is then filtered through a settling bag into a microaerosol. Once inhaled, larger particles

(>2 μm) deposit centrally in the trachea and pharynx; smaller particles (<0.5 μm) deposit in the distal tracheobronchial tree. Less than 10% of the aerosolized radioisotope is deposited within the lungs. Once in the lungs, ^{99m}Tc-DTPA diffuses across the alveolar membrane through the interstitium into the capillaries and is ultimately excreted by the kidneys. The biologic half-life of DTPA is 60 to 90 minutes, whereas the physical half-life of ^{99m}Tc is 6 hours. Airway turbulence caused by any obstructive lung disease results in more central deposition of particles, potentially compromising visualization of peripheral lung. The advantages of ^{99m}Tc-DTPA are that it is widely available and inexpensive and has a 140-keV photopeak, ideal for gamma camera imaging. A typical adult dose of nebulized ^{99m}Tc-DTPA is 30 mCi.

Perfusion

The goal of perfusion lung scanning is to distribute the radiopharmaceutical to pulmonary segments according to relative blood flow. This can be achieved using radiolabeled particles just larger than the diameter of capillaries (7–10 μm). Once injected intravenously, the particles travel through the right atrium, right ventricle, and then the pulmonary vascular bed, where they become trapped in the precapillary arterioles. Pulmonary segments with decreased or absent blood flow have reduced radiopharmaceutical delivery and trapping, resulting in a defect.

^{99m}Tc-macroaggregated albumin (MAA) is the most common radiopharmaceutical in current use. MAA is prepared by heat denaturation of human serum albumin. ^{99m}Tc-MAA is prepared by adding ^{99m}Tc-pertechnetate to a commercially available MAA kit. Of the radiolabeled particles, 90% measure between 10 and 100 μm. Particles larger than 150 μm should not be injected because they can obstruct arterioles. Typically, 200,000 to 500,000 particles are injected, and less than 0.1% of capillaries are temporarily occluded. A minimum of approximately 60,000 ^{99m}Tc-MAA particles must be injected to ensure reliable count statistics and image quality. The standard dose of ^{99m}Tc-MAA is 4 mCi, although larger doses are administered for heavier patients.

The biologic half-life of MAA particles in the lung is 2 to 12 hours. The MAA degrades over time and passes through the alveolar capillaries into the systemic circulation, where it is phagocytized by the reticuloendothelial system.

Scan Techniques

XENON-133 VENTILATION SCANNING

The patient is initially fitted with an airtight face mask. ^{133}Xe is inhaled from a closed shielded system. The patient is instructed to take a large breath and to hold it for as long as possible. A posterior projection 30-second wash-in or initial breath image of the lungs is obtained. The patient then rebreathes an air–^{133}Xe mixture. After 3 to 5 minutes of rebreathing, posterior, left posterior oblique, and right posterior oblique equilibrium images are obtained for 60 seconds each. The air–^{133}Xe mixture can be titrated with oxygen as needed. In the washout phase, the patient exhales the ^{133}Xe mixture into a charcoal trap. Serial posterior and lateral oblique 60-second washout images are obtained over a 5-minute interval. If possible, all images should be performed with the patient in an upright position. ^{133}Xe ventilation scanning should be performed in a negative pressure room with safe external ventilation.

TECHNETIUM-99m DTPA VENTILATION SCANNING

The patient inhales ^{99m}Tc-DTPA microaerosol for 3 to 5 minutes. This part of the examination should be performed with the patient in the supine position to minimize the normal apex to base gravity-induced ventilation gradient. After inhaling ^{99m}Tc-DTPA, the patient is imaged, preferably upright, in the anterior, posterior, right lateral, left lateral, right posterior oblique, left posterior oblique, right anterior oblique, and left anterior oblique positions for 500,000 counts each. One important advantage of ^{99m}Tc-DTPA ventilation scanning is that matching imaging projections as for perfusion scanning can be obtained. The exhaled aerosol is trapped in a filter that is stored to allow for decay until safe for disposal.

TECHNETIUM-99m MAA PERFUSION SCANNING

^{99m}Tc-MAA particles should be resuspended prior to injection by gentle agitation. The patient is injected in the supine position while taking slow deep breaths to facilitate lung expansion and reduce atelectasis. Blood should not be drawn into the syringe because aspirated blood may form clots, which become labeled by the ^{99m}Tc-MAA.

The patient is preferably imaged in the upright position using a large field of view, all-purpose gamma camera. Standard views in the anterior, posterior, right lateral, left lateral, right posterior oblique, left posterior oblique, right anterior oblique, and left anterior oblique positions of at least 500,000 counts each are obtained.

Importance of Sequence of Imaging

^{133}Xe ventilation scans should be obtained before perfusion lung scans because Compton scatter from the higher energy ^{99m}Tc-MAA photons (140 keV) down-scatters into the region of the 81-keV photopeak of the ^{133}Xe and would thus interfere with ventilation images.

A ^{99m}Tc aerosol ventilation lung scan should be performed after the perfusion lung scan. A standard dose of ^{99m}Tc-MAA is used, followed by a larger dose of ^{99m}Tc-DTPA (30 mCi); the rationale is that the higher activity of the ^{99m}Tc-DTPA scan will overwhelm any abnormalities present on the initial ^{99m}Tc-MAA scan. The historical practice of performing ^{99m}Tc-DTPA ventilation scan first, followed by ^{99m}Tc-MAA perfusion imaging, is no longer considered adequate.

Patient Preparation

A standard chest radiograph, preferably in both posterior-anterior and lateral projections, should be obtained within 24 hours of pulmonary scintigraphy. CT can substitute for chest radiography.

In patients with acute and symptomatic obstructive lung disease, bronchodilator therapy could be considered prior to lung scanning to reduce ventilation abnormalities that would result in a nondiagnostic study.

Contraindications to Pulmonary Scintigraphy

There are few absolute contraindications to the ventilation or perfusion phases of pulmonary scintigraphy. Allergy to human serum albumin products is a contraindication to perfusion imaging, but occurs very rarely.

A few conditions warrant precautionary measures during perfusion imaging. Patients with pulmonary hypertension have reduced pulmonary reserve, and patients with right-to-left shunts are at risk for intracranial microemboli. As such, these patients should be injected with fewer particles. The standard 4-mCi dose should be administered but with fewer particles, typically less than 150,000; this will often require reconstituting a fresh MAA kit with higher than standard ^{99m}Tc activity per particle. Alternatively, if lower than standard activity is administered, each perfusion view can be imaged for a longer time interval to achieve comparable counting statistics.

Children should also receive a reduced number of particles because they have fewer pulmonary arterioles. Specific guidelines for dosing children have been published by the European Society of Nuclear Medicine. A minimum of 10,000 particles should be administered.

Clinical Applications for Pulmonary Scintigraphy

Acute Pulmonary Embolism

The most important application for pulmonary scintigraphy is the detection of acute pulmonary emboli. Although CT has largely replaced pulmonary scintigraphy as the first-line diagnostic tool for diagnosing acute PE, pulmonary scintigraphy remains the modality of choice in patients for whom CT angiography is contraindicated, usually those with impaired renal function and allergy to iodinated contrast.

Comparison of Diagnostic Performance of Pulmonary Scintigraphy to CT Angiography

According to the original Prospective Investigation of Pulmonary Embolism Diagnosis (PIOPED I) trial data, a high-probability V/Q scan interpretation was associated with a sensitivity of 41% and specificity of 97% for detecting PE when compared to a pulmonary angiogram as the reference standard. If a scan was interpreted as either high or intermediate probability, the sensitivity improved to 82%, with a specificity of 52%. If a scan was interpreted as any category other than normal (including low probability), the sensitivity was 98%.

In the PIOPED II trial, comparing CT angiography to a composite standard, CT angiography was 83% sensitive and 95% specific in detecting PE. Combining CT venography increased the sensitivity from 83% to 90%. In practice, the diagnostic performance of any modality evolves with usage pattern and advances in technology. Diagnostic performance is also highly dependent on an individual radiologist's practice experience. As CT angiography continues to replace pulmonary scintigraphy as the preferred diagnostic study to diagnose PE by clinicians and radiologists, comfort with and proficiency at interpreting V/Q scans declines. It should be noted that a key advantage to CT angiography is that it can reveal coexisting or alternative causes that could explain a patient's symptoms.

As screening tools, both a diagnostic quality CT angiogram showing patent pulmonary arteries and normal or near-normal V/Q scans have comparable and high negative predictive values exceeding 95% for excluding PE.

Chronic Pulmonary Embolism

A chronic PE represents a distinct clinical entity from acute PE. Pulmonary scintigraphy is the diagnostic modality of choice for the diagnosis of chronic thromboembolic disease. Direct comparisons of multidetector CT and pulmonary scintigraphy have shown higher sensitivity (96%–97% vs. 51%). The diagnostic criteria for a chronic PE are identical to those for an acute PE.

V/Q Scans

QUANTITATIVE V/Q SCAN

Ventilation or perfusion can be quantified by drawing regions of interest around the upper, mid, and lower zones of each lung and calculating each zone's contributions to total lung activity using geometric mean calculations. Generally, this technique is used to estimate pulmonary function in a patient undergoing lung resection for lung carcinoma. The postoperative FEV_1 (forced expiratory volume in 1 second) can be estimated by multiplying the preoperative FEV_1 by the fractional perfusion supplying the nonresected lung regions. These data are important because many lung cancer patients have coexisting chronic lung disease. In the evaluation of the posttransplant lung, altered perfusion distribution or the development of matched ventilation perfusion defects may indicate transplant dysfunction and rejection.

NORMAL V/Q SCAN

A normal V/Q scan shows homogeneous and matched distribution of radiotracer on ventilation and perfusion images that outlines the shape of the lungs on radiograph (Fig. 12.1). There is expected cardiac, and sometimes hilar and aortic, impressions. A subtle base-to-apex gradient may be present because there is more basilar than apical lung parenchyma.

The ^{133}Xe parenchyma ventilation scan includes three phases—initial breath or wash-in, equilibrium, and washout. The wash-in images are often noisy because of relatively poor count statistics. Poorly ventilated lung will manifest as regions of low activity, which may fill in on equilibrium phase images. The distribution of ^{133}Xe activity on the equilibrium image represents aerated lung volume. The ^{133}Xe normally clears from the lungs within 3 minutes. Because the lung bases are better ventilated than the apices, the ^{133}Xe washes out of the bases faster than at the apices in a normal patient. Focal or diffuse retention of xenon is indicative of obstructive lung disease.

A normal ^{99m}Tc-DTPA aerosol scan often demonstrates activity within the trachea and the main stem bronchi in patients with obstructive lung disease. Swallowed ^{99m}Tc-DTPA aerosol activity can outline the esophagus and the stomach.

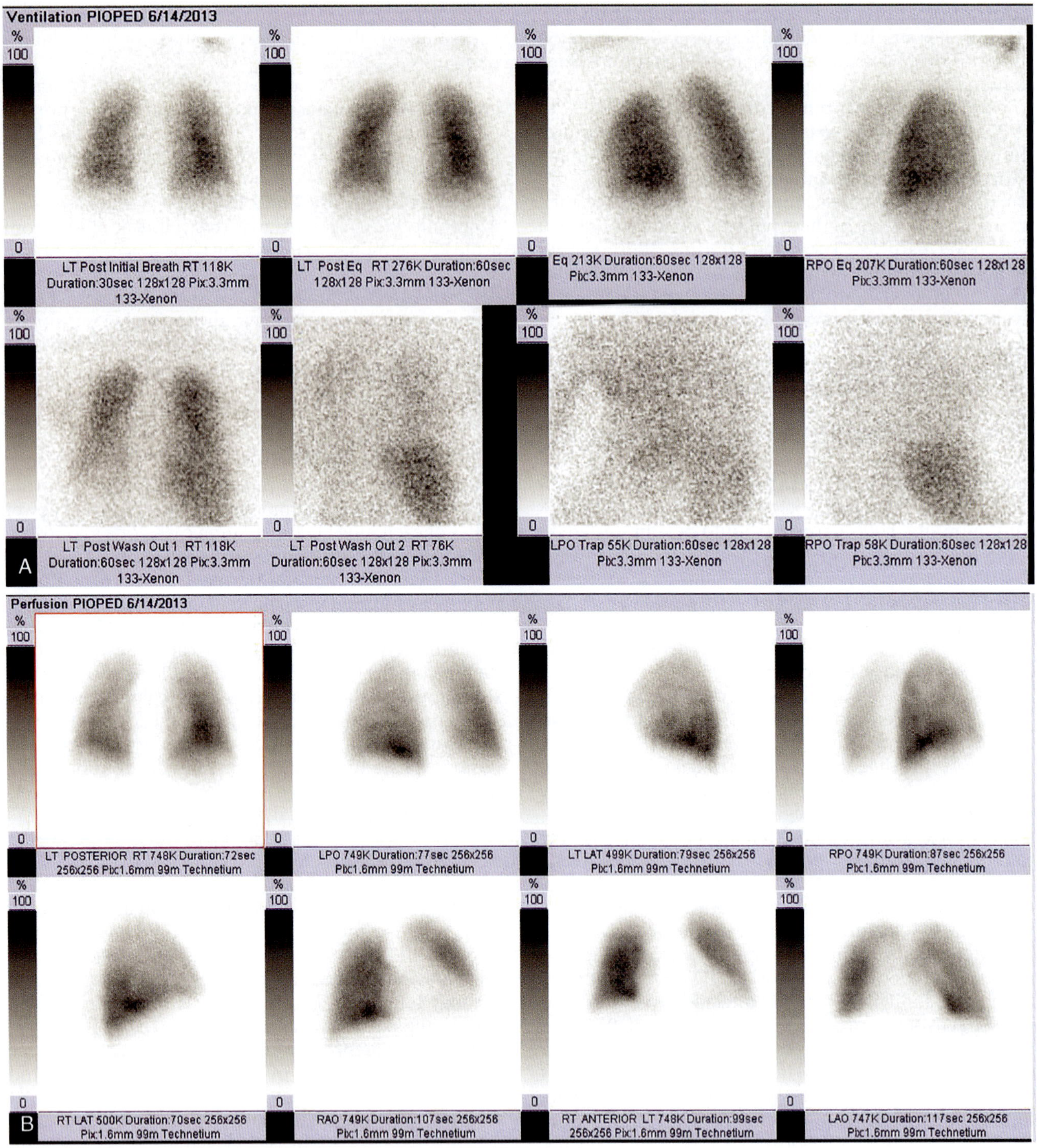

Figure 12.1 (A) Normal ^{81}Xe ventilation scan. Activity in the right upper quadrant abdomen is related to the deposition of ^{81}Xe in fatty liver. (B) Normal ^{99m}Tc-macroagreggated albumin perfusion scan.

APPROACH TO INTERPRETING THE ABNORMAL V/Q SCAN

The basis of pulmonary scintigraphy or V/Q scanning for PE is to detect a mismatch of pulmonary ventilation, which is relatively preserved, and pulmonary arterial perfusion, which is obstructed in the lung distal to a pulmonary artery embolus. Fundamentally, the interpretation of a perfusion defect rests on whether there is a matched defect on a ventilation image or radiograph that suggests an alternative explanation for the perfusion abnormality other than PE; if not, the scan has to be considered suspicious.

One consideration to bear in mind when comparing V/Q abnormalities to a standard radiograph is that V/Q images are obtained during tidal breathing, whereas chest radiographs are obtained at maximal inspiration. As a result, the lungs are smaller on the lung scan images than on radiographs. The reader should account for this difference in technique when deciding whether abnormalities are "matched" in size and shape.

ESTABLISHED CRITERIA FOR INTERPRETING V/Q SCANS

The first structured schema was published by Biello et al. in 1979 to standardize the interpretation of V/Q scans into low-, intermediate-, and high-probability categories. This schema was refined through the PIOPED study, a multiinstitutional trial designed to define evidence-based risk categories for PE. The PIOPED criteria stratified the risk of PE based on the number, size, shape, and distribution of perfusion defects and associated ventilation and radiographic findings. Based on these criteria, 13% of trial subjects had high-probability V/Q scans, 39% had intermediate, 34% had low, and 14% had normal or near-normal scans. A low-probability study conferred a less than 20% risk of PE, an intermediate-probability study conferred a 20% to 80% risk, and a high-probability study conferred a greater than 80% risk.

The PIOPED system posed several challenges for guiding clinical management because a risk of up to 20% for a low-probability scan was unacceptably high, and a range of 20% to 80% probability in the intermediate category was considered too broad to be prescriptive. Numerous revisions to the original PIOPED criteria have been proposed, including the modified PIOPED II criteria, a simplified classification system derived from the more recent PIOPED II data. The goal was to shift V/Q scan interpretations to high- and very low-probability categories and to add a nondiagnostic category. Specifically, the updated risk categories include the following:

1. Normal—that is, no perfusion defect (essentially excluding PE, irrespective of ventilation scan findings)
2. High probability of pulmonary emboli (positive predictive value [PPV], 87%) or
3. Very low probability (PPV, 6%)

See Table 12.1. All other V/Q scan appearances are considered nondiagnostic.

Causes and Implications of Diffusely Heterogeneous Pulmonary Perfusion Pattern

A diffusely heterogeneous pattern of pulmonary perfusion on a ^{99m}Tc-MAA perfusion scan can result from both technical and clinical factors. The most important technical factor is insufficient counts, usually related to insufficient particles due to partial extravasation of the dose. A low counting rate in the lungs and high counting rate at the injection site confirm a partially extravasated dose. Clinical entities that can contribute to a heterogeneous perfusion pattern include lymphangitic carcinomatosis and primary pulmonary hypertension. The distinction between primary pulmonary hypertension and pulmonary hypertension secondary to chronic thromboembolic disease is important because the latter may be treatable by anticoagulation and/or surgical thromboendarterectomy.

TABLE 12.1 Modified PIOPED II Criteria

FINDING	CATEGORY
Two or more large segmental defects Perfusion defect much larger than ventilation and radiographic abnormality	High probability
Nonsegmental perfusion abnormalities Perfusion defects smaller than corresponding radiographic abnormality Solitary triple-matched defect in the mid and upper lung zones One to three segmental perfusion defects (<25% segment) Moderate to large pleural effusion	Very low probability
All other findings	Nondiagnostic (low or intermediate probability)

Reverse Mismatch

Reverse ventilation-perfusion mismatches are ventilation defects without corresponding perfusion abnormalities. Reverse mismatches result from a failure of vasoconstriction that is usually induced by hypoxia in unventilated lung. This results in a functional right-to-left shunt because poorly oxygenated blood is never reoxygenated before returning to the systemic circulation. Mucus plugging is the most common cause of a reverse mismatch.

Examples are as follows. Typically, pulmonary emboli present as multiple segmental or wedge-shaped perfusion defects, with normal or near-normal ventilation and a clear radiograph (Fig. 12.2). It should be emphasized that pulmonary scintigraphy cannot confidently estimate the age of pulmonary emboli and therefore cannot reliably distinguish acute from chronic abnormalities.

While in the appropriate clinical setting, acute pulmonary emboli are the most common cause for segmental mismatched defects, but they are not the only cause. The most common alternative diagnosis is lung cancer. Pulmonary vasculature is preferentially occluded by mass effect from a mediastinal tumor or lymphadenopathy compared to the more rigid bronchi (Fig. 12.3). Old emboli are another consideration in the absence of prior studies for comparison. A list of additional differential diagnoses, most of which are exceedingly rare, is shown in Box 12.1.

Nonsegmental defects are those that do not correspond to segmental anatomy and are therefore unlikely to represent pulmonary emboli. Common causes of nonsegmental defects include pleural effusion, hilar lymphadenopathy, parenchymal masses, bullous lung disease, and atelectasis.

Underlying lung disease commonly confounds the interpretation of the V/Q scan. Regions of poorly ventilated lung, whether due to obstructive lung disease or pneumonia, are associated with reflexive pulmonary

BOX 12.1 Differential Diagnoses for Mismatched Defects

- Acute pulmonary embolus
- Chronic pulmonary embolus
- Fat or tumor embolus
- Central lung tumors
- Mediastinal or hilar lymphadenopathy
- Hypoplastic or aplastic pulmonary artery
- Swyer-James syndrome
- Postradiation therapy
- Vasculitis

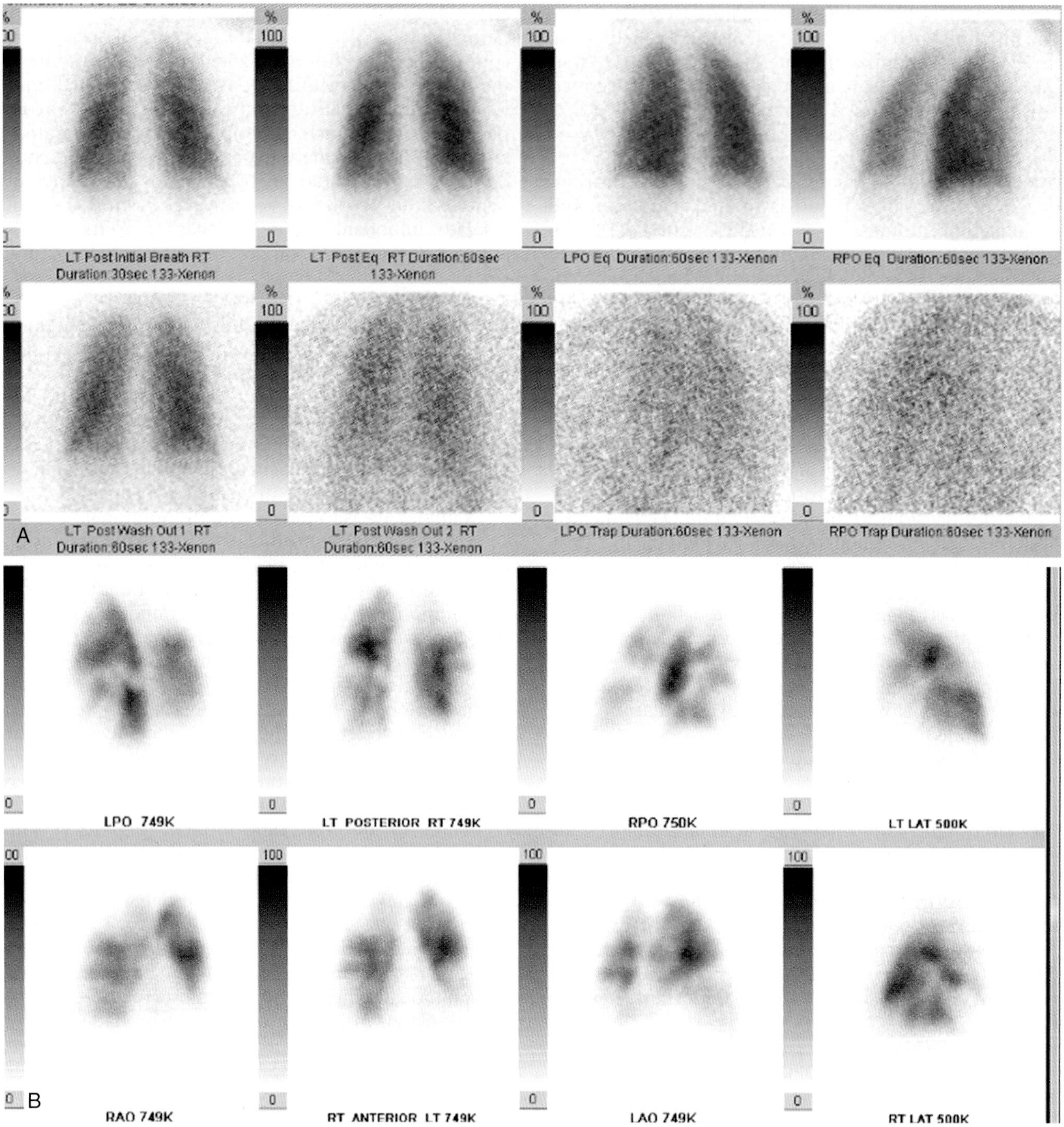

Figure 12.2 High-probability scan for pulmonary embolism. (A) ^{81}Xe ventilation scan shows normal ventilation. (B) ^{99m}Tc-macroaggregated albumin perfusion scan shows multiple segmental perfusion defects in both lungs.

arterial vasoconstriction, which may render the study uninterpretable for a pulmonary embolus. By the modified PIOPED II criteria, isolated triple-matched defects (abnormal perfusion with matching ventilation and chest x-ray abnormality) in the mid and lower lungs are nondiagnostic for PE (Fig. 12.4). In contrast, an isolated triple-matched defect in the upper lungs confers a very low probability for PE. The reason for this difference is epidemiologic, because basilar embolic disease is much more common than isolated mid and upper lung embolic disease.

A triple-matched defect must be distinguished from matched defects (abnormal perfusion with matching ventilation abnormality and normal or near-normal chest x-ray), which are associated with low and very low probabilities for pulmonary embolus.

Importantly, the terms *triple-matched* and *matched defect* require matching in both size and location. A perfusion defect that is clearly larger than the corresponding ventilation and radiographic abnormalities confers a high probability for PE because this appearance indicates an embolus with a distal perfusion defect associated with a subset of infarcted lung.

The Stripe Sign

The stripe sign is defined as preserved perfusion along the pleural surface on at least one projection. The sign suggests a cause other than an embolus because an embolus would be expected to result in obstructed perfusion extending to the subpleural lung. Although uncommonly present (<5% of V/Q scans), the stripe sign can be a helpful ancillary finding to help exclude pulmonary embolus. This sign is applicable only to immediately adjacent perfusion abnormalities and should not detract from the possibility of emboli as the cause for abnormalities elsewhere in either lung. The stripe sign is not specific for nonembolic causes, because it can be associated with reperfused lung previously obstructed by emboli.

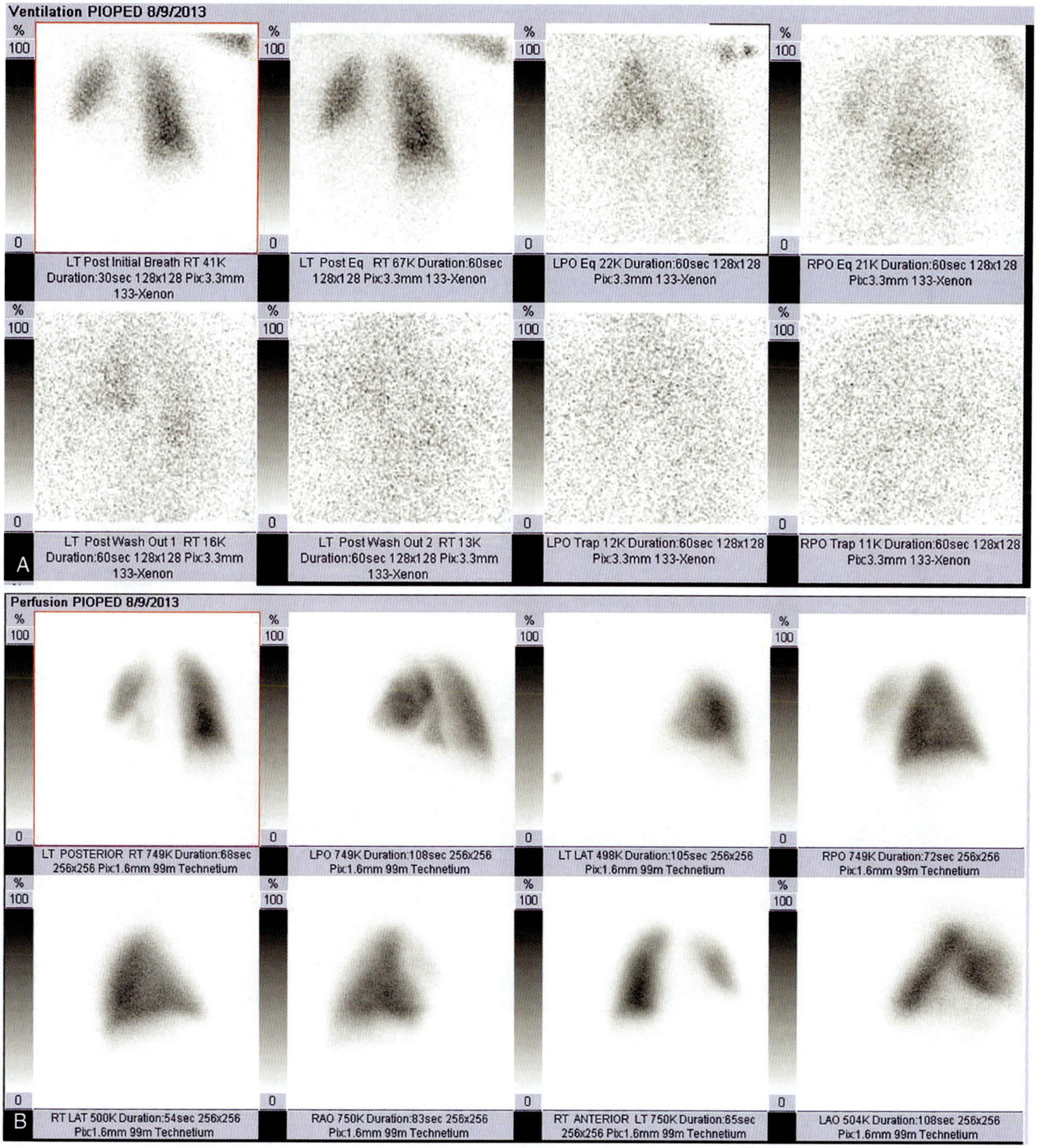

Figure 12.3 Nondiagnostic or intermediate probability scan for pulmonary embolism. (A) ^{81}Xe ventilation scan shows large defect in the left lower lung. (B) ^{99m}Tc-macroagreggated albumin perfusion scan shows matched defect in the left lower lung. *Continued*

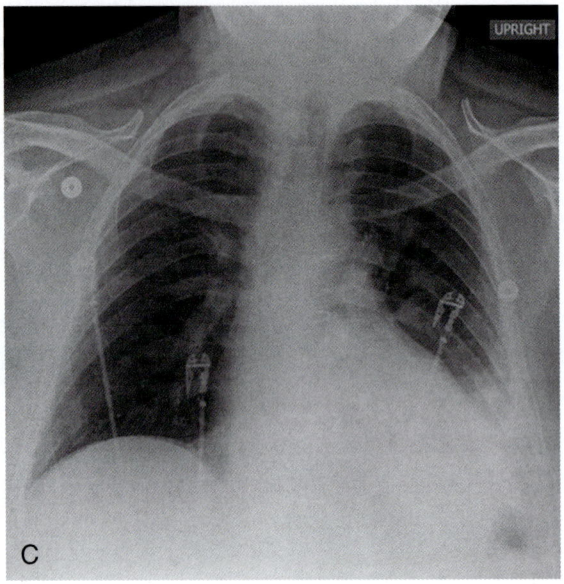

Figure 12.3, cont'd (C) Chest x-ray shows left lower lobe opacity in the territory of ventilation and perfusion abnormalities.

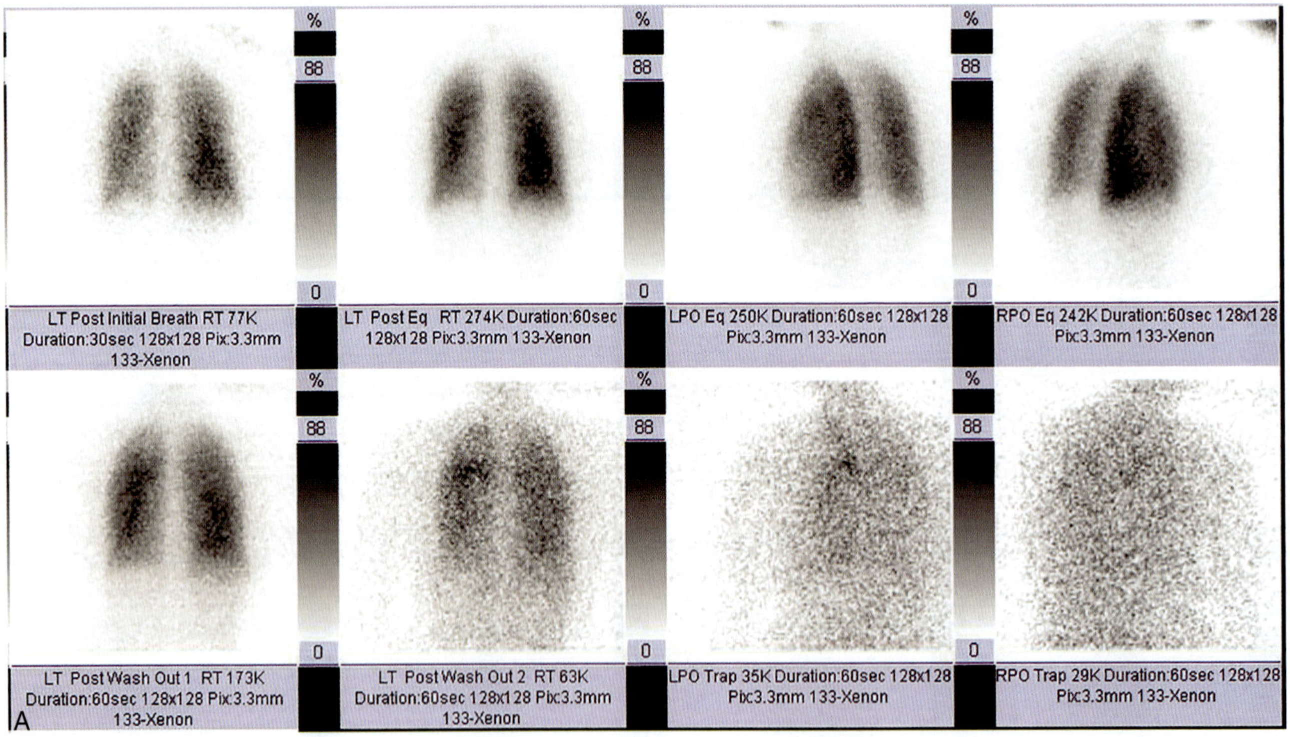

Figure 12.4 Sarcoidosis. (A) ^{81}Xe ventilation scan is normal.

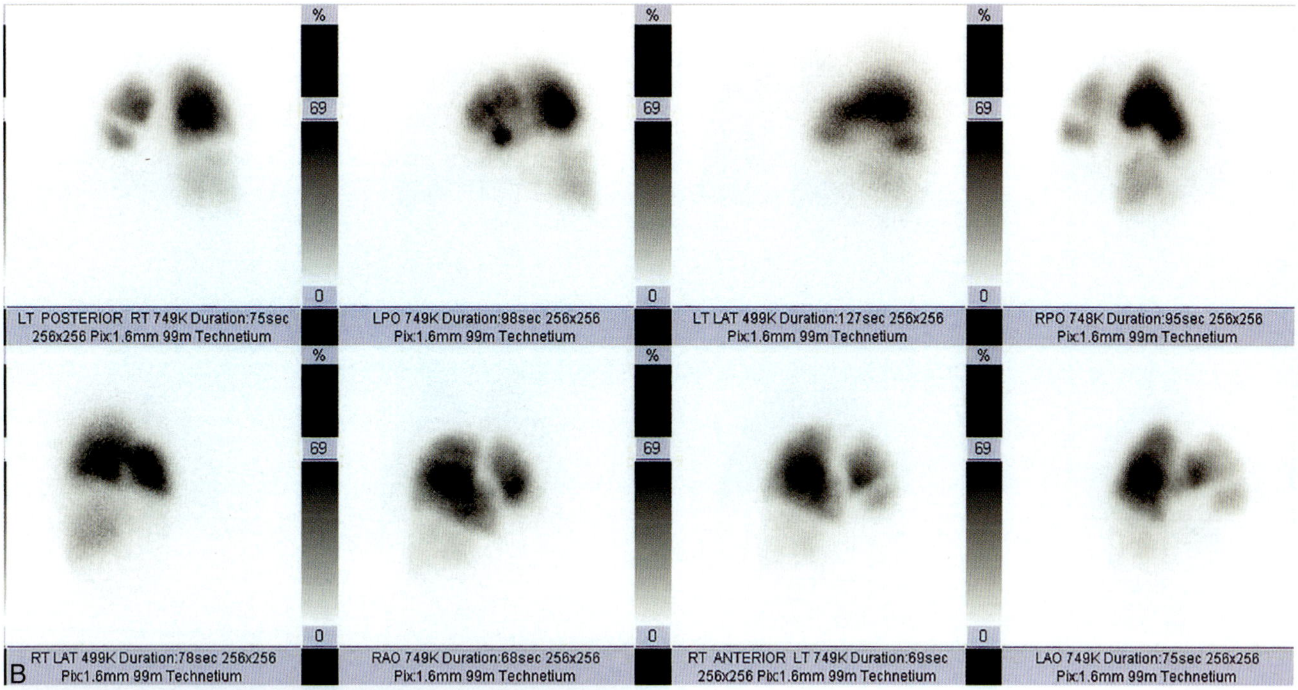

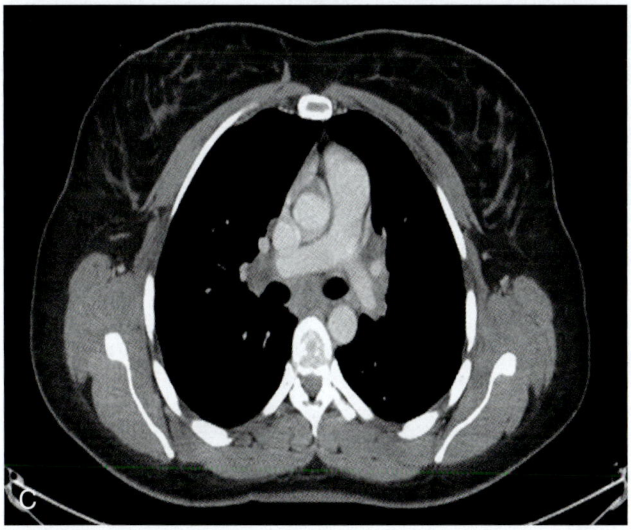

Figure 12.4, cont'd (B) ^{99m}Tc-macroagreggated albumin perfusion scan shows multiple mismatched defects in both lungs. (C) CT scan shows bilateral hilar lymphadenopathy that was pathology confirmed to represent sarcoidosis.

Interpreting the V/Q Scan in a Clinical Context

The predictive value of pulmonary scintigraphy is optimized when supported by clinical pretest likelihood of pulmonary embolus. The PIOPED study showed that combining imaging findings with a level of clinical suspicion substantially improved the predictive value of V/Q scanning. Of patients with high probability scans and a high clinical suspicion, 96% had emboli on pulmonary angiography. Of patients with low-probability scans and low clinical suspicion, 96% had no evidence of PE on angiography. A normal V/Q scan essentially excludes the presence of pulmonary emboli, even in the presence of associated clinical risk factors.

Important Incidental Imaging Findings

^{133}Xe is fat-soluble and deposits in fatty liver tissue. Hepatic accumulation is usually apparent during the washout phase of the ventilation scan and should not be mistaken for retention in the right lung base (see Fig. 12.1). The appearance is particularly prominent in patients with hepatic steatosis.

Any extrapulmonary activity on perfusion images should raise the possibility of the presence of free ^{99m}Tc–pertechnetate or a right-to-left shunt. Additional static imaging of the brain is indicated to evaluate for intracranial activity, a finding confirming a right-to-left shunt (Fig. 12.5). Patients with a right-to-left shunt will typically show punctate sites of radioactivity on whole-body imaging, reflecting the distribution of microemboli. Activity in the thyroid gland, stomach, and kidneys, which are usually visible on the original perfusion lung images, is usually the result of free ^{99m}Tc-pertechnetate (Fig. 12.6).

How to Recognize Technical Artifacts

Activity in the thyroid, salivary glands, and stomach can be present as the result of free ^{99m}Tc-pertechnetate.

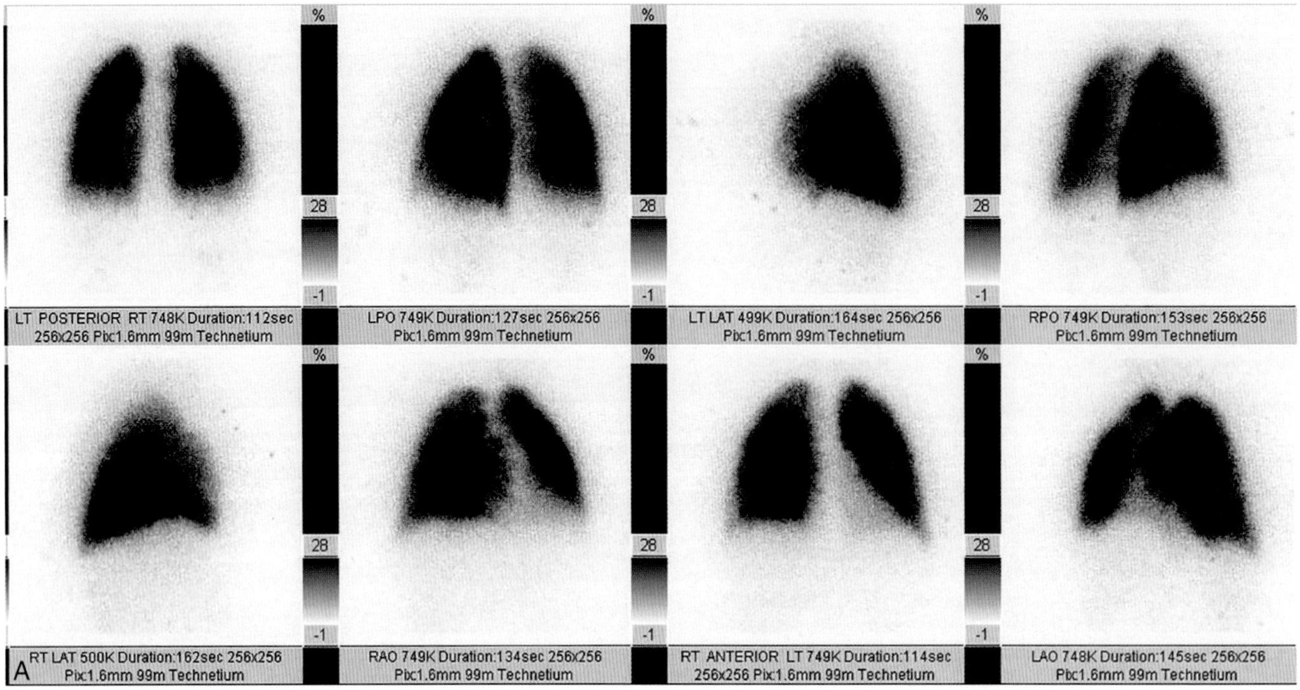

Figure 12.5 Right-to-left shunt. (A) ^{99m}Tc-macroagreggated albumin perfusion scan shows scattered punctate extrapulmonary foci of radiotracer. (B) Static imaging of the brain shows mottled intracranial distribution of radiotracer, confirming a right-to-left shunt.

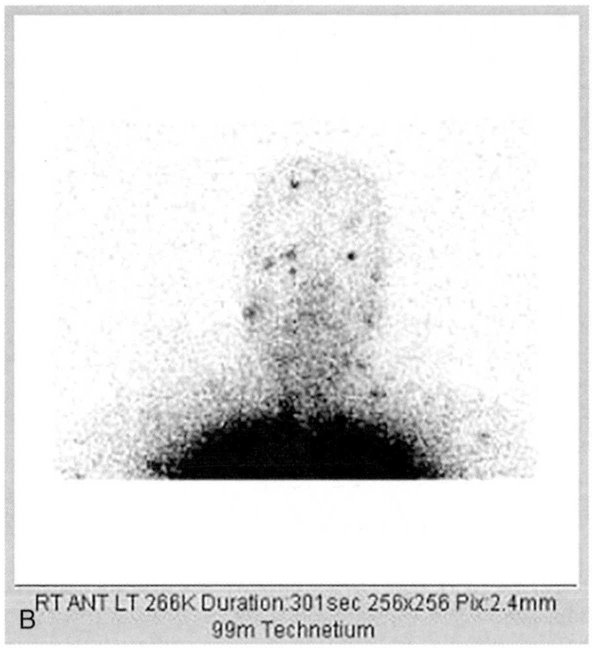

Injection of clumped ^{99m}Tc-MAA particles or labeled clot can result in multiple small focal hot spots scattered through the lungs (see Fig. 12.6). These could obscure perfusion defects, compromising the detection of emboli. If extensive, the study should be repeated the next day.

Esophageal activity can be seen on a DTPA aerosol scan as a result of swallowed activity.

Radiation Doses Associated With Pulmonary Scintigraphy

For ^{133}Xe ventilation imaging, the trachea receives a dose of 0.64 rad/mCi, the lungs a dose of 0.01 to 0.04 rad/mCi, and the whole body a dose of 0.001 rad/mCi. For ^{99m}Tc-DTPA aerosol imaging, the lungs receive an absorbed dose of 0.1 rad/mCi, the bladder wall a dose of 0.18 rad/mCi, and the entire body a dose of 0.01 rad/mCi. For ^{99m}Tc-MAA perfusion imaging, the lung is the critical organ and receives an absorbed dose of 0.15 to 0.5 rad/mCi. The whole-body and gonadal absorbed doses are 0.15 rad/mCi.

Radiation Risks During Pregnancy and Comparison of Dosimetry to CT Angiography

Both V/Q scanning and CT angiography expose the mother and fetus to ionizing radiation, although the level of exposure for both modalities is well below the accepted threshold for malformations or reduced intelligence (0.1 cGy).

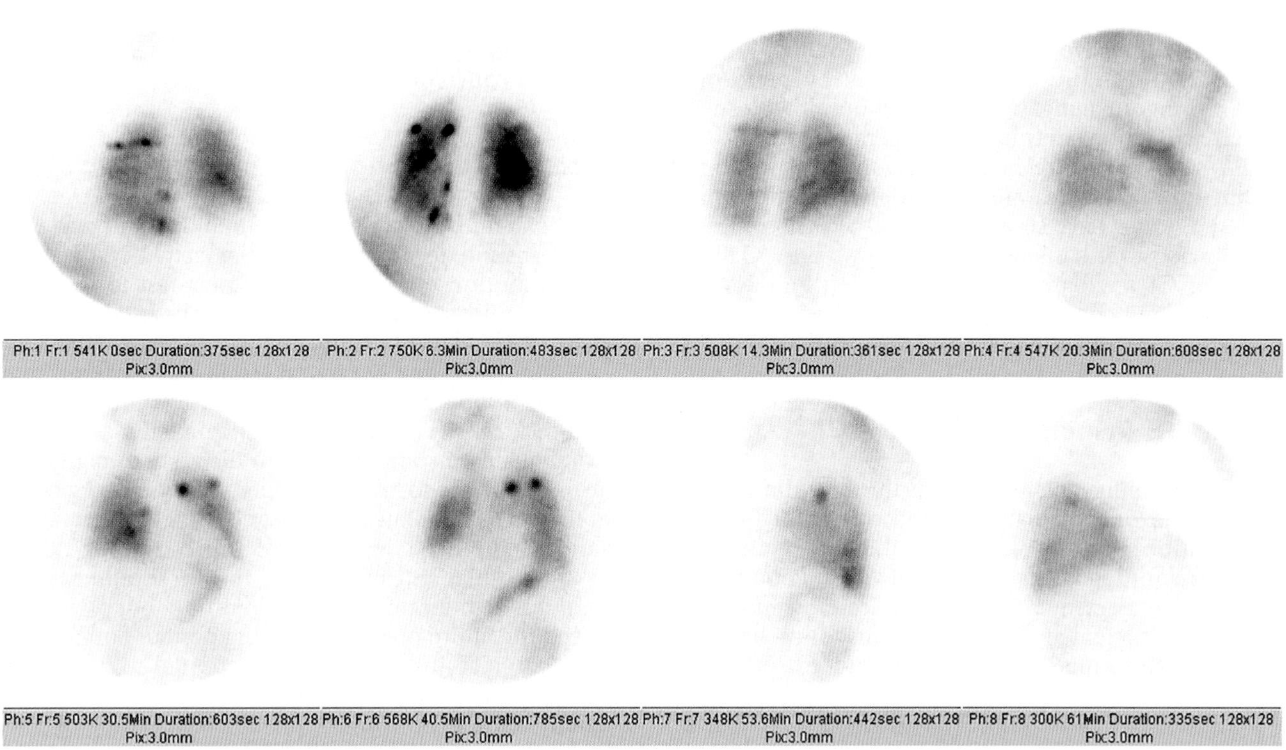

Figure 12.6 Free ^{99m}Tc-pertechnetate and clumped macroaggregated albumin (MAA) particles. Extrapulmonary distribution of radiotracer in the kidneys, stomach, and thyroid gland is indicative of free ^{99m}Tc-pertechnetate contamination. There are also foci of increased deposition in both lungs, consistent with clumped MAA particles.

Models of fetal radiation exposure from multislice CT angiography estimate an exposure range from 0.06 to 0.66 mGy. The exposure increases as the fetus enlarges and approaches the thoracic imaging field. The fetal exposure from V/Q scanning varies with the technique. Perfusion scanning contributes most of the radiation exposure and is estimated to be 0.48 mGy in the first trimester, 0.55 mGy in the second trimester, and 0.46 mGy in the third trimester. Radiation exposure to the breast is substantially higher in CT angiography (10–20 mGy) compared to V/Q scanning (0.6 mGy).

There is no consensus regarding the optimal imaging modality in the pregnant patient, and both the clinical context and patient preference must be considered when choosing appropriate diagnostic imaging. However, the fetus is considered to be more at risk than the mother, and minimizing fetal radiation exposure is often the primary focus in a desired pregnancy.

Strategies to Reduce Radiation Exposure

In pregnant patients, a perfusion scan only can be considered because coexisting lung disease is uncommon in this patient population. A PE can be excluded if the examination is normal. If the examination is abnormal but not diagnostic for embolism, a ventilation examination can be performed the next day.

The diagnostic accuracy of perfusion-only scintigraphy was recently appraised in the PISAPED study. Perfusion scans were independently attributed to one of four categories: (1) normal (no perfusion defects); (2) near-normal (impressions caused by enlarged heart, hila, or mediastinum seen in an otherwise normal scan); (3) abnormal, suggestive of PE (single or multiple wedge-shaped perfusion defects); and (4) abnormal, not suggestive of PE (single or multiple perfusion defects other than wedge-shaped). Using these criteria, the sensitivity achieved was 86% and the specificity was 93%. These criteria were further validated using the PIOPED II perfusion data. Applying the PISAPED criteria to those 889 perfusion scans yielded a sensitivity of 82% and specificity of 96%.

Guidelines for Breastfeeding Cessation

There are various published cessation times regarding diagnostic procedures involving radiopharmaceuticals. These provide guidance and are not regulatory requirements. The International Commission on Radiological Protection recommends cessation of breastfeeding for 12 hours following 4-mCi MAA perfusion imaging. No cessation is recommended following ^{133}Xe ventilation scanning alone.

In general, radiation exposure from diagnostic nuclear medicine procedures is expected to have no measurable consequences. Patient instructions should adhere to the ALARA principle (*a*s *l*ow *a*s *r*easonably *a*chievable) and common sense. Federal regulations (10 CFR 35.75) require that if the dose to a breastfeeding infant or child could exceed 100 mrem (1 mSv), assuming there was no interruption of breastfeeding, the licensee must give (1) guidance on the interruption or cessation of breastfeeding and (2) information on the consequences of failure to follow guidance.

Role for SPECT in V/Q Scanning

A few studies have shown that the accuracy of lung scans can be improved incrementally by performing SPECT lung imaging, with or without low-dose CT. SPECT ventilation scanning can be performed with ^{99m}Tc-DTPA aerosol and Technegas (ultrafine dispersion of technetium-labeled carbon; not available in the United States). Studies have shown that V/Q SPECT combined with low-dose CT has a higher sensitivity than V/Q SPECT alone or CT angiography for diagnosing PE. However, the number of clinical comparison studies is limited. At present, planar imaging remains the standard practice.

Part II: Principles of FDG PET

PET is a technique that reconstructs the three-dimensional distribution of radioactivity based on the high-energy annihilation photons (511 keV) that are emitted by positron-emitting radionuclides. PET allows noninvasive quantitative assessment of biochemical and functional processes. Integrated PET/CT systems offer both the metabolic information from PET and the anatomic information from the CT examination.

Radiotracer

The most commonly used PET radiotracer at present is 2-[fluorine-18]fluoro-2-deoxy-D-glucose. ^{18}F is produced in a cyclotron and has a half-life of 110 minutes. FDG accumulation in tissue is proportional to cellular glucose utilization. As a glucose analogue, FDG is transported by active glucose transport through the cell membrane into metabolically active cells and subsequently phosphorylated to ^{18}F-FDG-6-phosphate by hexokinase. Unlike glucose, ^{18}F-FDG-6-P-phosphate is not further metabolized and is therefore trapped inside the cell. FDG accumulation depends on both the blood supply of the tissue and its level of glycolytic metabolic activity. FDG is excreted by the genitourinary system and cannot be reabsorbed in proximal convoluted tubules.

Patient Preparation

Many patient factors, such as serum blood glucose level, blood insulin level, and muscular activity, affect the biodistribution of FDG. Patients must fast for 6 hours prior to radiotracer injection, to limit the following: (1) levels of circulating insulin that could drive FDG into skeletal muscle; and (2) serum blood glucose levels that could contribute to competitive inhibition of FDG uptake by tumor cells (Fig. 12.7). Diabetic patients, who have an attenuated insulin response to dietary serum glucose, are only required to fast for 4 hours. Ideally, blood glucose levels should be at fasting levels (<126 mg/dL), but many standard protocols allow levels up to 250 mg/dL. In general, regular and short-acting insulin should be held for at least 1 hour prior to FDG injection, but preferably during the entire prescribed fasting period. Long-acting basal coverage insulin has been reported to have little effect on the normal biodistribution of FDG. Strenuous activity should be limited for 24 hours prior to and immediately following radionuclide administration to limit muscle uptake of FDG.

Imaging Protocol

Once adequate patient preparation has been confirmed, a standard dose of 10 to 20 mCi of FDG is administered intravenously. Higher doses can be given for heavier patients to improve counting statistics and compensate for greater soft tissue attenuation. Speech should be minimized after injection to limit FDG uptake in the vocal cords; this is particularly important for patients referred for evaluation of a head and neck malignancy.

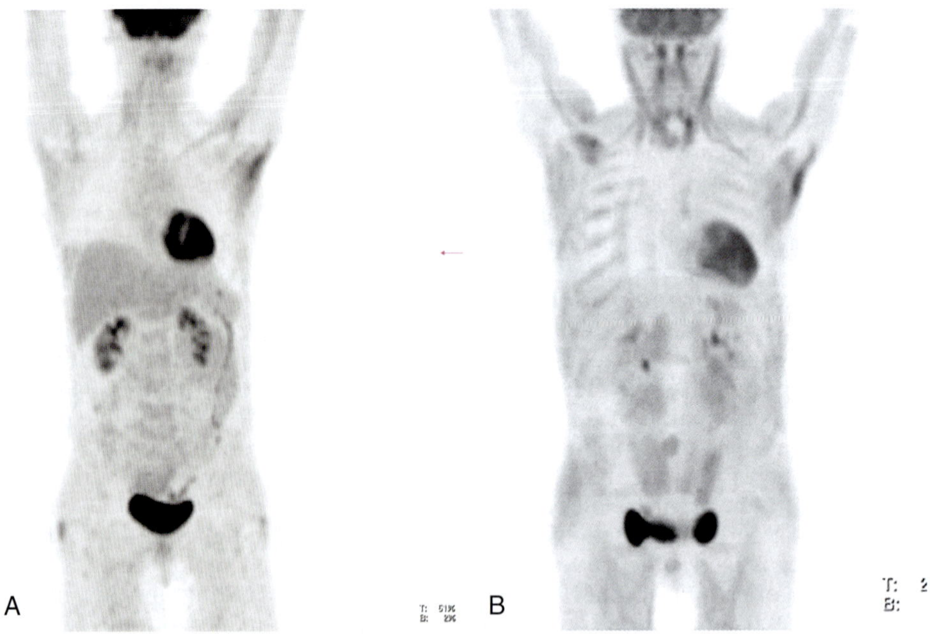

Figure 12.7 ^{18}F-fluorodeoxyglucose (FDG) biodistribution. (A) Normal distribution of FDG. (B) Altered biodistribution of FDG in the setting of food intake during the prescribed fasting period. Elevated levels of serum insulin drive FDG into skeletal muscle; the left ventricular myocardium is also intense.

Voiding of the bladder prior to imaging is helpful to limit high physiologic bladder activity that might obscure pelvic disease activity in the uterus, ovaries, or pelvic lymph nodes.

Whole-body imaging from the skull base to the upper thighs is initiated approximately 60 minutes after IV injection of FDG to allow time for the cellular uptake of FDG and clearance of FDG from the blood pool to decrease background activity. The arms at the side position is preferred for head and neck scanning, whereas the arms overhead position is preferred for body imaging. Scanning is performed during quiet tidal breathing. PET scanning is performed over 20 to 40 minutes, depending on the bed positions covered, number of acquisitions, and scanner speed.

An attenuation map must be applied to the PET images to compensate for the attenuation of detected photons. Reconstructed PET images are not interpretable without attenuation correction. Attenuation of either of the paired photons by absorption or scatter is greater in the presence of thicker intervening soft tissues. As a result, few photons from deep structures are detected. In contrast, the air-filled lungs contribute little to photon attenuation. Either a noncontrast transmission CT scan in combined PET/CT units or a positron-emitting rod source in stand-alone PET units can be used to create an attenuation map.

A separate diagnostic-quality CT, with or without IV contrast, may be performed with combined PET/CT systems. CT and PET images are reconstructed separately and then coregistered into composite images using image readout software.

Trajectory of PET Activity in Tumor Over Time

In general, PET imaging of tumor and infectious or inflammatory processes should occur no earlier than 45 minutes to allow for sufficient accumulation in lesions and viscera. Over time, uptake in lesions rises gradually, contributing to higher lesion-to-background ratios, although the change is not substantial enough to justify routine delayed imaging; greater decay of ^{18}F at later time points also makes delayed imaging challenging.

Common PET Artifacts

The attenuation correction process may introduce artifacts into the images. Misregistration artifacts can occur as a result of a mismatch between CT and PET lung volumes because the CT images are acquired during a single breath-hold and PET images are acquired during tidal breathing. If the CT is acquired in end-respiration, the so-called banana artifact, a zone of low activity above the liver, is apparent on PET/CT (Fig. 12.8). Patient movement, respiratory motion, cardiac pulsation, shifting bowel, and accumulating urine activity in the bladder can also contribute to misregistration artifacts. These artifacts can be resolved by comparing attenuation-corrected and attenuation-uncorrected PET image datasets.

High-density foreign objects and contrast agents can contribute artifacts when CT transmission data are used for attenuation correction. The Hounsfield units (HU) measured on CT images are scaled using a bilinear conversion to create an attenuation map for the higher energy PET photons (511 keV). Foreign objects, including dental implants, cardiac pacemakers, prosthetic valves, and surgical clips, have much higher density than biologic materials, with substantial attenuation of photons at CT energies but little attenuation of photons in PET. Applying an attenuation map derived from CT data results in the overestimation of PET emission activity. Similarly, IV and oral contrast can enhance the CT density in vessels and bowel by several hundred units and are not administered for attenuation correction CT scanning.

FDG Biodistribution in a Normal PET Scan

The challenge in PET interpretation is the differentiation of pathologic activity from normal and normal variant FDG activity. Organs with high basal metabolic activity show

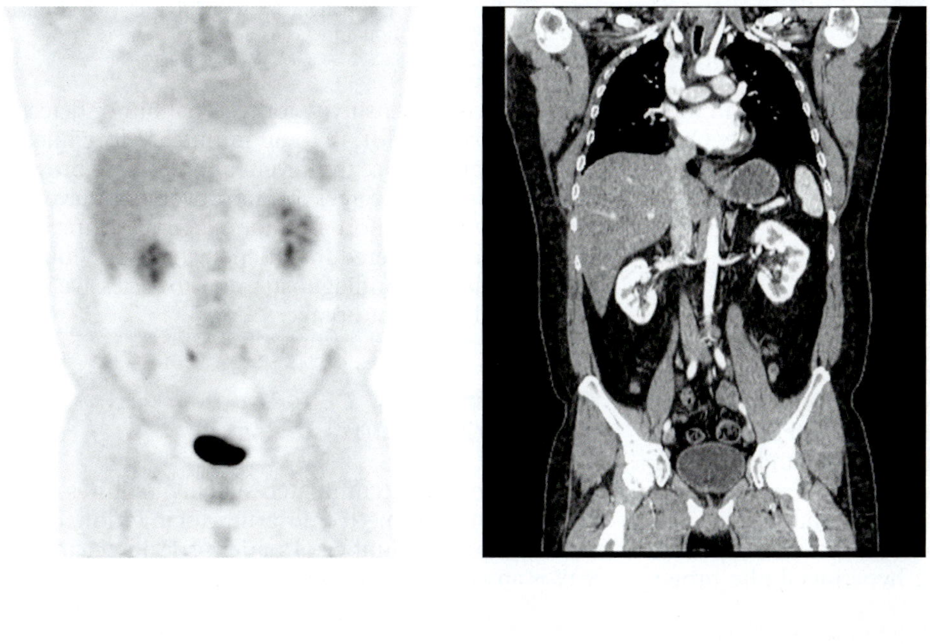

Figure 12.8 Banana artifact. The CT imaging for attenuation correction is acquired during end-expiration, whereas PET imaging is acquired during tidal breathing, resulting in a mismatch in lung volumes in the two datasets. An attenuation map corresponding to the dome of the liver is applied to the lower lungs on PET, resulting in overcorrection and a curvilinear band of low activity.

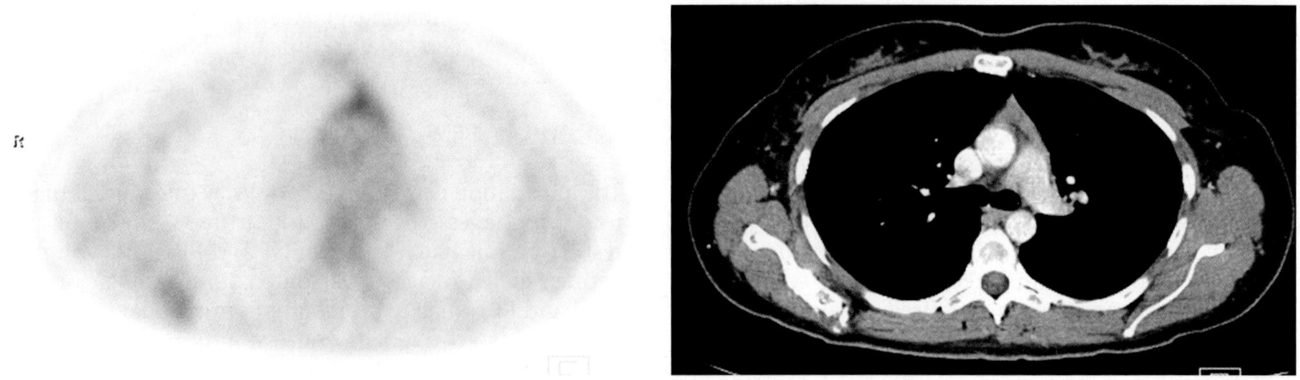

Figure 12.9 Normal thymus. Intense fluorodeoxyglucose uptake in a morphologically normal thymus gland in a pediatric patient is shown.

correspondingly high levels of FDG accumulation. Physiologic FDG uptake is highest in the brain. Myocardium can use both fatty acid and glucose as an energy source. Thus the uptake by myocardium largely depends on the metabolic state of the heart at the time of the injection, although, even among fasting patients, 20% will show intense left ventricular activity; high physiologic right ventricular and atrial activity is infrequently observed. Distribution of FDG to the gastrointestinal tract, liver, spleen, thymus, breast, salivary glands, vessels, and bone marrow is variable. High uptake localizing to morphologically normal thymic tissue can often be observed in children and young adults (Fig. 12.9). Thymic metabolic activity declines with age as thymic tissue involutes. Both the magnitude and distribution of physiologic bowel uptake vary widely; however, focal activity is suspicious for pathology. Uptake to the breasts is often low, but is higher during lactation and in the setting of hormone stimulation. Breast implants can result in increased uptake surrounding the implant. Activity of the lungs is low and typically does not exceed a standardized uptake value (SUV) of 1. Physiologic excretion of radiotracer is seen in the kidneys and renal collecting systems in patients with functional kidneys.

Low-level accumulation of FDG can be associated with interstitial body fluids, including pleural, peritoneal, and synovial fluids, although high-level activity should suggest a superimposed infectious, inflammatory, or malignant process.

Periarticular patterns of increased uptake can, in most cases, be attributed to degenerative joint disease. Occasional nonspecific focal uptake in the anterior rib ends may also be degenerative in cause. Muscle uptake, usually asymmetric, is common and is likely related to usage.

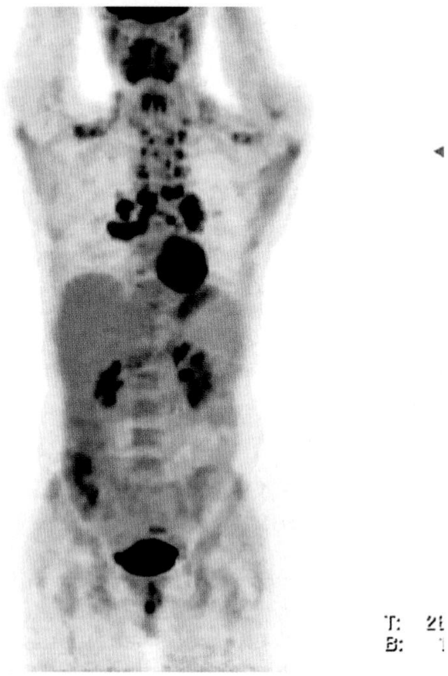

Figure 12.10 Hypermetabolic brown fat. There is intense fluorodeoxyglucose (FDG) uptake to the bilateral neck, supraclavicular, paraspinal, and axillary regions in the typical distribution of hypermetabolic brown fat. The patient has coexisting FDG-avid bilateral hilar and mediastinal nodal metastases.

Hypermetabolic Brown Fat

One common but occasionally problematic variant is FDG accumulation in the cervical and thoracic paraspinal, supraclavicular, axillary, and mediastinal regions localizing to fat (Fig. 12.10); the distribution is often asymmetric. This pattern usually occurs in cold weather and in young, thin patients. The uptake is related to the adrenergic stimulation of brown fat cells that may have originated as a primitive warming mechanism. Although the pattern is easy to recognize, FDG-avid hypermetabolic brown fat may decrease sensitivity for regional tumor detection. Warming patients for 30 to 60 minutes before injection is a common practice to prevent and decrease brown fat uptake. Variable degrees of improvement have been achieved with sedation and adrenergic-blocking agents and may be considered in patients whose previous scan was considered nondiagnostic due to excessive hypermetabolic brown fat uptake.

Quantitation of PET Activity With Standardized Uptake Value

Quantitation of accumulated activity requires precise knowledge of the injected dose, time of injection, imaging duration, and a number of patient-specific factors. The SUV is an estimate of relative uptake in a region of interest

(ROI), corrected for injected dose and patient weight. FDG distribution is very low in fat, which leads to higher values in tumor and normal tissues in heavier patients than in thin patients. As a result, correction for body weight is required; alternatively, lean body mass or body surface area can be used instead of body weight.

Volume averaging can artifactually lower SUVs because ROIs may include pixels from normal surrounding tissue in small tumors or from motion. Newer generation image analysis software allows the assessment of three-dimensional ROIs or volumes of interests. ROIs must be selected carefully to include only structures of interest.

When comparing serial examinations, imaging parameters should be similar to minimize the variability of SUVs. Despite standard imaging and patient preparation protocols, SUVs in normal tissues can vary by up to 35%.

Activity in a lesion can be reported in terms of the SUV_{max}, SUV_{mean}, or SUV_{peak}. The SUV_{max} is defined as the value of the most intense pixel in the ROI. Although SUV_{max} is the most reproducible parameter, it does not fully characterize the entirety of an abnormality and has limited statistical significance due to noise interference. The SUV_{mean} is an average of all counts in the ROI. The SUV_{peak} is calculated as an average of the counts from a small circular volume, usually 1 cm, surrounding the highest pixel. This technique is gaining popularity because it may more accurately represent maximal lesion metabolism compared to the SUV_{max}.

Clinical Applications

Increased consumption of glucose is a characteristic of many processes and is in part related to the overexpression of the glucose transporters and increased hexokinase activity. FDG accumulates indiscriminately at sites of high glycolytic metabolic activity in the body, allowing FDG PET to be a sensitive diagnostic tool for the detection and localization of a wide spectrum of pathologic processes. Currently, FDG PET is most widely used for oncologic applications; however, considerable overlap occurs between the FDG PET appearance of a tumor and benign infectious and inflammatory processes.

Oncology

Otto Warburg, a chemist, observed in the 1930s that the malignant transformation of cells is associated with an increased glycolytic rate. Increased glucose utilization by tumors is the basis of FDG PET imaging in oncology. Most common cancers demonstrate increased glucose uptake and are FDG avid. In general, higher FDG avidity is associated with higher grade and poorly differentiated tumors compared to lower grade and well-differentiated tumors.

The Centers for Medicare and Medicaid Services (CMS) has stratified applications of FDG PET for oncology into two main categories: initial and subsequent antitumor treatment strategies. The initial antitumor treatment strategy category includes assessment of primary tumors, initial staging, and localization of active tumor for biopsy planning (see Fig. 12.5). The subsequent antitumor treatment strategy category includes restaging, therapy monitoring, routine surveillance, and assessment for recurrence in the setting of elevated tumor markers (see Fig. 12.6). Recent literature reports have also cited the emerging application of PET for predicting the prognosis of malignancies based on SUVs.

Areas of tumor necrosis will have less FDG accumulation. This is often observed as absent activity centrally in very large masses. By defining areas of active tumor, PET scans can help direct biopsy for more reliable sampling. However, it is often not possible to differentiate a cavitary infectious process from a necrotic tumor on PET because both will have a photopenic center and a peripheral rim of increased activity.

Evaluation of lung cancer in solitary pulmonary nodules was the first clinical indication for FDG PET scanning in the United States to be approved by the CMS. If a solitary pulmonary nodule is a metastasis, whole-body PET can potentially detect the extrapulmonary primary cancer. FDG PET is reported to be 97% sensitive and 78% specific for the diagnosis of malignant pulmonary nodules. However, there is substantial overlap in SUVs between malignant nodules and benign processes, including tuberculosis, fungal infections, and sarcoidosis. Nevertheless, FDG PET–positive lesions should be considered malignant until proven benign (Fig. 12.11).

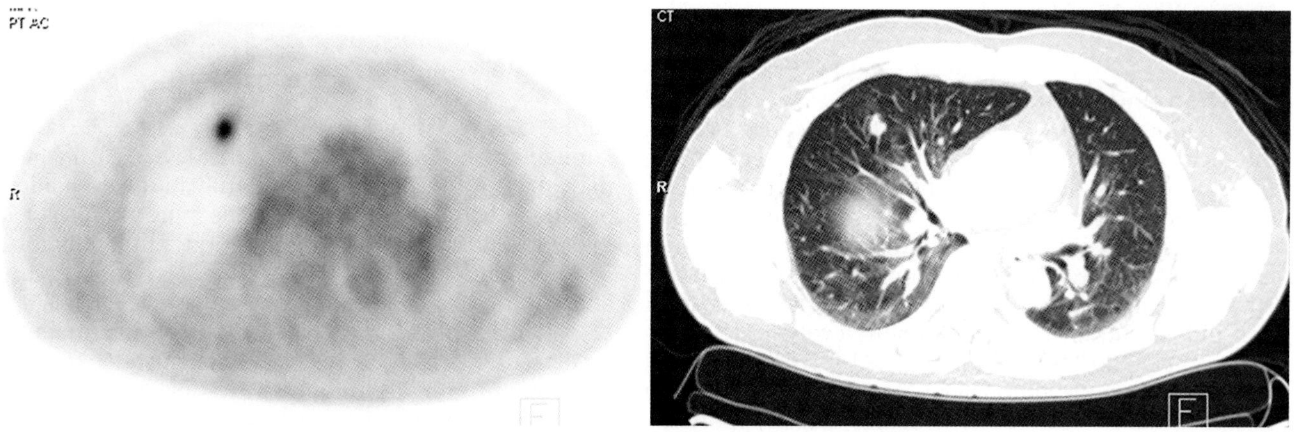

Figure 12.11 Solitary pulmonary nodule. There is intense fluorodeoxyglucose uptake to a right upper lobe pulmonary nodule that was confirmed to represent an adenocarcinoma at resection.

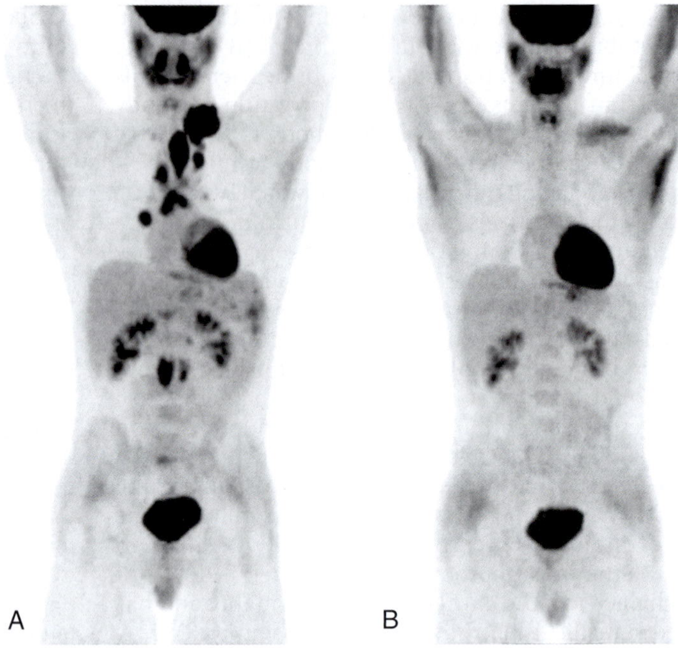

Figure 12.12 Lymphoma. (A) Initial staging of diffuse large B cell lymphoma shows widespread, intensely fluorodeoxyglucose (FDG)-avid supradiaphragmatic and infradiaphragmatic nodal disease. (B) Posttreatment PET imaging shows complete resolution FDG-avid lymphomatous disease.

FDG PET is less reliable for the characterization of small nodules (<1.5 cm) due to the effects of partial volume averaging and nodules of mixed solid and ground glass or predominantly ground glass CT morphology. The SUV_{mean} of a nodule may be artifactually lowered by smearing artifact produced by breathing during the prolonged acquisition of the PET scan. Respiratory gating and corrective algorithms for the PET data, based on CT images, can be used to enhance the accuracy of the SUV further but is not routinely performed for clinical studies. Lack of substantial FDG avidity to a nodule does not exclude malignancy, but suggests an indolent course. Nodules with no or only low level avidity can generally be followed if the patient has comorbidities that preclude treatment. Carcinoid tumors and adenocarcinoma in situ are two entities that often demonstrate little to no FDG avidity, despite their substantial size. It should be emphasized that the analysis of CT characteristics of the nodule is crucial in guiding management, and worrisome CT features should supersede reassuring PET features (Fig. 12.12)

Infection and Inflammation

FDG is not currently approved by the CMS for use in infection or inflammation imaging because large prospective studies with direct comparisons of PET with other diagnostic methods are lacking. More importantly, FDG PET imaging for infectious and inflammatory processes has thus far not been shown to improve health outcomes. However, the application of FDG PET for infection and inflammation imaging is rapidly evolving and, in practice, FDG PET is commonly used for this purpose at many institutions, although not necessarily as a first-line diagnostic tool. Indications with the most supportive evidence include evaluation of sarcoidosis, evaluation of vasculitides, and localization of a source in fever of unknown origin (FUO). Increased FDG uptake has also been reported in the lymph nodes, lung, and pleura-related inflammation in patients with occupational lung disease.

SARCOIDOSIS

The classic appearance of sarcoidosis on FDG PET imaging is intense uptake to hilar and mediastinal lymphadenopathy. FDG PET scanning can be helpful in distinguishing noncalcified inactive granulomas from active granulomas. FDG PET has also been advocated for monitoring the response to therapy.

EVALUATION OF VASCULITIDES

FDG PET has been used in the primary diagnosis of vasculitis when clinical symptoms are inconclusive and to evaluate the extent of disease involvement once the diagnosis is established. Although aortic wall uptake much higher than blood pool levels and similar to or exceeding the hepatic background is supportive of vasculitis, expert consensus criteria for the evaluation of vasculitis have not been established.

FEVER OF UNKNOWN ORIGIN

Limited prospective data indicate that FDG PET imaging may play a role as an adjunctive study in the evaluation of patients with FUO. The primary literature has suggested that FDG PET can localize infectious, inflammatory, and neoplastic processes with a high degree of certainty and contributes to the final diagnosis in 25% to 70% of patients with FUO. FDG PET can be instrumental in detecting occult processes not readily detected by anatomic imaging techniques, including chronic osteomyelitis, inflammatory bowel disease, and large-vessel vasculitis.

Timing of Posttreatment PET After Surgery or Radiation

FDG PET scanning after the completion of therapy should be performed at least 6 to 8 weeks after surgery and at least 8 to 12 weeks after radiation. The inflammatory changes associated with treatment are more likely to obscure sites of residual disease early following treatment and decline with time. Uptake associated with radiation pneumonitis parallels the CT evolution and is very intense during the acute phase; there may be persistent low-level activity associated with areas of chronic scarring.

Safety Considerations Following FDG PET Imaging

Breastfeeding Cessation

Cessation is not needed during breastfeeding following FDG PET imaging.

Contraindications to FDG PET Imaging

There are essentially no contraindications to FDG PET imaging. Although allergic reactions to FDG have been reported, they are extremely rare.

Radiation Exposure

The radiation dose for an FDG PET/CT examination must account for radiation exposure from both the PET and CT portions of the examination. The radiation dose for FDG PET is estimated to be 8 to 12 mSv for a standard 15-mCi dose. The radiation related to the CT portion of the examination varies with the application, imaging protocol, and CT system and can range from 1 mSv for a low-dose, nondiagnostic-quality CT scan obtained for attenuation correction purposes and up to 20 mSv for a multiphase, whole-body diagnostic CT scan with IV contrast.

Bibliography

PART I: PRINCIPLES OF PULMONARY SCINTIGRAPHY

Biello DR, Mattar AG, McKnight RC, Siegel BA. Ventilation-perfusion studies in suspected pulmonary embolism. *AJR Am J Roentgenol.* 1979;133(6):1033–1037.

Carvalho P, Lavender JP. The incidence and etiology of the ventilation/perfusion reverse mismatch defect. *Clin Nucl Med.* 1989;14:571–576.

Gutte H, Mortensen J, Jensen C, et al. Detection of pulmonary embolism with combined ventilation/perfusion SPECT and low dose CT: head-to-head comparison with CT-angiography. *J Nucl Med.* 2009;50(12):1987–1992.

Hartmann IJ, Hagen PJ, Melissant CF, Postmus PE, Prins MH. Diagnosing acute pulmonary embolism: effect of chronic obstructive pulmonary disease on the performance of D-dimer testing, ventilation/perfusion scintigraphy, spiral computed tomographic angiography, and conventional angiography. *Am J Respir Crit Care Med.* 2000;162:2232–2237.

International Commission on Radiological Protection. Radiation dose to patients from radiopharmaceuticals (addendum 2 to ICRP 53). *Ann ICRP.* 1998;28:1–126.

Palmer J, Bitzen U, Jonson B, Bajc M. Comprehensive ventilation/perfusion SPECT. *J Nucl Med.* 2001;42:1288–1294.

Scarsbrook AF, Bradley KM, Gleeson FV. Perfusion scintigraphy: diagnostic utility in pregnant women with suspected pulmonary embolic disease. *Eur Radiol.* 2007;17:2554–2560.

Schembri GP, Miller AE, Smart R. Radiation dosimetry and safety issues in the investigation of pulmonary embolism. *Semin Nucl Med.* 2010;40:442–454.

Schuemichen C. Pulmonary embolism: is multislice CT the method of choice? Against. *Eur J Nucl Med Mol Imaging.* 2005;32:107–112.

Sostman HD, Coleman RE, DeLong DM, Newman GE, Paine S. Evaluation of revised criteria for ventilation-perfusion scintigraphy in patients with suspected pulmonary embolism. *Radiology.* 1994;193:103–107.

Sostman HD, Gottschalk A. Prospective validation of the stripe sign in ventilation-perfusion scintigraphy. *Radiology.* 1992;184:455–459.

Sostman HD, Miniati M, Gottschalk A, Matta F, Stein PD, Pistolesi M. Sensitivity and specificity of perfusion scintigraphy combined with chest radiography for acute pulmonary embolism in PIOPED II. *J Nucl Med.* 2008;49:1741–1748.

The PIOPED Investigators. Value of the ventilation/perfusion scan in acute pulmonary embolism: results of the prospective investigation of pulmonary embolism diagnosis (PIOPED). *JAMA.* 1990;263:2753–2759.

Tunariu N, Gibbs SJ, Win Z, et al. Ventilation-perfusion scintigraphy is more sensitive than multidetector CTPA in detecting chronic thromboembolic pulmonary disease as a treatable cause of pulmonary hypertension. *J Nucl Med.* 2007;48:680–684.

van Beek EJ, Kuyer PM, Schenk BE, Brandjes DP, ten Cate JW, Buller HR. A normal perfusion lung scan in patients with clinically suspected pulmonary embolism. Frequency and clinical validity. *Chest.* 1995;108:170–173.

Webber MM, Gomes AS, Roe D, La Fontaine RL, Hawkins RA. Comparison of Biello, McNeil, and PIOPED criteria for the diagnosis of pulmonary emboli on lung scans. *AJR Am J Roentgenol.* 1990;154:975–981.

Wells PS, Ginsberg JS, Anderson DR, et al. Use of a clinical model for safe management of patients with suspected pulmonary embolism. *Ann Intern Med.* 1998;129:997–1005.

Worsley DF, Palevsky HI, Alavi A. Ventilation-perfusion lung scanning in the evaluation of pulmonary hypertension. *J Nucl Med.* 1994;35:793–796.

PART II: PRINCIPLES OF FDG PET

Antoch G, Freudenberg LS, Egelhof T, et al. Focal tracer uptake: a potential artifact in contrast-enhanced dual-modality PET/CT scans. *J Nucl Med.* 2002;43:1339–1342.

Bar-Shalom R, Yefremov N, Guralnik L, et al. Clinical performance of PET/CT in evaluation of cancer: additional value for diagnostic imaging and patient management. *J Nucl Med.* 2003;44:1200–1209.

Delbeke D, Coleman RE, Guiberteau MJ, et al. Procedure guideline for tumor imaging with 18F-FDG PET/CT 1.0. *J Nucl Med.* 2006;47:885–895.

Dizendorf E, Hany TF, Buck A, von Schulthess GK, Burger C. Cause and magnitude of the error induced by oral CT contrast agent in CT-based attenuation correction of PET emission studies. *J Nucl Med.* 2003;44:732–738.

Hillner BE, Siegel BA, Hanna L, et al. Impact of 18F-FDG PET used after initial treatment of cancer: comparison of the NOPR 2006 and 2009 cohorts. *J Nucl Med.* 2012;53(5):831–837.

Hillner BE, Siegel BA, Shields AF, et al. Impact of dedicated brain PET on intended patient management in participants of the NOPR. *Mol Imaging Biol.* 2011;13:161–165.

Hillner BE, Siegel BA, Shields AF, et al. The impact of PET on expected management during cancer treatment. *Cancer.* 2009;115:410–418.

Jacene HA, Leboulleux S, Baba S, et al. Assessment of interobserver reproducibility in quantitative FDG PET/CT measurements of tumor response to therapy. *J Nucl Med.* 2009;50(11):1760–1769.

Love C, Tomas MB, Tronco GG, Palestro CJ. FDG PET of infection and inflammation. *Radiographics.* 2005;25(5):1357–1368.

Nahmias C, Wahl LM. Reproducibility of SUV measurements determined by ^{18}F-FDG PET in malignancy tumors. *J Nucl Med.* 2008;49:1804–1808.

National Comprehensive Cancer Network. Clinical practice guidelines in oncology, version 1. 2013. http://www.nccn.org/professionals/physician_gls/pdf/cns.pdf. Accessed December 2014.

Schoder H, Erdi YE, Larson SM, Yeung HW. PET/CT: a new imaging technology in nuclear medicine. *Eur J Nucl Med Mol Imaging.* 2003;30:1419–1437.

Shankar LK, Hoffman JM, Bacharach S, et al. Consensus recommendations for the use of ^{18}F-FDG PET as an indicator of therapeutic response in National Cancer Institute (NCI) trials. *J Nucl Med.* 2006;47(6):1059–1066.

SECTION 3

Imaging Approach

CHAPTER 13
Introduction to Terminology

Sachin S. Saboo, Mukta D. Agrawal, Sandeep S. Hedgire, Robert Joodi, and Suhny Abbara

CHAPTER OUTLINE

■ Introduction

The focus of this chapter is to define terms used in cardiovascular and thoracic imaging and provide a basic framework for pattern recognition for problem solving in the clinical practice. The thoracic terms used in this book incorporate the recommendations of the Nomenclature Committee of the Fleischner Society published in 1984, 1996, and 2008 for thoracic radiography and computed tomography (CT). A few terms not included in the most recent Fleischner Society glossary of thoracic imaging terms are also defined. The updated terminology used in the cardiac and vascular imaging is also included.

■ Thoracic Terminology

Lung Parenchyma

Parenchyma: The gas-exchanging part of the lung is called the *lung parenchyma* and consists of the alveoli and their capillaries. On CT scans and radiographs, the lung parenchyma is the portion of the lung exclusive of visible pulmonary vessels and airways.

Lobe: Anatomically, lungs are divided into lobes, with the right lung typically consisting of three lobes and the left lung consisting of two lobes. Each lobe is enveloped by visceral pleura, except at the lung root (hilum) and in the presence of an incomplete interlobar fissure.

Segment: Anatomically, a segment refers to the lung lobe unit that is ventilated by a segmental bronchus, perfused by a segmental pulmonary artery, and drained by an intersegmental pulmonary vein. There are two to five segments per lung lobe.

Lobule, secondary pulmonary lobule, pulmonary lobule: A secondary pulmonary lobule (Fig. 13.1A) is a fundamental unit of the lung, and the smallest, surrounded by connective tissue septa and interlobular septa. It is an irregular polyhedron in shape and varies from 1 to 2.5 cm in size. Each is more developed in the periphery of lung and in the anterior, lateral, and paramediastinal portions of the upper and middle lobes. Each secondary pulmonary lobule is supplied by small bronchioles and a pulmonary artery branch that enters in the center of the lobule; it is also known as a *centrilobular* or *lobular core structure*. The interlobular septae are composed of connective tissue and contain pulmonary venules and lymphatic channels. One secondary pulmonary lobule contains 3 to 25 acini.

On thin section CT images, the secondary pulmonary lobule is composed of three primary components—the interlobular septa and septal structure, the centrilobular region and centrilobular structures, and the lobular parenchyma. In a normal lung, the pulmonary artery branch located in the center of secondary pulmonary lobule is visible (0.5–1.0 mm in diameter). However, a normally centrilobular bronchiole cannot be seen because of its thin wall (≈0.15 mm in diameter). The interlobular septa and septal structures are not usually visualized in the healthy lung (0.1 mm in the thickness) but are visible when thickened, such as in pulmonary edema and interstitial lung disease. Interlobular septa appear as thin linear opacities 10 to 20 mm in length between the secondary pulmonary lobules.

Lobular core structure: The lobular core structure at the center of secondary pulmonary lobule is composed of the centrilobular artery and preterminal bronchiole. The preterminal bronchiole branches into smaller

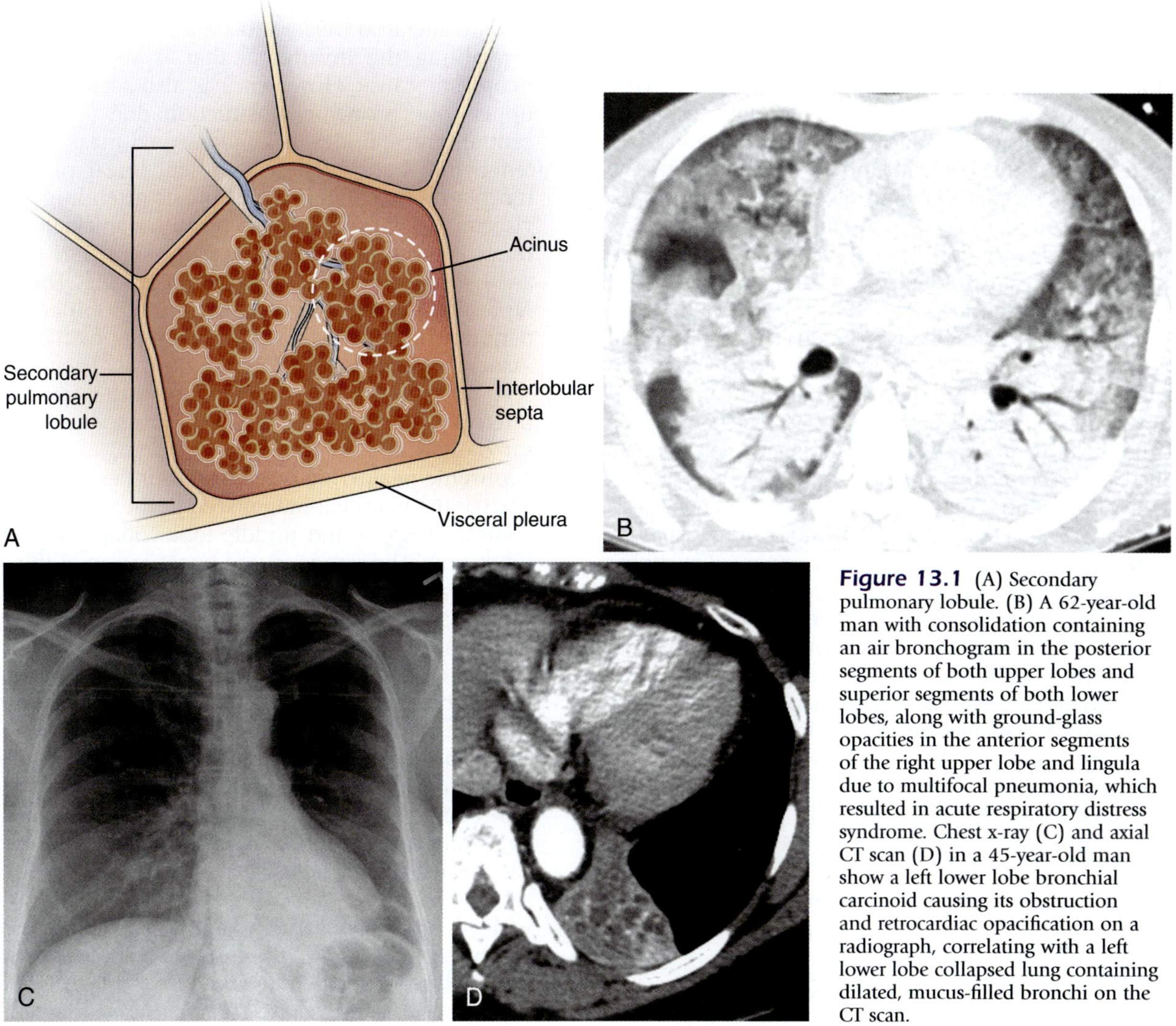

Figure 13.1 (A) Secondary pulmonary lobule. (B) A 62-year-old man with consolidation containing an air bronchogram in the posterior segments of both upper lobes and superior segments of both lower lobes, along with ground-glass opacities in the anterior segments of the right upper lobe and lingula due to multifocal pneumonia, which resulted in acute respiratory distress syndrome. Chest x-ray (C) and axial CT scan (D) in a 45-year-old man show a left lower lobe bronchial carcinoid causing its obstruction and retrocardiac opacification on a radiograph, correlating with a left lower lobe collapsed lung containing dilated, mucus-filled bronchi on the CT scan.

preterminal bronchioles, terminal bronchioles, and respiratory bronchioles.

Acinus: There are 3 to 25 acini in one secondary pulmonary lobule. A acinus is the portion of the lung distal to a terminal bronchiole, which is the last purely conducting airway. The acinus is supplied by first-order respiratory bronchioles and contains alveolar ducts and alveoli. Because the respiratory bronchiole is the largest airway that contains alveoli in their walls, an acinus is the biggest pulmonary unit in which all airways participate in gas exchange. An acinus is usually 6 to 10 mm in diameter. On thin section CT, an acinus is not visible unless filled with pathologic material (e.g., exudates), which appear as poorly defined nodular opacities. Hence, on a CT scan, the acinar nodules appear as multiple 6- to 10-mm rounded and ill-defined pulmonary opacities. Acinar nodules and air space nodules are almost equivalent terms.

Air space: Air space refers to the air-containing lung, which includes respiratory bronchioles; however, it excludes purely conducting airways, such as terminal bronchioles.

Consolidation: Pathologically, consolidation refers to an exudative or other air space and interstitial disease process resulting in alveolar air replacement and an opacified lung. On radiographs and CT scans, consolidation refers to an increase in lung attenuation causing obscuration of the margins of underlying pulmonary vessels and airway walls (see Fig. 13.1B). An air bronchogram may be present. The consolidation due to lipoid pneumonia shows decreased attenuation, and that related to pulmonary amiodarone toxicity has increased attenuation on CT and is helpful in narrowing the list of potential causes of the consolidation. Consolidation is nonspecific, with a wide differential diagnosis, so correlation with clinical and laboratory data is helpful.

Pneumonia: Pneumonia (see Fig. 13.1B) is an inflammatory condition of the air spaces and interstitium. Infective pneumonia is an exudative pathology of the air space resulting in consolidation, such as bacterial pneumonia. Noninfectious pneumonia is the result of pulmonary inflammation and fibrosis, such as idiopathic interstitial pneumonia.

Bronchopneumonia, lobular pneumonia: Bronchopneumonia is characterized by infectious bronchitis, bronchiolitis, suppurative peribronchiolar inflammation, and subsequent patchy consolidation involving one or more secondary pulmonary lobules. It spreads through the airways and leads to thick and tenacious secretions in the bronchi and bronchioles. On the radiograph, bronchopneumonia appears as a multifocal, peribronchial, or patchy consolidation often in multilobar distribution. On CT, it appears as ill-defined centrilobular and tree-in-bud nodular opacities and lobular consolidation.

Atelectasis, collapse: Atelectasis is reduced inflation of all or part of the lung that leads to volume loss. A common mechanism is resorption of air distal to the obstructed airway due to mucus plugging or a mass. The term *collapse* is used synonymously with atelectasis, especially with its increased severity and increased lung opacification. On radiographs and CT scans, the direct signs of atelectasis (see Fig. 13.1C, D) are a crowded pulmonary vasculature, crowded air bronchogram, and displacement of interlobar fissures. The indirect signs include pulmonary opacification, elevated diaphragm, ipsilateral shift of the heart and mediastinum, hilar displacement, compensatory hyperinflation of the adjacent lung, approximation of the ribs, and displaced pulmonary granulomas. Descriptively, atelectasis is classified into the following types: linear, subsegmental, segmental, lobar, or whole lung; rounded; and generalized or diffuse.

Linear atelectasis, discoid atelectasis, plate atelectasis: Linear atelectasis (Fig. 13.2A) is a focal subsegmental atelectasis with a linear shape that almost always abuts the pleura. It can be oriented in any plane from horizontal, oblique, to vertical, with a thickness ranging from a few millimeters to centimeters.

Luftsichel sign: The Luftsichel sign (from the German—*luft* means air, and *sichel* means sickle) is seen in left upper lung lobe collapse and occurs due to the upward and medial shift of the hyperexpanded superior segment of the left lower lobe, between the aortic arch and collapsed upper lobe. The collapsed left upper lobe moves anteriorly and superiorly to lie against the anterior chest wall; the hyperexpanded superior segment of the left lower lobe lies behind the upper lobe. On a radiograph (see Fig. 13.2B), the Luftsichel sign is characterized as a sharply marginated, crescentic, paraaortic hyperlucency extending from the apex of the left hemithorax to the left superior pulmonary vein and outlining the medial aspect of the collapsed left upper lobe. On a CT scan (see Fig. 13.2C), the collapsed left upper lobe is seen as a homogenous opacity lying anteriorly against the chest wall and mediastinum while the hyperexpanded superior segment of the lower lobe lies between the aortic arch medially and the collapsed upper lobe laterally, thus explaining the Luftsichel sign.

Golden S sign: The Golden S sign refers to right upper lobe collapse secondary to a centrally obstructing mass that is best seen on a frontal radiograph (see Fig. 13.2D) and CT scans. The collapsed upper lobe shifts cephalad and medially while the central mass expands the hilum. The term *inverted S sign of Golden* is derived from the configuration of a minor fissure with an upward lateral convexity and a caudal medial convexity resembling the inverted S that is suggestive of a neoplastic cause. However, it is also seen in a right upper lobe bronchus obstruction due to enlarged central lymph nodes or a mediastinal mass.

Parenchymal bands: These represent linear pleuroparenchymal opacities due to fibrosis extending to the visceral pleural surface, which is often thickened and retracted at the site of contact (see Fig. 13.2E). They are 1 to 3 mm thick and up to 5 cm long. They can represent contiguously thickened interlobular septa, peribronchovascular fibrosis, coarse scars, or atelectasis associated with lung or pleural fibrosis. They can be seen in patients with fibrosis and other causes of interstitial thickening such as asbestosis, silicosis, and sarcoidosis.

Juxtaphrenic peak: This is the tented or peaked appearance of the hemidiaphragm seen in the upper lobe or combined upper and middle lobe collapse or upper lobectomy. The sign is caused by retraction of the diaphragm at the inferior accessory fissure (most common), major fissure, or inferior pulmonary ligament.

On a frontal chest film, it appears as a small, sharply defined triangular opacity projecting upward from the highest point of the hemidiaphragm (see Fig. 13.2F).

Rounded atelectasis, folded lung syndrome, Blesovsky syndrome, atelectatic pseudotumor: This is a unique type of chronic peripheral lung collapse that develops as a result of pleural fibrosis and that can mimic lung carcinoma. It is usually seen following healing of an asbestos exposure–related exudative pleural effusion, with pleural fibrosis and adjacent lung collapse, but can be seen in other conditions as well. It is usually detected as an incidental finding on imaging. On a radiograph, a rounded atelectasis appears as a peripheral round, oval, or wedge-shaped, peripheral, masslike opacity, commonly in the posterior part of the lower lobe, with curvilinear opacities from the bronchi and vessels (comet tail sign) extending from the site of the rounded atelectasis toward the hilum. Adjacent pleural thickening and volume loss of the affected lobe are always present. CT better demonstrates the full extent of disease than a radiograph. On CT, a rounded atelectasis appears as a peripheral soft tissue density-enhancing mass, with smooth margins, except at the entry site of bronchi and vessel, and that forms an acute angle with the adjacent thickened pleura. The distortion and displacement of the converging bronchovasculature represent one of the diagnostic and commonly seen features (see Fig. 13.2G).

Infiltrate: This term was used on radiographs or CT scans to describe pulmonary opacification caused by air space or interstitial lung disease. Because the use of the term *infiltrate* is debatable, it is no longer recommended and has been widely replaced by other terminology. The term *opacity* with important qualifiers is preferred.

Parenchymal opacity: Parenchymal opacification means an increase in lung attenuation. It may or may not obscure underlying lung vasculature and airway walls.

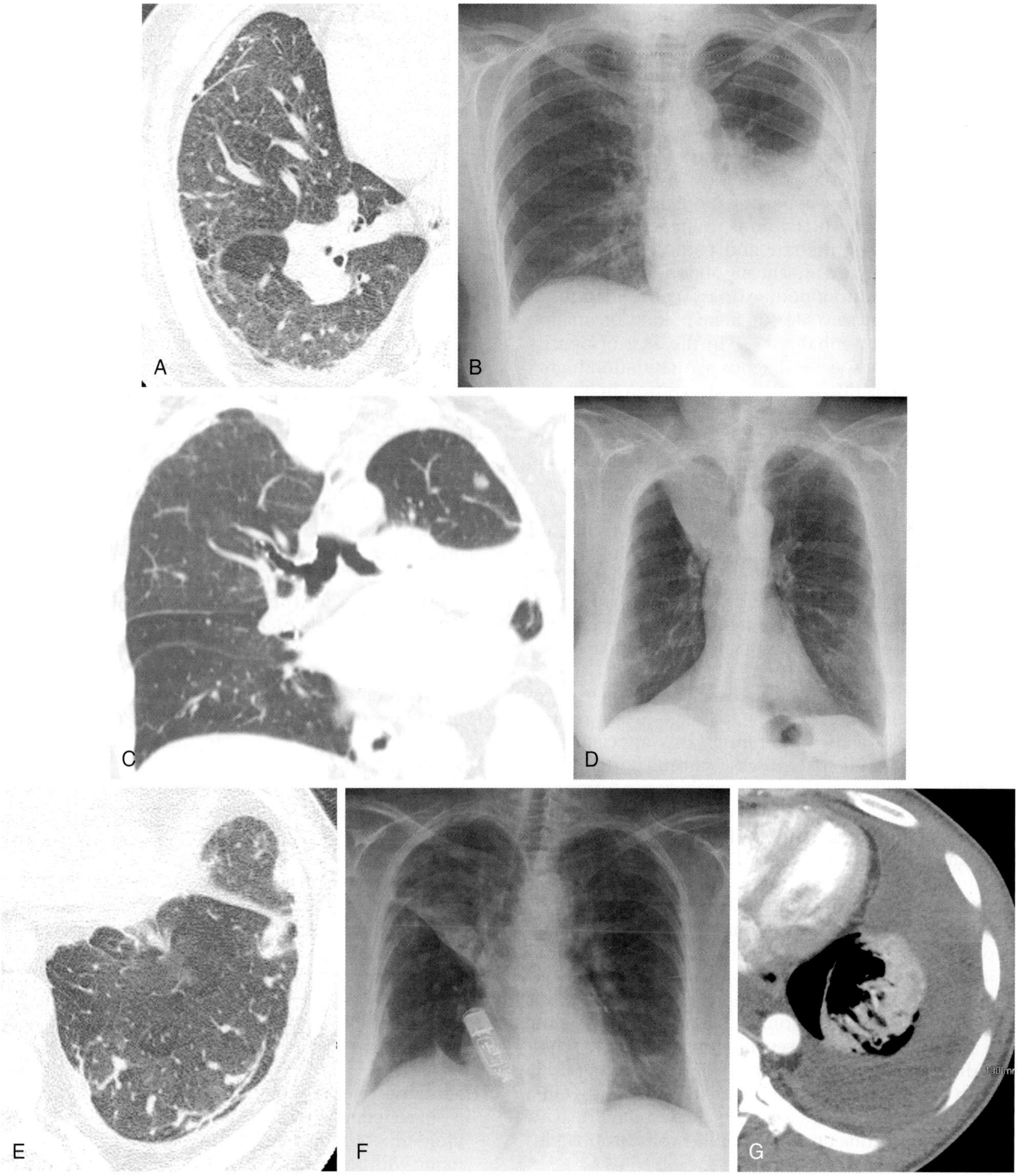

Figure 13.2 (A) Linear atelectasis, plate atelectasis, discoid atelectasis in a 61-year-old man with curvilinear parenchymal linear atelectasis in the right upper lobe. (B, C) Luftsichel sign. Chest x-ray (B) and coronal CT scan (C) in an 87-year-old man shows a left central bronchogenic carcinoma causing narrowing of the left upper lobe bronchus and resultant left upper lobe collapse, along with a hyperinflated left lower lobe in the form of the Luftsichel sign. Note the metastatic solid nodule in the hyperinflated left lower lobe. (D) Golden S sign in a 50-year-old man with collapse of the right upper lobe due to central obstructing squamous cell carcinoma of the lung, which gave rise to the Golden S sign. (E) Parenchymal band in a 61-year-old man with subpleural curvilinear parenchymal band related to prior asbestos exposure with adjacent pleural thickening. (F) Juxtaphrenic peak. (G) Rounded atelectasis in a 44-year-old man with enhancing rounded atelectasis in the left lower lobe along with empyema-related pleural thickening and pleural effusion in the left pleural cavity.

The more accurate terms are *consolidation* and *ground-glass opacity*. Consolidation is increased opacification of the lung, which obscures underlying vessels and lung architecture, except in the presence of an air bronchogram (see Fig. 13.2B). A ground-glass opacity is a subtle increase in lung attenuation, with a preserved margin of the underlying structures (see Fig. 13.2B).

Opacity: Opacity represents a focal increase in lung attenuation, thereby appearing more opaque than the surrounding area. It is a nonspecific term because it does not suggest the size and pathologic nature of the finding. It may represent any abnormality, including but not limited to a nodule, mass, consolidation, or ground-glass opacity. Measurement of lung attenuation on noncontrast-enhanced CT in the area of opacity can lead to the specific diagnosis. Attenuation higher than muscle is due to calcium deposition in a metastatic pulmonary calcification and pulmonary alveolar microlithiasis, talc powder deposits in talcosis, and iodine deposition of amiodarone toxicity. Attenuation less than muscle can be seen in lipoid pneumonia.

CT angiogram sign: The CT angiogram sign represents a finding in patients with consolidation on contrast-enhanced CT. It refers to the prominence of the contrast-opacified vessels in the consolidated lung (Fig. 13.3A). Although initially thought to be specific for bronchoalveolar carcinoma, it can be seen in pulmonary lymphoma and infectious and postobstructive pneumonia.

Ground-glass opacity: Ground-glass opacity (GGO) is a nonspecific term used to describe an increase in lung attenuation caused by a change in the relative proportions of air in the lung. This appearance is observed with air space disease causing partial filling of the alveoli with fluid, macrophages, neutrophils, or amorphous material, interstitial thickening due to inflammation, infiltration or fibrosis, partial alveolar collapse (atelectasis), and increased capillary blood volume. The degree of increase in lung opacity is not sufficient to obscure pulmonary vessels, as would be the case in pulmonary consolidation. Some active but potentially reversible processes that produce a GGO include pulmonary edema, pulmonary hemorrhage, alveolar proteinosis, and various causes of alveolitis and interstitial pneumonitis, whereas fibrosis is the leading cause of irreversible opacity. On a chest radiograph, a GGO appears as haziness of the lung, with indistinct bronchial or vascular markings. On a CT scan, it appears as a hazy increased lung opacity, without obscuring underlying bronchovascular margins (see Fig. 13.1B).

Mosaic perfusion, mosaic oligemia, mosaic attenuation pattern: The term *mosaic attenuation pattern* refers to an inhomogeneous lung opacity resulting in differing lung attenuation due to regional differences in lung perfusion on inspiratory CT. The causes are as follows: (1) occlusive vascular disease and vasculitis (see Fig. 13.3C); (2) obstructive airway disease (see Fig. 13.3B); or (3) mixed disease. Mosaic attenuation pattern is a more inclusive term than mosaic oligemia or mosaic perfusion. In mosaic perfusion, pulmonary vessels in low-attenuation lucent regions have a smaller caliber than in denser lung regions, thus differentiating them from a GGO. Redistribution of blood flow toward normal parts of the lung leads to increased attenuation of the uninvolved lung. Expiratory high-resolution computed tomography (HRCT) is useful in distinguishing mosaic perfusion due to airway disease from a vascular cause by demonstrating air trapping and sometimes thickened and dilated airways.

Head cheese sign: It represents the heterogeneous attenuation of the lung from a combination of mosaic perfusion and air trapping intermixed with the healthy lung. It is typically seen in hypersensitivity pneumonitis but has also been described in a few others, including sarcoidosis, atypical pneumonia, and respiratory bronchiolitis.

Crazy paving pattern: A crazy paving pattern refers to a GGO interspersed with a reticular pattern due to thickened interlobular septa or an intralobular interstitium (see Fig. 13.3D). Initially described in alveolar proteinosis, it can also be seen in various acute and subacute conditions, including atypical pneumonia, pulmonary hemorrhage, diffuse alveolar damage, and organizing pneumonia.

Air trapping: Air trapping represents abnormal retention of air within the lung or part of the lung due to airway obstruction. On end-expiratory CT, the areas of air trapping are more evident and appear as darker or more radiolucent compared to normal lung, which has relatively high attenuation. Comparison between inspiratory (see Fig. 13.3E) and expiratory CT (see Fig. 13.3F) is required to detect air trapping.

Air bronchogram: On a radiograph and CT scan, an air bronchogram is a pattern of air-filled bronchus on a background of surrounding high-attenuation lung due to consolidation or ground-glass opacification. On the radiograph, an air bronchogram with opacity reliably separates an intrapulmonary location from a pleural or mediastinal abnormality. The sign is particularly well seen on CT scans (see Fig. 13.1B) and indicates that proximal airways are patent but the alveolar space is filled (exudate, fluid, or cell), reduced (atelectasis), or a combination of both. The most common cause of an air bronchogram is the consolidation of various causative factors and pulmonary edema. It can also be seen in adenocarcinoma or marked interstitial lung expansion, as in lymphoma causing compression of the lung parenchyma, with patent airways.

Organizing pneumonia: Organizing pneumonia (OP) is characterized histologically by the presence of polyploid plugs of loose connective tissue and granulation tissue within the terminal or respiratory bronchioles, alveolar ducts, and alveoli, but with minimal or absent interstitial inflammation and fibrosis. OP is a relatively common condition accounting for approximately half of the cases of idiopathic interstitial pneumonia. Its idiopathic form is called *cryptogenic organizing pneumonia*. However, half of the histologic patterns of OP are secondary to conditions such as pulmonary infection, pulmonary infarction, hypersensitivity pneumonitis, collagen vascular disease, and a drug reaction.

On the radiograph, OP appears as patchy peripheral and basal consolidative opacities. On CT scans, the typical pattern is unilateral or bilateral, patchy, nonsegmental, often triangular or polygonal air space

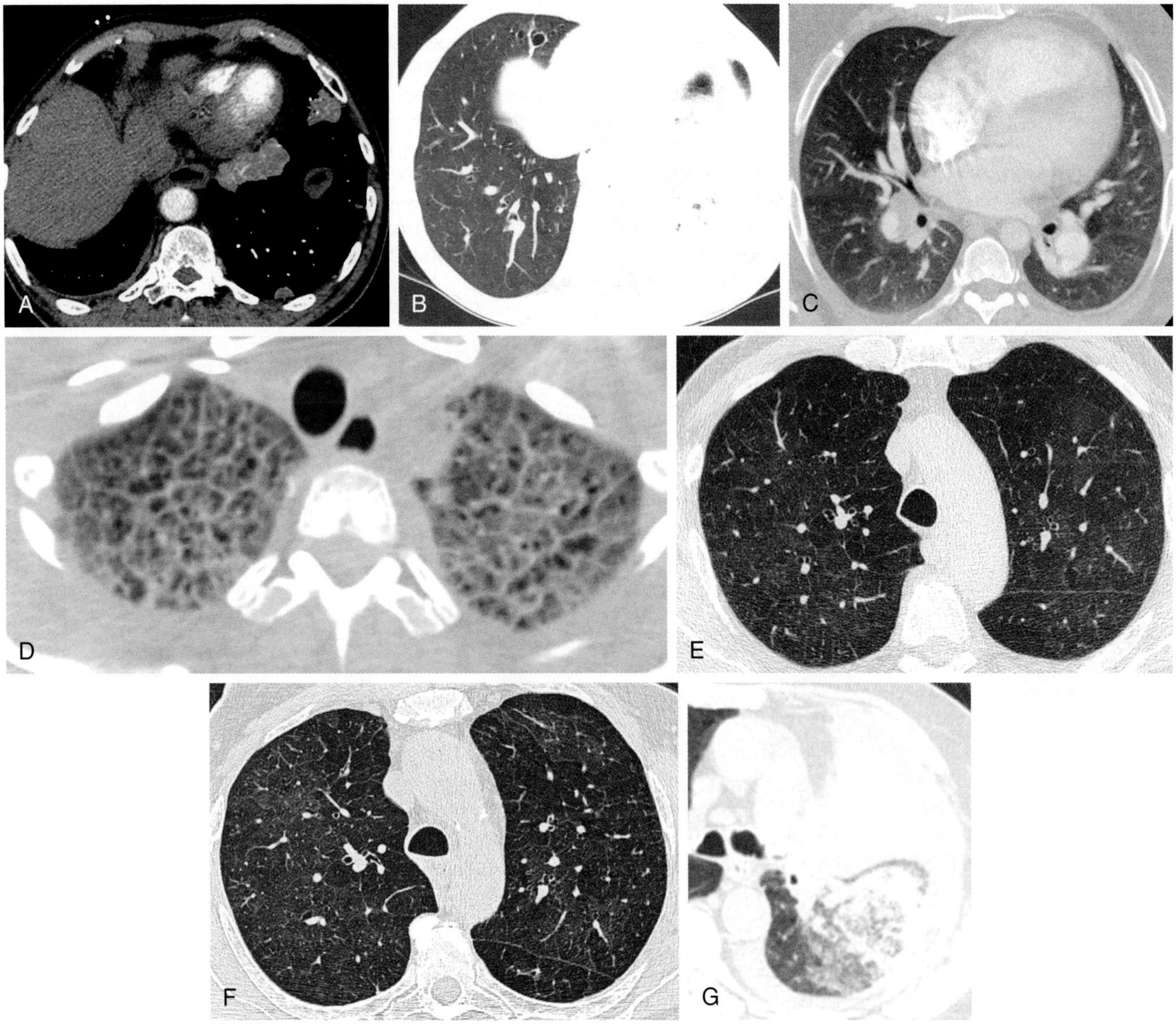

Figure 13.3 (A) A 50-year-old man with metastatic lung cancer causing multiple irregular enhancing nodular metastatic opacites in the left lung containing enhancing vessels suggestive of the CT angiogram sign. Note the right lower posterior pleural metastatic thickening. (B) In a 25-year-old man with cystic fibrosis, the CT scan reveals a mosaic attenuation pattern in the right lung due to cytomegalovirus-related small airway infection. Note the right middle lobe bronchiectasis, collapse consolidation of left lower lobe, and left pleural effusion. (C) A 50-year-old man with mosaic attenuation changes in both lungs due to pulmonary arterial hypertension. Note dilated pulmonary arteries. (D) A 50-year-old woman with an upper lobe, predominantly crazy paving pattern, and worsening hypoxia due to a combination of atypical pneumonia and pulmonary edema. The differential diagnosis include acute interstitial pneumonia, pulmonary edema, acute respiratory distress syndrome, and pulmonary hemorrhage. (E, F) Air trapping. Shown are extensive mosaic attenuation changes in both lungs on an inspiratory scan (E), with multiple patchy areas of air trapping on expiratory CT scans (F). The differential diagnoses include bronchiolitis obliterans, hypersensitivity pneumonitis, and chronic airway disease. (G) Organizing pneumonia in the left lower lobe in a 49-year-old man with distal left main bronchus carcinoma–related narrowing causing collapse of the left upper lobe and reversed halo sign (atoll sign) in part of the left lobe due to organizing pneumonia from a fungal infection.

consolidation in a subpleural and peribronchovascular distribution and often in the lower lobes (see Fig. 13.3G). An air bronchogram may be present. Scattered GGOs, centrilobular nodules, or a tree-in-bud pattern can also be seen. The lesions tend to progress and migrate over time. The differential diagnoses include bronchioalveolar carcinoma, lymphoma, vasculitis, and infections.

Diffuse alveolar damage: See acute interstitial pneumonia.

Pulmonary laceration: A pulmonary laceration is characterized by disruption of the lung parenchyma, resulting in a round or oval pulmonary cavity. The traumatic cavity may be filled with air (traumatic pneumatocele), blood (traumatic hematocele), or both (hematopneumatocele). Adjacent lung contusions are usually present, which obscure its identification on the radiograph. It is usually seen in children and young adults due to more flexibility of the chest wall. According to the mechanism, four CT patterns of lung injury (Fig. 13.4A) can be seen:

Type 1, compression rupture injury: Direct compression force results in laceration in a deep portion of the lung.

Type 2, compression shear injury: A severe sudden blow to the lower hemithorax results in the sudden shift of the lower lobes of the lung across the spine. These are usually paraspinal in location.

Type 3, rib penetration tear: This is peripheral in location, near a displaced rib fracture, and is associated with pneumothorax.

Type 4, adhesion tear: This is a laceration in the region of preexisting pleuroparenchymal adhesions and is usually diagnosed at surgery or autopsy.

Pulmonary contusion: Pulmonary contusion is the most common lung injury caused by blunt chest trauma. It is a traumatic alveolar injury with an alveolar hemorrhage, but without significant alveolar disruption. It usually occurs within 24 hours of injury, usually at the site of impact. On the radiograph, the typical imaging feature is a patchy, ill-defined consolidative opacity in the nonsegmental pattern. On CT scans, subpleural sparing (1–2 mm of clear parenchyma beneath the pleural surface) may be observed (Fig. 13.4A). CT is more sensitive for the detection of contusion because the contusion is seen immediately after injury on a CT scan but may not be seen until 6 hours after injury on a radiograph.

Interstitium

Interstitium: The pulmonary interstitium is the continuum of connective tissue throughout the lung and comprises three subdivisions:

1. The bronchovascular (axial) interstitium, surrounding and supporting the bronchi, arteries, and

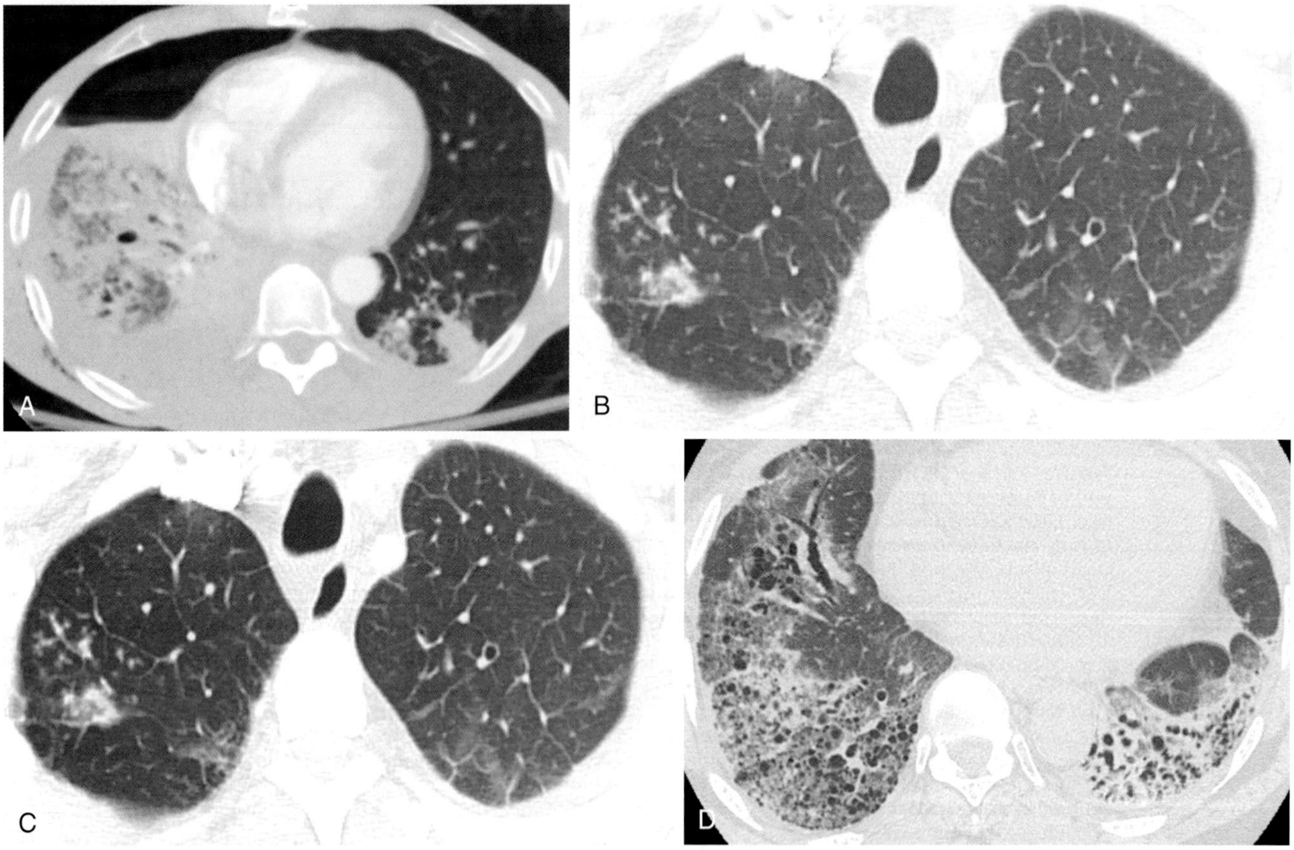

Figure 13.4 (A) Pulmonary laceration—a 56-year-old man with a motor vehicle collision–related right lower lobe contusion and laceration, patchy left lower lobe contusion related opacities, and a moderate-sized right hydropneumothorax. (B) Interlobular septal thickening, beaded septum sign, septal thickening in a 23-year-old man with cystic fibrosis. Note the ill-defined centrilobular opacities in the apices of both lungs with tree-in-bud opacities in the right apex proven to be from *Aspergillus* infection, along with mild bronchiectasis (not shown). The mild smooth interlobular septal thickening in both lung apices is due to associated pulmonary edema. (C) Subpleural curvilinear line—a 61-year-old woman with usual interstitial pneumonia (UIP)–related mild subpleural right upper lobe lines and bilateral subpleural reticular opacities. (D) Architectural distortion—a 66-year-old woman with UIP presenting with honeycombing reticular opacities, architectural distortion, traction bronchiectasis, bronchiolectasis, and mild ground-glass opacities predominantly in both lower lobes.

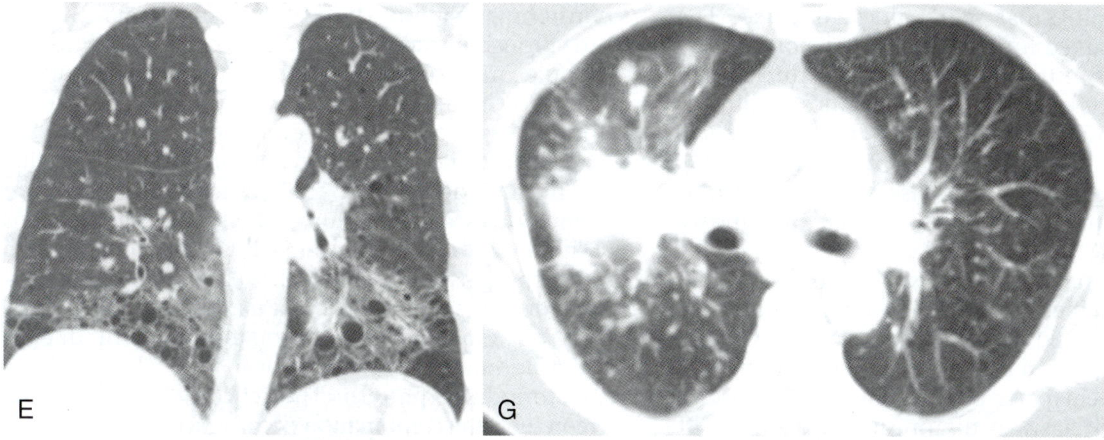

E G

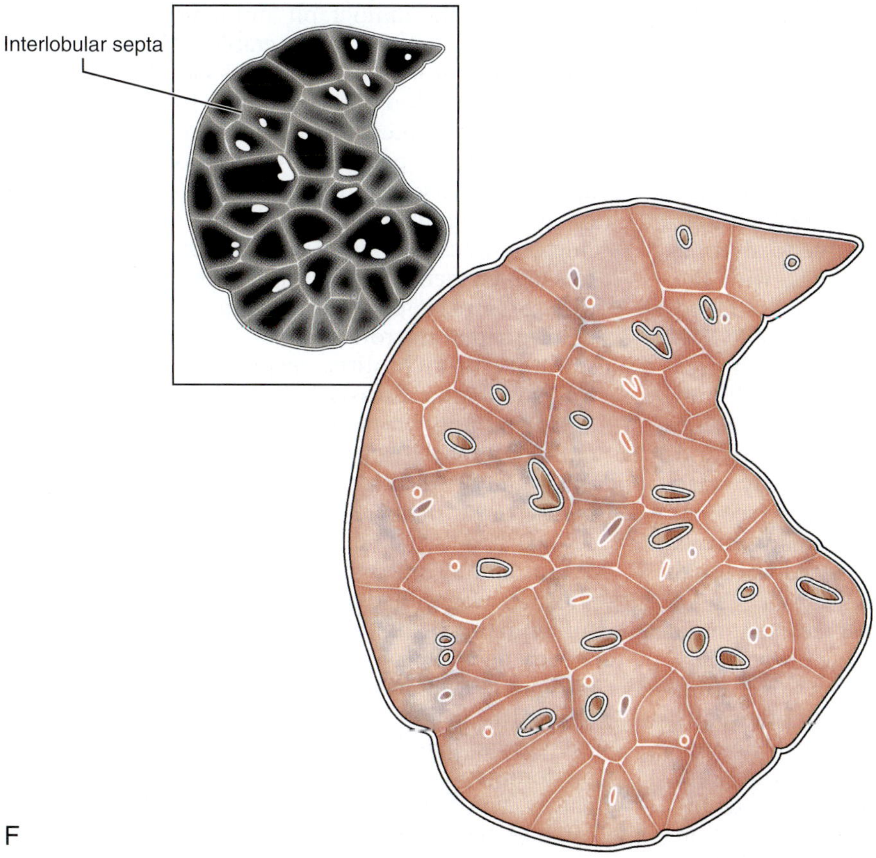

F

Figure 13.4, cont'd (E) Reticular pattern—a 40-year-old woman with lymphocytic interstitial pneumonia-related, bilateral lower zone, predominantly reticular pattern opacities caused by multiple lung cysts and reticulation. (F) Schematic illustration demonstrating perilobular pattern causing perilobular thickening. (G) Reticulonodular pattern—a 70-year-old woman with sarcoidosis; right upper lobe opacity is related to collapse consolidation due to chronic partial right and middle upper lobe, peribronchial, soft tissue causing narrowing, with resultant elevation of the right dome of the diaphragm and juxtaphrenic peak. Note the bilateral reticulonodular opacities in both lungs from sarcoidosis.

veins from the hilum to the level of the respiratory bronchiole

2. The parenchymal (acinar) interstitium, situated between the alveolar and capillary basement membrane
3. The subpleural connective tissue contiguous with the interlobular septa (see Fig. 13.4A)

Interlobular septum: See secondary pulmonary lobule.

Interlobular septal thickening, beaded septum sign, septal thickening: Thickening of the interlobular septum is easily recognized on HRCT. On a chest radiograph, they appear as a thin linear opacity at a right angle to and in contact with the lateral pleural surfaces near the lung bases (Kerley B lines). Kerley A lines seen in the upper lobes are 2- to 6-cm long thin lines, with the radial orientation toward the hilum. Recently, the anatomic descriptive term *interlobular septal lines* or *septal thickening* has gained preference over Kerley lines. On HRCT, the normal interlobular septum is not visible but, in several pathologic conditions, septal thickening is seen. Four different types of septal thickening are noted, based on the appearance and underlying cause. Pulmonary edema results in smooth septal thickening (see Figs. 13.3D and 13.4B). Infiltrative diseases, such as a tumor or tumor-like process, cause nodular septal thickening—a beaded septum sign of the lymphangitic spread of malignancy and sarcoidosis. Fibrotic conditions, such as interstitial fibrosis, cause irregular septal thickening (see Fig. 13.4C) and marked lung architecture distortion.

Intralobular lines, intralobular interstitial thickening: Intralobular lines are fine linear opacities within the secondary pulmonary lobule, which, when thickened, appear reticular or meshlike on HRCT (see Fig. 13.4C). These are seen in various disease processes, such as interstitial pulmonary fibrosis, alveolar proteinosis, and pulmonary hemorrhage.

Subpleural curvilinear line: This is seen on CT as a thin, nonspecific, curvilinear opacity, 1 to 3 mm in thickness, lying parallel to and less than 1 cm from the pleura (see Fig. 13.4C). It can be a normal finding when seen in the dependent parts of the lung and represents dependent atelectasis; it disappears on a prone CT scan. Curvilinear lines are also observed in fibrosis, pulmonary edema, and asbestosis.

Architectural distortion: This term refers to a distorted appearance of the lung due to the abnormal displacement of pulmonary structures, such as bronchi, vessels, fissures, or interlobular septa. It can be caused by diffuse or localized lung disease, particularly lung fibrosis (see Fig. 13.4D) or volume loss of the lung.

Honeycombing: Honeycombing occurs due to alveolar disruption and dilation of alveolar ducts, with the loss of acinar architecture. It represents destroyed and fibrotic lung tissue. Honeycombing on HRCT is characterized by the presence of peripheral, subpleural, air-filled cysts, typically between 3 and 10 mm in diameter. However, it may be as large as 2.5 cm, with clearly defined fibrous walls of 1 to 3 mm and arranged as a few clustered cysts in the early stage to multilayered cysts in the advanced stage (see Fig. 13.4D). It is a feature of established pulmonary fibrosis and is an important criterion for the diagnosis of usual interstitial pneumonia.

Reticular pattern, reticulation: On chest radiographs, a reticular pattern consists of innumerable linear opacities that resemble a mesh or net due to a summation effect (see Fig. 13.4E). A reticular pattern usually represents interstitial lung disease. It is a purely descriptive term, and several morphologic variations are seen, ranging from generalized interlobular septal thickening to intralobular lines to honeycomb lung destruction or parenchymal bands or irregular linear opacities. Reticular interstitial septal thickening can be smooth (pulmonary edema; see Fig. 13.4B), nodular (lymphangitic spread of malignancy, sarcoidosis), or irregular (fibrosis; see Fig. 13.4D).

Perilobular pattern: The perilobular region is composed of the structures that border the periphery of the secondary pulmonary lobule, which include the interlobular septa, visceral pleura, and vessels. Hence, the pulmonary disease occurring predominantly with the interlobular septa and periphery of the secondary pulmonary lobules has the perilobular pattern. On CT, the perilobular pattern is an ill-defined arcuate or polygonal bandlike opacity of thickness greater than that of thickened interlobular septa. These may be associated with ground-glass or consolidative opacities. The term is frequently used in the context of perilobular distribution of OP.

Centrilobular pattern: The centrilobular region represents the bronchiolovascular core of a secondary pulmonary lobule and consists of lesions that have an effect beyond the terminal bronchioles that center on the respiratory bronchioles or even the alveolar ducts. On CT, the centrilobular region appears as a small dotlike or linear opacity due to the intralobular artery in the center of a secondary pulmonary lobule, most evident within 1 cm of a pleural surface. Centrilobular disease patterns consist of (1) nodules, (2) tree-in-bud opacities due to small-airway disease (see Fig. 13.4B), or (3) an abnormal low attenuation pattern due to centrilobular emphysema.

Reticulonodular pattern: The reticulonodular pattern represents the combination of the reticular and nodular patterns on the radiograph and is usually the result of the intersection of innumerable lines, creating the effect of additional micronodules (see Fig. 13.2F and G). The dimension of the nodule is related to the size and number of linear or curvilinear components. (See also the reticular pattern.) The reticulonodular pattern appears on CT scans due to the simultaneous presence of reticular and micronodular patterns. On CT, the micronodules can be located in the center of the reticular elements, suggesting centrilobular micronodules, or superimposed on the linear opacities, suggesting septal micronodules.

Respiratory bronchiolitis, respiratory bronchiolitis–interstitial lung disease: Respiratory bronchiolitis (RB) and respiratory bronchiolitis–interstitial lung disease (RB-ILD) are part of a spectrum of smoking-related inflammatory diseases of the small airways and lungs. In the order of increasing severity, first is RB, then RB-ILD, and then desquamative interstitial pneumonia. Symptomatic smokers with RB-ILD histologically show an exaggerated form of RB, with more extensive inflammation and fibrosis. Chest radiographs are mostly normal in patients with RB or RB-ILD. HRCT findings in RB (Fig. 13.5A) and RB-ILD include poorly defined centrilobular nodules and patchy, multifocal, ground-glass opacities with mid and upper lung predominance, with or without accompanying areas of patchy centrilobular emphysema. Also, RB-ILD patients can have bronchial wall thickening and fibrosis-related reticular opacities.

Acute interstitial pneumonia: Acute interstitial pneumonia (AIP) is a fulminant disease of unknown cause, usually occurring in a previously healthy person. This is associated with the histologic pattern of diffuse alveolar damage. Chest radiographs show diffuse or lower lung zones with predominantly bilateral air space consolidation, with an air bronchogram or GGO. Honeycombing may be seen late in the disease. Findings are similar to other causes of acute respiratory distress syndrome (ARDS). On CT, the early exudative phase of AIP is characterized by bilateral, patchy, GGOs and consolidation, predominantly of the dependent lung and sometimes with a crazy paving pattern (see Fig. 13.5B). The later organizing phase of AIP is associated with distortion of bronchovascular bundles and traction bronchiectasis due to evolution to fibrosis. Areas of honeycombing

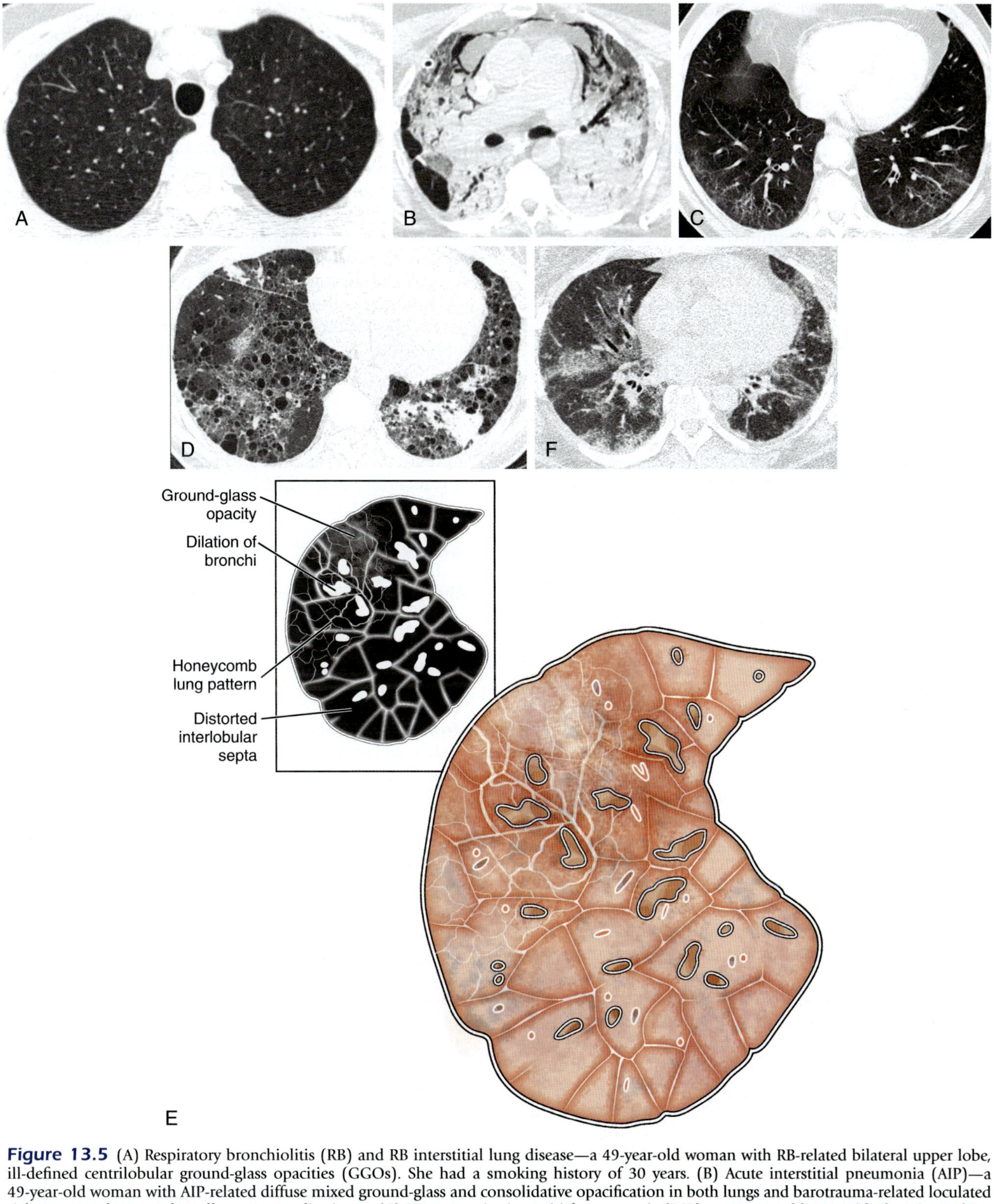

Figure 13.5 (A) Respiratory bronchiolitis (RB) and RB interstitial lung disease—a 49-year-old woman with RB-related bilateral upper lobe, ill-defined centrilobular ground-glass opacities (GGOs). She had a smoking history of 30 years. (B) Acute interstitial pneumonia (AIP)—a 49-year-old woman with AIP-related diffuse mixed ground-glass and consolidative opacification in both lungs and barotrauma-related loculated right pneumothorax and small pneumomediastinum. (C) Desquamative interstitial pneumonia (DIP)—a 70-year-old man with chronic smoking with DIP changes in the form of bilateral fine reticular and ill-defined GGOs with subpleural sparing. (D) Lymphoid interstitial pneumonia—a 40-year-old woman with dyspnea shows multiple focal round variable-sized, air-filled lucencies with thin walls in the lung parenchyma, with an apical basilar gradient with predominantly lower lobe involvement. Note the associated peribronchovascular consolidations in the lower lobes and inferior right middle lobe. These findings were proven to be due to lymphocytic interstitial pneumonitis, whereas the consolidations can occur because of superimposed infection, lymphoma, or organizing pneumonia. (E) Schematic illustration demonstrating various manifestations of usual interstitial pneumonia (UIP). However, ground glass-opacities are extremely rare in UIP. (F) Nonspecific interstitial pneumonia (NSIP)—a 48-year-old woman with hypoxemic respiratory failure and history of polymyositis. CT scan shows bilateral predominantly peribronchovascular and subpleural GGOs, interlobular and intralobular septal thickening with upper lobe predominance, and minimal traction bronchiectasis; no honeycombing seen. These findings were pathologically shown to be from a mixed type of NSIP.

are seen in the chronic phase occurring after 2 weeks in survivors.

Desquamative interstitial pneumonia: Desquamative interstitial pneumonia (DIP) is a rare interstitial lung disease primarily affecting smokers but can also be seen in various other conditions, such as occupational dust exposure, drug reaction, and infection. The predominant pathologic feature is the intraalveolar and distal airway accumulation of pigmented macrophages, with mild inflammation and minimal fibrosis. The macrophages are uniformly and diffusely distributed, unlike the bronchocentric distribution in RB-ILD. The chest radiographic appearances of DIP are nonspecific and reveal predominant GGOs in the lower lung zone. On HRCT, DIP is characterized by bilateral, patchy, GGOs, with subpleural and basal predominance (see Fig. 13.5C), air-filled cysts, centrilobular emphysema, mosaic perfusion, and mild reticular opacities. However, minimal honeycombing may also be present. It can be indistinguishable from RB-ILD.

Lymphoid interstitial pneumonia: Lymphoid interstitial pneumonia (LIP) is a rare interstitial pneumonia and is usually a secondary disease due to conditions such as Sjögren syndrome, HIV infection, and various immunodeficiency syndromes. It is characterized by diffuse infiltration of the interstitium by lymphocytes, plasma cells, and histiocytes and by diffuse peribronchiolar inflammation. The chest radiograph shows nonspecific bilateral reticular, reticulonodular, and air space opacities. On HRCT, diffuse, bilateral, GGOs, ill-defined centrilobular opacities, subpleural and peribronchovascular nodules, and thin-walled cystic spaces are the predominant findings (see Fig. 13.5D).

Usual interstitial pneumonia: Usual interstitial pneumonia (UIP) is the most common interstitial pneumonia and can be idiopathic or secondary to a drug reaction, asbestosis, or collagen vascular disease. UIP is characterized by temporal and spatial heterogeneity, with areas of normal lung alternating with interstitial inflammation and honeycombing (see Fig. 13.5E). The key findings are fibroblastic foci and fibroblastic destruction of the lung architecture, with macrocystic honeycombing. It has subpleural and basal lung zone predominance.

In the early stage, the radiograph is normal. In the advanced stage, the radiograph shows decreased lung volumes and predominant subpleural irregular reticular opacities in the lower zone and honeycombing. On HRCT, patchy, peripheral, and subpleural reticular opacities, traction bronchiectasis, macrocystic honeycombing with an apicobasal gradient, and areas of mild GGOs are highly suggestive of UIP (see Fig. 13.4D).

Idiopathic pulmonary fibrosis: Idiopathic pulmonary fibrosis (IPF) is a specific form of chronic, progressive, fibrosing interstitial pneumonia of unknown cause, limited to the lungs and associated with a histopathologic and/or radiologic pattern of UIP. On HRCT, IPF is characterized by the presence of bilateral, basal, peripheral subpleural reticular opacities associated with traction bronchiectasis (see Fig. 13.4D). Honeycombing is common and is critical for making a definitive diagnosis of IPF. Temporal and spatial heterogeneity due to old and active fibrotic processes and the presence of fibroblastic foci are pathologic characteristics of IPF.

Nonspecific interstitial pneumonia: Nonspecific interstitial pneumonia (NSIP) is a chronic interstitial lung disease characterized by interstitial inflammation and fibrosis. It can be idiopathic or due to connective tissue disorders, hypersensitivity pneumonitis, or a drug reaction. The characteristic histologic pattern of temporal and spatial homogeneous lung involvement distinguishes it from UIP.

On the radiograph, GGOs, predominantly in the lower lobes, along with reticular opacities, may be seen. HRCT findings include involvement of the lower lung lobes, but the sharp apicobasal gradient is absent. Bilateral symmetric patchy or subpleural GGOs with irregular linear or reticular opacities, with a relative subpleural dorsal lung sparing, and traction bronchiectasis are common findings. In advanced disease, traction bronchiectasis and patchy consolidation can be seen (see Fig. 13.5F).

Nodule

Solitary pulmonary nodule: A solitary pulmonary nodule (SPN) is a relatively well-defined, roughly spherical focal opacity, which is at least partially surrounded by the lungs, and is 3 cm or less in diameter (Fig. 13.6A–C). The most important first step is to determine that the nodule is truly solitary and arises from the lung. The differential diagnoses of SPN are extensive, and most fall under malignant and benign neoplasms and infectious granulomas. In a patient with SPN, a plain film or CT scan is used to determine the following: (1) morphologic features (e.g., margin, size, shape); (2) density or attenuation (e.g., solid, part solid, ground glass; fat, calcium, or contrast enhancement); and (3) growth rate.

Nodule: On a chest radiograph, a nodule appears as a rounded opacity, with a well- or ill-defined margin, 3 cm or less in diameter. A pseudonodule includes a rib lesion, skin lesion, or external device, anatomic variants, or a summation lesion that may mimic a pulmonary nodule on a radiograph. On a CT scan, a nodule is a rounded or irregular opacity, with well- or ill-defined margins and less than 3 cm in diameter. A nodule can be solid (homogenous soft tissue attenuation), nonsolid (ground-glass attenuation), or part solid (consisting of both soft tissue and ground-glass attenuation; see Fig. 13.6D). A nonsolid or ground-glass nodule (GGN) or GGO (see Fig. 13.6F) is defined as a well-defined or poorly defined localized nodular area of increased lung attenuation through which normal parenchymal structures, including airways and vessels, can be visualized. A part solid GGN is defined as a lesion containing a combination of both ground-glass and solid components, with the latter component obscuring the underlying lung architecture (see Fig. 13.6E). Purely solid nodules are defined as homogenous soft tissue attenuation lesions (see Fig. 13.6G).

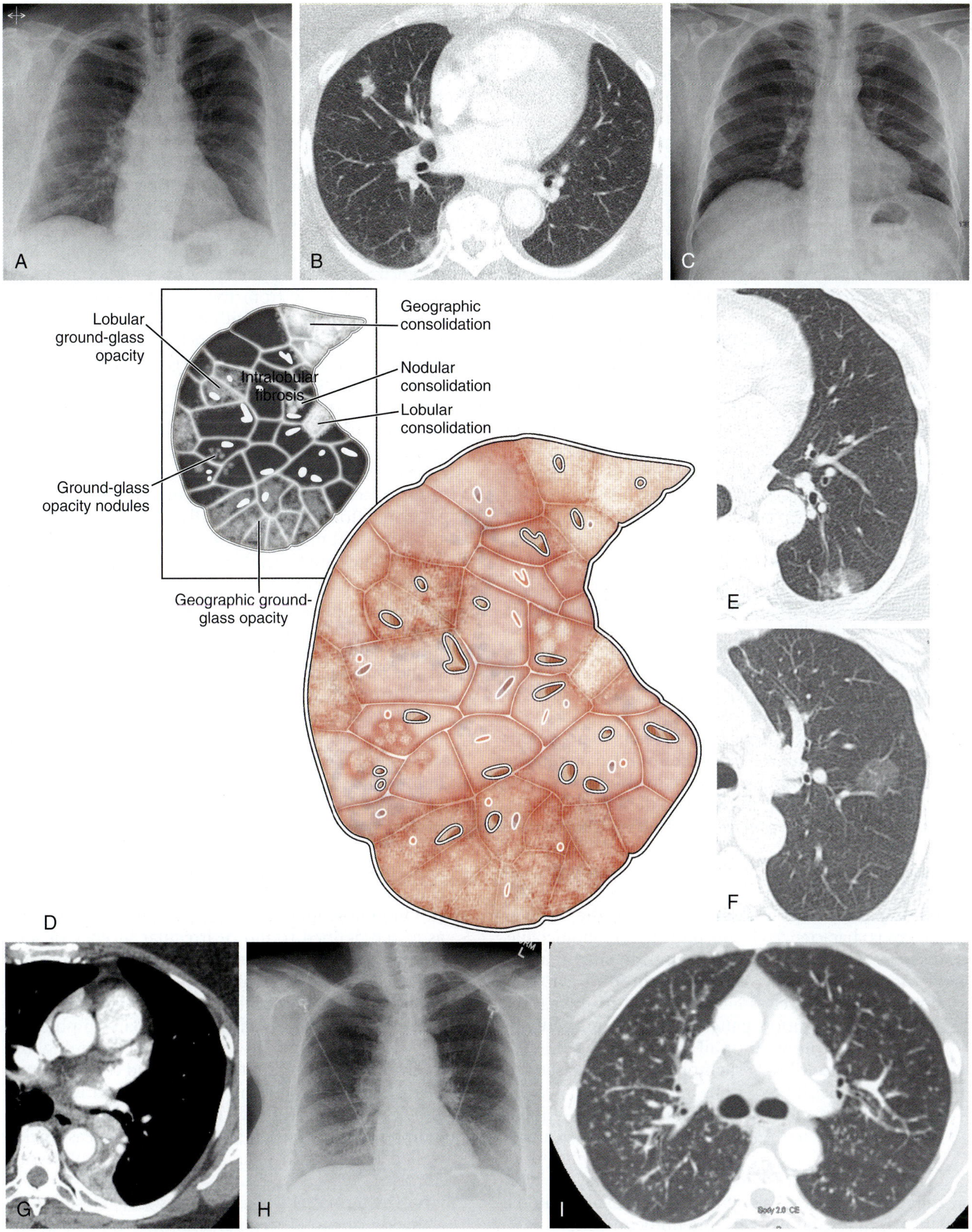

Figure 13.6 (A) Solitary pulmonary nodule. (B) A 61-year-old woman with stage I cervical cancer shows a faintly visualized nodular opacity in the right midzone overlapping the right anterior fourth rib, which correlates with the right middle lobe nodular opacity on the CT. Biopsy of this lesion revealed primary squamous cell carcinoma of the lung. (C) A 61-year-old man with a solitary nodular mass in the left midzone, which was confirmed to be a large 3.5-cm pulmonary arteriovenous malformation on the CT. (D) Schematic diagram showing various types of lung nodules and opacities. (E) A 63-year-old man with a 2.5-cm part solid nodule in the left lower lobe with a predominantly ground-glass component and a 0.7-cm solid component, which was biopsy-proven to be adenocarcinoma. (F) A 77-year-old man with a 2.3-cm ground-glass nodule in the left upper lobe, which was biopsy-proven to be adenocarcinoma. (G) A 63-year-old woman with a typical carcinoid presenting as a solid endobronchial nodule in the left lower lobe bronchus causing the left lower lobe to collapse; it contained mucus-filled dilated brochi. (H, I) A 58-year-old woman with diffuse miliary nodules in both lungs with centrilobular and subpleural distribution and enlarged mediastinal and bilateral hilar nodes, pathologically proven to be sarcoidosis. The differential diagnosis included tuberculosis, fungal infection, metastasis, and pneumoconiosis.

Micronodule: A micronodule is a discrete, small, round, focal opacity with a diameter of less than 5 mm, often less than 3 mm (see Fig. 13.6H, I). It has been recommended by the Fleischner Society that this term be reserved for describing nodules that are less than 3 mm in diameter.

CT halo sign: The CT halo sign refers to a halo of GGO surrounding a solid pulmonary nodule, mass, or consolidation. In leukemic patients with angioinvasive aspergillosis, the halo sign indicates hemorrhage surrounding a focal septic infarct. In patients with tumor, particularly adenocarcinoma or bronchoalveolar carcinoma, it reflects the presence of lepidic spread of the tumor. The CT halo sign is nonspecific and may also be seen in various other pulmonary infections, infarction, and vasculitis.

CT reverse halo sign, atoll sign: The CT reverse halo sign is a focal area of GGO surrounded by a crescentic or complete ring of denser opacity (at least 2 mm in thickness; see Fig. 13.3G). It was initially thought to be specific for cryptogenic OP but can be seen in other conditions, such as chronic eosinophilic pneumonia, various fungal and bacterial infections, infarct, and polyangiitis granulomatosis.

Feeding vessel sign: The feeding vessel sign refers to a small pulmonary artery leading directly to a pulmonary nodule. It is usually seen with hematogenous metastasis (see Fig. 13.3G), but can also be seen in septic emboli, infarcts, and an arteriovenous fistula. It is rare with primary lung tumors or benign lesions such as granulomas.

Miliary pattern: The miliary pattern refers to numerous tiny (<3 mm in diameter), discrete, rounded pulmonary nodules that are usually uniform in size, diffuse, and randomly distributed throughout the lungs (see Fig. 13.6H, I). This pattern of micronodules is characteristic of the hematogenous spread of tuberculosis and endemic fungi, metastatic disease, and pneumoconiosis. This pattern is seen on both CT and HRCT (Fig. 13.7A).

Nodular pattern: On a chest radiograph, the nodular pattern is characterized by the presence of innumerable, discrete, round opacities (2–10 mm in size) that are distributed widely and can be nonuniform. On a CT scan, nodules are classified according to their three anatomic distribution patterns as random, perilymphatic, or centrilobular or air space (see Fig. 13.7B).

Perilymphatic nodules: Perilymphatic nodules (see Fig. 13.7C) are distributed along the subpleural region, perihilar peribronchovascular interstitium, interlobar fissure, interlobular septa, and centrilobular regions. These nodules can be patchy and nonuniform in distribution with a tendency to cluster. They are typically seen in sarcoidosis, lymphangitic carcinomatosis, silicosis, and coal workers' pneumoconiosis.

Random nodules: Random nodules (see Fig. 13.6H, I) are diffuse in distribution, without restriction for particular anatomic structures. Similar to a lymphatic distribution, these can be centrilobular and subpleural in location but do not cluster. They are a result of hematogenous spread and are seen in miliary tuberculosis, miliary fungal disease, metastases, and septic embolization. They may have basal predominance and may be in proximity to a feeding vessel.

Centrilobular nodules: These nodules are limited to the centrilobular region, which is represented by the bronchovascular core of the secondary pulmonary lobule; they can reflect the presence of interstitial or air space abnormalities. They can be of soft tissue or ground-glass attenuation and may range from a few millimeters to about 1 cm in size. They are more diffuse and patchy in distribution and tend to surround small intralobular vessels and bronchi. These nodules spare the subpleural region, interlobular septa, and lung parenchyma near the interlobar fissure. They are found 5 to 10 mm away from the visceral pleural surface. Centrilobular nodules with a tree-in-bud pattern are usually seen in infectious bronchiolitis and aspiration, among many other causes (see Figs. 13.4B and 13.7E). Centrilobular GGNs without the tree-in-bud pattern are seen in conditions such as small airway infection (see Fig. 13.7D), RB, hypersensitivity pneumonitis, pulmonary edema, and Langerhans cell histiocytosis.

Air space, acinar nodule: Air space nodules represent a focal peribronchiolar inflammation or air space consolidation and are typically centrilobular in distribution, but may have a tree-in-bud pattern (see Fig. 13.7F). They are typically ill-defined nodules, ranging from a few millimeters to 1 cm in size, and can have solid or ground-glass attenuation. When the air space is filled with the byproduct of disease (e.g., pus, mucus, inflammatory infiltrate), individual acini may become visible on HRCT as poorly defined, centrilobular GGNs approximately 8 mm in diameter. They are the result of the endobronchial spread of tuberculosis, aspiration, infectious bronchiolitis, and diffuse panbronchiolitis.

Mass: A mass is any pulmonary, pleural, or mediastinal lesion that is larger than 3 cm in diameter, irrespective of the contour, border, or density of the lesion. Mass usually implies a solid or part solid opacity. CT allows superior morphologic assessment of a mass for its size, location, attenuation, margin, cavity, and other features (see Fig. 13.7G).

Cyst: On radiographs and CT scans, a lung cyst appears as a well-defined round or irregular lucency or low-attenuation parenchymal area, with a well-defined interface with adjacent lung parenchyma. They have a uniform or variable wall thickness less than 2 to 3 mm and occur without associated pulmonary emphysema (Fig. 13.8A). Pulmonary cysts are air-containing, but rarely they may contain fluid or a solid component. A cyst is a common finding in patients with lymphangioleiomyomatosis, Langerhans cell histiocytosis, and lymphocytic interstitial pneumonia, whereas thicker walled honeycomb cysts are present in pulmonary fibrosis.

Cavity: The term *cavity* is used to describe a lesion with a thicker or more irregular wall; it is created by the expulsion or drainage of a necrotic part of a pathologic lesion (nodule or mass) via the bronchial tree. On radiographs and CT scans, a cavity appears as an air-filled space within a pulmonary consolidation (see Fig. 13.8B), mass, or nodule. Both a cyst and cavity can have an air-fluid level. Cavity is not a synonym for an abscess or cyst.

Pseudocavity: A pseudocavity appears as an oval or round region of low attenuation in an area of lung

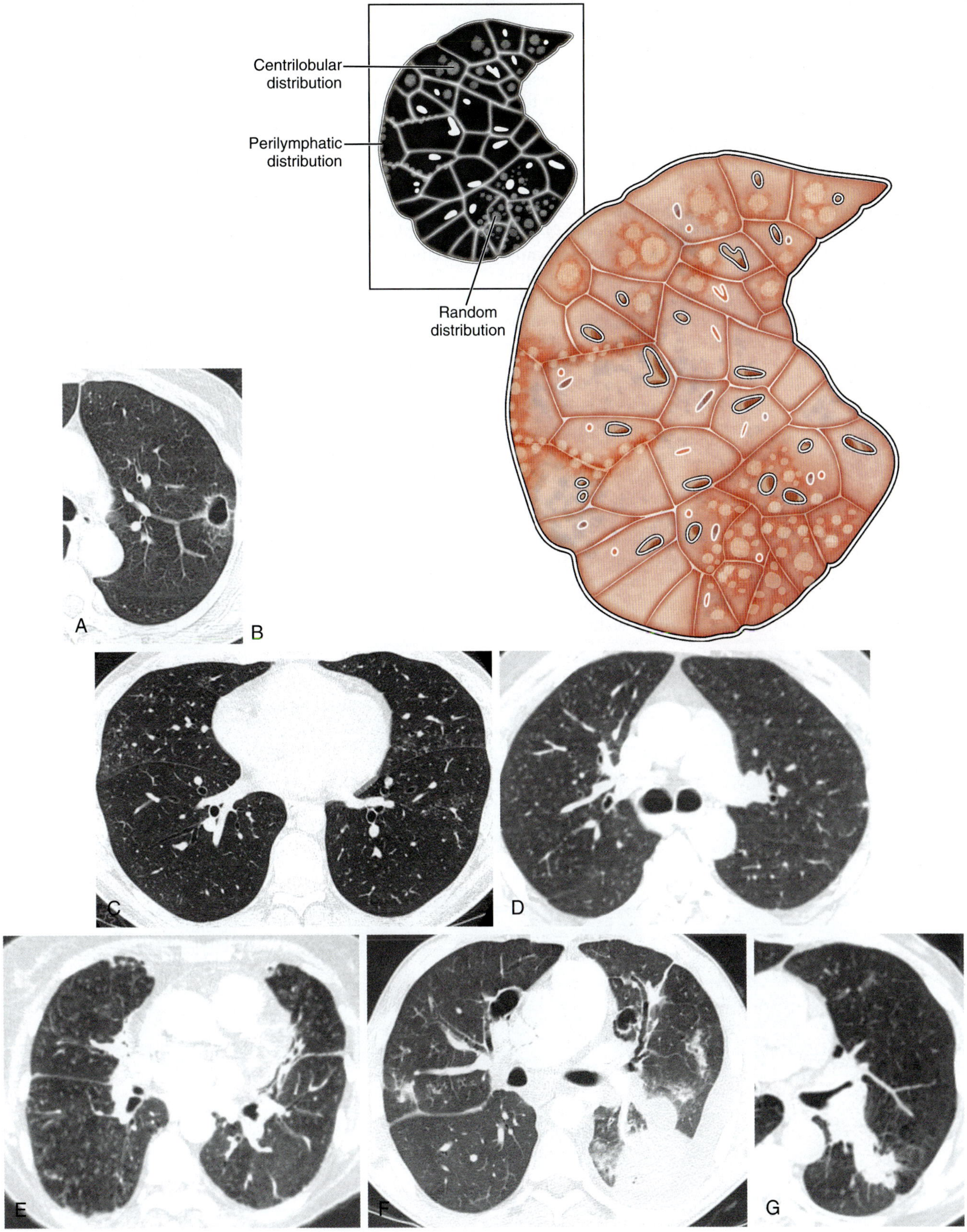

Figure 13.7 (A) Feeding vessel sign—a 63-year-old woman with chronic smoking history has a cavity lesion on CT scan with a thin irregular wall in the lingular lobe, a feeding vessel medially, and surrounding tiny nodularity. The differential diagnosis included primary or metastatic malignancy, fungal infection, and tuberculosis and was proven on endobronchial ultrasound to be squamous cell carcinoma. (B) Nodular pattern—schematic diagram of random, perilymphatic, and centrilobular nodules. (C) Perilymphatic nodules. A 32-year-old man with biopsy-proven pulmonary sarcoidosis shows numerous perilymphatic distributions of micronodules predominantly in the upper lobes along the peribronchovascular, centrilobular, and subpleural regions, along with patchy ground-glass opacities. (D) Centrilobular nodules—a 62-year-old man with numerous centrilobular nodules from the endobronchial spread of a bacterial infection. (E) A 62-year-old woman with bilateral cylindric bronchiectasis and bronchial wall thickening, with diffuse bilateral centrilobular and tree-in-bud nodules from endobronchial spread of a *Mycobacterium avium–intracellulare* infection. (F) 32-year-old man with cystic fibrosis presenting with peribronchovascular opacities, interlobular septal thickening, focal consolidations, tree-in-bud opacities, cylindrical and cystic bronchiectasis, and left-sided empyema. Empyema was due to streptococcus while the pulmonary infection was a combination of cytomegalovirus and aspergillus infection. (G) A 52-year-old man with squamous cell carcinoma of the left lower lobe presenting as an irregular, spiculated, 4.5-cm left lower lobe mass extending to the left hilum and involving the left lower lobe bronchus.

consolidation; it is a nodule or a mass that represents spared parenchyma, normal or ectatic bronchi, or focal emphysema, rather than actual cavitation. It is usually less than 1 cm in diameter and is seen in patients with adenocarcinoma (see Fig. 13.8D) and infectious pneumonia (see Fig. 13.8C).

Air crescent sign: Crescent-shaped air outlining or separating the wall of a cavity from the inner contained mass is termed an *air crescent sign*. The most common cause is aspergilloma (mycetoma) in a long-standing lung cavity (see Fig. 13.8E). The air crescent sign is also seen in an infarction of the lung, as in angioinvasive aspergillosis, cavitary carcinoma, blood clot in a cavity, hydatid disease, tuberculosis, and polyangiitis granulomatosis. The gravitational shift in the position of mass or nodule with change in position of the patient is strongly suggestive of aspergilloma rather than carcinoma.

Emphysema

Emphysema: Emphysema is a condition of the lung characterized by a permanent abnormal enlargement of air spaces distal to the terminal bronchiole, accompanied by the destruction of their walls, with no obvious lung fibrosis. However, recent studies have shown that some interstitial fibrosis may be present in emphysema due to cigarette smoking. On CT scans, the appearance of emphysema includes focal areas of abnormally decreased lung parenchymal attenuation, usually without visible walls (see Fig. 13.8F).

Centrilobular or centriacinar emphysema: Centrilobular emphysema predominantly affects respiratory bronchioles in the central portions of acini and therefore involves the central portion of a secondary lobule (see Fig. 13.8G). It is usually secondary to cigarette smoking and affects mainly the upper lobes. Centrilobular emphysema appears as diffusely distributed, multiple small, polka dot–like, round areas of low attenuation, ranging from a few millimeters to 1 cm in diameter, but usually with upper lobe predominance.

Panacinar or panlobular emphysema: This involves all the components of the acini more or less uniformly and therefore includes an entire pulmonary lobule. It is classically associated with an alpha-1-proteinase inhibitor (alpha-1-antitrypsin) deficiency and presents with diffuse or predominantly lower lobe involvement. On CT, panacinar emphysema appears as a generalized decrease in the pulmonary parenchyma attenuation, with a reduction in the caliber of blood vessels in the affected lung (see Fig. 13.8H). Its appearance of

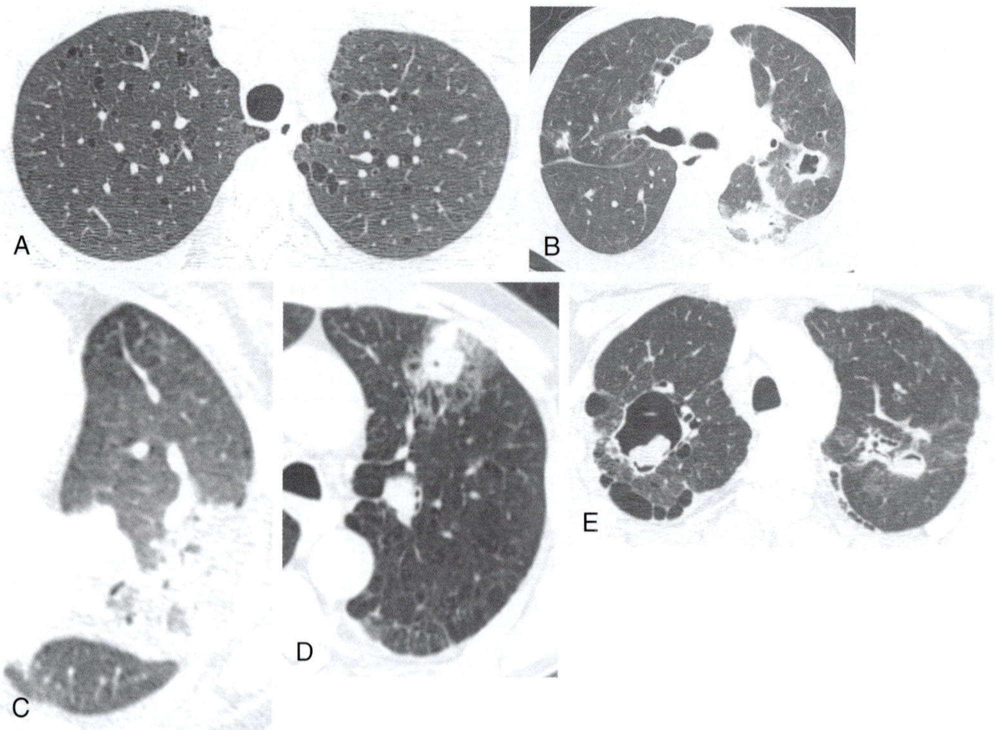

Figure 13.8 (A) Cyst—a 40-year-old woman with lymphocytic interstitial pneumonia has multiple, well-defined, round lucent cysts with a thin wall in both lungs. (B) Cavity—a 29-year-old man with cystic fibrosis with cavitary pneumonia and multifocal consolidation due to a staphylococcal infection. (C) Pseudocavity—a 50-year-old woman with left upper lobe consolidation, with an area of intervening spared parenchyma giving rise to a pseudocavitary sign. (D) A 60-year-old woman with adenocarcinoma of the lung presenting as a left upper lobe mass with a central, small, round air-filled focus due to an air- filled bronchiole giving a pseudocavitary appearance. (E) Air crescent sign—a 60-year-old woman with cavitary lesions in both upper lobes with dependent soft tissue densities and a crescent of surrounding air giving rise to the air crescent sign due to fungal mycetoma in the preexisting cavities from a prior mycobacterial infection.

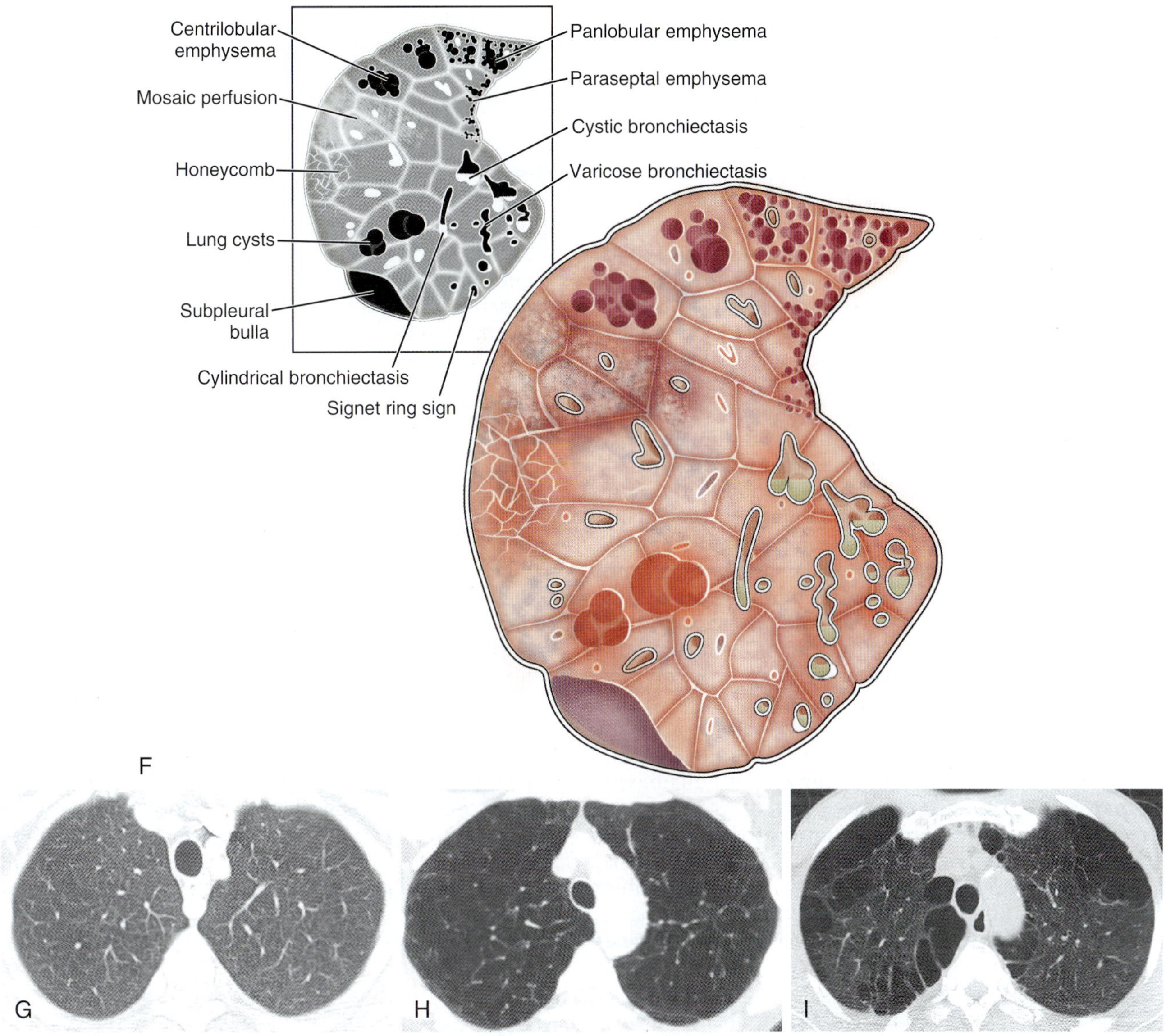

Figure 13.8, cont'd (F) Schematic illustration demonstrating various types of pulmonary emphysema, bronchiectasis, and air-filled lung lucencies and mosaic perfusion. (G) A 60-year-old chronic smoker with diffuse centrilobular emphysema. (H) Panacinar emphysema—a 59-year-old woman seen for a pretransplantation workup reveals panacinar or panlobular emphysema. (I) Paraseptal emphysema—a 60-year-old chronic smoker with diffuse paraseptal and centrilobular emphysema, along with subpleural apical bullae.

diffuse decreased attenuation without focal destruction may be indistinguishable from that of bronchiolitis obliterans.

Paraseptal emphysema: This predominantly affects a distal secondary pulmonary lobule, which comprises the alveolar ducts and sacs, and hence it is typically in the subpleural lung, with areas of lung destruction, often marginated by interlobular septa (see Fig. 13.8I). It can be an isolated phenomenon in young adults, often associated with spontaneous pneumothorax, or can be seen in older adults with centrilobular emphysema.

Bullae: By definition, a bulla is a sharply demarcated area of emphysema, 1 cm or more in diameter, with a wall that is less than 1 mm thick. It is usually subpleural in location, very thin-walled, and largest at the lung apices. On HRCT, other findings of emphysema usually are visible. Bullae are usually the manifestation of paraseptal emphysema, but are also seen in centrilobular emphysema (see Fig. 13.8I).

Bullous emphysema: In some patients with emphysema, bullae can be very large, resulting in significant compromise of respiratory function; this is termed *bullous emphysema*.

Bleb: A bleb is defined as a small gas-containing space within the visceral pleura or in the subpleural lung; it is typically less than 1 cm in diameter. On CT, a bleb appears as a thin-walled cystic air space contiguous with the pleura, generally at the lung apex. Considering the little clinical importance of differentiating a bleb from a bulla based on size, the use of this term by radiologists should be avoided and the term *bulla* used instead.

Paracicatricial, irregular emphysema, irregular air space enlargement: This type of emphysema typically occurs adjacent to localized parenchymal scars and diffuse pulmonary fibrosis and in the pneumoconiosis associated with progressive massive fibrosis.

Interstitial emphysema: Pulmonary interstitial emphysema is a rare entity in adults but occurs more commonly in neonates on mechanical ventilation. It is characterized by air dissecting within the pulmonary interstitium, typically along the peribronchovascular region, interlobular septa, and visceral pleura. In adults, interstitial emphysema is rarely seen radiographically and also uncommonly on CT. It appears as perivascular air or low-attenuating halos and small parenchymal or subpleural cysts.

Pneumatocele: A pneumatocele is a thin-walled, air-filled cystic space within the lung that typically occurs in association with acute infection, trauma, or hydrocarbon aspiration. It is usually transient and is commonly seen in patients with *Pneumocystis jiroveci* (previously *Pneumocystis carinii*) pneumonia in patients with AIDS (Fig. 13.9A), *Staphylococcus aureus* pneumonia, and other acute bacterial infections. Pathophysiologically, it is due to the combination of lung necrosis and air trapping. Radiologically, a pneumatocele can be differentiated from a lung abscess and pulmonary gangrene by the thin and uniform wall thickness of the round, thin-walled lung cystic space of a pneumatocele. However, it is hard to differentiate pneumatocele completely from a lung cyst or bulla based on the HRCT findings alone.

Progressive massive fibrosis, complicated pneumoconioses: Progressive massive fibrosis occurs in silicosis and coal workers' pneumoconiosis. A radiographic hallmark is nodules more than 1 cm in functionally impaired patients. It manifests as a conglomerate mass with a nodular periphery, calcifications, and air bronchogram, predominantly in the posterior third of the upper lobes of lungs. Paracicatricial emphysema and adjacent pleural thickening, in addition to background nodular opacities indicative of underlying pneumoconiosis, are common associated findings.

Pulmonary Vasculature

Pulmonary infarction: Typically, pulmonary infarctions appear as consolidative opacities predominantly in the lower lobes. On CT, a pulmonary infarct is a peripheral, subpleural, wedge-shaped, triangular, or dome-shaped consolidative opacity, without contrast enhancement, and may show central lucency. The consolidative opacity represents local hemorrhage, with or without central tissue necrosis.

Pulmonary blood flow redistribution: Pulmonary blood flow redistribution refers to any departure from the normal distribution of blood flow in the lung tissue, caused by an increase in pulmonary vascular resistance. On HRCT, a mosaic perfusion pattern is usually seen, with marked regional variation in attenuation of the lung parenchyma and disparity in the size of the segmental vessels. It manifests as a decrease in size and number of visible pulmonary vessels in one or more lung regions of lower attenuation and a corresponding increase in number and size of pulmonary vessels in parts of the lung with high attenuation.

Pleura

Split pleura sign: This refers to a smoothly thickened and enhancing outer parietal and inner visceral pleura enclosing the fluid in the pleural cavity. It is typically described in empyema but can be seen in loculated pleural fluid of any cause (see Fig. 13.9B).

Airways

Trachea: The trachea extends from the inferior cricoid cartilage (at the level of the sixth cervical vertebrae) to the carina (fifth thoracic vertebrae). It is 10 to 12 cm in length, and there are 16 to 22 horseshoe-shaped bands of hyaline cartilage supporting its anterior and lateral walls. A posterior tracheal membrane is thin and fibromuscular and supports the incomplete posterior portion of the tracheal ring. On CT, the normal trachea is round or oval, but it can appear horseshoe-shaped, triangular, or pear-shaped in some normal individuals.

Tracheal bronchus: A tracheal bronchus is an uncommon incidental anomaly in which an ectopic bronchus arises from the trachea above the level of the carina. It is commonly on the right side. It may cause recurrent upper lobe pneumonia. On CT, it appears as a small bronchus arising from the lateral wall of trachea, cephalad to the carina.

Saber-sheath trachea: Saber-sheath trachea refers only to the intrathoracic trachea, predominantly in men, and is a strong indicator of chronic obstructive pulmonary disease. It is characterized by a decreased coronal diameter of the intrathoracic trachea and increased sagittal diameter and is easy to visualize on CT (see Fig. 13.9C). On a frontal radiograph, a characteristic side-to-side narrowing of the tracheal lumen is visible, beginning at the thoracic inlet. On a lateral radiograph, the tracheal diameter appears normal or slightly increased, with the tracheal diameter on lateral film measuring 1.5 times that seen on a frontal film.

Tracheobronchomalacia: This refers to a focal or diffuse increase in compliance and excessive collapsibility of the trachea or bronchi due to the weakness of the wall. The diagnosis is based on >50% decrease in the airway lumen during expiration or coughing or a >70% decrease in cross-sectional area in expiration as compared to inspiration; it may result in lunate, crescentic, or frownlike narrowing of the lumen.

Bronchi: Bronchi are the conducting airways that contain cartilage in the walls.

Bronchioles: Bronchioles are the conducting airways without cartilage in the walls and are not visible on HRCT. The largest bronchiole is 3 mm in diameter, with 0.3-mm wall thickness. The terminal bronchiole is the last purely conducting airway, measuring 0.7 mm

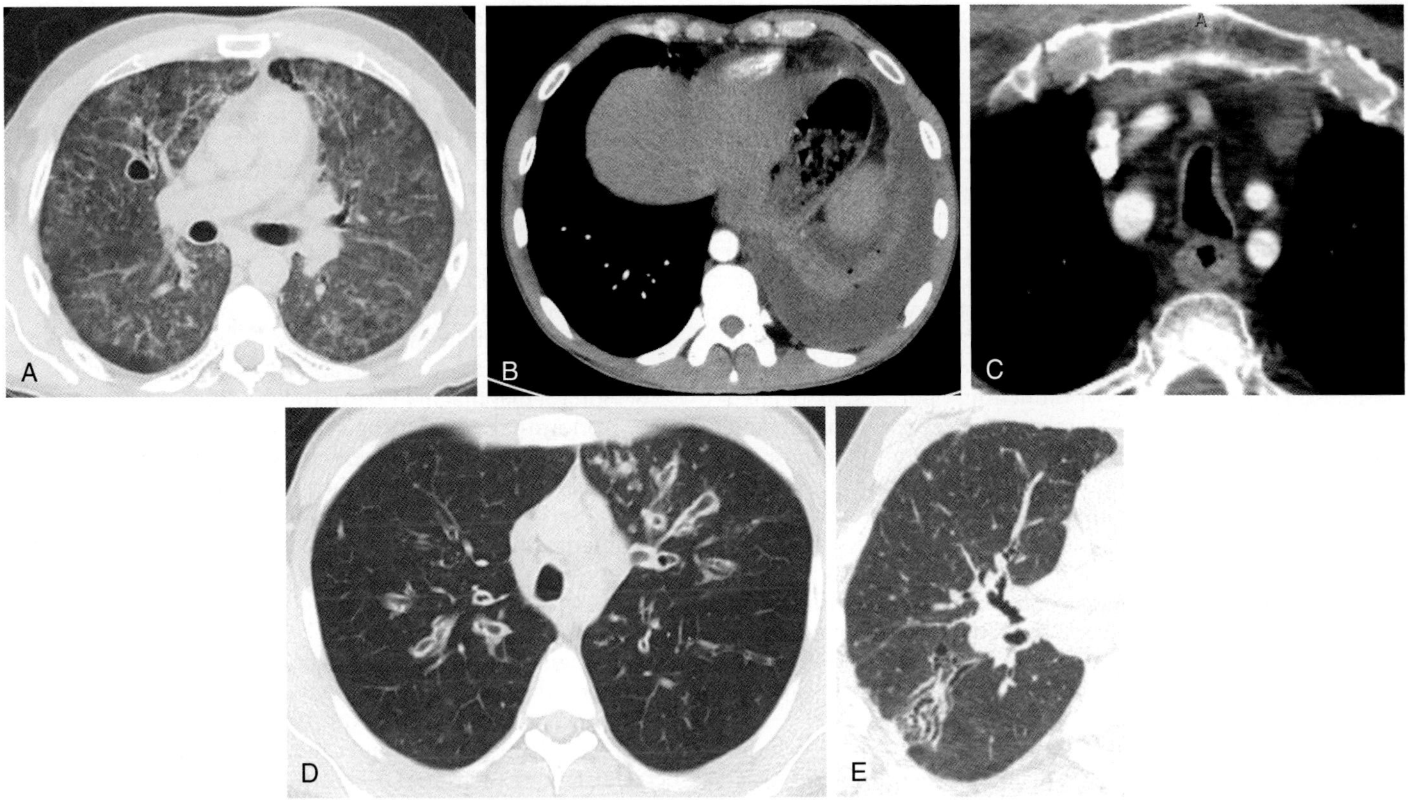

Figure 13.9 (A) Pneumatocele—a 60-year-old man with *Pneumocystis jiroveci* pneumonia presenting with diffuse ground-glass changes predominantly in both upper lobes, along with an air-filled pneumatocele in the right upper lobe. (B) Split pleura sign—a 30-year-old man with cystic fibrosis with a left-sided, moderate-sized pleural effusion with enhancing mildly thick-walled bordering pleura in the form of the split pleura sign. Note the left lower lobe bacterial pneumonia. (C) Saber-sheath trachea—a 65-year-old man with a saber-sheath trachea has an as ovoid structure with a smaller transverse diameter as compared to its sagittal diameter. (D) Bronchiectasis—a 35-year-old man with cystic fibrosis presenting with the signet ring sign and tram track sign due to cylindric bronchiectasis and diffusely thickened bronchial wall. Note the few tree-in-bud opacities due to chronic bronchial impactions. (E) A 55-year-old man with traction bronchiolectasis in the right lower lobe due to an old healed infection-related fibrosis.

in diameter, and gives rise to the respiratory bronchiole. The respiratory bronchiole branches into alveolar ducts and alveoli and is the largest bronchiole participating in gas exchange.

Bronchiolitis: Bronchiolitis is an infectious or noninfectious inflammation of the small airways (bronchioles). On CT scan, tree-in-bud opacities, centrilobular nodules, and bronchiolar wall thickening (see Fig. 13.4B) or mosaic attenuation (see Fig. 13.3B) with air trapping are seen. It is usually divided into cellular and constrictive or obliterative subtypes.

Exudative bronchiolitis, diffuse (Japanese) panbronchiolitis: Exudative bronchiolitis is a disease of unknown cause that is particularly common in Japanese and East Asian populations. On HRCT, ill-defined centrilobular nodules, tree-in-bud opacities, dilated, air-filled thick-walled bronchioles, mosaic lung attenuation, and air trapping are seen.

Tree-in-bud pattern: The term *tree-in-bud* refers to the presence of nodular and Y-shaped branching opacities, which resemble a branching or budding tree, and are seen in the lung periphery. Tree-in-bud nodules are due to the presence of mucus, pus, or fluid impaction of dilated thick-walled centrilobular bronchioles (the trunk and branches) and peribronchiolar inflammation (the buds) at the tips of the branches. This finding is seen in various small airway infections (see Fig. 13.3B), cystic fibrosis (see Fig. 13.4B), bronchiectasis, and panbronchiolitis.

Bronchocele, mucocele, mucoid impaction: A bronchocele is characterized by retained secretions in the dilated bronchi, with and without proximal bronchial obstruction, which can be congenital (e.g., bronchial atresia) or acquired (e.g., bronchogenic carcinoma, metastasis, carcinoid, allergic bronchopulmonary aspergillosis). On CT scan, a bronchocele appears as a tubular or branching opacity with retained mucus and with a finger-in-glove appearance.

Broncholith: A broncholith is a calcified peribronchial lymph node that has eroded into the lumen of the bronchus and is commonly seen in histoplasmosis or a tuberculous infection. On CT scan, a broncholith appears as a small calcified lesion, in or immediately adjacent to an airway. Distal obstructive changes in the form of atelectasis, mucoid impaction, and bronchiectasis can be seen.

Bronchiectasis: Bronchiectasis is defined as a localized or diffuse irreversible dilation of the bronchial tree (see Fig. 13.9D). It is commonly associated with acute, chronic, or recurrent infection. The causes of bronchiectasis include an immunodeficiency syndrome, abnormality of mucociliary clearance, congenital or genetic abnormality, chronic bronchial obstruction, allergic bronchopulmonary aspergillosis, and constrictive bronchiolitis in patients with a lung or marrow transplant. Based on morphology, there are three types—cylindric, varicose, and cystic. Classic CT findings include bronchial dilation, with a lumen diameter greater than that of the adjacent pulmonary artery (signet ring sign), horizontally oriented dilated bronchi (tram track sign), lack of tapering of bronchi, visibility of peripheral airways, and dilated airways within 1 cm of the costal pleura. Other associated findings include bronchial wall thickening, fluid- or mucus-filled tubular bronchi, Y-shaped or branching opacities, associated small airway disease–related mosaic attenuation, and centrilobular opacities. In patients with pulmonary fibrosis, traction bronchiectasis is seen (see Fig. 13.9E).

Bronchiolitis obliterans, constrictive obliterative bronchiolitis: Bronchiolitis obliterans (BO) is caused by peribronchiolar inflammation and fibrosis causing marked narrowing and obliteration of terminal and respiratory bronchioles. The causes of BO include prior infections, toxic fume inhalation, drug treatment (e.g., amiodarone, penicillamine, gold), collagen vascular disease, and transplantation.

On the radiograph, the finding is subtle and includes hyperinflation of the lung and reduction of lung vasculature, with or without bronchial wall thickening. On HRCT, areas of decreased lung attenuation with reduced-caliber pulmonary vessels, patchy mosaic attenuation, areas of air trapping on an expiratory scan, and bronchial wall thickening or bronchiectasis are seen. A predominantly unilateral finding of BO is known as *Swyer-James syndrome* or *McLeod syndrome*.

■ Vascular and Cardiac Terminology

Aorta

Aortic diameter: The maximum diameter of the aorta is measured from the external walls of the aorta, perpendicular to the long axis of flow and length of the aorta. The aortic measurements are made at the following sites:

1. Aortic sinuses of Valsalva
2. Sinotubular junction
3. Midascending aorta (midpoint in length between the sinotubular junction and proximal aortic arch at the level of the main pulmonary artery)
4. Proximal aortic arch (at the origin of the innominate artery)
5. Midaortic arch (between the left common carotid and left subclavian arteries)
6. Proximal descending thoracic aorta (begins at the isthmus, ≈2 cm distal to the left subclavian artery)
7. Middescending aorta (midpoint in length between the proximal descending and diaphragmatic aorta)
8. Aorta at diaphragm (2 cm above the celiac axis origin)
9. Abdominal aorta at the celiac axis origin

Normal measurement, levels of measurement: The normal reference values for the thoracic aorta are noted in Table 13.1.

True aneurysm: This is a permanent focal dilation of an artery, with at least a 50% increase in diameter compared with the expected standard diameter of the artery in question.

Pseudoaneurysm: This is a permanent focal dilation not composed of all the walls of an artery, with at least a 50% increase in diameter compared with the expected standard diameter of the artery in question (Fig. 13.10A).

Ectasia: This is an arterial dilatation with less than 50% increase in expected standard diameter of the normal artery.

Arteriomegaly: This is a diffuse arterial dilation involving multiple arterial segments, with an increase in diameter greater than 50% by comparison to the expected standard arterial diameter.

Coarctation: This is a focal or segmental narrowing of the descending aorta, just distal to the origin of the left subclavian artery at the insertion of the ductus arteriosus.

Pseudocoarctation: This is a congenital anatomic variant of the aortic arch and proximal descending aorta as a result of defective embryonic compression of the third through seventh dorsal aortic segments (less than expected). It results in a longer redundant aortic arch, with kinks at the level of the ligamentum arteriosum.

Atypical coarctation: This is a narrowing of the ascending or descending aorta at the level of the diaphragm or the abdominal aorta.

TABLE 13.1 Normal Reference Values for the Thoracic Aorta

THORACIC AORTA	RANGE OF REPORTED MEAN (cm)	REPORTED SD (cm)	ASSESSMENT METHOD
Root (female)	3.50–3.72	0.38	CT
Root (male)	3.63–3.91	0.38	CT
Ascending (female, male)	2.86	N/A	Chest x-ray
Middescending (female)	2.45–2.64	0.31	CT
Middescending (male)	2.39–2.98	0.31	CT
Diaphragmatic (female)	2.40–2.44	0.32	CT
Diaphragmatic (male)	2.43–2.69	0.27–0.40	CT, arteriography

SD, Standard deviation.

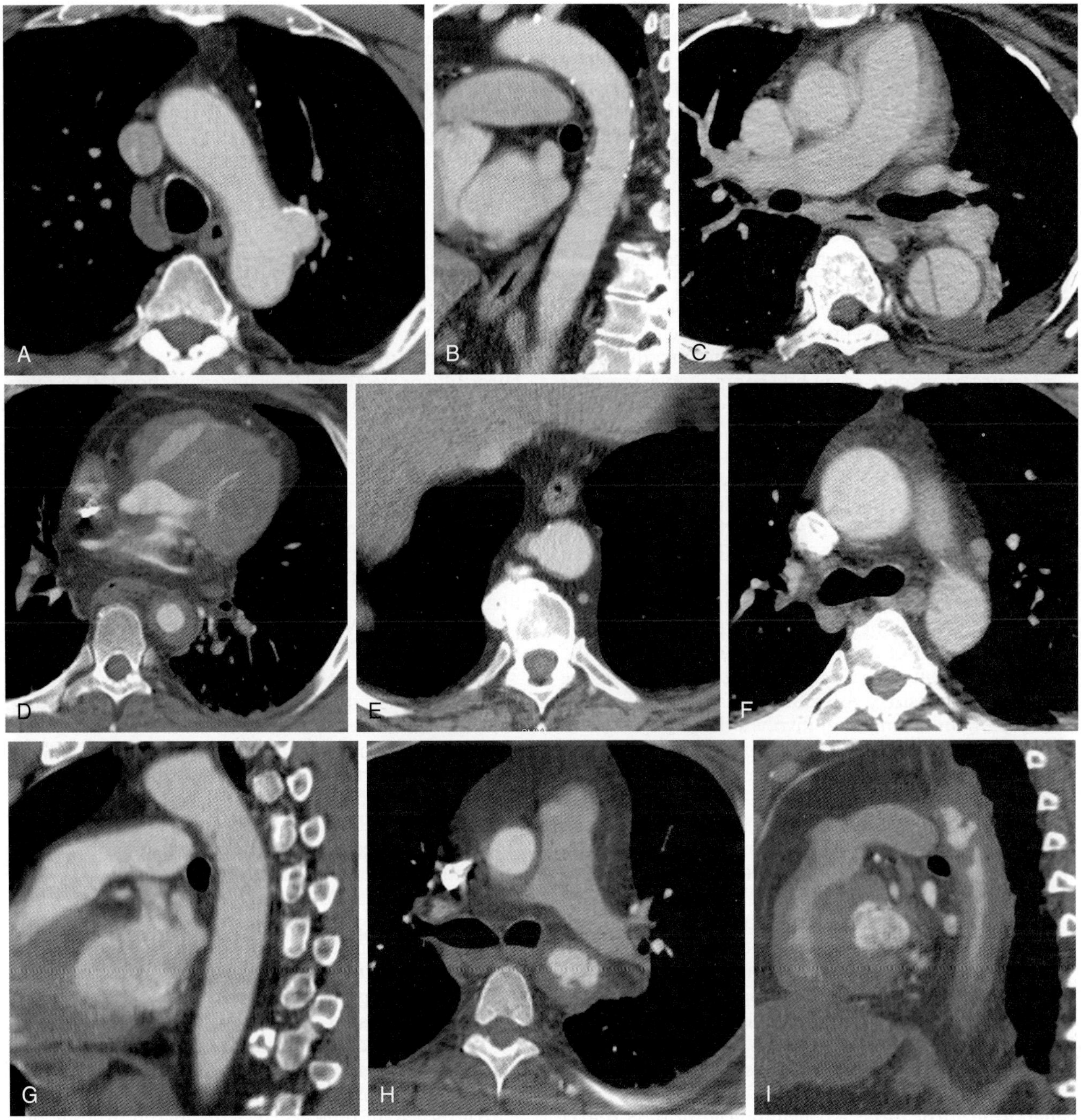

Figure 13.10 (A) Pseudoaneurysm—a 70-year-old man with a 1.9-cm aortic saccular pseudoaneurysm from the lateral wall of the aortic arch with intimal wall calcification likely related to sequelae of prior trauma. (B) Atheroma and its grades—a 61-year-old asymptomatic man with a simple atheroma, with intimal calcifications of the descending thoracic aorta and aortic arch. (C) Aortic dissection—a 55-year-old hypertensive man with type B aortic dissection appearing as an intimal flap and patent true and false lumens in the descending thoracic aorta. Note the adjacent small left pleural effusion and mild left periaortic atelectasis. (D) Intramural hematoma (IMH)—a 65-year-old hypertensive man with an IMH appearing as circumferential high density of the wall of descending thoracic aorta. (E) Penetrating aortic ulcer, CT thoracic aorta scan. A 61-year-old asymptomatic man with a penetrating aortic ulcer appearing as a 1.2-cm saccular contrast-filled, pseudoaneurysm-like outpouching from the right lateral wall of the lower descending thoracic aorta, with atherosclerotic wall thickening. (F, G) Minimal aortic injury—a 38-year-old man with intimal injury of the proximal descending aorta following trauma appearing as a thin focal filling defect in its lumen adjacent to the medial wall. (H, I) Traumatic aortic injury (TAI)—a 45-year-old man with an acute TAI appearing as a diffuse IMH in the descending thoracic aorta, with an irregular contour at the aortic isthmus in the form of a pseudoaneurysm, internal thrombus, and contained rupture.

Atheroma and its grades: The simplest lesions are usually reported as an atheroma or atheromatous plaque. When mobile components are seen attached to these plaques, the terms *ruptured plaque, mobile plaque, mobile debris,* and *superimposed thrombi* are used. Atheromatous plaques are graded from1 to 4, in progressive increase intimal wall thickness from normal (1–2 mm) to severe (>5 mm). Instead of the terms *mild, moderate,* and *severe,* some prefer the terms *small, moderate,* and *large* to quantify the plaques. The consensus statements from various societies have recommended classifying an aortic atheroma as simple (see Fig. 13.10B) or complex, based on the presence or absence of mobile components or ulceration(s). Although semiquantitative, these simple classifications—atheroma thickness, presence or absence of mobile components, presence or absence of ulceration—are relatively objective and reproducible.

Aortic dissection: Aortic dissection is defined as a tear in the intima of the aorta, with extension into the media creating a second or false lumen. The aortic dissection is described according to the Stanford (types A and B) or DeBakey (types I, II, and III) classification (see Fig. 13.10C). In the Stanford classification, type A dissections involve the ascending aorta; type B dissections spare the ascending aorta but involve the aortic arch and/or descending thoracic aorta, with the most common site of origin being just distal to the left subclavian artery. As per the DeBakey classification, in type I, an intimal flap involves the ascending and descending thoracic aorta, in type II, an intimal flap involves only the ascending thoracic aorta, and in type III, the intimal flap involves only the descending thoracic aorta.

Intramural hematoma: An intramural hematoma (IMH) is a variant of aortic dissection, usually produced by vasa vasorum rupture within the aortic media with a missing intimal flap, absent double channel, and lack of communication with the aortic lumen (see Fig. 13.10D). Typically, IMH appears as aortic wall thickening more than 0.5 cm in a crescentic or concentric pattern. The IMH is not a single entity but can be associated with several conditions, such as spontaneous (typical) and iatrogenic aortic dissection, penetrating ulcer, and aortic trauma.

Penetrating aortic ulcer: A penetrating aortic ulcer (PAU) is an ulceration of an atherosclerotic lesion that penetrates the internal elastic lamina into the aortic media. It presents as an ulcer or crater-like outpouching protruding beyond the aortic lumen in the aortic wall (see Fig. 13.10E).

Minimal aortic injury: Minimal aortic injury is an unclear term that has been used to refer to relatively small lesions. This term has been used to describe isolated intimal defects appearing as thin, linear, mobile intraluminal projections from the aortic wall, accompanied by minimal or no periaortic mediastinal hematoma, with a maintained diameter and external contour of the aorta (see Fig. 13.10F, G).

Traumatic aortic injury: Aortic injuries usually occur as a result of high-energy blunt trauma involving a rapid deceleration force. A traumatic aortic injury (TAI) is seen at the aortic isthmus in up to 90% of cases. The injury is graded as type I, intimal tear, type II, IMH, type III, pseudoaneurysm, and type IV, rupture (e.g., periaortic hematoma, free rupture; see Fig. 13.10H, I).

Traumatic aortic transection: This term refers to the disruption of all three layers of the aortic wall, commonly caused by sudden deceleration (typically from a high-speed motor vehicle accident or fall from a height; Fig. 13.11A). It results in a fusiform pseudoaneurysm with a smooth inner surface and an abrupt change in aortic diameter. The presence of a localized intravenous (IV) contrast leak outside the lumen of the aorta is an important sign of a contained transmural laceration, whereas free extravasation indicates a frank aortic rupture.

Ulcer-like projection: Ulcer-like projection (ULP) refers to an intimal disruption, with a widely communicating neck of >3 mm with the IMH. ULP is a strong predictor of adverse aorta-related events in patients with type B IMH.

Intramural blood pool: An intramural blood pool (IBP) is focal contrast pooling within the IMH that communicates with the intercostal lumbar artery on postcontrast CT or MRI scans (see Fig. 13.11B).

Bicuspid aortic valve–related aortopathy: A bicuspid aortic valve (BAV)–related aortopathy is aortic dilation and/or aortic dissection in patients with a BAV (see Fig. 13.11C–D). Approximately 50% of patients with BAV have dilation of the aortic root or ascending aorta.

Endoleak: An endoleak is defined as persistent blood flow in the aortic aneurysm sac outside the stent graft; it indicates a failure to exclude an aneurysm (see Fig. 13.11E) entirely. There are five types:

- Type 1: Inadequate seal at the proximal and distal graft attachment site
- Type 2: Retrograde aortic branch arterial blood flow into the aneurysm sac
- Type 3: Structural failure of an endograft (e.g., stent graft fractures, holes in the fabric, junctional separations)
- Type 4: Stent graft fabric porosity
- Type 5: Expansion of an aneurysm without a demonstrable endoleak; also called *endotension*

Aortitis: Aortitis represents inflammation of the aortic wall. Common causes include noninfectious inflammatory vasculitides, such as giant cell arteritis and Takayasu arteritis (see Fig. 13.11F). MRI, CT, and echocardiography demonstrate a homogeneous circumferential thickening of the aortic wall, with a uniform smooth internal surface.

Pulmonary Artery

Pulmonary arteriovenous malformation: A pulmonary arteriovenous malformation (AVM) represents abnormal communication between the pulmonary artery and vein, without an intervening capillary network (Fig. 13.12A). Other names include pulmonary arteriovenous fistulae, pulmonary arteriovenous aneurysms, cavernous angiomas of the lung, and pulmonary telangiectases.

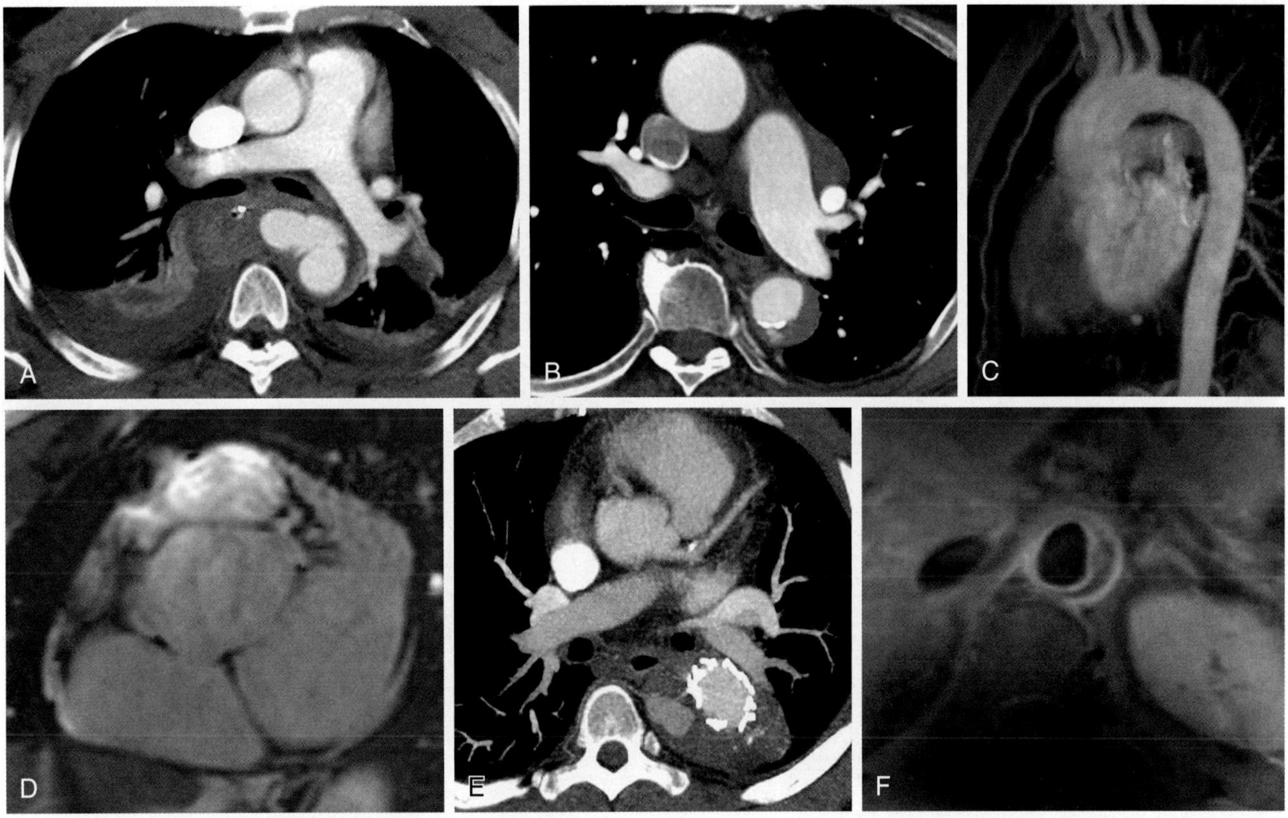

Figure 13.11 (A) Traumatic aortic transection—a 65-year-old man with traumatic aortic transection appearing as complete disruption of the anterior wall of the proximal descending thoracic aorta causing an irregular, contrast-filled pseudoaneurysm with an intramural hematoma (IMH) and a circumferential hematoma in the entire intrathoracic oesophagus. (B) Intramural blood pool (IBP)—a 49-year-old man with an IMH containing an IBP appearing as a focus of contrast in the posterior part, which appears to be connected medially with the intercostal artery. (C, D) Bicuspid aortic valve (BAV)–related aortopathy—a 36-year-old man with bicuspid valve–moderate aortic valve regurgitation and annuloaortic ectasia measuring up to 4.3 cm due to BAV-related aortopathy on the sagittal maximum intensity projection image from the postcontrast magnetic resonance angiography image. A short-axis steady-state free precession MRI reveals a BAV. (E) Endoleak—a 46-year-old man with a type II endoleak from the right fifth intercostal artery in the excluded aneurysmal dilated thrombosed descending thoracic aorta containing a fenestrated, patent aortic endoluminal stent graft. (F) Aortitis—a 56-year-old man with giant cell vasculitis presenting as a predominantly circumferential enhancing wall thickening of the upper abdominal aorta causing eccentric, mild, luminal narrowing.

Aneurysm: This is a focal, congenital, or acquired dilation of a pulmonary artery involving all three layers that is beyond its maximal normal caliber (on CT, >29 mm for the main pulmonary artery, >17 mm for the right interlobar pulmonary artery).

Bronchopulmonary sequestration: This is a nonfunctioning mass of lung tissue without normal communication with the tracheobronchial tree that receives its arterial blood supply from the systemic circulation (see Fig. 13.12B).

Pulmonary arterial hypertension: Pulmonary arterial hypertension (PAH) is defined as a mean pulmonary arterial pressure (mPAP) ≥25 mm Hg at rest or 30 mm Hg during exercise. An enlargement of the main pulmonary artery of more than 3 cm on CT or MRI suggests PAH. The assessment of PAH is reliably performed with right heart catheterization (see Fig. 13.12C).

Pulmonary embolism: A pulmonary embolism (PE) is an obstruction of the pulmonary artery or one of its branches by material (e.g., thrombus, tumor, air, fat) that originated elsewhere in the body (see Fig. 13.12D, E). In an acute PE, the embolus appears as a central filling defect with sharp interfaces with injected contrast agent and acute angles with the vessel wall. In chronic PE, the embolus is adherent to the vessel wall, with a peripheral location, that forms an obtuse angle.

Pulmonary artery atresia, pulmonary atresia, pulmonic stenosis: Atresia of the pulmonary valve resulting in an absent connection between the right ventricular outflow tract and pulmonary arteries has three subtypes. Pulmonary stenosis results in dilation of the left main pulmonary artery (see Fig. 13.12F, G).

Superior vena cava syndrome: A superior vena cava (SVC) syndrome is obstruction of blood flow through the SVC due to intraluminal, intramural, or extrinsic disease that causes nonopacification of the SVC, with or without collateral vessel formation. Obstruction can be caused by invasion or external compression of the SVC by a lung cancer, metastatic lymph node,

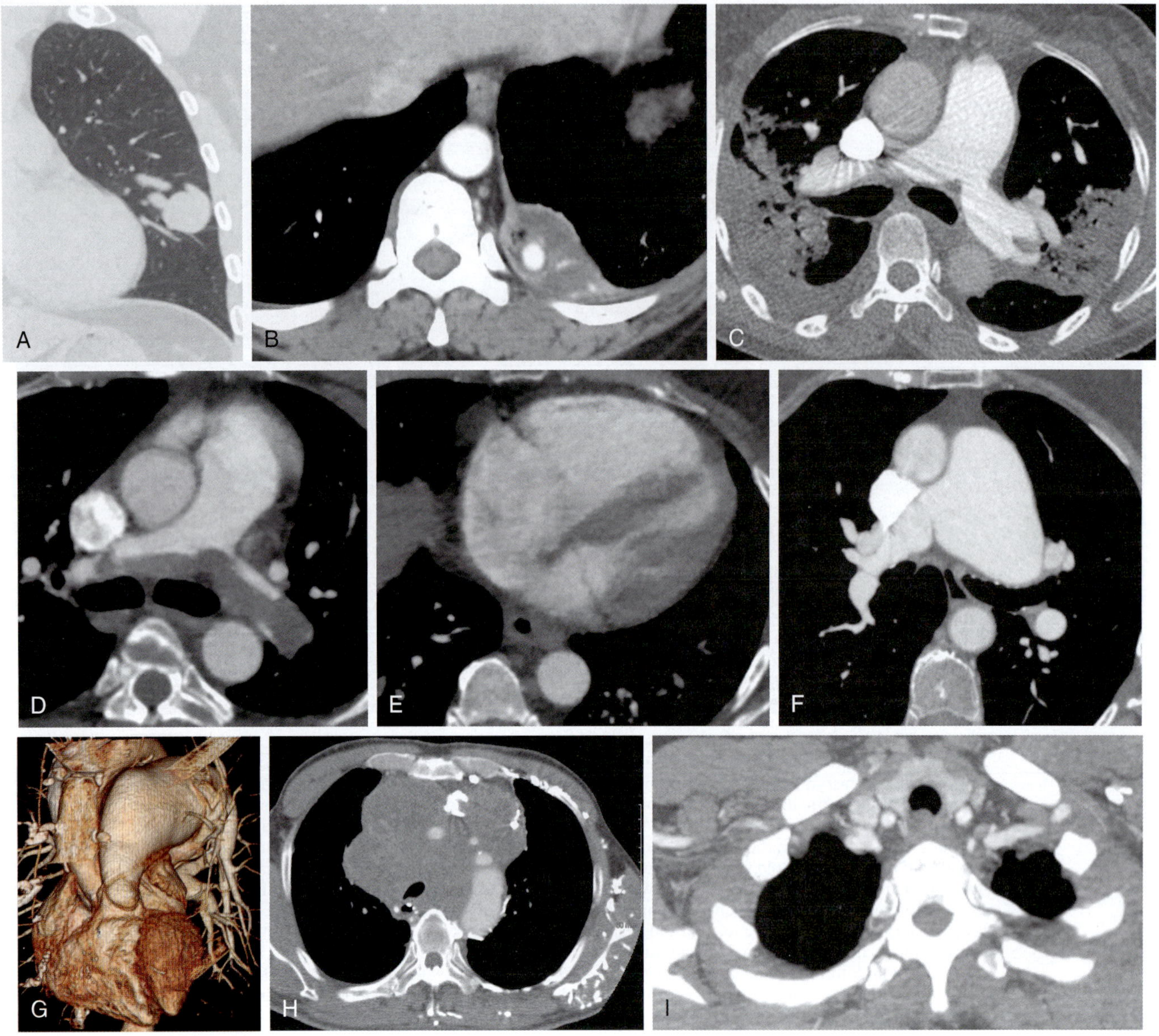

Figure 13.12 (A) Pulmonary arteriovenous malformation (AVM)—a 61-year-old man with a mass in the chest correlates with large 3.5-cm left upper lobe–enhancing lesion with a feeding artery and draining vein consistent with pulmonary AVM. (B) Bronchopulmonary sequestration—a 61-year-old man with an intralobar sequestration appearing as a large cystic fluid lesion with internal septae and a large-caliber supplying artery arising from the upper abdominal aorta and its draining vein to the left lower pulmonary vein. (C) Pulmonary arterial hypertension (PAH) in a 61-year-old man with usual interstitial pneumonia and consolidation due to adenocarcinoma in both upper lobes shows an enlarged main pulmonary artery, to 3.5 cm, consistent with PAH. (D, E) Pulmonary embolism—a 61-year-old man with a saddle pulmonary embolus extending across the bifurcation of the main pulmonary artery into both pulmonary arteries, with resultant acute right heart strain–related right ventricular enalrgement and interventricular septal flattenning. (F, G) Pulmonary valve stenosis—an 80-year-old woman with congenital stenosis of the pulmonary valve causing aneurysmal dilation of the main and left pulmonary arteries, with a normal-caliber right pulmonary artery. (H) Superior vena cava (SVC) syndrome—a 64-year-old man with shortness of breath and weight loss due to SVC syndrome from a small cell lung cancer–related large, lobulated, mediastinal mass surrounding and compressing the trachea, constricting the great vessels and invading the SVC and brachiocephalic veins, with resultant abundant chest wall and mediastinal collateral veins. (I) Thoracic outlet syndrome—a 55-year-old woman with a history of breast cancer has a short-segment bilateral subclavian artery; complete obliteration between the clavicle and first rib is suggestive of thoracic outlet syndrome.

lymphoma, mediastinal neoplasm, granulomatous disease, or SVC thrombosis (see Fig. 13.12H).

Thoracic outlet syndrome: This refers to a constellation of signs and symptoms that arise from compression of the brachial plexus and subclavian artery and vein within the confined space of the thoracic outlet of various structures, just above the first rib and behind the clavicle (see Fig. 13.12I). Synonyms include cervical rib syndrome, scalene anticus syndrome, costoclavicular syndrome, and hyperabduction syndrome.

Pulmonary Vein

Stenosis: This refers to the narrowing of a pulmonary vein. Primary pulmonary vein stenosis is congenital, whereas secondary pulmonary vein stenosis in adult patients is caused by a process such as a neoplasm, sarcoidosis, or fibrosing mediastinitis or from prior radiofrequency ablation for atrial fibrillation.

Varix: A varix, sometimes termed a *pulmonary venous aneurysm,* refers to a localized aneurysmal dilation of a pulmonary vein.

Scimitar syndrome, hypogenetic lung syndrome, congenital venolobar syndrome: Scimitar syndrome is a variant of a partial anomalous pulmonary venous connection in which part of or even the entire right lung drained by the right pulmonary veins connects anomalously to the inferior vena cava or portal vein. The other components include ipsilateral pulmonary parenchymal and arterial hypoplasia and an anomalous arterial supply of a portion of the right lower lobe (Fig. 13.13A).

Cardiac Terms

First-pass perfusion: This is a time-sensitive downstream transit of an extracellular contrast medium through the cardiac chambers and myocardium following administration of an IV medium. In a normal first-pass perfusion, the contrast agent shortens the T1 relaxation time and results in a high signal. In an abnormal first-pass perfusion, areas deprived of blood supply will appear as a hypointense signal (see Fig. 13.13B, C).

Late gadolinium enhancement: Late gadolinium enhancement (LGE) is abnormal ventricular wall enhancement on the delayed MRI scan, generally 5- to 15-minute delayed phase images (see Fig. 13.13D, E).

Myocardial infarction: A myocardial infarction (MI) is myocardial cell death secondary to a prolonged ischemic insult from a decreased supply of oxygenated blood. Subendocardial and variable transmural delayed hyperenhancement on MRI can be seen in both acute and chronic MIs (see Fig. 13.13D–E). However, wall thinning, regional or global wall motion abnormality, absent edema on T2-weighted images, linear myocardial calcification, or subendocardial fatty metaplasia on CT suggests a chronic MI (see Fig. 13.13F).

Myocardial stunning: Stunning refers to the delayed recovery of regional myocardial contractile function, despite the absence of irreversible damage and restoration of normal myocardial blood flow. This is not associated with LGE on MRI.

Myocardial hibernation: This is abnormal contractility of a thinned left ventricular wall at rest due to chronically reduced coronary blood flow that can be partially or completely restored to normal by improving blood flow or reducing oxygen demand.

Regional wall motion abnormality of ventricle: This includes akinesis, hypokinesis, and dyskinesis.

Akinesis: Akinesis refers to an absence of myocardial systolic thickening or contraction.

Hypokinesis: Hypokinesis refers to a reduction in myocardial systolic thickening or contraction.

Dyskinesis: Dyskinesis refers to absent systolic myocardial contraction, with paradoxic wall motion instead (see Fig. 13.13G).

Fatty metaplasia: Abnormal deposition of fat in the left ventricular subendocardium can be seen as a sequela of a prior MI or in the right ventricular wall in a setting of arrhythmogenic right ventricular dysplasia.

Myocardial thickening: Myocardial thickening refers to an end-diastolic myocardial thickness of 15 mm or more. Concentric left ventricular wall thickening is seen in long-standing hypertension and aortic valve stenosis, whereas asymmetric wall thickening is seen in asymmetric hypertrophic cardiomyopathy (see Fig. 13.13G, H).

Lipomatous hypertrophy of interatrial septum: Fat density on CT or signal intensity on MRI in an interatrial septum, with sparing of fossa ovalis, generally in a dumbbell shape and identical to nearby epicardial fat, with thickness >10 mm, is diagnostic of lipomatous hypertrophy of interatrial septum (Fig. 13.14A).

Myocardial segmentation and bull's eye model: The American Heart Association recommends myocardial segmentation referencing the long and short axes of the left ventricle (see Fig. 13.14B). The terms *basal, mid,* and *apex* refer to areas along the long axis of the ventricle (LV). With regard to the short-axis location, the basal and midcavity LV slices should be divided into six segments of 60 degrees each. An axially based version of this standard model, published by the Society of Cardiovascular Computed Tomography, is displayed in Fig. 13.14C, which has been altered to emulate CT angiography views more closely. In addition to combining the three standard invasive angiographic views into a single axial view, this model identifies a left posterolateral branch as segment 18 and a ramus intermedius branch as segment 17.

Cardiac thrombus: This represents an intracavitary filling defect within the cardiac chamber, separate from papillary muscle and trabeculae, and appears as a filling defect. Although identified with CT (see Fig. 13.14D) and echocardiography, long inversion recovery time, delayed-enhancement MRI is most sensitive for its assessment and differentiation from a cardiac mass (see Fig. 13.14E).

Pericardial effusion: This is an accumulation of fluid in the pericardial space, enclosed between the parietal and visceral layers of the pericardium more than the normal limits of 15 to 50 mL.

Pericardial effusion grades: Circumferential pericardial effusion can be graded based on the separation of the pericardial layers in diastole:

- **Minimal:** <5 mm of pericardial separation (corresponding to a fluid volume of 50–100 mL)
- **Small:** 5 to 10 mm of separation (corresponding to a fluid volume of 100–250 mL)
- **Moderate:** 10 to 20 mm of separation (corresponding to a fluid volume of 250–500 mL)
- **Large:** >20 mm separation (corresponding to a fluid volume >500 mL; see Fig. 13.14F)

Pericardial tamponade: This is increased intrapericardial pressure from an accumulation of large amounts of fluid, pus, blood, clots, or gas in the pericardial space.

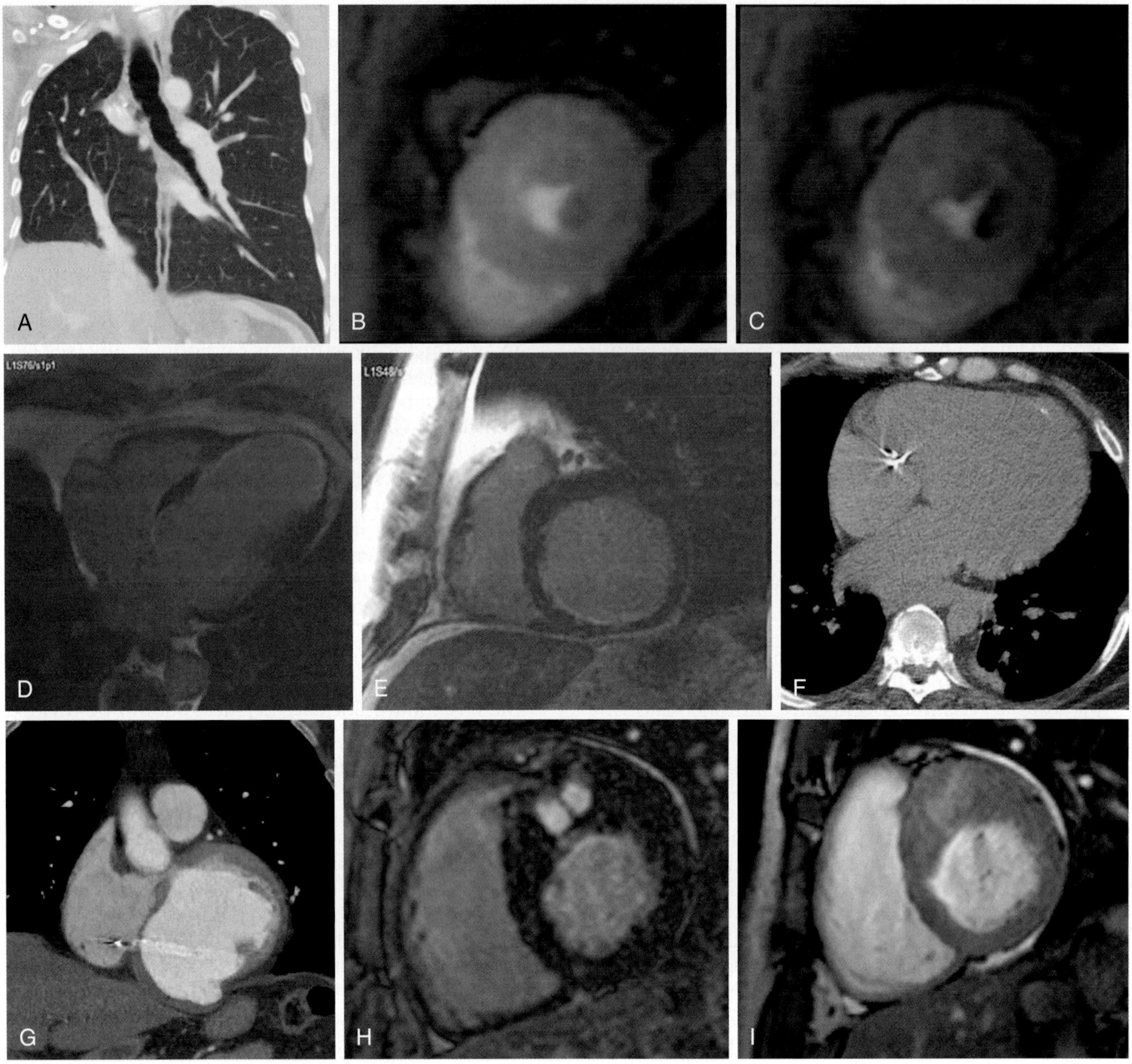

Figure 13.13 (A) Scimitar syndrome—a 49-year-old woman with an anomalous arterial supply of a portion of the right lower lobe without right pulmonary venous drainage to the left atrium; instead, drainage to the inferior vena cava, dextroposition of the heart due to right lung volume loss consistent with congenital pulmonary venolobar syndrome. Rest (B) and stress (C) cardiac MR perfusion images during regadenoson vasodilator stress protocol in a 51-year-old woman show moderate-sized reversible perfusion in the midinferolateral and midseptal segments, suggestive of flow-limiting coronary stenosis in the left circumflex artery, diagonal territory, and possibly in the septal left anterior descending (LAD) coronary artery territory as well. Late gadolinium enhancement (LGE)—shown are four-chamber (D) and short-axis (E) MR images in a 66-year-old man with abnormal subendocardial to midmyocardial LGE of the basal, mid, and apical septum and a true apex next to the mid and apical anterior walls (not shown) consistent with a large infarct in the distribution of the LAD coronary artery. (F) A 51-year-old man with linear calcification in the left ventricular apical myocardium from an old, chronic myocardial infarct. (G) Cardiac false aneurysm. A 78-year-old man with a saccular false aneurysm inferior from the mid to left ventricular cavity appearing as a contrast-filled outpouching of 5.3 cm extending inferiorly and causing a septal bulge and compression of the right ventricle. (H, I) Balanced steady-state free precession cardiac MR image in a 42-year-old man with hypertrophic obstructive cardiomyopathy reveals asymmetric, markedly thickened anterior and anterior septal walls of the basal left ventricular myocardium along with focal scar–related LGE consistent with asymmetric hypertrophic cardiomyopathy.

It can result in life-threatening rapid or gradual compression of the cardiac chambers and decreased cardiac output. The causes include infection, trauma, or myocardial rupture (see Fig. 13.14F).

Constrictive pericarditis: This is caused by a thickened fibrotic pericardium, with or without calcification (see Fig. 13.14G), that impedes normal diastolic filling of the left ventricle. It is best diagnosed by echocardiography or cine MRI with tagging (Fig. 13.15A, B).

Coronary artery: Recommended quantitative coronary artery stenosis grading (see Fig. 13.15C):

Normal: Absence of plaque and no luminal stenosis

Minimal: Plaque with <25% stenosis

Mild: 25%–49% stenosis

Moderate: 50%–69% stenosis

Severe: 70%–99% stenosis

Occluded: Complete obliteration of coronary artery lumen.

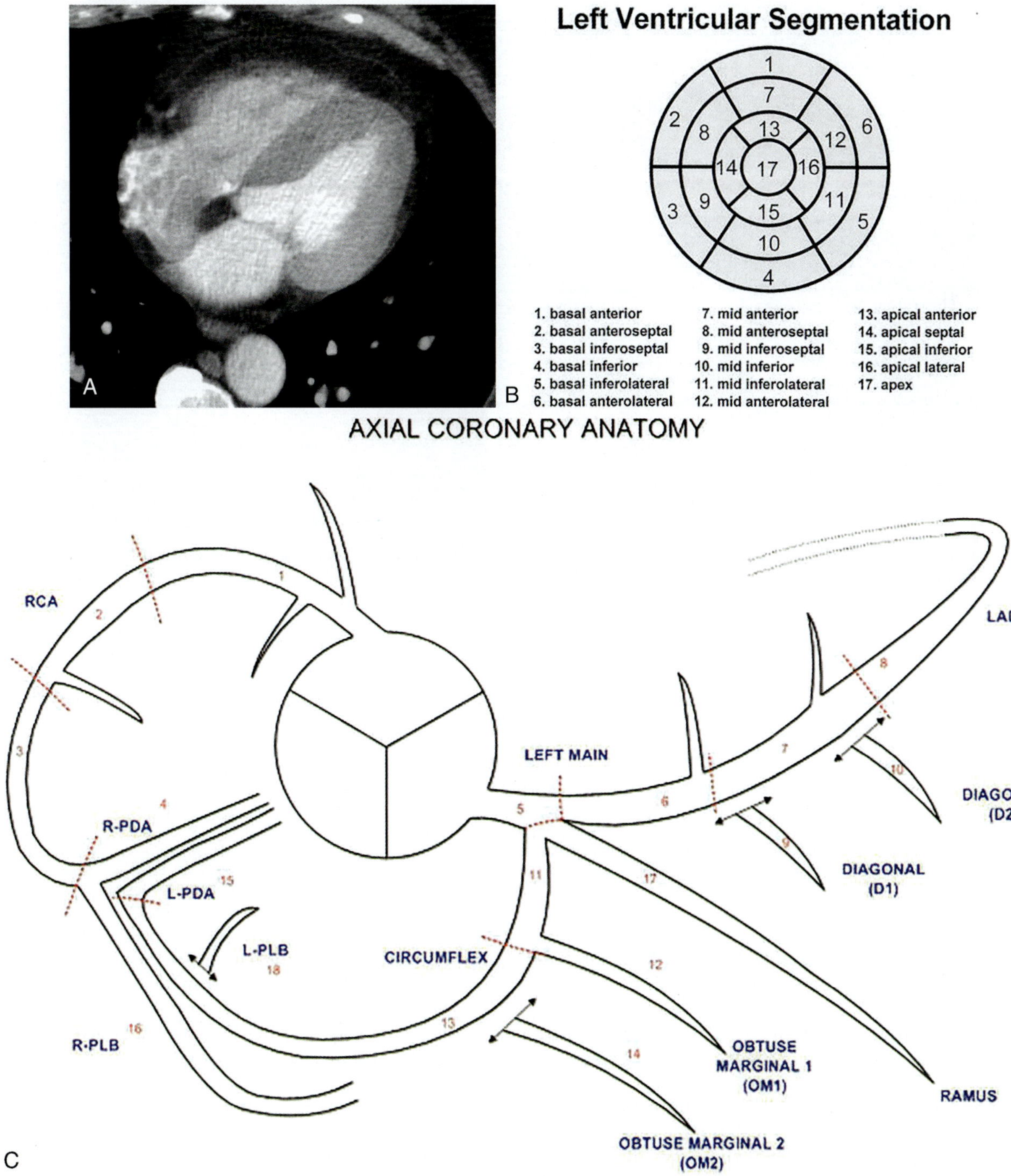

Figure 13.14 (A) A 66-year-old woman with a large, uniformly fat density mass in the region of the interatrial septum sparing the fossa ovalis is consistent with lipomatous hypertrophy of the interatrial septum. (B) Diagrammatic image of the 17-segment module of the American Heart Association. (C) Diagrammatic 18-segment modules of the Society of Cardiovascular Computed Tomography.

Continued

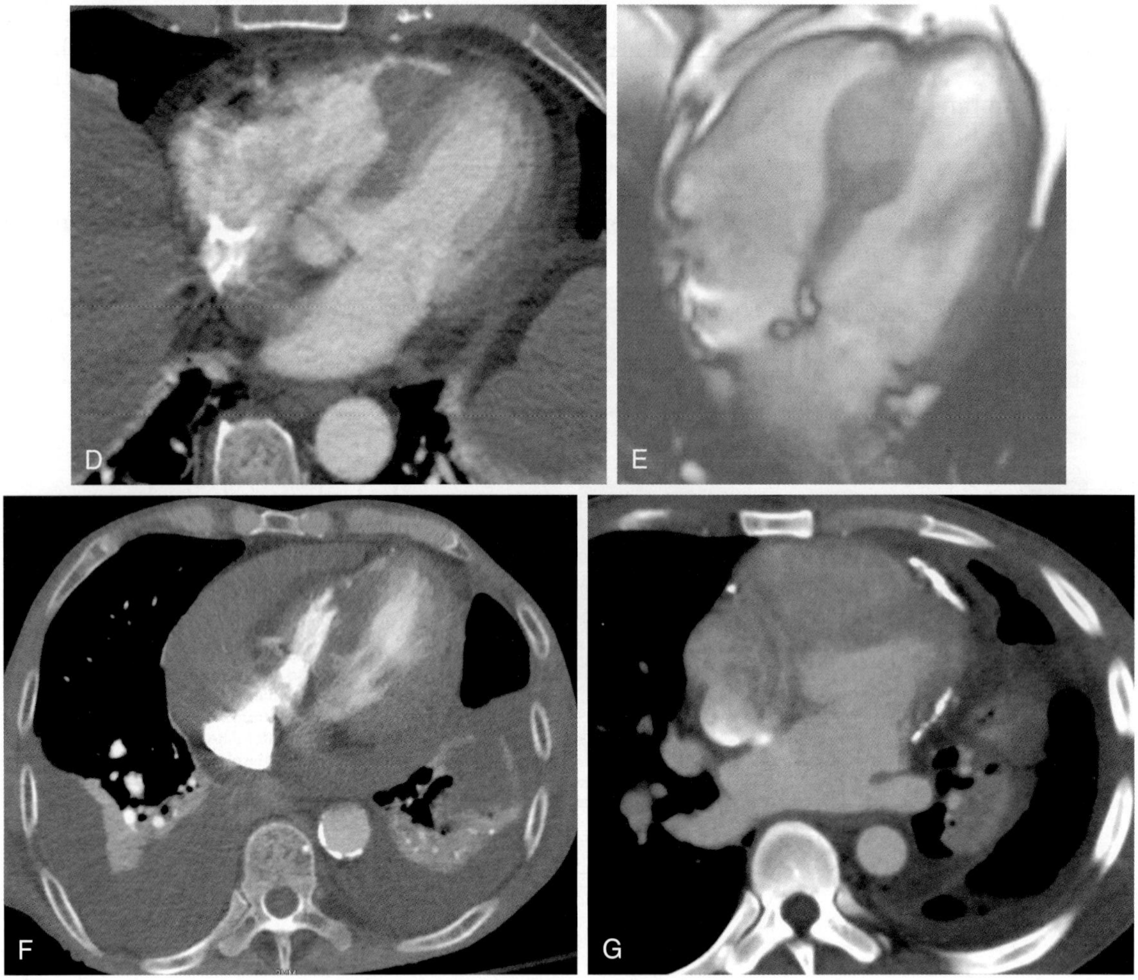

Figure 13.14, cont'd (D) Cardiac thrombus. This CT chest image shows a right ventricular thrombus in a 62-year-old woman with bilateral pulmonary emboli (not shown). (E) CT and MRI scans of a cardiac mass. This steady-state free precession four-chamber cardiac MR image of an 80-year-old man with carcinoid syndrome shows a mildly hyperintense carcinoid tumor involving the mid to apical interventricular septum causing a bulging focal mass in the right ventricle. (F) Pericardial tamponade. This axial CT scan of a 62-year-old woman with pericardial tamponade shows a large pericardial effusion causing a pressure effect on the right ventricle and dilated inferior vena cava (IVC). Note the bilateral pleural effusion. (G) This axial CT scan of a 44-year-old man with constrictive pericarditis shows linear pericardial calcification and a mildly dilated IVC, right atrium and right ventricle. Note the left hydropneumothorax and left lower lobe rounded atelectasis. *PDA*, Posterior descending artery; *PLB*, posterolateral branch; *RCA*, right coronary artery.

Plaques: Coronary artery plaques can be calcified (Hounsfield units >130), noncalcified (soft), or mixed. Plaque lesions containing 50% or more calcium are called *calcified* and less as *mixed*.

Myocardial bridge: This represents an abnormal intramyocardial course of a coronary artery segment (see Fig. 13.15D).

Coronary ectasia, aneurysm: This is a portion of a coronary artery that dilates to a diameter exceeding the adjacent segments or exceeds them by 1.5 times.

Coronary artery fistula: This is abnormal termination of a coronary artery resulting in communication between the coronary arteries and cardiac chambers (coronary cameral fistula) or other mediastinal vessels (coronary AVM).

Anomalous origin of the left coronary artery, Bland-White-Garland syndrome: An anomalous origin of the left coronary artery from the pulmonary artery (ALCAPA) results in a left-to-right shunt.

Anomalous origin of the right coronary artery from the pulmonary artery: An anomalous origin of the right coronary artery from the pulmonary artery (ARCAPA) is an extremely rare congenital coronary anomaly.

Coronary artery anomalies: This is a collective term for a diverse group of abnormalities involving an abnormal origin or course of the coronary artery. An interarterial course is the presence of a coronary artery between the aorta and pulmonary artery. Anomalous coronaries are prone to compression (often seen as slitlike ostium) from adjacent structures.

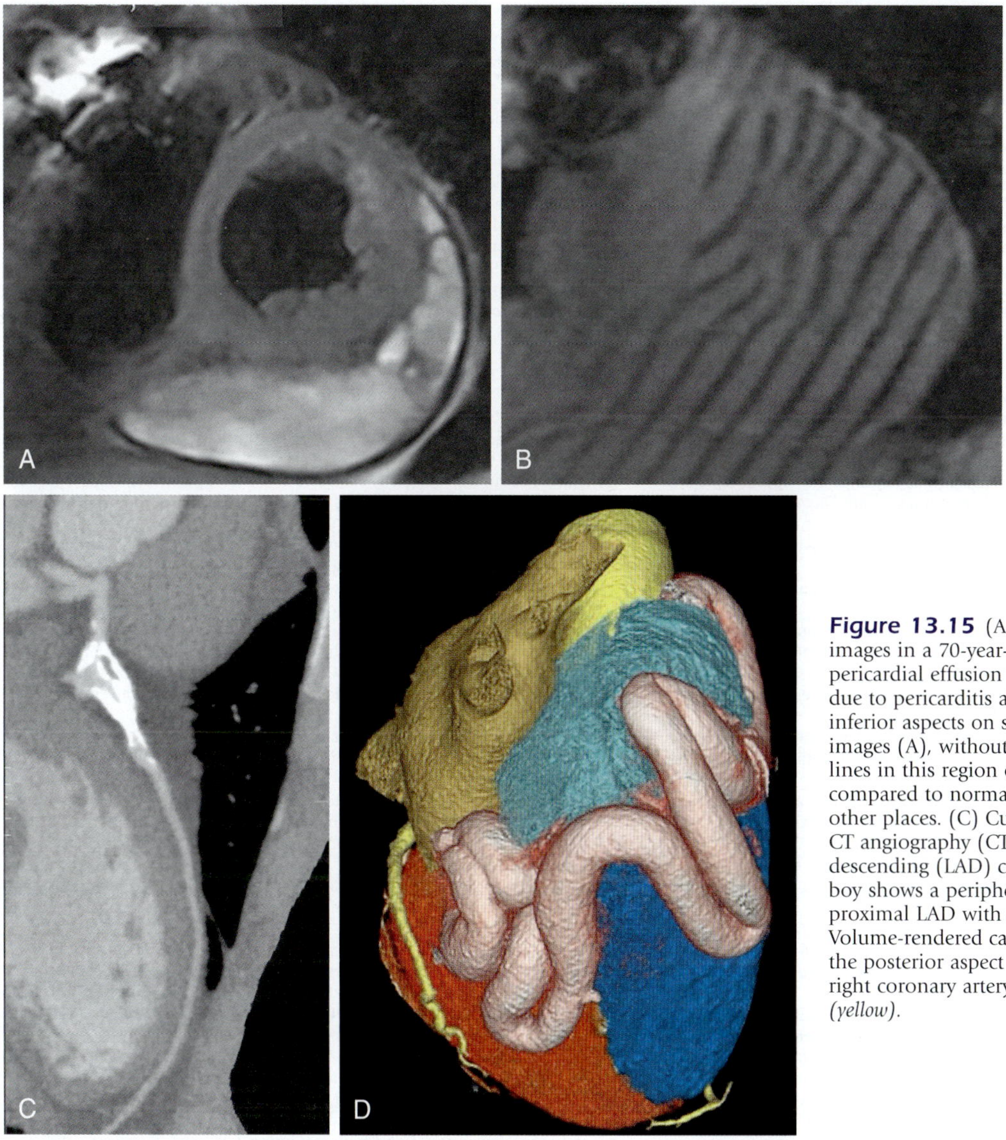

Figure 13.15 (A, B) Short-axis cardiac MR images in a 70-year-old man show loculated pericardial effusion with a thickened pericardium due to pericarditis along the left lateral and inferior aspects on short-axis T2 black blood images (A), without breaking the normal tagging lines in this region on the short-axis image (B) as compared to normal breaking of tagging lines at other places. (C) Curved multiplanar reformatted CT angiography (CTA) image of the left anterior descending (LAD) coronary artery in a 12-year-old boy shows a peripherally calcified aneurysm of the proximal LAD with a small thrombus. (D) Volume-rendered cardiac CTA image viewed from the posterior aspect in a 50-year-old man with a right coronary artery *(pink)* to right atrial fistula *(yellow)*.

Bibliography

Aberle DR, Gamsu G, Ray CS, et al. Asbestos-related pleural and parenchymal fibrosis: detection with high-resolution CT. *Radiology*. 1988;166:729–734.

Aberle DR, Gamsu G, Ray CS. High-resolution CT of benign asbestos-related diseases: clinical and radiographic correlation. *AJR Am J Roentgenol*. 1988;151:883–891.

Aberle DR, Hansell DM, Brown K, et al. Lymphangiomyomatosis: CT, chest radiographic, and functional correlations. *Radiology*. 1990;176:381–387.

Achenbach S, Moselewski F, Ropers D, et al. Detection of calcified and noncalcified coronary atherosclerotic plaque by contrast-enhanced, submillimeter multidetector spiral computed tomography: a segment-based comparison with intravascular ultrasound. *Circulation*. 2004;109:14–17.

Akira M, Kitatani F, Lee Y-S, et al. Diffuse panbronchiolitis: evaluation with high-resolution CT. *Radiology*. 1988;168:433–438.

Akira M, Yamamoto S, Yokoyama K, et al. Asbestosis: high-resolution CT-pathologic correlation. *Radiology*. 1990;176:389–394.

Aquino SL, Gamsu G, Webb WR, et al. Tree-in-bud pattern: frequency and significance on thin section CT. *J Comput Assist Tomogr*. 1996;20:594–599.

Arakawa H, Webb WR. Expiratory high-resolution CT scan. *Radiol Clin North Am*. 1998;36:189–209.

Austin JH, Müller NL, Friedman PJ, et al. Glossary of terms for CT of the lungs: recommendations of the nomenclature committee of the Fleischner Society. *Radiology*. 1996;200:327–331.

Azizzadeh A, Keyhani K, Miller CC 3rd, et al. Blunt traumatic aortic injury: initial experience with endovascular repair. *J Vasc Surg*. 2009;49:1403.

Bergin CJ, Müller NL. CT in the diagnosis of interstitial lung disease. *AJR Am J Roentgenol*. 1985;145:505–510.

Brauner MW, Grenier P, Mouelhi MM, et al. Pulmonary histiocytosis x: evaluation with high resolution CT. *Radiology*. 1989;172:255–258.

Bravo Soberon A, Torres Sanchez MI, Garcia Rio F, et al. High-resolution computed tomography patterns of organizing pneumonia [article in Spanish]. *Arch Bronconeumol*. 2006;42:413–416.

Bristow JD, Arai AE, Anselone CG, Pantely GA. Response to myocardial ischemia as a regulated process. *Circulation*. 1991;84:2580.

Caminati A, Cavazza A, Sverzellati N, et al. An integrated approach in the diagnosis of smoking-related interstitial lung disease. *Eur Respir Rev*. 2012;21:207–217.

Cerqueira MD, Weissman NJ, Dilsizian V, et al. Standardized myocardial segmentation and nomenclature for tomographic imaging of the heart: a statement for healthcare professionals from the cardiac imaging committee of the council on clinical cardiology of the American Heart Association. *Circulation*. 2002;105:539–542.

Chen D, Webb WR, Storto ML, et al. Assessment of air trapping using postexpiratory high-resolution computed tomography. *J Thorac Imaging*. 1998;13:135–143.

Churton T. Multiple aneurysms of the pulmonary artery. *Br Med J*. 1897;1:1223.

Colby TV, Swensen SJ. Anatomic distribution and histopathologic patterns in diffuse lung disease: correlation with HRCT. *J Thorac Imaging*. 1996;11:1–26.

Dodd JD, Souza CA, Müller NL. High-resolution MDCT of pulmonary septic embolism: evaluation of the feeding vessel sign. *AJR Am J Roentgenol*. 2006;187:623–629.

Eisenberg RL, Fleischner S. Ways to improve radiologists' adherence to Fleischner Society guidelines for management of pulmonary nodules. *J Am Coll Radiol*. 2013;10(6):439–441.

Falconer MA, Weddell G. Costoclavicular compression of the subclavian artery and vein. *Lancet*. 1943;2:539.

Feurestein IM, Archer A, Pluda JM, et al. Thin-walled cavities, cysts, and pneumothorax in *Pneumocystis carinii* pneumonia: further observations with histopathologic correlation. *Radiology.* 1990;174:697–702.
Franquet T, Giménez A, Bordes R, et al. The crazy-paving pattern in exogenous lipoid pneumonia: CT-pathologic correlation. *AJR Am J Roentgenol.* 1998;170: 315–317.
Fraser RS, Müller NL, Colman N, Paré PD. Pulmonary hypertension and edema. In: Fraser RS, Müller NL, Colman N, Paré PD, eds. *Diagnosis of Diseases of the Chest.* Philadelphia: Saunders; 1999:1935–1937.
Gaeta M, Volta S, Stroscio S, et al. CT "halo sign" in pulmonary tuberculoma. *J Comput Assist Tomogr.* 1992;16:827–828.
García Mónaco R, Bertoni H, Pallota G, et al. Use of self-expanding vascular endoprostheses in superior vena cava syndrome. *Eur J Cardiothorac Surg.* 2003;24:208.
Genereux GP. The end-stage lung: pathogenesis, pathology, and radiology. *Radiology.* 1975;116:279–289.
Genereux GP. The Fleischner lecture: computed tomography of diffuse pulmonary disease. *J Thorac Imaging.* 1989;4:50–87.
Gerber BL, Wijns W, Vanoverschelde JL, et al. Myocardial perfusion and oxygen consumption in reperfused noninfarcted dysfunctional myocardium after unstable angina: direct evidence for myocardial stunning in humans. *J Am Coll Cardiol.* 1999;34:1939.
Goldberg JB, Kim JB, Sundt TM. Current understandings and approach to the management of aortic intramural hematomas. *Semin Thorac Cardiovasc Surg.* 2014;26:123–131.
Goodman LR, Golkow RS, Steiner RM, et al. The right mid-lung window. *Radiology.* 1982;143:135–138.
Görich J, Rilinger N, Sokiranski R, et al. Treatment of leaks after endovascular repair of aortic aneurysms. *Radiology.* 2000;215:414.
Gotway MB, Lee ES, Reddy GP, et al. Low-dose, dynamic, expiratory thin-section CT of the lungs using a spiral CT scanner. *J Thorac Imaging.* 2000;15:168–172.
Grenier P, Maurice F, Musset D, et al. Bronchiectasis: assessment by thin-section CT. *Radiology.* 1986;161:95–99.
Grenier P, Valeyre D, Cluzel P, et al. Chronic diffuse interstitial lung disease: diagnostic value of chest radiography and high-resolution CT. *Radiology.* 1991;179:123–132.
Gruden JF, Webb WR, Naidich DP, et al. Multinodular disease: anatomic localization at thin-section CT—multireader evaluation of a simple algorithm. *Radiology.* 1999;210:711–720.
Gruden JF, Webb WR, Warnock M. Centrilobular opacities in the lung on high-resolution CT: diagnostic considerations and pathologic correlation. *AJR Am J Roentgenol.* 1994;162:569–574.
Gruden JF, Webb WR. Identification and evaluation of centrilobular opacities on high-resolution CT. *Semin Ultrasound CT MR.* 1995;16:435–449.
Hansell DM, Bankier AA, MacMahon H, et al. Fleischner Society: glossary of terms for thoracic imaging. *Radiology.* 2008;246:697–722.
Heitzman ER, Markarian B, Berger I, et al. The secondary pulmonary lobule: a practical concept for interpretation of radiographs. I. roentgen anatomy of the normal secondary pulmonary lobule. *Radiology.* 1969;93:507–512.
Heuvelmans MA, Oudkerk M. Management of subsolid pulmonary nodules in CT lung cancer screening. *J Thorac Dis.* 2015;7:1103–1106.
Hiratzka LF, Bakris GL, Beckman JA, et al. 2010 ACCF/AHA/AATS/ACR/ASA/SCA/SCAI/SIR/STS/SVM guidelines for the diagnosis and management of patients with thoracic aortic disease: a report of the American College of Cardiology Foundation/American Heart Association Task Force on Practice Guidelines, American Association for Thoracic Surgery, American College of Radiology, American Stroke Association, Society of Cardiovascular Anesthesiologists, Society for Cardiovascular Angiography and Interventions, Society of Interventional Radiology, Society of Thoracic Surgeons, and Society for Vascular Medicine. *Circulation.* 2010;121:e266–e369.
Hoeper MM, Bogaard HJ, Condliffe R, et al. Definitions and diagnosis of pulmonary hypertension. *J Am Coll Cardiol.* 2013;62:D42.
Hogg JC. Benjamin felson lecture. Chronic interstitial lung disease of unknown cause: a new classification based on pathogenesis. *AJR Am J Roentgenol.* 1991;156:225–233.
Hruban RH, Meziane MA, Zerhouni EA, et al. Radiologic-pathologic correlation of the CT halo sign in invasive pulmonary aspergillosis. *J Comput Assist Tomogr.* 1987;11:534–536.
Im JG, Itoh H, Shim YS, et al. Pulmonary tuberculosis: CT findings—early active disease and sequential change with antituberculous therapy. *Radiology.* 1993;186:653–660.
Itoh H, Murata K, Konishi J, et al. Diffuse lung disease: pathologic basis for the high-resolution computed tomography findings. *J Thorac Imaging.* 1993;8:176–188.
Johkoh T, Itoh H, Müller NL, et al. Crazy-paving appearance at thin-section CT: spectrum of disease and pathologic findings. *Radiology.* 1999;211:155–160.
Johkoh T, Müller NL, Ichikado K, et al. Perilobular pulmonary opacities: high-resolution CT findings and pathologic correlation. *J Thorac Imaging.* 1999;14:172–177.
Juan YH, Chatzizisis YS, Saboo SS, Newburger JW, Steigner ML. Hypoplastic left coronary artery with large collateral vessels from an ectatic right coronary artery: multimodality imaging-based diagnostic work-up. *Int J Cardiol.* 2014;172(3):e396–e397.
Juan YH, Saboo SS, Desai NS, Khandelwal K, Khandelwal A. Aortic intramural hematoma and hepatic artery pseudoaneurysm: unusual complication following resuscitation. *Am J Emerg Med.* 2014;32:107, e1–4.
Juan YH, Saboo SS, Keraliya A, Khandelwal A. Coronary strictures, intraluminal thrombus and aneurysms: unreported imaging appearance of ALCAPA syndrome post Takeuchi procedure. *Int J Cardiol.* 2015;186:291–293.
Juan YH, Saboo SS, Lin YC, Conner JR, Jacobson FL, Khandelwal A. Reverse halo sign in pulmonary mucormyosis. *QJM.* 2014;107:777–778.
Kalender WA, Fichte H, Bautz W, et al. Semiautomatic evaluation procedures for quantitative CT of the lung. *J Comput Assist Tomogr.* 1991;15:248–255.
Kalender WA, Rienmuller R, Seissler W, et al. Measurement of pulmonary parenchymal attenuation: use of spirometric gating with quantitative CT. *Radiology.* 1990;175:265–268.
Kemper AC, Steinberg KP, Stern EJ. Pulmonary interstitial emphysema: CT findings. *AJR Am J Roentgenol.* 1999;172:1642.
Kim SJ, Lee KS, Ryu YH, et al. Reversed halo sign on high-resolution CT of cryptogenic organizing pneumonia: diagnostic implications. *AJR Am J Roentgenol.* 2003;180:1251–1254.
Kitai T, Kaji S, Yamamuro A, et al. Impact of new development of ulcer-like projection on clinical outcomes in patients with type B aortic dissection with closed and thrombosed false lumen. *Circulation.* 2010;122: S74–S80.
Kuriyama K, Seto M, Kasugai T, et al. Ground-glass opacity on thin-section CT: value in differentiating subtypes of adenocarcinoma of the lung. *AJR Am J Roentgenol.* 1999;173:465–469.
Landing BH, Dixon LG. Congenital malformations and genetic disorders of the respiratory tract (larynx, trachea, bronchi, and lungs). *Am Rev Respir Dis.* 1979;120:151.
Lee JH, Park CM, Lee SM, Kim H, McAdams HP, Goo JM. Persistent pulmonary subsolid nodules with solid portions of 5 mm or smaller: their natural course and predictors of interval growth. *Eur Radiol.* 2016;26:1529–1537.
Lee KS, Primack SL, Staples CA, et al. Chronic infiltrative lung disease: comparison of diagnostic accuracies of radiography and low- and conventional-dose thin-section CT. *Radiology.* 1994;191:669–673.
Lee WA, Matsumura JS, Mitchell RS, et al. Endovascular repair of traumatic thoracic aortic injury: clinical practice guidelines of the Society for Vascular Surgery. *J Vasc Surg.* 2011;53:187.
Leipsic J, Abbara S, Achenbach S, et al. SCCT guidelines for the interpretation and reporting of coronary CT angiography: a report of the Society of Cardiovascular Computed Tomography guidelines committee. *J Cardiovasc Comput Tomogr.* 2014;8:342–358.
Lenoir S, Grenier P, Brauner MW, et al. Pulmonary lymphangiomyomatosis and tuberous sclerosis: comparison of radiographic and thin-section CT findings. *Radiology.* 1990;175:329–334.
Leung AN, Miller RR, Müller NL. Parenchymal opacification in chronic infiltrative lung diseases: CT-pathologic correlation. *Radiology.* 1993;188:209–214.
Liu H, Juan YH, Chen J, et al. Anomalous origin of one pulmonary artery branch from the aorta: role of MDCT angiography. *AJR Am J Roentgenol.* 2015;204:979–987.
Lucidarme O, Coche E, Cluzel P, et al. Expiratory CT scans for chronic airway disease: correlation with pulmonary function test results. *AJR Am J Roentgenol.* 1998;170:301–307.
Lynch DA, Gamsu G, Ray CS, et al. Asbestos-related focal lung masses: manifestations on conventional and high-resolution CT scans. *Radiology.* 1988;169: 603–607.
MacMahon H. Compliance with Fleischner Society guidelines for management of lung nodules: lessons and opportunities. *Radiology.* 2010;255:14–15.
Maisch B, Seferović PM, Ristić AD, et al. Guidelines on the diagnosis and management of pericardial diseases executive summary; the task force on the diagnosis and management of pericardial diseases of the European Society of Cardiology. *Eur Heart J.* 2004;25:587–610.
Majurin ML, Valavaara R, Varpula M, et al. Low-dose and conventional-dose high resolution CT of pulmonary changes in breast cancer patients treated by tangential field radiotherapy. *Eur J Radiol.* 1995;20:114–119.
Martin KW, Sagel SS, Siegel BA. Mosaic oligemia simulating pulmonary infiltrates on CT. *AJR Am J Roentgenol.* 1986;147:670–673.
Mayo JR, Webb WR, Gould R, et al. High-resolution CT of the lungs: an optimal approach. *Radiology.* 1987;163:507–510.
Miller WS. *The Lung.* Springfield, IL: Charles C Thomas; 1947:203.
Moore AD, Godwin JD, Müller NL, et al. Pulmonary histiocytosis x: comparison of radiographic and CT findings. *Radiology.* 1989;172:249–254.
Müller NL, Chiles C, Kullnig P. Pulmonary lymphangiomyomatosis: correlation of CT with radiographic and functional findings. *Radiology.* 1990;175: 335–339.
Müller NL, Miller RR. Diseases of the bronchioles: CT and histopathologic findings. *Radiology.* 1995;196:3–12.
Müller NL, Staples CA, Miller RR, et al. Disease activity in idiopathic pulmonary fibrosis: CT and pathologic correlation. *Radiology.* 1987;165:731–734.
Munk PL, Müller NL, Miller RR, et al. Pulmonary lymphangitic carcinomatosis: CT and pathologic findings. *Radiology.* 1988;166:705–709.
Murata K, Herman PG, Khan A, et al. Intralobular distribution of oleic acid-induced pulmonary edema in the pig: evaluation by high-resolution CT. *Invest Radiol.* 1989;24:647–653.
Murata K, Itoh H, Todo G, et al. Centrilobular lesions of the lung: demonstration by high-resolution CT and pathologic correlation. *Radiology.* 1986;161:641–645.

Murata K, Khan A, Herman PG. Pulmonary parenchymal disease: evaluation with high-resolution CT. *Radiology*. 1989;170:629–635.

Murayama S, Murakami J, Yabuuchi H, et al. Crazy paving appearance on high resolution CT in various diseases. *J Comput Assist Tomogr*. 1999;23:749–752.

Murch CR, Carr DH. Computed tomography appearances of pulmonary alveolar proteinosis. *Clin Radiol*. 1989;40:240–243.

Murphy JB. Cervical rib excision: collective review on surgery of cervical rib. *Clin John B Murphy*. 1916;5:227.

Nagpal P, Khandelwal A, Saboo SS, Bathla G, Steigner ML, Rybicki FJ. Modern imaging techniques: applications in the management of acute aortic pathologies. *Postgrad Med J*. 2015;91(1078):449–462.

Nagpal P, Saboo SS, Khandelwal A, Duran-Mendicuti MA, Abbara S, Steigner ML. Traumatic right atrial pseudoaneurysm. *Cardiovasc Diagn Ther*. 2015;5:141–144.

Naidich DP. High-resolution computed tomography of cystic lung disease. *Semin Roentgenol*. 1991;26:151–174.

Naidich DP, Bankier AA, MacMahon H, et al. Recommendations for themanagement of subsolid pulmonary nodules detected at CT: a statement from the Fleischner Society. *Radiology*. 2013;266(1):304–317.

Naidich DP, McCauley DI, Khouri NF, et al. Computed tomography of bronchiectasis. *J Comput Assist Tomogr*. 1982;6:437–444.

Naidich DP, Zerhouni EA, Hutchins GM, et al. Computed tomography of the pulmonary parenchyma: part 1. Distal air-space disease. *J Thorac Imaging*. 1985;1:39–53.

Nguyen ET, Silva CI, Seely JM, Chong S, Lee KS, Müller NL. Pulmonary artery aneurysms and pseudoaneurysms in adults: findings at CT and radiography. *AJR Am J Roentgenol*. 2007;188:W126–W134.

Ochsner A, Gage M, DeBakey M. Scalenus anticus (Naffziger) syndrome. *Am J Surg*. 1935;28:669–695.

Osborne DR, Effmann EL, Hedlund LW. Postnatal growth and size of the pulmonary acinus and secondary lobule in man. *AJR Am J Roentgenol*. 1983;140: 449–454.

Primack SL, Hartman TE, Hansell DM, et al. End-stage lung disease: CT findings in 61 patients. *Radiology*. 1993;189:681–686.

Primack SL, Hartman TE, Lee KS, et al. Pulmonary nodules and the CT halo sign. *Radiology*. 1994;190:513–515.

Raad RA, Suh J, Harari S, Naidich DP, Shiau M, Ko JP. Nodule characterization: subsolid nodules. *Radiol Clin North Am*. 2014;52:47–67.

Rajiah P, Desai MY, Kwon D, Flamm SD. MR imaging of myocardial infarction. *Radiographics*. 2013;33(5):1383–1412.

Raskin SP. The pulmonary acinus: historical notes. *Radiology*. 1982;144:31–34.

Reid L. The secondary pulmonary lobule in the adult human lung, with special reference to its appearance in bronchograms. *Thorax*. 1958;13:110–115.

Reid L, Simon G. The peripheral pattern in the normal bronchogram and its relation to peripheral pulmonary anatomy. *Thorax*. 1958;13:103–109.

Remy-Jardin M, Beuscart R, Sault MC, et al. Subpleural micronodules in diffuse infiltrative lung diseases: evaluation with thin-section CT scans. *Radiology*. 1990;177:133–139.

Remy-Jardin M, Degreef JM, Beuscart R, et al. Coal worker's pneumoconiosis: CT assessment in exposed workers and correlation with radiographic findings. *Radiology*. 1990;177:363–371.

Remy-Jardin M, Giraud F, Remy J, et al. Importance of ground-glass attenuation in chronic diffuse infiltrative lung disease: pathologic-CT correlation. *Radiology*. 1993;189:693–698.

Remy-Jardin M, Remy J, Deffontaines C, et al. Assessment of diffuse infiltrative lung disease: comparison of conventional CT and high-resolution CT. *Radiology*. 1991;181:157–162.

Remy-Jardin M, Remy J, Giraud F, et al. Computed tomography assessment of ground-glass opacity: semiology and significance. *J Thorac Imaging*. 1993;8: 249–264.

Remy-Jardin M, Remy J, Wallaert B, et al. Subacute and chronic bird breeder hypersensitivity pneumonitis: sequential evaluation with CT and correlation with lung function tests and bronchoalveolar lavage. *Radiology*. 1993;198:111–118.

Ren H, Hruban RH, Kuhlman JE, et al. Computed tomography of inflation-fixed lungs: the beaded septum sign of pulmonary metastases. *J Comput Assist Tomogr*. 1989;13:411–416.

Ridge CA, Hobbs BD, Bukoye BA, et al. Incidentally detected lung nodules: clinical predictors of adherence to Fleischner Society surveillance guidelines. *J Comput Assist Tomogr*. 2014;38:89–95.

Robinson TE, Leung AN, Moss RB, et al. Standardized high-resolution CT of the lung using a spirometer-triggered electron beam CT scanner. *AJR Am J Roentgenol*. 1999;172:1636–1638.

Saboo SS, Juan YH, Khandelwal A, George E, Steigner ML, Landzberg M. Rybick FJ. MDCT of congenital coronary artery fistulas. *AJR Am J Roentgenol*. 2014;203(3):W244–W252.

Sanders RJ, Hammond SL, Rao NM. Diagnosis of thoracic outlet syndrome. *J Vasc Surg*. 2007;46:601.

Sloan RD, Cooley RN. Congenital pulmonary arteriovenous aneurysm. *Am J Roentgenol Radium Ther Nucl Med*. 1953;70:183.

Smyth PT, Edwards JE. Pseudocoarctation, kinking or buckling of the aorta. *Circulation*. 1972;46:1027–1032.

Snider GL. Interstitial pulmonary fibrosis. *Chest*. 1986;89(suppl):115–121.

Snider GL. Pathogenesis and terminology of emphysema. *Am J Respir Crit Care Med*. 1994;149:1382–1383.

Snider GL, Kleinerman J, Thurlbeck WM, et al. The definition of emphysema: report of a National Heart, Lung, and Blood Institute, division of lung diseases workshop. *Am Rev Respir Dis*. 1985;132:182–185.

Spodick DH. Pericardial diseases. In: Braunwald E, Zipes DP, Libby P, eds. *Heart Disease: A Textbook of Cardiovascular Medicine*. Vol. 2. 6th ed. Philadelphia: Saunders; 2001:1823–1876.

Stein MG, Mayo J, Müller N, et al. Pulmonary lymphangitic spread of carcinoma: appearance on CT scans. *Radiology*. 1987;162:371–375.

Stern EJ, Webb WR. Dynamic imaging of lung morphology with ultrafast high-resolution computed tomography. *J Thorac Imaging*. 1993;8:273–282.

Stern EJ, Webb WR, Gamsu G. Dynamic quantitative computed tomography: a predictor of pulmonary function in obstructive lung diseases. *Invest Radiol*. 1994;29:564–569.

Stern EJ, Webb WR, Weinacker A, et al. Idiopathic giant bullous emphysema (vanishing lung syndrome): imaging findings in nine patients. *AJR Am J Roentgenol*. 1994;162:279–282.

Thurlbeck WM. *Chronic Airflow Obstruction in Lung Disease*. Philadelphia: Saunders; 1976.

Tuddenham WJ. Glossary of terms for thoracic radiology: recommendations of the nomenclature committee of the Fleischner Society. *AJR Am J Roentgenol*. 1984;143:509–517.

Ujita M, Renzoni EA, Veeraraghavan S, et al. Organizing pneumonia: perilobular pattern at thin-section CT. *Radiology*. 2004;232:757–761.

Uyama T, Monden Y, Harada K, et al. Pulmonary varices: a case report and review of the literature. *Jpn J Surg*. 1988;18(3):359–362.

Webb WR. High-resolution CT of the lung parenchyma. *Radiol Clin North Am*. 1989;27:1085–1097.

Webb WR. High-resolution computed tomography of obstructive lung disease. *Radiol Clin North Am*. 1994;32:745–757.

Webb WR. Radiology of obstructive pulmonary disease. *AJR Am J Roentgenol*. 1997;169:637–647.

Webb WR. Thin-section CT of the secondary pulmonary lobule: anatomy and the image—the 2004 Fleischner lecture. *Radiology*. 2006;239:322–338.

Webb WR, Müller NL, Naidich DP. Standardized terms for high-resolution computed tomography of the lung: a proposed glossary. *J Thorac Imaging*. 1993;8:167–175.

Webb WR, Stein MG, Finkbeiner WE, et al. Normal and diseased isolated lungs: high-resolution CT. *Radiology*. 1988;166:81–87.

Webb WR, Stern EJ, Kanth N, Gamsu G. Dynamic pulmonary CT: findings in healthy adult men. *Radiology*. 1993;186:117–124.

Weibel ER. Looking into the lung: what can it tell us? *AJR Am J Roentgenol*. 1979;133:1021–1031.

Weibel ER, Taylor CR. Design and structure of the human lung. In: Fishman AP, eds. *Pulmonary Diseases and Disorders*. 2nd ed. New York: McGraw-Hill; 1988:11–60.

Westcott JL, Cole SR. Traction bronchiectasis in end-stage pulmonary fibrosis. *Radiology*. 1986;161:665–669.

Worthy SA, Müller NL. Small airway diseases. *Radiol Clin North Am*. 1998;36:163–173.

Wright IS. The neurovascular syndrome produced by hyperabduction of the arms. The immediate changes produced in 150 normal controls, and the effects on same persons of prolonged hyperabduction of the arms, as in sleeping, and in certain occupations. *Am Heart J*. 1945;29:1.

Wright JL, Tazelaar HD, Churg A. Fibrosis with emphysema. *Histopathology*. 2011;58:517–524.

Wu MT, Wang YC, Huang YL, et al. Intramural blood pools accompanying aortic intramural hematoma: CT appearance and natural course. *Radiology*. 2011;258:705–713.

Xanthos T, Giannakopoulos N, Papadimitriou L. Lipomatous hypertrophy of the interatrial septum: a pathological and clinical approach. *Int J Cardiol*. 2007;121:4–8.

Yoshimura H, Hatakeyama M, Otsuji H, et al. Pulmonary asbestosis: CT study of subpleural curvilinear shadow. Work in progress. *Radiology*. 1986;158:653–658.

Zerhouni E. Computed tomography of the pulmonary parenchyma: an overview. *Chest*. 1989;95:901–907.

Zerhouni EA, Naidich DP, Stitik FP, et al. Computed tomography of the pulmonary parenchyma: part 2. Interstitial disease. *J Thorac Imaging*. 1985;1:54–64.

Zompatori M, Poletti V, Battista G, et al. Bronchiolitis obliterans with organizing pneumonia (BOOP), presenting as a ring-shaped opacity at HRCT (the atoll sign). A case report. *Radiol Med (Torino)*. 1999;97:308–310.

Zwirewich CV, Mayo JR, Müller NL. Low-dose high-resolution CT of lung parenchyma. *Radiology*. 1991;180:413–417.

CHAPTER 14

Differential Diagnosis Based on Imaging Findings

Adam Bernheim, Carol C. Wu, and Subba R. Digumarthy

CHAPTER OUTLINE

■ Air Space Disease

Acute Consolidation

Air space consolidation results when alveoli are filled with material that attenuates the x-ray beam more than the surrounding lung parenchyma. When encountered in the acute setting, air space consolidation on imaging has a differential diagnosis (Table 14.1).

Chronic Consolidation

When air space consolidation persists on imaging studies over several weeks to months, the differential diagnosis shifts away from pneumonia, which typically has a more acute presentation, with subsequent resolution. Infectious, inflammatory, and neoplastic causes should be considered when chronic air space consolidation is encountered (Fig. 14.1), and the most common entities are outlined in Table 14.2.

■ Pulmonary Nodules

Solitary Pulmonary Nodule

The differential diagnosis of a solitary pulmonary nodule on chest radiography or CT is broad, but more than 95% of the time the nodule is an infectious granuloma (Fig. 14.2), malignant neoplasm (primary or metastatic), or benign tumor (e.g., a hamartoma). Nodule size, shape, density, calcification pattern, degree of contrast enhancement, fluorodeoxyglucose (FDG) avidity, and rate of growth are key imaging characteristics that when combined with clinical factors (e.g., patient age, immune status, clinical history) help narrow the differential diagnosis. Ultimately, this combination of factors may indicate a

TABLE 14.1 Differential Diagnosis of Acute Consolidation

DIAGNOSIS	COMMENTS
Infectious pneumonia	Alveoli are filled with pus or inflammatory fluid; fever and leukocytosis are often present
Aspiration of gastric contents	There is a predilection for gravity-dependent lung segments; Mendelson syndrome refers to chemical pneumonitis from aspiration during obstetric anesthesia
Alveolar pulmonary edema	Cardiomegaly and pleural effusions may be present; acute respiratory distress syndrome may be considered in severe cases
Pulmonary hemorrhage	Consider pulmonary contusion in the setting of trauma; there may be a history of anticoagulation or bleeding diathesis
Pulmonary infarction	Risk factors for pulmonary embolism are present; consolidation is peripheral and is more likely in the lower lobes

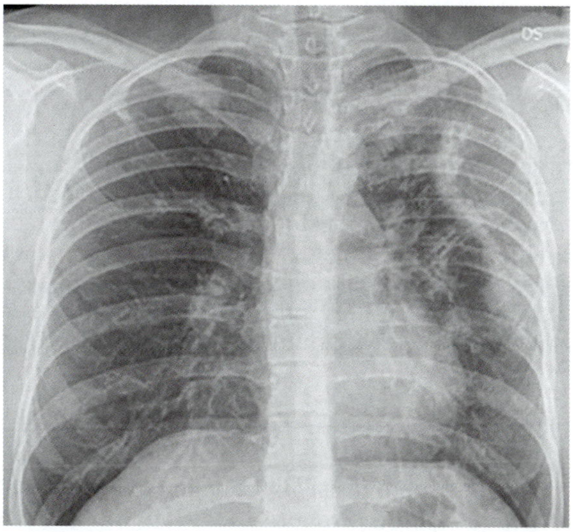

Figure 14.1 Frontal chest radiograph of a 33-year-old woman with chronic eosinophilic pneumonia demonstrates focal peripheral air space consolidation in the left upper lung zone, which persisted on multiple studies.

TABLE 14.2 Differential Diagnosis of Chronic Consolidation

DIAGNOSIS	COMMENTS
Organizing pneumonia	Reverse halo sign seen in up to 20%; consolidation typically responds to steroid therapy
Chronic eosinophilic pneumonia	Often elevated eosinophils in bronchoalveolar lavage fluid and peripheral blood; upper lobe predominant consolidation; typically responds to steroid therapy
Poorly treated infection	May be due to suboptimal antibiotic choice or resistance; also consider fungal and mycobacterial infection
Adenocarcinoma	Air bronchograms may be seen
Sarcoidosis	Confluent granulomatous nodules may mimic consolidation
Lymphoma	Usually derived from bronchus-associated lymphoid tissue; air bronchograms may be seen
Lipoid pneumonia	Demonstrates areas of fat attenuation; generally indolent course
Churg-Strauss syndrome	Nearly all patients have asthma and eosinophilia

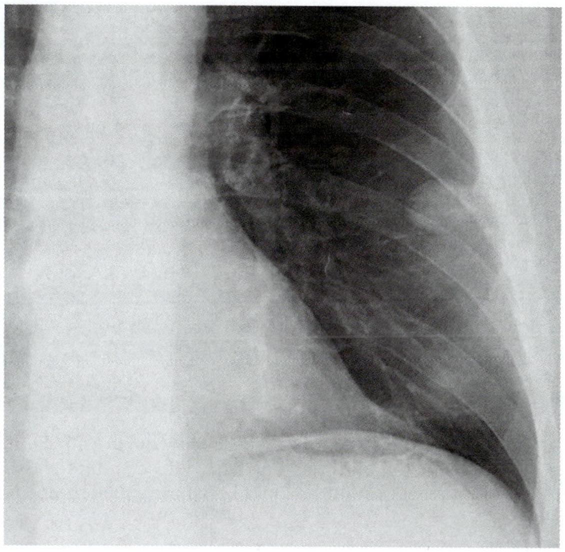

Figure 14.2 Coned down frontal chest radiograph of a 70-year-old man with malaise and fatigue reveals a solitary, well-circumscribed pulmonary nodule overlying the lateral left middle lung zone. Surgical resection and pathologic analysis demonstrated the nodule to be a histoplasmoma.

nodule's likelihood of benignity versus malignancy or even provide a specific diagnosis. There are many possible causes of a solitary pulmonary nodule (Table 14.3).

Multiple Pulmonary Nodules

Centrilobular Distribution

Diseases that involve the centrilobular bronchioles, pulmonary arterioles, or lymphatics may produce multiple centrilobular nodules. These nodules characteristically are evenly spaced from one another and spare the interlobular septa and pleural surfaces (Fig. 14.3). Nodules in this distribution may be solid or of ground-glass attenuation, and the most common entities producing this pattern are outlined in Table 14.4. If the nodules are branching, with a V or Y shape, it is termed a *tree-in-bud pattern.*

Perilymphatic Distribution

On CT imaging, diseases that involve the perilymphatic channels are typically subpleural and are along bronchovascular bundles, interlobular septae, and fissures. Unlike centrilobular nodules, nodules with a perilymphatic

TABLE 14.3 Differential Diagnosis of Solitary Pulmonary Nodule

DIAGNOSIS	COMMENTS
Granuloma	May be other calcified granulomas or calcified lymph nodes; likelihood dependent on where patient has lived (far more common in Midwestern United States)
Lung cancer	Calcification seen in 6%–7%; most lung cancers double in volume every 1–18 months
Metastasis	Patients with melanoma, testicular cancer, or sarcoma more likely to have a solitary metastasis than primary lung cancer
Intrapulmonary lymph node	Often found along fissures or in a subpleural location; morphology may be triangular, oval, round, or trapezoidal
Pulmonary nodule mimic	Consider clothing artifact (button), nipple shadow, skin or chest wall lesion, healing rib fracture, and enostosis in a rib
Hamartoma	Fat within a nodule nearly pathognomonic; popcorn calcification sometimes present
Pulmonary carcinoid	Location generally more central; can enhance avidly; high false-negative rate on FDG PET imaging
Infection (nongranulomatous)	Round pneumonia, septic embolus, or abscess
Mesenchymal or neural tumor	Consider fibroma, chondroma, lipoma, or neurofibroma
Arteriovenous malformation	Feeding artery and draining vein; multiple in hereditary hemorrhagic telangiectasia
Inflammatory nodule	Rheumatoid nodule or granulomatosis with polyangiitis

FDG, Fluorodeoxyglucose; *PET*, positron emission tomography.

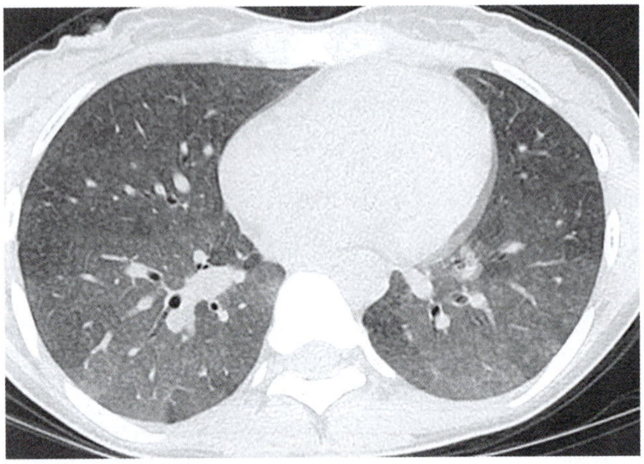

Figure 14.3 Axial CT scan of a 35-year-old woman with subacute hypersensitivity pneumonitis demonstrates diffuse ground-glass centrilobular nodules, with scattered areas of hypoattenuation due to air trapping.

distribution are generally unevenly spaced from one another. There are several diagnostic considerations for nodules with a perilymphatic distribution (Table 14.5).

Random Distribution

Multiple pulmonary nodules that are diffusely distributed and without architectural predominance—that is, lack a centrilobular or peribronchovascular distribution—are likely random. These nodules may be variable in number and density, and often the underlying pathophysiologic mechanism is hematogenous dissemination. There are several diagnoses to consider when pulmonary nodules are found to have a random distribution (Table 14.6).

Calcified Pulmonary Nodules

A variety of disease entities can present with multiple calcified pulmonary nodules, with causes that include neoplastic, infectious, metabolic, and inhalational factors (Fig. 14.4). Clinical history and the size, appearance, and distribution of the nodules can add specificity. The most common entities producing multiple calcified pulmonary nodules are outlined in Table 14.7.

Cavitary Pulmonary Nodules

A cavitary lung nodule usually contains air, but may also contain blood, pus, or debris. A cavitary nodule has a definite wall with thickness of at least 4 mm and should not be confused with a cyst, which is a thin-walled, air-containing lesion. Chest radiography may identify cavitary nodules, although CT offers increased sensitivity and provides improved lesion localization and characterization. There are several entities to consider when cavity pulmonary nodules are encountered (Table 14.8).

■ Pulmonary Masses

Anterior Mediastinal Masses

Because the anterior mediastinum houses the thymus, lymph nodes, vessels, and fat, masses that arise in this space originate from these structures. These masses may be recognized as mediastinal widening on a frontal radiograph or as loss of the retrosternal clear space on a lateral radiograph, but they are best evaluated on

TABLE 14.4 Differential Diagnosis of Multiple Nodules With Centrilobular Distribution

DIAGNOSIS	COMMENTS
Hypersensitivity pneumonitis	Ground-glass nodules; exposure to organic antigen identified in 50%; air trapping usually present
Respiratory bronchiolitis	Upper lobe predominant ground-glass nodules; history of cigarette smoking
Pulmonary arterial hypertension; pulmonary capillary hemangiomatosis; pulmonary veno-occlusive disease	Ground-glass nodules; due to pulmonary edema and/or hemorrhage; dilated main pulmonary trunk
Metastatic calcification	Upper lobe ground-glass nodules ± calcification; hypercalcemia
Endobronchial infection, bronchopneumonia	Solid or ground-glass ± tree-in-bud opacities; bacterial, viral, or fungal causes
Follicular bronchiolitis	Solid or ground-glass nodules ± tree-in-bud opacities; immunosuppression or connective tissue disease
Pneumoconioses	Solid centrilobular nodules; especially siderosis and coal workers' pneumoconiosis
Langerhans cell histiocytosis	Upper lobe predominant solid or ground-glass nodules; early in disease course; history of cigarette smoking

TABLE 14.5 Differential Diagnosis of Multiple Nodules With Perilymphatic Distribution

DIAGNOSIS	COMMENTS
Pulmonary sarcoidosis	Concomitant symmetric hilar and mediastinal lymph nodes; patients commonly between 20 and 40 years of age
Silicosis and coal workers' pneumoconiosis	Nodules range from 1–10 mm in diameter; nodules have an upper lobe and posterior distribution
Lymphangitic carcinomatosis	Adenocarcinoma (lung and breast) most common cause; associated pleural effusions are common
Nodular pulmonary amyloidosis	Patients usually in sixth decade of life and often asymptomatic; lower lobe and peripheral distribution often appreciated
Lymphocytic interstitial pneumonia	Associated with HIV (in children) and Sjögren syndrome; scattered thin-walled perivascular cysts often present

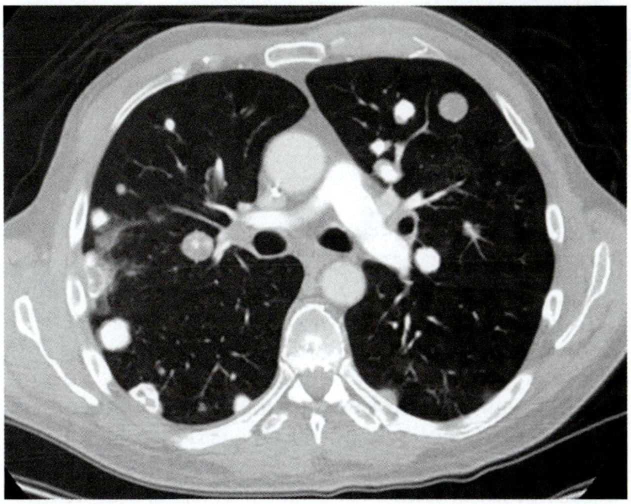

Figure 14.4 Axial CT scan of a 60-year-old man with chondrosarcoma metastases demonstrates multiple calcified pulmonary nodules.

TABLE 14.6 Differential Diagnosis of Multiple Nodules With Random Distribution

DIAGNOSIS	COMMENTS
Hematogenous metastases	Lower lobe predominance; metastases may be small in size, as from thyroid cancer, or may be large (cannonball), as from seminoma
Fungal infection	Can be miliary or larger; histoplasmosis, blastomycosis, and coccidioidomycosis; aspergillosis or zygomycosis in the immunocompromised
Miliary tuberculosis	May be seen in primary or postprimary infection; miliary nodules imply active infection and poor prognosis
Septic emboli	Peripheral and lower lobe predominance ± cavitation
Adenocarcinoma of lung	Rarely presents as multiple nodules in a random distribution
Rheumatoid necrobiotic nodules	Nodules wax and wane with rheumatoid arthritis activity; miliary nodularity occurs early, prior to pulmonary fibrosis
Amyloidosis	Nodules may cavitate and/or show calcification
Granulomatosis with polyangiitis	Nodules ± cavitation
Benign metastasizing leiomyoma	Often a history of hysterectomy for uterine leiomyomas; nodules enhance with contrast and may cavitate

cross-sectional imaging (Fig. 14.5). The most common masses arising in the anterior mediastinum are outlined in Table 14.9.

Middle Mediastinal Masses

The middle mediastinum is bounded by the thoracic inlet superiorly, the diaphragm inferiorly, the pericardium anteriorly, and the posterior tracheal wall (or, according to

TABLE 14.7 Differential Diagnosis of Multiple Calcified Pulmonary Nodules

DIAGNOSIS	COMMENTS
Chronic granulomatous disease	Tuberculosis and histoplasmosis most common; may be associated findings such as calcified lymph nodes
Metastatic disease	History of sarcoma or medullary thyroid cancer; mucinous adenocarcinoma metastases may calcify; treated choriocarcinoma metastases may calcify
Pneumoconioses	Particularly silicosis and coal workers' pneumoconiosis
Healed varicella pneumonia	Generally 2–3 mm in size; diffuse distribution
Pulmonary alveolar microlithiasis	Sandlike calcifications, often ≈1 mm in size; lower lobe predominant
Metastatic calcification	Upper lobe predominant; centrilobular ground-glass nodules; hypercalcemia
Pulmonary amyloidosis	May be associated with tracheobronchial amyloidosis
Multiple chondromas	One component of the Carney triad—paragangliomas, gastrointestinal stromal tumors, pulmonary chondromas

TABLE 14.8 Differential Diagnosis of Cavitary Pulmonary Nodules

DIAGNOSIS	COMMENTS
Pneumonia and lung abscess	Typically from *Staphylococcus aureus, Pseudomonas aeruginosa*, or *Klebsiella pneumoniae;* tuberculosis and fungal pneumonia also cavitate
Metastases	Usually a primary squamous or transitional cell carcinoma; nodules often have round, well-demarcated borders
Primary lung cancer	Squamous cell carcinoma most likely to cavitate; cavitation most likely when mass is >3 cm
Pulmonary emboli	Lower lobe and peripheral distribution; septic emboli cavitate more commonly than bland emboli
Granulomatosis with polyangiitis	Cavitation occurs in nearly 50% of patients with nodules; nodule size variable; may be associated with consolidation
Rheumatoid lung nodules	Occur in <1% of rheumatoid arthritis patients; more common in men and in upper and middle lung zones
Congenital lesions	Congenital pulmonary airway malformation; pulmonary sequestration

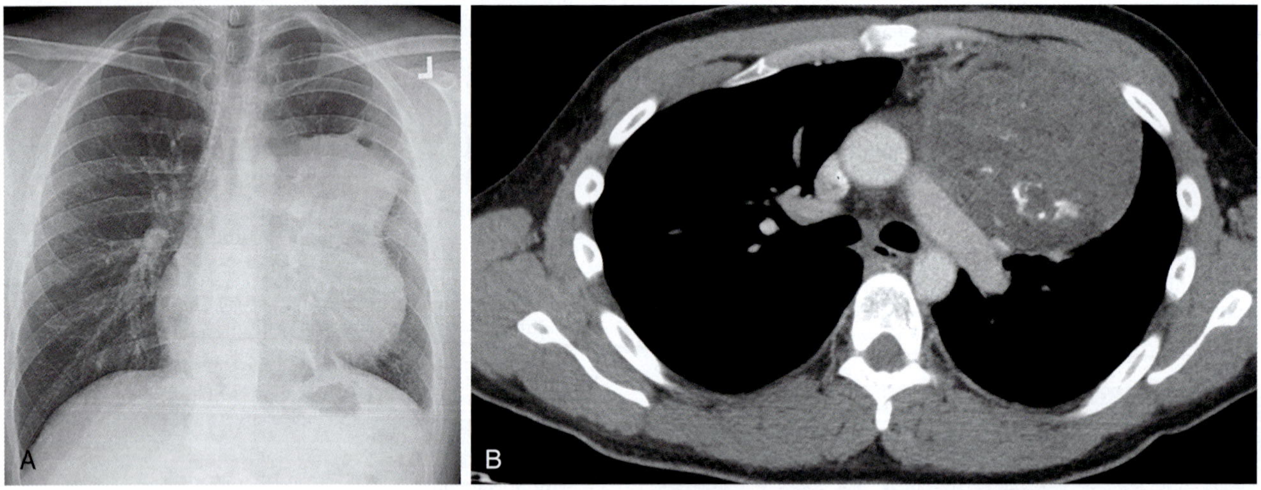

Figure 14.5 (A) Frontal chest radiograph of a 28-year-old man demonstrates a large mediastinal mass. (B) Axial CT scan demonstrates a large, heterogeneous, anterior mediastinal mass that contains foci of calcification and fat. Biopsy proved the mass to be an immature teratoma.

some authors, the esophagus) posteriorly. It contains the trachea, azygos vein, vena cavae, aortic arch, pulmonary vessels, lymph nodes, and (according to some authors) the esophagus. It also contains the phrenic, vagus, and left recurrent laryngeal nerves. Radiographic findings suggestive of a middle mediastinal mass include widening of the paratracheal stripe, convexity of the aortopulmonary window, displacement of the azygoesophageal recess to the right, and appearance of a left pseudoparavertebral line. Several masses arise in the middle mediastinum (Table 14.10).

Posterior Mediastinal Masses

Neurogenic tumors are the most common cause of a posterior mediastinal mass (Fig. 14.6), comprising 75% of primary posterior mediastinal neoplasms. Neurogenic tumors usually arise from peripheral nerves or sympathetic ganglia; the most likely tumor type is dependent on the patient's age. Nonneoplastic masses in the posterior mediastinum include esophageal masses, duplication cysts, paraspinal abscess, and other types, the most common of which are presented in Table 14.11.

TABLE 14.9 Differential Diagnosis of Anterior Mediastinal Mass

DIAGNOSIS	COMMENTS
Thymic masses	Thymoma, thymic carcinoma, thymolipoma, thymic cyst; rarely, thymic carcinoid or thymic lymphoma
Lymphoma or lymphadenopathy	Lymphoma more common in younger patients; adenopathy from metastases or granulomatous disease
Germ cell tumors	More likely to contain fat and/or calcification; more likely to maintain a midline anatomic position
Thyroid masses	Substernal thyroid goiter usually continuous with thyroid; thyroid adenoma and carcinoma less common
Vascular masses	Ascending aortic aneurysm
Congenital cysts	Bronchogenic cyst or lymphangioma
Neural tumors	Arise from vagus or phrenic nerve
Foramen of Morgagni hernia	Sometimes demonstrated on fluoroscopic studies

TABLE 14.10 Differential Diagnosis of Middle Mediastinal Mass

DIAGNOSIS	COMMENTS
Foregut duplication cyst	Includes esophageal duplication and bronchogenic cysts; usually contains simple fluid
Lymphoma or lymphadenopathy	Lymphoma more common in younger patients; adenopathy from metastases or granulomatous disease
Vascular abnormality	Aortic aneurysm may present as a middle mediastinal mass; right-sided aortic arch may appear as a "mass"
Hiatus hernia	May be sliding, paraesophageal, or mixed hernia; may be retrocardiac air-fluid level on chest radiography
Pulmonary artery enlargement	Seen in pulmonic stenosis or pulmonary artery hypertension
Pericardial cyst	May change in shape with inspiration and patient position; may be congenital or result from prior pericarditis
Tracheal lesions	Intrinsic and extrinsic lesions occupy middle mediastinum
Germ cell tumors	Rarely in middle mediastinum (more common anteriorly); often contain fat and/or calcification
Neural tumors	Arise from vagus, phrenic, or left recurrent laryngeal nerve

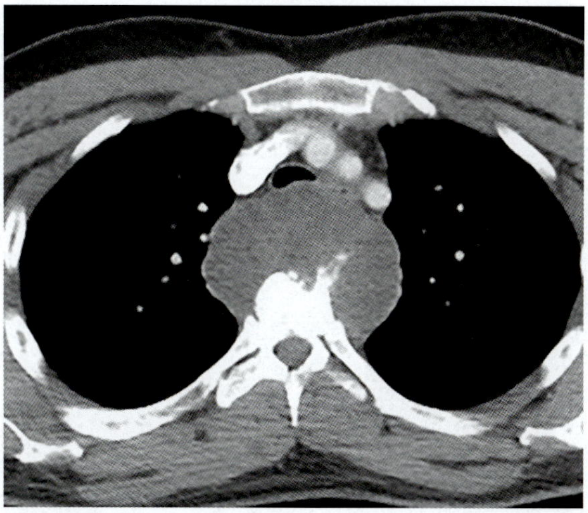

Figure 14.6 Axial CT scan of a 31-year-old man with neck and chest discomfort demonstrates a large posterior mediastinal soft tissue mass—in this case, a chordoma, extending from the thoracic vertebral column.

TABLE 14.11 Differential Diagnosis of Posterior Mediastinal Mass

DIAGNOSIS	COMMENTS
Neurogenic nerve sheath tumor	Schwannomas and neurofibromas are benign; malignant peripheral nerve sheath tumors in neurofibromatosis patients
Neurogenic sympathetic ganglion tumor	Neuroblastoma in young children; ganglioneuroma affects older children and young adults
Nonneurogenic tumor	Includes chordoma and pheochromocytoma
Descending aortic aneurysm	Vascular origin apparent on cross-sectional imaging
Esophageal mass	May be benign such as leiomyoma; malignancies include squamous cell carcinoma and adenocarcinoma
Paraspinal abscess	Bacterial, fungal, or tuberculous causes most common
Extramedullary hematopoiesis	History of hemoglobinopathy or bone marrow infiltration; smooth, lobulated, and often bilateral paraspinal masses
Lateral thoracic meningocele	75% of cases associated with neurofibromatosis; continuity of cerebrospinal fluid between meningocele and thecal sac
Duplication cyst	Neurenteric cyst or esophageal duplication cyst; usually fluid attenuation on CT unless infected or hemorrhagic
Lymphoma or lymphadenopathy	Usually accompanied by enlarged lymph nodes elsewhere

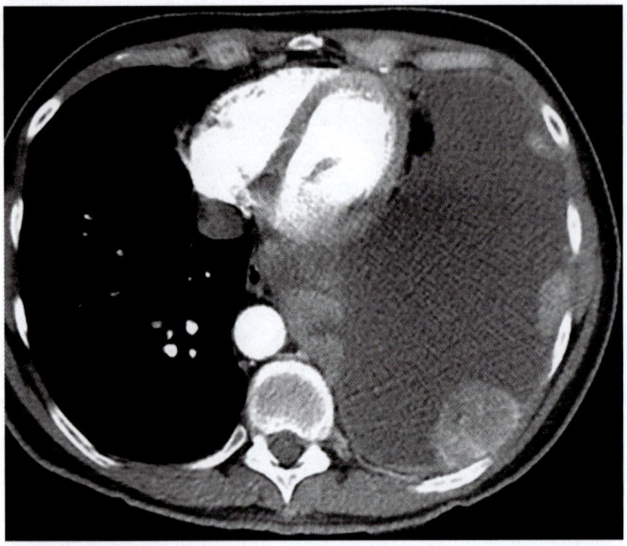

Figure 14.7 Axial CT scan of a 54-year-old man with malignant mesothelioma (mixed type) demonstrates a large left pleural effusion, with multiple enhancing solid pleural masses.

Pleural Masses

When a pleural mass is encountered, it is critical to delineate its location correctly as within the pleural space because this leads to a particular differential diagnosis. Imaging characteristics and clinical information can then be integrated to narrow the differential diagnosis. Chest radiography and CT are the standard modalities used for the evaluation of pleural masses (Fig. 14.7), but MRI plays a supplemental role. There are several diagnoses to consider when a mass has been localized to the pleural space (Table 14.12).

TABLE 14.12 Differential Diagnosis of Pleural Mass

DIAGNOSIS	COMMENTS
Metastatic pleural disease	Commonly adenocarcinoma (lung, breast, ovarian); common site for spread of invasive thymoma
Malignant mesothelioma	Calcified pleural plaques from asbestos often present; may invade chest wall, diaphragm, or mediastinum
Solitary fibrous tumor of pleura	May change position on serial studies if pedunculated; hypoglycemia and/or hypertrophic osteoarthropathy
Loculated pleural fluid (pseudotumor)	Pleural effusion, empyema, hemothorax
Pleural lipoma	Fat attenuation in well-defined, convex pleural mass; usually asymptomatic and incidentally discovered
Pleural lymphoma	Accounts for 0.3% of non-Hodgkin lymphoma cases; chronic pleural inflammation is risk factor
Chest wall mass invading pleural space	Examples: Askin tumor or Ewing sarcoma
Splenosis	History of trauma or surgery; demonstrates uptake on sulfur colloid scintigraphy

Cardiophrenic Angle Masses

The normal cardiophrenic angle is filled with a small amount of fat, but a number of disease entities, both superior and inferior to the diaphragm, are differential diagnostic considerations when a mass is identified in this location. When a cardiophrenic angle mass is discovered by conventional radiography, cross-sectional imaging with CT is valuable for narrowing the differential diagnosis or, in some cases, for identifying one specific diagnosis (Fig. 14.8). Several masses occur in the cardiophrenic angle (Table 14.13).

TABLE 14.13 Differential Diagnosis of Cardiophrenic Angle Mass

DIAGNOSIS	COMMENTS
Epicardial fat pad	More common in overweight patients; large fat pad associated with increased cardiovascular risk
Pericardial cyst	Fluid-filled lesion with well-defined borders and smooth wall; low signal on T1-weighted MRI and high signal on T2-weighted MRI
Morgagni hernia	More common on right side; presence of omental vessels confirms diagnosis on CT
Lymphadenopathy	As in the setting of lymphoma or metastatic disease
Pericardial fat necrosis	Benign idiopathic condition presents with pleuritic chest pain; more common on the left side
Thymic tumors	May be benign (thymolipoma) or malignant (thymoma)
Cardiophrenic space varices	Associated signs of portal hypertension are present

■ Thoracic Masses: Fat-Containing Masses

A fat-containing mass in the chest can sometimes be suggested by a somewhat diminished density on chest radiography, but CT and MRI can confirm the presence of fat within a mass. The definitive identification of fat within a thoracic mass is helpful because it suggests a particular differential diagnosis, which can be further narrowed based on lesion location, clinical information, and other imaging characteristics. There are several

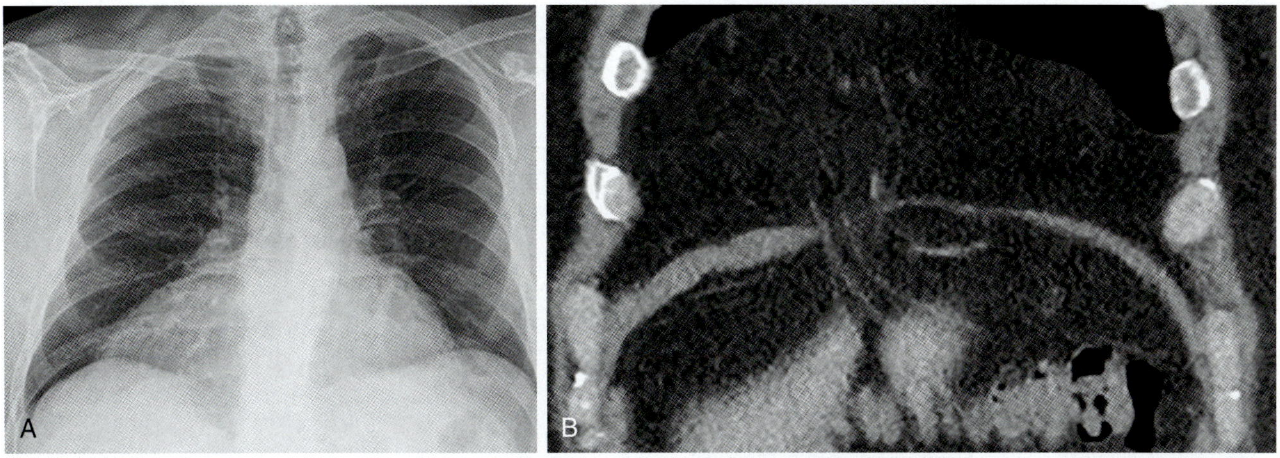

Figure 14.8 (A) Frontal chest radiograph of a 52-year-old man demonstrates a right cardiophrenic angle mass. (B) Coronal-reformatted CT scan demonstrates this patient to have a Morgagni diaphragmatic hernia.

fat-containing masses that are commonly encountered in the chest (Table 14.14).

TABLE 14.14 Differential Diagnosis of Fat-Containing Mass

DIAGNOSIS	COMMENTS
Pulmonary hamartoma	Accounts for 6% of pulmonary nodules; fat identified on CT in approximately 50% of cases
Lipoma	Well-circumscribed mesenchymal tumor from adipose tissue; mediastinal, pleural, cardiac, or intrapulmonary location
Teratoma	Heterogeneous mass often with fat and/or calcification; accounts for 15% of anterior mediastinal masses
Thymolipoma	2%–9% of all thymic neoplasms; appears on CT scan as fatty tissue admixed with thymic tissue
Diaphragmatic hernia	Abdominal fat within a Morgagni or Bochdalek hernia
Metastatic disease	Primary tumor may be liposarcoma or renal cell carcinoma
Lipoid pneumonia	Results from chronic aspiration of mineral or vegetable oils; association with neuromuscular or esophageal abnormalities
Mediastinal lipomatosis	Excessive unencapsulated mediastinal fat; associated with obesity and steroid administration
Extramedullary hematopoiesis	Posterior mediastinal (often bilateral paravertebral) location; may contain fat when underlying anemia has been treated
Liposarcoma	Rare primary mediastinal or cardiac tumor
Lipoblastoma	Rare tumor found in infancy and early childhood; mediastinal or paravertebral location

■ Lymphadenopathy

Calcified Lymphadenopathy

Although infectious granulomatous disease accounts for most incidentally detected calcified lymph nodes encountered on a routine basis, particularly in patients from endemic locations, there are several other causes of calcified lymph nodes that should be considered. Sarcoidosis, silicosis, treated lymphoma, and metastases from certain primary malignancies (Fig. 14.9) are among the additional possibilities. Combining the clinical history with other imaging findings will help the radiologist narrow the differential diagnosis when calcified lymph nodes are identified (Table 14.15).

Low-Attenuation Lymphadenopathy

When thoracic lymphadenopathy is of diminished attenuation, it is important to recognize because it suggests underlying intranodal necrosis or cystic degeneration, which is suggestive of certain diagnoses. It is also important for the radiologist to be aware of mimics of low-attenuation lymph nodes, which include fluid in pericardial recesses, mediastinal bronchogenic cysts, and cisterna chyli, which may mimic a posterior diaphragmatic lymph node. There are a number of entities to consider that produce low-attenuation lymph nodes in the chest (Table 14.16).

Bilateral Hilar Lymphadenopathy

When hilar lymph nodes that measure more than 10 mm in the short-axis dimension are discovered, it is important to assess whether these lymph nodes are unilateral,

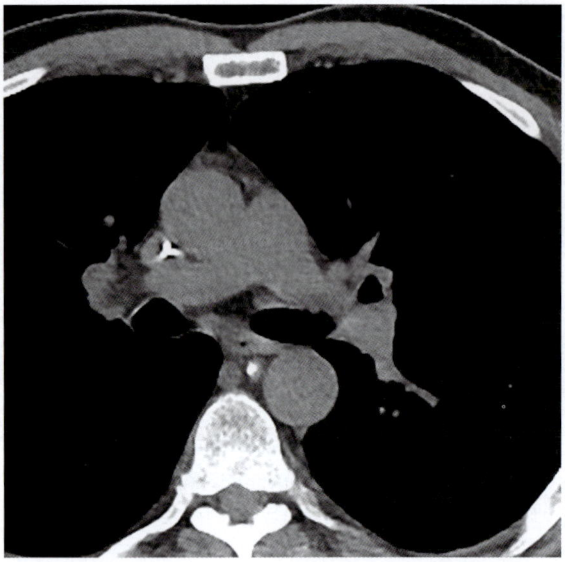

Figure 14.9 Axial CT scan of a 48-year-old man with rectal adenocarcinoma demonstrates a calcified metastatic lymph node.

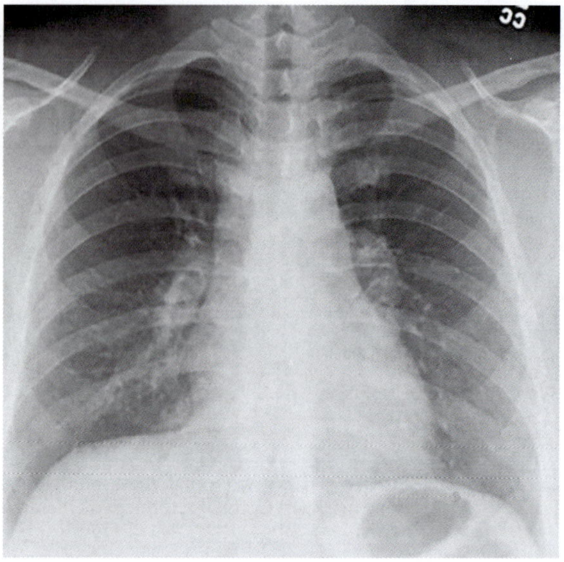

Figure 14.10 Frontal chest radiograph of a 29-year-old woman with sarcoidosis demonstrates bilateral symmetric hilar lymphadenopathy.

TABLE 14.15 Differential Diagnosis of Calcified Lymphadenopathy

DIAGNOSIS	COMMENTS
Granulomatous disease	Usually tuberculosis or histoplasmosis; calcifications often complete rather than focal
Sarcoidosis	Nodal calcification reported in up to 50% of patients; calcified lymph nodes rarely in eggshell pattern
Silicosis	Calcified lymph nodes in eggshell pattern seen in 3%–6%
Treated lymphoma	Mean time from radiotherapy to calcification is 3 months
Metastases	In setting of mucinous colonic or ovarian adenocarcinoma; also seen in thyroid carcinoma and osteosarcoma
Castleman disease	Lymph node(s) enhance intensely with contrast; lymph nodes often FDG-avid on PET/CT imaging
Pneumocystis pneumonia	Occasionally causes hilar, mediastinal lymph nodes to calcify
Amyloidosis	Pulmonary nodules also usually present
Scleroderma	Lymph node calcification very rare

FDG, Fluorodeoxyglucose; *PET*, positron emission tomography.

bilaterally asymmetric, or bilaterally symmetric (Fig. 14.10). It is also important to differentiate lymph node enlargement on radiography from pulmonary arterial enlargement. There is overlap with some entities that typically create asymmetric hilar lymphadenopathy that produces symmetric lymphadenopathy, and vice versa, but in general it is nonetheless helpful to make this distinction because, when combined with other findings, it can narrow the differential diagnosis (Table 14.17).

TABLE 14.16 Differential Diagnosis of Low-Attenuation Lymphadenopathy

DIAGNOSIS	COMMENTS
Metastatic disease	Often of squamous cell histology; consider lung, testicular, or ovarian primary tumor
Infectious lymphadenopathy	Mycobacterial disease should in particular be considered; fungal infection may also be considered
Whipple disease	Small bowel involvement nearly always present; lung involvement in 35%–50% of cases
Lymphoma	Rarely results in low-attenuation lymphadenopathy

TABLE 14.17 Differential Diagnosis of Symmetric Hilar Lymphadenopathy

DIAGNOSIS	COMMENTS
Sarcoidosis	Typically symmetric adenopathy, 30%–50% of patients asymptomatic; without (stage I) or with (stage II) parenchymal abnormality
Lymphoma	May also be a cause of unilateral hilar lymphadenopathy; systemic symptoms (fever, night sweats) are common
Metastases	Typically renal cell carcinoma and testicular cancer
Silicosis	Lymph nodes may be calcified, sometimes in eggshell pattern; associated with upper lobe lung nodules and/or opacities
Castleman disease	Chronic, low-grade lymphoproliferative disorder; lymph nodes may intensely enhance with intravenous contrast
Infection	Typically unilateral, but bilateral hilar adenopathy possible; consider fungal infection such as histoplasmosis

■ Airways

Tracheal Narrowing

The normal intrathoracic trachea measures approximately 20 mm in diameter in men and 17 mm in women. Tracheal narrowing may be focal or diffuse, and the differential diagnosis includes diseases with a broad range of causes (Fig. 14.11). Treatment options for tracheal narrowing depend on the cause and location of the narrowing, but include tracheal dilation via bronchoscopy, tracheal stent placement, and tracheal resection with reconstruction. The most common non-neoplastic entities producing tracheal narrowing are provided in Table 14.18.

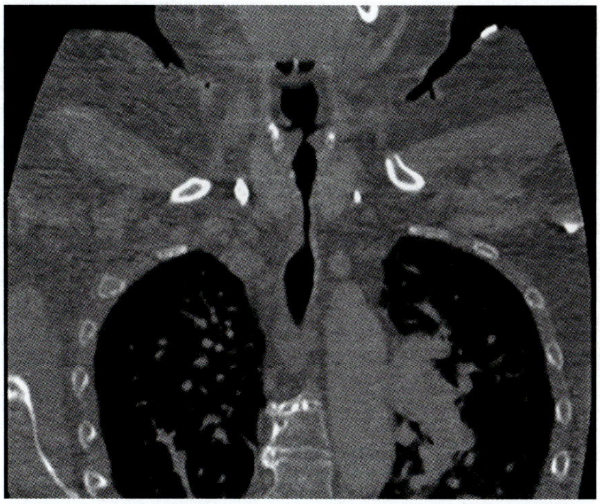

Figure 14.11 Coronal reformatted CT scan of a 52-year-old woman demonstrates focal tracheal narrowing following previous endotracheal intubation.

Tracheal Dilation

The tracheal diameter normally increases slightly with age but, when the tracheal diameter exceeds 26 mm in coronal diameter in men or 23 mm in women, it is considered dilated. Tracheal widening may be focal (as in the case of a tracheocele or following endotracheal intubation injury) or diffuse (Fig. 14.12). Some causes of tracheal dilation such as relapsing polychondritis are also causes of tracheal narrowing. There are many common causes of localized and diffuse tracheomegaly (Table 14.19).

Bronchiectasis

Bronchiectasis refers to pathologic and irreversible dilation of bronchi. Bronchiectasis may be cylindric, varicose, or cystic in its morphology. Chest radiographs are usually abnormal in the setting of bronchiectasis, but CT scans show the presence and extent of airway dilation to far better advantage. There are several disease categories that may result in bronchiectasis (Table 14.20).

■ Distribution of Disease

Upper Lung Distribution

A combination of gravity, differences in ventilation and perfusion, lymphatic flow, metabolism, and mechanics creates a situation whereby certain diseases have a predilection to affect the upper lungs preferentially. This distribution is best recognized on chest radiography and coronal-reformatted CT imaging (Fig. 14.13). There are several commonly encountered entities that produce an upper lung distribution of disease (Table 14.21).

TABLE 14.18 Differential Diagnosis of Tracheal Narrowing

DIAGNOSIS	COMMENTS
Postintubation stricture	Risk factor—prolonged intubation with high cuff location
Saber-sheath trachea	Fixed narrowing only in the transverse dimension; seen in men with chronic obstructive pulmonary disease
Relapsing polychondritis	Airway collapse seen on expiration (tracheomalacia); smooth tracheal wall thickening, sparing the posterior membrane; cartilage of nose and ears also affected
Postinfectious stricture	Granulation tissue and fibrosis is a response to infection; consider rhinoscleroma or other granulomatous infections
Wegener granulomatosis	Circumferential tracheal narrowing; predominantly affects subglottic trachea
Tracheobronchopathia osteochondroplastica	Osteocartilaginous nodules spare posterior trachea
Sarcoidosis	Affects upper trachea in 1%–3% of sarcoidosis patients
Tracheobronchial amyloidosis	Circumferential tracheal narrowing; intraluminal nodules and/or diffuse airway calcification
Extrinsic compression	Causes include enlarged thyroid, mediastinal lymphadenopathy, dilated or tortuous vessels

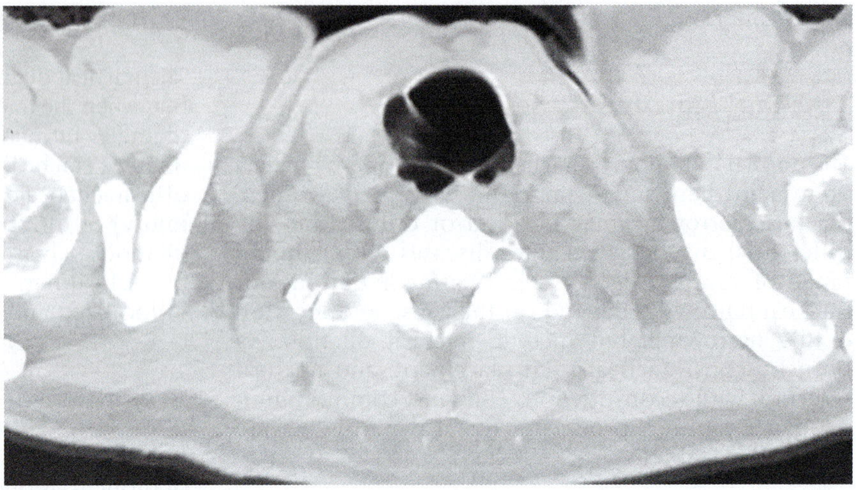

Figure 14.12 Axial CT scan of a 72-year-old man with Mounier-Kuhn syndrome demonstrates a dilated trachea measuring 4.4 × 4.0 cm at the level of the thoracic inlet, with intraluminal secretions.

TABLE 14.19 Differential Diagnosis of Tracheal Dilation

DIAGNOSIS	COMMENTS
Mounier-Kuhn syndrome	Associated with recurrent respiratory tract infections; trachea has corrugated outline and forms sacculations
Pulmonary fibrosis	Particularly from sarcoidosis, tuberculosis, and radiation; tracheal dilation usually mild
Endotracheal tube cuff damage	Most common in patients who have had tracheostomy; also a cause of focal tracheal stenosis
Inherited connective tissue disorders	Marfan syndrome, Ehlers-Danlos syndrome, or cutis laxa
Chronic obstructive pulmonary disease	Chronic bronchitis and emphysema
Cystic fibrosis	Tracheal widening accompanied by bronchiectasis; associated with recurrent respiratory tract infections
Relapsing polychondritis	Posterior membranous tracheal wall is spared; also a cause of tracheal narrowing

TABLE 14.20 Differential Diagnosis of Bronchiectasis

DIAGNOSIS	COMMENTS
Postinfectious bronchiectasis	Often focal in recurrent aspiration and/or pneumonia; mycobacterial infection a common cause
Postobstructive bronchiectasis	Cause may be endobronchial tumor or foreign body
Cystic fibrosis	Upper lung bronchiectasis
Asthma	Cylindric bronchiectasis, with air trapping
Allergic bronchopulmonary aspergillosis	Central cystic bronchiectasis with mucus plugging
Immotile cilia syndrome	Middle and lower lobe bronchiectasis; situs inversus seen in 50% of cases
Congenital causes	Williams-Campbell syndrome and Mounier-Kuhn syndrome; yellow nail syndrome in patients with discolored nails
Traction bronchiectasis	Results from fibrotic lung surrounding an airway; may be seen in fibrotic sarcoidosis, radiation fibrosis, idiopathic pulmonary fibrosis

Lower Lung Distribution

There are a number of diffuse lung diseases that preferentially affect the lower lobes, with relative sparing of the upper lungs (Fig. 14.14). This distribution can be helpful in both including and excluding considerations from a differential diagnosis list. Coronal-reformatted CT imaging may help one appreciate the distribution of disease to better advantage. The most common entities producing a lower lobe predominant distribution of disease are outlined in Table 14.22.

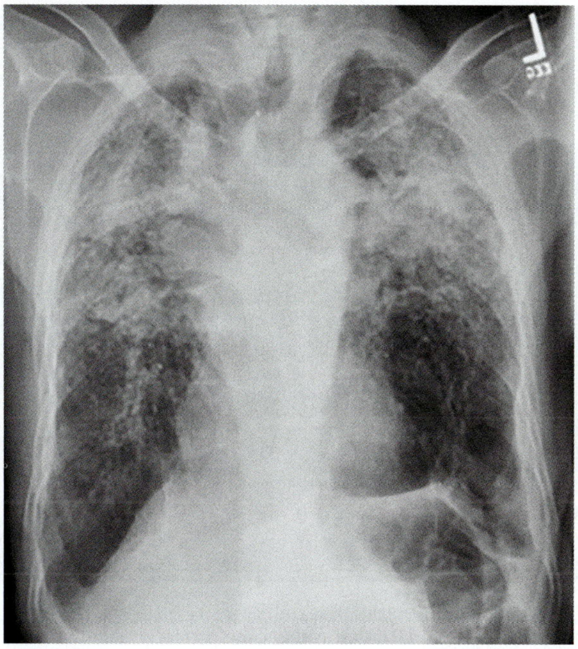

Figure 14.13 Frontal chest radiograph of a 63-year-old man with silicosis reveals bilateral upper lung zone opacities with associated architectural distortion, hilar retraction, and volume loss.

■ Miscellaneous Considerations

Unilateral Hyperlucent Hemithorax

A unilateral hyperlucent hemithorax on chest radiography can be the result of abnormality in the pulmonary parenchyma, pleural space, or chest wall (Fig. 14.15) or may be related to technical factors. Consideration of the clinical history and other radiologic findings may help narrow the differential diagnosis or identify the specific cause in some cases, and CT may be recommended in other cases for further clarification. There are many entities that could cause a unilateral hyperlucent hemithorax (Table 14.23).

Opacified Hemithorax

Complete opacification of an entire hemithorax on a frontal chest radiograph carries a relatively short differential diagnosis (Table 14.24), but it is often critical for the radiologist to use clinical information and associated radiographic findings to identify the underlying pathophysiology correctly. This is because the proper

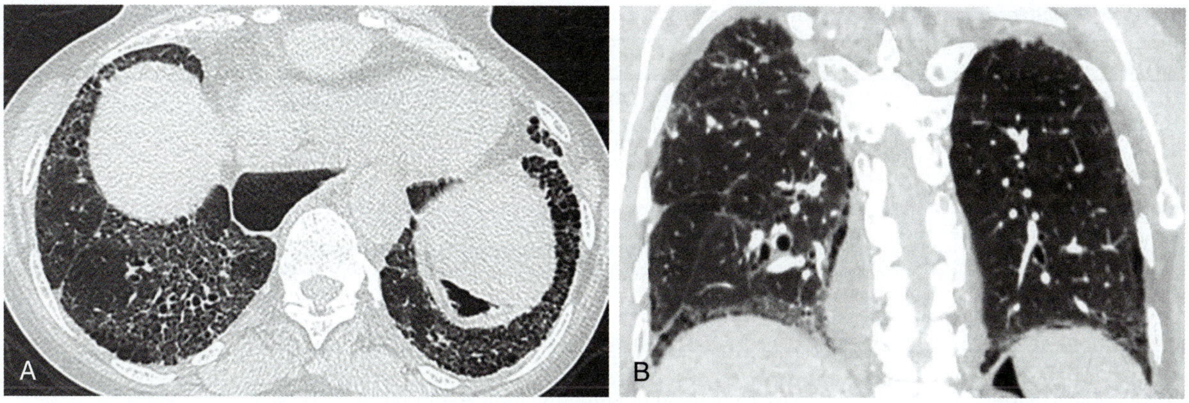

Figure 14.14 (A) Axial CT scan of a 58-year-old man with scleroderma demonstrates pulmonary fibrosis with honeycombing, reticulation, architectural distortion, and traction bronchiectasis in the lower lobes. Also note the dilated esophagus. (B) Coronal CT reconstruction scans from a study 5 years later in the same patient demonstrate the lower lung zone predilection.

TABLE 14.21 Differential Diagnosis of Upper Lung Distribution of Disease

DIAGNOSIS	COMMENTS
Centrilobular and paraseptal emphysema	Caused by cigarette smoking; bullous emphysematous changes may also be present
Langerhans cell histiocytosis	Mostly in smokers; nodules and bizarre-shaped cysts
Pneumoconioses	Particularly silicosis and coal workers' pneumoconiosis; occupational history central to diagnosis
Cystic fibrosis	Mucociliary clearance most impaired in the upper lobes; bronchiectasis and bronchial wall thickening common
Hypersensitivity pneumonitis	Centrilobular ground-glass nodules in subacute stage
Tuberculosis	Recurrent (postprimary) infection affects the upper lobes; cavitary nodules and asymmetric adenopathy common
Sarcoidosis	Perilymphatic nodules or opacities; bilateral hilar and mediastinal lymphadenopathy
Metastatic pulmonary calcification	Calcium deposits in alkaline environment of upper lobes; often a history of hyperparathyroidism or renal failure
Anklyosing spondylitis	Pleuropulmonary findings in 1%–2% of patients; spinal ankylosis precedes lung disease

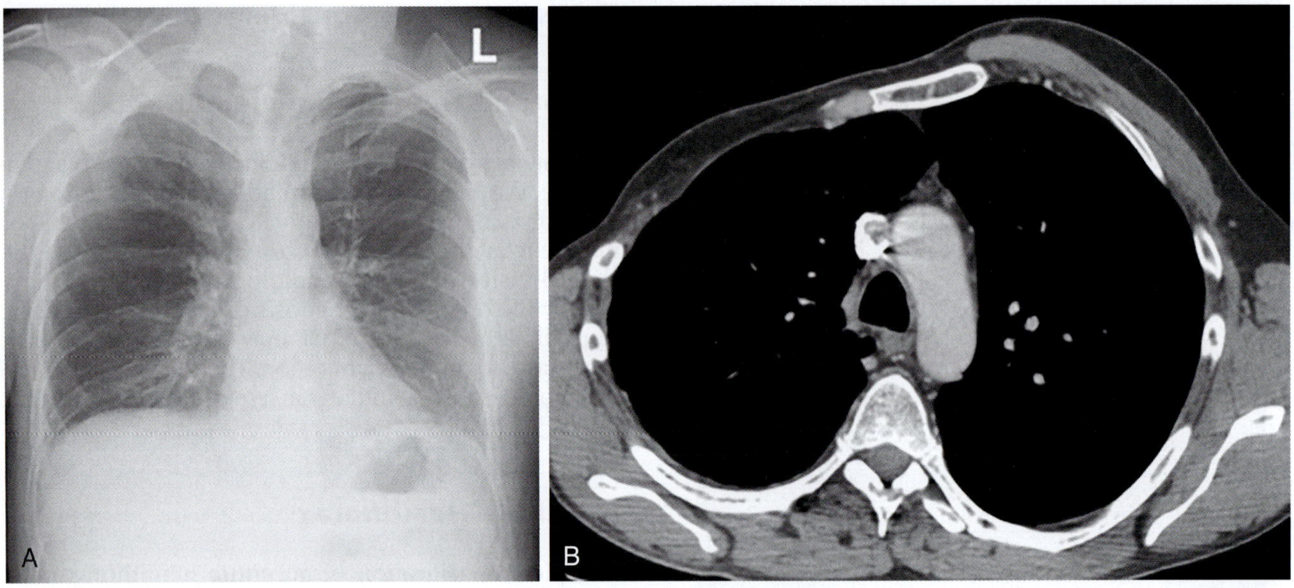

Figure 14.15 (A) Frontal chest radiograph of a 52-year-old man demonstrates subtle diffuse increased lucency of the right hemithorax as compared with the left side. (B) Axial CT scan in the same patient demonstrates congenital absence of the right pectoralis musculature, consistent with Poland syndrome.

TABLE 14.22 Differential Diagnosis of Lower Lung Distribution of Disease

DIAGNOSIS	COMMENTS
Aspiration pneumonia	More common on the right side; posterior segments of upper lobes also commonly affected
Usual interstitial pneumonia pattern	As in idiopathic pulmonary fibrosis or asbestosis; peripheral honeycombing a strongly suggestive feature
Hematogenous metastases	Distribution due to greater lower lobe blood flow
Hematogenous infection	Miliary tuberculosis or miliary fungal infection; septic (and bland) emboli also more common in lower lobes
Nonspecific interstitial pneumonia pattern	May be related to drug toxicity or connective tissue disease
Panacinar emphysema	History of alpha-1-antitrypsin deficiency; history of intravenous methylphenidate
Idiopathic bronchiectasis	Likely the result of prior aspiration and/or pneumonia events
Bronchiectasis in Kartagener syndrome	Associated with situs inversus

TABLE 14.23 Differential Diagnosis of Unilateral Hyperlucent Hemithorax

DIAGNOSIS	COMMENTS
Radiologic technique	May be due to factors such as patient rotation or low kilovoltage
Emphysema	Bullous emphysema—may be unilateral or asymmetric
Asymmetric chest wall soft tissue	Congenital absence of pectoralis muscle (Poland syndrome); follows unilateral mastectomy
Extrapulmonary air collection	Pneumothorax or subcutaneous emphysema
Contralateral increased density	Such as from layering contralateral pleural effusion
Bronchial obstruction	Endobronchial lung cancer, broncholith, or foreign body; expiratory chest radiograph shows unchanged lung volume
Bronchiolitis obliterans	Such as in Swyer-James syndrome; hemithorax may be small, with ipsilateral mediastinal shift
Pulmonary embolism	Due to oligemia (Watermark sign) in acute or chronic pulmonary embolism
Congenital lobar hyperinflation	More common on left side

TABLE 14.24 Differential Diagnosis of Opacified Hemithorax

DIAGNOSIS	COMMENTS
Atelectasis of entire lung	Ipsilateral mediastinal shift and elevated hemidiaphragm; underlying cause often main stem endobronchial lesion
Large pleural effusion	Contralateral mediastinal shift; pleural fluid can be blood (hemothorax) or pus (empyema)
Pneumonia of an entire lung	No significant mediastinal shift; air bronchogram may be present
Postpneumonectomy appearance	Evidence of surgery (surgical clips and fifth rib resection); ipsilateral mediastinal shift
Large pulmonary, pleural, or chest wall mass	Examples include mesothelioma and Ewing sarcoma; no significant mediastinal shift or mild contralateral shift
Pulmonary hypoplasia or agenesis	Ipsilateral mediastinal shift

treatment and optimal outcome are often contingent on reaching the correct diagnosis.

Cystic Lung Disease

Pulmonary cysts measure more than 1 cm, contain air or occasionally fluid, and have a recognizable wall. Although a few lung cysts may be seen in otherwise normal (particularly older) patients, the presence of many cysts suggests a primary cystic lung disease (Fig. 14.16). It is also important to distinguish true cystic lung disease from emphysema, bullous change, and honeycombing. True primary cystic lung disease is seen in several entities (Table 14.25).

Pneumomediastinum

Extraluminal air in the mediastinum, or pneumomediastinum, must be differentiated from pneumopericardium, a medial pneumothorax, subcutaneous emphysema, and Mach bands. A pneumomediastinum may originate from the tracheobronchial tree, lungs, or esophagus (Fig. 14.17), or it may track from the neck or abdomen. Causes range from benign to life-threatening conditions, and both clinical features and radiologic findings are helpful in determining the cause and appropriate treatment. There are a number of common causes of pneumomediastinum (Table 14.26).

Elevated Hemidiaphragm

When both sides of the diaphragm are elevated, the cause is usually diminished lung volumes (poor patient inspiration or restrictive pulmonary disease) or symmetric intraabdominal disease (e.g., ascites). An elevated hemidiaphragm (Fig. 14.18), however, has a more specific differential diagnosis (Table 14.27).

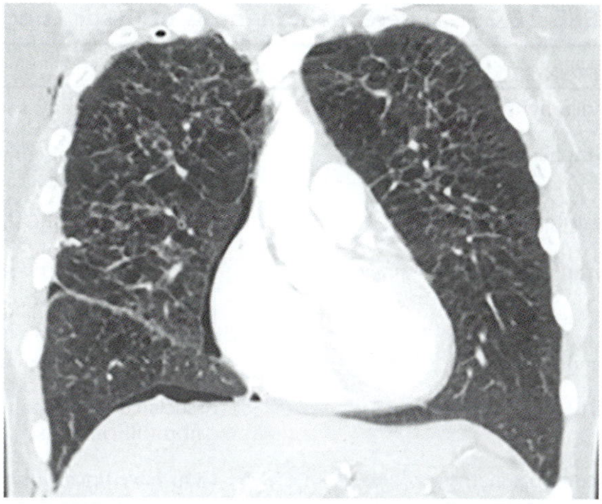

Figure 14.16 Coronal CT reconstruction image of a 31-year-old woman with pulmonary Langerhans cell histiocytosis demonstrates innumerable irregularly shaped cysts, with relative sparing of the costophrenic angles, in addition to a small right pneumothorax.

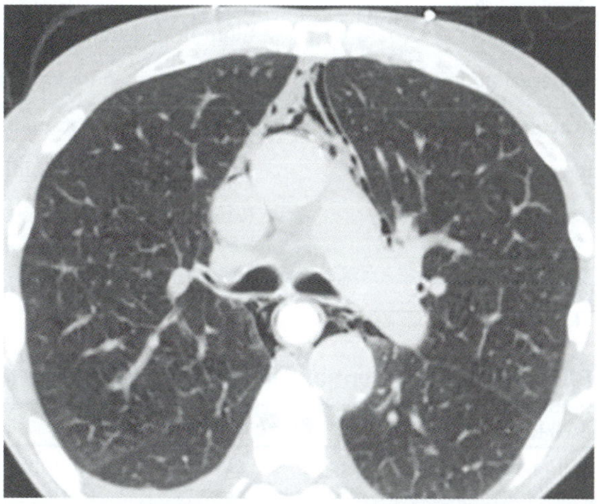

Figure 14.17 Axial CT scan of a 70-year-old man demonstrates pneumomediastinum due to esophageal perforation following endoscopy.

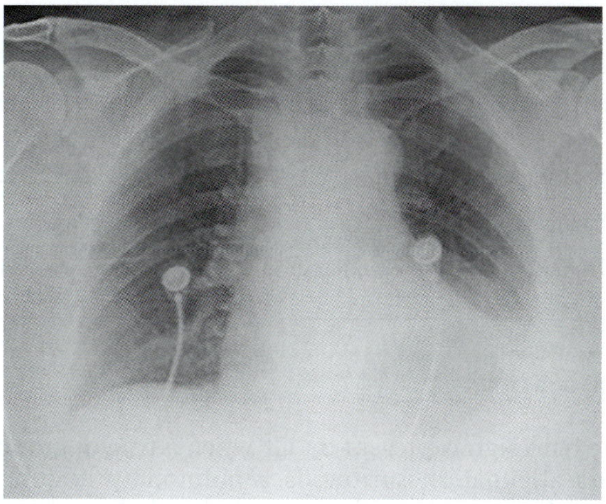

Figure 14.18 Frontal chest radiograph of a 59-year-old woman demonstrates left hemidiaphragmatic elevation in this patient with left phrenic nerve paralysis. A fluoroscopic study in this patient demonstrated paradoxic left hemidiaphragmatic motion with breathing (positive sniff test).

TABLE 14.25 Differential Diagnosis of Cystic Lung Disease

DIAGNOSIS	COMMENTS
Langerhans cell histiocytosis	History of cigarette smoking; more irregularly shaped cysts in upper lobes ± nodules
Lymphangioleiomyomatosis	Affects women of childbearing age; round regular cysts in all lobes ± pleural effusions; associated with tuberous sclerosis
Multiple pneumatoceles	Seen from prior infection, trauma, or hydrocarbon inhalation
Lymphoid interstitial pneumonia	History of connective tissue disease or HIV infection; cysts are perivascular in location
Cystic metastases	Includes colonic adenocarcinoma and endometrial sarcoma
Papillomatosis	Associated with human papillomavirus infection
Birt-Hogg-Dubé disease	Associated with renal cell carcinoma and oncocytoma; cutaneous manifestations include fibrofolliculomas
Neurofibromatosis	Cysts have upper lobe predominance; may see mediastinal neurofibromas or lateral meningoceles

TABLE 14.26 Differential Diagnosis of Pneumomediastinum

DIAGNOSIS	COMMENTS
Asthma	Common cause in younger patients; peribronchiolar thickening may also be seen
Trauma	Blunt or penetrating trauma involving trachea or esophagus
Esophageal perforation	May be from endoscopy or vomiting (Boerhaave syndrome); usually left pleural effusion is present
Tracheobronchial perforation	May be from laceration, bronchoscopy, or tracheostomy
Surgery	Neck, thoracic, or abdominal surgery; free abdominal air may track into mediastinum
Barotrauma	Patients on positive pressure ventilation (e.g., as in acute respiratory distress syndrome); may also be seen in divers (drop in atmospheric pressure)
Infection	Consider histoplasmosis and tuberculosis; retropharyngeal infection can spread to cause mediastinitis

TABLE 14.27 Differential Diagnosis of Elevated Hemidiaphragm

DIAGNOSIS	COMMENTS
Diaphragmatic eventration	Weakness and thinning of the diaphragm; no paradoxic motion on fluoroscopy (negative sniff test)
Diminished lung volume	Includes causes such as atelectasis or pulmonary hypoplasia; prior lobectomy recognized by rib defects and surgical clips
Subpulmonic pleural effusion	Represents only apparent (not actual) diaphragm elevation; dome of the diaphragm more lateral than normal; ipsilateral decubitus positioning can confirm diagnosis
Phrenic nerve paralysis	Causes include lung cancer, mediastinal mass, or iatrogenesis; fluoroscopy demonstrates paradoxic motion (sniff test)
Abdominal disease	Consider subphrenic abscess or mass and Chilaiditi syndrome; ultrasound best test for confirming subphrenic abscess
Diaphragmatic hernia	May be due to Morgagni or Bochdalek hernia
Diaphragmatic tumor	Consider mesothelioma, lipoma, and fibroma; serial radiographs may show growth with time
Traumatic diaphragmatic rupture	Other signs of chest and/or abdominal trauma are evident; liver herniation may simulate elevated right hemidiaphragm

Halo Sign

The halo sign is present on CT when a ring of ground-glass attenuation surrounds a pulmonary nodule or mass. In most cases, the ground-glass halo represents alveolar hemorrhage. The sign was initially described as a specific finding in the setting of angioinvasive aspergillosis but it has since been established that there are many other causes of a halo sign (Table 14.28).

Reverse Halo Sign

The reverse halo sign, also known as the *atoll sign,* refers to a central focus of ground-glass attenuation surrounded by denser consolidation that forms a crescentic or circular perimeter. The central ground-glass opacity often correlates histopathologically with inflammation and/or debris within alveolar spaces. The sign is important because, when recognized, the radiologist can integrate clinical and

TABLE 14.28 Differential Diagnosis of Halo Sign

DIAGNOSIS	COMMENTS
Angioinvasive aspergillosis	Immunocompromised patient; results in pulmonary infarction, necrosis, and hemorrhage
Pulmonary metastases	Consider melanoma, angiosarcoma, and choriocarcinoma; consider squamous cell histology from any primary source
Granulomatosis with polyangiitis	Bilateral nodules that may cavitate; may be associated tracheal abnormalities such as tracheal stenosis
Kaposi sarcoma	Ill-defined nodules with peribronchovascular distribution; mucocutaneous lesions usually present
Atypical infection	Described with mycobacterial and fungal infection; also described with viral pneumonia from CMV and HSV
Adenocarcinoma in situ	Ground-glass halo represents tumor infiltration; pseudocavitation (internal bubbly lucencies) may be present
Septic embolism	Lower lung distribution
Pulmonary endometriosis	Abnormality may wax and wane with menstrual cycle

CMV, Cytomegalovirus; *HSV*, herpes simplex virus.

TABLE 14.29 Differential Diagnosis of Reverse Halo Sign

DIAGNOSIS	COMMENTS
Cryptogenic organizing pneumonia	Subacute to chronic pulmonary opacities that may migrate; distribution may be peribronchovascular or peripheral; seen in about 20% of patients
Fungal pneumonia	Consider invasive aspergillosis or mucormycosis; consider paracoccidioidomycosis in South American patients
Nonfungal pneumonia	Consider tuberculosis and *Pneumocystis* infection
Granulomatosis with polyangiitis	Bilateral nodules that may cavitate; tracheal abnormalities may also be present
Pulmonary infarction	Lower lung and peripheral distribution
Sarcoidosis	Symmetric hilar and mediastinal lymphadenopathy; nodules with a perilymphatic distribution
Pulmonary malignancy	Rarely seen in primary lung cancer and metastatic disease
Lymphomatoid granulomatosis	Multiple nodules that may cavitate and peripherally enhance; association with Epstein-Barr virus infection

other imaging data to narrow the differential diagnosis or even suggest one specific diagnosis (Table 14.29).

Bibliography

Bejvan S, Godwin D. Pneumomediastinum: old signs and new signs. *AJR Am J Roentgenol.* 1996;166:1041–1048.

Bharty S, Prakash B, Agarwal M. Opaque hemithorax: re-visiting the causes. *Internet J Pulmonary Med.* 2013;14(1).

Boitsios G, Bankier A, Eisenberg R. Diffuse pulmonary nodules. *AJR Am J Roentgenol.* 2010;194(5):W354–W366.

Cantin L, Bankier A, Eisenberg R. Multiple cystlike lung lesions in the adult. *AJR Am J Roentgenol.* 2010;194(1):W1–W11.

Dynes M, White E, Fry W. Imaging manifestations of pleural tumors. *Radiographics.* 1992;12:1191–1201.

Elicker B, Webb W. *Fundamentals of High-Resolution Lung CT: Common Findings, Common Patterns, Common Diseases, and Differential Diagnosis.* Philadelphia: Lippincott Williams and Wilkins; 2013.

Falconer M, Collins D, Feeney J. Mounier-Kuhn syndrome in an older patient. *Age Ageing.* 2008;37:115–116.

Gaerte S, Meyer C, Winer-Muram H. Fat-containing lesions of the chest. *Radiographics.* 2002;22:S61–S78.

Gawne-Cain M, Hansell D. The pattern and distribution of calcified mediastinal lymph nodes in sarcoidosis and tuberculosis: a CT study. *Clin Radiol.* 1996;51(4):263–267.

Gruden J, Webb W, Warnock M. Centrilobular opacities in the lung on high-resolution CT: diagnostic considerations and pathologic correlation. *AJR Am J Roentgenol.* 1994;162:569–574.

Hansell D, Lynch D, McAdams H. *Imaging Diseases of the Chest.* London: Elsevier Mosby; 2010.

Juanpere S, Canete N, Ortuno P. A diagnostic approach to the mediastinal masses. *Insights Imaging.* 2013;4:29–52.

Khan A, Al-Jahdali H, Allen C. The calcified lung nodule: what does it mean? *Ann Thorac Med.* 2010;5:67–79.

Kim N, Han J. Pathologic review of cystic and cavitary lung diseases. *Korean J Pathol.* 2012;46(5):407–414.

Lee Y, Choi Y, Lee K. CT halo sign: the spectrum of pulmonary diseases. *Br J Radiol.* 2005;78(933):862–865.

Muller N, Silva I. *High-Yield Imaging: Chest.* Philadelphia: Saunders; 2010.

Nemec S, Bankier A, Eisenberg R. Pulmonary hyperlucency in adults. *AJR Am J Roentgenol.* 2013;200:W101–W115.

Nemec S, Bankier A, Eisenberg R. Upper lobe-predominant diseases of the lung. *AJR Am J Roentgenol.* 2013;W222–W237.

Pineda V, Andreu J, Caceres J. Lesions of the cardiophrenic space: findings at cross-sectional imaging. *Radiographics.* 2007;27:19–32.

Prince J, Duhamel D, Levin D. Nonneoplastic lesions of the tracheobronchial wall: radiologic findings with bronchoscopic correlation. *Radiographics.* 2002;22:S215–S230.

Reed J. *Chest Radiology: Plain Film Patterns and Differential Diagnoses.* Philadelphia: Elsevier; 2011.

Rubinowitz A, Antin-Ozerkis D, Hanna S. Imaging and differential diagnosis of chronic air-space consolidation. *Clin Pulm Med.* 2009;16(1):33–44.

Stern E, Gurney J. *Expert Differential Diagnosis: Chest.* Altona, Manitoba, Canada: Amirsys Inc.; 2011.

Strollo D, Rosado de Christenson M, Jett J. Primary mediastinal tumors—tumors of the middle and posterior mediastinum. *Chest.* 1997;112(5):1344–1357.

Suwatanapongched T, Gierada D. CT of thoracic lymph nodes—part II: diseases and pitfalls. *Br J Radiol.* 2006;79:999–1006.

Whitten C, Khan S, Munneke G. A diagnostic approach to mediastinal abnormalities. *Radiographics.* 2007;657–671.

SECTION 4

Entities by Pathologic Category

CHAPTER 15
Congenital and Developmental Diseases of the Lungs and Airways

Matthew Gilman

CHAPTER OUTLINE

Introduction

Congenital lung disease in the adult patient is rare. However, some congenital lung diseases can cause clinical symptoms for which patients undergo imaging, or these diseases may be incidentally discovered on imaging performed for other reasons. Although encountering congenital lung disease on imaging is very uncommon, the imaging appearance is often very characteristic, allowing the radiologist to make a specific diagnosis. Knowledge of the imaging and relevant clinical features is helpful for the radiologist to make the correct diagnosis and direct these patients to appropriate clinical care.

Imaging Modalities

- Chest radiography
- CT of the chest and CT angiography (CTA)
- Thoracic MRI and MR angiography (MRA)
- Digital subtraction catheter angiography
- Imaging algorithm

Chest Radiography

In patients with congenital lung disease, the chest radiograph is frequently the initial examination performed. A typical scenario is a patient referred for chest radiography for productive cough, dyspnea, chest pain, or fever who is discovered to have a congenital lung abnormality. The clinical symptoms observed may or may not be related to the congenital lung disease. Although the chest radiograph may be suggestive for a particular congenital lung disease, cross-sectional imaging (CT or MRI) is usually required to confirm the diagnosis and to evaluate for associated abnormalities.

After the diagnosis is established, the chest radiograph may be used to monitor the stability of the lesion and evaluate for complications such as superimposed infection if clinical symptoms arise. If the patient is to undergo surgical resection, the patient may undergo chest radiography during the preoperative workup.

Chest CT and CT Angiography

CT of the chest is the most common modality used to evaluate and diagnose congenital lung disease. Due to the high spatial resolution of chest CT, it is well suited to illustrate the nature and anatomic considerations of congenital lung lesions. This includes evaluation of the anatomic location, extent of the lesion, nature of the lesion, bronchial supply, arterial supply, and venous drainage. CT angiography (CTA) is useful in cases that are vascular in nature or have important vascular anatomy. The bolus timing of the CTA should be determined by the suspected vascular supply of the lesion. For example, for lesions suspected to be of pulmonary artery origin (e.g., a pulmonary arteriovenous malformation), a bolus timing technique timed to peak enhancement of the pulmonary arteries (similar to the CT pulmonary embolism protocol) may be chosen. For lesions suspected to be of systemic arterial origin (e.g., a bronchopulmonary sequestration), a bolus timing technique timed to the descending aorta may be chosen.

Thoracic MRI and MR Angiography

MRI of the chest can also be used to evaluate congenital lung lesions, especially for younger patients in whom radiation is an important clinical concern. However, MRI is not as useful for evaluation of the lung and airways. Therefore, chest CT with IV contrast is usually chosen as the initial modality for evaluation of adult patients with suspected congenital lung disease.

However, thoracic MRI excels at evaluation of cystic lesions in the mediastinum. Therefore, thoracic MRI may be used as the primary imaging modality for the evaluation of suspected mediastinal foregut duplication cysts, such as bronchogenic or esophageal duplication cysts. Mediastinal MRI is very useful as a problem-solving technique in patients with a suspected cystic mediastinal lesion on CT but for whom the measured CT attenuation values are not diagnostic for a cyst. MRI is an excellent modality to differentiate cystic and solid lesions. MRI of the thorax performed pre- and post-gadolinium, with subtraction of precontrast from the postcontrast signal, can detect even a subtle enhancing component.

MR angiography (MRA) is sometimes used to define the arterial supply of a lung or mediastinal lesion when the arterial supply is suspected to be of systemic origin. To ensure adequate spatial resolution and avoid respiratory or cardiac motion artifacts, thoracic MRA requires meticulous technique, particularly for smaller vessels. For these reasons, and for evaluation of the airways, chest CTA is usually preferred due to its higher spatial resolution, speed, and ease of imaging.

Catheter Angiography

Catheter angiography can also be used to define the arterial supply, venous drainage, and general vascularity of a congenital lung lesion. Catheter angiography is most often used as a problem-solving technique in patients in whom the vascular anatomy requires further definition prior to surgical resection. Occasionally, congenital lung lesions are embolized as a primary therapy or prior to surgical resection. In these circumstances, angiography will be performed prior to embolization.

■ Diseases

Bronchopulmonary Sequestration

A bronchopulmonary sequestration is a mass of abnormal lung tissue that lacks normal communication with the tracheobronchial tree. The mass usually consists of abnormal, nonfunctioning lung tissue that derives its arterial supply from a systemic artery rather than a pulmonary artery. The systemic artery may be a single systemic artery or multiple arteries most commonly arising from the descending aorta, but may arise from the abdominal aorta, celiac artery, splenic artery, or rarely an intercostal artery. The identification of the systemic artery is a key feature for diagnosis of bronchopulmonary sequestration on imaging (Fig. 15.1A–D).

Types of Sequestration

There are two types of bronchopulmonary sequestration that are differentiated by their pleural covering and venous drainage. Intralobar sequestration is more common, comprising 75% of sequestrations, and the sequestered lung tissue is located within the visceral pleura of the affected lobe. Therefore an intralobar sequestration may communicate through collateral air drift with the normally aerated lung of the affected lobe. In extralobar sequestration, the sequestered lung tissue is enclosed within its own pleural envelope. This unique pleural covering precludes communication with other parts of the lung. The presence of air within the sequestration indicates that the lesion is most likely an intralobar sequestration because intralobar sequestrations can communicate with the lung through collateral air drift, whereas the extralobar sequestration is enclosed and should not contain air.

The venous drainage of intralobar and extralobar sequestration is sometimes a differentiating feature but is not universally consistent. The venous drainage of intralobar sequestrations tends to be to pulmonary veins, whereas the venous drainage of extralobar sequestrations tends to be to systemic veins, such as the azygous vein, hemiazygos vein, or inferior vena cava (IVC).

Imaging Appearance

Intralobar sequestrations may present as a solid mass or cystic mass. Cystic intralobar sequestrations may contain air cysts, fluid cysts, or both air- and fluid-filled cysts and there may be air-fluid levels (see Fig. 15.1E–H).

Rarely, an intralobar sequestration may present as a focal area of hyperinflated lung. Extralobar sequestration typically presents as a solid vascular mass in the lung base, near the hemidiaphragm (Fig. 15.2). In all cases of sequestration, a systemic artery is present, and normal bronchial communication is absent.

Complications

The most common complication of intralobar bronchopulmonary sequestration is superinfection. This complication is unique to intralobar sequestration due to the potential collateral air drift or fistulous communication of the sequestration with other parts of the lung. Extralobar sequestrations rarely become infected because they are completely enclosed. Deciding whether an infection is present may be difficult on imaging. However, if there is prior imaging, any new consolidation or air-fluid levels may suggest superimposed infection.

Other rare complications of intralobar sequestrations may include hemoptysis, hemothorax, and high-output cardiac failure from left-to-right or left-to-left shunting. Rare complications of extralobar sequestration include hemothorax, infarction, torsion, and high-output failure from shunting.

Goals of Imaging

The goals of imaging are to identify the feeding artery and its origin because identification of the artery is essential to the diagnosis and potential management. It is also important to identify if there is more than one feeding artery for a surgeon who may be planning a surgical resection.

Identify the venous drainage if possible. This may suggest whether the lesion is intralobar or extralobar and is also important information for a surgeon.

Delineate the extent of the lesion. Identify the full anatomic extent of the lesion, the lobe involved, and

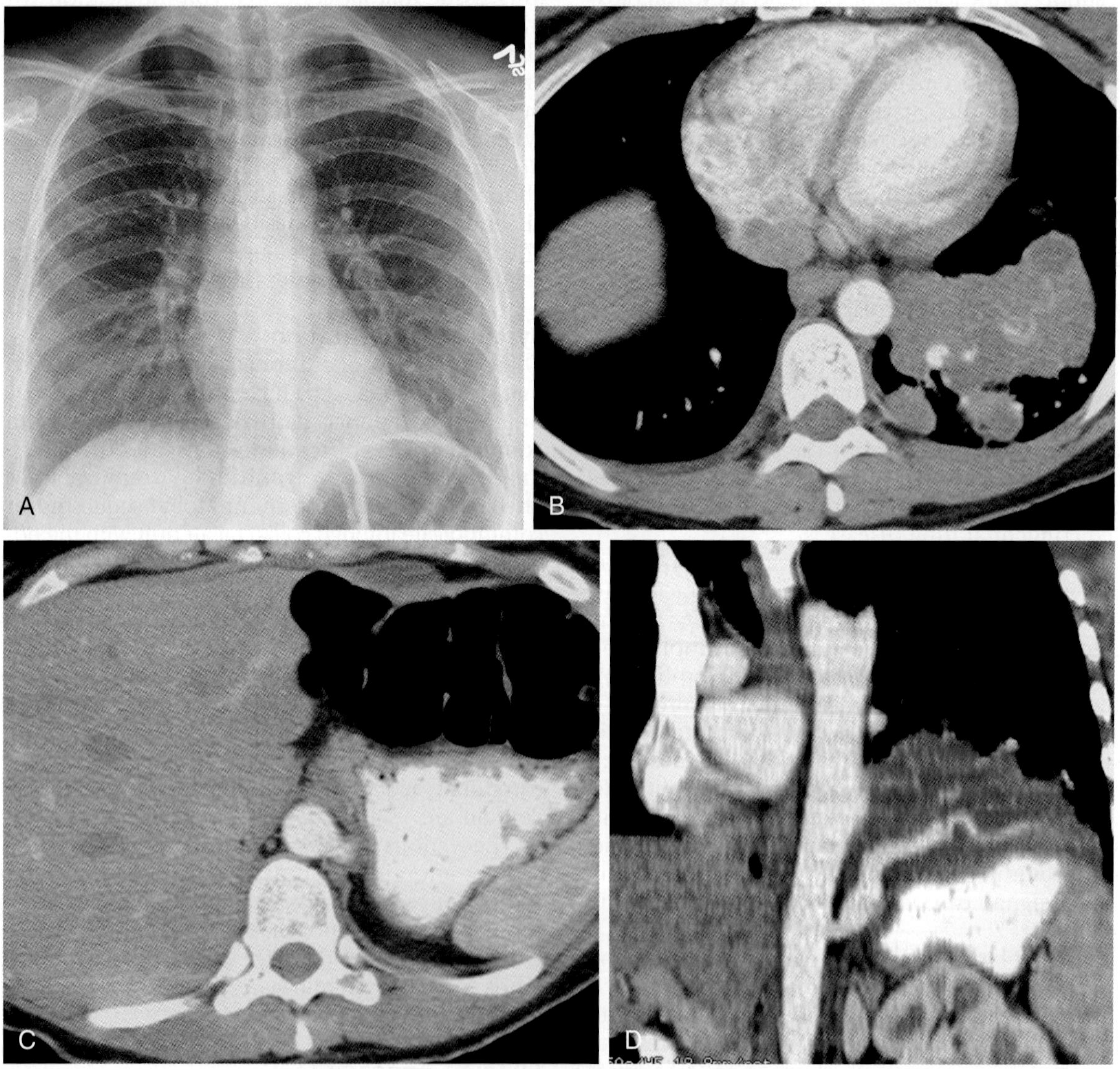

Figure 15.1 Intralobar sequestration. (A) Posteroanterior chest radiograph shows a left lower lobe mass. (B, C) Axial contrast-enhanced CT scans in the same patient as in (A) shows a low-attenuation mass and a large vessel supplying the mass originating from the descending aorta. (D) Oblique multiplanar CT reformation from the same patient as in (A–C) shows a large systemic artery originating from the descending aorta.

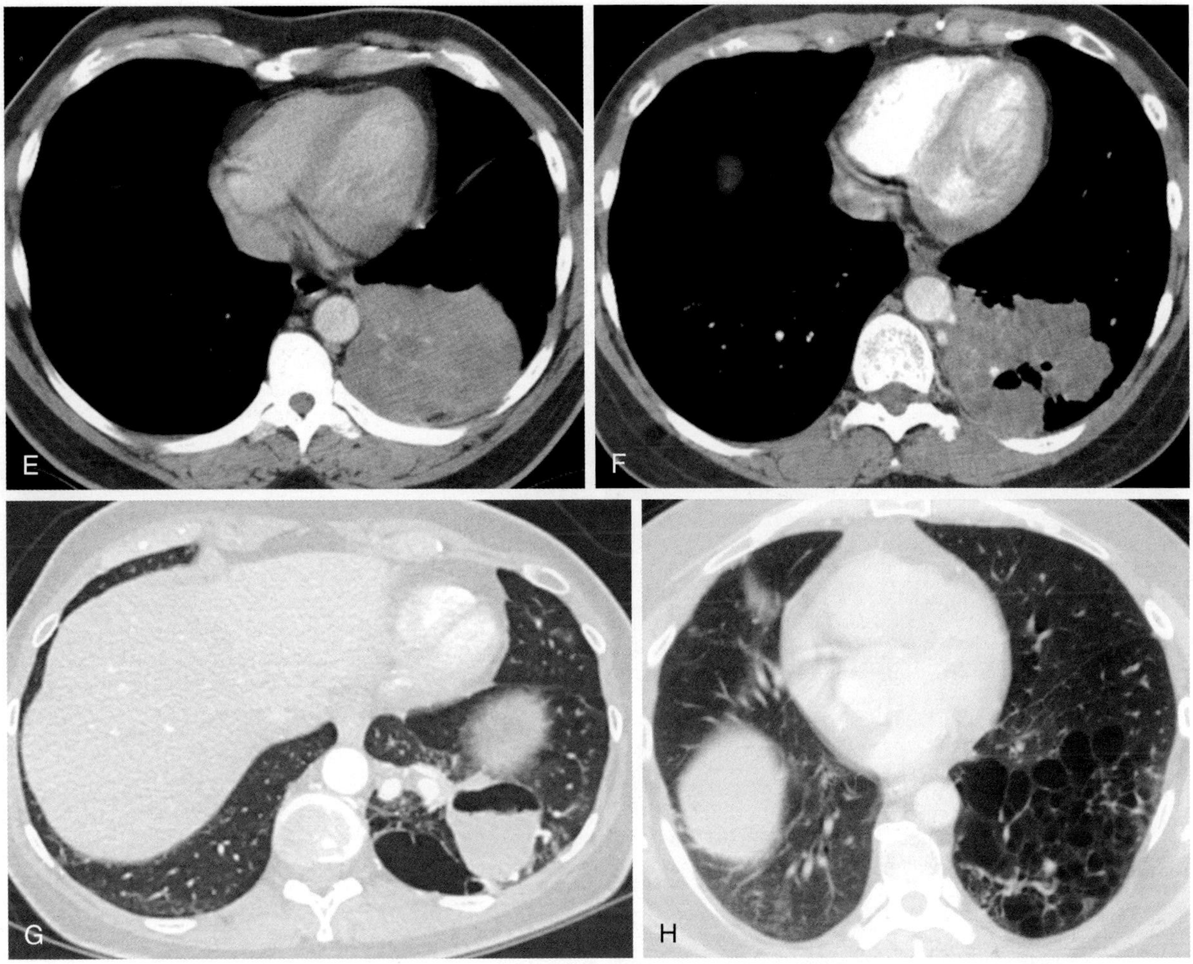

Figure 15.1, cont'd (E–H) Different patients showing the varied appearance of pulmonary sequestration from a solid mass (E), fluid-containing cysts (F), air-fluid levels in cysts (G), to air-filled cysts (H).

whether there is any involvement below the diaphragm. Extralobar sequestrations have a higher incidence of an ectopic location.

Describe any features that may suggest a complication, such as superimposed infection.

Differential Diagnosis

1. It is important to distinguish sequestration from a malignancy such as a primary lung malignancy or metastasis. These would usually be differentiated by identification of the systemic arterial supply. Extremely rarely, a malignancy may occur in conjunction with a sequestration and may be suggested by an increasing or enhancing mass within the lesion.
2. Systemic arterial supply to normal lung may arise from hypertrophy in chronic inflammation, chronic pulmonary embolism, or the absence of an interlobar or segmental pulmonary artery. The diagnosis of a sequestration requires the concurrent absence of normal bronchial communication to the affected lung parenchyma in addition to the systemic arterial supply.
3. Certain congenital lung diseases may have a systemic arterial supply to portions of the lung in the absence of bronchopulmonary sequestration. These diseases have normal bronchial communication to the affected lung.

Treatment

Bronchopulmonary sequestration is usually excised by open thoracotomy or video-assisted thoracic surgery. This may be a segmentectomy or lobectomy, depending on the anatomy of the lesion. Transcatheter embolization has been used in select cases, with variable success.

Congenital Pulmonary Airway Malformation

Congenital pulmonary airway malformations (CPAMs) comprise a spectrum of airway malformations (hamartomas) that involve various portions of the tracheobronchial tree. CPAMs were previously referred to as *congenital cystic adenomatoid malformations* (CCAMs), but the name of the disease has been changed because not all these lesions are adenomatoid or cystic. The classification scheme for CPAMs has also been expanded, and there are now five types of CPAM based

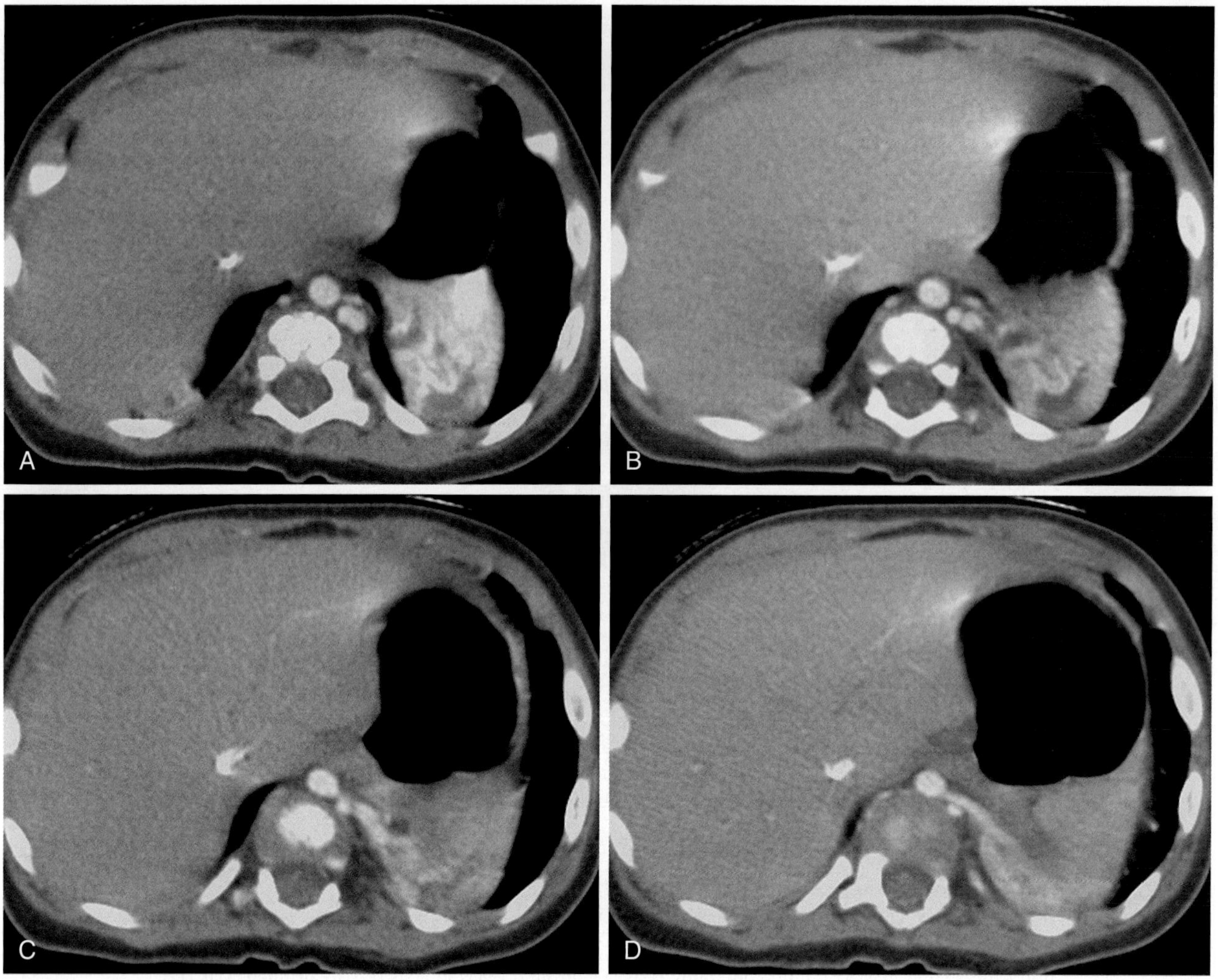

Figure 15.2 Extralobar sequestration. (A–D) Axial images from contrast-enhanced CT show a vascular airless mass in the left lower lobe, with systemic arterial supply and systemic venous drainage to the hemiazygos vein.

on the pathologic site of origin of the lesion in the tracheobronchial tree:

Type 0: Airway malformations of the proximal tracheobronchial tree
Type 1: Airway malformations of bronchial or bronchiolar origin (large cyst lesion)
Type 2: Airway malformations of bronchiolar origin (the small cyst lesion)
Type 3: Airway malformations of bronchiolar or alveolar duct origin (the adenomatoid lesion)
Type 4: Airway malformations of distal acinar or alveolar origin (the unlined cyst lesion)

Imaging Appearance

Usually CPAMs present early in life but have been reported in adult patients. At imaging, CPAMs usually present as a cystic mass (Fig. 15.3), but occasionally appear solid. If the largest cyst is >2.5 cm, these tend to be type 1 CPAMs. If the cysts are <2.5 cm or the lesion is solid, it is difficult to predict the subtype of CPAM. The diagnosis of a CPAM in an adult patient is controversial due to overlap of the imaging features of CPAM and lung injury or repair, which may result in cystic lesions or pneumatoceles. Usually, CPAMs have normal arterial and venous connections, differentiating CPAM from bronchopulmonary sequestration.

Complications

The classic presentation of CPAM is respiratory distress in a newborn patient. In older patients, CPAM may present as recurrent pneumonia in the region of a multicystic lesion on CT. Less commonly, patients may present with spontaneous pneumothorax, and there is a rare association with adenocarcinoma (especially for type 1 CPAM).

Differential Diagnosis

The following are part of the differential diagnosis for a CPAM:

1. Postinflammatory cystic lesion. This may be difficult to differentiate from CPAM, making the diagnosis of CPAM in adult patients controversial.
2. Bronchopulmonary sequestration. This would be distinguished by the presence or absence of a systemic artery supplying the lesion.

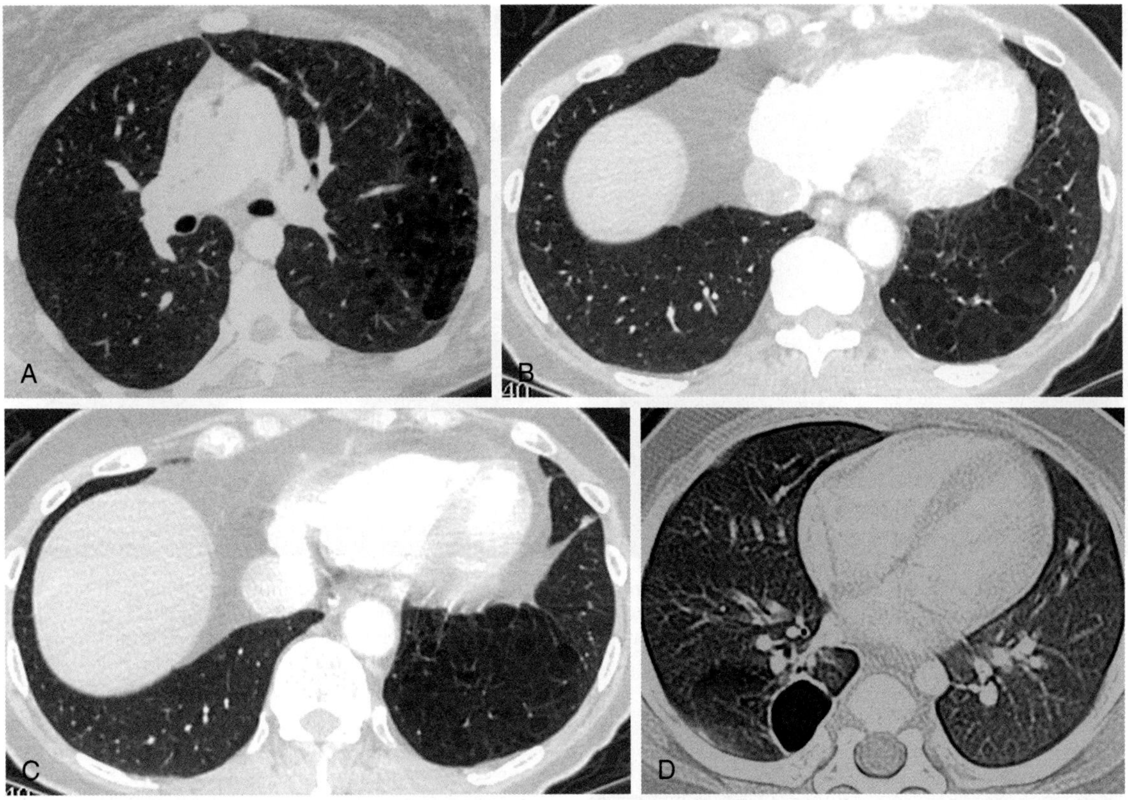

Figure 15.3 Congenital pulmonary airway malformation (CPAM). (A) Axial CT scan shows a multicystic mass in the left upper lobe in an adult patient with known CPAM from birth. (B, C) Multicystic lesion in the left lower lobe consistent with a type 2 CPAM. (D) Cyst in the right lower lobe was a type 2 CPAM on resection.

3. Cystic malignancy, such as adenocarcinoma or cystic metastasis. The cysts associated with CPAM typically have thin walls. Thickening or irregularity of the wall of a cyst should raise concern for a cystic malignancy or a superimposed malignancy.
4. Bullous emphysema, cystic lung disease, or emphysema. This is usually diffuse and involves both lungs.

Congenital Lobar Overinflation

Congenital lobar overinflation (CLO) is the result of the congenital partial obstruction of a bronchus, with progressive overinflation of the affected lobe. It has been postulated that there is a ball valve obstruction with overinflation during inspiration and distal air trapping in expiration. The result is progressive overinflation of the affected lobe. In about 50% of cases, the cause is unknown, but known causes include mucosal flaps, deficient cartilage, airway stenosis or malacia, and an extrinsic mass (bronchogenic cyst, a vessel such as patent ductus arteriosis, or vascular ring). The classic presentation is respiratory distress in infancy, and only 5% of cases present after the age of 6 months.

Imaging Appearance

On chest radiography, CLO presents as overinflation of a lobe, usually the left upper lobe (41%), right middle lobe (34%), or right upper lobe (21%). There is displacement of the mediastinum away from the affected lobe, depression of the diaphragm, and compressive atelectasis in the adjacent lobe (Fig. 15.4A). In the postnatal period, the lobe may be filled with amniotic fluid, which clears in days.

On chest CT, there is severe lobar overinflation. There will be increased volume within the affected lobe, hyperlucency, attenuation of pulmonary vessels, and a contralateral mediastinal shift (see Fig. 15.4B). Atelectasis may also be seen in the unaffected lobe. CT confirms lobar overinflation and excludes the radiographic differential considerations of hypoplasia, proximal interruption of the pulmonary artery, or scimitar syndrome. CT may also reveal an underlying cause.

Foregut Duplication Cysts: Bronchogenic and Esophageal Duplication Cysts

A bronchogenic cyst is a congenital lesion thought to be secondary to abnormal budding of the embryonic foregut. The separated focus of tracheal-bronchial tissue fails to develop further, resulting in a cyst. Two-thirds of bronchogenic cysts occur in the mediastinum and one-third occur in the lung. Connection with a bronchus is unusual, but may occur if the lesion becomes infected or is instrumented.

Esophageal duplication cysts occur due to abnormal esophageal development and recanalization. Due to the

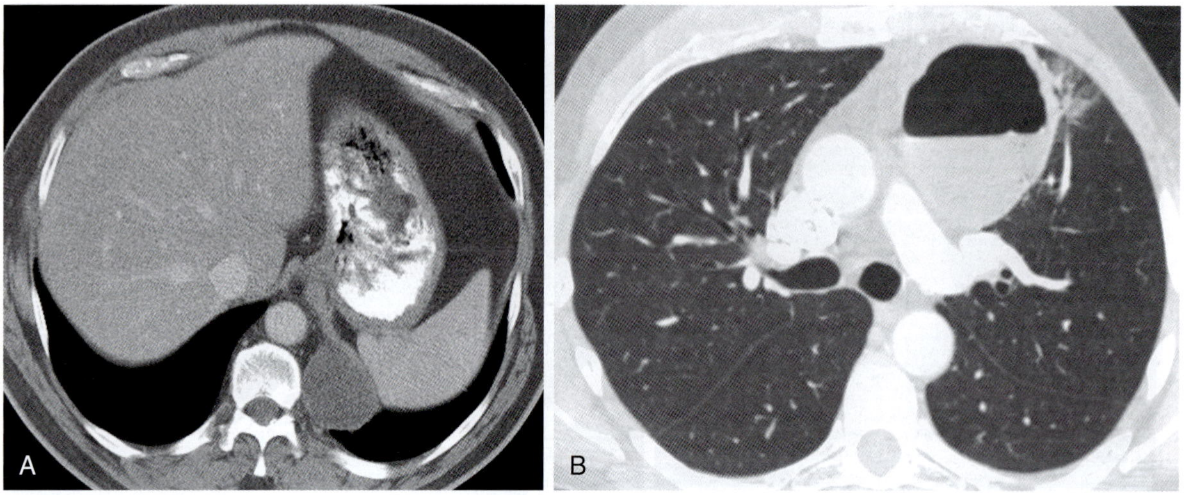

Figure 15.7 Bronchogenic cysts. (A) Axial contrast-enhanced CT scan shows a low-attenuation mass in the medial left lower lobe, which was an intrapulmonary bronchogenic cyst on resection. (B) Cystic mass with internal air-fluid level, mildly thickened wall, and adjacent ground-glass opacity, which was an infected bronchogenic cyst.

Differential Diagnosis

1. If an FDC presents as a soft tissue attenuation mass on CT, the differential would include lymphadenopathy, benign tumor, and malignancy. Thoracic MRI is very helpful in these cases and distinguishes a cyst from a solid lesion.
2. In the anterior mediastinum, the differential may include thymic cyst, cystic thymoma, and teratoma.
3. If a bronchogenic cyst occurs in the lung, the differential may include a hydatid cyst, lung mass, necrotic tumor, lung abscess, and hamartoma.

Scimitar Syndrome

Scimitar syndrome (also known as *venolobar syndrome*) is a group of disorders of lung and vascular development that occur together. The most consistent features of scimitar syndrome are an anomalous pulmonary venous return and pulmonary hypoplasia exclusively affecting the right lung.

Characteristic Feature of Scimitar Syndrome on Imaging

Identification of the anomalous vein is the characteristic feature of scimitar syndrome, typically draining to the infradiaphragmatic IVC between the right atrium and hepatic veins. Less commonly, the anomalous vein may connect to the hepatic vein, portal vein, azygous vein, coronary sinus, or right atrium. The anomalous pulmonary venous return of the right lung may be complete or partial.

Additional Disorders That Can Occur in Scimitar Syndrome

Additional disorders of lung and vascular development may occur in scimitar syndrome. The right lung is usually smaller in size due to pulmonary hypoplasia, which may be mild or severe. Patients may also have a bilateral left-sided bronchial branching pattern, horseshoe lung, airway diverticula, bronchiectasis, and/or bronchopulmonary sequestration. The arterial supply to the right lung is often abnormal. In about 50% of cases, the right pulmonary artery is reduced in size or absent. Systemic arterial supply to the right lung may also be present, originating from the abdomen or descending aorta. Cardiac malformations occur in 25% of patients, with atrial septal defect being the most common. Ventricular septal defect, tetralogy of Fallot, patent ductus arteriosis, aortic coarctation, left-sided superior vena cava, and pulmonary stenosis may also occur.

Imaging Appearance

On a chest radiograph, the right lung is usually smaller in size, with a small appearance of the right hilum. The diagnosis is suggested by identification of the characteristic so-called scimitar vein adjacent to or crossing the right atrium (Fig. 15.8A). When the degree of pulmonary hypoplasia is severe, the vein may be difficult to identify. Associated abnormalities such as bronchiectasis may be seen.

On chest CT, the diagnosis is confirmed by identification of the anomalous pulmonary vein (see Fig. 15.8B–E). Instead of returning to the left atrium, part or all of the pulmonary venous return of the right lung connects to an anomalous vein, usually inserting to the IVC below the right atrium. Hypoplasia of the right lung is usually present, which may be mild or severe. The associated abnormalities are as described above.

Differential Diagnosis

Diseases that result in dextroposition of the heart may appear similar to scimitar syndrome on a chest radiograph. In these cases, the anomalous vein will not be present

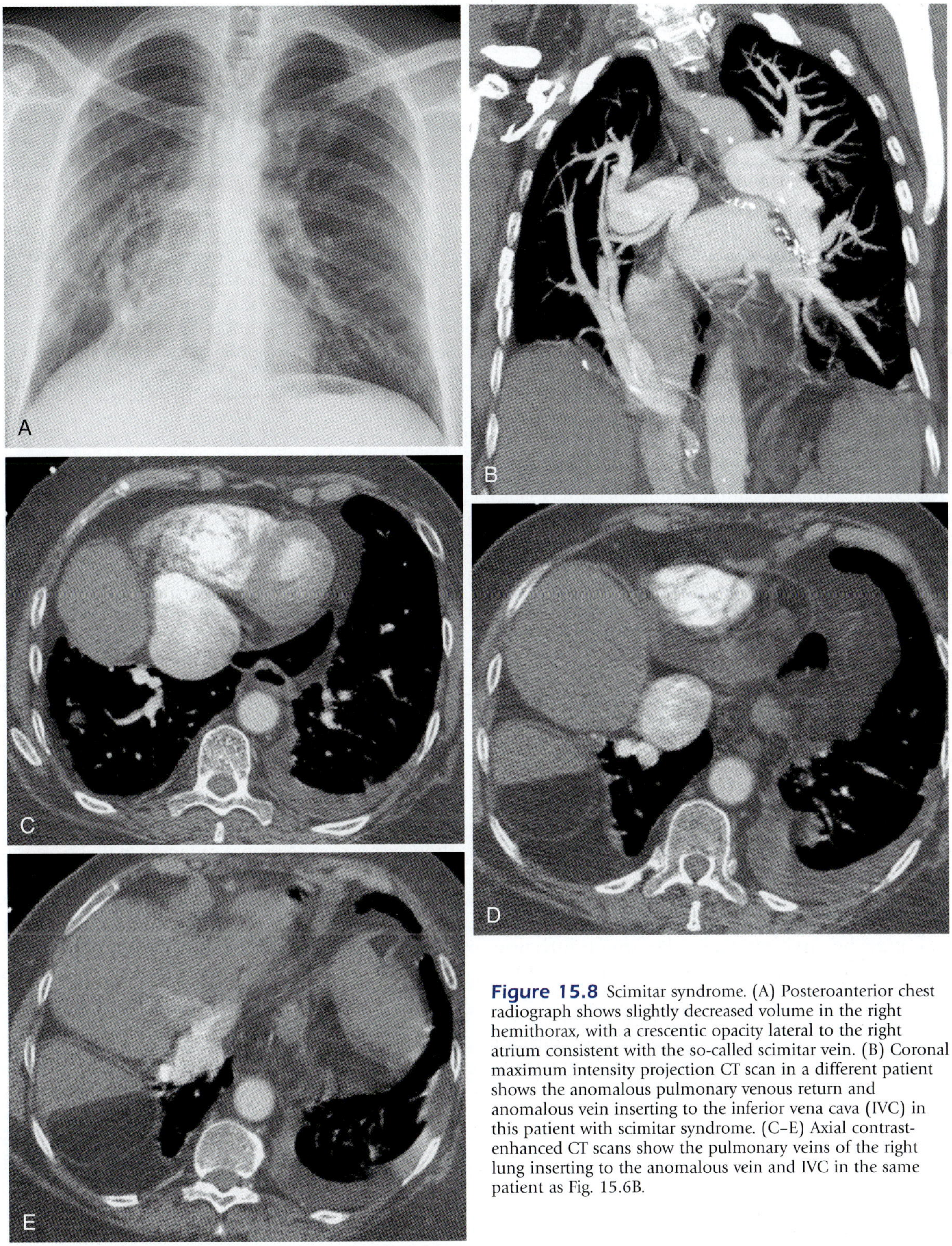

Figure 15.8 Scimitar syndrome. (A) Posteroanterior chest radiograph shows slightly decreased volume in the right hemithorax, with a crescentic opacity lateral to the right atrium consistent with the so-called scimitar vein. (B) Coronal maximum intensity projection CT scan in a different patient shows the anomalous pulmonary venous return and anomalous vein inserting to the inferior vena cava (IVC) in this patient with scimitar syndrome. (C–E) Axial contrast-enhanced CT scans show the pulmonary veins of the right lung inserting to the anomalous vein and IVC in the same patient as Fig. 15.6B.

or will be lateral to or overlying the right atrium. These diseases may include the following:

1. Dextrocardia
2. Proximal interruption of the pulmonary artery
3. Hypoplasia of the right lung (without anomalous venous drainage)
4. Swyer-James syndrome
5. Volume loss from atelectasis, endobronchial lesion, or foreign body in the airway

Complications

Most patients are asymptomatic and require no treatment. Some patients experience recurrent infection due to airway diverticula, bronchiectasis, and airway stenosis. Patients could also present with symptoms of volume overload from large left-to-right shunting. If treatment is required due to symptoms, this may involve reimplantation of the anomalous vein to the left atrium.

Proximal Interruption of the Pulmonary Artery

Proximal interruption of the pulmonary artery occurs when the central pulmonary artery is completely absent or terminates within 1 cm of its origin. However, the pulmonary arteries within the lung are intact and are supplied by systemic arterial collaterals. Proximal interruption usually occurs on the right, most often opposite to the side of the aortic arch. Left-sided proximal interruption (with a right aortic arch) has a higher incidence of associated congenital heart disease, especially tetralogy of Fallot.

Imaging Appearance

On a chest radiograph, the affected lung is usually decreased in volume compared to the unaffected lung. There is an ipsilateral mediastinal shift and elevation of the hemidiaphragm associated with the smaller size of the affected lung. The affected hilum is usually small in size, with no identifiable central pulmonary artery (Figs. 15.9A and 15.10A). In patients with vigorous intercostal artery collaterals, rib notching may occur.

On chest CT, the affected pulmonary artery is completely absent or terminates within 1 cm of its origin (see Figs. 15.9B and 15.10B). Collateral flow to the affected lung, with prominent systemic arterial collaterals, such as the bronchial arteries, intercostal arteries, internal mammary arteries, or phrenic arteries, may be seen (see Figs. 15.9B–C and 15.10B). The venous drainage of the affected lung is normal, distinguishing this disorder from scimitar syndrome.

On chest CT lung windows, a common finding is serrated pleural thickening and subpleural parenchymal bands (see Fig. 15.9D). Occasionally, transpleural intercostal arteries may be seen crossing the pleura to the lung. Mosaic attenuation of the lung may also be seen.

Complications

Patients may be asymptomatic. Recurrent infection, decreased exercise tolerance, and dyspnea are most common if symptoms do occur. Patients may also experience hemoptysis, occasionally life-threatening hemoptysis from vigorous collaterals. Patients may also develop bronchiectasis. Pulmonary hypertension is the most important prognostic feature for these patients and occurs in up to 25% of patients.

Differential Diagnosis

1. Scimitar syndrome. The major differentiation on imaging is the absence of an anomalous pulmonary vein in proximal interruption of the pulmonary artery.
2. Pulmonary hypoplasia. The central pulmonary artery may be smaller but will be intact.
3. Other causes for volume loss. These include atelectasis, endobronchial lesion, and a foreign body.

Pulmonary Arteriovenous Malformation

A pulmonary arteriovenous malformation (PAVM) refers to a direct communication of a pulmonary artery and vein, without an intervening capillary bed. PAVMs are multiple in 33% of cases and up to one-third to two-thirds of cases are associated with Osler-Weber-Rendu syndrome. PAVMs are usually congenital but can also be acquired in patients with congenital heart disease (e.g., patients with Glenn or Fontan shunts), chronic liver disease, or infection (e.g., tuberculosis, actinomycosis). Enlargement of the vascular sac over time is common, occasionally with rapid enlargement.

Types of Pulmonary Arteriovenous Malformations

Simple arteriovenous malformations are most frequent, consisting of lesions with one feeding pulmonary artery and one draining pulmonary vein. Complex PAVMs are less common (20%) and consist of lesions with one or more feeding pulmonary arteries or draining pulmonary veins. Due to the multiplicity of vessels, these are more difficult to treat.

Clinical Manifestations

When PAVMs are small, the patient may be asymptomatic. When PAVMs enlarge or are multiple, the right-to-left shunt may become more significant, and patients may develop hypoxemia, embolic complications (stroke or cerebral abscess), polycythemia, or, rarely, pulmonary hemorrhage. It is important when imaging patients with known or suspected PAVM to clear the IV tubing and injectors of all air to avoid the potential for systemic air embolism. For routine IV infusions, an IV filter is often used on IV tubing to avoid an air embolism.

Imaging Appearance

On a chest radiograph, a PAVM may appear as a pulmonary nodule or nodules (Fig. 15.11A). It may be possible to suggest a PAVM if feeding or draining vessels are visible; however, cross-sectional imaging will be required for confirmation.

On pre- and postcontrast images, a PAVM will appear as a homogeneously enhancing vascular sac isoattenuating to a pulmonary artery, with feeding pulmonary artery (or arteries) and draining pulmonary vein(s); (see Fig. 15.11B–F). The draining vein is usually enlarged. The PAVMs may be single or multiple.

Differential Diagnosis

1. Pulmonary artery pseudoaneurysm. See later section, "Pitfalls of Imaging Congenital Lung Diseases."
2. Granuloma. Occasionally, a granuloma can exist with a converging pulmonary artery and vein, giving the appearance of an arteriovenous malformation. See later section, "Pitfalls of Imaging Congenital Lung Diseases."
3. Nodules from other causes (e.g., carcinoid tumor, metastasis). These would not have a feeding artery or draining vein.

Bronchial Atresia

In bronchial atresia, there is focal atresia or stenosis of a bronchus, which may occur in a lobar, segmental, or subsegmental bronchus close to its point of origin. It

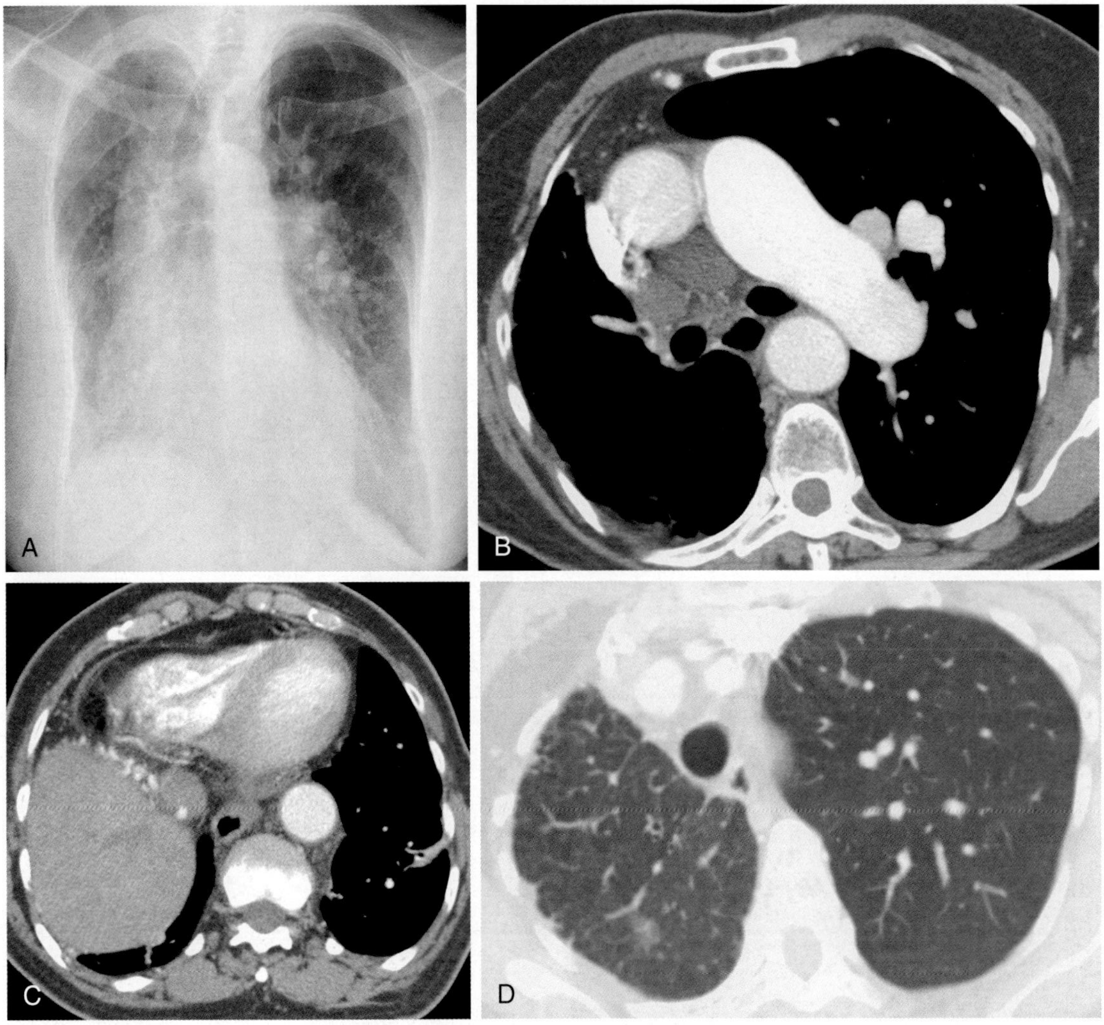

Figure 15.9 Proximal interruption of the right pulmonary artery. (A) Posteroanterior chest radiograph shows reduced volume in the right hemithorax, a small right hilum, decreased vascularity in the right lung, and a left aortic arch. (B, C) Axial contrast-enhanced CT scan shows complete absence of the right pulmonary artery and prominent systemic artery collateral flow in the right internal mammary and right phrenic arteries. (D) Axial CT scan in the lung window shows serrated pleural thickening, a common finding in proximal interruption of the pulmonary artery.

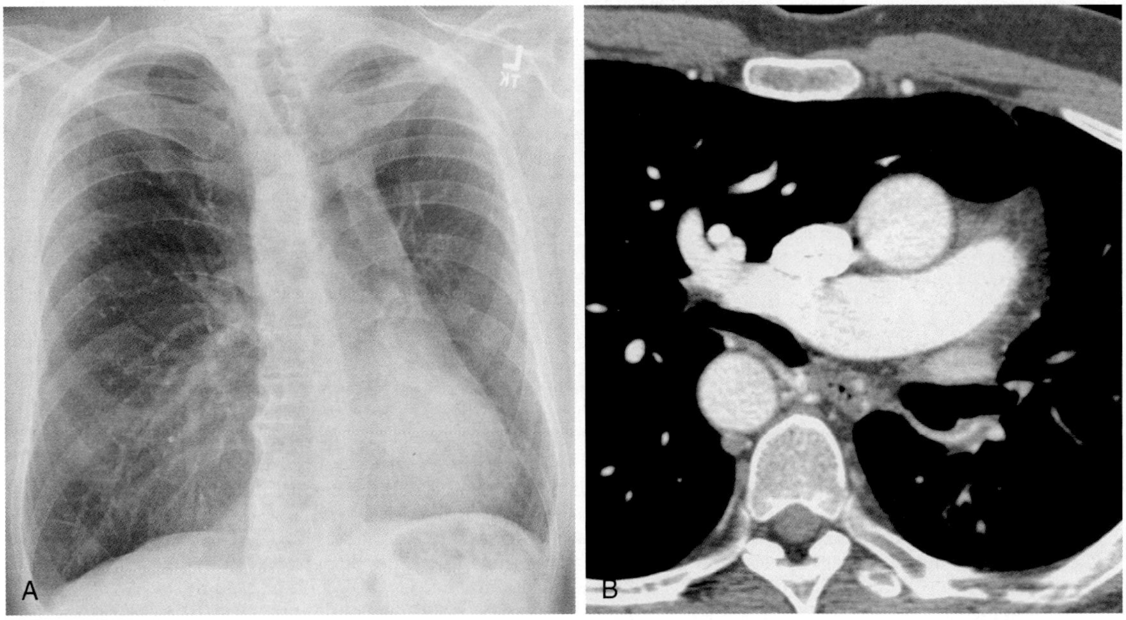

Figure 15.10 Proximal interruption of the left pulmonary artery. (A) Posteroanterior chest radiograph shows decreased volume in the left hemithorax, decreased vascularity in the left lung, decreased size of the left hilum, and a right-sided aortic arch. (B) Contrast-enhanced axial CT scan shows complete absence of the left pulmonary artery and systemic collateral flow in the bronchial and left internal mammary arteries.

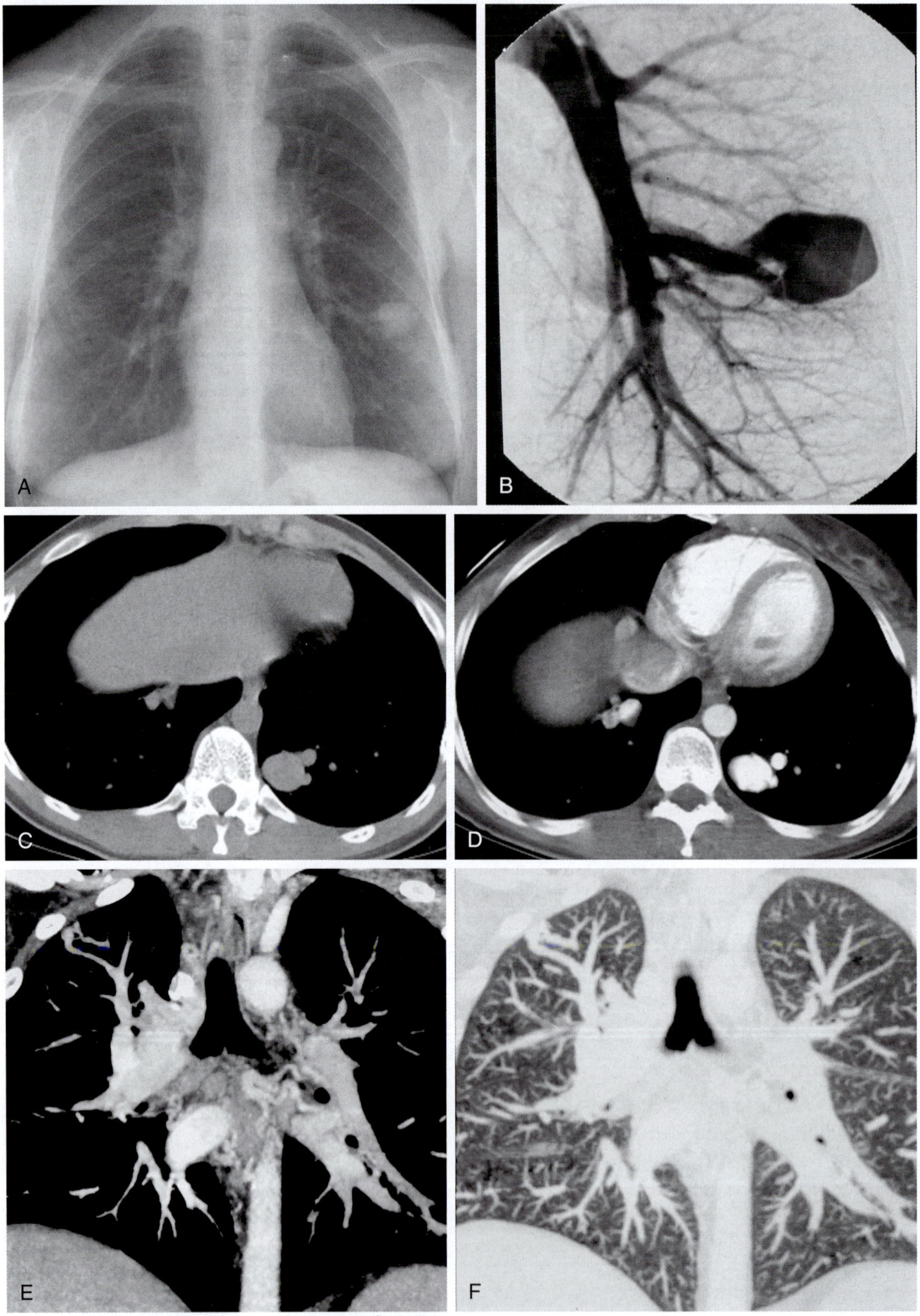

Figure 15.11 Pulmonary arteriovenous malformation (PAVM). (A, B) Posteroanterior chest radiograph and digital subtraction angiogram in the same patient show a rounded opacity with one feeding artery and one dilated draining vein, consistent with PAVM. (C, D) Pre- and postcontrast axial chest CT angiography scans of the pulmonary arteries show pulmonary arterial enhancement in bilateral PAVMs in this patient with Osler-Weber-Rendu syndrome. (E, F) Coronal maximum intensity projection CT scan shows a right upper lobe arteriovenous malformation, with a feeding artery and dilated draining vein. This was an acquired arteriovenous malformation after a Fontan procedure for congenital heart disease.

may occur secondary to prenatal interruption of bronchial arterial flow or disordered bronchial development. Distal to the point of atresia, the bronchial tree is patent and accumulates mucus (mucocele), which is a characteristic imaging feature seen on radiography and CT. The lung distal to the point of atresia becomes hyperinflated, likely secondary to collateral air drift between the normally ventilated portions of the lung and the lung distal to the point of atresia. The most common locations are the upper lobes and right middle lobe.

Imaging Appearance

On a chest radiograph, the characteristic finding is identification of the mucocele, which presents as an ovoid, branching, central mass (Fig. 15.12A). Occasionally, hyperlucency may be seen on a chest radiograph of the lung, distal to the point of atresia.

On chest CT, the mucocele will be a hypodense lesion consistent with mucus, which does not enhance after IV contrast (see Fig. 15.12B and C). Distal to the point of atresia and the mucocele, there is characteristic segmental hyperinflation (see Fig. 15.12D).

Differential Diagnosis

1. Obstructing tumor or foreign body. Occasionally, an obstructing tumor (e.g., carcinoid tumor) or foreign body could result in a mucocele and distal hyperinflation. It will be important to exclude an endobronchial lesion or an enhancing lesion in the airway proximal to the mucocele.
2. Vascular malformation. This may have a similar branching appearance on noncontrast imaging but would enhance postcontrast and lack the typical distal segmental hyperinflation.

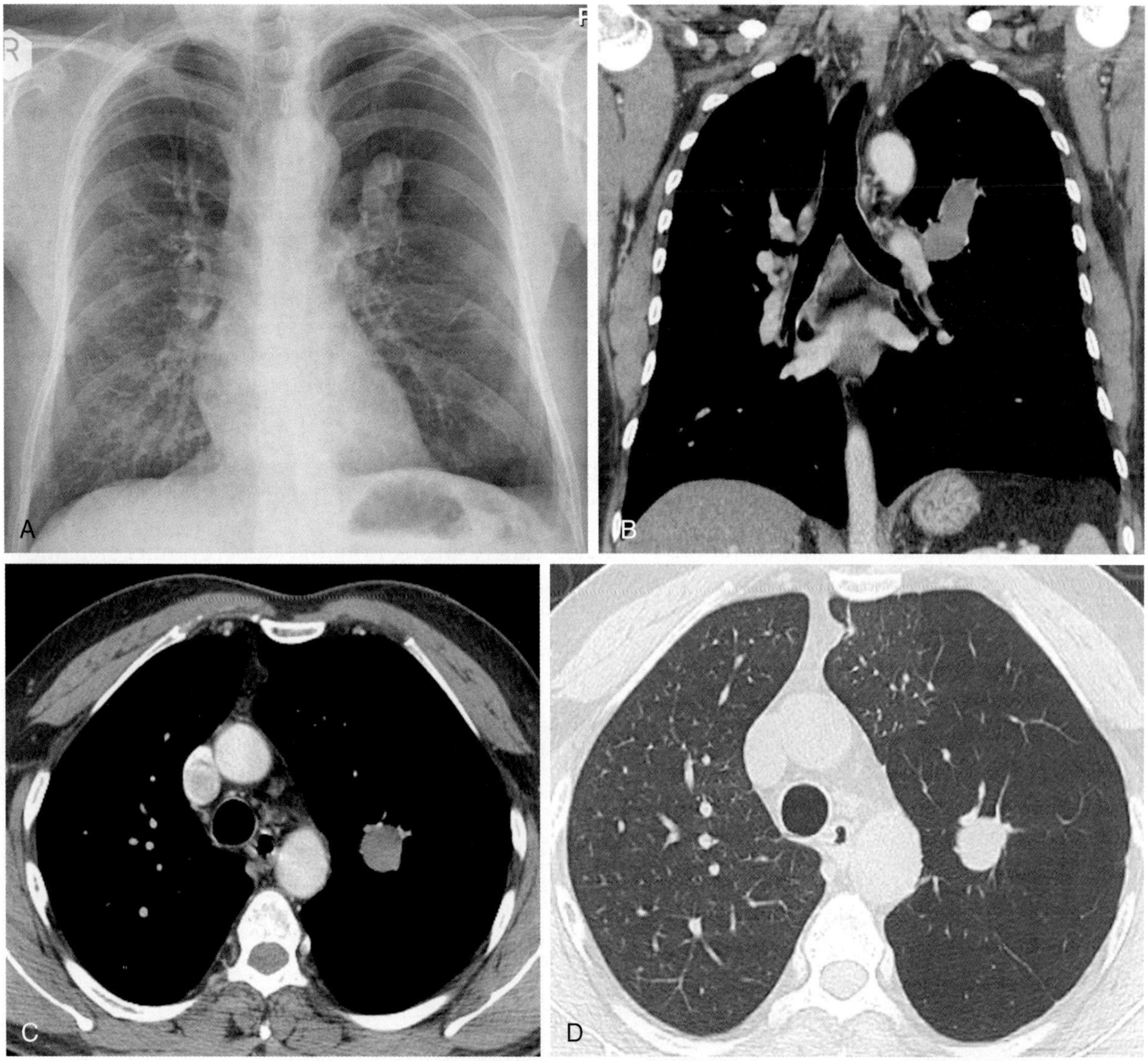

Figure 15.12 Bronchial atresia. (A) Posteroanterior chest radiograph shows a tubular mass extending from the left hilum, with left upper lobe hyperinflation. (B, C) Coronal multiplanar reformatted and axial contrast-enhanced CT images show a nonenhancing tubular mass consistent with a mucocele in the apicoposterior segment of the left upper lobe. (D) Axial CT scan in lung windows shows the mucocele and characteristic air trapping in the distal segment, in this case the apicoposterior left upper lobe. (Courtesy Dr. Rathachai Kaewlai.)

3. Other disorders with mucoid impaction (e.g., allergic bronchopulmonary aspergillosis). These will lack the characteristic segmental hyperinflation and would usually have additional areas of bronchiectasis and mucus plugging.

Tracheal Bronchus

A tracheal bronchus occurs when there is an ectopic origin of an upper lobe bronchus from the trachea (Fig. 15.13). The tracheal bronchus is usually right-sided, with a left-sided tracheal bronchus much less common. The most common appearance of a tracheal bronchus is the ectopic origin of a right upper lobe bronchus from the right lateral wall of the trachea, within 2 cm of the carina.

A tracheal bronchus may be classified as displaced or supernumerary. A displaced tracheal bronchus occurs when a segmental or subsegmental bronchus arises from the trachea instead of its normal position in the tracheobronchial tree. Thus, in effect, the right upper lobe airways are missing a single branch, which arises from an ectopic position in the trachea. A supernumerary tracheal bronchus occurs when a tracheal bronchus originates from the trachea and there is an otherwise normal branching pattern of the right upper lobe. A true so-called pig bronchus or bronchus suis occurs when the entire airway supply of the right upper lobe arises from the trachea instead of the right main bronchus.

Clinical Significance

A tracheal bronchus is often an incidental asymptomatic finding. However, a tracheal bronchus may be associated with disease, including recurrent infection and bronchiectasis. If a patient is to undergo a pulmonary resection or bronchoscopy, knowledge of the variant bronchial anatomy is very helpful to the surgeon or interventional physician. The lung supplied by a tracheal bronchus could also be subject to atelectasis in the setting of endotracheal intubation or mucus plugging.

Accessory Cardiac Bronchus

The accessory cardiac bronchus (ACB) is a blind-ending supernumerary bronchus arising from the medial wall of the distal right main bronchus or bronchus intermedius in the region of the right upper lobe bronchus (Fig. 15.14A–B). It is directed toward the pericardium and is thus referred to as a *cardiac bronchus*. The ACB varies in length; the longer ACBs are occasionally associated with rudimentary alveolar tissue, known as a *cardiac lobe* (see Fig. 15.14C).

Clinical Significance

Usually the ACB is an incidental, asymptomatic finding on chest CT of no clinical significance. Knowledge of an ACB is important to avoid diagnosis of an airway disease such as airway disruption associated with trauma, surgery, or infection. A focal outpouching of the airway associated with trauma or infection will often have an associated adjacent pneumomediastinum and inflammatory changes. Pathologically, the ACB contains cartilage in the wall, whereas diverticula and fistula do not.

■ Problem-Solving Issues

Differentiating Bronchopulmonary Sequestration From Other Congenital Lesions on Imaging

The imaging appearance of bronchopulmonary sequestration may overlap with other forms of congenital lung disease. A bronchopulmonary sequestration may present as a solid mass, a cystic mass (containing air, fluid, or air-fluid levels), or a region of hyperlucent hyperinflated lung parenchyma. The main diagnostic feature for bronchopulmonary sequestration is the presence of a systemic artery arising from the aorta (or other systemic artery in the chest or upper abdomen), which supplies pulmonary tissue lacking normal bronchial communication.

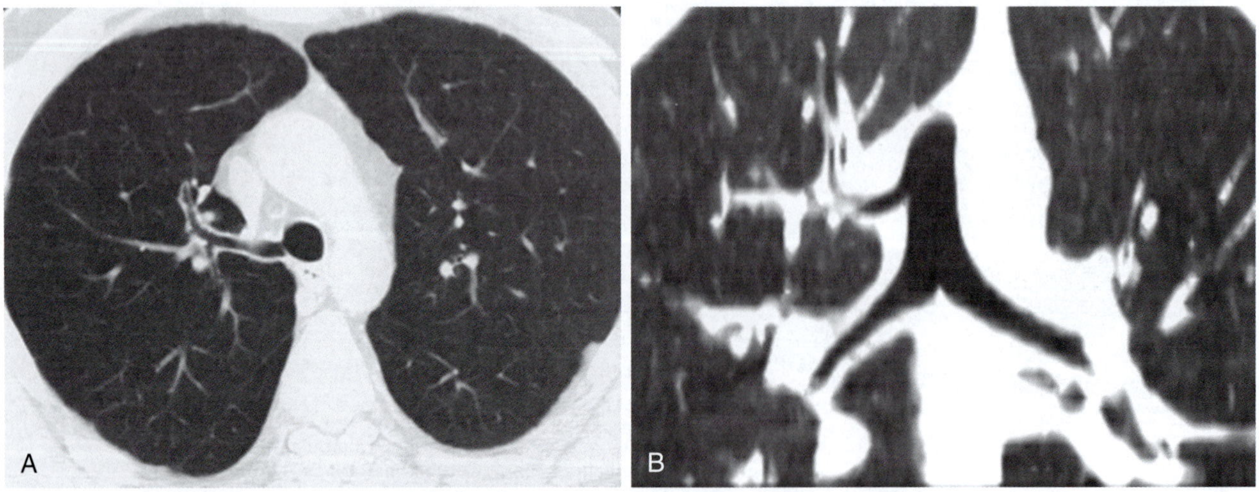

Figure 15.13 Tracheal bronchus. (A, B) Axial and coronal multiplanar reformatted CT images show that the entire bronchial supply of the right upper lobe originates from the right lateral wall of the trachea rather than the right main bronchus. This is a true *pig bronchus* or *bronchus suis*.

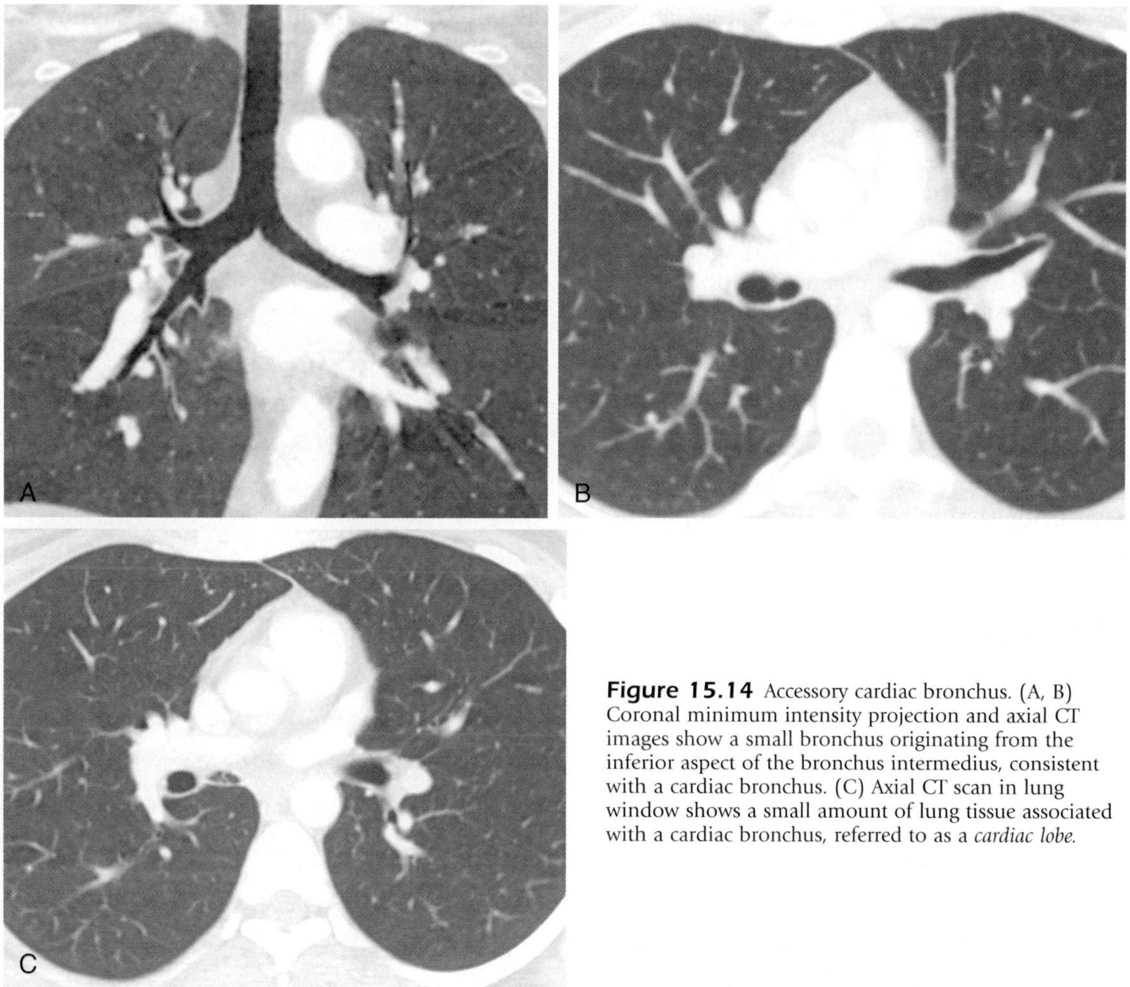

Figure 15.14 Accessory cardiac bronchus. (A, B) Coronal minimum intensity projection and axial CT images show a small bronchus originating from the inferior aspect of the bronchus intermedius, consistent with a cardiac bronchus. (C) Axial CT scan in lung window shows a small amount of lung tissue associated with a cardiac bronchus, referred to as a *cardiac lobe*.

Determining Whether the Presence of a Systemic Artery Suggests a Bronchopulmonary Sequestration

Systemic arterial supply to the lung can be found in acquired and congenital pulmonary diseases other than bronchopulmonary sequestration. A systemic arterial supply to the lung may be acquired in response to chronic inflammation or pulmonary artery obstruction. This includes diseases such as chronic pulmonary embolism and Takayasu arteritis. Some congenital lung diseases such as scimitar syndrome or proximal interruption of the pulmonary artery may also have a systemic arterial supply to the lung in the absence of bronchopulmonary sequestration.

An anomalous systemic artery may also supply normal lung in the absence of other congenital or acquired pulmonary diseases. The lung supplied by the systemic artery will be normal in appearance and have normal bronchial connections. The anomalous systemic artery often supplies the basilar portions of the lung and is sometimes found distal to an absent interlobar or segmental lower lobe pulmonary artery.

In the setting of congenital lung disease, the presence of a systemic artery is usually considered to be caused by bronchopulmonary sequestration when the supplied lung lacks a normal connection with the bronchial tree. Disagreement exists as to whether other forms of congenital lung disease with a systemic arterial supply but intact bronchial connections should be referred to as a *bronchopulmonary sequestration*. In this case, it is best to refer to the lesion as in the *spectrum of bronchopulmonary sequestration*, along with a detailed description of all findings, including arterial, venous, bronchial, and parenchymal findings.

When to Suspect Superimposed Infection

Regions of abnormal lung in congenital lung disease may become superinfected and may be why the patient presents to imaging. The presence of consolidation, fluid, or air-fluid levels within the affected lung parenchyma raises the possibility of infection. Prior imaging showing a new or increase in consolidation, fluid, or air-fluid levels is most helpful in diagnosing superimposed infection, but prior imaging is not always available. If prior cross-sectional imaging is not available, be certain to look for and compare to prior chest radiographs, which may also answer questions regarding changes over time.

In the context of bronchogenic and esophageal duplication cysts, the presence of air, an air-fluid level, thick enhancing wall, or surrounding inflammatory changes suggests the possibility of infection.

Distinction of a Congenital Mediastinal Cyst From a Solid Mass or Lymphadenopathy

Mediastinal cysts are usually able to be diagnosed correctly as a cyst due to low CT attenuation values, between 0 and 20 HU. Occasionally, the CT attenuation value may be higher, approaching that of soft tissue (40–70 HU). It may not be possible to diagnose a spherical mass seen on CT alone as a cyst, and additional imaging may be required to exclude a soft tissue mass or enlarged lymph node. In these cases, mediastinal MRI can be diagnostic. The MRI appearance of the FDC is described earlier (see "Imaging Appearance" under "Foregut Duplication Cysts").

Difficult to Categorize or Hybrid Lesions

Congenital bronchopulmonary foregut malformations represent a spectrum of diseases that are interrelated. In some patients, the imaging and even the pathology of the lesion may exhibit features of more than one congenital disease entity. These combinations are referred to as *hybrid lesions*. The most common hybrid lesion is the combination of sequestration and a type 2 CPAM. Other hybrid lesions may include an FDC near a sequestration or may include a CLO or CPAM combined with a bronchogenic cyst, tracheal bronchus, or bronchial atresia.

To address the difficulty in categorizing such lesions, some have proposed using generic terminology, such as *congenital thoracic malformation*. In such cases, it is better to detail the important imaging features completely and not insist on one specific disease categorization.

Poland Syndrome

Poland syndrome is a congenital chest wall defect characterized by partial or complete absence of the pectoralis major and minor muscles. Almost invariably, the disorder is unilateral; however, the bilateral absence of the pectoralis muscles has been rarely reported. Associated agenesis or hypoplasia of the latissimus dorsi, serratus anterior, and external oblique muscles may also be seen. Additional chest wall abnormalities associated with Poland syndrome include hypoplasia, partial agenesis, and fusion of consecutive ribs, which may lead to significant depression of the anterior chest wall, resulting in contralateral pectus carinatum. Absence of the costal cartilages of ribs 2, 3, and 4 or 3, 4, and 5 may lead to an anterior chest wall defect. Hand abnormalities have been described as part of Poland syndrome, including shortness of the fingers (brachydactyly), fused fingers (syndactyly), or a combination of both (brachysyndactyly), with the middle phalanx most often affected. Of all patients presenting with syndactyly, 10% will have Poland syndrome. An ipsilateral decrease in nipple size, superior displacement of the nipple, and hypoplasia of subcutaneous tissues may also occur.

Imaging Appearance

On a chest radiograph, the primary manifestation of Poland syndrome is unilateral hyperlucency in the affected hemithorax, which may be a subtle radiographic finding (Fig. 15.15A). When detected, the diagnosis can be more strongly suggested when the ipsilateral axillary fold

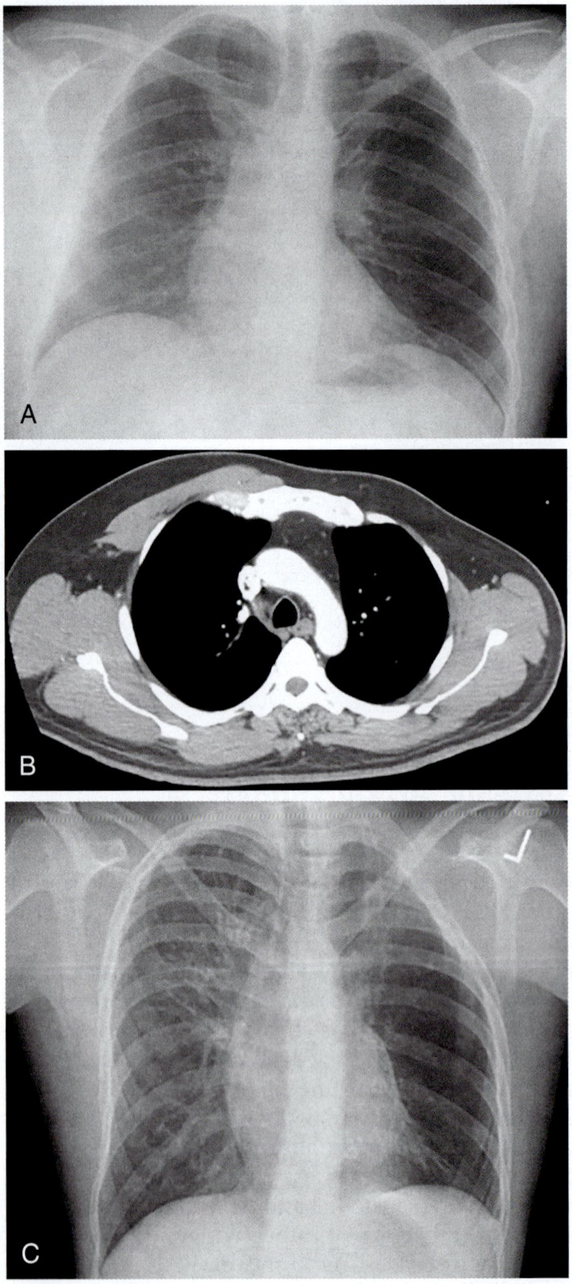

Figure 15.15 Poland syndrome. (A) Chest radiograph shows unilateral hyperlucency in the left hemithorax. (B) A follow-up chest CT scan shows complete absence of the left pectoralis major and minor muscles. (C) Chest radiograph in a different patient with left-sided Poland syndrome shows hyperlucency in the left hemithorax. There is a normal right axillary fold and absence of a left axillary fold on the affected side. Associated abnormalities of ribs 1–5 are seen in the left chest. Incidental note is also made of an unrelated bronchiectasis.

normally created by the pectoralis major muscle is absent (see Fig. 15.15C). In general, cross-sectional imaging with CT or MRI of the thorax is required to confirm the diagnosis. The pathognomonic finding on CT or MRI is the complete or partial absence of the pectoralis major and minor muscles (see Fig. 15.15B). If present, the associated rib abnormalities and chest wall defect may also be observed (see Fig. 15.15C). Occasionally, the rib and pectoralis muscle defects may be associated with an anterior lung hernia.

Differential Diagnosis

On chest radiography, the main differential diagnosis for Poland syndrome includes lung disease, pulmonary vascular disease, chest wall abnormality, pleural abnormality, or imaging artifact. Imaging artifacts such as grid misalignment could lead to asymmetric opacity when comparing one lung to the other. Asymmetric chest wall thickness and soft tissue can also result in unilateral hyperlucency from decreased ipsilateral chest wall thickness (e.g., mastectomy) or increased contralateral chest wall thickness (e.g., chest wall mass, hematoma, breast implant). In a similar fashion, asymmetric pleural disease could also result in asymmetric opacity, such as a contralateral posterior pleural effusion or asymmetric posterior pleural thickening. An increased volume or retention of air in the affected hemithorax could also create unilateral hyperlucency (e.g., Swyer-James-McLeod syndrome, CLO, asymmetric emphysema, large pneumothorax). Rarely, air trapping from an endobronchial foreign body or carcinoid tumor could lead to diffuse air trapping and a hyperinflated lung. Diseases that diminish pulmonary vascularity could also lead to a unilaterally hyperlucent hemithorax, including a large central pulmonary embolus (Westermark sign), proximal interruption of the pulmonary artery, and scimitar syndrome.

If unilateral hyperlucency is observed on chest radiography and Poland syndrome is suspected, examination of the axillary folds can be helpful. If there is a normal axillary fold in the contralateral axilla but asymmetric absence of a similar axillary fold in the affected hemithorax, this suggests the diagnosis of hypoplasia of the pectoralis muscles and Poland syndrome (see Fig. 15.15C). On chest CT or MRI, hypoplasia or absence of the pectoralis muscle is clearly established, and the other differential considerations for unilateral hyperlucency are excluded.

■ Pitfalls of Imaging Congenital Lung Diseases

In some cases of bronchopulmonary sequestration, the diagnostic systemic artery is small or inconspicuous on imaging. In cases in which the systemic artery is small, or if noncontrast chest CT is initially performed, the person performing the imaging needs to be aware of the possibility of a bronchopulmonary sequestration and to look carefully for the systemic artery. In addition, it is important to identify if there are multiple systemic arteries. Unless contraindicated, contrast-enhanced chest CT should be used to evaluate bronchopulmonary sequestration.

Due to the overlap in the imaging appearance of CPAM and acquired postinfectious or postinflammatory lesions of the lung, it is not always possible to know if a cystic lung lesion is acquired or congenital. In such case, a differential may be given.

Malignancy can mimic or occur in conjunction with congenital lesions. Rarely, type 1 CPAMs are associated with the later development of adenocarcinoma. Some lung and mediastinal malignancies are cystic in nature and may appear similar to a nonmalignant cystic lung lesion. Rarely, a congenital lung lesion could develop a superimposed malignancy within it. The presence of malignancy should be suspected if a cyst wall is thickened, irregular, or nodular or shows increased thickness or nodularity over time. For any lesion, the presence of an increasing or enhancing internal nodule or mass raises the possibility of malignancy. In the mediastinum, certain tumors can also be cystic and overlap with FDCs. For example, in the anterior mediastinum, cystic thymomas or teratomas may occur. Findings suspicious for cystic neoplasm include a thickened wall, mural nodularity, internal septations, and cyst complexity.

Certain diseases can mimic the appearance of a PAVM. Sometimes, a granuloma can be associated with a converging pulmonary artery and vein. A calcified granuloma can be diagnosed if the nodule is recognized as calcified on a noncontrast or virtual noncontrast (dual-energy) chest CT scan. This is why a precontrast examination is often useful on the initial chest CT in a patient with suspected arteriovenous malformation to avoid confusing a calcified granuloma with a contrast-enhanced arteriovenous malformation. After IV contrast, a noncalcified granuloma would not enhance to the same degree as the adjacent pulmonary arteries and would appear as a soft tissue nodule rather than an avidly enhancing pulmonary artery. Pulmonary artery pseudoaneurysms should also not be confused with PAVMs. A pseudoaneurysm will appear as an enhancing saccular outpouching from a pulmonary artery, without a draining vein.

Proximal interruption of the right pulmonary artery and scimitar syndrome can appear very similar on a chest radiograph. Care should be taken to interrogate the region of the right heart for the presence or absence of the anomalous "scimitar" vein. Cross-sectional imaging with chest CT or MRI is usually performed for confirmation and evaluation of associated anomalies.

In scimitar syndrome, if the degree of pulmonary hypoplasia is severe, the anomalous draining vein may be obscured. In these cases, it may not be possible to suggest scimitar syndrome on chest radiography, and cross-sectional imaging with CT or MRI would be required.

Bibliography

Berrocal T, Madrid C, Novo S, Gutiérrez J, Arjonilla A, Gómez-León N. Congenital anomalies of the tracheobronchial tree, lung, and mediastinum: embryology, radiology, and pathology. *Radiographics*. 2004;24(1):e17.

Biyyam DR, Chapman T, Ferguson MR, Deutsch G, Dighe MK. Congenital lung abnormalities: embryologic features, prenatal diagnosis, and postnatal radiologic-pathologic correlation. *Radiographics*. 2010;30(6):1721–1738.

Castañer E, Gallardo X, Rimola J, et al. Congenital and acquired pulmonary artery anomalies in the adult: radiologic overview. *Radiographics*. 2006;26(2): 349–371.

Frazier AA, Rosado de Christenson ML, Stocker JT, Templeton PA. Intralobar sequestration: radiologic-pathologic correlation. *Radiographics*. 1997;17(3): 725–745.

Garcia-Peña P, Coma A, Enríquez G. Congenital lung malformations: radiological findings and clues for differential diagnosis. *Acta Radiol*. 2013;54(9):1086–1095.

Ghaye B, Szapiro D, Fanchamps JM, Dondelinger RF. Congenital bronchial abnormalities revisited. *Radiographics*. 2001;21(1):105–119.

Godwin JD, Tarver RD. Scimitar syndrome: four new cases examined with CT. *Radiology*. 1986;159(1):15–20.

Hellinger JC, Daubert M, Lee EY, Epelman M. Congenital thoracic vascular anomalies: evaluation with state-of-the-art MR imaging and MDCT. *Radiol Clin North Am*. 2011;49(5):969–996.

Langston C. New concepts in the pathology of congenital lung malformations. *Semin Pediatr Surg*. 2003;12(1):17–37.

Lee EY, Boiselle PM, Cleveland RH. Multidetector CT evaluation of congenital lung anomalies. *Radiology*. 2008;247(3):632–648.

Lee EY, Dorkin H, Vargas SO. Congenital pulmonary malformations in pediatric patients: review and update on etiology, classification, and imaging findings. *Radiol Clin North Am*. 2011;49(5):921–948.

Lee EY, Tracy DA, Mahmood SA, Weldon CB, Zurakowski D, Boiselle PM. Preoperative MDCT evaluation of congenital lung anomalies in children: comparison of axial, multiplanar, and 3D images. *AJR Am J Roentgenol*. 2011;196(5): 1040–1046.

Miyake H, Hori Y, Takeoka H, Takuma M, Kawagoe T, Mori H. Systemic arterial supply to normal basal segments of the left lung: characteristic features on chest radiography and CT. *AJR Am J Roentgenol*. 1998;171(2):387–392.

Newman B. Congenital bronchopulmonary foregut malformations: concepts and controversies. *Pediatr Radiol*. 2006;36(8):773–791.

Rosado-de-Christenson ML, Frazier AA, Stocker JT, Templeton PA. From the archives of the AFIP. Extralobar sequestration: radiologic-pathologic correlation. *Radiographics*. 1993;13(2):425–441.

Ryu DS, Spirn PW, Trotman-Dickenson B, et al. HRCT findings of proximal interruption of the right pulmonary artery. *J Thorac Imaging*. 2004;19(3):171–175.

Sakai S, Murayama S, Soeda H, et al. Unilateral proximal interruption of the pulmonary artery in adults: CT findings in eight patients. *J Comput Assist Tomogr*. 2002;26(5):777–783.

Shimohira M, Hara M, Kitase M, et al. Congenital pulmonary airway malformation: CT-pathologic correlation. *J Thorac Imaging*. 2007;22(2):149–153.

Stocker JT. Congenital pulmonary airway malformation: a new name for and an expanded classification of congenital cystic adenomatoid malformations of the lung. *Histopathology*. 2002;41(suppl):424–431.

Walker CM, Wu CC, Gilman MD, Godwin JD, Shepard JA, Abbott GF. The imaging spectrum of bronchopulmonary sequestration. *Curr Probl Diagn Radiol*. 2014;43(3):100–114.

Zylak CJ, Eyler WR, Spizarny DL, Stone CH. Developmental lung anomalies in the adult: radiologic pathologic correlation. *Radiographics*. 2002;22(Spec No): S25–S43.

CHAPTER 16
Infection

Christopher M. Walker and Subba R. Digumarthy

CHAPTER OUTLINE

Introductory Considerations

Diagnostic imaging is used in the detection of thoracic infections, identifying complications associated with infection, and differentiating noninfectious from infectious diseases. Chest radiography and computed tomography (CT) comprise the primary modalities used in diagnosis, with ultrasound, nuclear medicine, and magnetic resonance imaging (MRI) used in select cases. Suggesting a specific organism is generally not possible in the immunocompetent patient presenting with thoracic infection. Imaging is usually able to suggest a specific pathogen in patients with known human immunodeficiency virus (HIV) infection or in patients with other forms of immunosuppression, such as bone marrow transplant (BMT) recipients. Thoracic infection is broadly categorized into three separate categories:

1. Infection in the immunocompetent host
2. Infection in the immunocompromised host with HIV
3. Infection in the immunocompromised host without HIV

Epidemiology

Pneumonia and influenza are the eighth leading cause of death in the United States. An estimated 1.23 million hospital admissions yearly are attributable to pneumonia. Pneumonia affects all ages and genders, but tends to be more severe and deadly in the very young and very old. Pneumonia is caused by bacteria, viruses, fungi, and parasites, as well as following the inhalation of food, liquid, gas, and dust.

Symptoms

Bacterial pneumonia may have a rapid and sudden onset with symptoms of high fever, productive cough, sweats, and shaking chills. Occasionally, bacterial pneumonia may have a gradual course with less severe symptoms. The symptoms of influenza and viral pneumonia are similar and include fever, dry cough, headache, weakness, and muscle aches.

Pathogenesis

Pathogens may gain access to the respiratory system in a variety of ways, ultimately leading to infection. The most common route of spread is via the tracheobronchial tree, usually by inhalation of aerosolized organisms or, less commonly, aspiration of secretions. Less common routes are via direct spread from infected mediastinal or hilar lymph nodes or extension of an infection from an adjacent organ, such as a liver abscess or perforated esophagus. Infection may also gain access to the lungs through the pulmonary vasculature occurring with infective endocarditis, bacteremia, or infected central venous catheters.

Most hospital-acquired infections occur via aspiration of oropharyngeal pathogens or leakage of secretions containing pathogenic bacteria around the endotracheal tube cuff. Infected biofilm surrounding the endotracheal tube may also be important in the pathogenesis of ventilator-associated pneumonia. Inhalation or direct inoculation of organisms into the lungs, hematogenous dissemination, and bacterial spread from the gastrointestinal tract are less common patterns of spread in hospitalized patients.

Diagnosis

Pneumonia is determined to be present clinically when a chest radiograph shows new or increasing consolidation and clinical evidence that the consolidation is of infectious origin. Clinical features suggestive of infectious origin of consolidation include fever (≥38 °C), purulent secretions, and leukocytosis or leucopenia. Pathogen-directed therapy is advised and may be obtained by Gram staining and culture of sputum, blood cultures, testing for *Legionella* and pneumococcal urinary antigens, and multiplex polymerase chain reaction (PCR) assays for *Mycoplasma pneumoniae, Chlamydia pneumoniae,* and respiratory viruses, as well as other pathogens, as indicated by the patient's exposure history or specific risk factors. Procalcitonin is a peptide precursor produced by cells in the intestine and lungs and is a useful marker to differentiate bacterial from nonbacterial infections and other noninfectious causes of inflammation. A procalcitonin level does not generally rise in patients with viral or noninfectious causes of inflammation. The serum procalcitonin concentration is a helpful marker of bacterial sepsis, and a low concentration (<0.1 μg/L) can support a decision to withhold or discontinue antibiotics.

In one large study of 2706 adults diagnosed with pneumonia, almost one-third initially had a normal chest radiograph. In these patients, the absence of consolidation should not supersede clinical judgment and empiric therapy because many of these patients will develop bacteremia, with associated increased mortality.

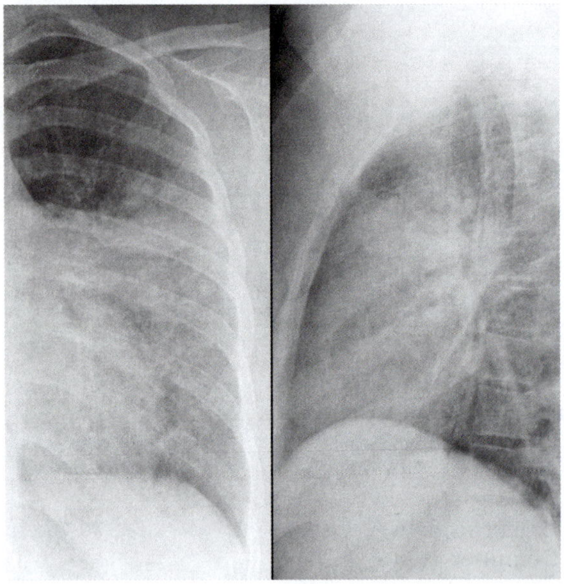

Figure 16.1 Community-acquired pneumococcal pneumonia. A composite image with posteroanterior *(left)* and lateral *(right)* chest radiographs shows lingular consolidation obscuring the left heart border (silhouette sign).

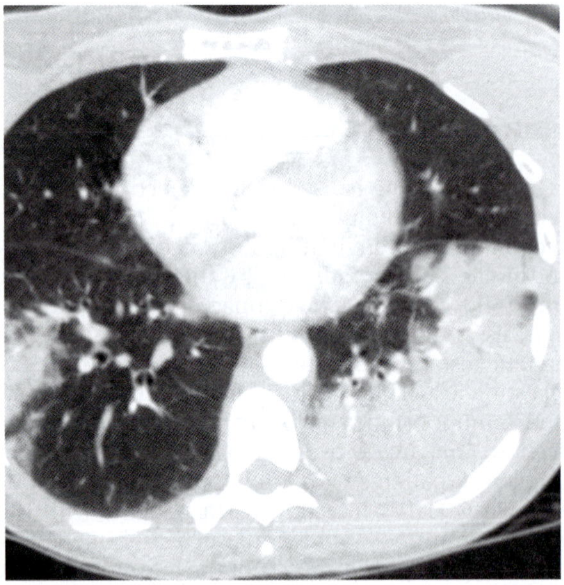

Figure 16.2 Hospital-acquired *Klebsiella* pneumonia. This axial contrast-enhanced CT scan shows left greater than right lower lobe consolidation, compatible with pneumonia. Hospital-acquired pneumonia develops 48 hours or later in a patient in a hospital and is the second most common nosocomial infection.

Definitions

Pneumonia is broadly divided into infection that is acquired in the community and infection acquired by hospital or nursing home patients. Multidrug-resistant (MDR) organisms are more common in hospital or health care–associated pneumonia.

Community-Acquired Pneumonia

Community-acquired pneumonia (CAP) is pneumonia manifesting in a patient who has not been recently hospitalized and who has had no regular exposure to the health care system (Fig. 16.1). *Pneumococcus* is the most common bacterial pathogen responsible for CAP, but its incidence has been declining with the use of the pneumococcal vaccination and with decreased rates of cigarette smoking. Other causes of CAP include *Haemophilus influenzae, Staphylococcus aureus, Moraxella catarrhalis, Pseudomonas aeruginosa,* viruses, and other gram-negative bacteria. Despite exhaustive testing, no organism is found in about 50% of cases.

Hospital-Acquired Pneumonia

Hospital-acquired pneumonia (HAP) is pneumonia manifesting 48 hours or more after a hospital admission, usually caused by bacterial pathogens (Fig. 16.2). HAP is associated with a high morbidity and mortality and is the second most common nosocomial infection in the United States, trailing only urinary tract infection. HAP increases a hospital stay by 7 to 9 days and increases the total cost by approximately $40,000/patient. Common pathogens include gram-positive cocci such as *S. aureus* and gram-negative organisms, including *P. aeruginosa, Klebsiella pneumoniae, Escherichia coli,* and *Actinobacter* spp. Rates of polymicrobial infection appear to be rising, especially in patients with acute respiratory distress syndrome (ARDS).

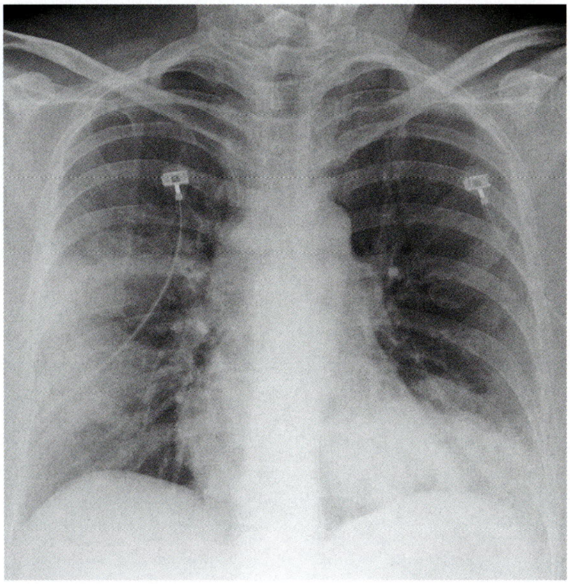

Figure 16.3 Health care–associated pneumococcal pneumonia. This posteroanterior chest radiograph shows multifocal consolidation in this nursing home patient with fever and cough.

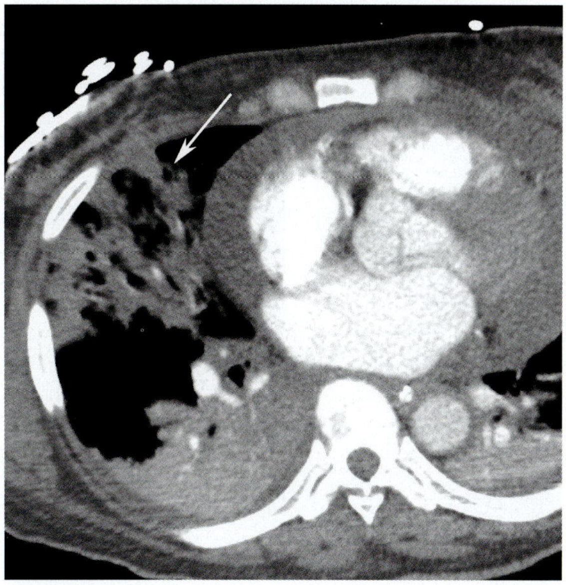

Figure 16.4 Ventilator-associated pneumonia. This axial contrast-enhanced CT scan shows multifocal consolidation involving the right middle, right lower, and left lower lobes. Note heterogeneity of the right lower lobe consolidation and low density of the right middle lobe consolidation *(arrow)*.

Health Care–Associated Pneumonia

Health care–associated pneumonia (HCAP) is pneumonia manifesting in a patient who was recently hospitalized for 20 or more days in the preceding 90 days of infection, resided in a nursing home or long-term care facility, received recent intravenous antibiotic therapy, chemotherapy, or wound care within the preceding 30 days of infection, or attended a hospital or hemodialysis clinic (Fig. 16.3).

Ventilator-Associated Pneumonia

Ventilator-associated pneumonia (VAP) is pneumonia manifesting 48 to 72 hours following recent endotracheal intubation (Fig. 16.4). VAP occurs in about 9% to 27% of intubated patients, with about 50% of all cases occurring within the first 4 days of ventilation.

■ Patterns of Infection

Pulmonary infections may affect the pulmonary parenchyma (pneumonia), the small airways (bronchiolitis), and the central airways (tracheobronchitis). Pneumonia is often subdivided into lobar pneumonia, bronchopneumonia, and interstitial pneumonia, although differentiating among these different patterns is often difficult and usually unreliable in suggesting a specific pathogen.

Lobar Pneumonia

Lobar pneumonia usually starts as a unilateral peripheral opacity that progresses to homogeneous consolidation, often bounded by an interlobar fissure (Fig. 16.5) or the hemidiaphragm. Lobar pneumonia is most common with infection by *Streptococcus pneumoniae*, *K. pneumoniae*, and *Legionella pneumophila*. Lower lobe pneumonia may manifest the spine sign on the lateral chest radiograph, which represents a paradoxic increased density of the lower thoracic spine (Fig. 16.6). There are often air bronchograms (Fig. 16.7) within the consolidation, and the infection tends to cross bronchopulmonary segments. It uncommonly affects the entire lobe due to the early initiation of antibiotic therapy. Occasionally, there may be copious amounts of inflammatory exudates, which cause bulging or displacement of fissures (i.e., bulging fissure sign; Fig. 16.8). Although typically described with

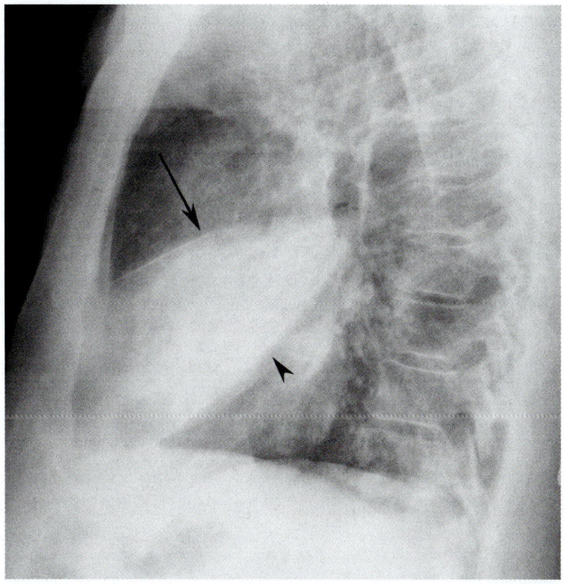

Figure 16.5 Right middle lobe pneumococcal pneumonia. This lateral chest radiograph shows right middle lobe consolidation bounded by the minor fissure superiorly *(arrow)* and the right major fissure inferiorly *(arrowhead)*.

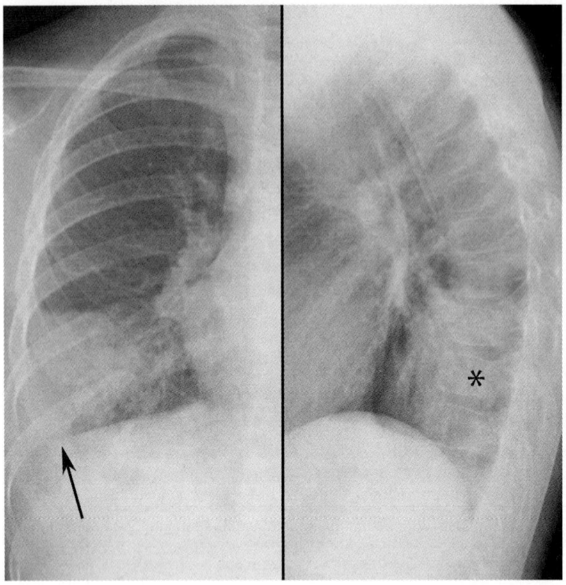

Figure 16.6 Spine sign in right lower lobe pneumonia. This composite image with a posteroanterior chest radiograph *(left)* and lateral chest radiograph *(right)* shows right lower lobe consolidation obscuring the lateral and posterior right hemidiaphragm *(arrow)*. Note the increased density overlying the lower thoracic spine *(asterisk)* on the lateral radiograph, which represents the spine sign.

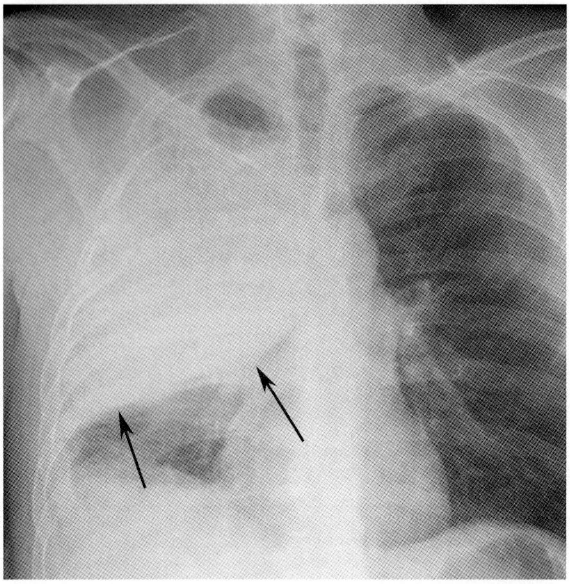

Figure 16.8 Bulging fissure sign in *Klebsiella* pneumonia. This posteroanterior chest radiograph shows right upper lobe consolidation causing inferior displacement *(arrows)* of the right major and minor fissures.

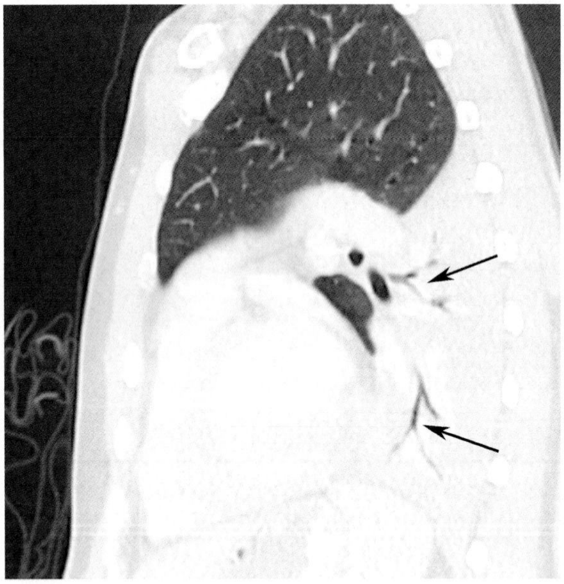

Figure 16.7 Air bronchogram in left lower lobe pneumonia. This sagittal contrast-enhanced CT scan shows left lower lobe consolidation, with multiple branching, air-filled tubular bronchi *(arrows)*. Air-filled bronchi become visible on imaging (air bronchogram sign) when they are surrounded by consolidated lung.

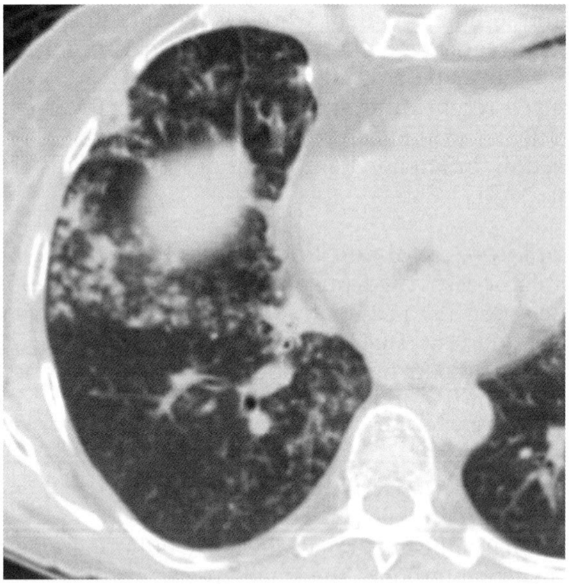

Figure 16.9 Bronchopneumonia caused by *Staphylococcus aureus*. This axial nonenhanced CT scan shows patchy right lower and middle lobe nodular opacities and tree-in-bud opacities.

K. pneumoniae, the bulging fissure sign is usually seen with *S. pneumoniae* owing to its greater prevalence.

Bronchopneumonia

Bronchopneumonia begins with infection of the distal airways, which eventually extends into the adjacent alveoli (Fig. 16.9). Lobules are often first affected in a patchy fashion and may be initially limited to one or a few bronchopulmonary segments before progressing to multifocal bilateral consolidation. Air space nodules or acinar nodules represent infection of distal bronchioles and surrounding alveoli and manifest as 5- to 10-mm ill-defined centrilobular nodules. There are often associated branching V- and Y-shaped opacities that are referred to as the *tree-in-bud sign* (Fig. 16.10). Bronchopneumonia is most common with infection by *S. aureus*, gram-negative organisms, anaerobic bacteria, and *L. pneumophila*.

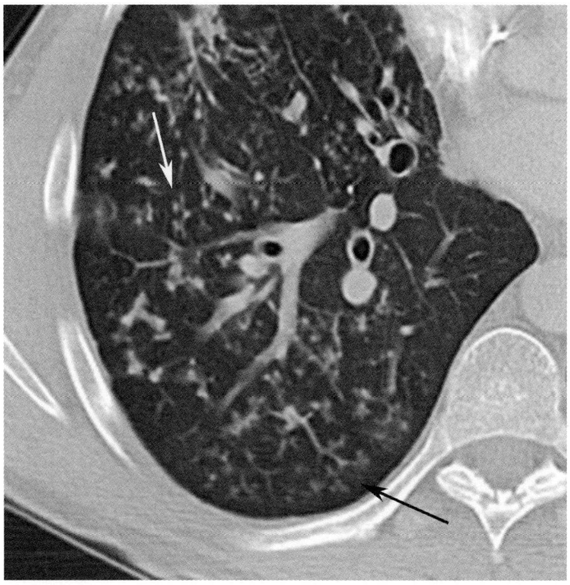

Figure 16.10 Tree-in-bud opacities in a patient with cystic fibrosis. This axial nonenhanced CT scan shows multiple branching V- and Y-shaped opacities *(arrows)* representing the tree-in-bud sign, which is most commonly seen with infectious bronchiolitis or aspiration. Note mild bronchiectasis and bronchial wall thickening, typical of cystic fibrosis.

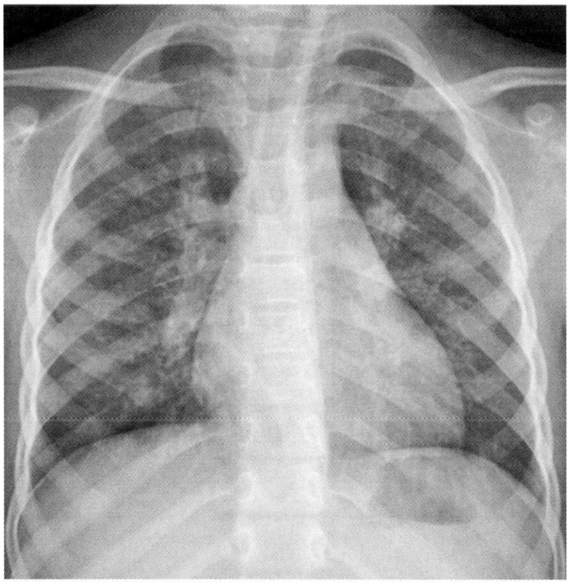

Figure 16.11 Viral bronchiolitis secondary to respiratory syncytial virus infection. This anteroposterior chest radiograph shows bilateral perihilar bronchial thickening, with reticulation typical of a viral infection or reactive airway disease.

Interstitial Pneumonia and Bronchiolitis

Reticulonodular and nodular opacities are the most common interstitial manifestations of pneumonia and generally are the radiographic manifestation of bronchial wall thickening (Fig. 16.11) and cellular bronchiolitis on CT. The individual nodules are too small to visualize on radiography but manifest as small nodular opacities when multiple overlapping nodules summate (Fig. 16.12). The radiographic appearance may mimic that of interstitial

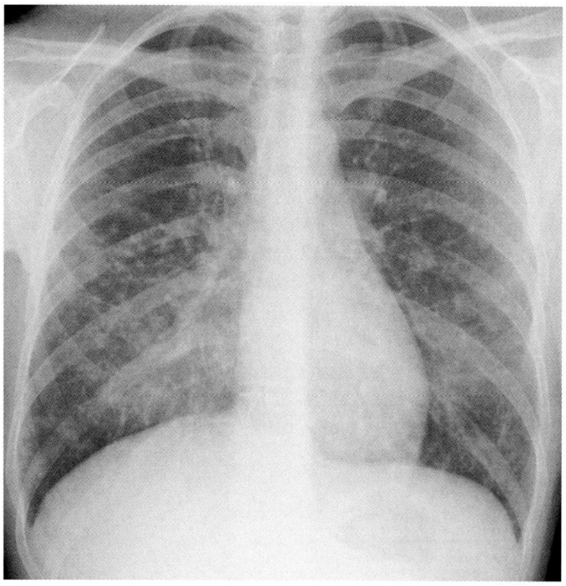

Figure 16.12 Varicella pneumonia. This posteroanterior chest radiograph shows multiple bilateral nodular opacities and bronchial wall thickening, typical of interstitial pneumonia. An interstitial pattern of pneumonia is most common with atypical organisms, including viruses, mycoplasma, and pneumocystis.

edema (Fig. 16.13A). On CT, interstitial pneumonia manifests as cellular bronchiolitis with tree-in-bud opacities, centrilobular nodules, bronchial wall thickening, and ground-glass opacities (Fig. 16.14; see Fig.16.13B). Consolidation is less commonly visualized. Mosaic attenuation (see Fig. 16.14) is common and represents air trapping caused by small airway inflammation and obstruction. Interstitial pneumonia is usually caused by atypical organisms, including viruses, mycoplasma, and *Pneumocystis jirovecii*.

Tracheobronchitis

Primary infection of the trachea and central bronchi is generally caused by viruses and usually affects young children. The principle cause is croup, which manifests as the steeple sign of subglottic narrowing on anteroposterior radiography of the neck (Fig. 16.15). Viral tracheobronchitis in adults is uncommonly imaged and, very rarely, will be superinfected by bacteria.

The most common manifestations of bronchitis include linear or tramlike opacities emanating from the hila on chest radiography. The primary CT manifestations include bronchial wall thickening, mosaic lung attenuation related to air trapping, and bronchial plugging. Patients are often managed conservatively in the absence of consolidation.

Uncommonly, *Aspergillus*, tuberculosis, or *Candida* may affect the trachea and central bronchi in an immunocompromised patient. The most common manifestations of infection include focal airway wall thickening or plaques, which may be of high attenuation. Occasionally, wall thickening is diffuse and circumferential (Fig. 16.16), mimicking other diseases such as amyloidosis and polyangiitis with granulomatosis (formerly Wegener granulomatosis).

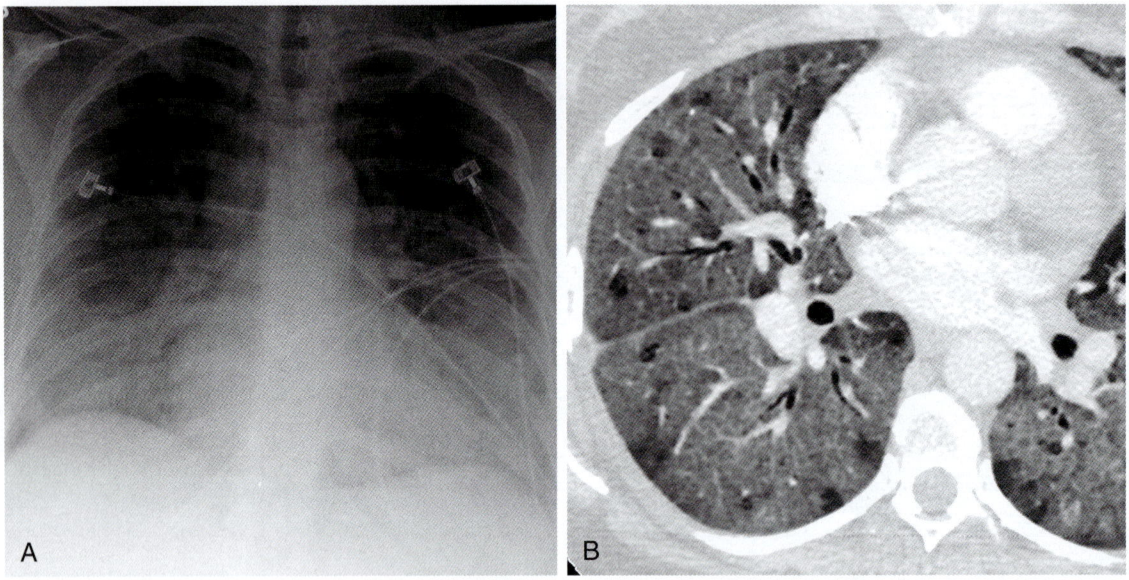

Figure 16.13 Mycoplasma pneumonia in a 47-year-old woman. (A) This anteroposterior chest radiograph shows diffuse perihilar and basal predominant opacities with indistinct vasculature, an appearance that could be mistaken for pulmonary edema. (B) Contrast-enhanced CT scan shows diffuse bilateral ground-glass opacities, with interlobular septal and intralobular interstitial thickening (crazy paving sign). Ground-glass opacities have a large differential diagnosis including infection by atypical organisms such as mycoplasma, *Pneumocystis jirovecii*, and viruses.

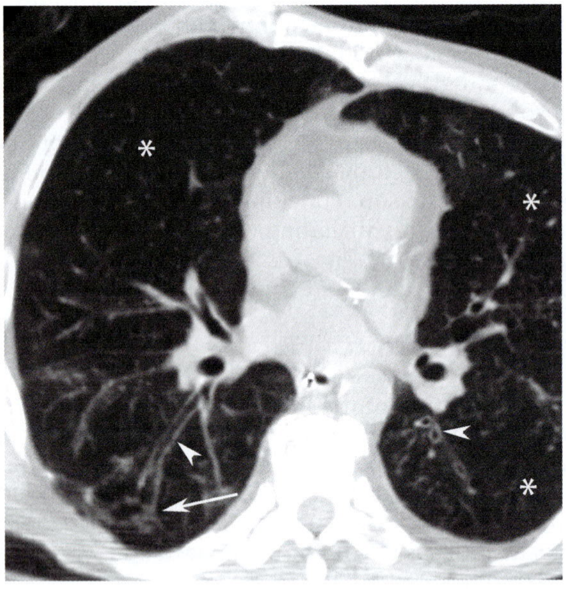

Figure 16.14 Viral pneumonia caused by parainfluenza. This axial nonenhanced CT scan shows bilateral bronchial wall thickening *(arrowheads)*, patchy ground-glass opacities, and tree-in-bud opacities *(arrow)*. Note focal areas of decreased lung attenuation *(asterisks)* representing mosaic attenuation due to small airway infection and secondary air trapping.

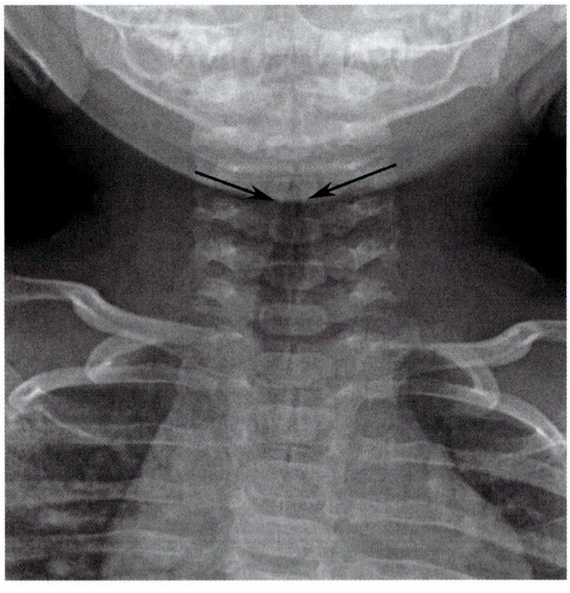

Figure 16.15 Viral croup with steeple sign. This anteroposterior radiograph of the upper airway shows subglottic tracheal narrowing, with an inverted V configuration *(arrows)*. (Courtesy Dr. Sherwin Chan, Kansas City, MO.)

Hematogenous Spread of Infection

Hematogenous spread of bacterial infection usually occurs in intravenous drug users (IVDUs) or in patients with infected central catheters. The most common manifestation is multiple mid and lower lung zone poorly defined nodules and wedge-shaped consolidations (Fig. 16.17). The nodules are usually located in the lung periphery and many undergo central cavitation over a period of several days. The nodules are often closely associated with pulmonary vasculature, which has been termed the *feeding vessel sign* (see Fig. 16.17B). This pattern of spread is usually found with infections caused by staphylococcal species, usually *S. aureus*. Uncommonly, multiple septic emboli occur in patients with thrombophlebitis of the internal or external jugular vein resulting from an oropharyngeal infection from *Fusobacterium necrophorum*.

This constellation of findings is termed *Lemierre syndrome* (Fig. 16.18).

Hematogenous spread of fungal infection is uncommon and usually affects immunocompromised individuals. It manifests with a miliary pattern on radiography and CT, which represents innumerable small (<3 mm), randomly distributed pulmonary nodules throughout both lungs, often with a mid and lower lung zone predominance (Fig. 16.19). Miliary spread of infection is most common with *Mycobacterium tuberculosis* as well as endemic fungi such as *Histoplasma capsulatum* and *Coccidioides immitis*.

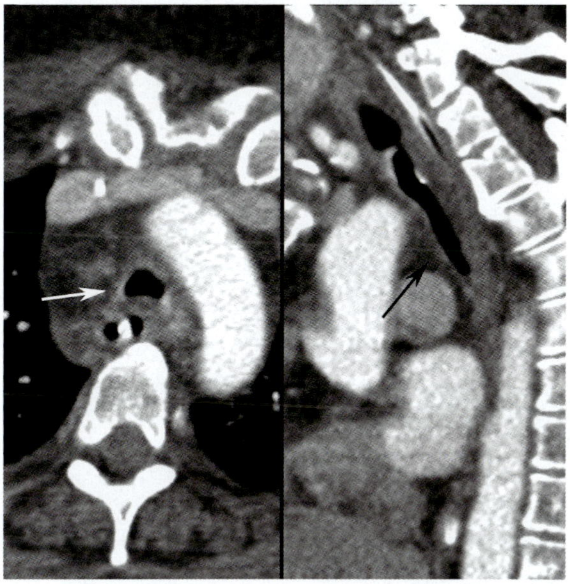

Figure 16.16 Candidal tracheitis in a patient with underlying immunosuppression. This composite image with axial *(left)* and sagittal *(right)* contrast-enhanced CT scans shows diffuse, circumferential tracheal wall thickening *(arrows)*. The differential diagnosis is broad, but infections such as fungal infection or tuberculosis should be considered in patients with underlying immunosuppression.

Patterns of Infection That Suggest a Specific Organism or Narrow the Differential Diagnosis

Cavitation

Cavitation within focal or diffuse consolidation usually indicates the presence of necrotizing infection. A reasonable differential diagnosis can be constructed by looking at the distribution of infection and whether or not the patient is immunosuppressed. Cavitation within a previously diagnosed pneumonia is most common in patients infected with *S. aureus* (Fig. 16.20), gram-negative bacteria, or anaerobes. New cavitation predisposes the patient to pneumothorax.

A cavitary upper lobe lesion, often with signs of volume loss in a patient with signs and symptoms of infection, represents *M. tuberculosis* infection until proven otherwise (Fig. 16.21). On CT, there are often associated tree-in-bud opacities and other small centrilobular nodules, which represent endobronchial spread of infection (Fig. 16.22). Atypical mycobacterial infection may manifest in an identical manner and is usually seen in alcoholics or those with chronic obstructive pulmonary disease (COPD; Fig. 16.23). A right upper lobe cavitary process that develops over weeks to months may be the initial manifestation of semiinvasive *Aspergillus* infection (also known as *chronic necrotizing aspergillosis*). This infection commonly affects patients with relative immunosuppression, such as alcoholics, patients on low-dose corticosteroids, diabetics, or patients with COPD. It first manifests as upper lobe consolidation, which progresses to cavitation and eventually lung destruction over weeks to months (Fig. 16.24). The consolidation often abuts thickened

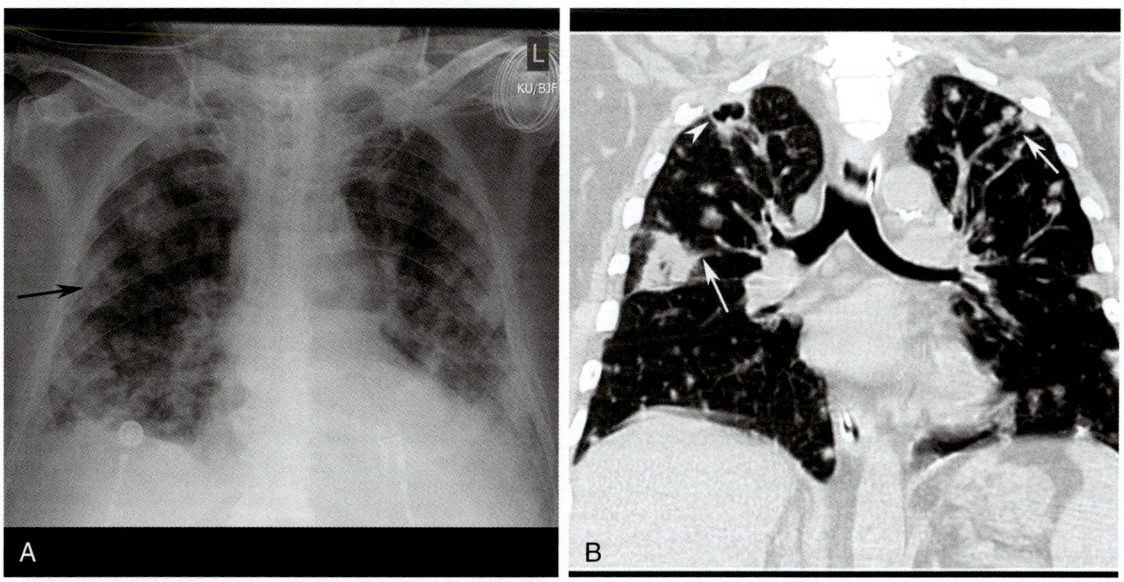

Figure 16.17 Septic embolism related to intravenous drug use. (A) Anteroposterior chest radiograph shows multiple bilateral nodules, some with internal lucency *(arrow)* suggestive of cavitation. (B) Coronal nonenhanced CT scan shows multiple bilateral pulmonary nodules, many manifesting the feeding vessel sign *(arrows)*. Note the right upper lobe cavitary nodule *(arrowhead)*.

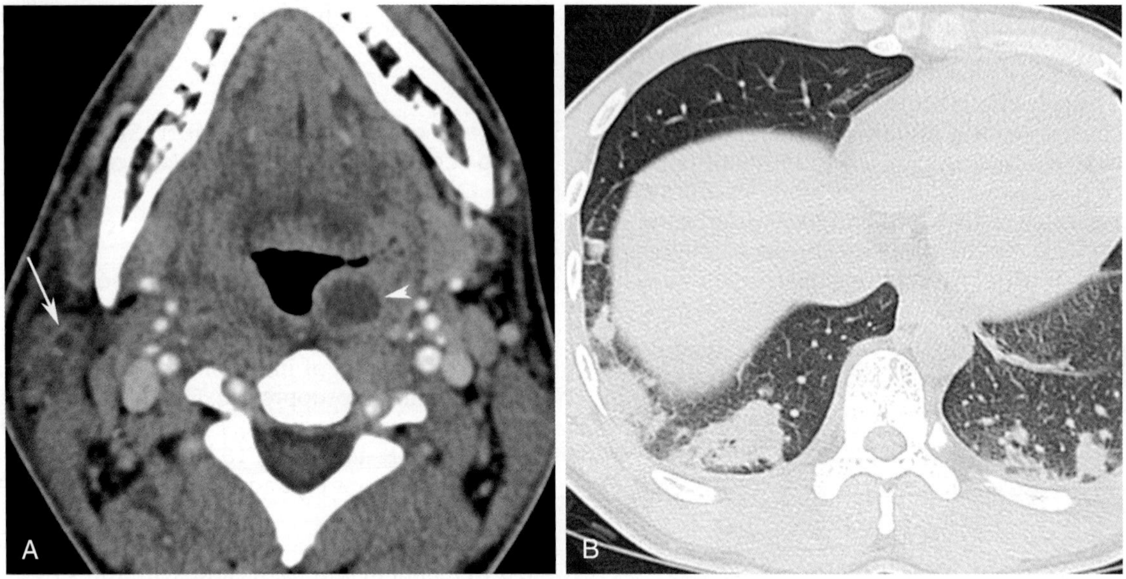

Figure 16.18 Lemierre syndrome. (A) Axial contrast-enhanced neck CT scan shows a left peritonsillar abscess *(arrowhead)* and right external jugular vein thrombosis *(arrow)*. (B) Axial nonenhanced CT scan shows lower lobe, wedge-shaped peripheral consolidation and pulmonary nodules consistent with septic emboli with infarction.

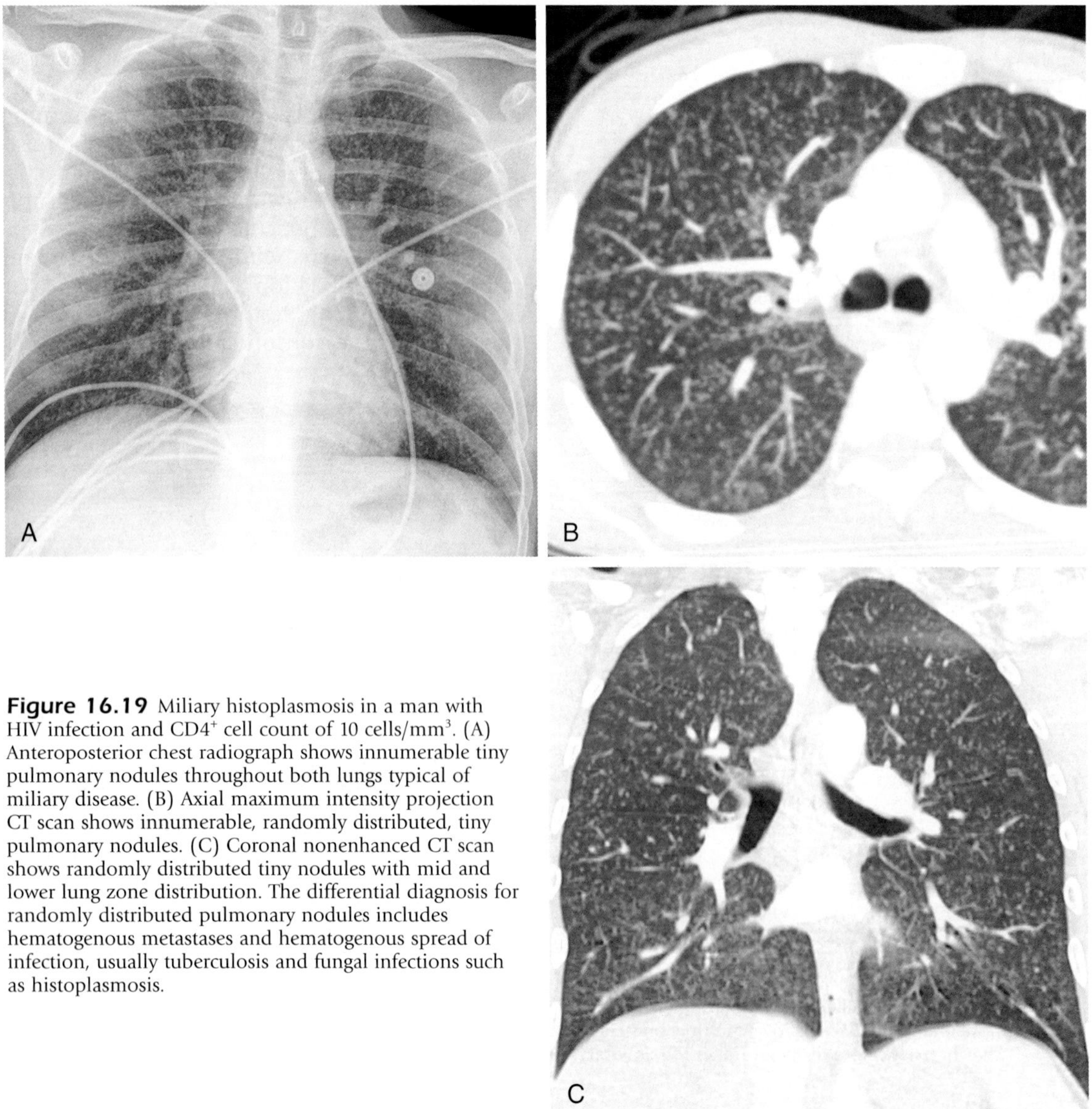

Figure 16.19 Miliary histoplasmosis in a man with HIV infection and $CD4^+$ cell count of 10 cells/mm^3. (A) Anteroposterior chest radiograph shows innumerable tiny pulmonary nodules throughout both lungs typical of miliary disease. (B) Axial maximum intensity projection CT scan shows innumerable, randomly distributed, tiny pulmonary nodules. (C) Coronal nonenhanced CT scan shows randomly distributed tiny nodules with mid and lower lung zone distribution. The differential diagnosis for randomly distributed pulmonary nodules includes hematogenous metastases and hematogenous spread of infection, usually tuberculosis and fungal infections such as histoplasmosis.

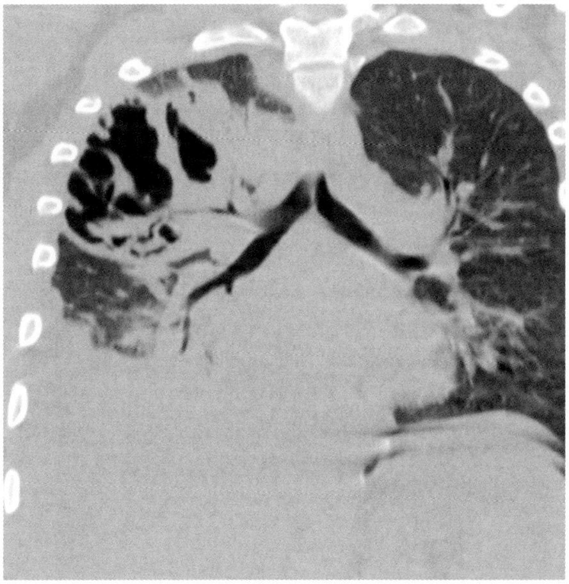

Figure 16.20 Necrotizing right upper lobe pneumonia from methicillin-resistant *Staphylococcus aureus*. Coronal nonenhanced CT scan shows right upper lobe consolidation, with underlying cavitation consistent with necrotizing pneumonia.

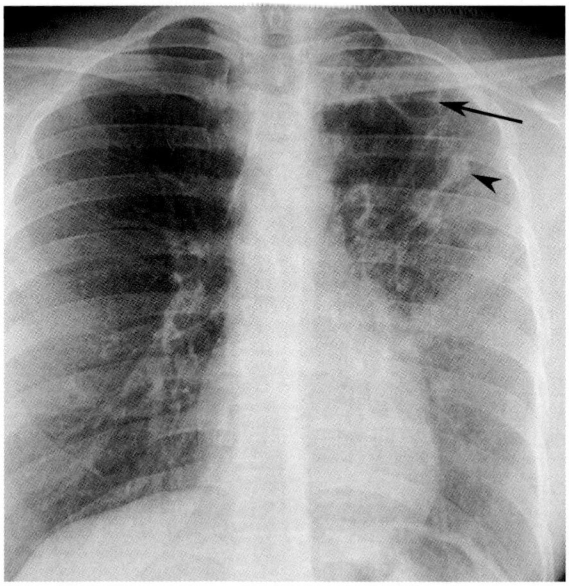

Figure 16.21 Reactivation tuberculosis infection. This posteroanterior chest radiograph shows left upper lobe nodular opacities *(arrowhead)*, cavitation *(arrow)*, and volume loss. This represents tuberculosis infection until proven otherwise.

pleura, and there may be high-attenuation fungal strands within the cavitary lesion.

Cavitation occurring in an immunosuppressed patient suggests a different differential diagnosis. Cavitary nodules in a recently neutropenic patient usually indicate the presence of an invasive fungal infection, often aspergillosis (Fig. 16.25). Less common infectious causes of cavitation include mucormycosis, *Cryptococcus*, and *Nocardia*. Cavitary nodules in an IVDU or patient with an infected central catheter often represent septic pulmonary embolism (Fig. 16.26).

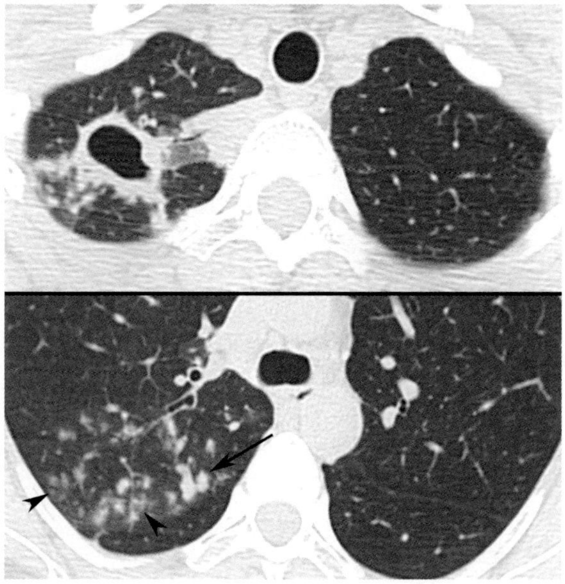

Figure 16.22 Reactivation tuberculosis with endobronchial spread of infection. This composite image of two axial nonenhanced CT images at the level of the lung apices *(upper image)* and carina *(lower image)* shows a cavitary right upper lobe nodule. Note distant smaller solid nodules *(arrow)*, ill-defined ground-glass nodules, centrilobular micronodules, and tree-in-bud opacities *(arrowheads)* indicating endobronchial spread of infection.

Nodules and Masses

Nodules and/or masses are uncommon manifestations of infection in immunocompetent patients. When present, they are most common with endemic fungal infections, such as histoplasmosis or coccidiomycosis. Importantly these types of infection tend to mimic and are often initially diagnosed as primary lung cancer (Fig. 16.27). Important clues to the diagnosis of a fungal infection include the presence of small satellite nodules around a larger dominant nodule or mass, exposure history, and ipsilateral hilar/mediastinal lymphadenopathy out of proportion to the size of the nodule or mass.

Nodules and/or masses are more common manifestations of infection in immunocompromised patients, especially in patients with neutropenia. Single or multiple pulmonary nodules in a patient with neutropenia are generally fungal infection until proven otherwise, usually angioinvasive aspergillosis. Less common infectious causes of pulmonary nodules in an immunocompromised patient include mucormycosis, *Cryptococcus*, tuberculosis, and *Nocardia* (Fig. 16.28).

CT Halo and Reverse Halo Signs

The CT halo sign represents a ground-glass opacity surrounding a central nodule or mass. The finding is highly suggestive of infection by angioinvasive aspergillosis in a patient with febrile neutropenia (Fig. 16.29). In this setting, the ground-glass opacity halo represents pulmonary hemorrhage surrounding the nodule of infarcted lung.

The reverse halo sign is a CT finding of central ground-glass opacity surrounded by a rim of consolidation. The sign was originally described in organizing pneumonia but has subsequently been identified in numerous other

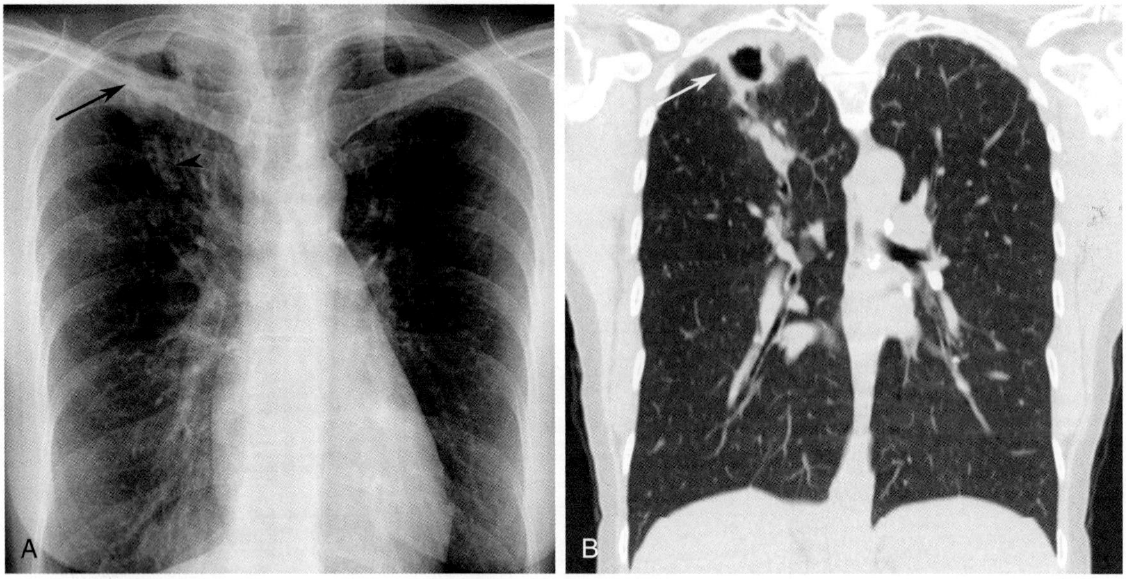

Figure 16.23 *Mycobacterium kansasii* infection mimicking reactivation tuberculosis. (A) Posteroanterior chest radiograph and coronal nonenhanced CT scan (B) show hyperinflated lung volumes with a cavitary right upper lobe nodule *(arrows)* with adjacent nodular opacities *(arrowheads)*. This appearance represents reactivation tuberculosis infection until proven otherwise. Atypical mycobacterial infection may appear similar and is most common in patients with chronic obstructive pulmonary disease or alcoholism.

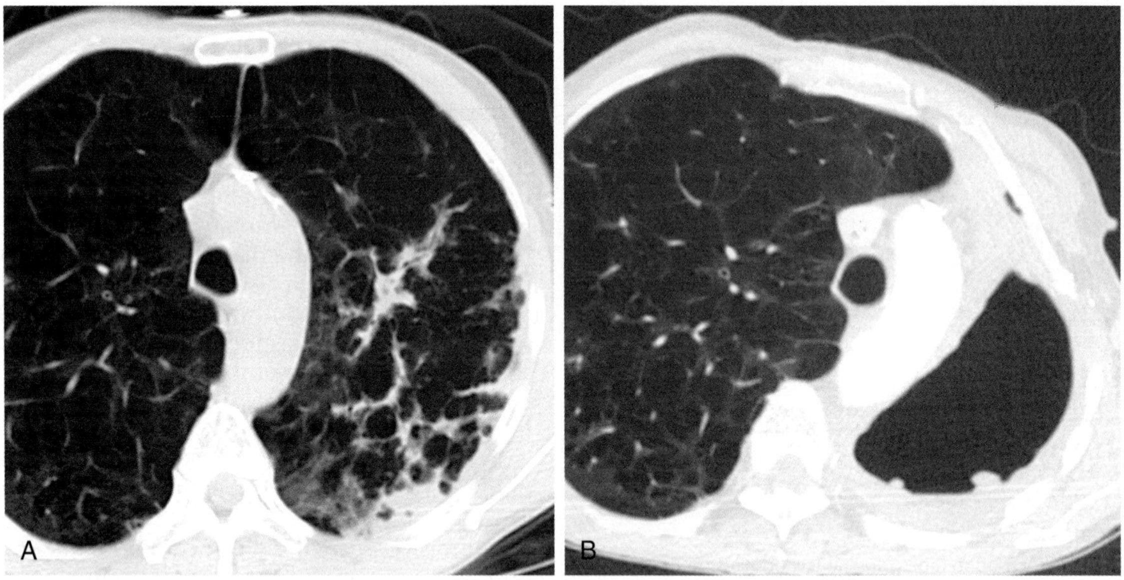

Figure 16.24 Semiinvasive *Aspergillus* infection. (A) Axial nonenhanced CT (NECT) scan shows severe emphysema and patchy left upper lobe nodular opacities. (B) Axial NECT scan obtained 1 year later shows complete destruction of the left upper lobe, with volume loss and thickened nodularity within the left upper lobe cavity likely representing mycetoma formation.

conditions. In a patient with febrile neutropenia or other form of immunosuppression, the reverse halo sign is suggestive of an invasive fungal infection, such as *Mucor* or *Aspergillus* (Fig. 16.30).

Lymphadenopathy

Visible lymphadenopathy on chest radiography is uncommon and is usually only seen with certain pathogens. The most common causative organisms include *M. tuberculosis* (Fig. 16.31) and endemic fungal infections, such as histoplasmosis and coccidioidomycosis. Uncommon causes of lymphadenopathy on chest radiography include *Pasteurella tularensis* (tularemia), *Yersinia pestis* (plague), and *Bacillus anthracis* (inhalational anthrax).

Mildly enlarged lymph nodes (>1 cm short-axis diameter) are commonly seen by CT in patients with bacterial pneumonia, occurring in over 50% of patients with pneumococcal pneumonia or an empyema. Enlarged

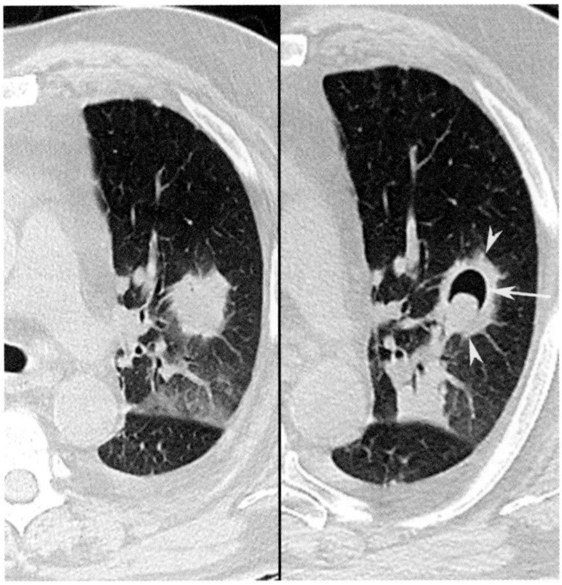

Figure 16.25 Angioinvasive aspergillosis with air crescent sign. This composite image of two axial nonenhanced CT images obtained at the time of neutropenic fever *(left)* and following granulocyte recovery *(right)* show a left upper lobe nodule that has undergone cavitation *(arrow)* consistent with the air crescent sign. The nodule within the cavity represents infarcted lung tissue that is separated from hemorrhagic but viable lung tissue *(arrowheads)*.

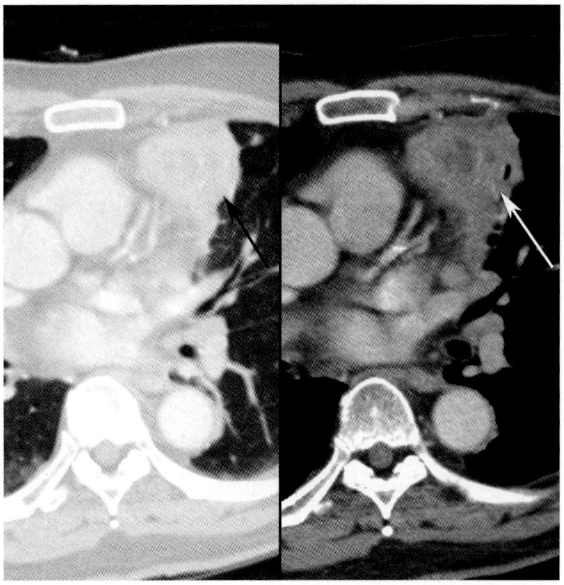

Figure 16.27 Coccidioidomycosis infection initially misdiagnosed as lung cancer. This composite image of an axial contrast-enhanced CT scan in the lung window *(left)* and soft tissue window *(right)* shows a heterogeneously enhancing left upper lobe mass *(arrow)*, which is centrally necrotic. The appearance closely mimics primary lung cancer. Fungal infection should always be considered as a diagnostic consideration in patients who have recently traveled to or originated from endemic areas.

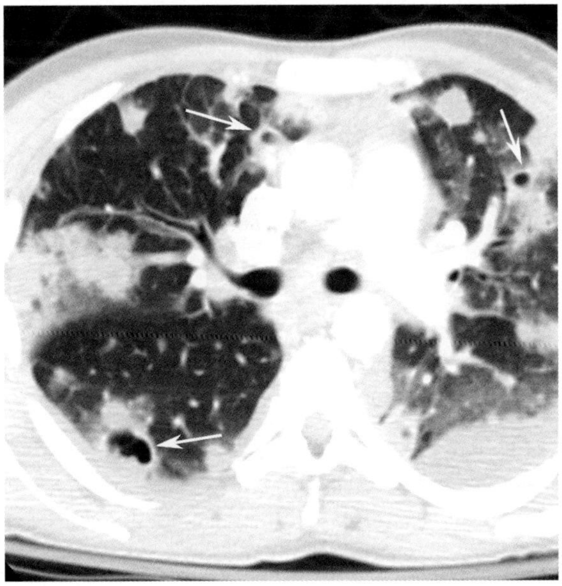

Figure 16.26 Septic embolism in an intravenous drug user. This axial nonenhanced CT scan shows cavitary pulmonary nodules *(arrows)* and noncavitary peripherally distributed pulmonary nodules, typical of septic embolism.

lymph nodes with low-attenuation centers (e.g., necrotic lymph nodes) are uncommon and are usually seen with mycobacterial infection (including atypical mycobacterial organisms), as well as infection from endemic fungal organisms (Fig. 16.32). High-attenuation lymph nodes reflecting intranodal hemorrhage have been described with inhalational anthrax.

Tree-in-Bud Sign

The small bronchioles are generally invisible on standard CT because of their small size and thin walls. When small airways become filled with mucus, pus, or debris, they become visible as branching V- and Y-shaped structures, said to resemble a budding tree (tree-in-bud sign). Tree-in-bud opacities characteristically spare the subpleural lung, including parenchyma adjacent to interlobar fissures (Fig. 16.33). The tree-in-bud sign almost universally indicates the presence of infection or, less commonly, aspiration. Although it may be caused by many different kinds of infection, tree-in-bud opacities generally are seen with bacterial or viral infections. If tree-in-bud opacities are associated with middle lobe and lingular predominant bronchiectasis, atypical mycobacterial infection is the usual cause of the opacities. Tree-in-bud opacities associated with diffuse bronchiectasis are most common in patients with cystic fibrosis, immunodeficiencies, allergic bronchopulmonary aspergillosis, and primary ciliary dyskinesia. Consolidation and tree-in-bud opacities are most common in bacterial pneumonia and aspiration. Dependent distribution of tree-in-bud opacities and esophageal abnormalities are usually associated with aspiration.

Migratory Pulmonary Opacities

Migratory pulmonary opacities may be present in a variety of conditions, including parasitic infections. Patients often have a history of recent travel to or emigration from an endemic area. The presence of peripheral blood eosinophilia is a helpful secondary clue suggesting the diagnosis.

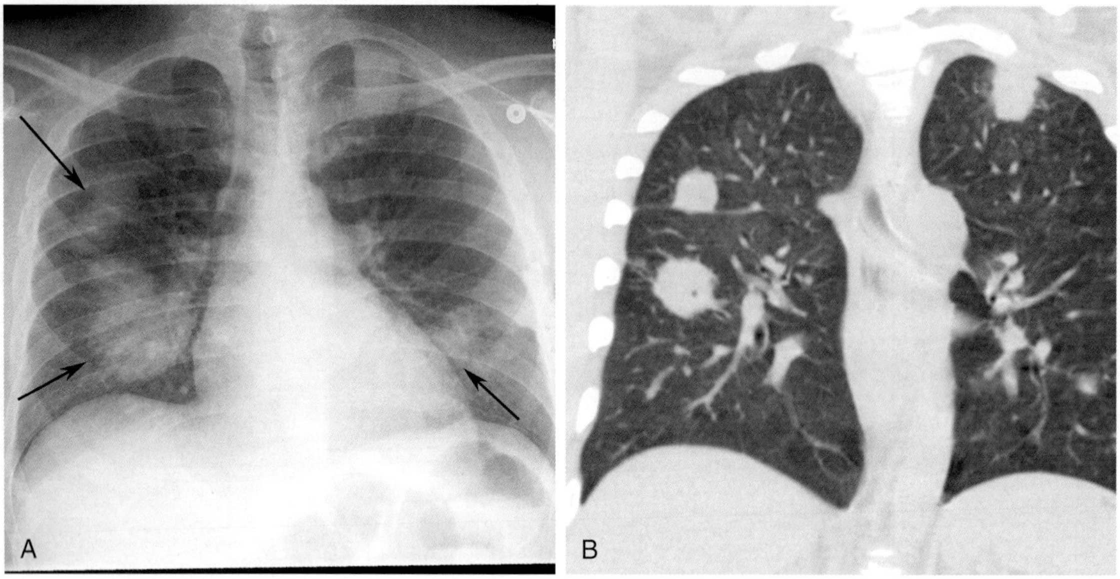

Figure 16.28 Nocardial and cryptococcal infection in a renal transplant patient. (A) Posteroanterior chest radiograph shows multiple bilateral pulmonary nodules and masses *(arrows)*. (B) Coronal nonenhanced CT scan shows bilateral pulmonary nodules. Considerations for multiple nodules or masses in a solid organ transplant recipient include infections (e.g., fungal organisms and *Nocardia*), posttransplantation lymphoproliferative disorder, and metastatic disease.

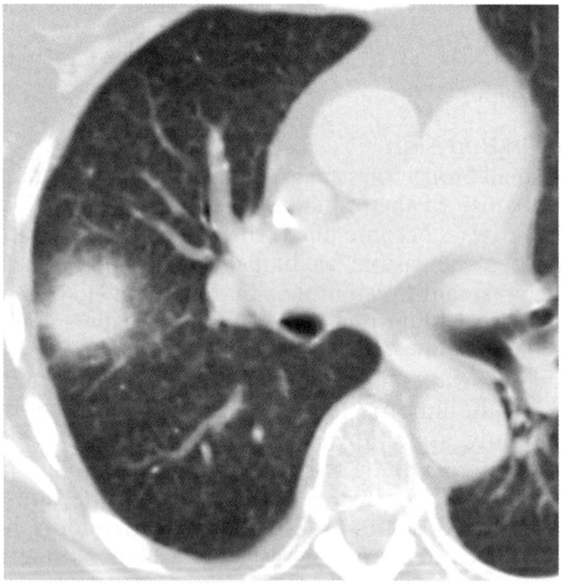

Figure 16.29 Halo sign in angioinvasive *Aspergillus* infection. This axial nonenhanced CT scan shows a right upper lobe nodule with a surrounding ground-glass opacity halo. In a febrile neutropenic patient, the halo sign around a pulmonary nodule is highly suggestive of angioinvasive *Aspergillus* infection.

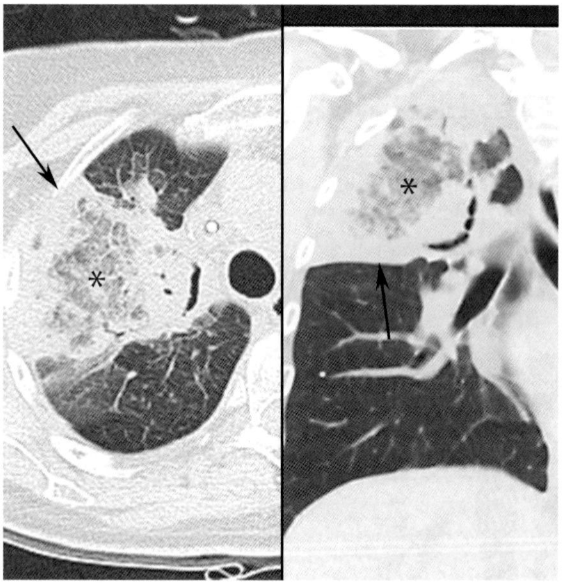

Figure 16.30 Reverse halo sign in angioinvasive *Aspergillus* infection. This composite image of an axial nonenhanced CT (NECT) scan *(left)* and coronal NECT scan *(right)* shows a right upper lobe masslike opacity with peripheral consolidation *(arrows)* and central ground-glass opacity *(asterisks)*. In a patient with neutropenic fever, this is highly suggestive of angioinvasive fungal infection, usually from *Aspergillus* or *Mucor.*

■ Complications of Infection

Lung Necrosis and Pulmonary Abscess

In a patient with pneumonia, the presence of inhomogeneous enhancement or cavitation is suggestive of a necrotizing infection. Occasionally, the bacterial pneumonia will be of a low enough density that it is difficult to differentiate it from adjacent pleural effusion (Fig. 16.34). Necrotizing pneumonia is more common with certain infections, including *S. aureus*, gram-negative bacteria, and anaerobes. Cavitation may also be seen in invasive fungal infections, including aspergillosis and mucormycosis.

A lung abscess characteristically manifests with an air-fluid level on radiography and CT and makes acute angles with the adjacent pleural surface. The wall of a

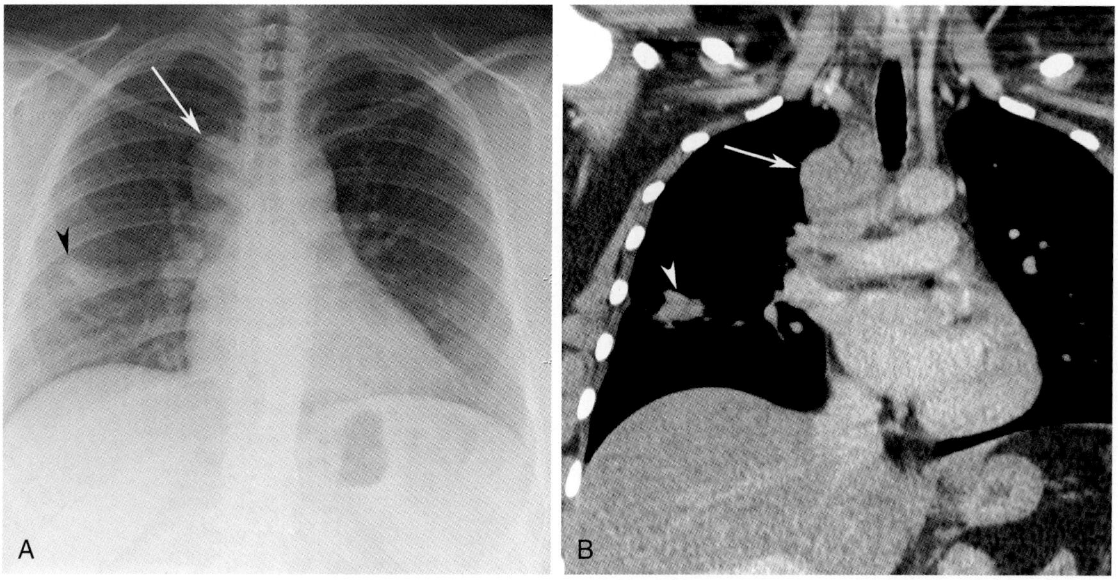

Figure 16.31 Primary tuberculosis infection. (A) Posteroanterior chest radiograph shows a nodular opacity *(arrowhead)* in the right upper lobe and extensive thickening of the right paratracheal stripe *(arrow)*. (B) Coronal contrast-enhanced CT scan shows a right upper lobe nodule *(arrowhead)* and extensive right paratracheal lymphadenopathy *(arrow)*. The degree of lymphadenopathy is out of proportion to the size of the nodule, which raises the possibility of a fungal infection or primary tuberculosis infection.

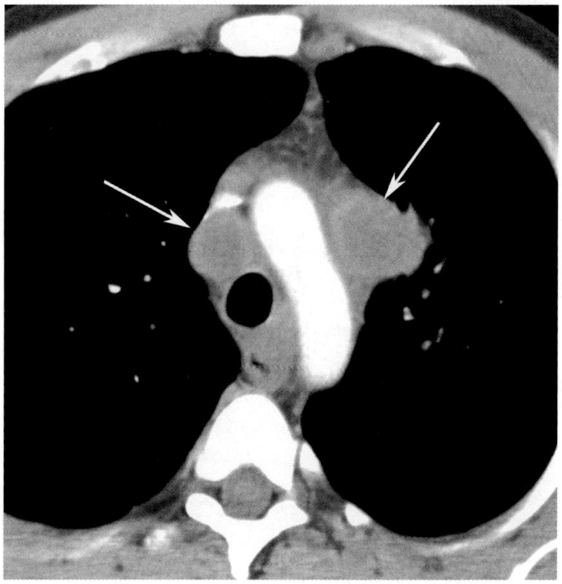

Figure 16.32 Tuberculosis infection with necrotic mediastinal lymph nodes. This axial contrast-enhanced CT scan shows right paratracheal and paraaortic lymphadenopathy *(arrows)*. Note the low density within the center of the lymph nodes, reflecting central necrosis.

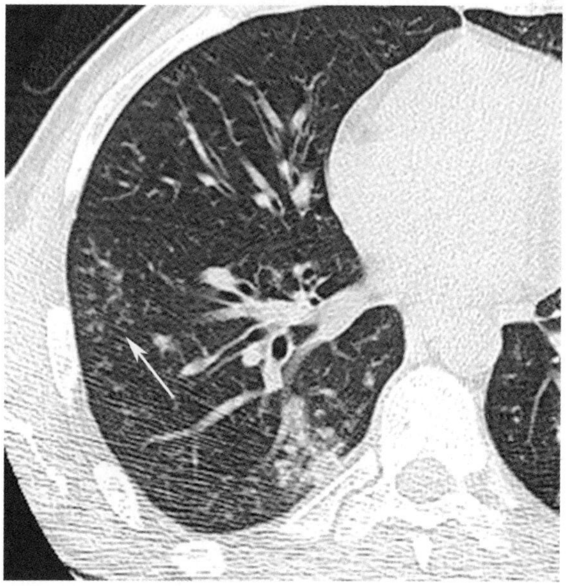

Figure 16.33 Tree-in-bud opacities from airway invasive *Aspergillus* infection in a neutropenic patient. This axial nonenhanced CT scan shows multiple right lower lobe branching V- and Y-shaped structures *(arrow)* and nodular consolidation.

lung abscess is often thick and irregular. In contrast to empyema, the length of the air-fluid level is similar on both the posteroanterior and lateral radiographs due to the roughly spherical shape of a lung abscess (Fig. 16.35). In contrast, empyema typically is lenticular in configuration, and therefore the air-fluid level length is different when comparing the posteroanterior and lateral projections (Fig. 16.36). Lung abscess is usually seen following aspiration or in patients with septic emboli. The most common causative organisms include *S. aureus, K. pneumoniae*, and anaerobes. Treatment is medical, often with prolonged antibiotic therapy.

Parapneumonic Effusion and Empyema

Pneumonia may irritate the adjacent visceral pleura, causing increased capillary permeability and an exudative pleural effusion (simple parapneumonic effusion), which occurs in 20% to 40% of hospitalized patients with

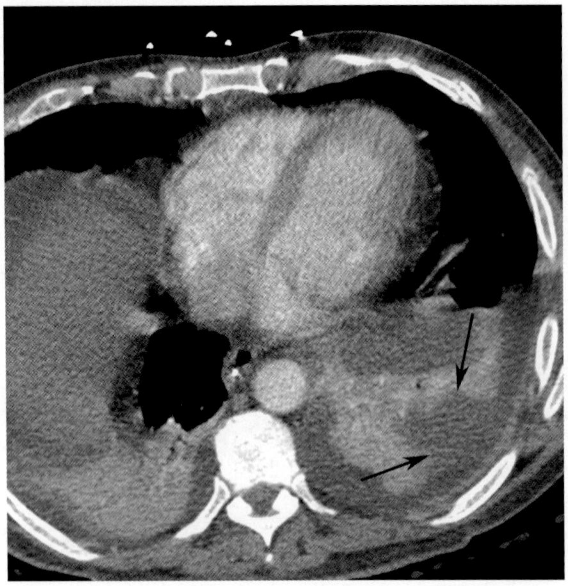

Figure 16.34 Left lower lobe pneumonia. This axial contrast-enhanced CT scan shows hypoenhancing left lower lobe consolidation *(arrows)* in a patient with pneumonia. The consolidated lung closely approximates the density of the adjacent parapneumonic effusion.

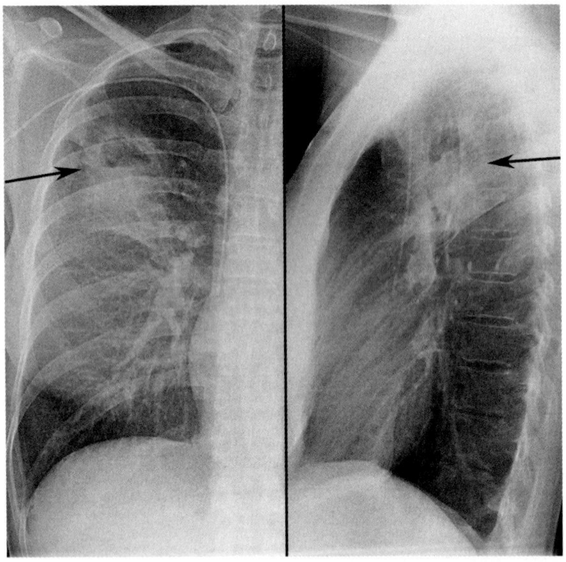

Figure 16.35 Lung abscess. This composite image of a posteroanterior *(left)* and lateral *(right)* chest radiograph shows an irregularly defined right upper lobe cavitary lesion, with an air-fluid level. The air-fluid level *(arrows)* is of equal length on the orthogonal radiographic projections, typical of a lung abscess.

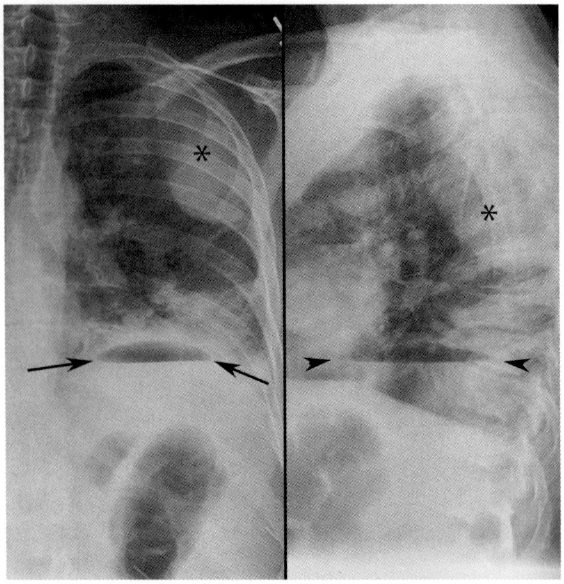

Figure 16.36 Multiloculated empyema. This composite image of a posteroanterior *(left)* and lateral *(right)* chest radiograph shows a multiloculated left pleural effusion *(asterisks)*. Note the air-fluid level, which is longer on the lateral projection *(arrowheads)* when compared to its length on the frontal projection *(arrows)*.

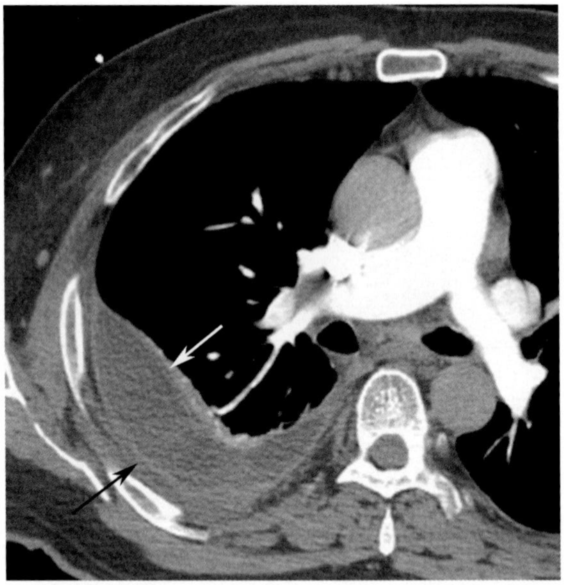

Figure 16.37 Split pleural sign in empyema. This axial contrast-enhanced CT scan shows a right pleural effusion manifesting the split pleura sign, with enhancement of the visceral pleura *(white arrow)* and parietal pleura *(black arrow)*.

pneumonia. At this stage, the parapneumonic effusion is generally free-flowing and culture-negative and has a normal pH and glucose level. If the patient deteriorates and does not seek appropriate medical therapy, the parapneumonic effusion may progress to the fibropurulent stage (empyema).

Parapneumonic effusion manifests as a small to moderate-sized pleural effusion, usually with adjacent pneumonia. There is occasionally thickening and enhancement of the pleura on CT. The most common appearance of empyema is a small to large pleural effusion, which is often seen adjacent to pneumonia. Importantly, empyema may be a late manifestation, and pneumonia may be absent or inconspicuous. About 50% of all empyemas manifest the split pleural sign, which represents parietal and visceral pleural thickening and enhancement that surround the pleural fluid collection (Fig. 16.37). Loculated pleural fluid may manifest as nondependent pleural fluid or scalloping of pleural fluid contours. The presence of air within the pleural fluid collection is presumptive evidence of a bronchopleural fistula in the absence of recent intervention (Fig. 16.38).

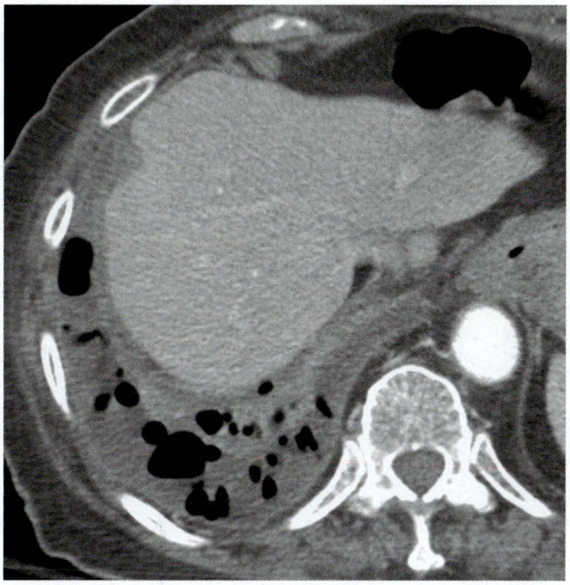

Figure 16.38 Empyema with bronchopleural fistula. This axial contrast-enhanced CT scan shows a multiloculated right pleural effusion, with several foci of air. In the absence of recent intervention, the presence of air is presumptive evidence of a bronchopleural fistula.

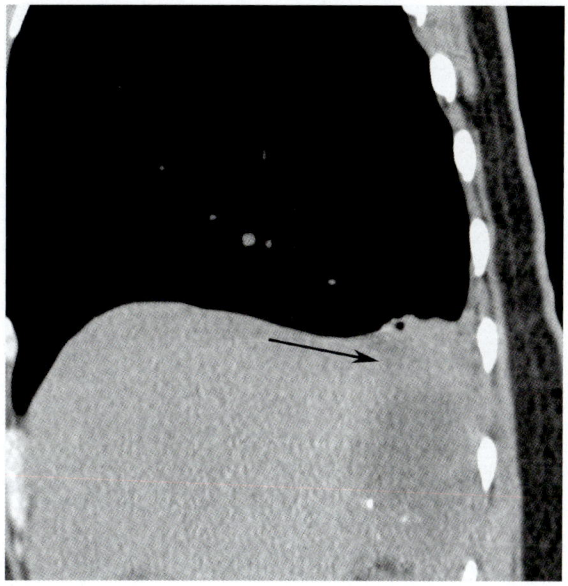

Figure 16.40 Thoracic actinomycosis invading through the right hemidiaphragm into the liver. This sagittal nonenhanced CT scan shows right lower lobe consolidation, with extension into the right hepatic lobe through the right hemidiaphragm *(arrow)*.

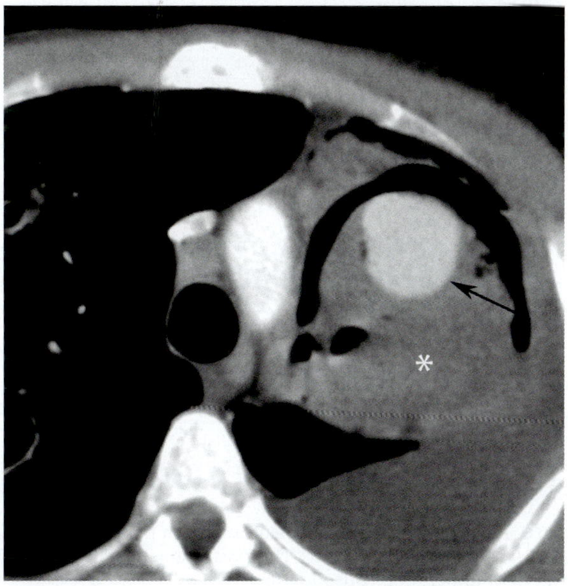

Figure 16.39 Rasmussen aneurysm associated with cavitary tuberculosis infection. This axial contrast-enhanced CT scan shows a large left upper lobe pulmonary artery pseudoaneurysm *(arrow)* associated with a pulmonary cavity. High attenuation *(asterisk)* within the cavity is due to hemorrhage.

Pseudoaneurysm and Bronchial Artery Dilation

Pulmonary artery pseudoaneurysm is an uncommon complication of pulmonary infection and is typically associated with cavitary tuberculosis infection (Rasmussen aneurysm). The pseudoaneurysm develops when cavitary infection leads to weakening of an adjacent pulmonary artery wall (Fig. 16.39). Life-threatening hemoptysis is a common presenting symptom.

Bronchial artery hypertrophy and dilation occur in patients with chronic inflammatory conditions of the lungs and airways, such as cavitary lung infection and bronchiectasis. The bronchial artery dilation is thought to occur from angiogenic growth factor release, including vascular endothelial growth factor (VEGF). Bronchial artery dilation is most common with chronic infections, including tuberculosis and nontuberculous mycobacteria and fungal infections, such as mycetoma. Patients with bronchial artery dilation are at an increased risk for fatal hemoptysis.

Chest Wall or Diaphragm Invasion

There are several organisms that have a propensity to spread across the chest wall or diaphragm through fascial and connective tissue barriers. The organisms responsible for this type of behavior are remembered by the BATMAN mnemonic because the superhero Batman tends to break through barriers:

B: Blastomycosis
A: Actinomycosis (Fig. 16.40)
T: Tuberculosis
M: Mucormycosis (Fig. 16.41)
A: Aspergillosis
N: *Nocardia*

■ Infections in Immunocompromised Hosts

Infection is the most common cause of pulmonary complications in the immunocompromised host.

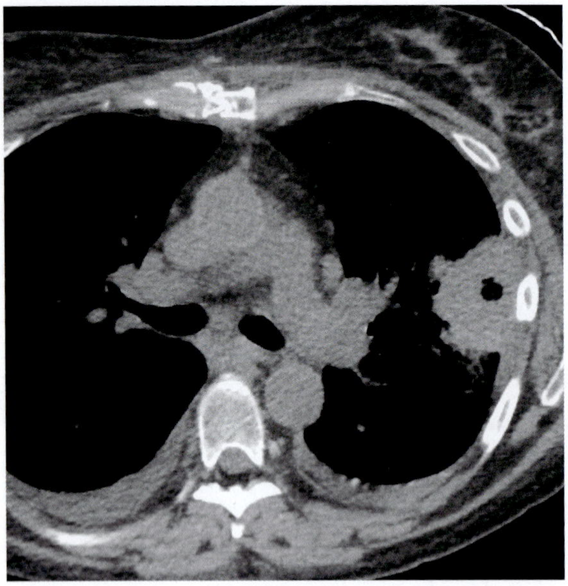

Figure 16.41 Mucormycosis invading chest wall. This axial nonenhanced CT scan shows a peripheral left upper lobe mass, with central low attenuation. At surgery, the infection had invaded the pleura and chest wall.

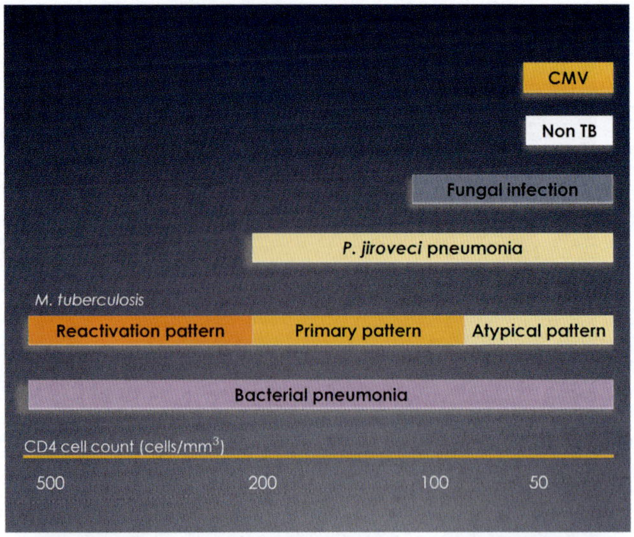

Figure 16.42 Chart highlighting most common infections in patients with HIV, depending on the patient's $CD4^+$ cell count. *CMV,* Cytomegalovirus; *TB,* tuberculosis.

Knowledge of the patient's level of immunosuppression, as well as the time from transplantation, is helpful in suggesting a specific pathogen or narrowing the differential diagnosis sufficiently. There are six principal types of immunodeficiencies that can be congenital or acquired that predispose the patient to specific infection risks:

1. Phagocyte defects (primarily bacterial and fungal organisms such as *S. aureus, K. pneumoniae, E. coli,* and *Aspergillus*)
2. Antibody-mediated B lymphocyte defects (primarily bacterial organisms such as *S. pneumoniae, S. aureus, H. influenzae,* and *P. aeruginosa*)
3. Cell-mediated T lymphocyte defects (e.g., AIDS patients at risk for bacterial, viral, fungal, and parasitic infections)
4. Corticosteroid use (at risk for all types of infection)
5. Hyposplenism or splenectomy patients (encapsulated bacteria such as *S. pneumoniae, Salmonella typhi,* and *H. influenzae*)
6. Complement system defects

HIV and AIDS

The respiratory system is the most frequent site of infection in patients with HIV and is an important cause of patient morbidity and mortality. At the end of 2016, the UNAIDS estimated there were 36.7 million people living with HIV worldwide. The causes of pulmonary infection have changed over the past decades due to increased awareness, antiretroviral therapy (ART), and prophylaxis against *P. jirovecii* pneumonia (PJP). The cause of infection can often be predicted by looking at the patient's $CD4^+$ cell count (Fig. 16.42) and is grouped according to the following:

1. $CD4^+$ cell count >200 cells/mm^3
2. $CD4^+$ cell count of 100–200 cells/mm^3
3. $CD4^+$ cell count <100 cells/mm^3

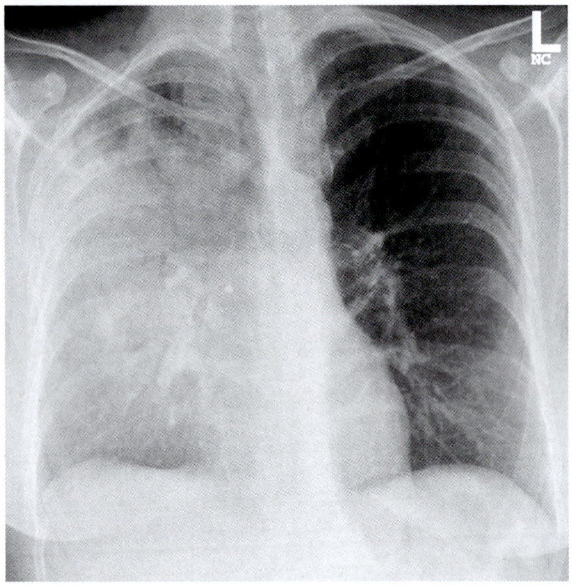

Figure 16.43 Pneumococcal pneumonia in a patient with HIV and $CD4^+$ cell count of 295 cells/mm^3. This posteroanterior chest radiograph shows right upper lobe consolidation.

$CD4^+$ CELL COUNT

$CD4^+$ CELL COUNT >200 CELLS/mm^3. Bacterial pneumonia is the most common infection in patients with HIV, with patients having a 10- to 25-fold higher rate of pneumonia compared with the general population. The incidence of bacterial pneumonia increases with a decreasing $CD4^+$ cell count, with about 80% of all cases occurring in patients with a cell count <400 cells/mm^3. The most common pathogens include *S. pneumoniae, H. influenzae, S. aureus,* and *P. aeruginosa*. The most common appearance is a lobar or bronchopneumonia pattern of disease (Fig. 16.43). Multifocal reticular or reticulonodular opacities are also a common manifestation of bacterial pneumonia in patients with HIV. Recurrent bacterial pneumonia is considered an AIDS-defining illness.

HIV infection is the single greatest risk factor for developing tuberculosis, with approximately one-third of all HIV-infected patients having coexistent *M. tuberculosis* infection. Tuberculosis infection may occur with any $CD4^+$ cell count but is more likely to manifest with a postprimary pattern in patients with a $CD4^+$ cell count >200 cells/mm^3 (Fig. 16.44). Primary pattern of disease with consolidation and lymphadenopathy may also occur in patients who are newly infected with tuberculosis (Fig. 16.45).

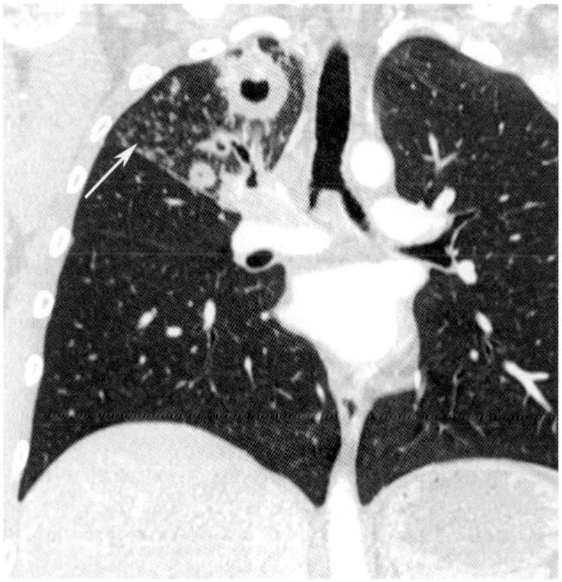

Figure 16.44 Reactivation tuberculosis infection with endobronchial spread. This coronal contrast-enhanced CT scan shows multiple right upper lobe cavitary lesions, with adjacent centrilobular micronodules *(arrow)* representing endobronchial spread of infection.

$CD4^+$ CELL COUNT OF 100–200 CELLS/mm^3. Despite prophylaxis, *Pneumocystis* pneumonia remains the most common opportunistic infection and AIDS-defining illness. It commonly affects noncompliant patients or is a first manifestation of HIV infection in patients with a $CD4^+$ cell count <200 cells/mm^3. Patients are generally severely hypoxic. Chest radiography demonstrates a reticular or interstitial pattern of disease (Fig. 16.46). The most common manifestation on CT is diffuse ground-glass opacities, often with a perihilar and upper lung zone predominance (Fig. 16.47). Pleural effusions are rare, but pneumatoceles may complicate up to one-third of cases (Fig. 16.48). As previously stated, tuberculosis can occur at any $CD4^+$ cell count, but disseminated disease or atypical patterns of reactivation disease are more likely in patients with a $CD4^+$ cell count <200 cells/mm^3.

Focal consolidation in an HIV patient with a $CD4^+$ cell count <200 cells/mm^3 may represent bacterial pneumonia or tuberculosis infection manifesting in a primary pattern of disease. Normal chest radiographs are common in HIV patients, with subsequently proven pulmonary disease occurring in 10% to 39% of patients with proven *Pneumocystis* pneumonia and 14% of patients with proven tuberculosis. Therefore, chest CT should be considered for symptomatic HIV patients with a normal chest radiograph.

$CD4^+$ CELL COUNT <100 CELLS/mm^3. Patients with a very low $CD4^+$ cell count are at risk for many opportunistic infections including *Pneumocystis* pneumonia, *Nocardia*, cytomegalovirus (CMV), tuberculosis, nontuberculous mycobacterial infection, endemic fungal infection, *Cryptococcus*, and toxoplasmosis. *Cryptococcus* usually results in disseminated disease most commonly affecting the central nervous system (CNS) and lungs. The imaging appearance consists of a solitary pulmonary nodule or multiple pulmonary nodules (see Fig. 16.28).

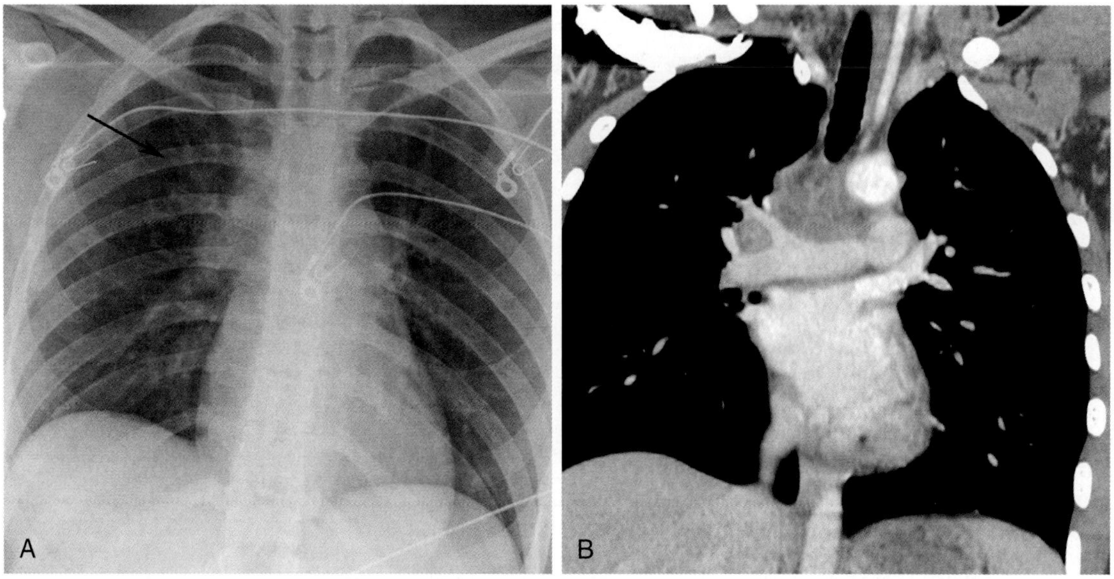

Figure 16.45 Primary tuberculosis infection with extensive lymphadenopathy. Posteroanterior chest radiograph (A) and coronal contrast-enhanced CT scan (B) show patchy right upper lobe nodular opacities *(arrow)*, with extensive right hilar and right paratracheal lymphadenopathy. Note central low attenuation within the lymph nodes, indicating the presence of necrosis.

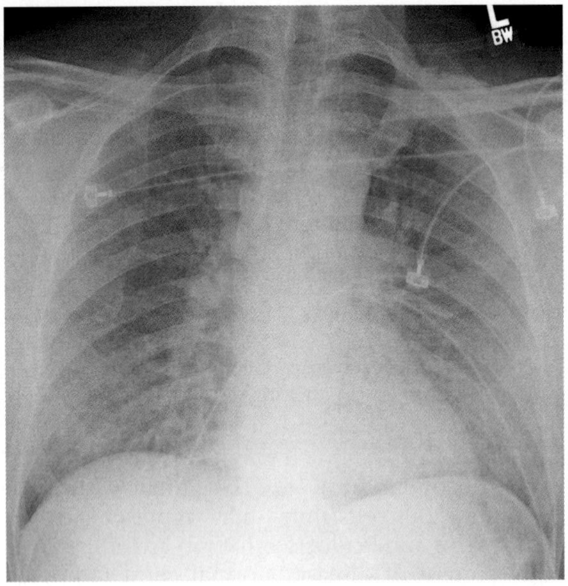

Figure 16.46 *Pneumocystis* pneumonia in HIV-positive man with profound hypoxia. This posteroanterior chest radiograph shows diffuse bilateral hazy lung opacities.

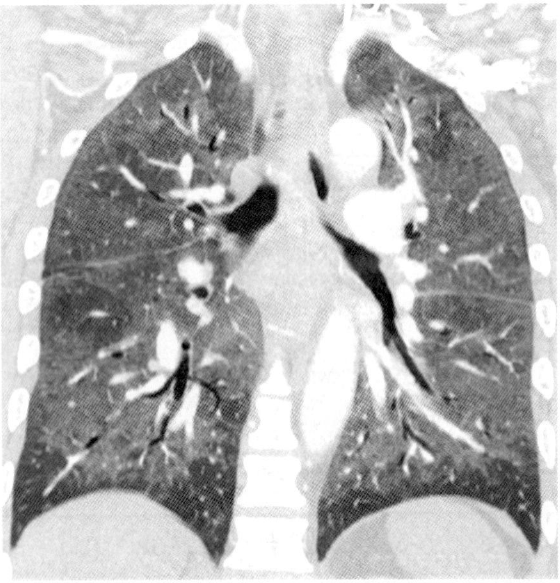

Figure 16.47 *Pneumocystis jirovecii* pneumonia (PJP). This coronal contrast-enhanced CT scan shows bilateral ground-glass opacities, with relative sparing of the lung bases. This is the most common manifestation of PJP.

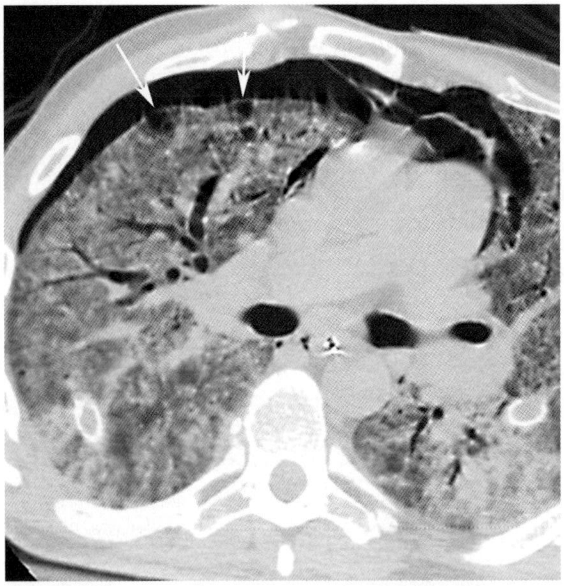

Figure 16.48 *Pneumocystis jirovecii* pneumonia with pneumothorax and pneumomediastinum. This axial nonenhanced CT scan shows bilateral ground-glass opacities, consolidation, and small cysts *(arrows)*. There is pneumomediastinum and small bilateral pneumothoraces secondary to cyst rupture.

A surrounding ground-glass opacity halo (CT halo sign) is seen in about 40% of patients. Endemic fungal infection is usually caused by histoplasmosis, coccidioidomycosis, and blastomycosis organisms. Infection may be newly acquired or may be reactivation of a latent infection. Disseminated infection with a miliary pattern is common (see Fig. 16.19). Nocardial infection is uncommon due to prophylaxis against *P. jirovecii* and usually only occurs in a patient with an extremely low $CD4^+$ cell count and in patients who do not take PJP prophylactic medications. It usually manifests with multifocal consolidation, nodules, or masses, all of which may cavitate. Toxoplasmosis is the most common parasitic disease in patients with HIV. Toxoplasmosis generally causes CNS disease, with pneumonia being the second most common manifestation.

Nontuberculous mycobacterial infection is generally disseminated at presentation and usually only affects AIDS patients with an extremely low $CD4^+$ cell count (<50 cells/mm^3). The most common manifestation is mediastinal lymphadenopathy, which often demonstrates central low attenuation, indicating necrosis. CMV pneumonitis is uncommon and usually affects patients with an extremely low $CD4^+$ cell count (<50 cells/mm^3). The most common manifestations include focal or diffuse ground-glass opacity, patchy consolidation, small centrilobular nodules, and septal thickening.

Patients with opportunistic infection and extremely low $CD4^+$ cell counts are at risk for immune reconstitution inflammatory syndrome (IRIS) with the initiation of ART. The manifestations of IRIS are numerous and should be considered in a patient with acute exacerbation of symptoms following initiation of ART. The most common manifestations include diffuse ground-glass opacities or consolidation, mediastinal and hilar lymphadenopathy, which is often centrally necrotic, and miliary or centrilobular nodules. The manifestations of IRIS vary depending on the underlying opportunistic infection. The most common infections associated with IRIS include tuberculosis, nontuberculous mycobacterial infection, PJP, and viral infections such as CMV or herpes simplex virus infection.

Bone Marrow Transplantation Infections

Infections in stem cell transplant recipients are more likely to occur at certain time points following transplantation and can be divided into three groups:

1. Preengraftment period (0–30 days)
2. Early posttransplantation period (31–100 days)
3. Late posttransplantation period (>100 days)

PREENGRAFTMENT PERIOD (0–30 DAYS)

Neutropenia is the primary risk factor for infection immediately after stem cell transplantation, before hematopoiesis resumes. Bacterial infections are uncommon, likely due to empiric antibiotic use at the earliest signs of infection. The most common infections in this period are fungal infections, usually from *Aspergillus* and, less commonly, *Candida* and *Mucor*. *Aspergillus* is usually angioinvasive or airway invasive, manifesting with multiple pulmonary nodules, often with a surrounding ground-glass opacity halo (CT halo sign, as seen in Fig. 16.29).

EARLY POSTTRANSPLANTATION PERIOD (31–100 DAYS)

Aspergillosis, respiratory syncytial virus (RSV) pneumonia, and CMV pneumonia are the most common pulmonary infections in the early posttransplantation period. *Pneumocystis* pneumonia is uncommon due to widespread prophylaxis but may be seen in noncompliant patients. CMV infection is usually due to the reactivation of a latent virus or by infusion of CMV-positive blood products or marrow at the time of transplantation.

Idiopathic pneumonia syndrome occurs in 10% of patients and is a diagnosis of exclusion. It manifests with diffuse bilateral lung opacities and respiratory failure, with diffuse alveolar damage. Importantly, no infectious organisms are recovered at the time of bronchoscopy or via blood cultures. However, the 1-year survival rate is poor, with only 15% of patients surviving. The cause is unclear; it has been theorized to be a manifestation of graft-versus-host disease (GVHD), toxicity of chemotherapy medications, or undiagnosed infection.

LATE POSTTRANSPLANTATION PERIOD (>100 DAYS)

Pulmonary complications continue to decline in the late posttransplantation period as both humoral and cell-mediated immunity recover. About 50% of all transplant recipients develop GVHD, which requires treatment with corticosteroids. GVHD predisposes patients to developing infection due to abnormalities in the mucosal membranes, bone marrow, and reticuloendothelial system. Patients with GVHD are at the highest risk for developing bacterial infections but may also develop infection by fungi (*Aspergillus* and *Mucor*) and viruses (RSV, varicella zoster, parainfluenza, adenovirus).

SOLID ORGAN TRANSPLANTATION

Nosocomial infections related to hospitalization are the most common types of infection within the first month following transplantation. Bacterial pathogens are most common and usually are a consequence of endotracheal tube ventilation.

Opportunistic infections are most common within the first 6 months following transplantation because immunosuppressive doses are typically at their highest levels. The incidence of *Nocardia* infection has declined, affecting less than 2% of patients, which is likely due to widespread prophylactic therapy for PJP (Fig. 16.49). Reactivation of *M. tuberculosis* is uncommon in developed countries, occurring in 0.5% to 2% of patients in the United States and Europe. CMV is the most common viral cause of pneumonia, usually occurring 1 to 3 months after transplantation (Fig. 16.50). Fungal infection is most commonly caused by *Aspergillus* and usually occurs within the first 6 months following transplantation. PJP infection is uncommon due to widespread prophylactic therapy. The most common infections after 6 months are from community-acquired pathogens, usually bacteria.

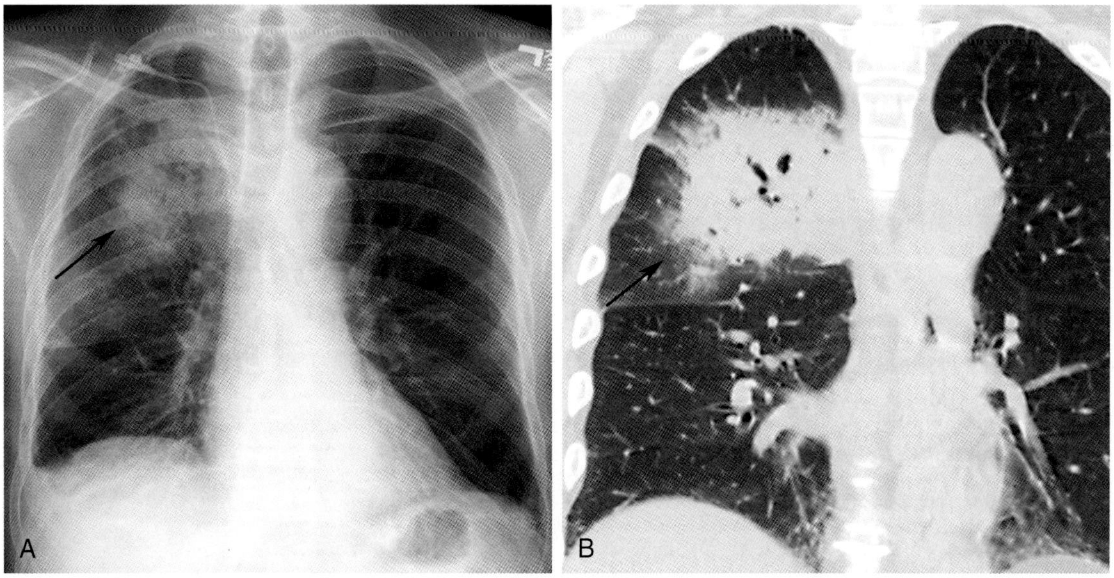

Figure 16.49 *Nocardia* infection in a renal transplant recipient. (A) posteroanterior chest radiograph shows right upper lobe consolidation *(arrow)*. (B) Coronal nonenhanced CT scan shows a right upper lobe masslike opacity with surrounding ground-glass opacity *(arrow)*.

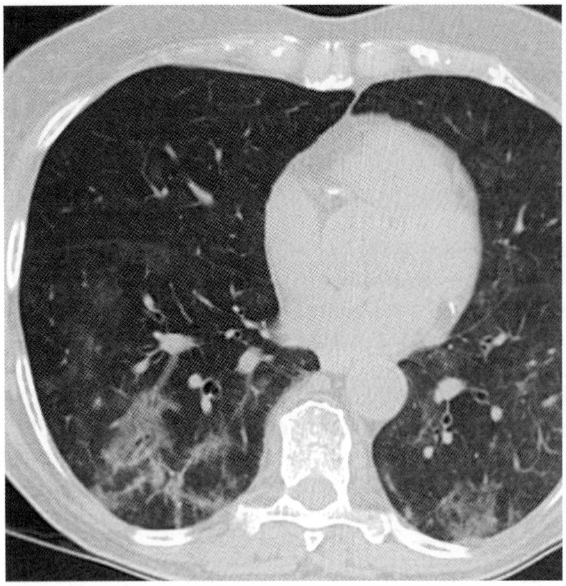

Figure 16.50 Cytomegalovirus pneumonia in a renal transplant recipient. This axial nonenhanced CT scan shows peribronchial consolidation and ground-glass opacities, with bronchial wall thickening.

Bibliography

Burrill J, Williams CJ, Bain G, Conder G, Hine AL, Misra RR. Tuberculosis: a radiologic review. *Radiographics*. 2007;27(5):1255–1273.

Chou SH, Prabhu SJ, Crothers K, Stern EJ, Godwin JD, Pipavath SN. Thoracic diseases associated with HIV infection in the era of antiretroviral therapy: clinical and imaging findings. *Radiographics*. 2014;34(4):895–911.

Coy DL, Ormazabal A, Godwin JD, Lalani T. Imaging evaluation of pulmonary and abdominal complications following hematopoietic stem cell transplantation. *Radiographics*. 2005;25(2):305–317.

Cunha BA. The atypical pneumonias: clinical diagnosis and importance. *Clin Microbiol Infect*. 2006;12(suppl 3):12–24.

Escuissato DL, Gasparetto EL, Marchiori E, et al. Pulmonary infections after bone marrow transplantation: high-resolution CT findings in 111 patients. *AJR Am J Roentgenol*. 2005;185(3):608–615.

Franquet T, Lee KS, Müller NL. Thin-section CT findings in 32 immunocompromised patients with cytomegalovirus pneumonia who do not have AIDS. *AJR Am J Roentgenol*. 2003;181(4):1059–1063.

Franquet T, Müller NL, Giménez A, Guembe P, de La Torre J, Bagué S. Spectrum of pulmonary aspergillosis: histologic, clinical, and radiologic findings. *Radiographics*. 2001;21(4):825–837.

Franquet T. Imaging of pulmonary viral pneumonia. *Radiology*. 2011;260(1):18–39.

Gasparetto EL, Escuissato DL, Davaus T, et al. Reversed halo sign in pulmonary paracoccidioidomycosis. *AJR Am J Roentgenol*. 2005;184(6):1932–1934.

Kanne JP, Godwin JD, Franquet T, Escuissato DL, Müller NL. Viral pneumonia after hematopoietic stem cell transplantation: high-resolution CT findings. *J Thorac Imaging*. 2007;22(3):292–299.

Kanne JP, Yandow DR, Meyer CA. Pneumocystis jiroveci pneumonia: high-resolution CT findings in patients with and without HIV infection. *AJR Am J Roentgenol*. 2012;198(6):W555–W561.

Kanne JP, Yandow DR, Mohammed TL, Meyer CA. CT findings of pulmonary nocardiosis. *AJR Am J Roentgenol*. 2011;197(2):W266–W272.

Ketai L, Alrahji AA, Hart B, Enria D, Mettler F. Radiologic manifestations of potential bioterrorist agents of infection. *AJR Am J Roentgenol*. 2003;180(3):565–575.

Ketai L, Jordan K, Marom EM. Imaging infection. *Clin Chest Med*. 2008;29(1):77–105.

Ketai LH, Williamson MR, Telepak RJ, et al. Hantavirus pulmonary syndrome: radiographic findings in 16 patients. *Radiology*. 1994;191(3):665–668.

Marchiori E, Müller NL, Soares Souza A, Escuissato DL, Gasparetto EL, Franquet T. Pulmonary disease in patients with AIDS: high-resolution CT and pathologic findings. *AJR Am J Roentgenol*. 2005;184(3):757–764.

Martinez S, McAdams HP, Batchu CS. The many faces of pulmonary nontuberculous mycobacterial infection. *AJR Am J Roentgenol*. 2007;189(1):177–186.

Martínez S, Restrepo CS, Carrillo JA, et al. Thoracic manifestations of tropical parasitic infections: a pictorial review. *Radiographics*. 2005;25(1):135–155.

McAdams HP, Rosado-de-Christenson ML, Lesar M, Templeton PA, Moran CA. Thoracic mycoses from endemic fungi: radiologic-pathologic correlation. *Radiographics*. 1995;15(2):255–270.

McAdams HP, Rosado-de-Christenson ML, Templeton PA, Lesar M, Moran CA. Thoracic mycoses from opportunistic fungi: radiologic-pathologic correlation. *Radiographics*. 1995;15(2):271–286.

Miller WT, Mickus TJ, Barbosa E, Mullin C, Van Deerlin VM, Shiley KT. CT of viral lower respiratory tract infections in adults: comparison among viral organisms and between viral and bacterial infections. *AJR Am J Roentgenol*. 2011;197(5):1088–1095.

Musher DM, Thorner AR. Community-acquired pneumonia. *N Engl J Med*. 2014;371(17):1619–1628.

Rossi SE, Franquet T, Volpacchio M, Giménez A, Aguilar G. Tree-in-bud pattern at thin-section CT of the lungs: radiologic-pathologic overview. *Radiographics*. 2005;25(3):789–801.

CHAPTER 17

Neoplasms of the Lung and Airways

Brett W. Carter, Girish S. Shroff, and Carol C. Wu

CHAPTER OUTLINE

Introduction

Primary lung cancer is the leading cause of cancer-related mortality worldwide and accounts for more deaths than the next three malignancies combined—pancreatic, colorectal, and pancreatic cancer in men; breast, colorectal, and pancreatic cancer in women. In 2017, it was estimated that 222,500 new cases would be diagnosed, with 155,870 deaths expected from the disease. Lung cancers are generally divided into two types, non–small cell lung carcinoma (NSCLC), which accounts for 85% of all lung cancers, and small cell lung carcinoma (SCLC), which represents 15% of all lung cancers. NSCLC primarily includes adenocarcinoma and squamous cell carcinoma, as well as less common tumors such as large cell carcinoma, sarcomatoid carcinoma, and spindle cell sarcoma. SCLC is an aggressive malignancy and the most common primary pulmonary neuroendocrine neoplasm.

Lung Neoplasms

Imaging of Lung Cancer

Diagnostic imaging plays a key role in the identification, characterization, and staging of lung cancer. Suspicious pulmonary lesions may be initially identified on chest radiography because the modality is widely available and relatively inexpensive. However, there are significant limitations of radiography, including the inability to detect small nodules and other abnormalities, poor delineation of primary tumor and nodal status, and the inability to evaluate for extrathoracic disease. It has been reported that approximately 12% to 30% of lung cancers are missed on chest radiography. Multidetector computed tomography (MDCT) is the primary imaging modality used to evaluate pulmonary nodules and masses, characterize primary tumors, and detect intrathoracic and extrathoracic lymphadenopathy and metastatic disease. Limitations of MDCT include inferiority to MRI in the visualization of mediastinal and chest wall invasion and inferiority to fluorodeoxyglucose (FDG)–positron emission tomography (PET)/CT in the evaluation of nodal and metastatic disease. MRI is not routinely used in the evaluation of lung cancer, but is complementary to conventional imaging techniques. Advantages of MRI include the ability to evaluate the status of the intrathoracic vasculature when there are contraindications to contrast-enhanced MDCT (e.g., renal failure, severe contrast allergy) and improved evaluation of the mediastinum and chest wall compared to MDCT. Limitations of MRI include inherent problems with imaging the chest, although improved MR techniques have resulted in decreased scan times and diminished respiratory and cardiac motion. PET/CT has demonstrated an improved ability to assess for intrathoracic and extrathoracic lymphadenopathy and metastatic disease, assess response to therapy, and detect residual and/or recurrent disease. Important restrictions of PET/CT include limited characterization of the primary tumor, limited evaluation of mediastinal and chest wall invasion, and false-positives and false-negatives, which can result in misinterpretation.

BOX 17.1 IASLC/ATS/ERS Classification of Lung Adenocarcinoma

Preinvasive lesions
Atypical adenomatous hyperplasia
Adenocarcinoma in situ
- Nonmucinous
- Mucinous
- Mixed nonmucinous/mucinous

Minimally invasive adenocarcinoma
- Nonmucinous
- Mucinous
- Mixed nonmucinous/mucinous

Invasive adenocarcinoma
- Lepidic predominant
- Acinar predominant
- Papillary predominant
- Micropapillary predominant
- Solid predominant with mucin production

Variants of invasive adenocarcinoma
- Invasive mucinous adenocarcinoma
- Colloid
- Fetal
- Enteric

ATS, American Thoracic Society; *ERS*, European Respiratory Society; *IASLC*, International Association for the Study of Lung Cancer.

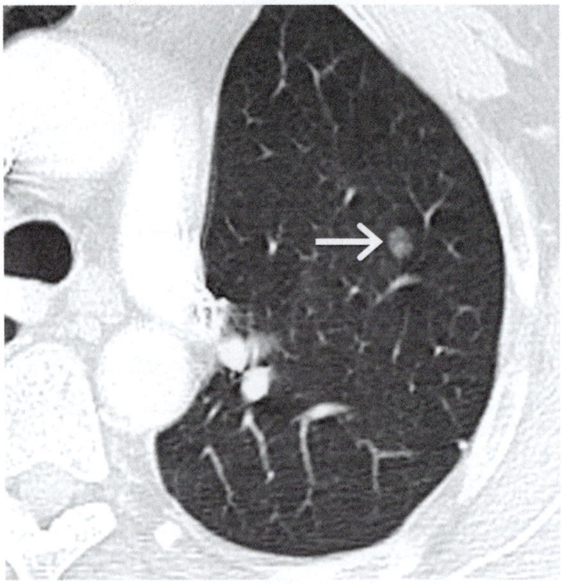

Figure 17.1 Collimated contrast-enhanced axial CT scan of a 64-year-old man with a history of adenocarcinoma of the left upper lobe status post–left upper lobectomy demonstrates a 9-mm ground-glass nodule *(arrow)* in the left lower lobe. Wedge resection revealed atypical adenomatous hyperplasia.

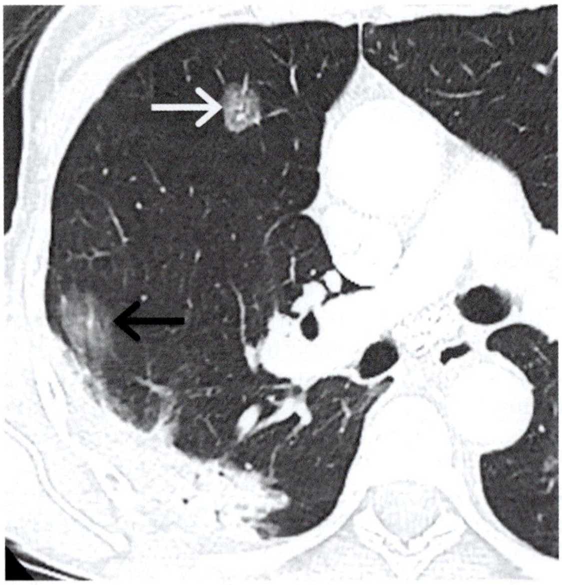

Figure 17.2 Collimated contrast-enhanced axial CT scan of a 68-year-old woman with a history of adenocarcinoma of the right lower lobe treated with chemoradiation therapy demonstrates a part solid nodule *(white arrow)* in the right middle lobe and a ground-glass nodule (*black arrow*) in the right lower lobe. Biopsy of these nodules revealed adenocarcinoma in situ.

Malignant Neoplasms

Adenocarcinoma

Adenocarcinoma is the most common subtype of NSCLC and represents a spectrum of malignant epithelial neoplasms characterized by glandular differentiation or mucus production. It is more common in women than in men and is associated with smoking in 46% of cases. Adenocarcinoma includes a wide variety of patterns and differentiation. An updated classification system was introduced in 2011 by a joint working group of the International Association for the Study of Lung Cancer (IASLC), American Thoracic Society (ATS), and European Respiratory Society (ERS) emphasizing the correlation among pathology, imaging, and clinical topics such as diagnosis, treatment, and prognosis (Box 17.1). This new system eliminated the term *bronchioloalveolar carcinoma* (BAC) and grouped lesions into the following categories: (1) preinvasive lesions; (2) atypical adenomatous hyperplasia; (3) adenocarcinoma in situ; (4) minimally invasive adenocarcinoma; (5) invasive adenocarcinoma; (6) invasive adenocarcinoma; and (7) variants of invasive adenocarcinoma.

Atypical adenomatous hyperplasia (AAH) represents a small proliferation of atypical type II pneumocytes, Clara cells, and respiratory bronchioles measuring ≤5 mm. On MDCT, AAH manifests as a focal ground-glass nodule, typically measuring ≤5 mm, although they may range up to 12 mm in size (Fig. 17.1). Adenocarcinoma in situ (AIS), formerly referred to as BAC, represents adenocarcinoma with pure lepidic growth, no evidence of nuclear atypia, and no evidence of stromal, vascular, or pleural invasion. Nonmucinous, mucinous, and mixed types have been described, although the nonmucinous type represents the majority of adenocarcinomas. On MDCT, AIS appears as a ground-glass, solid, or part solid nodule typically measuring ≤3 cm. These nodules may demonstrate slightly higher attenuation than AAH (Fig. 17.2). Minimally invasive adenocarcinomas (MIAs) are characterized by lepidic predominant growth and invasion of ≤5 mm. On MDCT, MIAs usually manifest as a part solid nodule with a predominant ground-glass component and a solid component measuring ≤5 mm (Fig. 17.3). Invasive adenocarcinomas are characterized by lepidic predominant spread and invasion of ≥5 mm. Acinar predominant, papillary predominant, micropapillary predominant, and solid predominant with mucin production types have been described. On MDCT, invasive adenocarcinomas manifest as a solid or part solid nodule, with a predominantly solid component (Fig. 17.4). Local invasion of the pleura, chest wall, or diaphragm may be present. Other findings include air bronchograms, internal lucent regions, and masslike consolidation. Multiple pulmonary nodules, masses, and/or regions of consolidation may be present. PET/CT is most effective at staging and restaging aggressive tumors such as invasive adenocarcinomas. Other malignancies such as AIS and MIA may demonstrate little to no FDG uptake, which may be due to poor cellularity or slow cellular proliferation (Fig. 17.5).

Squamous Cell Carcinoma

Squamous cell carcinoma (SCC) is the second most common subtype of NSCLC and accounts for 25% to

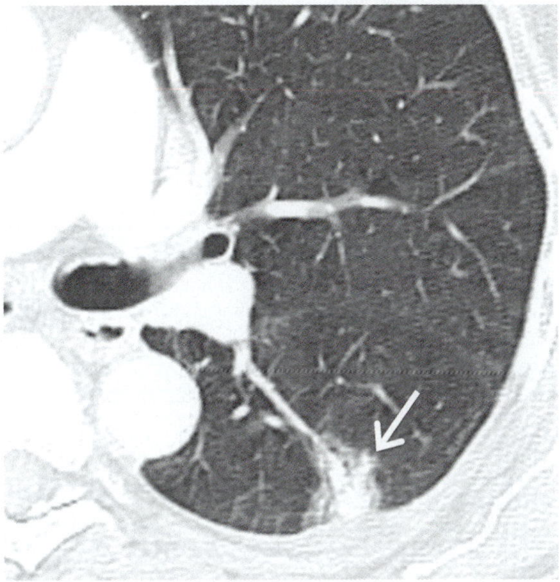

Figure 17.3 Collimated contrast-enhanced axial CT scan of a 73-year-old woman demonstrates a part solid nodule *(arrow)* in the left lower lobe, with both ground-glass and solid components. A left lower lobectomy was performed and revealed minimally invasive adenocarcinoma.

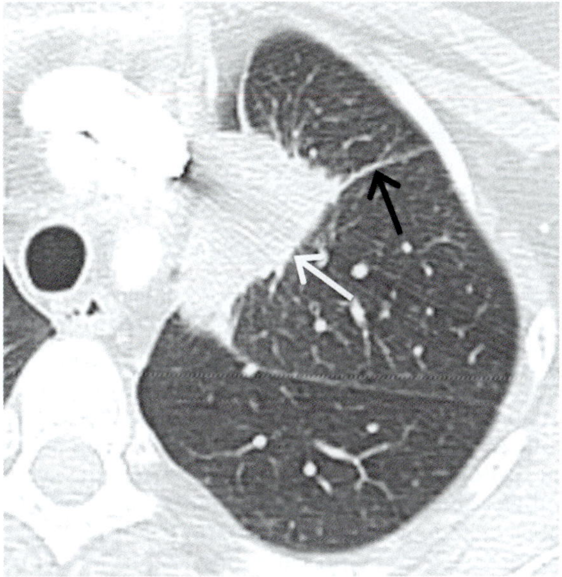

Figure 17.4 Collimated contrast-enhanced axial CT scan of a 43-year-old woman demonstrates a solid mass *(white arrow)* with irregular and spiculated margins in the left upper lobe. Note the presence of pleural tags *(black arrow)*. Biopsy revealed invasive adenocarcinoma.

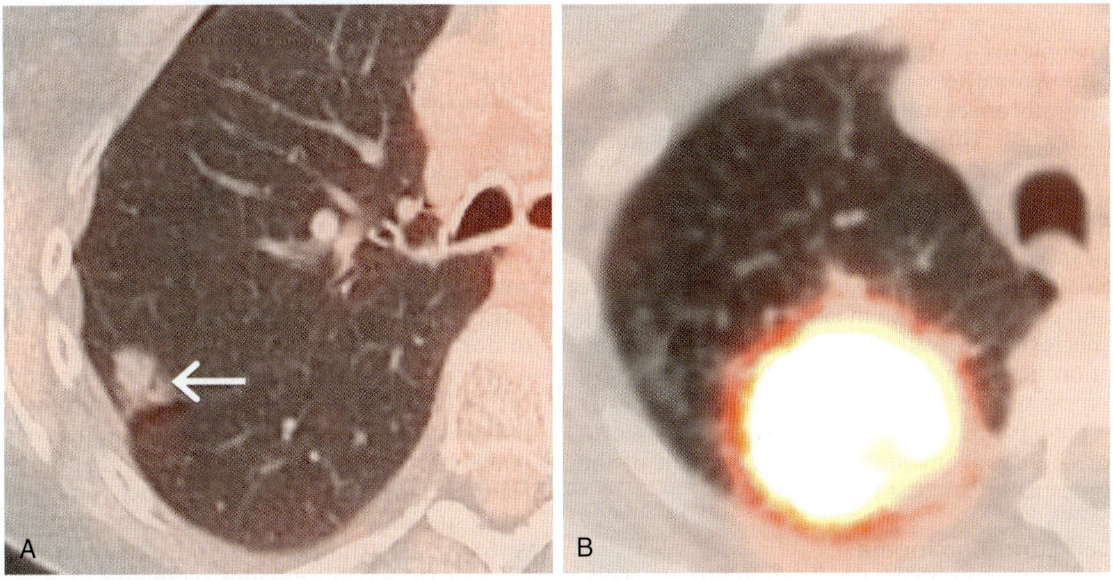

Figure 17.5 FDG-PET/CT of adenocarcinoma. (A) Collimated axial fused PET/CT image of a 52-year-old woman demonstrates a lobular nodule in the right lower lobe *(arrow)* with FDG uptake similar to that of the adjacent chest wall soft tissues. Biopsy revealed minimally invasive adenocarcinoma. (B) Collimated axial fused PET/CT image of a 67-year-old woman with a large soft tissue mass in the right lower lobe that is markedly FDG-avid. Biopsy revealed invasive adenocarcinoma.

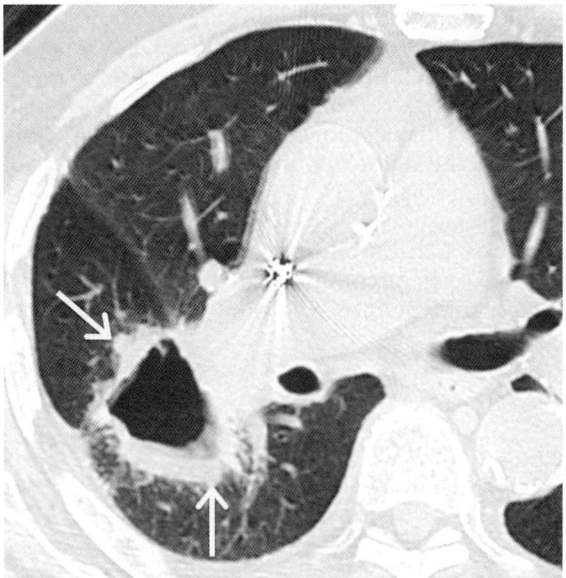

Figure 17.6 Collimated contrast-enhanced axial CT scan of a 92-year-old man demonstrates a large, thick-walled, cavitary mass *(arrows)* in the right lower lobe. Biopsy revealed squamous cell carcinoma of the lung.

30% of all lung cancers. It is strongly associated with smoking, and 50% of tumors develop in current or former smokers. SCC is more common in men than women. Four histopathologic variants have been described—papillary, small cell, clear cell, and basaloid—and 7% to 10% of patients are asymptomatic. Clinical symptoms are more likely to be present when lesions are centrally located and in an advanced stage of disease. When present, symptoms most commonly reported include cough, dyspnea, hemoptysis, and fever. Paraneoplastic syndromes such as hypercalcemia due to secretion of a parathyroid hormone–like substance may be present. SCCs arising in the lung apices, also referred to as *Pancoast tumors,* can result in neuropathic pain due to involvement of the brachial plexus or Horner syndrome due to involvement of the sympathetic chain.

SCC typically arises from large bronchi in the central aspect of the chest. Thus, on MDCT, most SCCs manifest as a centrally located nodule or mass. An endobronchial component may be present, and postobstructive atelectasis and/or pneumonia may be visible. Alternatively, tumors may appear as a peripherally located nodule or mass, with lobulated or spiculated margins. Cavitation may be present and is more common in larger lesions (Fig. 17.6). Central necrosis and wall thickening may be present. Calcification has been reported in 13% of lesions. On PET/CT, most tumors demonstrate FDG uptake greater than the mediastinal background. MRI can be used to assess for chest wall invasion and involvement of the brachial plexus in Pancoast tumors (Fig. 17.7).

Large Cell Lung Carcinoma

Large cell lung carcinoma (LCLC) represents a heterogeneous group of neoplasms that account for 5% to 10% of all lung cancers. LCLC encompasses several malignancies, including giant cell carcinoma, basaloid large cell carcinoma, clear cell carcinoma, lymphoepithelioma-like

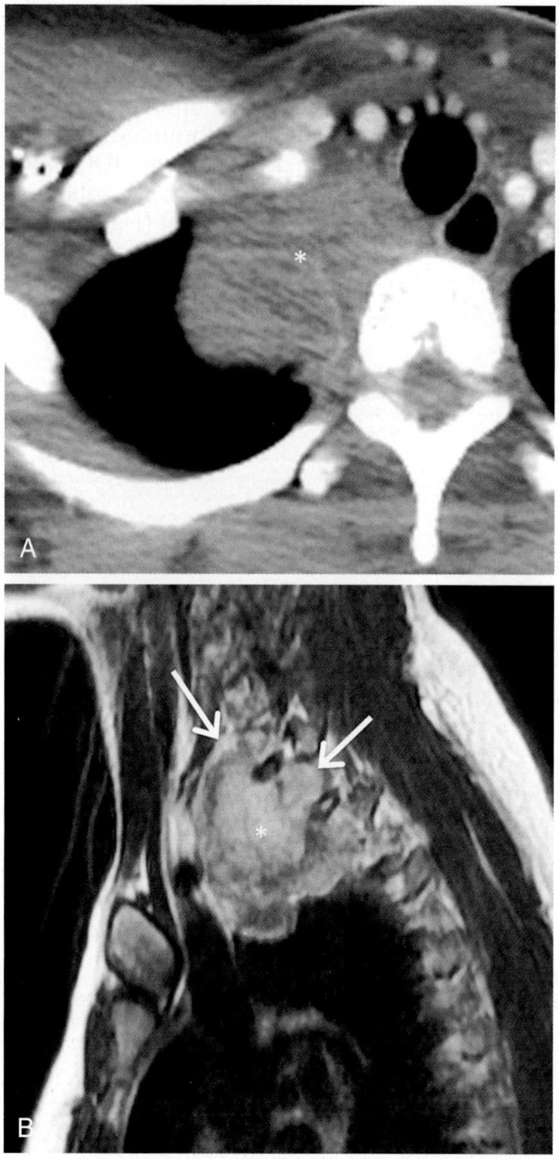

Figure 17.7 Pancoast tumor with chest wall invasion. (A) Collimated contrast-enhanced axial CT scan of a 19-year-old woman shows a soft tissue mass *(asterisk)* in the right lung apex, representing a primary Pancoast tumor. (B) Sagittal T2-weighted MR image of the same patient demonstrates invasion of the right chest wall *(arrows)* by the tumor *(asterisk)*.

carcinoma, large cell carcinoma with rhabdoid phenotype, and large cell neuroendocrine carcinoma (LCNEC). LCLC has been described as a diagnosis of exclusion in that tumor cells lack histopathologic features that would otherwise classify the lesion as an SCLC or specific subtype of NSCLC. LCNEC is one of the most clinically significant LCLCs and represents a high-grade neuroendocrine malignancy characterized by neuroendocrine histologic features. Most LCNECs occur in men with a history of heavy smoking, and the mean age at the time of diagnosis is 65 years. Clinical symptoms include chest pain, hemoptysis, cough, and other symptoms such as dyspnea, weight loss, and fever. Unlike SCC, paraneoplastic syndromes are rare.

On MDCT, LCNEC is usually indistinguishable from other lung cancers. Lesions usually appear as a large

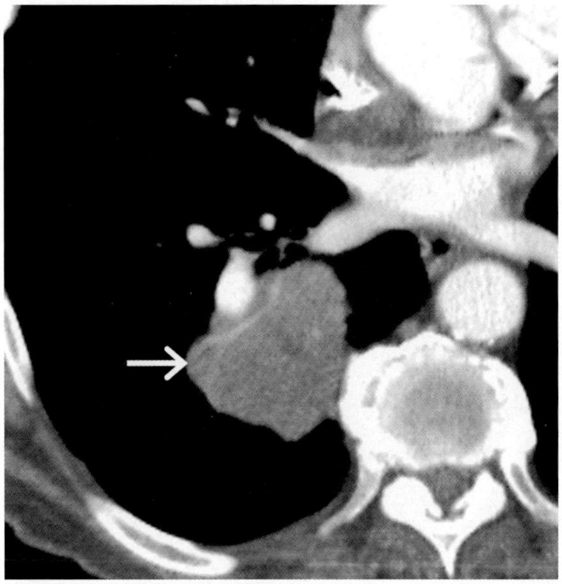

Figure 17.8 Collimated contrast-enhanced axial CT scan of a 74-year-old man demonstrates a large soft tissue mass *(arrow)* in the right lower lobe. Note the presence of internal vascularity. Biopsy revealed large cell neuroendocrine carcinoma.

mass in the peripheral aspect of the chest, ranging in size from 13 to 92 mm (Fig. 17.8). Only one-fifth of lesions are centrally located. Most tumors demonstrate lobular margins, although tumors with spiculated borders have been described. The attenuation of LCNEC has been described as similar to that of chest wall musculature. Following the administration of IV contrast, tumors demonstrate varying degrees of enhancement. Heterogeneous or peripheral enhancement may be seen in the setting of necrosis. Calcification is an infrequent finding and has been reported in less than 9% of cases. LCNEC typically demonstrates increased FDG uptake on PET/CT, and the modality is used for staging and restaging purposes.

Small Cell Lung Carcinoma

SCLCs account for approximately 13% to 15% of all lung cancers and are the most common primary pulmonary neuroendocrine neoplasm. SCLC has the strongest association with cigarette smoking, which is responsible for approximately 95% of cases of SCLC. In general, SCLC is much more aggressive than NSCLC and has a greater propensity for the early development of widespread metastases. SCLC has traditionally been staged with the Veterans Administration Lung Study Group (VALSG) systems, which divide SCLC into limited stage (LS) and extensive stage (ES) based on radiation treatment planning. However, the IASLC has recommended that the current seventh edition of the American Joint Committee on Cancer (AJCC) tumor-node-metastasis (TNM) staging system for lung cancer be used to stage SCLC.

Because 90% to 95% of SCLCs arise from lobar or main bronchi, most SCLCs are located within the central aspect of the chest and manifest as a mediastinal (92%) or hilar (84%) lymphadenopathy or pulmonary lesion (Fig. 17.9). Postobstructive atelectasis and/or pneumonia may be seen in these patients. MDCT can be useful in revealing the presence and extent of mediastinal invasion. In 68% of patients, encasement of mediastinal structures such as the trachea, esophagus, heart, and vessels, including the superior vena cava, is evident (Fig. 17.10). Intratumoral calcification has been reported in 23% of patients. A small group of patients with SCLC (<5%) may have a peripheral pulmonary nodule without associated lymphadenopathy.

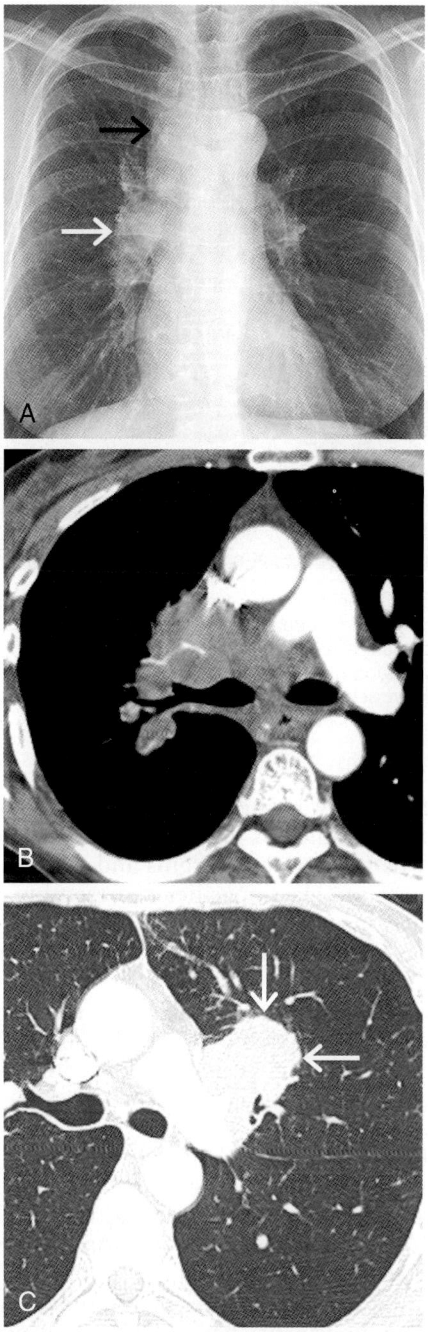

Figure 17.9 Manifestations of small cell lung carcinoma (SCLC). (A) Posteroanterior chest radiograph of a 52-year-old woman presenting with chest pain demonstrates thickening of the right paratracheal stripe *(black arrow)* and convexity of the right hilum *(white arrow)* suggestive of lymphadenopathy. (B) Collimated contrast-enhanced axial CT scan of the same patient confirms the presence of a soft tissue mass in the right hilum and mediastinal lymphadenopathy. Biopsy revealed SCLC. (C) Collimated contrast-enhanced axial CT scan of a 52-year-old man with SCLC demonstrates a soft tissue mass *(arrows)* in the medial left upper lobe, with lobular margins representing the primary tumor.

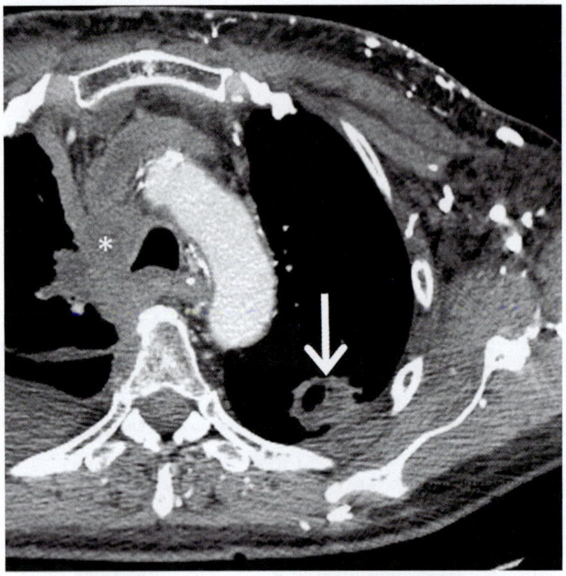

Figure 17.10 Superior vena cava obstruction due to small cell lung carcinoma (SCLC). Collimated contrast-enhanced axial CT scan of a 52-year-old man with SCLC demonstrates soft tissue in the right paratracheal region *(asterisk)* obliterating the superior vena cava. Note the collateral vessels in the left chest wall and mediastinum. A cavitary metastasis *(arrow)* is present in the left lung.

These peripherally located tumors usually manifest as well-defined nodules or masses that are homogeneous and demonstrate lobular margins and spiculation. Surrounding ground-glass opacities, representing edema or hemorrhage, may be identified. Unusual manifestations of SCLC on MDCT include consolidation, air space opacities, and lymphangitic carcinomatosis. On PET/CT, most SCLCs demonstrate markedly increased FDG uptake due to high metabolic activity. PET/CT has been shown to stage patients more accurately than conventional imaging and can be used for restaging purposes.

Carcinoid

Carcinoid tumors are neuroendocrine neoplasms that are typically found in the gastrointestinal tract; however, 20% to 30% of all carcinoids arise from the respiratory tract, and these neoplasms represent 1% to 2% of all primary lung cancers. Carcinoid tumors are classified based on mitotic activity—typical (low grade) and atypical (intermediate grade). Most neoplasms are typical carcinoids, which are well-differentiated neoplasms with neuroendocrine features measuring ≥5 mm and exhibiting less than 2 mitoses/10 high-power field (HPF) or 2 mm^2 and no necrosis. Typical carcinoids are less aggressive, and 13% of patients present with lymph node involvement. Atypical carcinoid tumors account for 10% to 16% of carcinoids, are characterized by 2 to 10 mitoses/HPF or necrosis, and are more aggressive, and more patients (57%) present with lymph node involvement.

Typical and atypical carcinoids demonstrate similar features on imaging studies. The most common finding on chest radiography is a well-defined hilar or perihilar nodule or mass. In general, carcinoids are more common in the right lung than in the left lung. The average size is 3 cm, with a range of 2 to 5 cm, although atypical carcinoids tend to be larger than typical carcinoids and are more likely to be located in the lung periphery. Associated findings, such as postobstructive atelectasis and/or pneumonia, may be present. MDCT usually demonstrates a soft tissue nodule that is often closely associated with an airway. In some cases, the tumor may be entirely endoluminal or partially endoluminal. Punctate, eccentric, or diffuse patterns of calcification have been reported in 30% of cases. Associated findings such as postobstructive atelectasis and/or pneumonia, mucoid impaction, bronchiectasis, or air trapping may be present. Carcinoid tumors may demonstrate enhancement following the administration of IV contrast (Fig. 17.11). PET/CT is of limited utility in the evaluation of carcinoids because

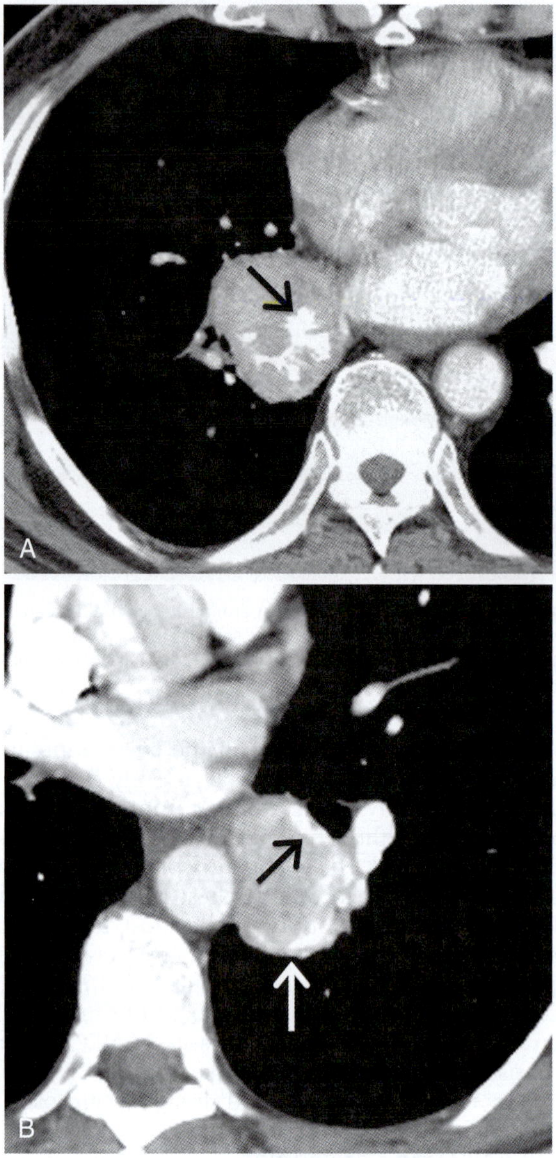

Figure 17.11 Imaging manifestations of carcinoid. (A) Collimated contrast-enhanced axial CT scan of a 70-year-old man demonstrates a soft tissue mass in the right lower lobe, with eccentric calcification *(arrow)*. Biopsy revealed carcinoid. (B) Collimated contrast-enhanced axial CT scan of a 46-year-old woman demonstrates a carcinoid tumor in the left lower lobe *(white arrow)* with extensive peripheral enhancement and vascularity *(black arrow)*.

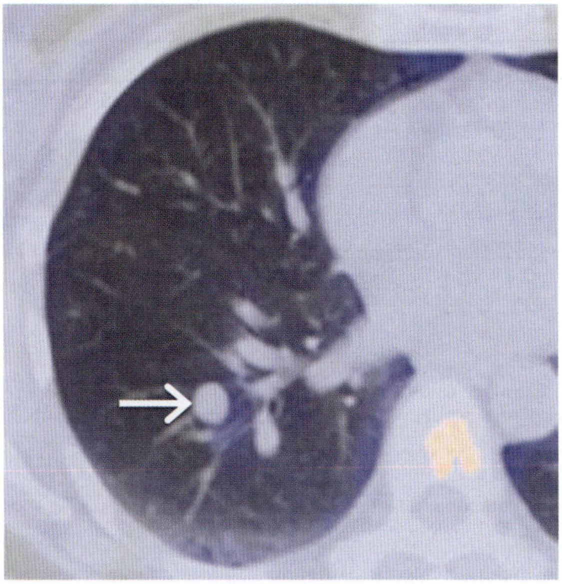

Figure 17.12 Collimated axial fused PET/CT image of a 47-year-old woman with a history of breast cancer demonstrates a well-circumscribed nodule *(arrow)* in the right lower lobe. FDG uptake within the nodule is similar to background. Biopsy revealed typical carcinoid.

tumors may demonstrate little to no FDG uptake, and a high false-negative rate has been reported (Fig. 17.12).

BOX 17.2 Veterans Administration Lung Study Group Staging System

Limited Stage
Confined to single radiation port
Confined to ipsilateral mediastinum
Ipsilateral mediastinal or supraclavicular lymph nodes

Extensive Stage
Disease not confined to single radiation port
Contralateral mediastinal or supraclavicular lymph nodes
Malignant pleural or pericardial effusion
Metastatic disease

BOX 17.3 Modified Veterans Administration Lung Study Group Staging System

Limited Stage
Confined to single radiation port
Ipsilateral mediastinal or supraclavicular lymph nodes
Contralateral mediastinal or supraclavicular lymph nodes
Ipsilateral pleural effusion (regardless of cytology)

Extensive Stage
Disease not confined to single radiation port
Metastatic disease

Lung Cancer Staging

The IASLC has recommended that the current eighth edition of the AJCC TNM staging system be used to stage NSCLC, SCLC, and bronchopulmonary carcinoid. Traditionally, SCLC has been staged with the VALSG and modified VALSG systems, which divide SCLC into LS and ES based on radiation treatment planning.

VALSG and Modified VALSG Staging Systems

Although it has been recommended that the TNM system replace the VALSG staging systems for the staging of SCLC, a brief review of the latter is beneficial because they are still commonly used in clinical practice. In the original VALSG system, LS-SCLC was characterized by tumor involvement limited to one hemithorax (with or without local extension) and no distant extrathoracic metastatic disease (Box 17.2). Regional and ipsilateral supraclavicular lymph nodes were considered to be LS-SCLC if these groups could be included in a single safe and adequate radiation port. ES-SCLC applied to all other patients; this included specific features such as malignant pleural and pericardial effusions, contralateral hilar or supraclavicular lymph nodes, and metastatic disease that could not be treated in a single radiation port. In 1989, the IASLC proposed key changes to the VALSG system (Box 17.3), the most significant of which included contralateral mediastinal and supraclavicular lymph nodes and ipsilateral pleural effusions (benign and malignant, regardless of cytology) into LS-SCLC. ES-SCLC disease was defined as disease beyond that of LS-SCLC. A retrospective study at one institution indicated that the IASLC system had better prognostic value than the VALSG system. In clinical practice, features of the VALSG and IASLC staging systems are often combined. For example, LS-SCLC can include contralateral mediastinal and ipsilateral supraclavicular lymph node involvement. However, certain findings, such as contralateral supraclavicular or hilar lymph node involvement, remain controversial, and clinical management is typically based on the ability to include these regions in a safe and adequate radiation port.

TNM System

The eighth edition of the AJCC TNM staging system has made key changes to the system based on significant differences in 5-year survival, as determined by the IASLC Lung Cancer Staging Project. Highlights of the eighth edition of the TNM staging system will be discussed here; the complete scheme is outlined in Table 17.1.

One of the key changes made in the eighth edition included the further subdivision of primary lung cancers into tumor (T) descriptors based on size. The analysis of the new database showed significant separation of T1 tumors from T2 lesions based on a threshold size of 3 cm, as well as a progressive reduction in patient survival for each 1-cm threshold (≤1 cm, >1–2 cm, >2–3 cm, >3–4 cm, >4–5 cm, >5–6 cm, >6–7 cm, and >7 cm). T1 lung cancers are subdivided into three groups at 1-cm thresholds, including T1a lesions measuring ≤1 cm, T1b nodules measuring >1 and ≤2 cm, and T1c tumors measuring >2 and ≤3 cm. T2 lesions have been subdivided into two groups, including T2a tumors measuring >3 and ≤4 cm

TABLE 17.1 Eighth Edition of the TNM Staging System (TNM-8)

T DESCRIPTOR	DEFINITION
TX	Primary tumor cannot be assessed or tumor proven by the presence of malignant cells in sputum or bronchial washings but not visualized by imaging or bronchoscopy.
T0	No evidence of primary tumor
Tis	Carcinoma in situ
T1	Tumor ≤ 3 cm in greatest dimension, surrounded by lung or visceral pleura, without bronchoscopic evidence of invasion more proximal than the lobar bronchus
T1a	Tumor ≤ 1 cm in greatest dimension
T1b	Tumor > 1 cm and ≤ 2 cm in greatest dimension
T1c	Tumor > 2 cm and ≤ 3 cm in greatest dimension
T2	Tumor > 3 cm and ≤ 5 cm or tumor with any of the following features: involvement of a main bronchus regardless of distance from the carina; invasion of the visceral pleura; partial or complete lung atelectasis or pneumonitis
T2a	Tumor > 3 cm and ≤ 4 cm in greatest dimension
T2b	Tumor > 4 cm and ≤ 5 cm in greatest dimension
T3	Tumor > 5 cm or directly invading any of the following structures: parietal pleura, chest wall, phrenic nerve, parietal pericardium, or separate tumor nodule(s) in the same lobe as the primary lesion
T4	Tumor measuring >7 cm that invades any of the following structures: mediastinum, diaphragm, heart, great vessels, trachea, recurrent laryngeal nerve, esophagus, vertebral body, carina; or separate tumor nodule(s) in a different lobe of the same lung.
N DESCRIPTOR	**DEFINITION**
NX	Lymph nodes cannot be assessed.
N0	No regional lymph nodes
N1	Ipsilateral peribronchial and/or hilar lymph nodes and intrapulmonary nodes; includes lymph nodes affected by direct extension
N2	Ipsilateral mediastinal and/or subcarinal lymph node(s)
N3	Contralateral mediastinal, contralateral hilar, ipsilateral or contralateral scalene, or supraclavicular lymph node(s)
M DESCRIPTOR	**DEFINITION**
M0	No metastases
M1	Presence of metastasis
M1a	Intrathoracic metastases: separate tumor nodule(s) in contralateral lung; malignant pleural effusion or pleural thickening, nodules, or masses; malignant pericardial effusion or pericardial thickening, nodules, or masses
M1b	Single extrathoracic metastasis in single distant organ
M1c	Multiple extrathoracic metastases in single or multiple distant organs

and T2b lesions measuring >4 and ≤5 cm. Lung cancers measuring >5 cm and ≤7 cm are classified as T3 tumors, and those measuring >7 cm are classified as T4 lesions.

Other significant modifications to the T descriptor include the grouping of lung cancers resulting in atelectasis of a lobe or the entire lung as T2 disease, the grouping of lung cancers involving a main bronchus regardless of distance from the carina as T2 disease, reclassification of diaphragmatic invasion as T4 disease (previously T3 disease), and elimination of mediastinal pleural invasion as a descriptor. No changes were made to lymph node descriptors in the eighth edition. However, metastatic disease was further subdivided into M1a, M1b, and M1c components based on the location of metastases. For example, intrathoracic metastatic disease, including contralateral tumor nodules and pleural or pericardial metastases, is designated M1a. Extrathoracic metastatic disease is classified as M1b disease if there is a solitary metastasis or a single distant organ is involved and is classified as M1c disease if there are multiple metastases in one or more distant organs.

Molecular Profiling

The improved molecular and genetic characterization of lung cancer has revealed certain driver mutations that may confer susceptibility or resistance to specific treatments. Some of the most common driver mutations in NSCLC include epidermal growth factor receptor (*EGFR*), Kirsten rat sarcoma virus (*KRAS*), and anaplastic lymphoma kinase (*ALK*) mutations, which are almost always mutually exclusive. Never-smokers with lung adenocarcinoma have the highest incidence of certain mutations, such as *EGFR* and *ALK*. Activation of *EGFR* by EGF leads to cellular growth, proliferation, and decreased apoptosis, and these mutations are more common in adenocarcinomas, Asian patients, female patients, and never-smokers. The most common *EGFR* mutations include deletion in exon 19 and a point mutation in exon 21. The *ALK* gene codes for a receptor tyrosine kinase and is fused to the echinoderm microtubule-associated, protein-like 4 (*EML4*) gene, producing the *EML4-ALK* fusion oncogene in 3% to 7% of patients with NSCLC. The *EML4-ALK* fusion oncogene (or *ALK* rearrangement) promotes cell growth and proliferation and is more likely to be seen in younger patients who are light smokers or never-smokers with adenocarcinoma of the lung. The *KRAS* gene codes for RAS proteins, guanosine nucleotide binding proteins located at the inner surface of the plasma membrane that are involved in the transduction of growth signals from receptor tyrosine kinases (RTKs). *KRAS* accounts for most of the RAS mutations, are present in 25% to 40% of NSCLCs, and are more common in whites, current or former smokers, and adenocarcinomas.

Benign Neoplasms

Hamartoma

Hamartoma is the most common benign pulmonary neoplasms and is composed of connective tissue containing cartilage and varying amounts of fat, smooth muscle, bone, and lymphovascular structures. Approximately 6% of all solitary pulmonary nodules identified on imaging studies represent hamartomas. Most lesions are identified in patients in the sixth decade of life, and the incidence is two or three times greater in men than women. Most hamartomas are detected incidentally on radiographs or MDCT performed for other reasons. These tumors are characterized by slow growth, and malignant transformation is incredibly rare.

The most common appearance of hamartoma on MDCT is a well-circumscribed solitary pulmonary nodule or mass, with smooth or lobular borders in the lung periphery. Calcification is more common as lesions increase in size and is much better visualized on MDCT than radiography. The characteristic "popcorn" configuration of calcification is only present in 10% to 15% of cases. Internal fat (−40 to −120 Hounsfield units on MDCT) is present in 60% of cases. The identification of internal fat and calcium is typically considered diagnostic of hamartoma (Fig. 17.13). Following the administration of IV contrast, heterogeneous enhancement is typical. Regions of internal enhancing septations may be present. Although features on MDCT are typically sufficient to make the diagnosis, lesions may be visible on MRI. Hamartomas are typically of intermediate signal intensity on T1-weighted imaging and high signal intensity on T2-weighted imaging. Following the administration of IV contrast, enhancement of the capsule and internal septations may be present. On PET/CT, approximately 20% of lesions demonstrate FDG uptake; larger lesions tend to be more FDG-avid than smaller lesions.

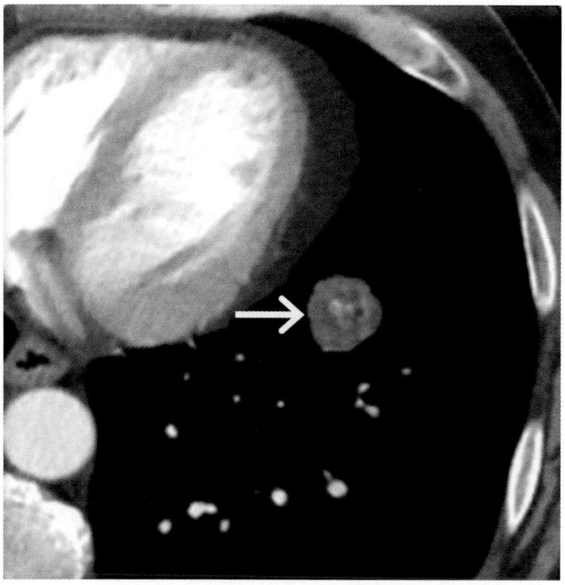

Figure 17.13 Collimated contrast-enhanced axial CT scan of a 39-year-old woman demonstrates a left lower lobe nodule with internal fat and calcification *(arrow)*, characteristic of a pulmonary hamartoma.

■ Airway Neoplasms

Tumors of the tracheobronchial tree are uncommon, accounting for 2% of all respiratory malignancies in the United States, with an estimated incidence of 1/1,000,000 individuals. Neoplasms affecting the bronchi are 400 times more common than tracheal tumors. Most (90%) of tracheal tumors in adults are malignant, whereas most in children are benign. Clinical symptoms reported at the time of presentation are typically nonspecific and may include stridor, wheezing, adult-onset asthma, hemoptysis, and recurrent pneumonia. Because of the relative rarity of these tumors and nonspecific symptoms, diagnosis is often delayed.

Imaging of Airway Neoplasms

Radiography is typically the initial radiologic examination that is performed when patients present with respiratory symptoms; careful evaluation of the trachea and proximal bronchial air columns is essential to detect abnormalities. However, only 18% to 28% of tracheal tumors are visible on radiography. The most common findings include a lobular or rounded opacity in the tracheal or bronchial air columns. Postobstructive atelectasis or pneumonia may be present. Endoluminal lesions may produce a ball valve mechanism and resultant hyperinflation and air trapping. Chronic airway obstruction may lead to regions of bronchiectasis or bronchiolectasis.

MDCT is the imaging modality of choice, optimally demonstrates the presence and extent of disease, and can be used for surgical planning. MDCT has the advantages of fast acquisition times and widespread availability, and imaging of the entire tracheobronchial tree can be performed in seconds. Nonspecific findings such as endoluminal lesions and airway wall thickening may be identified. Features such as extraluminal extension, mediastinal invasion, and irregular margins suggest malignancy, whereas well-circumscribed margins suggest a benign lesion. Several specific imaging features can be used to narrow the differential diagnosis, including fat, calcification, and enhancement. When fat is present, hamartoma, lipoma, and liposarcoma should be included in the differential diagnosis. In the setting of internal calcification, hamartoma, carcinoid, chondroma, and chondrosarcoma should be included. When enhancement is present, carcinoid, hypervascular metastases from

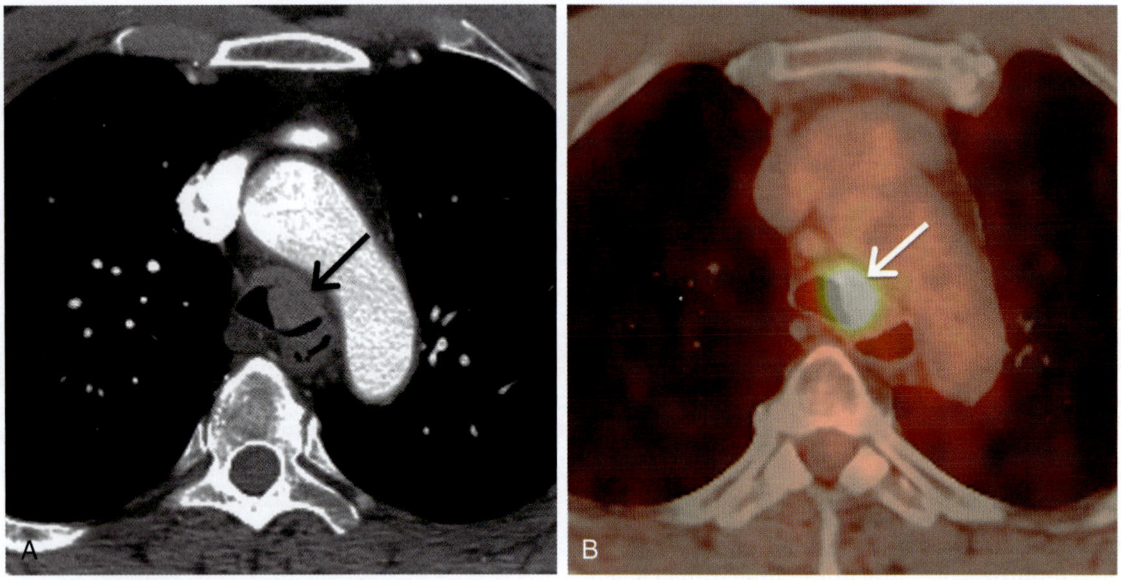

Figure 17.14 Squamous cell carcinoma of the trachea. (A) Collimated contrast-enhanced axial CT scan demonstrates thickening of the anterior wall of the trachea and an adjacent soft tissue mass *(black arrow)*. (B) Collimated axial fused PET/CT image of the same patient shows marked FDG uptake in the lesion *(white arrow)*, typical of squamous cell carcinoma.

primary malignancies such as thyroid and renal cell carcinomas, melanoma, choriocarcinoma, and hemangioma should be considered.

Two-dimensional (2D) multiplanar reconstruction (MPR) images and three-dimensional (3D) reconstruction images can be used to provide additional information. 2D MPRs can improve delineation of the craniocaudal extent of tumor and can be used to obtain accurate measurements from a tumor to important anatomic landmarks. 3D volume rendering or virtual bronchoscopy provides an endoluminal perspective, the advantages of which include the evaluation of patients in whom bronchoscopy is contraindicated due to comorbidities and bronchoscopes cannot be advanced secondary to an obstructing tumor.

With the advent of MDCT with MPRs, there is no distinct advantage to using MRI. The long acquisition times associated with most studies may be difficult for those with respiratory symptoms. However, it can be useful for follow-up imaging of children and young adults by limiting cumulative radiation doses.

FDG-PET/CT has been increasingly used in the evaluation of a wide variety of neoplasms. The presence and extent of FDG uptake in airway neoplasms depend on tumor histology because highly malignant tumors such as SCC demonstrate intense FDG uptake, but more indolent lesions such as carcinoid demonstrate little to no FDG uptake. PET/CT effectively stages patients by demonstrating metastatic disease and can provide guidance for tissue biopsy.

Malignant Airway Neoplasms

Squamous Cell Carcinoma

SCC is the most common primary malignancy of the trachea and constitutes approximately 50% of all tracheal malignancies. It is strongly associated with cigarette smoking and typically affects men 50 to 60 years of age. Nearly 40% of patients develop synchronous or metachronous malignancies of the head and neck or lung. Mediastinal lymphadenopathy and/or pulmonary metastases are present in one-third of patients at the time of diagnosis.

The most common appearance of SCC on MDCT is a polypoid intraluminal mass, the borders of which may be highly variable and demonstrate smooth, lobular, or irregular characteristics (Fig. 17.14). Although tumors may arise from any portion of the tracheobronchial tree, there is preference for the posterior wall of the lower two-thirds of the trachea. Lesions may be confined to the affected portion of the airway or result in extraluminal extension into the adjacent mediastinum and affect structures such as the esophagus. These cases may be complicated by the development of a tracheoesophageal fistula. Alternatively, SCC may manifest as airway wall thickening, which can be focal or circumferential. SCCs typically demonstrate increased FDG uptake on PET/CT (see Fig. 17.14).

Adenoid Cystic Carcinoma

Adenoid cystic carcinomas are the second most common primary malignancy of the trachea and arise from the submucosal minor salivary glands. Unlike SCCs, there is no association with cigarette smoking. Men and women are affected equally and patients are typically diagnosed in the fourth decade of life. Regional lymph nodes are affected in approximately 10% of patients at the time of diagnosis.

The most common imaging manifestation of adenoid cystic carcinoma is a focal intraluminal soft tissue mass. Alternatively, tumors can result in diffuse or circumferential thickening of airway walls, which may or may not result in luminal stenosis (Fig. 17.15). The lower trachea

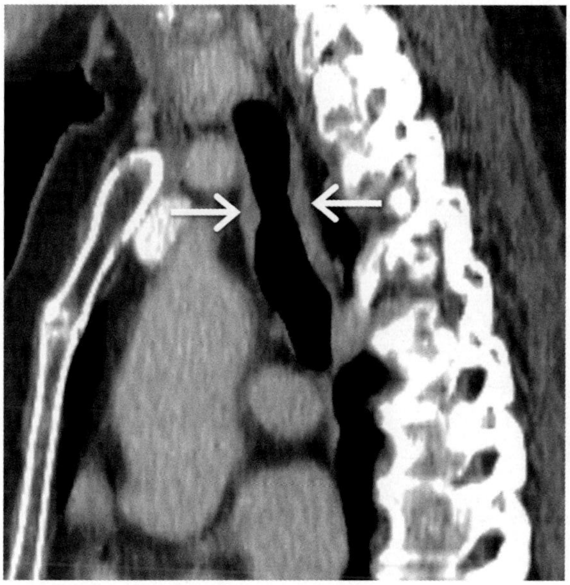

Figure 17.15 Sagittal reformatted image from a contrast-enhanced CT scan demonstrates irregular thickening of the anterior and posterior walls *(arrows)* of the trachea. Biopsy revealed adenoid cystic carcinoma.

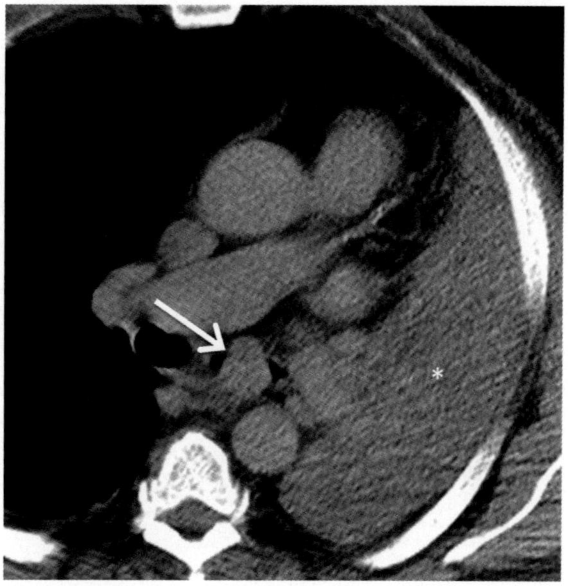

Figure 17.16 Collimated noncontrast axial CT scan of a 51-year-old man demonstrates a soft tissue mass *(arrow)* in the left main bronchus and complete atelectasis of the left lung *(asterisk)*. Endobronchial biopsy revealed mucoepidermoid carcinoma.

and main bronchi are the most commonly affected regions. Because of the tendency for adenoid cystic carcinoma to result in submucosal and perineural spread, the full extent of disease can be underestimated on cross-sectional imaging; thus sagittal and coronal MPR imaging is effective at demonstrating the longitudinal spread of tumor. Adenoid cystic carcinoma commonly shows extraluminal extension. Because most tumors demonstrate slow growth, FDG uptake on PET/CT can be highly variable, with one study showing a maximum standardized uptake value (SUV_{max}) of 3.7 to 3.8. High-grade tumors tend to demonstrate greater FDG uptake.

Mucoepidermoid Carcinoma

Mucoepidermoid carcinomas are rare primary malignancies of salivary gland origin that represent 0.1% to 0.2% of all pulmonary neoplasms. Metastatic disease is present in 10% of patients at the time of diagnosis. Patients younger than 40 years are most frequently affected.

The most common imaging appearance of mucoepidermoid carcinoma is an intraluminal soft tissue nodule with mild to marked heterogeneous enhancement following the administration of IV contrast. Thus these lesions may be indistinguishable from carcinoid tumors on MDCT. Punctate internal calcifications have been reported in up to 50% of cases. Although any portion of the tracheobronchial tree can be affected, 45% arise from the central airways (the main bronchi more commonly than the trachea) and 55% arise from the distal airways (usually a segmental bronchus; Fig. 17.16). Variable FDG uptake on PET/CT has been reported; low-grade tumors tend to result in mild FDG uptake, whereas high-grade tumors show high FDG uptake.

Carcinoid

Carcinoid tumors are the most common endobronchial neoplasm diagnosed in young adults; most patients present during the fourth decade of life. Men and women are affected equally. Carcinoid tumors are neuroendocrine tumors that are classified based on mitotic activity—typical (low grade) and atypical (intermediate grade). Clinically, patients may present with paraneoplastic syndromes related to the secretion of adrenocorticotropic hormone (ACTH) or serotonin.

Carcinoid tumors may manifest as postobstructive atelectasis or pneumonia resulting from the endobronchial location of these lesions. On MDCT, an intraluminal soft tissue mass with smooth or lobulated margins is the most common appearance. Typical carcinoids tend to be centrally located in the main, lobar, or segmental bronchi, whereas atypical carcinoids tend to develop in the lung periphery. The iceberg phenomenon has been described, in which large lesions may manifest as hilar or perihilar masses with a large extraluminal component and a small intraluminal component. Carcinoid tumors may demonstrate intense enhancement following the administration of IV contrast (Fig. 17.17). Internal calcification has been described in up to 20% of cases. Lesions demonstrate variable uptake on FDG-PET/CT. In general, FDG uptake is lower than in other tracheobronchial malignancies, and tumors may demonstrate no FDG uptake or uptake less than that of the mediastinal background.

Sarcomas and Lymphoma

Sarcomas and lymphomas represent an uncommon, heterogeneous group of malignancies that may involve the tracheobronchial tree. The most common types of sarcoma include spindle cell sarcoma, chondrosarcoma, leiomyosarcoma, fibrosarcoma, and synovial sarcoma. A wide variety of primary lymphomas, including Hodgkin lymphoma and various non-Hodgkin lymphomas, the latter of which include mucosa-associated lymphoid tissue (MALT), anaplastic large cell, unspecified T cell, mantle

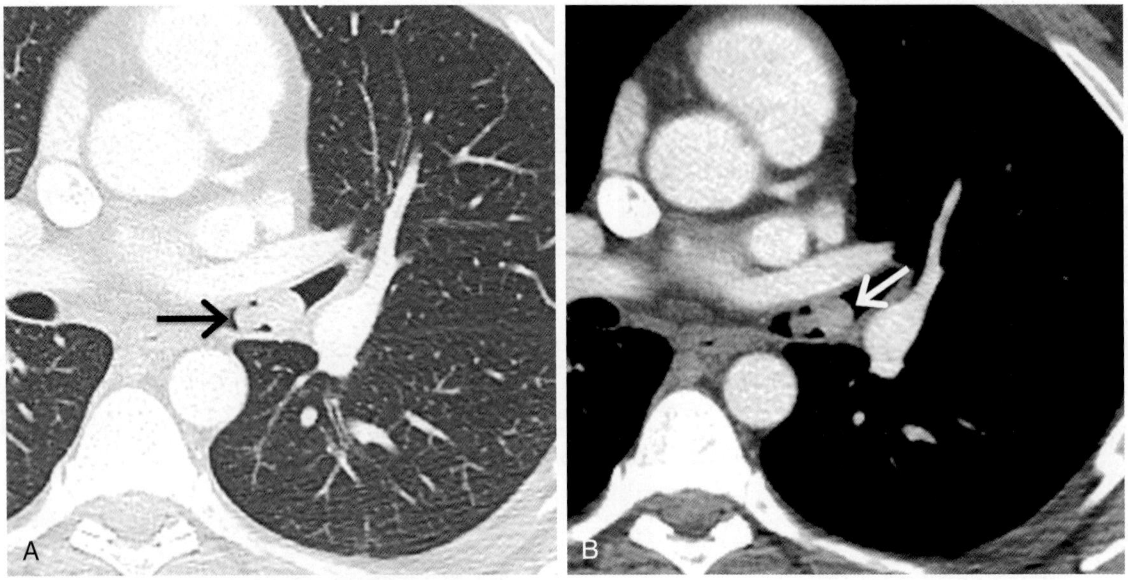

Figure 17.17 Endobronchial carcinoid tumor. (A) Collimated contrast-enhanced axial CT scan on lung windows demonstrates a bilobed lesion *(black arrow)* in the left main bronchus. (B) Collimated contrast-enhanced axial CT scan of the same patient on soft tissue windows shows marked enhancement of a portion of the lesion *(white arrow)*. Biopsy revealed carcinoid tumor, which was entirely endoluminal at the time of resection.

cell, B cell, lymphocytic, diffuse large histiocytic, and diffuse large cell immunoblastic lymphomas, have been described. In general, histopathologic analysis is necessary to differentiate sarcomas and lymphomas from other primary airway malignancies. Patients may be asymptomatic or may present with dyspnea, cough, wheezing or stridor, and hoarseness. Hemoptysis may complicate sarcomas but is only rarely reported with lymphoma.

The most common finding on chest radiography is a lobulated or rounded opacity in the tracheal or bronchial air columns. Nonspecific findings such as atelectasis or recurrent or nonresolving pneumonia may be the only radiographic abnormality. On MDCT, sarcomas usually manifest as intraluminal soft tissue masses, although extraluminal extension into the mediastinum or lung may occur. The presence of stippled or amorphous internal calcification suggests chondrosarcoma, although it is important to remember that benign lesions such as carcinoid, hamartoma, and chondroma may demonstrate calcification and are much more common. Lymphoma typically results in a solitary intraluminal soft tissue nodule or mass. Alternatively, lobulated thickening of the affected airway, representing submucosal infiltration, may be the predominant finding.

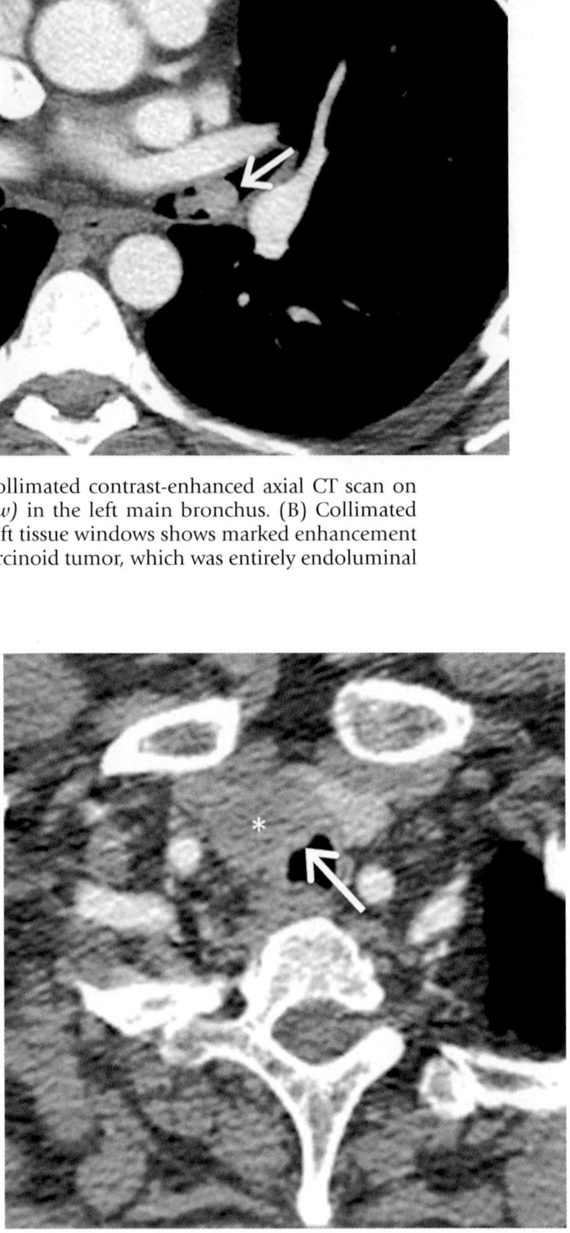

Figure 17.18 Collimated contrast-enhanced axial CT scan demonstrates a hypodense lesion in the right thyroid lobe representing medullary thyroid carcinoma *(asterisk)*. Note the invasion of the right and anterior aspects of the adjacent trachea *(arrow)*.

Metastatic Disease

Metastases affecting the airways are more common than primary tumors and may be the result of direct invasion or hematogenous spread. Tumors that tend to spread directly through to the airways include primary malignancies of the larynx, thyroid gland, lung, mediastinum, and esophagus. Tumors that tend to spread hematogenously include melanoma, sarcoma, and colorectal, breast, and lung cancers.

Direct invasion of the trachea manifests as a primary tumor extending into the airways, with an intraluminal mass and/or airway thickening (Fig. 17.18). Destruction of tracheal or bronchial cartilage may be present. These lesions may be complicated by tracheoesophageal or bronchoesophageal fistulas. For hematogenous metastases, the imaging characteristics of metastases typically mirror those of the primary tumor. For example, vascular tumors such as melanoma and renal cell carcinoma may demonstrate intense enhancement following the administration of IV contrast.

Benign Airway Neoplasms

Squamous Cell Papilloma and Tracheobronchial Papillomatosis

Squamous cell papilloma is the most common benign neoplasm of the tracheobronchial tree and is composed of a core of fibrovascular tissue surrounded by stratified squamous epithelium. Men are affected more than women, and the mean age at the time of diagnosis is 51 years. Papillomas are associated with cigarette smoking. These lesions may be found in the solitary form as a papilloma or tracheobronchial papillomatosis when multiple lesions are present. Tracheobronchial papillomatosis is the result of infection with human papilloma virus types 6 and 11, typically acquired from an affected mother during vaginal delivery.

The most common imaging manifestation of squamous cell papilloma is a solitary small nodule projecting into the airway lumen, without extraluminal extension (Fig. 17.19). Most papillomas are present in a lobar bronchus, whereas involvement of a main bronchus or the trachea is less common. Malignant transformation has been described. Tracheobronchial papillomatosis manifests as multiple intraluminal polypoid nodules of various size that usually occur in the trachea. The central airways are involved in 5% of cases, and the small airways and lungs are involved in less than 1%. When it spreads to the lungs, nodules may cavitate and demonstrate air-fluid levels. These nodules typically present in the posterior half of the chest. Malignant transformation to SCC can occur.

Hamartoma and Lipoma

Hamartomas are benign neoplasms consisting of cartilage, fat, bone, smooth muscle cells, and connective tissue; 1.4% to 3% of hamartomas are endobronchial lesions,

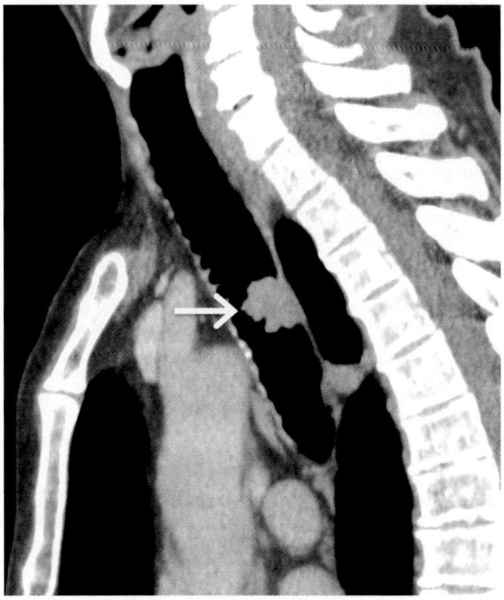

Figure 17.19 Sagittal reformatted image from a contrast-enhanced CT scan demonstrates a soft tissue mass *(arrow)* with lobular margins arising from the posterior wall of the trachea. Biopsy revealed solitary papilloma.

and neoplasms involving the trachea are even less common. Men are more commonly affected than women, and the median age at the time of diagnosis is 62 years. Hamartomas of the airway typically contain less fat and more cartilaginous components than parenchymal hamartomas. The most common manifestation of hamartoma is an exophytic, polypoid, or sessile mass with smooth margins. The presence of fat and/or internal calcification on MDCT suggests the diagnosis. MRI may be beneficial in some scenarios because the fat components demonstrate high signal intensity on T1- and T2-weighted imaging.

Lipomas are rare tumors that arise from the submucosal adipose tissue of the tracheobronchial tree. These lesions are slightly more common in men than women and are typically seen in patients 60 years of age. Lipomas demonstrate fat attenuation on MDCT and signal intensity on T1- and T2-weighted MRI. In most cases, the identification of fat is enough to suggest the diagnosis.

Hemangioma

Hemangiomas of the trachea are classified as benign neoplasms of mesenchymal origin and usually occur in children. Specifically, capillary hemangioma is the most common subglottic mass in children. On MDCT, hemangiomas manifest as well-marginated, soft tissue masses located in the posterior or posterolateral aspect of the subglottic trachea. Involvement of the distal airways is much less common.

Glomus Tumor

Glomus tumor is an uncommon soft tissue neoplasm that usually occurs in the extremities, but may also affect the airways. It represents a neoplastic proliferation of smooth muscle arising from the glomus body. Although glomus tumors may mimic carcinoid tumors histologically, immunohistochemical stains readily differentiate between these entities. Glomus tumors are more common in men than women by a ratio of 2:1 to 7:1. These lesions are classified based on biologic activity, and most are benign. The World Health Organization has divided them into benign glomus tumors, malignant glomus tumors, and glomus tumors of uncertain malignant potential. On MDCT, the most common imaging feature is a polypoid nodule or mass in the trachea that arises from the airway wall, usually the posterior wall of the lower two-thirds of the trachea (Fig. 17.20). Tumor may demonstrate marked enhancement on contrast-enhanced CT and mimic vascular tumors such as carcinoid and hypervascular metastases.

Myofibroblastic Tumor

Myofibroblastic tumor is an uncommon primary tumor that usually affects the lungs but has been described in the airways. It is known by a number of other names such as inflammatory pseudotumor and plasma cell granuloma and typically affects children and young adults. Histologically, these tumors are composed of myofibroblastic spindle cells, an inflammatory infiltrate of plasma cells, lymphocytes, and eosinophils. It has low to intermediate malignant potential, and the prognosis is excellent in the setting of complete tumor resection.

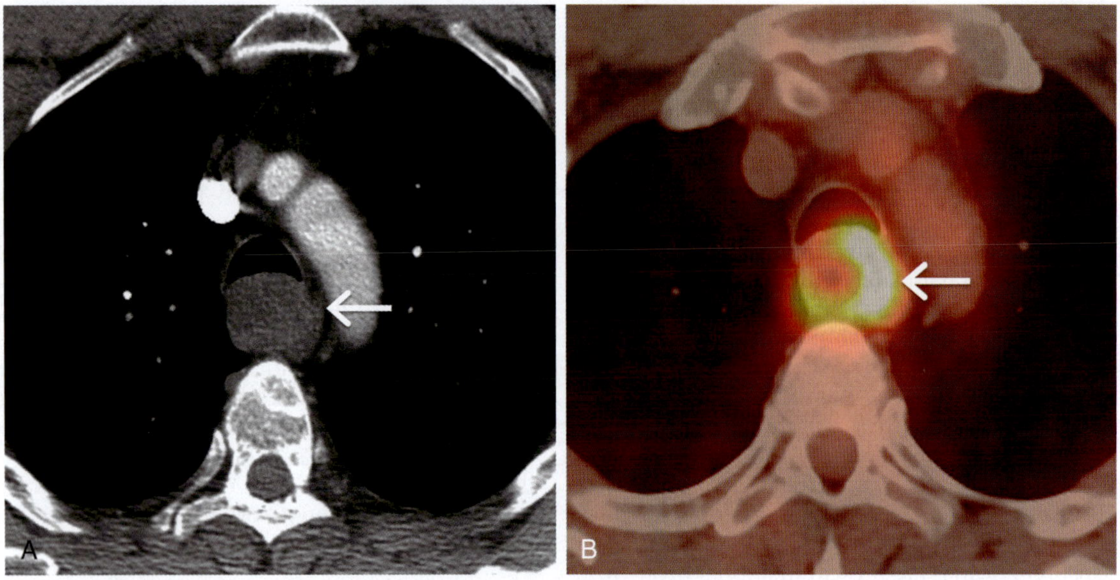

Figure 17.20 Glomus tumor of the trachea. (A) Collimated contrast-enhanced axial CT scan demonstrates a large soft tissue mass *(arrow)* arising from the trachea. (B) Collimated axial fused PET/CT of the same patient shows increased FDG uptake in the peripheral aspect of the lesion *(arrow)*. Biopsy revealed primary glomus tumor.

On MDCT, these lesions manifest as well-circumscribed polypoid endotracheal or endobronchial soft tissue nodules or masses.

Conclusion

Worldwide, lung cancer remains the leading cause of cancer-related mortality. Therefore it is imperative that the radiologist understand specific concepts regarding lung cancer, from imaging manifestations based on tumor subtype to overall staging, to guide appropriate management. Although neoplasms of the airways are, in contrast, relatively uncommon, the radiologist plays an essential role in identifying and characterizing these lesions to facilitate further imaging and treatment.

Bibliography

American Cancer Society (ACS). *Cancer Facts and Figures*. Atlanta: ACS; 2017.

Austin JH, Garg K, Aberle D, et al. Radiologic implications of the 2011 classification of adenocarcinoma of the lung. *Radiology*. 2013;266(1):62–71.

Backhus L, Puneet B, Bastawrous S, et al. Radiographic evaluation of the patient with lung cancer: surgical implications of imaging. *Curr Probl Diagn Radiol*. 2013;42(3):84–98.

Benson RE, Rosado-de-Christenson ML, Martínez-Jiménez S, et al. Spectrum of pulmonary neuroendocrine proliferations and neoplasms. *Radiographics*. 2013;33(6):1631–1649.

Carter BW, Glisson BS, Truong MT, et al. Small cell lung carcinoma: staging, imaging, and treatment considerations. *Radiographics*. 2014;34(6):1707–1721.

Carter BW, Wu CC, Khorashadi L, et al. Multimodality imaging of cardiothoracic lymphoma. *Eur J Radiol*. 2014;83(8):1470–1482.

Chan BA, Hughes BG. Targeted therapy for non-small cell lung cancer: current standards and the promise of the future. *Transl Lung Cancer Res*. 2015;4:36–54.

Dean CW, Speckman JM, Russo JJ. AIRP best cases in radiologic-pathologic correlation: adenoid cystic carcinoma of the trachea. *Radiographics*. 2011;31(5):1443–1447.

Eberhardt WEE, Mitchell A, Crowley J, et al. The IASLC lung cancer staging project: proposals for the revision of the M descriptors in the forthcoming eighth edition of the TNM classification of lung cancer. *J Thorac Oncol*. 2015;10(11):1515–1522.

Ferretti GR, Bithigoffer C, Righini CA, et al. Imaging of tumors of the trachea and central bronchi. *Thorac Surg Clin*. 2010;20(1):31–45.

Gainor JF, Varghese AM, Ou SH, et al. ALK rearrangements are mutually exclusive with mutations in EGFR or KRAS: an analysis of 1,683 patients with non-small cell lung cancer. *Clin Cancer Res*. 2013;19:4273–4281.

Goldstraw P, Chansky K, Crowley J, et al. The IASLC lung cancer staging project: proposals for revision of the TNM stage groupings in the forthcoming (eighth) edition of the TNM classification for lung cancer. *J Thorac Oncol*. 2016;11(1):39–51.

Javidan-Nejad C. MDCT of trachea and main bronchi. *Radiol Clin North Am*. 2010;48:157–176.

Kang EY. Large airway diseases. *J Thorac Imaging*. 2011;26(4):249–262.

Kim SA, Um SW, Song JU, et al. Bronchoscopic features and bronchoscopic intervention for endobronchial hamartoma. *Respirology*. 2010;15(1):150–154.

Kligerman S. The clinical staging of lung cancer through imaging: a radiologist's guide to the revised staging system and rationale for the changes. *Radiol Clin North Am*. 2014;52(1):69–83.

Lee KS, Boiselle PM. Update on multidetector computed tomography imaging of the airways. *J Thorac Imaging*. 2010;25:112–124.

Miller WT. Value of clinical history. *AJR Am J Roentgenol*. 1990;155(3):653–654.

Nair A, Klusmann MJ, Jogeesvaran KH, et al. Revisions to the TNM staging of non-small cell lung cancer: rationale, clinicoradiologic implications, and persistent limitations. *Radiographics*. 2011;31(1):215–238.

Park CM, Goo JM, Lee HJ, et al. Tumors in the tracheobronchial tree: CT and FDG PET features. *Radiographics*. 2009;29:55–71.

Pirker R, Filipits M. Targeted therapies in lung cancer. *Curr Pharm Des*. 2009;15:188–206.

Rami-Porta R, Bolejack V, Crowley J, et al. The IASLC lung cancer staging project: proposals for the revisions of the T descriptors in the forthcoming eighth edition of the TNM classification for lung cancer. *J Thorac Oncol*. 2015;10:990–1003.

Rami-Porta R, Bolejack V, Giroux DJ, et al. The IASLC lung cancer staging project: the new database to inform the eighth edition of the TNM classification of lung cancer. *J Thorac Oncol*. 2014;9(11):1618–1624.

Savas P, Hughes B, Solomon B. Targeted therapy in lung cancer: IPASS and beyond, keeping abreast of the explosion of targeted therapies for lung cancer. *J Thorac Dis*. 2013;5:S579–S592.

Suda K, Tomizawa K, Mitsudomi T. Biological and clinical significance of KRAS mutations in lung cancer: an oncogenic driver that contrasts with EGFR mutation. *Cancer Metastasis Rev*. 2010;29:49–60.

Travis WD, Brambilla E, Noguchi M, et al. International Association for the Study of Lung Cancer/American Thoracic Society/European Respiratory Society international multidisciplinary classification of lung adenocarcinoma. *J Thorac Oncol*. 2011;6(2):244–285.

Wu CC, Shepard JA. Tracheal and airway neoplasms. *Semin Roentgenol*. 2013;48(4):354–364.

Questions

1. What is the most common histologic subtype of lung cancer?
   A. Small cell
   B. Squamous cell
   C. Adenocarcinoma
   D. Large cell
   Answer: C
2. What is the appearance of AAH on MDCT?
   A. Solid pulmonary nodule
   B. Nonsolid (ground-glass) pulmonary nodule
   C. Part solid pulmonary nodule
   D. Consolidation
   Answer: B
3. In the eighth edition of the TNM staging system (TNM-8), what is the tumor descriptor for complete lung atelectasis?
   A. T1
   B. T2
   C. T3
   D. T4
   Answer: B
4. What is the most common primary malignancy of the trachea?
   A. SCC
   B. Adenoid cystic carcinoma
   C. Carcinoid
   D. Lymphoma
   Answer: A

CHAPTER 18
Smoking-Related Lung Diseases

Lindsay E. Wright, Paul von Herrmann, and Stephen B. Hobbs

CHAPTER OUTLINE

Introduction

The deleterious effects of smoking tobacco have been established for decades and largely began with the 1964 Surgeon General's Report, which linked smoking to the development of bronchogenic carcinoma. Since then, smoking tobacco has been causally linked to diseases of nearly every organ system in the body. Specific pulmonary diseases linked to smoking include bronchogenic carcinoma, chronic bronchitis, and chronic obstructive pulmonary disease, as well as a variety of other interstitial lung diseases.

Determining Who Needs Imaging

Usually, patients with a history of smoking present with acute or chronic dyspnea related to their smoking-induced cardiopulmonary disease. Clinical signs and symptoms, along with the physical examination, can often help ascertain whether the cause is cardiac or pulmonary; however, this distinction is not always apparent. In these cases, the use of imaging can help establish the cause, as well as any related complications.

Appropriate Modalities in These Disease Processes

Imaging is frequently used in patients with confirmed or suspected smoking-related lung diseases, first to establish or confirm the diagnosis and second to evaluate the extent of disease. The most common first-line imaging examination in the evaluation of acute or chronic dyspnea is chest radiography, largely due to its low cost, low radiation exposure, and wide availability. There are a number of smoking-related diseases that can be identified on a chest radiograph; however, a negative radiograph does not exclude diffuse disease. Depending on the interpretation of the radiograph and the symptoms of the patient, proceeding to CT of the chest without IV contrast, using both thin section acquisition and a high-resolution filter, is frequently appropriate (commonly referred to as *high-resolution CT* [HRCT]). As part of the HRCT examination, expiratory CT imaging is useful for the evaluation of the small airway component of obstruction. CT of the chest with IV contrast is often not indicated unless there is suspected mediastinal or hilar adenopathy or if there is suspicion of a pulmonary embolism as a compounding factor in the patient's dyspnea.

Chronic Obstructive Pulmonary Disease

Chronic obstructive pulmonary disease (COPD) is defined by the Global Initiative for Chronic Lung Disease as "a disease state characterized by airflow limitation that is not fully reversible" and is validated by decreased airflow at forced expiration. This is secondary to a combination of airway disease, referred to as *obstructive bronchitis*, and lung tissue parenchymal destruction, known as *emphysema*.

The major site of resistance in COPD is the small airways (airways <2 mm in internal diameter), although the entire airway is typically involved. Small airways vary from large airways in that they lack cartilage and contain a greater percentage of smooth muscle. Small airways are generations 8 to 14 of airway branching. The airflow reduction in the small airways is thought to be secondary to narrowing of the small airways from inflammation, fibrosis, and mucus plugging. The most significant contributor to airflow obstruction is mucous metaplasia.

Small airway inflammation following exposure to cigarette smoke precedes tissue destruction, fibrosis, and clinically detectable airflow obstruction. On the cellular level, this is thought to be secondary to migration of the $CD8^+$ T lymphocytes inducing apoptosis and necrosis of epithelial and endothelial cells, which ultimately leads to the parenchymal destruction seen in COPD.

Currently, the diagnosis and assessment of severity of COPD predominantly involve pulmonary function tests (PFTs). PFTs are sometimes limited in their assessment because they are difficult to interpret in the presence of concomitant lung pathology. Additionally, they primarily provide an assessment of global lung function and are limited in determining any information regarding regional heterogeneity or quantification of emphysema versus small airway disease. Imaging with HRCT can provide additional diagnostic information and is substantially more sensitive than spirometry for detecting emphysema.

Classification of COPD falls into three primary categories—emphysema-predominant COPD, airway-predominant COPD (bronchitis and bronchiolitis), and mixed. The CT-based classification is based on the morphologic appearance of pathologic changes relating to airflow limitation—that is, the presence or absence of emphysema, bronchial wall thickening, and evidence of bronchiolitis. This categorization is somewhat limited given that the relative contributions of emphysema and airway disease vary among patients, as well as their correlation with symptomatology. The CT appearance can vary dramatically among patients with a similar degree of airflow limitation.

■ Emphysema

Different Types of Emphysema

Emphysema is defined histologically as the abnormal permanent enlargement of the air spaces distal to the respiratory bronchioles, with destruction of the septal walls. On CT, this presents with regions of low density (i.e., decreased CT attenuation) surrounded by normal lung parenchyma. Depending on the distribution of these low-density changes relative to the secondary pulmonary lobule, the pattern of emphysema can be characterized as centrilobular, panlobular (panacinar), or distal acinar (paraseptal). A fourth type of emphysema is sometimes described but refers to emphysema associated with scarring, without a distinct relationship to the secondary pulmonary lobule (cicatricial).

Centrilobular emphysema is manifested by central destruction of the secondary pulmonary lobular parenchyma, which surrounds the pulmonary artery. Centrilobular emphysema is the most common type of smoking-related emphysema and, like many inhalational injuries, is upper lung predominant.

Uniform destruction of the secondary pulmonary lobule is seen in panlobular emphysema. Panlobular emphysema appears as a generalized decrease in CT attenuation; however, it is predominantly in the lower lobes. Pulmonary vessels in the affected areas are typically reduced in caliber. Panlobular emphysema is most characteristically seen with alpha-1-antitrypsin deficiency, although it can also been seen in severe, end-stage, smoking-related emphysema and other rare causes, such as IV methylphenidate (Ritalin) abuse or hypocomplementemic urticarial vasculitis syndrome.

Distal acinar (paraseptal) emphysema is a subtype of panlobular emphysema, which is localized to the parenchyma adjacent to the visceral pleural surface. It is usually in the upper lobes and is frequently seen in association with centrilobular emphysema in smokers.

The association between emphysema and airflow limitation is explained by a decrease in elastic recoil of the airway. Normal airways have a certain degree of elastic recoil that maintains airway patency, which is lost in patients with COPD because of the destruction of the lung parenchyma. Combined with the loss of elastic recoil of the airways, the hyperinflation characteristic of emphysema compresses and further obstructs the small airways.

Distinguishing the Types of Emphysema on Imaging

Evaluation of COPD by a standard posteroanterior and lateral chest radiographs is easily obtained, inexpensive, and involves minimal radiation. Typical findings for detection of emphysema on chest radiographs include the following (Fig. 18.1):

1. Increased radiolucency of lung fields
2. Flattening of the diaphragms
3. Pruning of the peripheral vasculature
4. Increased retrosternal airspace
5. Widening of the intercostal spaces
6. Narrowed and more vertical cardiac silhouette

Historically, the application of these criteria has had mixed results in correlation with the histopathologic diagnosis of emphysema. However, a recent study has demonstrated that both experienced and inexperienced readers are able to identify moderate and severe emphysema with over 90% sensitivity, so chest radiographs do retain some clinical utility in the diagnosis and quantification of emphysema. Nevertheless, it is generally agreed that the accuracy of chest radiographs for detecting early emphysema is limited.

Additionally, distinguishing the types of emphysema on chest radiographs is limited. Radiographs can highlight the craniocaudal distribution of emphysema, with centrilobular emphysema related to smoking typically being upper lung predominant and panlobular emphysema being lower lung predominant (Fig. 18.2; also see

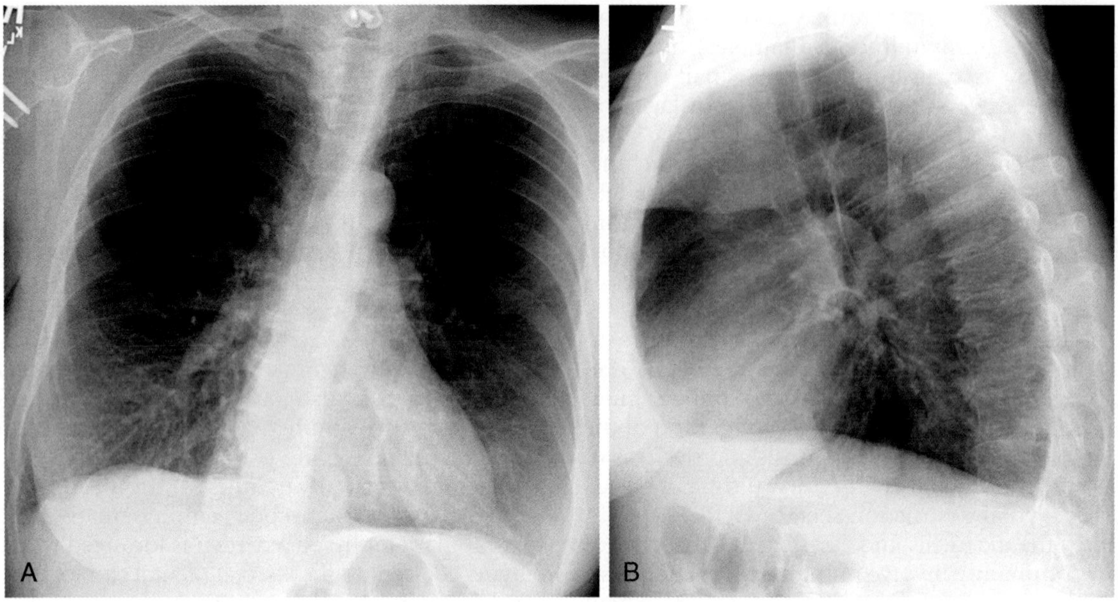

Figure 18.1 Centrilobular emphysema on chest radiographs. (A) On the frontal radiograph, the findings of centrilobular emphysema can be subtle. There is moderate upper lung hyperlucency and decreased upper lung vascular markings. (B) On the lateral radiograph, there is mild diaphragmatic flattening and increased retrosternal clear space.

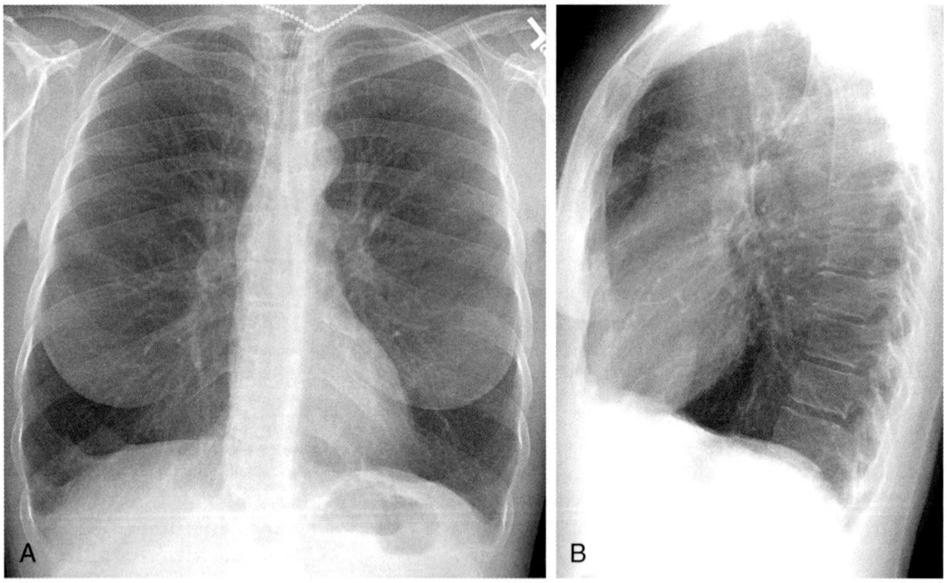

Figure 18.2 Panlobular emphysema on chest radiographs. (A) On the frontal radiograph, findings include lower lung hyperlucency and decreased vascular markings. (B) On the lateral radiograph, the diaphragms are markedly flattened, and lower lung hyperlucency is pronounced.

Fig. 18.1). The detection of paraseptal emphysema is generally limited to identifying larger peripheral blebs and bullae.

In contrast to radiographs, the evaluation of emphysema by CT is standard (Fig. 18.3). The detection and quantification of emphysema on CT can be performed through both visual pattern analysis and, more objectively, by lung density measurements. Visual detection and quantification involve a global and regional qualitative assessment and a subjective grading of severity. This type of visual assessment has been shown in multiple studies to correlate with histopathology, lung function, and response to therapeutic intervention.

Centrilobular emphysema is characterized on HRCT by multiple small, round to polygonal areas of low attenuation (Fig. 18.4). These are frequently situated near the center of the secondary pulmonary lobule, with the centrilobular artery at the center. Most of these areas should have no discernible wall, although thin walls can sometimes be seen related to fibrosis or adjacent septal interstitium. As the disease progresses, the emphysema will become more confluent, with bullae formation and involvement of the entire secondary pulmonary lobule (Fig. 18.5). Despite the mimic appearance of this advanced centrilobular emphysema with panlobular emphysema, mentioning panlobular emphysema in a radiology

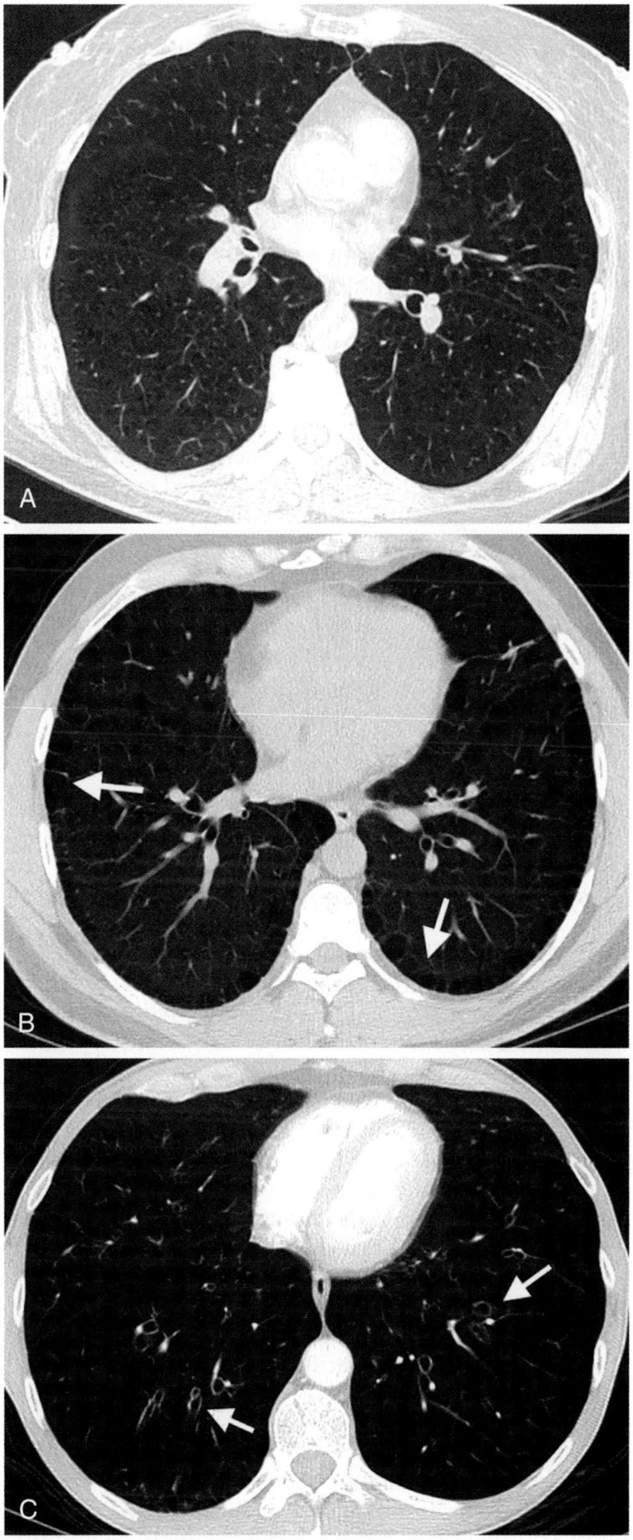

Figure 18.3 Types of emphysema on axial CT scans. (A) Centrilobular emphysema. Numerous areas of low attenuation in the center of the secondary pulmonary lobule, with surrounding normal parenchyma, result in an appearance of low-attenuation holes in the lung. (B) Paraseptal emphysema, characteristic subpleural location *(arrows)*. (C) Panlobular emphysema. Confluent low attenuation of the entire secondary pulmonary lobule results in diffuse low attenuation. There is also a degree of lower lung bronchiectasis, typical of alpha-1-antitrypsin deficiency *(arrows)*.

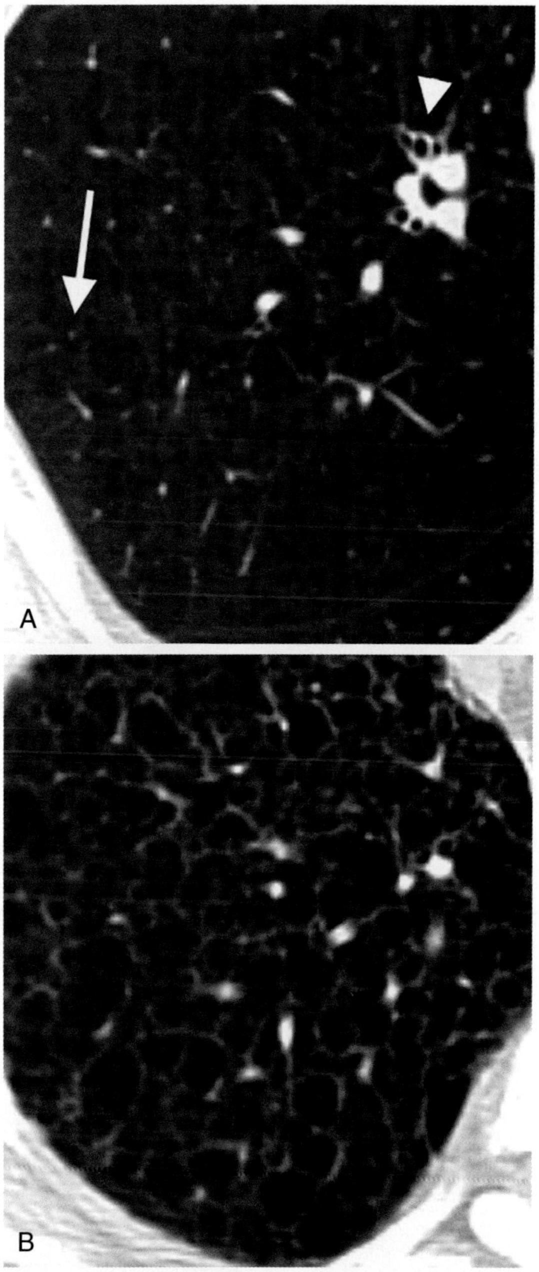

Figure 18.4 Centrilobular emphysema on axial CT scan versus pulmonary cysts. (A) Coned image of centrilobular emphysema. A low-attenuation area is greatest in the center of the pulmonary lobule, with the corresponding centrilobular artery identified *(arrow)*. Also note the bronchial wall thickening *(arrowhead)* frequently seen in smokers (but nonspecific and found in other causes of inflammatory airway disease). (B) Coned image of pulmonary cystic disease. Rounded areas of low attenuation all have well-defined walls and no discrete relation to the secondary pulmonary lobule.

report should not occur unless one specifically wants a referring clinician to consider alpha-1-antitrypsin deficiency; this is because some equate the two entities with each other.

Panlobular emphysema results from a much more uniform destruction of the secondary pulmonary lobule, resulting in a more diffuse low attenuation of the lung parenchyma and hyperinflation (see Fig. 18.3). Early cases may be missed entirely without close evaluation and a high degree of suspicion. Note that bronchiectasis is

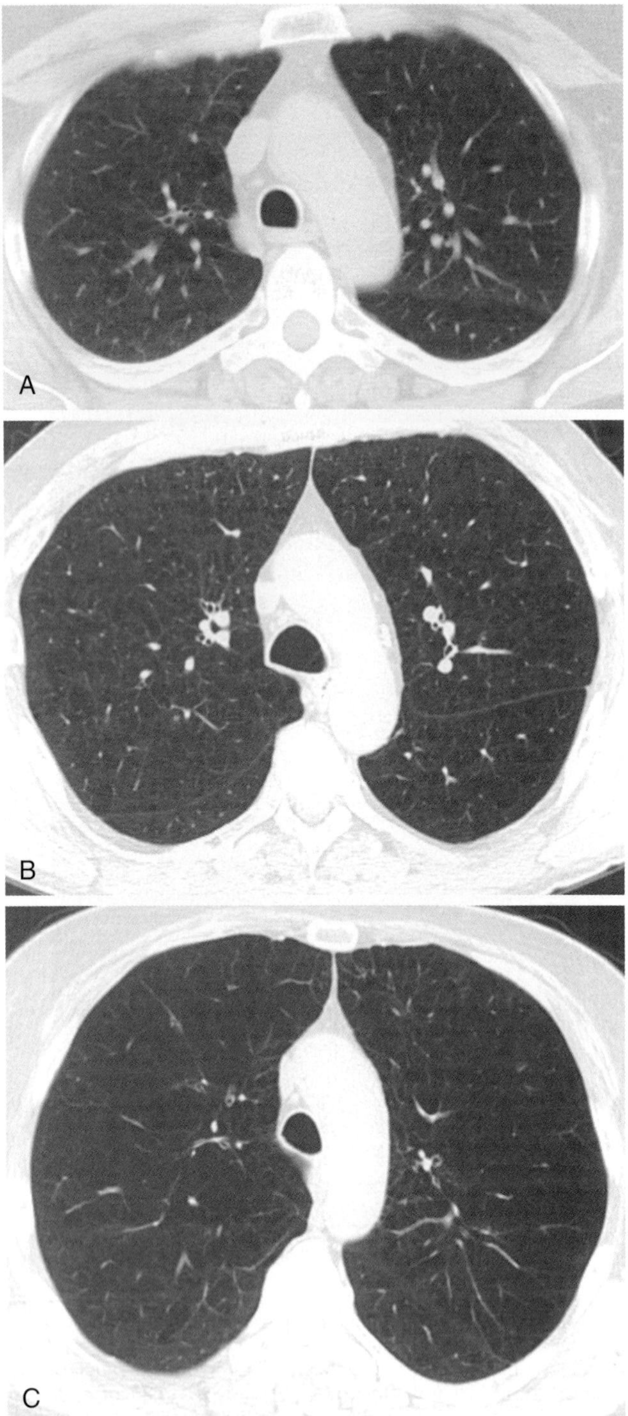

Figure 18.5 Qualitative severity of centrilobular emphysema on axial CT. Mild (A), moderate (B), and severe (C) centrilobular emphysema related to smoking. Note the increasing degree of confluence, with the severe emphysema being indistinguishable from panlobular emphysema (see Fig. 18.3C) except by clinical history and craniocaudal distribution.

common in cases of alpha-1-antitrypsin deficiency, likely related to repeat infections, at least in part.

Paraseptal emphysema on CT often has visible walls corresponding with interlobular septa due to the subpleural location (see Fig. 18.3). Bullae are areas of paraseptal emphysema larger than 1 cm in diameter, which can be seen in isolation or in association with other causes of emphysema.

More recent studies have attempted to quantify emphysema using CT densimetry parameters, such as relative low-attenuation area and the percentile of the frequency attenuation distribution. Low-attenuation regions of −950 Hounsfield units or less on thin section CT correlate well with PFTs. The anatomic distribution of low-attenuation regions should also be considered when performing quantitative analysis of these regions on CT because they may help clarify the pathophysiology.

Of note, the distribution of emphysema with regard to the lobes is important to recognize and comment on because of surgical options for treatment. Lung volume reduction surgery (LVRS) is a treatment option for patients with end-stage emphysema and preserved exercise tolerance. In these patients, CT is a critical preoperative step in determining surgical candidacy—specifically, diagnosing the emphysema as nonhomogeneous (upper lung predominant) is paramount (Fig. 18.6). In effect, this means that the emphysema needs to be most severe in the area of lung to be resected (the upper lobes). If the lungs are affected more diffusely, then surgical resection is of no benefit.

Smoking-Related Diffuse Lung Disease

Pulmonary Langerhans Cell Histiocytosis

Langerhans cell histiocytosis (LCH) is a disorder of abnormal proliferation and infiltration of Langerhans cells into various organs. Pulmonary involvement has been historically known as histiocytosis X and associated with systemic disorders of histiocytes, such as eosinophilic granuloma, Letterer-Siwe disease, and Hand-Schüller-Christian disease. Pulmonary involvement in these LCH disorders is not common but, when it occurs, it tends to present in children, is not associated with a smoking history, and follows a more aggressive clinical course, with a worse prognosis. Today, pulmonary LCH (PLCH) is recognized as a variant of LCH that almost solely affects adult smokers.

PLCH is thought to be an uncontrolled immune reaction to a presenting antigen, commonly associated with smoking, although there have been reports of PLCH developing in response to other pulmonary irritants. Langerhans cells are almost exclusively located within the subendothelium of the tracheobronchial tree. The cells are a primary immune defense against inhaled antigens. Once activated by an antigen, they stimulate an immune response and increase lymphocyte production.

Imaging Findings

Characteristic features of PLCH on chest imaging are a combination of nodules that cavitate and evolve to cysts over time (Fig. 18.7). There is a predominant distribution in the mid and upper lung zones, with sparing of the lung bases and general preservation of lung volumes. Nodules and some cystic lesions may be occasionally

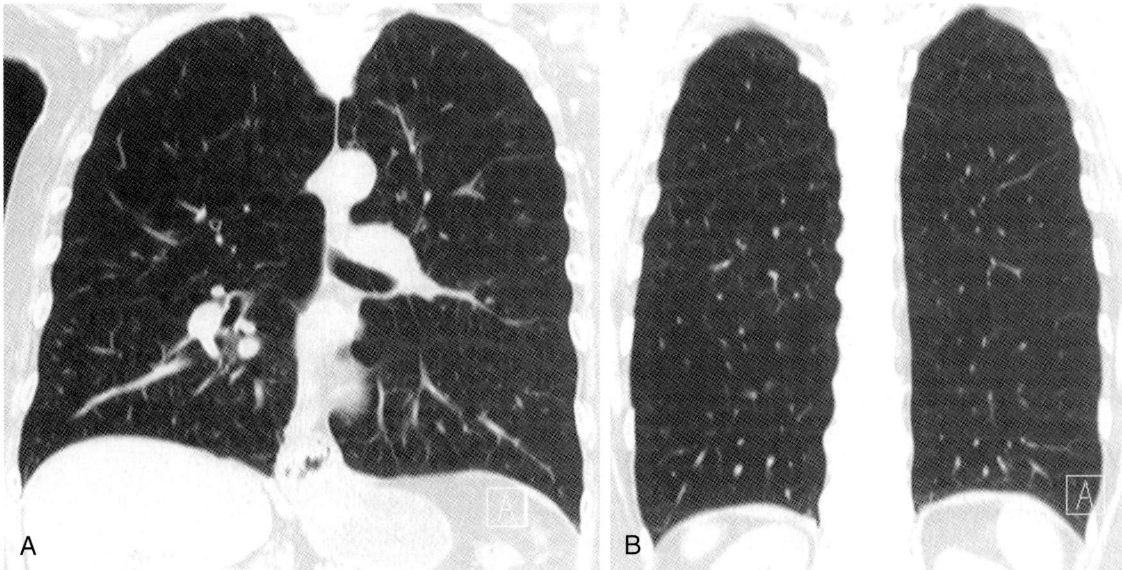

Figure 18.6 CT for evaluation of lung volume reduction surgery (LVRS). (A) A coronal CT image of the chest demonstrates upper lung predominant emphysema, making this patient an ideal candidate for LVRS. (B) A coronal CT scan of the chest demonstrates a much more diffuse centrilobular emphysema related to smoking. This patient is not ideal for LVRS.

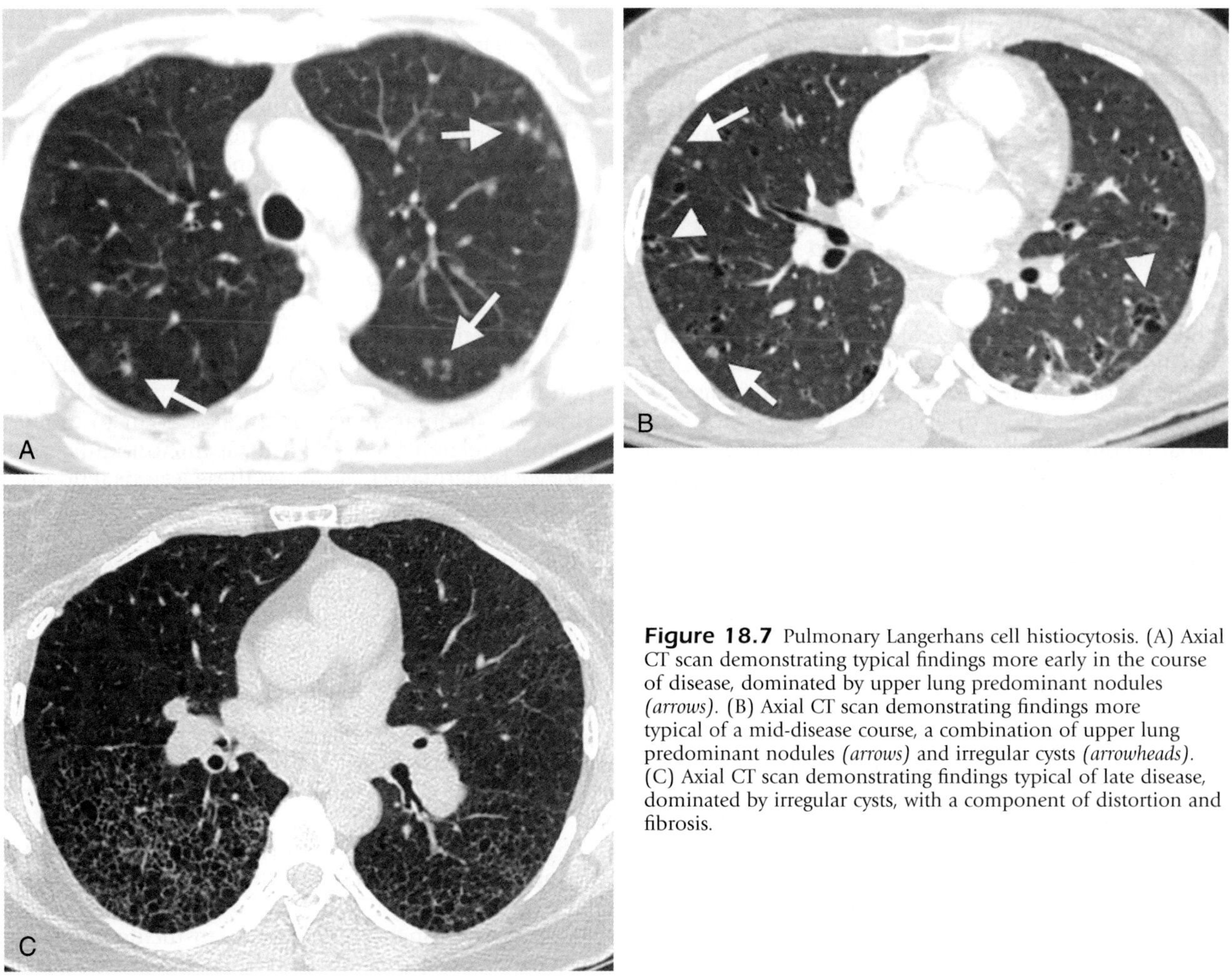

Figure 18.7 Pulmonary Langerhans cell histiocytosis. (A) Axial CT scan demonstrating typical findings more early in the course of disease, dominated by upper lung predominant nodules *(arrows)*. (B) Axial CT scan demonstrating findings more typical of a mid-disease course, a combination of upper lung predominant nodules *(arrows)* and irregular cysts *(arrowheads)*. (C) Axial CT scan demonstrating findings typical of late disease, dominated by irregular cysts, with a component of distortion and fibrosis.

identified on chest radiographs but are best appreciated on HRCT.

In the acute or early phase of the disease, small nodules predominate (see Fig. 18.7A). Histologically, the nodules are composed of immune cells and fibroblasts that form a granuloma. Because these granulomas form in the subendothelium of the bronchi, the nodules will appear centrilobular, peribronchial, or bronchiolar in location on HRCT. These nodules tend to have irregular, poorly defined borders, although occasionally they may appear well defined and smooth. The nodules are generally small (<5 mm), but may be up to 1 cm.

With disease progression, the inflammation from the continued immune response results in destruction of the bronchiolar walls and the normal adjacent lung parenchyma, causing bronchiolar dilation. This results in cavitation of the nodules and the appearance of irregularly shaped cysts on HRCT and as a reticulonodular pattern on a chest radiograph (see Fig. 18.7B). At this point in the disease, it is common to see a combination of cysts and nodules, which is considered diagnostic for PLCH. Over time, the cystic appearance dominates, with regression of nodular lesions. The cysts may even appear confluent and bullous-like.

End-stage disease is characterized by bizarre and irregularly shaped cysts, with a mild degree of fibrotic architectural distortion, which may cause further dilation of the bronchial tree (see Fig. 18.7C). The combination of fibrosis and cystic changes often counteracts each other, resulting in little change in the lung volumes, which are normal or slightly increased. With advanced disease, patients may develop pulmonary artery hypertension, leading to enlarged pulmonary arteries on imaging.

Distinguishing Pulmonary Langerhans Cell Histiocytosis From Other Cystic and Nodular Diseases

The appearance of both cysts and centrilobular nodules in the upper and mid lung zones is considered nearly pathognomonic. When imaging findings are limited only to nodules or only to cysts, the differential diagnosis may include other lung diseases (see below). However, the sparing of the posterior costophrenic angles is highly characteristic of PLCH and can be useful as a distinguishing feature (Fig. 18.8).

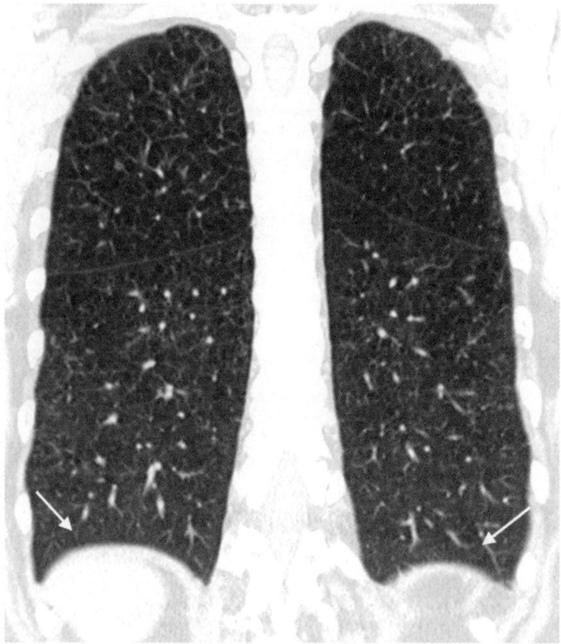

Figure 18.8 Pulmonary Langerhans cell histiocytosis. This coronal CT scan demonstrates typical sparing of the costophrenic angles *(arrows)*, even late in the disease course of this patient.

NODULAR-ONLY LUNG DISEASE

PLCH has a characteristic distribution in the mid and upper lungs, with sparing of the lung bases, that helps distinguish it from other nodular lung diseases. Pulmonary nodules caused by hematogenous spread (metastasis and disseminated infection) have a diffuse distribution through the lungs. Other nodular diseases that may initially present predominantly in the mid and upper lungs include sarcoidosis, lymphangitic carcinomatosis, and some pneumoconioses, such as coal workers' pneumoconiosis or silicosis. However, these diseases tend to have a perilymphatic distribution that characteristically involves the fissures and pleura instead of the centrilobular-predominant distribution seen in PLCH. Additional characteristics such as associated lymphadenopathy, septal thickening, and florid pulmonary fibrosis are often present with these other diseases, unlike PLCH.

CYSTIC LUNG DISEASE

The lung volumes in PLCH are generally preserved to slightly increased. In comparison, honeycomb cystic changes of usual interstitial pulmonary fibrosis are subpleural and basilar in location and are surrounded by fibrotic changes, with associated volume loss. Lymphangioleiomyomatosis (LAM) is a cystic lung disease that is uniformly distributed throughout both lungs, with involvement of the costophrenic angles, as opposed to PLCH, which spares these areas. LAM cysts are generally uniform in size and shape; PLCH cysts may be bizarrely shaped and of different sizes. Furthermore, solid, upper lung preponderant, centrilobular nodules would be unusual in LAM but common in PLCH. However, nodular opacities can also occur in tuberous sclerosis–related LAM (multifocal micronodular pneumocyte hyperplasia), although these lesions tend not to have basilar sparing or centrilobular prominence, as in PLCH. Lymphocytic interstitial pneumonia (LIP) often manifests as cysts and, occasionally, nodules secondary to lymphocytic infiltration of the parenchyma. However, the nodules are ill-defined and lower lung predominant. Additionally, the cysts tend to be lower lung predominant and perivascular in location. Adult patients with LIP almost always have an underlying diagnosis of Sjögren syndrome, although immunodeficiency and Castleman disease are other secondary causes of LIP.

Respiratory Bronchiolitis and Respiratory Bronchiolitis–Interstitial Lung Disease

Respiratory bronchiolitis (RB) is an incidental asymptomatic disease that presents in patients who smoke.

Patients with RB have normal pulmonary function. RB is caused by pigmented laden macrophages accumulating in the first- and second-degree bronchioles and alveoli, with a mild degree of chronic inflammation in the bronchiolar walls. In some patients, usually males 30 to 40 years of age with a heavy smoking history (30 or more pack-years), RB progresses so that there are respiratory signs or symptoms of chronic lung disease—respiratory bronchiolitis–interstitial lung disease (RB-ILD).

Patients with RB-ILD develop symptoms such as dyspnea and cough, with abnormal pulmonary function. Like RB, RB-ILD histologically has pigmented macrophages in the secondary pulmonary lobules and peribronchiolar inflammation. The difference is the greater severity of disease seen in RB-ILD compared to RB. Because of this, RB and RB-ILD are considered to be different points in the spectrum of the same disease process.

Smoking cessation and, sometimes, steroid therapy are the main treatments for RB-ILD. The prognosis is generally good, and imaging findings often stabilize or improve.

Imaging Findings

Chest radiographs are not sensitive for RB or RB-ILD and often appear normal. Occasionally, nonspecific reticulonodular opacities can be seen. On HRCT, the predominant findings in RB and RB-ILD are ground-glass centrilobular nodules and focal patches of centrilobular ground-glass opacities, caused by the accumulation of macrophages in the bronchioles and alveoli (Fig. 18.9). These findings are more extensive in RB-ILD than in RB, with greater amounts of centrilobular nodules and more diffuse ground-glass opacities. Pulmonary findings in RB and RB-ILD have a mid and upper lung zone predominance. There is often concurrent centrilobular emphysema. Imaging alone cannot definitively distinguish between RB and RB-ILD; histologic findings and clinical symptomatology are important in making the diagnosis of RB-ILD.

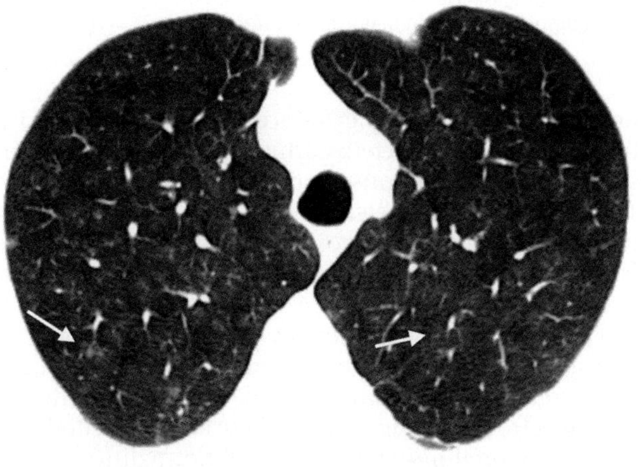

Figure 18.9 Respiratory bronchiolitis (RB) and respiratory bronchiolitis–interstitial lung disease (RB-ILD). This axial CT scan demonstrates typical centrilobular ground-glass nodules found in RB and RB-ILD *(arrows)*. As the disease progresses, these can become more confluent, but the distinction between RB and RB-ILD is a clinical one based on symptomatology, not on radiographic findings. The differential would include hypersensitivity pneumonitis based on radiology alone.

Distinguishing Respiratory Bronchiolitis–Interstitial Lung Disease From Other Causes of Centrilobular Nodules

Centrilobular ground-glass nodules and patchy ground-glass opacities, with a clinical history of heavy smoking and pulmonary function abnormalities, are highly suggestive of RB-ILD. Subacute hypersensitivity pneumonitis is frequently the primary differential consideration in the nonacute setting. The presence of significant expiratory air trapping is more suggestive of hypersensitivity pneumonitis but can be seen in either disease. More importantly, smoking appears to be protective against hypersensitivity pneumonitis, making the clinical history critical for distinction between these two processes.

Desquamative Interstitial Pneumonia

Definition

Desquamative interstitial pneumonia (DIP) is an interstitial pneumonia that is strongly associated with smoking (60%–90% of cases). DIP tends to occur in men (2 : 1 male-to-female ratio) at about 40 years of age. Nonsmoking-related cases of DIP have been attributed to a variety of conditions, including infection, connective tissue disease, environmental exposures, and idiopathic causes.

In the clinical context of smoking, DIP is considered to be part of the spectrum of RB and RB-ILD. Analogous to RB-ILD, pigmented macrophages accumulate in the secondary pulmonary lobules of the lungs with DIP and induce local inflammation. However, in DIP, the macrophages tend to accumulate diffusely in the alveoli rather than the bronchiolocentric accumulation identified in RB-ILD. One study has found that there is a greater amount of interstitial fibrosis and eosinophilic infiltration in patients with DIP compared to cases of RB-ILD. There was no histologic or imaging difference between cases of smoking- and nonsmoking-related DIP. It has been suggested that the nonsmoking-related cases of DIP may further evolve into a nonspecific idiopathic pneumonia (NSIP)–like pattern of fibrosis.

Imaging Findings

In patients with DIP, chest radiographs may show nonspecific hazy and ill-defined opacities, especially in the lower lungs. On HRCT, ground-glass opacities are the predominant finding (Fig. 18.10). The imaging findings are caused by the diffuse pattern of macrophage infiltration into the alveoli. Unlike most other smoking or inhalational lung disease, the subpleural and lower lungs tend to be the most affected. HRCT may reveal changes of fibrosis, such as small thin-walled cysts and thickening of the alveolar septa, which can look like reticular or irregular linear opacities. Honeycombing is uncommon.

The imaging findings in DIP frequently overlap with those of RB-ILD, NSIP, hypersensitivity pneumonitis, and atypical infection. The clinical scenario and, when necessary, lung biopsy, allow for a more definitive diagnosis.

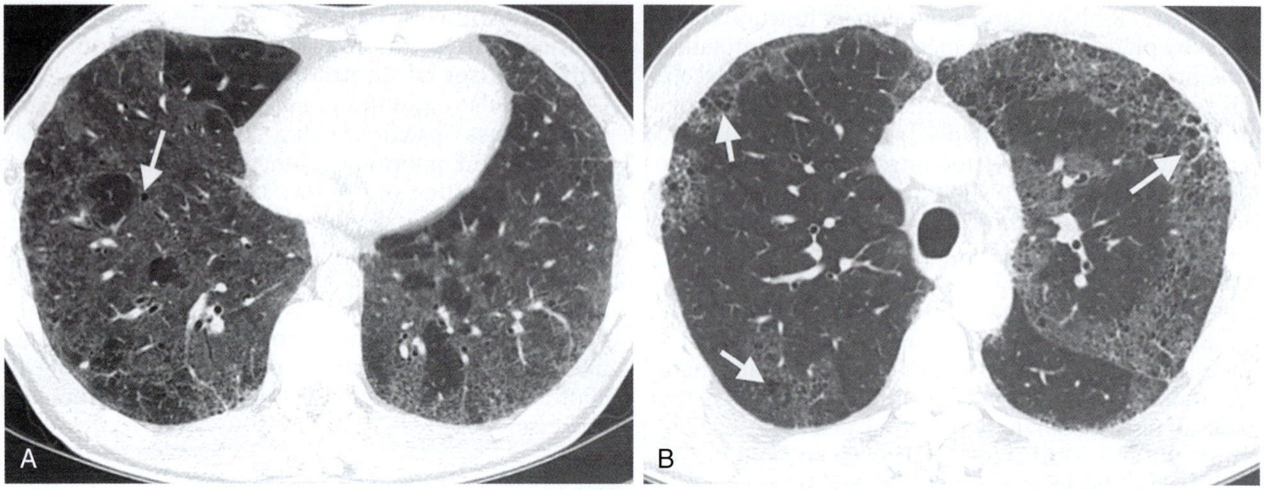

Figure 18.10 Desquamative interstitial pneumonia (DIP). (A, B) Axial CT scans demonstrating typical findings of DIP, with lower lung predominant ground-glass opacities and variable areas of architectural distortion and fibrosis. Note that small cysts in the areas of ground-glass opacities are frequently but not always seen *(arrows)*.

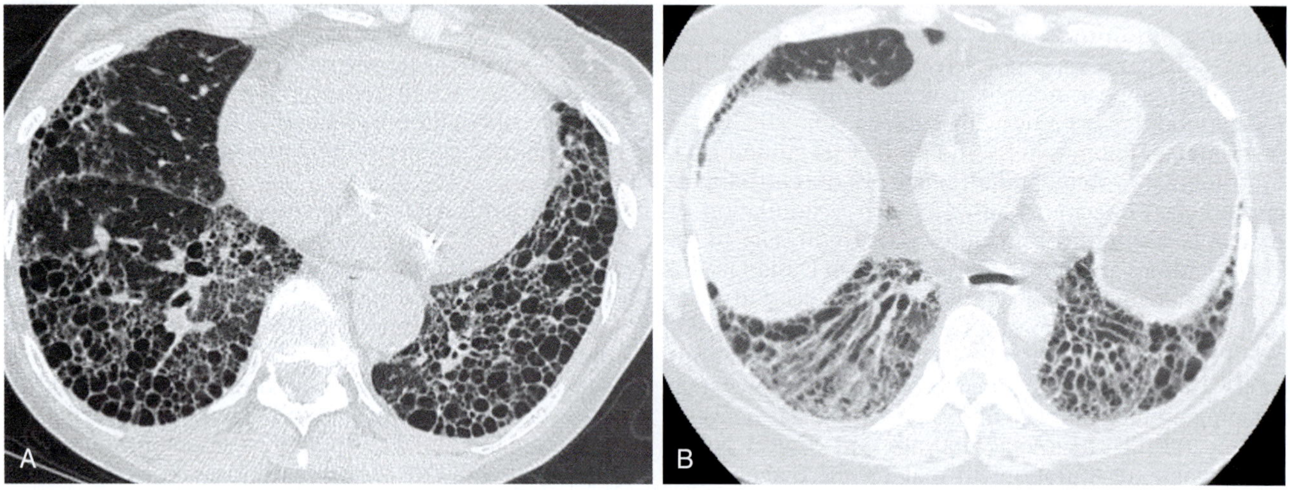

Figure 18.11 Fibrosing interstitial pneumonias. (A) Axial CT scans demonstrating the typical subpleural and lower lung predominant reticular abnormality, with honeycomb cyst formation seen in the usual interstitial pneumonia pattern. (B) Axial CT scans demonstrating the typical lower lung but more bronchovascular distribution of architectural distortion and traction bronchiectasis seen in nonspecific interstitial pneumonia.

Fibrosing Interstitial Pneumonias

The fibrosing interstitial pneumonias have had an increasingly recognized correlation with smoking. The manifestation can include the usual interstitial pneumonia (UIP) pattern or the NSIP pattern. There is a high prevalence of fibrosis in smokers, with some studies demonstrating an increased risk of developing fibrosis, with an odds ratio of 1.6. Smoking may have a negative effect on survival in patients with fibrosis relative to fibrosis in nonsmokers, so identification of a UIP or NSIP pattern in the setting of smoking is important.

Usual Interstitial Pneumonia

UIP is the morphologic pattern associated with the clinical syndrome of interstitial pulmonary fibrosis. Interstitial pulmonary fibrosis is usually seen in men older than 50 years and, although its direct link to smoking has been debated, there is clearly evidence of an association. UIP morphology is characterized histologically by different stages of fibrotic lesions, termed *temporal heterogeneity*. There is also spatial heterogeneity, with areas of normal lung interspersed with fibrosis and honeycombing. There is a lower lung predominance, termed an *apicobasilar gradient*.

Early in the disease course, chest radiographs can appear normal, with more advanced disease presenting as decreased lung volumes and subpleural reticular opacities from fibrosis. On CT, there are subpleural and lower lung predominant reticular abnormalities, with a predilection for honeycomb cyst formation (Fig. 18.11A).

Nonspecific Idiopathic Pneumonia

The NSIP pattern of idiopathic interstitial pneumonia is characterized by temporal and spatial homogeneity of fibrosis and inflammation, in contrast to the

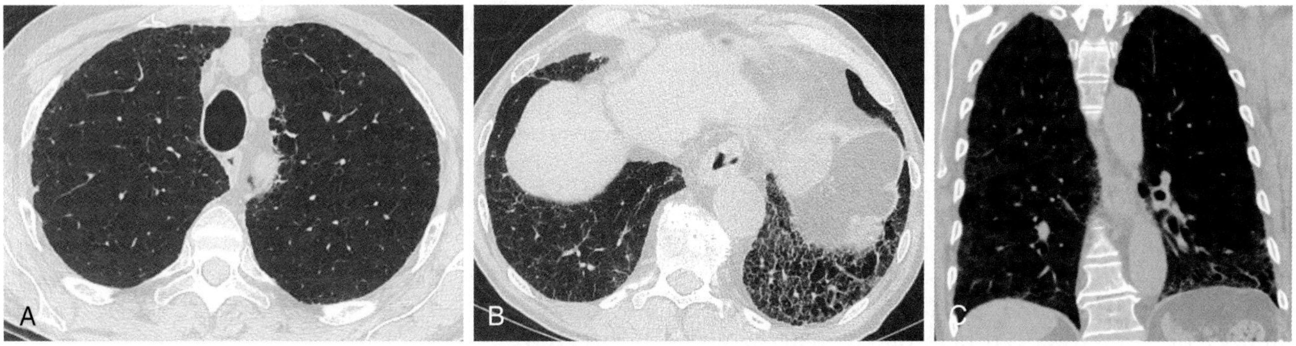

Figure 18.12 Combined pulmonary fibrosis and emphysema. Axial (A, B) and coronal (C) CT scans demonstrating the typical combination of upper lung predominant centrilobular emphysema, with lower lung fibrosis. The fibrosis can be in a pattern of nonspecific interstitial pneumonia or usual interstitial pneumonia and, as such, has varying degrees of traction bronchiectasis, reticular abnormality, ground-glass opacity, and honeycomb cyst formation. This case is dominated by reticular abnormality and traction bronchiectasis, greatest in the left lower lobe.

heterogeneous UIP pattern. The NSIP pattern is often associated with collagen vascular diseases, drug exposures, hypersensitivity pneumonitis, or sometimes smoking.

As with many of the interstitial diseases, early radiographs may appear normal. In later stages, there may be lower lung ground-glass opacities or consolidation with volume loss due to fibrosis. CT scans in NSIP tend to demonstrate patchy ground-glass opacities, with intralobular reticulations in a peribronchovascular distribution resulting in traction bronchiectasis (see Fig. 18.11B). Honeycombing is mild when present, in distinction to the large honeycomb cysts seen in UIP.

Combined Pulmonary Fibrosis and Emphysema

Pulmonary fibrosis with coexisting emphysema had been regarded as coincidental until relatively recently, when the syndrome of combined pulmonary fibrosis and emphysema (CPFE) was proposed. Patients with CPFE tend to be male smokers (>40 pack-year history) and in their sixth or seventh decade of life.

Clinical features include dyspnea, preservation of lung volumes, hypoxemia with exertion, and decreased carbon monoxide diffusion capacity. There is an increased mortality in these patients, often due to the association of precapillary pulmonary hypertension, which is estimated to be in as many as 50% of CPFE patients. The prognosis for CPFE is also worse than for emphysema or interstitial pulmonary fibrosis alone, with a 5-year survival rate of 55%. Additional studies are currently being performed to delineate this syndrome, its features, and possible treatment options better.

Radiographically, emphysema (paraseptal, centrilobular, or bullous) is identified in the upper lung zones, with basilar pulmonary fibrosis (Fig. 18.12). The pulmonary fibrosis seen in CPFE may include honeycombing, traction bronchiectasis, reticular opacities, or ground-glass opacities (UIP or NSIP patterns). Most are associated with UIP-type fibrosis, although there may be an association with other interstitial lung diseases, such as DIP and NSIP.

Acute Eosinophilic Pneumonia

Acute eosinophilic pneumonia (AEP) is a type of acute interstitial pneumonia characterized by the following: (1) onset of acute fever; (2) progressive hypoxemia; (3) bilateral diffuse pulmonary infiltrates; (4) increased eosinophils in bronchoalveolar lavage fluid (>25%); and (5) no known causes of other eosinophilic pneumonia, such as drugs or parasitic infections. In several studies, AEP has been associated with new or increased cigarette smoking. Other cases have been linked to environmental exposures, although in most cases a distinct cause has not been not identified. AEP is a type of acute lung injury, and histologic findings demonstrate diffuse and organizing alveolar damage.

Findings on chest radiography include bilateral air space and interstitial opacities that may progress to frank consolidation, reticular opacities (from septal thickening), and pleural effusions. On CT, there are patchy to confluent areas of ground-glass opacities, consolidation, thickening of both interlobular septa and bronchovascular bundles, and pleural effusions (Fig. 18.13). Findings can overlap those of pulmonary edema, acute respiratory distress syndrome (ARDS), other infections, and hemorrhage. Peripheral and upper lung predominance can be a clue in some cases of eosinophilic pneumonia. Bronchoalveolar lavage should be suggested to look for eosinophilia in the appropriate setting. AEP generally shows complete and frequently rapid resolution with steroid treatment.

■ Problem-Solving Issues

Distinguishing Emphysema From Cystic Lung Disease

Emphysema is a common finding in smokers and frequently coexists with other smoking-related diseases and lung injury. It can be difficult to separate cystic disease from emphysematous changes, especially in cases where both may be present, such as in PLCH. The key differentiation is that cysts are surrounded by a wall, whereas emphysema, by definition, is the destruction of parenchyma, causing air space enlargement that presents as areas of ill-defined low attenuation but without a discrete wall (see Fig. 18.4). Because the parenchymal destruction occurs around the bronchovascular bundle, vessels can be seen crossing emphysematous spaces. In cystic lung diseases, the cysts occur in the parenchyma and will be adjacent to the bronchovascular bundles; therefore, vessels typically do not cross a true lung cyst. Distinguishing paraseptal emphysema from honeycomb cysts can be challenging. Both the distribution and number of cystic rows can help differentiate between paraseptal emphysema and honeycomb cysts. Paraseptal emphysema tends to be apical in distribution, whereas honeycombing associated with UIP will be basilar predominant. The emphysematous changes in paraseptal emphysema tend to form a single subpleural row without a large degree of architectural distortion, whereas advanced honeycombing consists of multiple rows of well-defined cysts, with significant associated reticular abnormalities (Fig. 18.14).

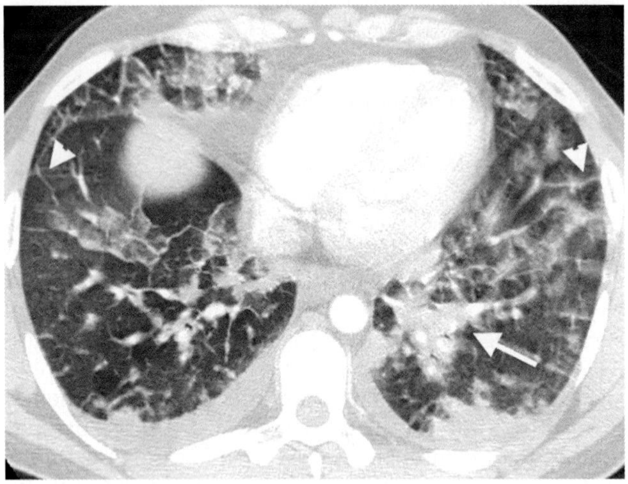

Figure 18.13 Acute eosinophilic pneumonia (AEP). This axial CT scan of AEP shows areas of patchy ground-glass opacity, bronchovascular consolidation *(arrow)*, interlobular septal thickening *(arrowheads)*, and small pleural effusions. The imaging appearance mimics that of acute left-sided heart failure.

Other Complications of Smoking

Infection

The lungs are directly exposed to a number of pathogens daily, and the respiratory epithelium plays an important role in host defense. Cigarette smoking is known to cause an increased risk of bacterial and viral infection due to a breakdown in the pulmonary immune response and the ability to protect against pathogens. The mechanism of increased infection in smokers includes structural lung changes and the alteration of immune responses, which allow pathogens the opportunity to breach normal protective immune responses and cause both respiratory and systemic diseases. Structural changes to lung parenchyma include decreased mucociliary clearance, increased peribronchiolar inflammation and fibrosis, respiratory epithelial damage, and increased permeability of the mucosa. Cigarette smoking also directly affects the humoral and cell-mediated immune response, including decreased levels and impaired function of immune cells and signaling cascades. Cigarette smokers have been shown to have an increased risk of influenza, tuberculosis, the common cold, Legionnaires' disease, pneumococcal pneumonia, and varicella pneumonia, among others. This increased risk is also seen in patients exposed to second-hand smoke. Several studies have also shown an increased incidence of meningococcal disease, bronchitis, and otitis media in children exposed to second-hand smoke.

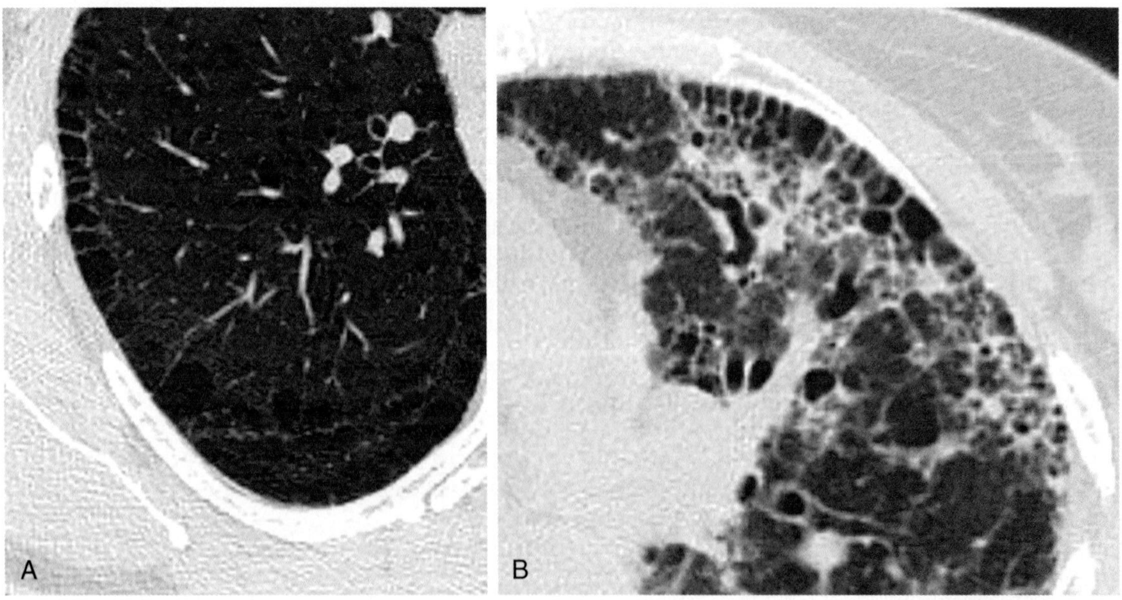

Figure 18.14 Honeycomb cysts versus paraseptal emphysema. On axial CT, the emphysematous changes in paraseptal emphysema (A) tend to form a single subpleural row, with little architectural distortion, whereas honeycombing (B) consists of well-defined cysts stacked as progressive subpleural layers as the disease progresses, with significant associated reticular abnormality.

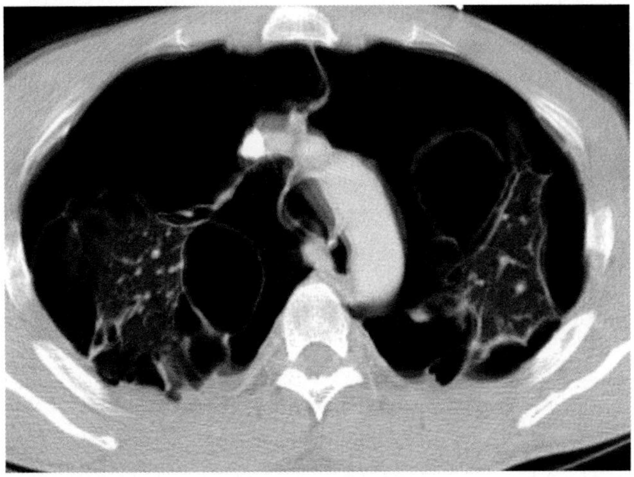

Figure 18.15 Pneumothorax. This axial CT scan demonstrates bullous emphysema with bilateral pneumothoraces. The presence of subpleural blebs and bullae significantly increases the risk of pneumothorax from rupture of these peripheral lesions.

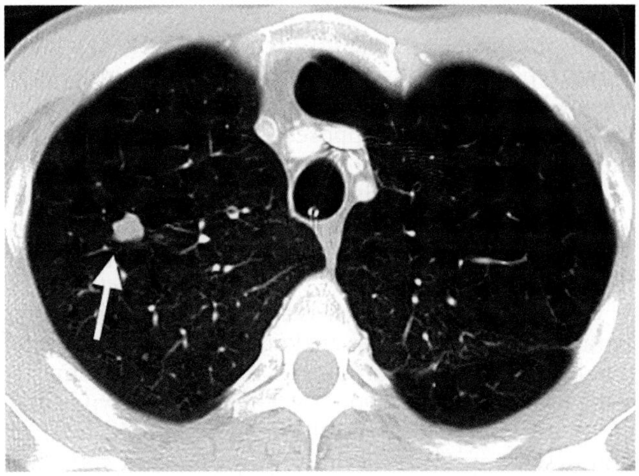

Figure 18.16 Emphysema and lung cancer. This axial CT scan demonstrates a right upper lobe nodule *(arrow)* in the setting of emphysema. Smoking significantly increases the risk of bronchogenic carcinoma, and nodules such as this warrant close scrutiny and possible biopsy based on lung cancer screening guidelines.

Hemorrhage

Hemorrhage can be a secondary consequence of smoking from underlying smoking-induced lung disease, such as lung cancer. Smoking may also increase the risk of hemorrhage in patients with other baseline pulmonary diseases, such as patients with Goodpasture syndrome.

Pneumothorax

Pneumothorax is a known complication of smoking-related lung disease. The incidence of pneumothorax in PLCH alone has been reported to be as high as 25%. Many studies have demonstrated an increased risk of spontaneous pneumothorax in smokers verse nonsmokers. Spontaneous pneumothorax is associated with airway obstruction, a common condition in long-term smokers with COPD, and subpleural blebs (Fig. 18.15). The risk of pneumothorax is dose-related and therefore increases with increased exposure to cigarette smoke.

Lung Cancer

According to the American Cancer Society, lung cancer is the leading cause of cancer-related deaths in men and women. Smoking is implicated in 80% to 90% of cases of lung cancer (Fig. 18.16). Men who smoke are 23 times more likely, and women who smoke are 13 times more likely, to develop lung cancer than nonsmokers. Numerous carcinogens in tobacco smoke predispose smokers to the development of lung cancer and make smoking an important risk factor for lung cancer. In addition to direct carcinogenic effects, the long-term chronic inflammation associated with smoking-related lung diseases increases patients' risk of developing cancer.

Chest radiography is ineffective for lung cancer screening. In 2013, the US Preventive Services Task Force (USPSTF) found that screening with low-dose CT is beneficial in reducing the mortality associated with lung cancer. The USPSTF criteria for lung cancer screening include the following:

1. Current or former smoker (former smokers having quit in the past 15 years)
2. Age, 55 to 80 years
3. 30+ pack-year smoking history
4. No health condition that substantially limits life expectancy
5. Willingness to undergo curative lung surgery

Pitfalls

Respiratory Motion Limits Evaluation for Nodules in the Setting of Smoking and Emphysema

Even in healthy patients, micronodules can be missed due to slice selection and respiratory motion. In cases in which the image is complicated by smoking-related parenchymal changes and distortion, micronodules are easily missed or misdiagnosed. Keeping the underlying lung changes in mind and using maximum intensity projection (MIP) images may be useful.

Other Causes of Emphysema in Addition to Smoking

Smoking is undoubtedly the most common cause of emphysema, but emphysema is not synonymous with smoking and can occur in nonsmokers (10% of all cases of emphysema). Smoking-related emphysema typically occurs in the sixth to eighth decades of life, with an upper lung predominance, as discussed above. The onset of emphysema due to other, nonsmoking causes has a variable distribution in the lungs and occurs earlier, with many congenital forms beginning in infancy. Genetic, infectious, and environmental factors have all been associated with emphysema in the absence of a smoking history.

Alpha-1-antitrypsin deficiency is a well-proven cause of emphysema in nonsmokers (3% of emphysema cases) and can expedite the onset of emphysema in smokers with this deficiency. Patients may have no detectable levels of alpha-1-antitrypsin, deficient levels of alpha-1-antitrypsin, or dysfunctional alpha-1-antitrypsin. Insufficient levels of serum alpha-1-antitrypsin result in various degrees of unopposed elastase activity in the lungs. Increased elastase activity causes the destruction of lung tissue and results in the appearance of emphysematous changes. The emphysema is apparent in the fourth to fifth decades of life, with a basilar and panacinar distribution. It is associated with liver dysfunction.

Other genetic causes such as connective tissue disorders or rare hereditary diseases are known to result in emphysema. Connective tissue diseases associated with emphysema include Marfan syndrome, Ehlers-Danlos syndrome, and cutis laxa. The onset of emphysema is in infancy. Emphysema in Ehlers-Danlos syndrome and cutis laxa are panacinar in appearance, whereas patients with Marfan syndrome develop apical bullae. Errors of metabolism seen with Salla disease and Menkes syndrome are rare genetic causes of emphysema.

Some reports have implicated HIV and other chronic infections with emphysematous changes; the cause is not completely understood but is suspected to be the destruction of normal lung parenchyma associated with a chronic inflammatory response. Small airway disease and hyperinflation as a direct cause of infection has been demonstrated in the case of Swyer-James or MacLeod syndrome and resulting constrictive bronchiolitis. Inhaled environmental pollutants and dust can cause emphysema, likely due to chronic inflammation and an increased immune response.

IV drug abuse has been associated with basilar, panacinar, and bullous emphysema, particularly IV injection of methylphenidate (Ritalin) and talc-containing substances. The proposed mechanism of action is damage to the pulmonary arteries from insoluble substances in the drug. Emphysematous changes are seen in as many as 2% of IV drug abusers.

Emphysema Complicates Evaluation of Other Common Lung Diseases

In the presence of emphysema, the diagnostic appearance of common acute lung diseases such as pneumonia or edema may be altered. Normal patterns of consolidation and air space opacities are distorted and can mimic fibrotic and cystic changes. For example, the pattern of cardiogenic edema can be altered to become more lower lung predominant due to compensatory vasoconstriction in the areas most severely affected by emphysema (generally the upper lungs). The presence of large bullae can confound the evaluation of infection for evidence of cavitation due to the more frequent presence of air-fluid levels in patients with preexisting emphysema.

Bibliography

Arcavi L, Benowitz NL. Cigarette smoking and infection. *Arch Intern Med.* 2004;164(20):2206–2216.

Bak SH, Lee HY. Overlaps and uncertainties of smoking-related idiopathic interstitial pneumonias. *Int J Chron Obstruct Pulmon Dis.* 2017;12: 3221–3229.

Bok GH, Kim YK, Lee YM, et al. Cigarette smoking-induced acute eosinophilic pneumonia: a case report including a provocation test. *J Korean Med Sci.* 2008;23(1):134–137.

Churg A, Müller NL, Wright JL. Respiratory bronchiolitis/interstitial lung disease: fibrosis, pulmonary function, and evolving concepts. *Arch Pathol Lab Med.* 2010;134(1):27–32.

Desai SR, Ryan SM, Colby TV. Smoking-related interstitial lung diseases: histopathological and imaging perspectives. *Clin Radiol.* 2003;58(4):259–268.

Dyer DS, Khan AR, Mohammed T-L, et al. ACR appropriateness criteria on chronic dyspnea: suspected pulmonary origin. *J Thorac Imaging.* 2010;25(2): W21–W23.

Galvin JR, Franks TJ. Smoking-related lung disease. *J Thorac Imaging.* 2009; 24(4):274–284.

Hansell D, Lynch DH, McAdams P, et al. *Imaging of Diseases of the Chest.* 5th ed. St. Louis: Mosby; 2010:451–459.

Hobbs S, Lynch D. The idiopathic interstitial pneumonias: an update and review. *Radiol Clin North Am.* 2014;52(1):105–120.

Humphrey LL, Deffebach M, Pappas M, et al. Screening for lung cancer with low-dose computed tomography: a systematic review to update the US preventive services task force recommendation. *Ann Intern Med.* 2013;159(6): 411–420.

Iwasawa T, Takemura T, Ogura T. Smoking-related lung abnormalities on computed tomography images: comparison with pathological findings. *Jpn J Radiol.* 2018;36(3):165–180.

Jawad H, Walker CM, Wu CC, Chung JH. Cystic interstitial lung diseases: recognizing the common and uncommon entities. *Curr Probl Diagn Radiol.* 2014;43(3):115–127.

Kim HJ, Lee KS, Johkoh T, et al. Pulmonary Langerhans cell histiocytosis in adults: high-resolution CT-pathology comparisons and evolutional changes at CT. *Eur Radiol.* 2011;21(7):1406–1415.

Kurashima K, Hoshi T, Takaku Y, et al. Changes in the airway lumen and surrounding parenchyma in chronic obstructive pulmonary disease. *Int J Chron Obstruct Pulmon Dis.* 2013;8:523–532.

Lee P, Gildea TR, Stoller JK. Emphysema in nonsmokers: alpha 1-antitrypsin deficiency and other causes. *Cleve Clin J Med.* 2002;69(12):928–929.

Lynch DA. Imaging of small airways disease and chronic obstructive pulmonary disease. *Clin Chest Med.* 2008;29(1):165–179, vii.

Miniati M, Monti S, Stolk J, et al. Value of chest radiography in phenotyping chronic obstructive pulmonary disease. *Eur Respir J.* 2008;31(3):509–515.

Moyer VA, US Preventive Services Task Force. Screening for lung cancer: U.S. Preventive services task force recommendation statement. *Ann Intern Med.* 2014;160(5):330–338.

Oh CK, Murray LA, Molfino NA. Smoking and idiopathic pulmonary fibrosis. *Pulm Med.* 2012;2012:808260.

Seely JM, Salahudeen S, Cadaval-Goncalves AT, et al. Pulmonary Langerhans cell histiocytosis: a comparative study of computed tomography in children and adults. *J Thorac Imaging.* 2012;27(1):65–70.

Stewart JI, Criner GJ. The small airways in chronic obstructive pulmonary disease: pathology and effects on disease progression and survival. *Curr Opin Pulm Med.* 2013;19(2):109–115.

Takahashi M, Fukuoka J, Nitta N, et al. Imaging of pulmonary emphysema: a pictorial review. *Int J Chron Obstruct Pulmon Dis.* 2008;3(2):193–204.

Tuder RM, Yoshida T, Arap W, Pasqualini R, Petrache I. State of the art. Cellular and molecular mechanisms of alveolar destruction in emphysema: an evolutionary perspective. *Proc Am Thorac Soc.* 2006;3(6):503–510.

Vassallo R. Diffuse lung diseases in cigarette smokers. *Semin Respir Crit Care Med.* 2012;33(5):533–542.

CHAPTER 19
Interstitial Lung Disease

Christopher Lee and Jonathan H. Chung

CHAPTER OUTLINE

Introduction

Interstitial lung disease (ILD) refers to a broad category of diffuse parenchymal lung diseases characterized by inflammation and/or fibrosis of the lungs. Patients invariably present with dyspnea of varying time course and severity. Patients are often hypoxemic, and pulmonary function tests typically demonstrate a restrictive pattern, with reduced diffusing capacity. The term *interstitial lung disease* is somewhat of a misnomer because many ILDs also involve the alveolar spaces. To date, more than 150 ILDs have been described. Imaging, particularly high-resolution computed tomography (HRCT), plays a pivotal role in the evaluation, diagnosis, and monitoring of ILD. In this chapter, we begin by discussing the imaging modalities and techniques used to evaluate ILD. We then describe the idiopathic interstitial pneumonias (IIPs), which are a subset of ILDs of unknown cause but with distinct clinicopathologic descriptions. Of the various IIPs, we spend the most time discussing usual interstitial pneumonia because it is the most common IIP and has the most detailed diagnostic criteria. Other common ILDs, including sarcoidosis, hypersensitivity pneumonitis (HP), pneumoconioses, and ILDs associated with collagen vascular diseases, are discussed elsewhere in this text. Finally, we conclude with a brief summary of emerging knowledge on the genetics of pulmonary fibrosis.

Appropriateness of Imaging Modalities

Appropriate Modalities in Suspected Interstitial Lung Disease

Chest radiography is one of the initial screening tests for ILD due to its wide availability, low cost, and low radiation exposure to the patient. Posteroanterior and lateral chest radiographs are commonly ordered for patients with dyspnea. However, early manifestations of ILD are difficult to perceive on chest radiographs. In fact, chest radiographs are normal in up to 15% of patients with ILD. And, even in cases of advanced ILD, it can be challenging to characterize radiographic findings and formulate a differential diagnosis.

CT is the imaging modality of choice for the evaluation of ILD. More specifically, HRCT, in which images are reconstructed with thin sections and high spatial frequency algorithms, is recommended to image the lung interstitium optimally and characterize parenchymal abnormalities. Since its introduction over 30 years ago, HRCT has emerged as an indispensable diagnostic tool in the evaluation of patients with suspected ILD.

MRI has limited utility in the evaluation of ILD. MRI suboptimally images the lungs due to the inherent absence of proton density in the aerated lungs, as well as increased susceptibility artifact from extensive air–soft tissue interfaces. However, due to the concern of cumulative radiation exposure in patients with chronic pulmonary disease, MRI has been used in lieu of CT at some centers to monitor certain patient populations. For example, MRI surveillance of patients with cystic fibrosis has been well reported in the literature.

Standard CT Protocol for Interstitial Lung Disease Assessment

The standard HRCT protocol for ILD assessment includes an inspiratory scan with the patient in the supine position, an inspiratory scan in the prone position, and an expiratory scan in the supine position. In the current multidetector CT (MDCT) era, these scans are typically performed helically, with whole-lung volumetric acquisition. However, the prone and expiratory scans may be performed with individual axial scans at spaced (1–4 cm) intervals if radiation exposure is a concern. The HRCT protocol may be tailored to the clinical indication. For example, the prone scan may be omitted in patients without suspected ILD or with advanced lung disease. However, in a busy clinical practice, these modifications to the HRCT protocol may prove to be challenging.

Rationale for Including Prone Images

The supine inspiratory HRCT is adequate for diagnosis in most cases. However, prone images can be valuable in detecting subtle or early ILD. Subsegmental atelectasis is often present in the dependent lungs in normal individuals, appearing as dependent subpleural densities or lines. These findings, unfortunately, can mimic those of early lung ILD. However, on prone scanning, the posterior subsegmental atelectasis resolves due to increased posterior lung aeration, whereas true subpleural disease remains visible (Fig. 19.1). As mentioned previously, in patients with advanced ILD, prone images may be omitted because subtle dependent opacities no longer pose a diagnostic dilemma.

Rationale for Including Expiratory Images

Expiratory scanning is a useful adjunct to the inspiratory scan in the evaluation of patients with suspected small airways or obstructive lung disease. Air trapping is diagnosed by identifying areas of relative lucency on expiratory images that maintain the same attenuation as on the corresponding inspiratory images (Fig. 19.2). Air trapping on expiratory HRCT has been shown to correlate with obstructive deficits on pulmonary function testing. Although air trapping is not a prominent component of most ILDs, the presence of air trapping may occasionally

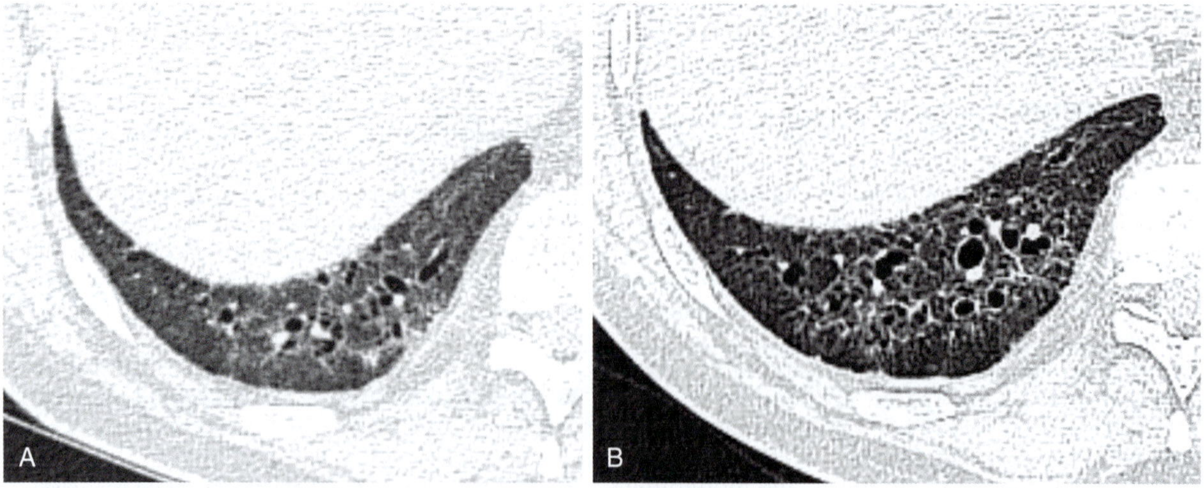

Figure 19.1 Supine (A) and prone (B) images of the right lower lobe from high-resolution chest CT demonstrate the relative difference in appearance of the dependent portion of the lung. Note that the dependent lung is better inflated during the prone image (B) as opposed to the supine image (A), with decrease in atelectasis in the right lower lobe that manifests as mild diffuse ground-glass abnormality on the supine image (A). Also, subpleural sparing and bronchiectasis are much more evident on the prone image (B) than on the supine image (A).

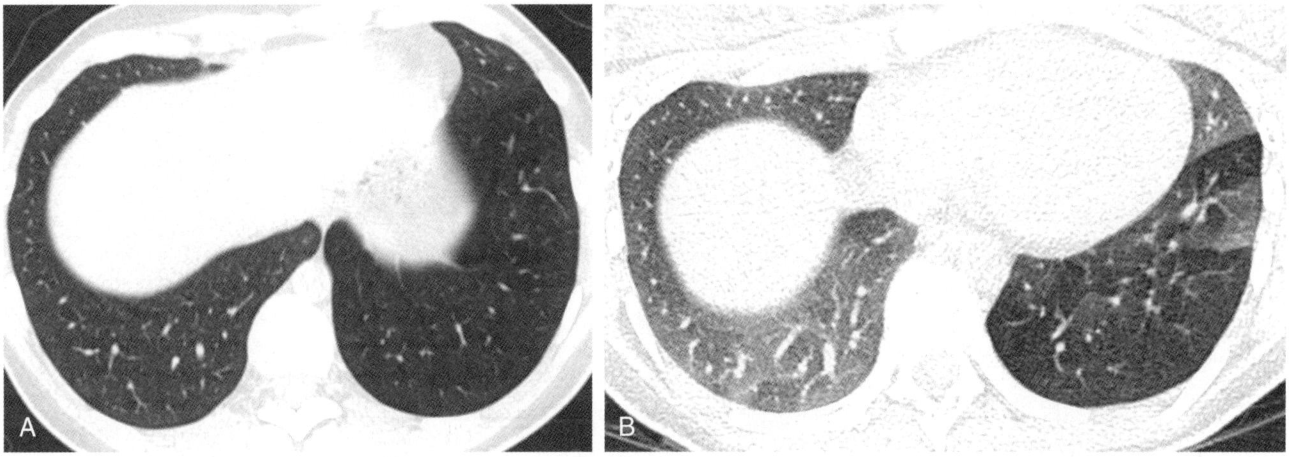

Figure 19.2 (A) Inspiratory image from high-resolution chest CT scan demonstrates relative hyperlucency and paucity of vessels of the left lower lobe compared to other portions of the lungs. (B) Expiratory image demonstrates marked air trapping throughout the left lower lobe.

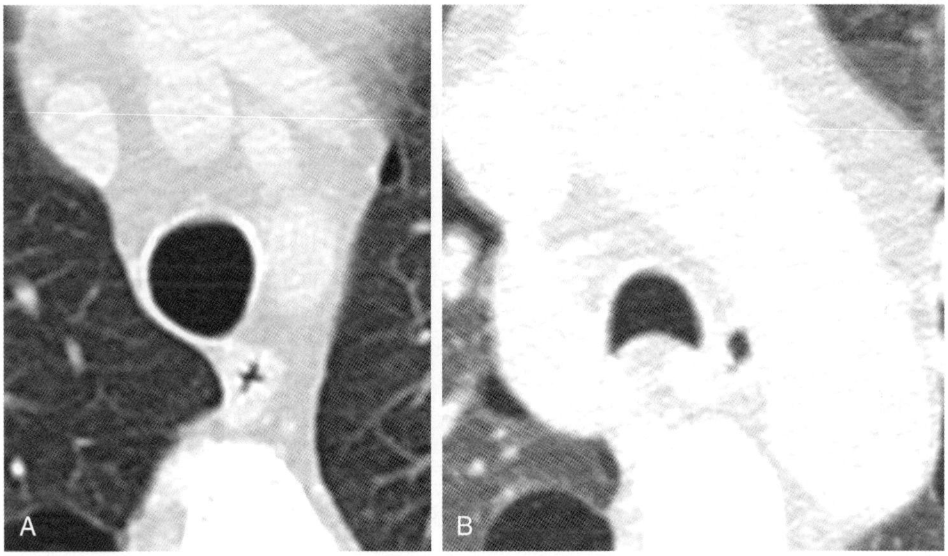

Figure 19.3 Inspiratory (A) and expiratory (B) images from chest CT scans demonstrate the typical appearance of the trachea during different phases of the respiratory cycle. During inspiration, the trachea is typically convex throughout its margins and has an oval shape. During expiration, the posterior aspect of the trachea composed primarily of the trachealis muscle and connective tissue bows anteriorly.

aid in the differential diagnosis. Moreover, the cause of the patient's symptoms may be due to obstructive lung disease rather than restrictive ILD. Consequently, we recommend that expiratory scans be routinely acquired in every patient's initial HRCT assessment.

Ensuring That CT Images Were Acquired in Expiration

Expected CT findings during expiration include an increase in lung attenuation, decrease in cross-sectional lung area, and reduction in airway size. Of these, reduction in airway size, particularly the trachea, is most useful in determining if the patient performed an adequate expiratory maneuver. During inspiration, the trachea maintains a round or elliptic shape. During expiration, the trachea assumes more of a crescent shape as the membranous posterior wall bows anteriorly (Fig. 19.3). The mean cross-sectional area of the trachea can decrease by up to half of its area on inspiration. If the tracheal morphology and area do not change between inspiratory and expiratory scans, the patient may not have reached an adequate level of expiration. On the other hand, obliteration of the tracheal lumen during expiration is diagnostic of flaccidity of the supporting tracheal cartilage, known as *tracheomalacia.*

■ Usual Interstitial Pneumonia

Usual interstitial pneumonia (UIP) is a chronic fibrosing interstitial pneumonia in which there is a spatially and temporally heterogeneous distribution of normal lung, interstitial inflammation, fibrosis, and honeycomb change (Fig. 19.4). A characteristic histologic lesion is the fibroblastic focus, which represents an aggregate of proliferating fibroblasts and myofibroblasts. UIP represents the histopathologic pattern associated with idiopathic pulmonary fibrosis (IPF). UIP/IPF is the most common IIP, accounting for 50% to 60% of cases. It is important to make the diagnosis of UIP because IPF has a poor prognosis, with a median survival of less than 5

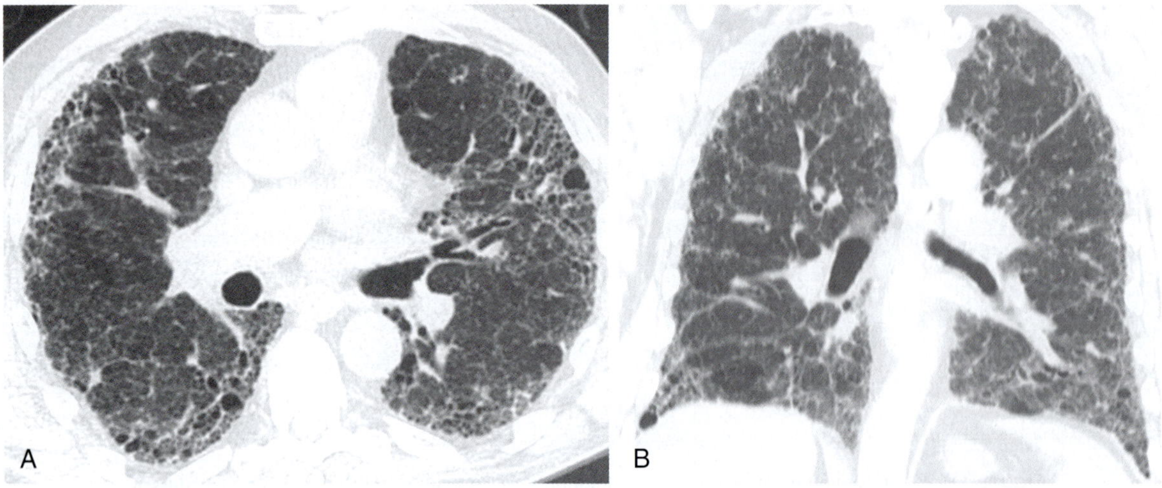

Figure 19.4 Axial (A) and coronal (B) images from high-resolution chest CT scans demonstrate the typical appearance of usual interstitial pneumonia pattern of pulmonary fibrosis. There is subpleural and basal predominant pulmonary fibrosis characterized by reticulation, traction bronchiectasis, traction bronchiolectasis, architectural distortion, and subpleural honeycombing.

TABLE 19.1 UIP Classification on HRCT

UIP PATTERN	PROBABLE UIP PATTERN	INDETERMINATE FOR UIP PATTERN	ALTERNATIVE DIAGNOSIS PATTERN
Subpleural and basal predominant; heterogeneous distribution	Subpleural and basal predominant; heterogeneous distribution	Subpleural and basal predominant	CT features: cysts, marked mosaic attenuation, predominant GGO, profuse micronodules, centrilobular nodules, nodules, consolidation
Honeycombing with or without traction bronchiectasis/ bronchiolectasis	Reticular pattern with traction bronchiectasis/ bronchiolectasis	Subtle reticulation; may have mild GGO or distortion	Distribution: peribronchovascular, perilymphatic, upper or mid-lung
	May have mild GGO	CT features or distribution of fibrosis that do not suggest any specific etiology	Other: pleural plaques, dilated esophagus, distal clavicular erosions, extensive lymph node enlargement, pleural effusions or thickening

GGO, Ground-glass opacification; *HRCT,* high-resolution CT; *UIP,* usual interstitial pneumonia.
Modified from Raghu G, Remy-Jardin M, Myers JL, et al. Diagnosis of idiopathic pulmonary fibrosis. An official ATS/ERS/JRS/ALAT clinical practice guideline. *Am J Respir Crit Care Med.* 2018;198:e44–e68.

years after the time of diagnosis. Unlike other ILDs, IPF does not respond to conventional corticosteroid and/or immunomodulator therapy. Moreover, given recent US Food and Drug Administration (FDA) approval of medications shown to slow functional decline in IPF patients, accurate diagnosis is paramount.

Clinical Causes

The differential diagnosis for UIP consists of IPF (majority of cases in most clinics), connective tissue diseases, drug toxicity, chronic HP, and pneumoconioses. Although IPF is the most common cause of UIP, it is a diagnosis of exclusion and should only be made when other possible causes of UIP and ILD have been excluded.

Classification System on HRCT

In 2011 the American Thoracic Society, European Respiratory Society, Japanese Respiratory Society, and Latin American Thoracic Association published an evidence-based consensus statement on the diagnosis and management of IPF. In 2018, the same organizations published revisions of the original recommendations. The updated document established four categories of HRCT patterns in patients with suspected IPF: (1) UIP; (2) probably UIP; (3) indeterminate for UIP; and (4) alternative diagnosis. The radiologist reading these scans should make every effort to classify the HRCT findings as one of these four patterns.

Establishing Definite Diagnosis on HRCT

According to the 2018 updated guidelines, the features that are required to make a diagnosis of a UIP pattern on HRCT are (1) subpleural and basal predominant; distribution is often heterogeneous; and (2) honeycombing with or without peripheral traction bronchiectasis or bronchiolectasis (Table 19.1). A number of studies have shown that a UIP pattern on HRCT is highly predictive of a histopathologic UIP pattern. In patients with suspected IPF who do not have identifiable causes of ILD, fulfillment of these HRCT criteria is diagnostic of IPF and obviates the need for surgical lung biopsy.

Importance of Honeycombing

Honeycombing is critical to make a definitive diagnosis of a UIP pattern on HRCT. Honeycombing appears as clustered cystic air spaces with well-defined walls, typically subpleural in location. If honeycombing is absent but other features of UIP are present, the HRCT findings are best classified as a "probable UIP" pattern. In a patient with high pretest probability of IPF (over 60 years of age, no signs of connective tissue disease, no exposure history, or pertinent medication history), a presumptive diagnosis of IPF can be made with a probable UIP pattern on CT, decreasing the importance of CT honeycombing from a diagnostic standpoint. Several studies have also shown that patients without honeycombing (probable UIP or indeterminate for UIP pattern) have a longer survival than those with honeycombing (UIP pattern).

HRCT Findings Suggestive of Alternative Diagnosis

HRCT findings that are suggestive of an alternative diagnosis include upper or mid-lung predominance, peribronchovascular or perilymphatic predominance, predominant ground-glass abnormality, profuse nodules, discrete cysts, marked mosaic attenuation/air trapping, and consolidation. Other findings suggestive of an alternative diagnosis include pleural plaques (indicating possible asbestosis), dilated esophagus or distal clavicular erosions (indicating connective tissue disease), extensive lymph node enlargement, pleural effusions, and pleural thickening. If any of these features are present in a patient with suspected IPF, the HRCT findings should be classified as "alternative diagnosis," and surgical lung biopsy should again be considered. This does not necessarily mean that the diagnosis is not UIP, however, as there are a substantial number of cases that have an alternative diagnosis pattern on HRCT but are shown to have a UIP pattern on surgical lung biopsy and are eventually diagnosed as IPF.

Atypical Appearance on HRCT

An atypical HRCT appearance of UIP, either an indeterminate for UIP or an alternative diagnosis pattern on HRCT but a UIP pattern on histopathology, is fairly common. In one study of 55 biopsy-proven UIP cases, 62% of these cases were considered to have a low probability of representing UIP. Of these atypical UIP cases, the most common first-choice diagnoses based on HRCT were nonspecific interstitial pneumonia (NSIP), chronic HP, and sarcoidosis. Often, HRCT demonstrates peripheral basal-predominant reticular and ground-glass opacities with traction bronchiectasis but without significant honeycombing, an appearance commonly associated with fibrotic NSIP (Fig. 19.5).

HRCT Features and Diagnosis of Pulmonary Fibrosis

HRCT features of pulmonary fibrosis include irregular pulmonary parenchymal interfaces, traction bronchiectasis and bronchiolectasis, regional volume loss, and honeycombing. Honeycombing is the most specific sign of fibrotic lung disease and results from alveolar disruption and dilation of bronchioles and alveolar ducts, with the creation of clustered, cystic air spaces lined by bronchiolar epithelium.

In the absence of honeycombing, pulmonary fibrosis can still be diagnosed by the presence of the other findings. There are often irregular interfaces at the edges of pulmonary vessels or bronchi, along the interlobar fissures, and along the peripheral pleural surfaces of the lungs. Traction bronchiectasis represents bronchial dilation in areas of pulmonary fibrosis secondary to the traction effect of the fibrous tissue on the bronchial walls. The bronchi often demonstrate an irregular or varicose morphology (Fig. 19.6). In the extreme lung periphery of these patients, a dilated airway likely reflects traction

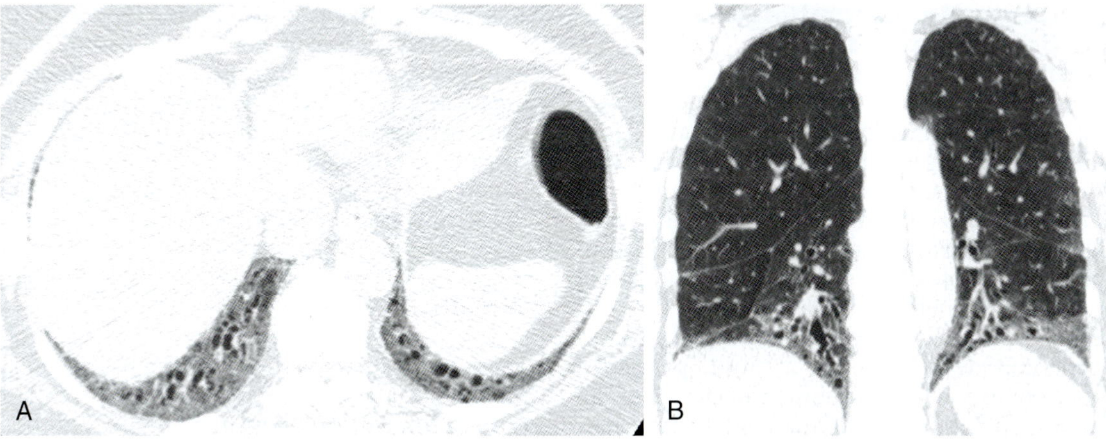

Figure 19.5 Axial (A) and coronal (B) images from high-resolution chest CT scans demonstrate basal predominant pulmonary fibrosis in this patient with known nonspecific interstitial pneumonia characterized by ground-glass opacity, reticulation, and traction bronchiectasis.

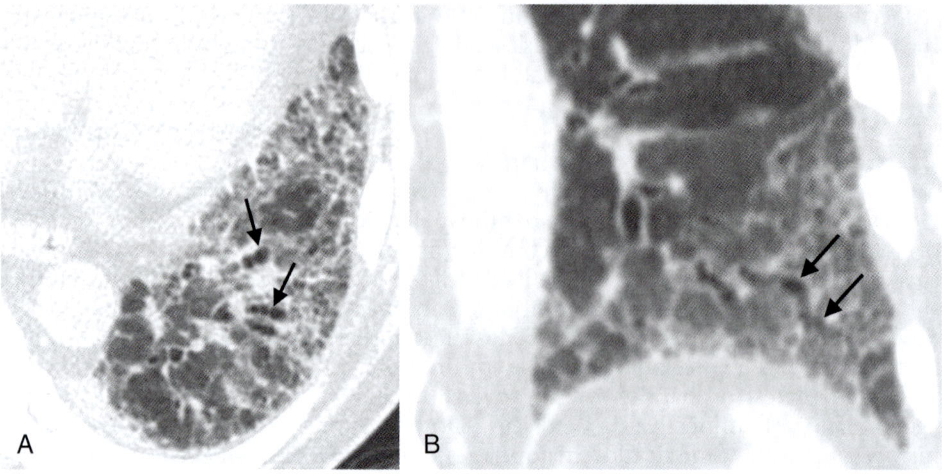

Figure 19.6 Axial (A) and coronal (B) images of the left lower lobe from high-resolution chest CT demonstrate basal predominant pulmonary fibrosis. In the setting of pulmonary fibrosis, traction bronchiectasis often takes on a varicoid pattern *(arrows)*.

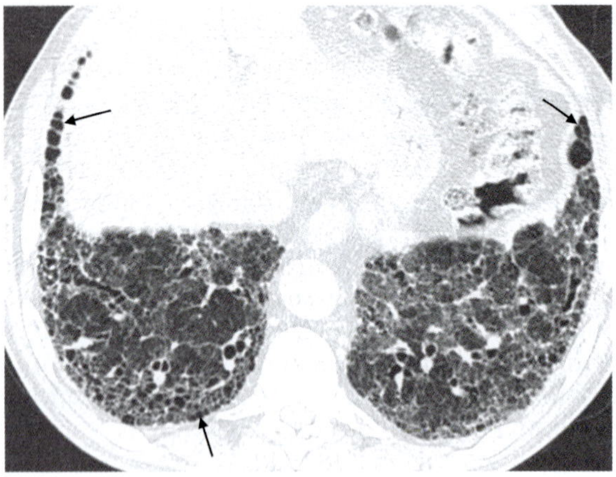

Figure 19.7 Axial image from high-resolution chest CT scan demonstrates peripheral predominant pulmonary fibrosis with focal areas of subpleural honeycombing *(arrows)*.

bronchiolectasis. Over time, pulmonary fibrosis causes progressive volume loss, which is manifested by crowding of bronchovascular structures in areas of disease involvement and retraction of the fissures.

Differentiating Honeycombing From Traction Bronchiolectasis and Paraseptal Emphysema

On HRCT, honeycombing appears as cystic air spaces, several millimeters to several centimeters in diameter, with well-defined walls and predominating in a subpleural location (Fig. 19.7). Honeycomb cysts typically share walls and occur in multiple layers, although early honeycombing may manifest as a single layer of subpleural cysts.

Paraseptal emphysema represents distal acinar air space enlargement and destruction. As a result, paraseptal emphysema appears as subpleural lucencies that can mimic honeycombing. However, there are several characteristics that can distinguish paraseptal emphysema from honeycombing. Paraseptal emphysema usually occurs in a single subpleural layer, predominates in the upper lobes, and is usually associated with centrilobular emphysema (Fig. 19.8). On the other hand, honeycombing tends to occur in several layers, predominates in the lung bases, and is typically associated with architectural distortion or other features of fibrosis. Occasionally, paraseptal emphysema and honeycombing may coexist in the same patient, usually in the setting of combined pulmonary fibrosis and emphysema (CPFE).

Traction bronchiolectasis can be distinguished from honeycombing by carefully examining contiguous HRCT sections and observing continuity and branching of bronchi and bronchioles rather than discrete honeycomb cysts; sagittal and coronal reformations may demonstrate characteristic airway morphology better. Furthermore, traction bronchiolectasis is typically located a few millimeters or more from the pleura, whereas honeycomb cysts are immediately adjacent to the pleura.

Acute Exacerbation

Acute exacerbation of UIP is the clinical scenario in which a patient with UIP/IPF develops acute respiratory worsening not secondary to an identifiable cause, such as pulmonary embolism, congestive heart failure, or infection (e.g., *Pneumocystis* pneumonia). This occurs in 5% to 10% of IPF patients/year, and the prognosis is very poor, with mortality exceeding 60%. Histopathologically, acute exacerbation represents diffuse alveolar damage and/or organizing pneumonia superimposed on UIP. HRCT demonstrates bilateral ground-glass opacities and/or consolidations superimposed on the preexisting UIP pattern (Fig. 19.9). Acute exacerbation can also occur in the setting of NSIP.

Pitfalls

There are several pitfalls in making the diagnosis of UIP on HRCT. Acute interstitial infiltration or inflammation can sometimes be confused for pulmonary fibrosis because intralobular interstitial thickening can be seen in infiltrative, inflammatory, and fibrotic lung disease. It is important to look for associated findings when intralobular

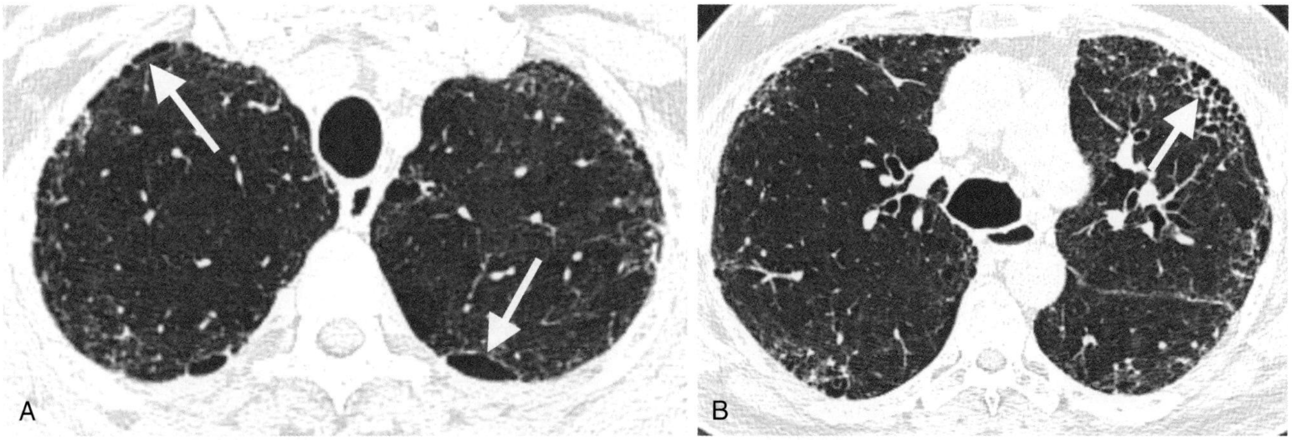

Figure 19.8 (A) Axial chest CT scan through the upper lobes demonstrates rows of cystic spaces within the subpleural lung *(arrows)* without adjacent reticulation or substantial ground-glass abnormality, consistent with paraseptal emphysema. Mild fibrotic changes are noted within the other portions of the lungs. (B) More inferiorly, this axial chest CT scan demonstrates clustered cystic spaces *(arrow)* within the anterior left upper lobe with adjacent reticulation, ground-glass abnormality, and mild thickening of some of the cystic wall spaces, consistent with subpleural honeycombing.

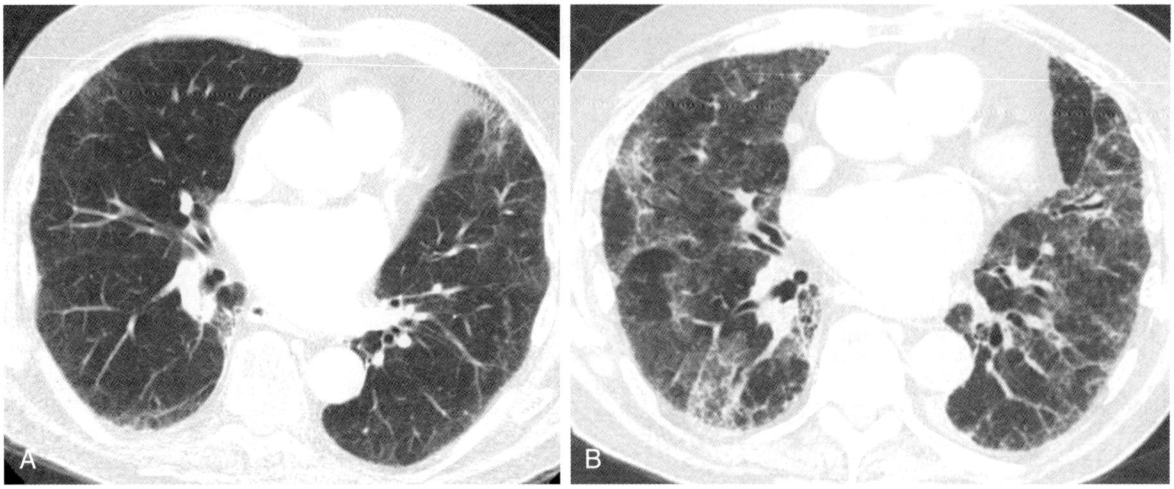

Figure 19.9 (A) Axial image from chest CT scan at baseline demonstrates mild peripheral predominant pulmonary fibrosis. (B) During an acute exacerbation of the patient's pulmonary fibrosis, this axial image from the chest CT scan at that time demonstrates diffuse ground-glass opacity superimposed on pulmonary fibrosis, most consistent with diffuse alveolar damage histology.

interstitial thickenings or reticular opacities are present. If there are associated ground-glass opacities, the reticulations may represent infiltrative or inflammatory disease (Fig. 19.10). On the other hand, if there is associated traction bronchiectasis or honeycombing, reticulations likely reflect pulmonary fibrosis.

Traction bronchiectasis should be distinguished from bronchiectasis secondary to chronic inflammation. Compared to inflammatory bronchiectasis, traction bronchiectasis typically lacks significant wall thickening or mucoid impaction (Fig. 19.11). Most importantly, traction bronchiectasis should be accompanied by other findings of fibrosis, such as irregular reticular opacities, honeycombing, architectural distortion, and volume loss.

Another pitfall in diagnosing UIP on HRCT is the belief that honeycombing must be present in all UIP cases. The prevalence of honeycombing in UIP actually varies widely. Honeycombing has been reported in 24% to 91% of patients who have UIP/IPF. In early or mild UIP, honeycombing may be minimal. And, as mentioned earlier, an atypical HRCT appearance of UIP often resembles NSIP, with minimal to no honeycombing. It is important to remember that if other HRCT features of UIP are present, despite the absence of honeycombing, the findings may still be classified as a probable UIP and that biopsy may not be necessary in patients with a high likelihood of an IPF diagnosis.

Due to the relatively high prevalence of atypical UIP, HRCT findings are highly specific but only moderately sensitive in making the diagnosis of UIP. Reported sensitivity ranges from 48% to 78%; specificity ranges from 90% to 98%. Diagnostic HRCT features of UIP are only present in 50% to 70% of cases. Thus, in the absence of a UIP or proable UIP pattern on HRCT, surgical lung biopsy is recommended, and diagnosis should be made based on multidisciplinary discussion.

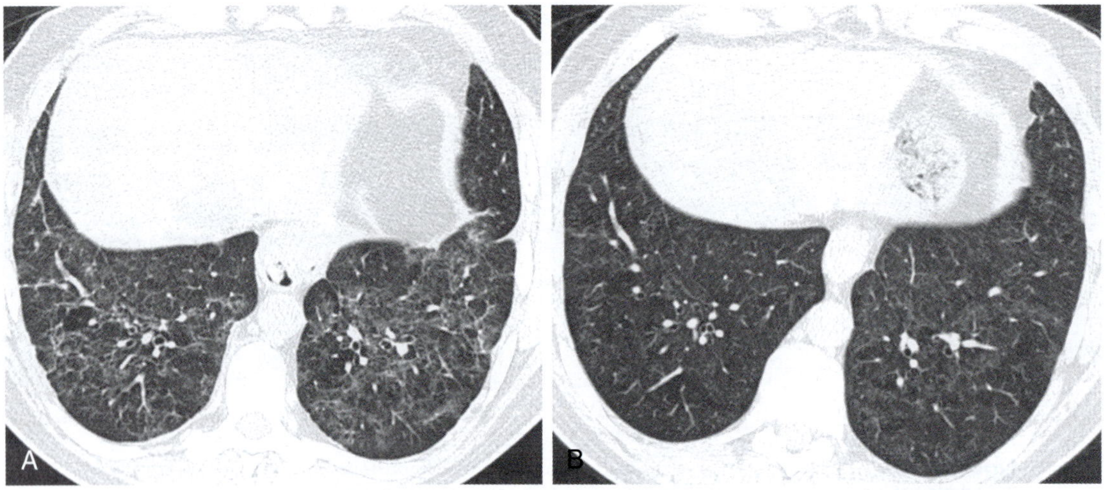

Figure 19.10 (A) Axial image from chest CT scan at initial presentation demonstrates diffuse ground-glass abnormality, reticulation, and bronchial dilation suggestive of interstitial lung disease. (B) On follow-up imaging 6 months later, this demonstrates near-complete resolution of ground-glass opacity, reticulation, and bronchial dilation. Initial CT findings were thought to have been related to an acute aspiration event.

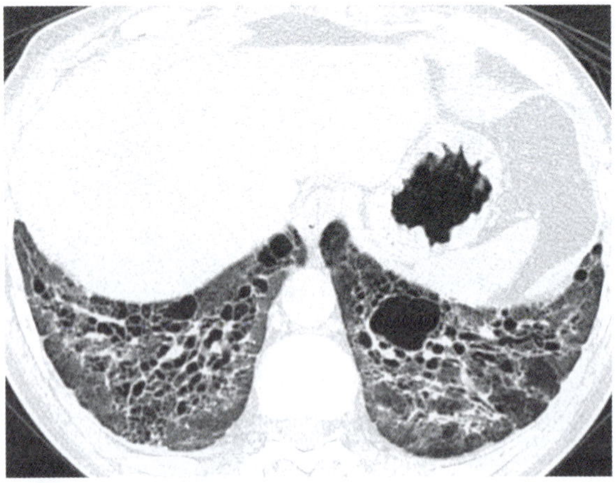

Figure 19.11 Axial image from high-resolution chest CT scan demonstrates extensive traction bronchiectasis, with mild superimposed ground-glass opacity and reticulation within the lower lobes. Note that the areas of traction bronchiectasis do not demonstrate substantial degree of mucus plugging or asymmetric inflammatory bronchial wall thickening.

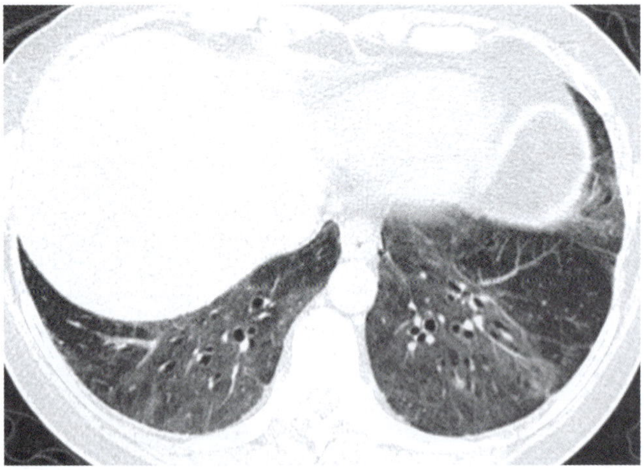

Figure 19.12 Axial image from high-resolution chest CT scan demonstrates extensive ground-glass abnormality and traction bronchiectasis at the lung bases with minimal reticulation in this patient with known nonspecific interstitial pneumonia.

Nonspecific Interstitial Pneumonia

NSIP is a chronic IIP in which there is a spatially and temporally homogeneous distribution of interstitial inflammation and/or fibrosis. The histology of NSIP may range from a predominantly inflammatory process (cellular NSIP) to a predominantly fibrotic process (fibrotic NSIP). In actual practice, however, fibrotic NSIP is far more common than cellular NSIP. The presence of fibrosis is associated with a worse prognosis. The median survival of fibrotic NSIP is 6 to 14 years after diagnosis, whereas survival of cellular NSIP, particularly if treated, is excellent. Regardless of the degree of inflammation or fibrosis, patients with NSIP have a much better prognosis than those with UIP. Therefore, it is critical that patients are correctly diagnosed with NSIP and not erroneously labeled with IPF/UIP, which unfortunately occurs far too often in the community.

Clinical Causes

Unlike UIP, NSIP is usually a manifestation of other diseases, such as collagen vascular diseases (particularly scleroderma), HP, drug toxicity, and diffuse alveolar damage. Some believe that almost all cases of NSIP are secondary to an underlying condition. Therefore, idiopathic NSIP should be diagnosed only when secondary causes have been meticulously worked up and excluded.

Appearance on HRCT

The most common HRCT finding of NSIP is bilateral ground-glass opacities, occurring in nearly all cases (Fig. 19.12). Irregular reticular opacities with associated traction bronchiectasis and bronchiolectasis are present in approximately 75% of cases, usually in the setting of

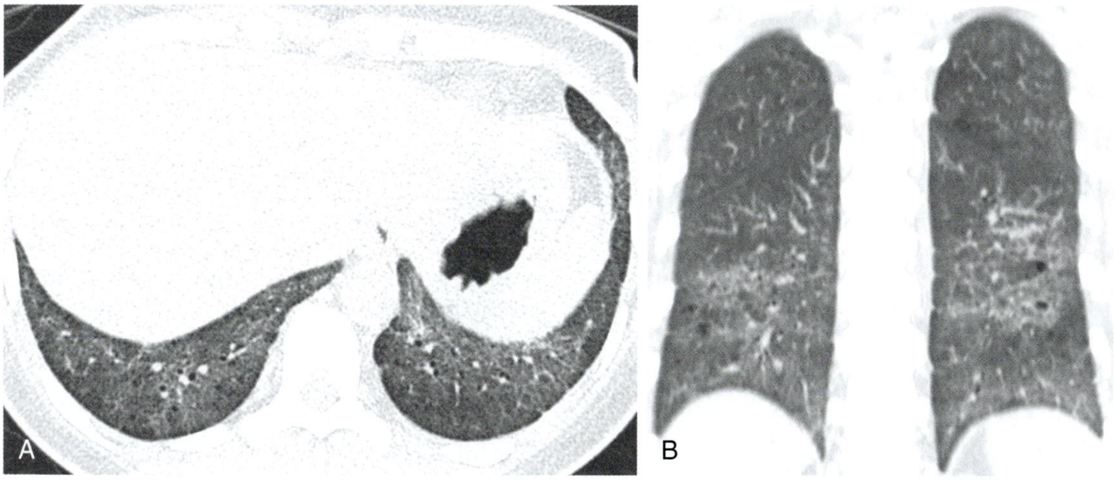

Figure 19.13 Axial (A) and coronal (B) images from high-resolution chest CT scans demonstrate extensive ground-glass abnormality, reticulation, and traction bronchiectasis at the lung bases with relative subpleural sparing in this patient with known nonspecific interstitial pneumonia. Subpleural sparing is a powerful differentiator of nonspecific interstitial pneumonia from usual interstitial pneumonia.

TABLE 19.2 Summary of Characteristic HRCT Features of Interstitial Lung Diseases

DISEASE	DISTRIBUTION	PREDOMINANT HRCT PATTERNS
Usual interstitial pneumonia	Subpleural, basal	Reticular opacities, honeycombing, traction bronchiectasis
Nonspecific interstitial pneumonia	Peripheral, subpleural sparing common, peribronchovascular, basal	Ground-glass opacities, reticular opacities, traction bronchiectasis
Organizing pneumonia	Subpleural, peribronchial	Consolidation, ground-glass opacities, perilobular opacities
Acute interstitial pneumonia	Diffuse	Ground-glass opacities, consolidation
Respiratory bronchiolitis–interstitial lung disease	Upper lobes	Ground-glass opacities, centrilobular nodules
Desquamative interstitial pneumonia	Subpleural, basal	Ground-glass opacities, cysts
Lymphoid interstitial pneumonia	Lower lung, peribronchovascular	Ground-glass opacities, centrilobular nodules, subpleural nodules, cysts
Pleuroparenchymal fibroelastosis	Subpleural, upper lobes	Pleural thickening, consolidation

HRCT, High-resolution CT.

fibrotic NSIP. Honeycombing is seen in a minority of cases and, if present, tends to be mild. When ground-glass opacities are not accompanied by reticulations, traction bronchiectasis, and honeycombing, the findings suggest a predominantly cellular NSIP.

The ground-glass and reticular opacities typically have a basal and peripheral predominance, although a peribronchovascular distribution is also common. Relative sparing of the immediate subpleural lung has been reported in up to 64% of cases but, in our experience, this occurs in a minority of cases (Fig. 19.13). When present, however, subpleural sparing is highly suggestive of NSIP as opposed to UIP, which invariably affects the lung periphery most severely.

Differentiating NSIP From HP From UIP

The HRCT appearances of UIP and NSIP are somewhat variable and often overlap, which can render an accurate diagnosis of either disease difficult. We find a useful strategy in differentiating these two entities, as well as in the overall evaluation of ILD, is to determine the predominant HRCT pattern present (Table 19.2). If ground-glass opacities are the prevailing HRCT feature, NSIP is more likely than UIP. However, if reticular opacities and honeycombing are the predominant pattern, UIP is the likely diagnosis. As mentioned earlier, the presence of subpleural sparing is characteristic of NSIP. Recall that a definitive diagnosis of a UIP pattern on HRCT can only be made when both subpleural and basal predominance and honeycombing are present. The vast majority of cases of probable UIP pattern on CT will be UIP on pathology, though not as high as in clear UIP patterns on CT. If HRCT demonstrates an indeterminate for UIP pattern or alternative diagnosis pattern, surgical lung biopsy is often required as the imaging pattern is often not specific for a single non-UIP diagnosis.

Although the typical HRCT findings of subacute HP frequently allow for a confident diagnosis, the HRCT manifestations of chronic HP often mimic those of UIP or NSIP. However, if centrilobular nodules, mosaic attenuation, and/or air trapping are present, chronic HP is more likely than UIP or NSIP. Furthermore, chronic HP may be upper lung preponderant and, even if it is lower lung preponderant, often spares the lung bases and costophrenic angles, whereas UIP and NSIP characteristically involve the extreme lung bases most severely (Fig. 19.14).

Pitfalls

Patients with NSIP often demonstrate gradual progression of fibrosis on HRCT, although the overall HRCT pattern still resembles that of NSIP. However, it is important to note that a significant minority of patients progress, so that their follow-up HRCT assumes more of a UIP pattern over time (Fig. 19.15). Within this context, if the patient is imaged at an institution that does not have access to his or her prior imaging, the patient may be misdiagnosed as having UIP/IPF. This scenario underscores the importance of evaluating historical imaging in patients with NSIP and, in fact, all ILDs, because HRCT findings at initial presentation may offer the best characterization of the patient's disease.

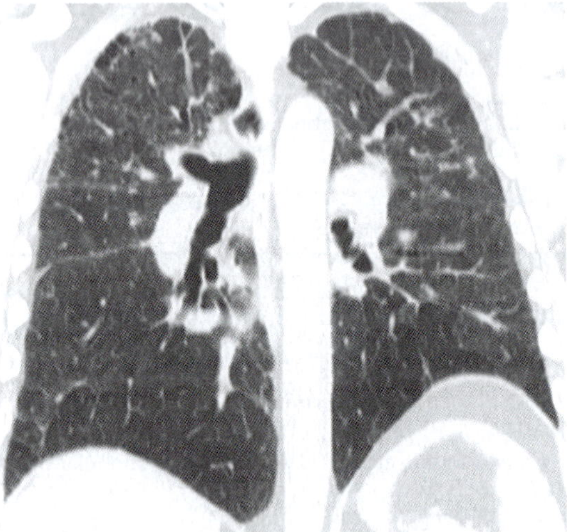

Figure 19.14 Coronal image from high-resolution chest CT scan demonstrates upper lung predominant pulmonary fibrosis characterized by reticulation, traction bronchiectasis and bronchiolectasis, mild architectural distortion, and subpleural honeycombing in this patient with known hypersensitivity pneumonitis from chronic bird exposure. Upper lung preponderance is a helpful differentiator of hypersensitivity pneumonitis from usual interstitial pneumonia and nonspecific interstitial pneumonia.

■ Organizing Pneumonia

Organizing pneumonia (OP) is a subacute IIP characterized histologically by granulation tissue within the alveolar ducts and alveoli, with chronic inflammation of the surrounding lung parenchyma. Granulation tissue polyps may also be present within the bronchioles, which is why this condition has also been referred to as *bronchiolitis obliterans organizing pneumonia* (BOOP). However, involvement of the air spaces is the dominant feature of this disease process; consequently, *organizing pneumonia* is the favored terminology. It is important to make the diagnosis of OP because most patients respond favorably to corticosteroid therapy, although relapse is common.

Clinical Causes

OP frequently occurs secondary to systemic disease or preexisting lung disease. Some of the common causes include collagen vascular diseases, inflammatory bowel disease, inhalational injury, HP, drug toxicity, pulmonary infection, aspiration, and radiation pneumonitis. When no underlying cause is identified, the condition is termed *cryptogenic organizing pneumonia* (COP).

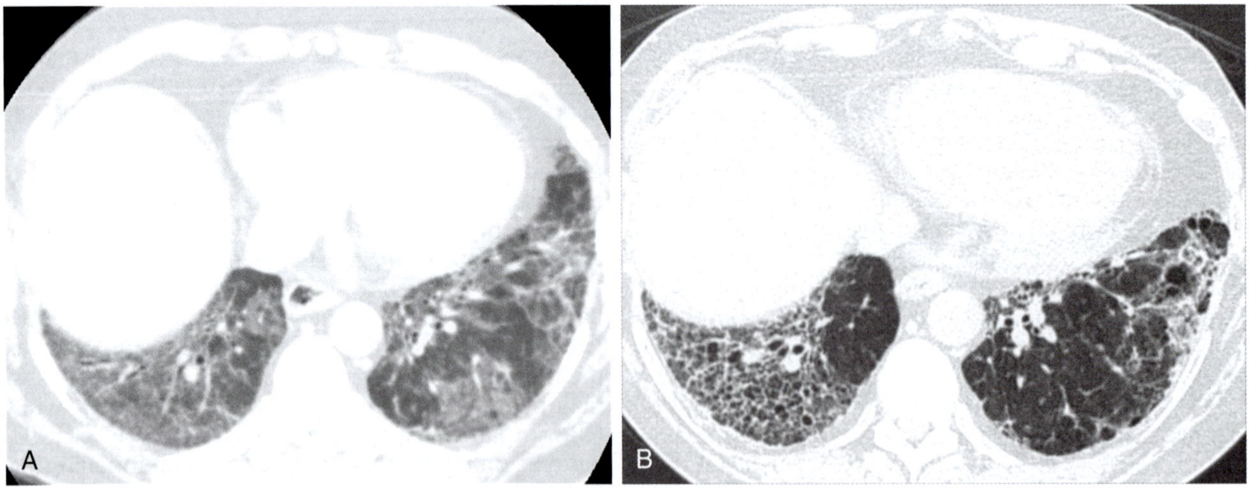

Figure 19.15 (A) Axial CT image from noncontrast chest CT scan demonstrates basal ground-glass opacity and reticulation consistent with nonspecific interstitial pneumonia. (B) Follow-up CT examination 2.5 years later demonstrates peripheral predominant pulmonary fibrosis characterized by reticulation, traction bronchiectasis, and early subpleural honeycombing, now much more suggestive of a usual interstitial pneumonia pattern.

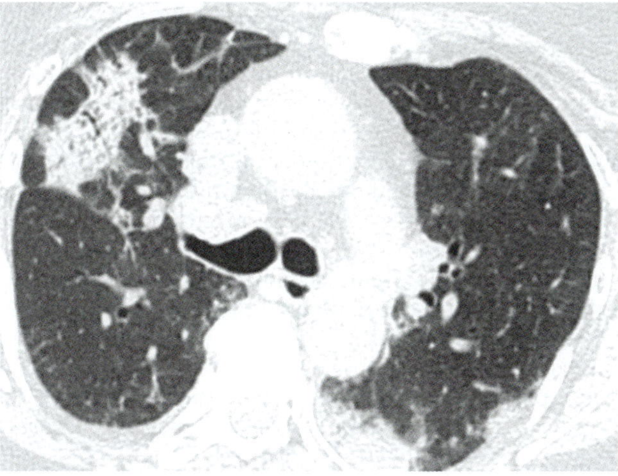

Figure 19.16 Axial image from noncontrast chest CT scan demonstrates focal consolidation within the right upper and left lower lobes consistent with organizing pneumonia.

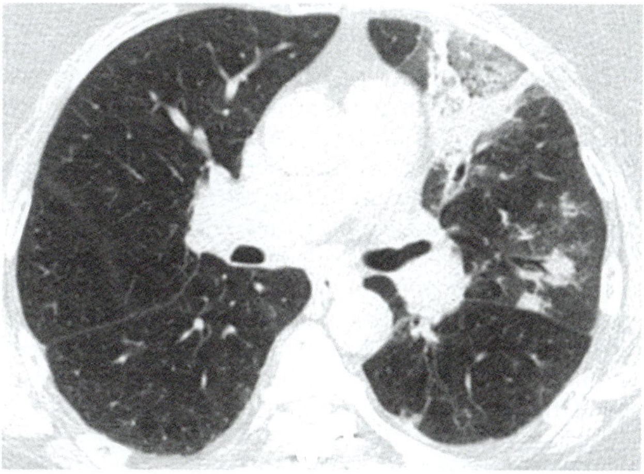

Figure 19.18 Axial image from noncontrast chest CT scan demonstrates the reversed halo sign (also referred to as the *atoll sign*) within the left upper lobe, highly suggestive of organizing pneumonia. The reversed halo sign is defined as a central focus of ground-glass opacity with a surrounding rim of consolidation.

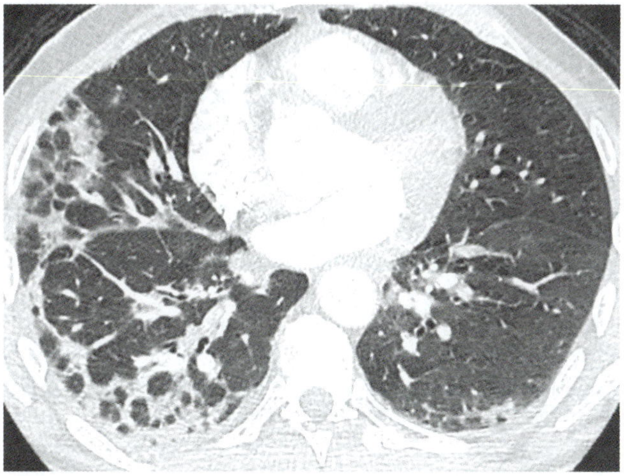

Figure 19.17 Axial image from noncontrast chest CT scan demonstrates perilobular pattern of consolidation within the right lower lobe, highly suggestive of organizing pneumonia. Organizing pneumonia was confirmed on biopsy.

Appearance on HRCT

The most common HRCT manifestation of COP is patchy bilateral consolidations, occurring in 80% to 90% of cases, with a subpleural and/or peribronchial predominance (Fig. 19.16). Ground-glass opacities are also present in most cases, usually in association with areas of consolidation. Perilobular opacities, defined as ill-defined linear opacities along the periphery of secondary pulmonary lobules, are also frequently present (Fig. 19.17). Bronchial wall thickening or dilation in the affected lung regions is commonly encountered. OP secondary to preexisting lung disease, such as pneumonia or aspiration, is often unilateral or localized to the region of previous lung disease, rather than bilateral and diffuse, as in the case of COP.

Less common findings include ill-defined centrilobular nodules, larger nodules or masses, a crazy paving pattern of ground-glass opacities with superimposed septal thickening, and central ground-glass opacity with a peripheral rim or crescent of consolidation, referred to as the *atoll sign* or *reversed halo sign* (Fig. 19.18). Although most frequently associated with COP, the reversed halo sign can also occur secondary to other conditions, such as infection, sarcoidosis, granulomatosis with polyangiitis, pulmonary infarct, and lymphomatoid granulomatosis.

Differentiating Cryptogenic Organizing Pneumonia From Chronic Eosinophilic Pneumonia

The primary differential considerations in a patient with subacute respiratory symptoms and peripheral consolidations on imaging are COP and chronic eosinophilic pneumonia (CEP). Clinically, it is not difficult to distinguish the two conditions, because most patients with CEP have asthma and peripheral eosinophilia. There are also differences in the HRCT appearances of these diseases. The consolidations in COP often demonstrate a peribronchial distribution, whereas consolidations in CEP tend to be more strictly peripheral (Fig. 19.19). Additionally, nodules are present in a significant minority of patients with COP, but rarely occur in those with CEP.

■ Acute Interstitial Pneumonia

Acute interstitial pneumonia (AIP) is a fulminant acute IIP that manifests histopathologically as diffuse alveolar damage. The histologic features of AIP are indistinguishable from those of acute respiratory distress syndrome; thus AIP is often referred to as *idiopathic acute respiratory distress syndrome*. The prognosis of AIP is poor, with most patients rapidly developing respiratory failure and dying within 6 months of presentation.

Appearance on HRCT

The HRCT appearance of AIP varies according to the time course of the disease process. In the early exudative phase of AIP, HRCT findings consist of bilateral patchy ground-glass opacities, with dependent and basilar predominant consolidations (Fig. 19.20). A crazy paving pattern of ground-glass opacities with superimposed septal thickening is also frequently seen. In the later organizing stage of AIP, HRCT typically demonstrates architectural distortion and traction bronchiectasis indicative of fibrosis (see Fig. 19.20). In chronic cases, AIP can progress to a pattern similar to that of fibrotic NSIP or even UIP with honeycombing.

■ Respiratory Bronchiolitis–Interstitial Lung Disease

Respiratory bronchiolitis (RB) is a common incidental finding in cigarette smokers. It is the most common manifestation of smoking-related lung disease. On histology, RB is characterized by numerous pigmented macrophages filling respiratory bronchioles, alveolar ducts, and alveoli. Most smokers with RB are asymptomatic. However, a small percentage of smokers with RB are symptomatic and are thus referred to as having respiratory bronchiolitis–interstitial lung disease (RB-ILD). In addition to pigmented smokers' macrophages, patients with RB-ILD typically demonstrate patchy peribronchiolar and alveolar wall inflammation on histology. When the inflammation becomes more diffuse, the condition is termed desquamative interstitial pneumonia (DIP; discussed further in the next section). RB-ILD has a good prognosis, with smoking cessation resulting in symptomatic improvement in the vast majority of cases.

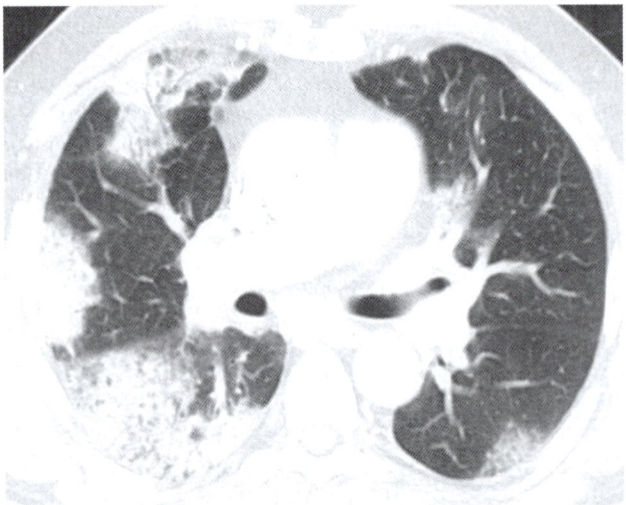

Figure 19.19 Axial image from noncontrast chest CT scan demonstrates focal areas of peripheral lung consolidation in this patient with pathologically proven chronic eosinophilic pneumonia.

Appearance on HRCT

HRCT characteristics of RB-ILD consist of patchy ground-glass opacities and ill-defined centrilobular nodules, with an upper lobe predominance (Fig. 19.21). Reticular opacities reflecting mild fibrosis are also present in a small percentage of cases. Associated findings include bronchial wall thickening and upper lobe predominant emphysema. In clinical practice, RB-ILD can be diagnosed without surgical lung biopsy based on a significant smoking history, characteristic HRCT findings, and the presence of smokers' macrophages in the bronchoalveolar lavage fluid.

Differentiating RB-ILD From Subacute HP

Both RB-ILD and subacute HP demonstrate ill-defined centrilobular nodules on HRCT. The centrilobular nodules in subacute HP are usually more diffuse than those in RB-ILD, which tend to predominate within the upper lobes. Clinical differentiation of these two diseases is typically straightforward because HP usually affects nonsmokers, whereas RB-ILD almost exclusively involves smokers.

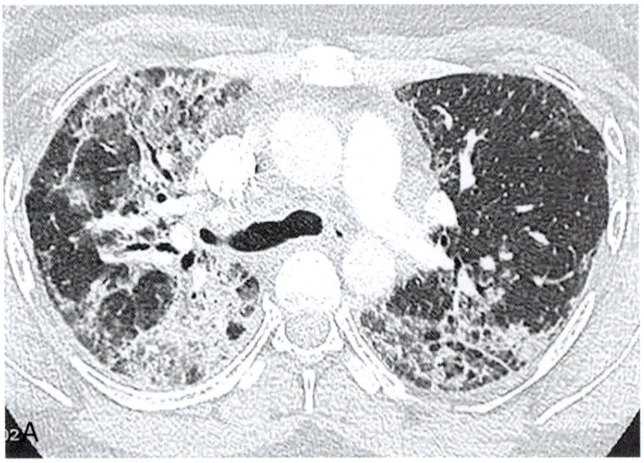

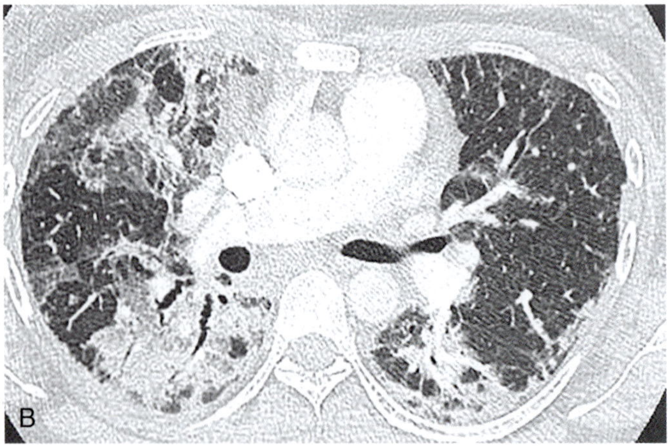

Figure 19.20 (A and B) Axial images in this contrast-enhanced chest CT demonstrate right greater than left ground-glass opacity in this patient with acute interstitial pneumonia. The presence of mild bronchiectasis within the right lower suggests early fibrosis, which is not uncommon in this setting of diffuse alveolar damage histology.

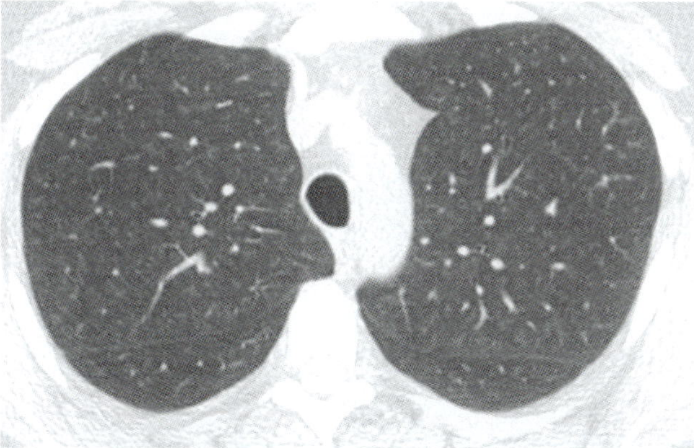

Figure 19.21 Axial image from noncontrast chest CT demonstrates diffuse centrilobular ground-glass nodularity in this patient with a long smoking history, consistent with respiratory bronchiolitis.

Desquamative Interstitial Pneumonia

As mentioned above, RB-ILD and DIP are part of the spectrum of smoking-related ILD, with histologic differentiation based on the extent and distribution of pigmented macrophage accumulation and associated peribronchiolar and alveolar wall inflammation. DIP typically demonstrates more diffuse involvement of the air spaces than RB-ILD. Interestingly, the correlation between smoking and DIP is not as strong as between smoking and RB-ILD because up to 10% of patients with DIP do not have a significant smoking history. The prognosis of DIP is poorer than that of RB-ILD, with a significant minority of patients not responding to smoking cessation and corticosteroid therapy.

Appearance on HRCT

The most common HRCT manifestation of DIP is confluent, bilateral, ground-glass opacities, with a subpleural and basal predominance (Fig. 19.22). Thin-walled, air-filled cysts—not to be confused with honeycombing—may be present within the areas of ground-glass opacity. Similar to RB-ILD, reticular opacities reflecting mild fibrosis may be seen, and centrilobular emphysema is often encountered. In patients who do not respond to therapy, the ground-glass opacities may increase and be accompanied by further signs of fibrosis, including mild honeycombing.

Differentiating DIP From RB-ILD and NSIP

DIP can be distinguished from RB-ILD on HRCT by the presence of more extensive ground-glass opacities and a lower lung predilection. Discrete centrilobular nodules are rarely visualized in DIP. However, because RB-ILD and DIP are part of the spectrum of smoking-related ILD, the distinction between these two conditions is somewhat arbitrary. In fact, RB-ILD often coexists with DIP in the same patient.

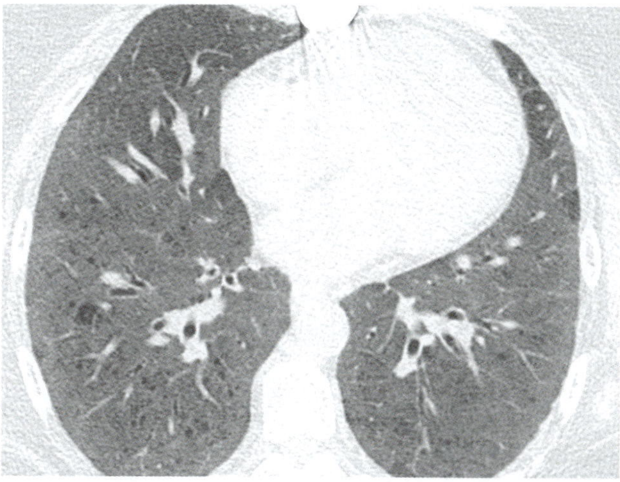

Figure 19.22 Axial image from noncontrast chest CT scan demonstrates diffuse ground-glass abnormality with superimposed small innumerable cysts. Imaging findings are highly suggestive of desquamative interstitial pneumonia in this patient with a smoking history.

The HRCT appearances of DIP and cellular NSIP are very similar, and distinction between these two entities likely relies on correlating the HRCT findings with a significant smoking history. Fibrotic NSIP, on the other hand, may be distinguished from DIP by the increased conspicuity of irregular reticular opacities and traction bronchiectasis, as well as by the presence of subpleural sparing. Unfortunately, a minority of cases of DIP may progress to a fibrotic phase, at which point differentiation of this entity from NSIP may be difficult if not impossible.

Rare Idiopathic Interstitial Pneumonias

Lymphoid Interstitial Pneumonia

Lymphoid interstitial pneumonia (LIP) is a benign lymphoproliferative disorder characterized histologically by a dense interstitial lymphoid infiltrate consisting predominantly of polyclonal lymphocytes. Most cases of LIP are secondary to other conditions, usually Sjögren syndrome (discussed elsewhere in this text). However, idiopathic LIP can rarely occur, which allows for the classification of LIP as an IIP.

HRCT characteristics of LIP include bilateral ground-glass opacities, ill-defined centrilobular nodules, subpleural nodules, interlobular septal thickening, peribronchovascular thickening, and thin-walled cysts (Figs. 19.23 and 19.24). When the lung cysts are extensive, LIP can be differentiated from other cystic lung diseases, such as lymphangioleiomyomatosis and pulmonary Langerhans cell histiocytosis, by the presence of accompanying ground-glass opacities and ill-defined centrilobular nodules, which are rare in these other entities. Moreover, the cysts in LIP are usually basilar predominant and peribronchovascular in distribution.

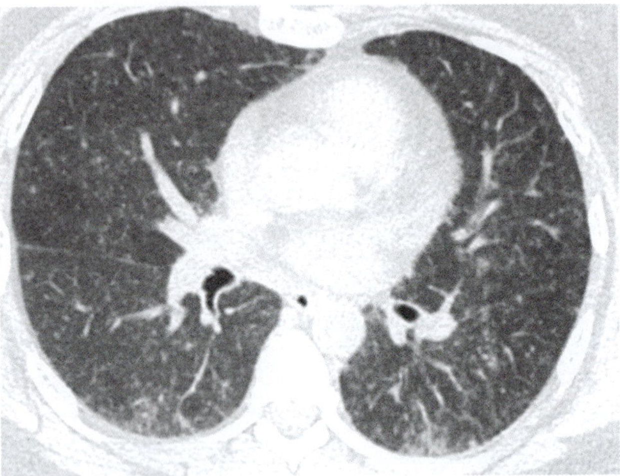

Figure 19.23 Axial image from noncontrast chest CT scan demonstrates diffuse ground-glass abnormality as well as mild micronodularity with clustering along the fissures in this patient with pathologically proven lymphoid interstitial pneumonia.

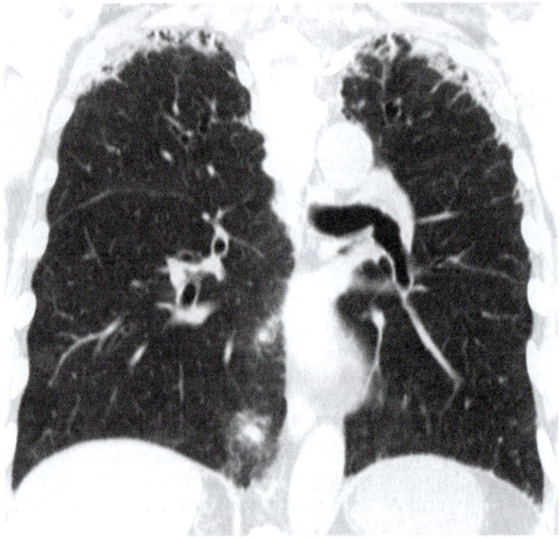

Figure 19.25 Coronal image from noncontrast chest CT scan demonstrates exuberant biapical pleural and parenchymal fibrosis in this patient with idiopathic pleuroparenchymal fibroelastosis.

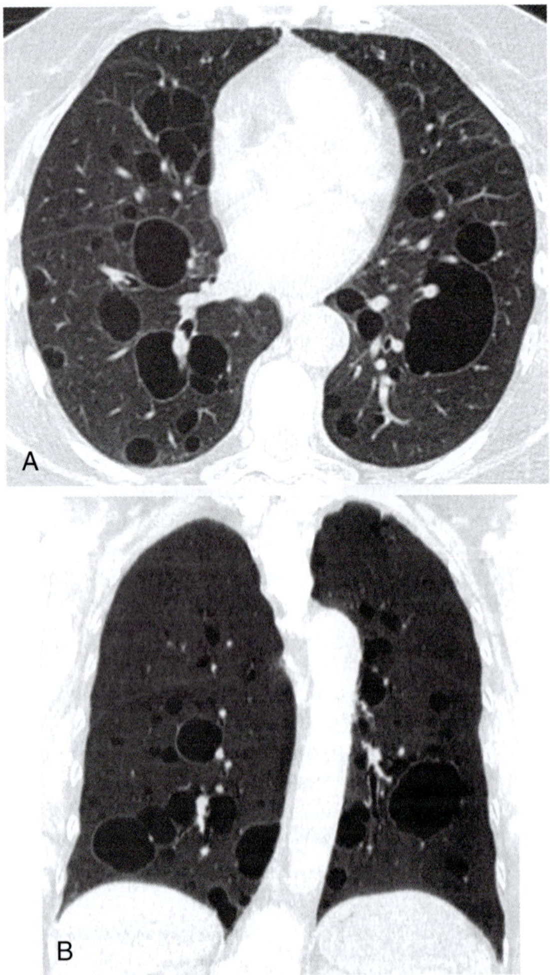

Figure 19.24 Axial (A) and minimum intensity projection coronal (B) images from noncontrast chest CT scan demonstrate bronchovascular predominant diffuse cystic lung disease consistent with lymphoid interstitial pneumonia in this patient with known Sjögren syndrome.

Pleuroparenchymal Fibroelastosis

Pleuroparenchymal fibroelastosis (PPFE) is a rare condition that was newly recognized as a distinct IIP in the 2013 revision of the American Thoracic Society–European Respiratory Society classification of the IIPs. On histology, PPFE consists of fibrosis involving the pleura and subpleural lung parenchyma, predominantly affecting the upper lobes. HRCT typically demonstrates irregular pleural thickening and dense subpleural consolidations, with associated traction bronchiectasis, architectural distortion, and upper lobe volume loss (Fig. 19.25).

Genetics of Pulmonary Fibrosis

Familial Pulmonary Fibrosis

Familial pulmonary fibrosis is defined as fibrotic lung disease, usually IPF, affecting two or more members of the same primary biologic family. Familial IPF and sporadic IPF are often histologically indistinguishable. Familial pulmonary fibrosis is likely transmitted via an autosomal dominant mechanism, although identification of responsible genes is still ongoing. Although the CT appearance of familial pulmonary fibrosis has not been well delineated, there is some evidence that suggests that those with familial pulmonary fibrosis more often have a non-UIP pattern of pulmonary fibrosis (not peripheral and basilar predominant).

Link Between Genetics and Pulmonary Fibrosis

Although millions of people are exposed to factors known to cause pulmonary fibrosis, only a small proportion of those at risk for the development of pulmonary fibrosis

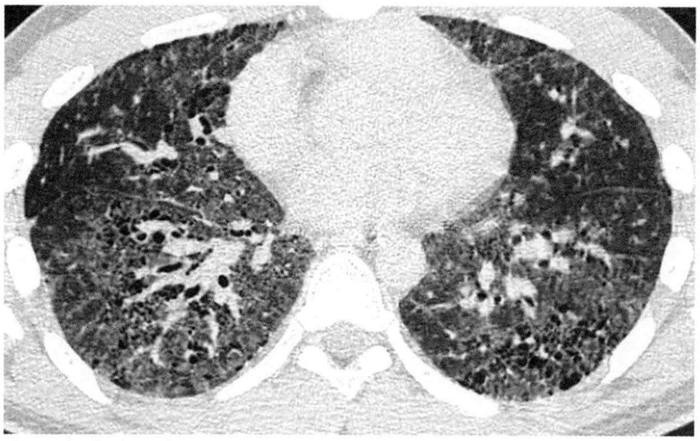

Figure 19.26 Axial image from noncontrast chest CT demonstrates mild ground-glass opacity, reticulation, and traction bronchiectasis with mild subpleural honeycombing in this patient with Hermansky-Pudlak syndrome. (Courtesy Dr. Brett W. Carter, MD Anderson Cancer Center, Houston.)

actually develop the disease. Clearly, underlying genetic factors and host susceptibility make some individuals more likely to develop pulmonary fibrosis than others. Recent research has indicated that genetic abnormalities at specific loci play a major role in the development of pulmonary fibrosis in a substantial minority of patients; some have estimated that up to 20% of pulmonary fibrosis cases may have an associated genetic component. The genetic mutation that has been most often replicated and with the highest signal in the setting of pulmonary fibrosis is the rs35705950 single-nucleotide polymorphism (SNP), a promoter site of an airway mucin gene (*MUC5B*), although many other genetic mutations have been associated with pulmonary fibrosis (e.g., surfactant protein C, surfactant protein A2, telomerase). The phenotype in the *MUC5B* mutation (dominant minor allele) is that of a UIP pattern, with peripheral and basilar preponderance. However, those with a mutation at *MUC5B* have an improved prognosis relative to those without mutation at this genetic locus.

A well-known genetic cause of pulmonary fibrosis discussed in the literature is Hermansky-Pudlak syndrome (Fig. 19.26), which is transmitted in an autosomal recessive manner. This condition has gained notoriety for its relatively high prevalence in the Puerto Rican community (especially in the northwest, where up to 1/1800 individuals are affected) as well as its typical phonotypic constellation of findings. Affected patients manifest with some combination of oculocutaneous albinism, bleeding diathesis, pulmonary fibrosis, neutropenia, and/or granulomatous colitis. The pulmonary fibrosis pattern in this condition is relatively nonspecific and is characterized by zonally diffuse and axially peripheral predominant reticulation reticulation, bronchiectasis, honeycombing, and peribronchovascular thickening.

Bibliography

Chung JH, Chawla A, Peljto AL, et al. CT scan findings of probable usual interstitial pneumonitis have a high predictive value for histologic usual interstitial pneumonitis. *Chest.* 2015;147:450–459.

Chung JH, Cox CW, Montner SM, et al. CT features of the usual interstitial pneumonia pattern: differentiating connective tissue disease-associated interstitial lung disease from idiopathic pulmonary fibrosis. *AJR Am J Roentgenol.* 2018;210:307–313.

Elliot TL, Lynch DA, Newell JD Jr, et al. High-resolution computed tomography features of nonspecific interstitial pneumonia and usual interstitial pneumonia. *J Comput Assist Tomogr.* 2005;29:339–345.

Lynch DA, Sverzellati N, Travis WD, et al. Diagnostic criteria for idiopathic pulmonary fibrosis: a Fleischner Society White Paper. *Lancet Respir Med.* 2018;6:138–153.

Raghu G, Collard HR, Egan JJ, et al. An official ATS/ERS/JRS/ALAT statement: idiopathic pulmonary fibrosis: evidence-based guidelines for diagnosis and management. *Am J Respir Crit Care Med.* 2011;183:788–824.

Raghu G, Remy-Jardin M, Myers JL, et al. Diagnosis of idiopathic pulmonary fibrosis. An official ATS/ERS/JRS/ALAT clinical practice guideline. *Am J Respir Crit Care Med.* 2018;198:e44–e68.

Richeldi L, Wilson KC, Raghu G. Diagnosing idiopathic pulmonary fibrosis in 2018: bridging recommendations made by experts serving different societies. *Eur Respir J.* 2018;52:pii1801485.

Silva CI, Muller NL, Lynch DA, et al. Chronic hypersensitivity pneumonitis: differentiation from idiopathic pulmonary fibrosis and nonspecific interstitial pneumonia by using thin-section CT. *Radiology.* 2008;246:288–297.

CHAPTER 20

Occupational and Inhalational Lung Diseases

Christian W. Cox and Lara A. Walkoff

CHAPTER OUTLINE

Introduction

In many ways, the challenges related to occupational and environmental lung disease imaging reflect the challenges for all of radiology. The best imaging interpretation relies heavily on the appropriate imaging selection for the particular indication and access to patient history and clinical evaluation. The decision between ordering chest radiography, CT, MRI, or PET can absolutely make the difference for the correct diagnosis or treatment. Knowledge of the patient's exposure history and relative timing of symptoms plays a critical role in diagnostic considerations. Table 20.1 provides a quick reference for more common occupational and environmental lung diseases seen in practice matched with the associated typical occupational or environmental setting. At other times, the occupational lung disease may have characteristic manifestations that can be incidentally recognized on studies performed for other indications. Making sure that those imaging diagnoses enter into the patient's medical history and overall care plan is important, but can be challenging. Many diagnoses require multidisciplinary coordination and interaction. Multidisciplinary conferences, ideally including the pulmonologist, occupational and environmental medicine physician, radiologist, and pathologist, provide necessary interactions to weigh the various clinical, laboratory, imaging, and pathology data appropriately, as well as determine the best course for disease surveillance and management. Finally, the radiologist's knowledge and experience in the various imaging manifestations and complications of disease contribute to the patient's appropriate workup, diagnosis, and treatment.

In other ways, the imaging of occupational and environmental lung disease presents several unique challenges. Some arise from the long history of occupational lung disease imaging. Although screening and surveillance of occupational lung disease with chest radiography have provided a wealth of knowledge about various exposures, the ongoing reliance on chest radiography for diagnosis limits imaging sensitivity for identifying subtle but real disease. Another challenge for radiology arises from the

TABLE 20.1 Occupational and Environmental Lung Diseases Matched With Common Associated Exposure Settings

DISEASE	ASSOCIATED OCCUPATIONAL OR ENVIRONMENTAL EXPOSURE
Asbestos-related disease	Shipyards, manufacturing, mining, pipe stripping, demolition
Silicosis	Foundries, sandblasting, hard rock mining, ceramics construction, stone cutting, grinding
Chronic beryllium disease	Ceramics, dentistry, aerospace industry, nuclear weapons and reactors, fluorescent light bulb manufacturing
Coal workers' pneumoconiosis	Coal mining
Hypersensitivity pneumonitis	Farming, hot tubs, avian exposures, household water damage, humidifiers, machine operators, paint refinishers

success of mitigating occupational lung diseases in developed nations. Strict government oversight of workplace environment and public awareness of environmental exposures have decreased some inhalational lung diseases in the developed nations, but a highly mobile world population and constant immigration results in the sporadic presentation of unexpected occupational and environmental lung diseases to all radiology practices. Finally, the constant evolution of industrial practices and environmental conditions challenges the radiologist by causing an ongoing broadening of occupational and environmental lung disease while reintroducing well-known pneumoconioses in new settings.

Imaging Modalities

Imaging plays a key role in the screening, diagnosis, surveillance, and management of occupational and environmental lung diseases. The most commonly used modalities include chest radiography (often used as a screening tool) and chest CT. Chest CT is critical for the diagnosis, surveillance, and management of symptomatic patients with an occupational exposure history, as well as for patients with a known pneumoconiosis. CT is the primary modality used to evaluate the type of involvement, extent of involvement, and pulmonary complications of occupational and environmental exposures. For example, chest CT is useful for following the progression of fibrosis and evaluating for potential bronchogenic carcinoma because there is a well-established causal relationship between several of the pneumoconioses and pulmonary malignancy. In most cases, the greater the exposure, the higher the risk of malignancy. Bronchogenic carcinoma is estimated to develop in 20% to 25% of asbestos workers with heavy exposure. Many individuals affected by occupational and environmental lung diseases also smoke tobacco products. Tobacco smoke and asbestos exposure together carry an increased risk of malignancy that is synergistic in increasing the risk of developing lung cancer. Studies have demonstrated a 92-fold or greater increase in lung cancer risk when exposed to both tobacco smoke and asbestos compared to individuals exposed to neither substance. Also, the reported typical latency period for complications of pneumoconioses ranges between 10 and 40 years, so ongoing imaging at regular intervals can be common.

Patients Who Need Radiologic Screening

No well-defined screening guidelines exist for pneumoconioses, and protocols vary by type of exposure and organization. In summary, anyone with respiratory symptoms and/or a significant exposure history could benefit from imaging. The National Institute for Occupational Safety and Health (NIOSH) administers a free voluntary medical screening that must be offered to coal mine workers by their employers as part of the Coal Workers' Health Surveillance Program. A component of this medical screening consists of a baseline radiograph, subsequent radiographs 3 years later, and, if abnormalities are detected, 2 years later. The Agency for Toxic Substances and Disease Registry (ATSDR) endorses a chest radiograph as a first-line screening for asbestos-related lung disease. If the radiograph is abnormal or inconclusive, and there is an exposure history, a repeat radiograph in subsequent years is recommended. Lateral and/or oblique radiographs are recommended for pleural changes. The ATSDR does not propose chest CT as a screening tool. CT is only advocated in situations in which pulmonary function test results suggest disease without corresponding radiographic abnormality or in cases of indeterminate findings on a chest radiograph. The ATSDR also notes that CT may assist in differentiating pleural plaques from soft tissue densities and cancer from round atelectasis when findings are indeterminate on chest radiograph.

Determining Which Imaging Techniques and Protocols Are Best

For decades, chest radiography has been the primary screening tool for occupational and environmental lung diseases in the United States and worldwide. The advantages of a chest radiograph include low cost, low radiation dose, and availability. Unfortunately, it has been well established that chest radiographs are insensitive for the detection of pneumoconioses, especially the early changes of occupational lung diseases and ground-glass opacities. As many as 10% to 15% of patients with proven asbestosis have normal chest radiographs. In addition to being insensitive, abnormalities demonstrated on chest radiographs are also nonspecific. For example, cigarette smoking can result in many of the same radiographic abnormalities as occupational lung diseases.

Numerous studies have demonstrated that CT is more sensitive for the detection and classification of pulmonary abnormalities associated with occupational and environmental lung disease; however, it is also more costly and confers a higher radiation dose. The most appropriate CT imaging protocol includes image acquisition in both the prone and supine positions, which can be beneficial in differentiating between basilar fibrosis and atelectasis. Likewise, obtaining images in both the inspiratory and expiratory phases of the respiratory cycle can provide evidence of air trapping and small airway disease.

The National Lung Screening Trial (NLST) demonstrated that low dose high-resolution CT (HRCT) decreases mortality from lung cancer in high-risk individuals (smokers and former smokers), although this study did not specifically investigate populations with occupational and environmental exposures. Research has suggested the benefit of screening asbestos-exposed, high-risk individuals with low-dose CT, but more investigation will be required before formal recommendations can be outlined.

Similar to the International Labor Organization (ILO) classification system for radiographs, grading systems for screening HRCT for occupational lung disease have been proposed. A CT classification system would provide a standardized method for evaluating CT images in occupational and environmental lung disease in a systematic, semiquantitative, and reproducible way. In one study in which such a system was used, reliability (as measured by interreader agreement) was deemed satisfactory. Although this type of classification system has been discussed, it has not been verified on a large scale and is not currently in widespread use.

New image reconstruction techniques have also allowed for ultralow-dose CT scans that have comparable sensitivity to standard radiation dose CT scans in detection of asbestos-related diseases. Some of these ultralow-dose CT scans have radiation doses comparable to a two-view chest radiograph. Ultralow-dose CT potentially has a future role in pneumoconiosis screening but has not yet been validated. The sensitivity for the detection of other pneumoconioses other than asbestos-related disease remains unknown. As an example, Fig. 20.1 demonstrates a case of unsuspected subtle asbestos-related pleural disease identified by low-dose lung cancer screening CT.

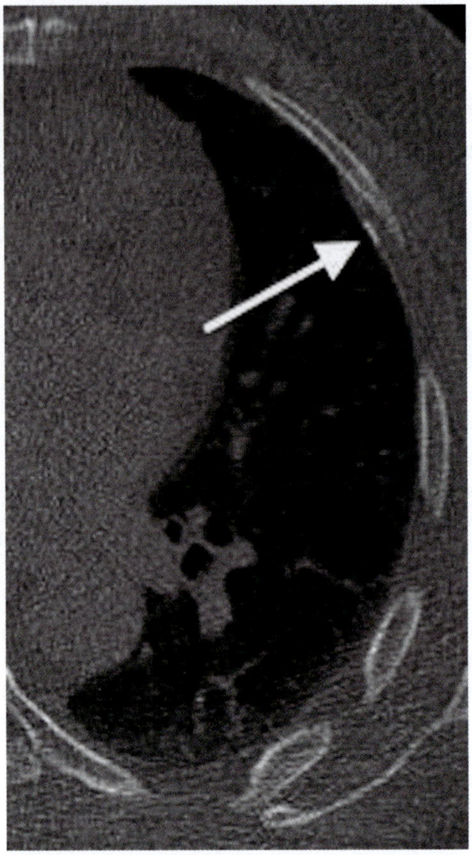

Figure 20.1 Partially calcified asbestos-related pleural plaques *(arrow)* were present bilaterally on lung cancer screening on a low-dose chest CT scan in a 72-year-old man with a 50 to 70 pack-year history of smoking and no known significant asbestos exposure.

International Labor Organization Classification of Radiographs

The ILO classification system for radiographs was designed over 60 years ago for the purposes of codifying radiographic abnormalities of pneumoconioses in a simple, reproducible manner for statistical, research, and epidemiologic purposes. It classifies abnormalities based on posteroanterior chest radiograph appearance only. The grading is based on comparison to a set of standard radiographs. Criteria for grading include technical quality, parenchymal abnormalities, pleural abnormalities, and additional abnormalities. Parenchymal abnormalities include opacity type, profusion (the number of small rounded or irregular opacities, which are further subclassified), and extent. The interpreter is instructed not to consider any additional information (e.g., exposure history) when determining the classification. In 2011 the ILO released a classification system for digital radiographs that allows for side-by-side comparison of standards with the current examination on a digital workstation. Not only are digital radiographs more accurate for the classification of abnormalities, they also have the added benefit of reduced radiation dose when compared with conventional radiographs.

Unfortunately, the ILO classification has limitations, including the lack of specificity. An abnormal classification does not necessarily indicate lung disease or the presence of pneumoconiosis, and approximately 5% of patients with an "abnormal" classification have not had any occupational exposure.

A and B Readers

The ILO conducts a course and examination for physicians using the ILO classification system. Trained readers have demonstrated less interobserver variability in classification compared with untrained physicians. It designates the terms *A reader* for a physician who has completed the ILO course and *B reader* for one who has passed the accompanying examination. B readers must be recertified every 4 years to maintain B reader status.

Imaging Occupational and Environmental Lung Diseases

Role of PET/CT

The role of PET/CT is somewhat controversial. Several studies have demonstrated that PET/CT can be helpful in distinguishing benign and malignant imaging features. For example, atypical round atelectasis and pleural plaques, which could be equivocal for malignancy on

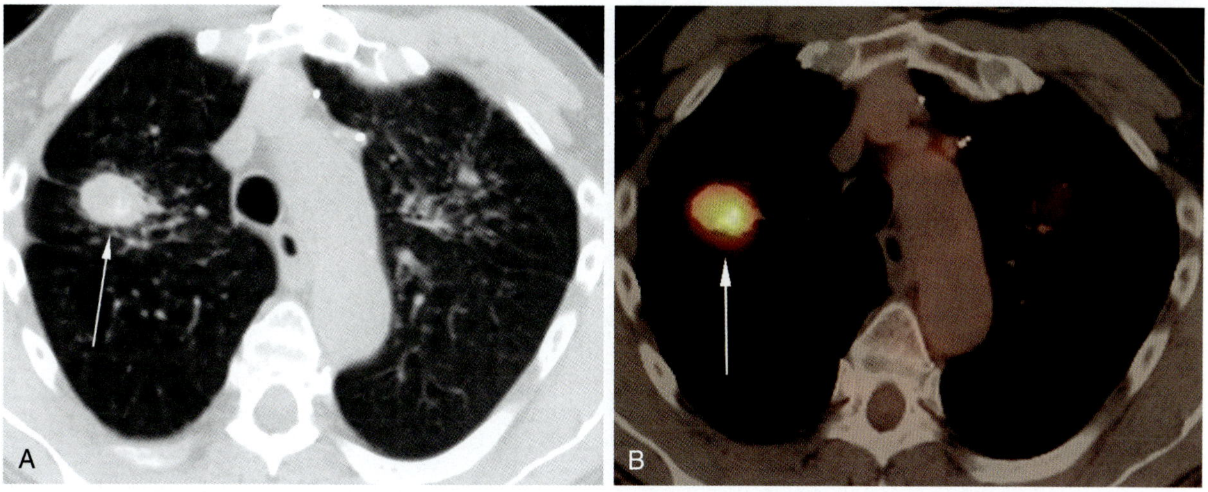

Figure 20.2 Progressive massive fibrosis in a 75-year-old man with a history of hard rock mining. (A) On CT, a unilateral right upper lobe conglomerate mass is present *(arrow)*, with subtle central calcification on a background of silicotic nodules. (B) Subsequent fused PET/CT image demonstrates associated increased FDG uptake (standard uptake value = 7.3) within the mass *(arrow)*, which remained stable for 3 years, consistent with progressive massive fibrosis. Although FDG uptake is a concerning feature, benign lesions can also be metabolically active.

CT, are not usually fluorodeoxyglucose (FDG)-avid on PET/CT, whereas malignancy characteristically is FDG-avid. Additionally, there have been case reports of the utility of PET/CT in distinguishing progressive massive fibrosis from pulmonary malignancy. However, there have also been reports to the contrary, with cases of FDG-avid, nonmalignant lung nodules in patients with pneumoconioses (Fig. 20.2). The potential role of PET/CT in the distinction of intrapulmonary malignancy from changes associated with occupational and environmental lung diseases is in the process of being elucidated. PET/CT plays an important role in increasing the conspicuity of nodal and extrathoracic metastases in patients with known malignancy and in cases of suspected recurrent mesothelioma, where PET/CT has been shown to be more specific than contrast-enhanced CT.

Role of MRI

At this time, MRI does not have an established role in the imaging algorithm for the workup of occupational and environmental lung diseases. Some research has suggested that MRI is equally as or more sensitive than CT in detecting malignancy in the setting of asbestos-related pleural disease. Although MRI has the benefit of no ionizing radiation, which can be a concern in individuals who require serial follow-up CT examinations, it is much more costly, time-consuming, and usually not as accessible.

Imaging Approach

Role of the Radiologist

Radiologists play an instrumental role in the diagnosis, surveillance, and management of individuals with suspected occupational and environmental lung diseases. Imaging is one component of a multidisciplinary effort in diagnosis and treatment. In addition to imaging, a workup usually includes detailed medical, exposure, and occupational histories (including a smoking history), physical examination, and pulmonary function tests. Radiologists also have the opportunity to add value in cases where an occupational and environmental lung disease was not initially suspected and may suggest this cause in the differential diagnosis. With the increased use of HRCT and ever-expanding insights into the patterns of pulmonary disease, such an occurrence is becoming more commonplace.

Consideration of Occupational and Environmental Lung Diseases

Many occupational and environmental lung diseases can present with imaging features that overlap with other entities, so it is important that they be considered, regardless of exposure history. Pneumonoconioses can share imaging features with hypersensitivity pneumonitis (HP), organizing pneumonia, usual interstitial pneumonia (UIP), nonspecific interstitial pneumonia (NSIP), and sarcoidosis. For example, many cases of pulmonary sarcoidosis can appear similar to chronic beryllium disease (CBD). A case series of patients initially diagnosed with sarcoidosis demonstrated CBD in over one-third of cases on re-review. Thus when sarcoidosis is suggested, CBD should at least be considered as a diagnostic possibility.

Asbestos-Related Disease

Relying on a Clinical History of Exposure

A provided indication of asbestos exposure for an imaging study is the exception rather than the rule, with most cases of asbestos-related pleural disease being recognized incidentally on a chest radiograph or CT scan.

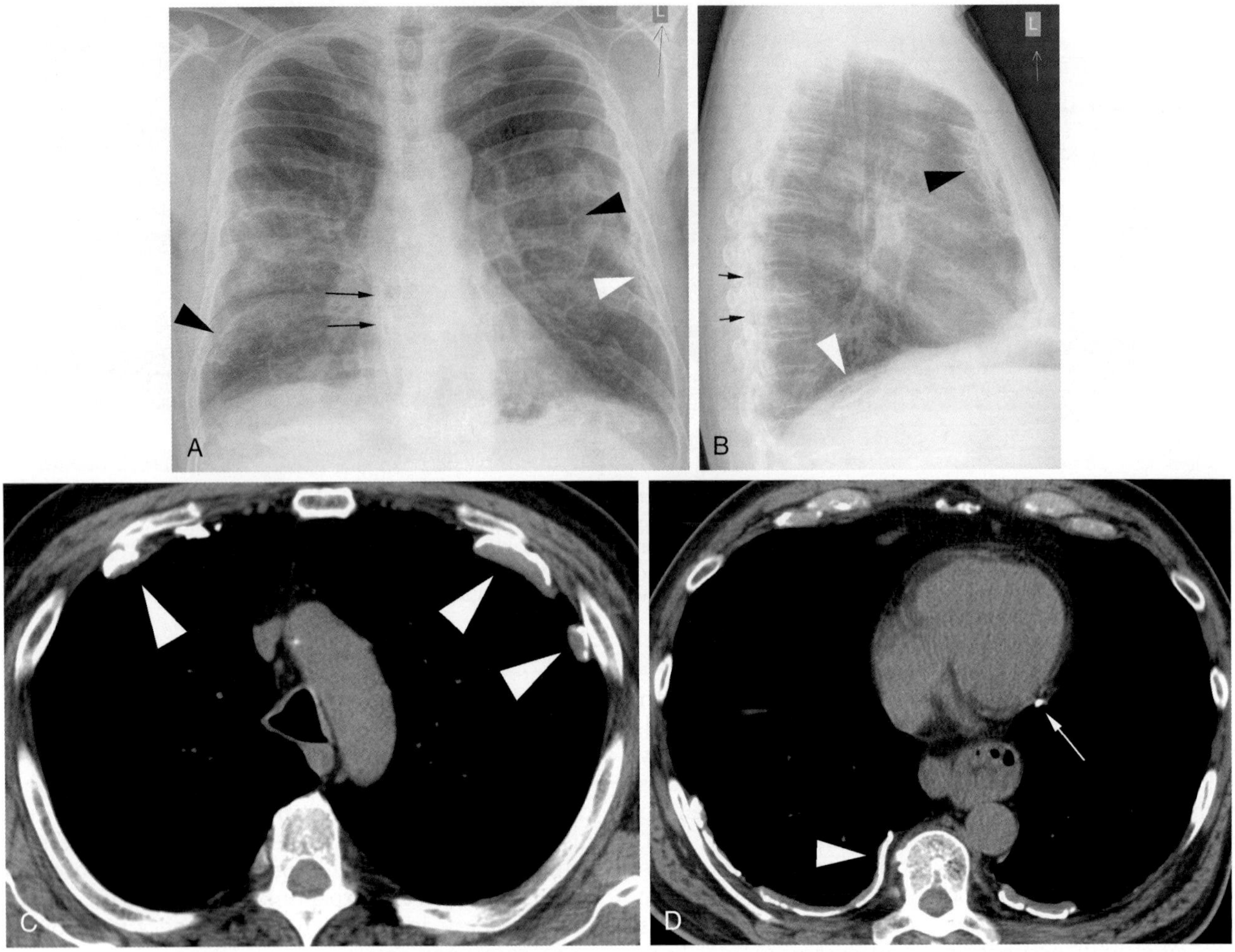

Figure 20.3 Asbestos-related pleural disease in a 74-year-old man. (A) Frontal chest radiograph demonstrates extensive en face pleural plaques. The undulating borders *(black arrowheads)* produce the classic holly leaf appearance. Pleural plaques in profile are seen along the lateral lungs *(white arrowheads)* and along the mediastinum *(black arrows)*. (B) Lateral chest radiograph better demonstrates the characteristic appearance of calcified plaques in profile along the anterolateral upper lobes *(black arrowhead)* and posterior lower lobes *(black arrows)*. In profile, plaques are also seen along the diaphragms *(white arrowhead)*. Selected chest CT in mediastinal window in the same patient reveals anterior plaques underlying ribs (C) and plaques along the posterior lung *(white arrowheads)* and mediastinum *(white arrow)* in (D).

Pleural plaques are the most common imaging abnormality associated with asbestos exposure. The characteristic findings are bilateral calcified pleural plaques, predominantly along the anterolateral upper lobes, posterior and diaphragmatic lower lobes, and mediastinum. Usually, asbestos-related pleural plaques overlie the ribs and involve the parietal pleural; however, visceral pleural thickening does occur and is associated with round atelectasis or an abnormality in the underlying lung parenchyma. The well-defined undulating contour of the pleural plaque has been said to bear a resemblance to a holly leaf when viewed en face on a posteroanterior chest radiograph (Fig. 20.3). Calcification within the plaques is identified on 10% to 15% of chest radiographs and is more common with increasing chronicity of pleural disease. Along the diaphragm, pleural plaques have a plateau appearance that may help differentiate plaques from eventration of the diaphragm.

At other times, asbestos-related pleural disease is subtle and can overlap in radiographic appearance with other thoracic abnormalities. For example, en face anterior pleural plaques may mimic a pulmonary nodule and can be assigned greater concern than necessary if additional evidence of pleural disease is not recognized. Alternatively, normal extrapleural fat has the potential to be mistaken for pleural plaque on a chest radiograph.

Just as in asbestos-related pleural disease, asbestosis on chest CT is often found in the absence of reported asbestos exposure. Asbestosis is the development of fibrosing interstitial pneumonia secondary to the inhalation of asbestos fibers. Almost all patients who develop asbestosis have associated pleural disease on HRCT. The severity of the asbestosis is directly related to the dose of asbestos exposure. Like many occupational lung diseases, the diagnosis is usually based on a combination of findings, including imaging appearance, pulmonary function tests, physical examination, and exposure history.

Chest radiograph findings associated with asbestosis include fine, irregular linear or reticular opacities with a basilar predilection. As the fibrosis progresses an

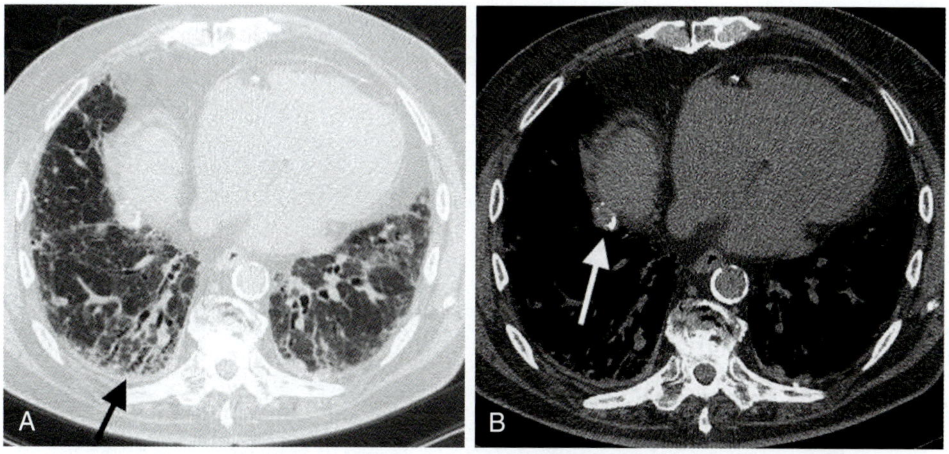

Figure 20.4 Asbestosis on chest CT. (A) Lung window demonstrates basilar peripheral predominant reticular opacities, with peripheral traction bronchiolectasis *(black arrow)* in the right lower lobe. (B) Mediastinal window at the same level reveals a calcified pleural plaque along the right hemidiaphragm *(white arrow)*.

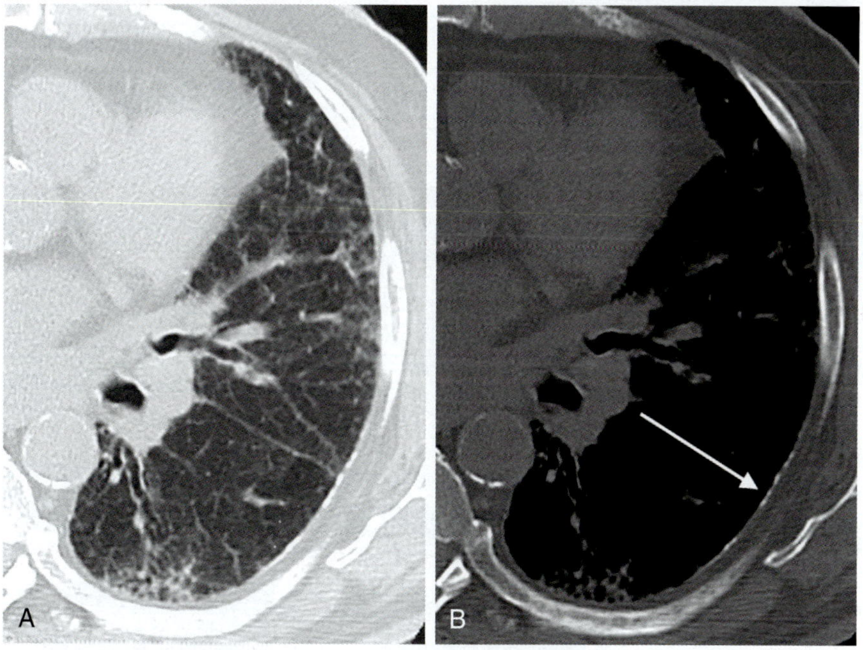

Figure 20.5 Fibrosing interstitial pneumonia with possible usual interstitial pneumonia pattern. (A) High-resolution CT chest image in lung window demonstrates patchy, peripheral, coarse reticular opacities greatest along the posterior left lower lobe. (B) When the contrast window level and width are adjusted for calcification (close to the bone window), the thin bands of pleural calcification *(arrow)* seen bilaterally become more apparent and confirm asbestosis as the cause of pulmonary fibrosis.

irregular shaggy appearance of the cardiomediastinal silhouette and diaphragm may be noted. Chest radiography is insensitive for the detection of asbestosis, especially early findings, and it is estimated that from 60% to 80% of patients with evidence of asbestosis on HRCT will have a normal chest radiograph.

Asbestosis manifests on HRCT as a fibrosing interstitial pneumonia. The appearance is not specific, however, but when present in the setting of pleural plaques, it strongly suggests asbestosis (Fig. 20.4). Fibrosis has a predilection for the peripheral lower lobes. Other characteristic findings include subpleural dotlike opacities, curvilinear subpleural lines, interlobular septal thickening, traction bronchiectasis, parenchymal bands, and honeycombing. The curvilinear subpleural lines are one of the earliest manifestations of asbestosis. Honeycombing is a feature of late-stage disease, although is not present in most cases.

Therefore, even in the absence of known asbestos exposure, every case of fibrosing interstitial pneumonia needs to be closely inspected for evidence of asbestos-related pleural disease to direct the clinical workup toward asbestosis. These pleural plaques can be very subtle, with only focal thickening or minimal calcification along the bilateral pleura, and may require manually adjusting the CT contrast window level and width for best visualization (Fig. 20.5). Recognizing the CT findings of asbestos exposure can obviate the need for lung biopsy in otherwise indeterminate cases. In contrast, unilateral pleural calcification has a differential diagnosis and does not necessarily indicate the presence of asbestosis in the setting of pulmonary fibrosis.

Length of the Latency Period for Asbestos-Related Pleural and Lung Diseases

The official 2004 statement of the American Thoracic Society, "Diagnosis and Initial Management of Nonmalignant Disease Related to Asbestos," stated that asbestos-related pleural plaques are "rare within 20 years" of exposure. Additionally, the statement noted that "Chronic

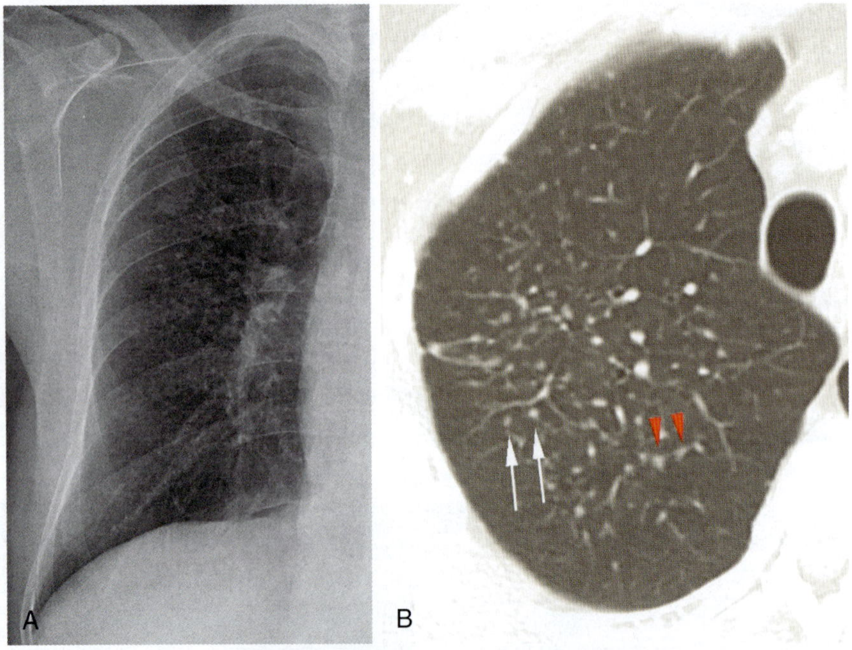

Figure 20.6 Simple silicosis in a 71-year-old miner. (A) Nodular pattern on chest radiograph with upper lobe predominance. (B) The following CT scan in the lung window demonstrates upper lobe nodularity, which is primarily centrilobular *(white arrows)* but does have some perilymphatic nodules studding a septum *(red arrowheads)*.

severe pleuritic pain is rare with asbestos-related pleural disease." More recent literature covering asbestos exposure in the mining of vermiculite in Libby, Montana, however, has redefined the expected behavior of asbestos-related pleural disease. In 2010, Larson et al. published a retrospective study of imaging changes in workers exposed to Libby amphibole, a unique mixture of asbestiform amphibole found in Libby, Montana. Radiographs of workers over time revealed a shorter latency period for circumscribed pleural plaques, with a median of 8.6 years. Consequently, imaging of some individuals in their late 20s and early 30s demonstrated pleural disease. Likewise, Black et al. described five example cases to illustrate the earlier and more aggressive manifestation of pleural disease with exposure to Libby amphibole. Each patient experienced rapid deterioration of pulmonary function in the setting of aggressive pleural disease and severe chest pain.

Pleural effusions in the setting of asbestos exposure are less common than pleural plaques, but are typically one of the earliest radiographic manifestations, presenting within 10 years of exposure. On the other hand, asbestosis generally presents 10 to 20 years after exposure, and mesothelioma can have a latency period of over 40 years.

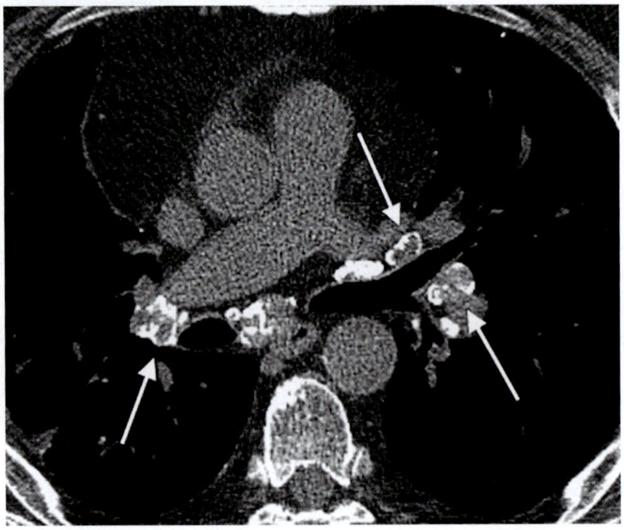

Figure 20.7 Eggshell calcification of bilateral hilar lymph nodes *(arrows)* with additional calcified mediastinal lymph nodes on chest CT in silicosis. This patient also happened to have rheumatoid arthritis in the setting of Caplan syndrome.

Silicosis and Coal Workers' Pneumoconiosis

Classifying Silicosis and Coal Workers' Pneumoconiosis

In general, silicosis and coal workers' pneumoconiosis (CWP) are divided into simple and complicated forms differentiated by the presence of pulmonary fibrosis. In the simple form, silicosis and CWP produce a similar upper lobe predominant nodular pattern on chest radiography and CT (Fig. 20.6). Chest CT better demonstrates the earlier centrilobular distribution of upper lobe nodularity, which may appear more perilymphatic as the disease progresses. Patients with these pneumoconioses often develop mediastinal and hilar lymphadenopathy, which may or may not calcify. An eggshell pattern of intrathoracic lymph node calcification (Fig. 20.7) is characteristic but not pathognomonic, and alternative patterns of lymph node calcification may be seen.

As disease severity progresses, complicated silicosis or CWP develops, with pulmonary fibrosis. Generally, upper lobe nodularity begins to coalesce until conglomerate masses form, called *progressive massive fibrosis*, as shown in Fig. 20.8. Radiographically, the hila retract superiorly secondary to upper lobe volume loss, often with characteristic posterior upper lobe masslike opacities on lateral chest radiographs. Chest CT scans also demonstrate upper

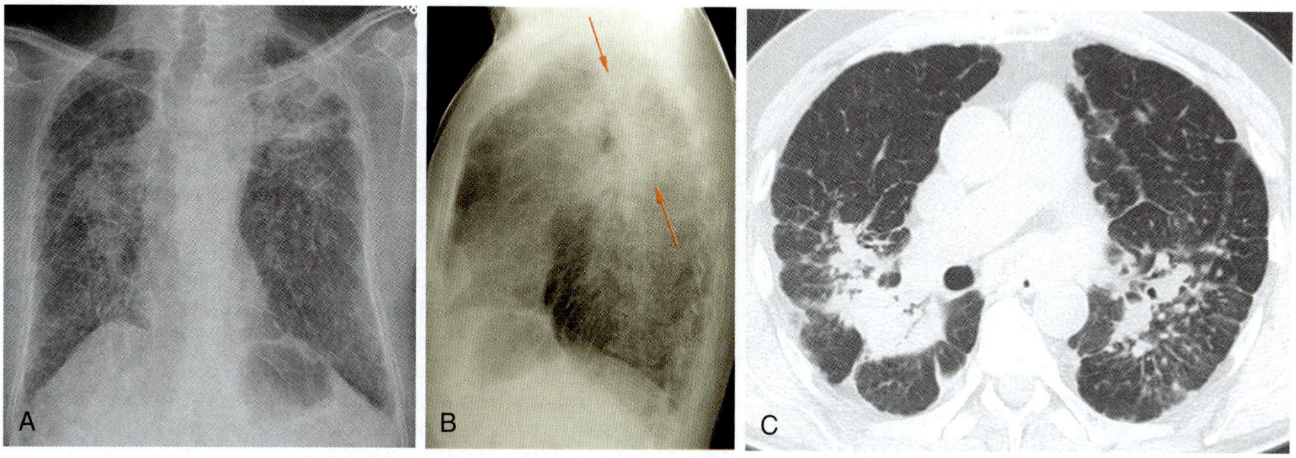

Figure 20.8 Progressive massive fibrosis from silicosis: 69-year-old miner with conglomerate fibrosis in the posterior upper lobes on frontal (A) and lateral (B) chest radiographs *(arrows)*. Note the superior hilar retraction on the frontal view from the upper lobe volume loss. (C) Chest CT in lung window on the same patient demonstrates the degree of architectural distortion associated with the posterior upper lobe progressive massive fibrosis.

lobe masslike fibrosis, commonly with a characteristic posterior upper lobe swirled appearance. When signs and symptoms of simple or complicated silicosis manifest less than 10 years from exposure, the disease is referred to as *accelerated*.

Finally, heavy dust exposure may produce acute silicosis or silicoproteinosis. In this setting, patients present in less than 4 years following exposure with evidence of centrilobular nodularity, ground-glass opacities, consolidations, and/or crazy paving on medical imaging. Acute silicosis almost invariably results in fulminant disease, with rapid deterioration, respiratory failure, and potentially death.

Effect of Regulation of Workplace Air Quality on Silicosis and Coal Workers' Pneumoconiosis

Several specific work populations have demonstrated a significant risk for pneumoconiosis, despite the well-known risk of disease in the setting of dust exposure. As particular countries legislate more extensive regulation of workplace exposures, risky industrial practices may be "exported" to less regulated countries. In Turkey, workers were exposed to high levels of silica dust exposure related to denim sandblasting, with little or no significant respiratory protection. The substantial dust load often resulted in accelerated or acute silicosis. Many of these denim-sandblasting workers subsequently developed end-stage lung disease by their 20s with reported deaths from respiratory failure as early as 18 years of age. In a 4-year follow-up study of patients, almost 96% of the sandblasters available for reimaging demonstrated evidence of silicosis on radiographs.

Even developed nations have reported new groups at risk for silicosis. Spanish workers installing quartz conglomerate countertops in private residences experienced an outbreak of silicosis related to quartz cutting without adequate respiratory precautions. Many of the affected workers presented with symptoms requiring CT for definitive characterization as silicosis. In the United States, similar cases have been described in tile cutting in private residences. Also in the United States, studies following US cases of CWP have identified a recent relative increase in pneumoconiosis to include an increase in the number of progressive massive fibrosis cases, despite regulations limiting dust levels below specific standards.

■ Chronic Beryllium Disease

Differentiating Chronic Beryllium Disease From Other Pneumoconioses

Like silicosis and CWP, chronic beryllium disease (CBD) arises in the setting of respirable dust exposure, but unlike the others, CBD is dependent on individual susceptibility rather than on the quantity of dust exposure. The desk worker at the nuclear plant may develop CBD, whereas individuals working directly with alloys containing beryllium may not. Therefore any symptomatic worker in industries related to beryllium exposure (see Table 20.1) should be screened for potential CBD. The immunologic component of disease results in a useful diagnostic test for CBD, the beryllium lymphocyte proliferation test, and, with a positive test result, together with an appropriate exposure history and medical imaging findings, a confident diagnosis of CBD can be made.

The thoracic imaging and pathologic appearance of CBD is usually identical to that of sarcoidosis, and, as stated above, a significant number of individuals diagnosed with sarcoidosis may be reclassified as having CBD when a complete exposure history and beryllium proliferation test are obtained. As such, the imaging findings of CBD include an upper lobe nodularity with perilymphatic distribution that may coalesce into conglomerate masses. Additionally, symmetric hilar and mediastinal lymphadenopathy, with or without calcification, may be present (Fig. 20.9). In a minority of cases, CBD may manifest similarly to HP on imaging, demonstrating more ground-glass abnormality than nodularity.

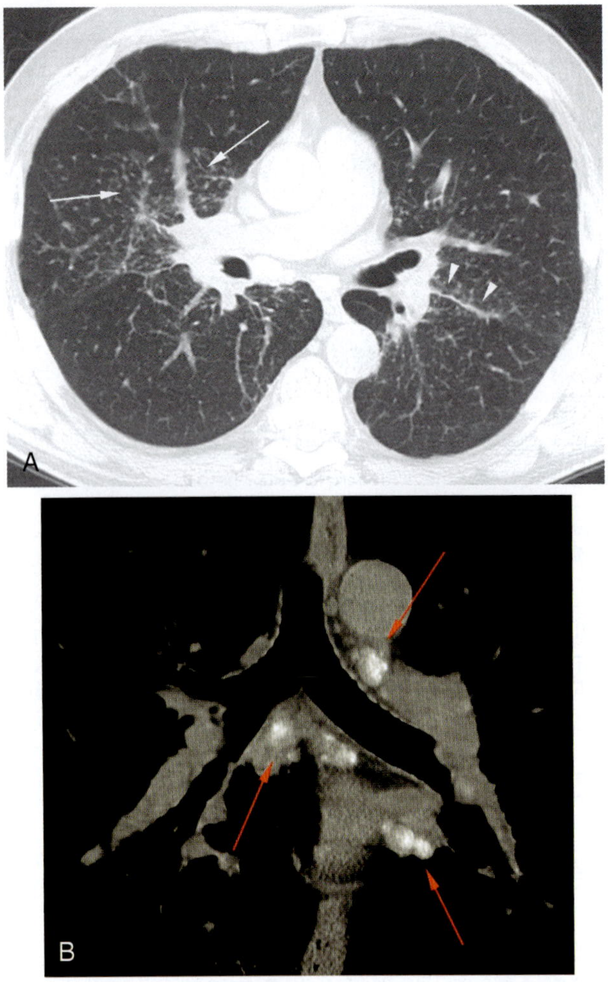

Figure 20.9 Chronic beryllium disease in a 68-year-old nuclear power plant worker. (A) Axial chest CT image in lung window shows characteristic perilymphatic nodularity to include studding of the bronchovascular bundle *(white arrows)* and left fissure *(white arrowheads)* identical to sarcoidosis. (B) When reconstructed in the coronal plane and soft tissue window, the typical amorphous calcified lymph nodes in the mediastinum and hila are seen *(red arrows)*.

Hypersensitivity Pneumonitis

Excluding Hypersensitivity Pneumonitis if No Clear Exposure Is Identified

Unfortunately, up to 50% of patients with HP will not have a clear cause. As listed in Table 20.1, many potential occupational and environmental exposures can result in HP, but the most common exposures can be linked to bird antigens, mycobacteria, fungus, or molds. Some less common exposures include chemicals such as isocyanate paints or plastics, animals such as rodents, and plants such as soybeans or coffee.

Although a history of being a pigeon breeder certainly helps narrow the differential diagnosis during imaging interpretation, the imaging characteristics play an equally important role. HP produces a combination of pneumonitis and cellular bronchiolitis, which results in CT findings of poorly defined centrilobular nodularity, ground-glass opacities, mosaic attenuation, and air trapping. Commonly, several or all of these findings may be present. For example, mixed ground-glass opacity and mosaic attenuation interspersed between regions of normal lung comprises the so-called head cheese sign and is characteristic, but not pathognomonic, of HP. Occasionally, the affected patient may present in a more acute setting, in which patchy areas of consolidation and ground-glass opacity similar to noncardiogenic pulmonary edema may be seen on a radiograph or CT scan. When pulmonary fibrosis develops, HP is characterized as chronic. Studies of chronic HP have revealed a common pattern of midlung and upper lung predominant pulmonary fibrosis, although fibrosis can be basilar and mimic a UIP pattern (Fig. 20.10). In these cases, mosaic attenuation and air trapping can be an important differentiating feature suggesting HP. In fact, air trapping in three or more lobes is inconsistent with a UIP pattern by the American Thoracic Society, European Respiratory Society, Japanese Respiratory Society, and Latin American Thoracic Association criteria because this finding is significantly related to the presence of HP. This emphasizes that a complete CT evaluation of fibrosing interstitial pneumonia includes inspiratory and expiratory series. Additional CT findings in the setting of HP include emphysema and scattered cysts.

The greatest challenge in the diagnosis of HP occurs when there is discordance between clinical, imaging, and pathologic findings, or no particularly characteristic finding is present on any test. Idiopathic pulmonary fibrosis and sarcoidosis are common competing diagnoses in these situations, and multidisciplinary discussions are critical to determine ongoing patient workup and care and to avoid contradictory and confusing communication with the patient.

Less Common Occupational Exposures

Similarity of Imaging Patterns of Occupational and Environmental Lung Diseases

Many of the occupational and environmental lung diseases present with similar imaging patterns to those already described. For example, stannosis (tin oxide), talcosis (inhaled), and siderosis (iron; Fig. 20.11) all overlap with imaging findings of silicosis and CWP, demonstrating upper lobe predominant nodularity. Other newly recognized exposures such as humidifier detergent lung and dug well lung are actually forms of HP.

Other new or less common occupational and environmental lung diseases can manifest the full gamut of possible imaging appearances. Ardystil syndrome resulting from aerosolized ink causes organizing pneumonia, with areas of consolidation on CT. Flavor workers' lung secondary to artificial flavoring added to popcorn causes obliterative bronchiolitis, with mosaic attenuation and air trapping found on CT. Some exposures, such as indium–tin oxide, hard metal, and flock, can have more complicated and less specific CT patterns that include ground-glass opacities, poorly defined nodules, and fibrosis. Therefore occupational and environmental lung

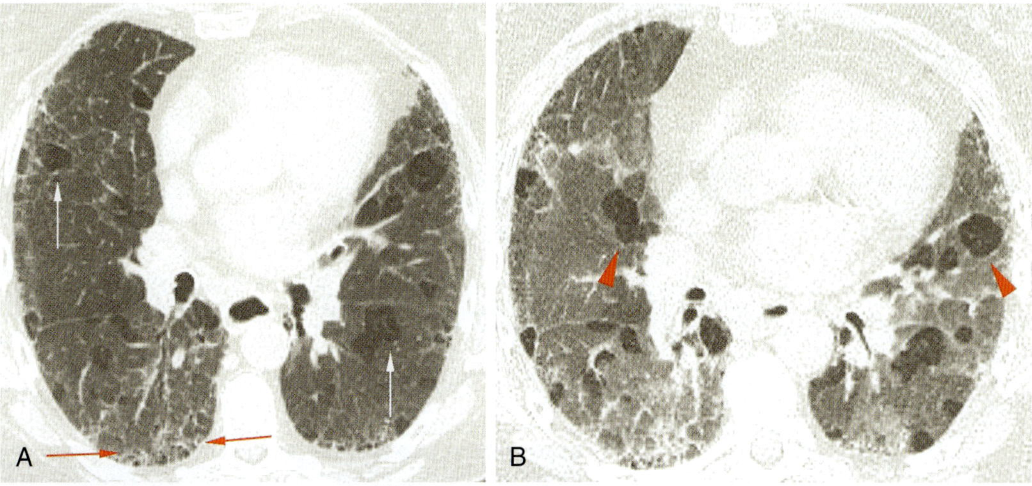

Figure 20.10 Lower lobe predominant fibrosis *(red arrows)* in hypersensitivity pneumonitis in a 68-year-old woman with multiple birds at home. (A) Note the characteristic lobular mosaic attenuation *(white arrows)* on inspiratory imaging and air trapping *(red arrowheads)* on expiratory imaging (B).

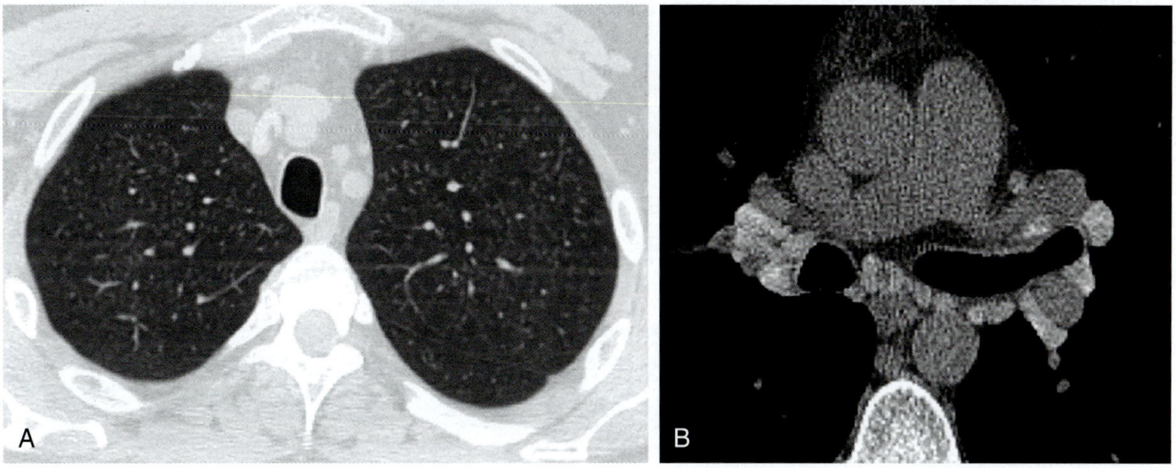

Figure 20.11 Siderosis in a welder. (A) Diffuse centrilobular, poorly defined nodules are present, in addition to hyperdense mediastinal and hilar lymphadenopathy (B) secondary to iron deposition.

diseases should be included in the differential for any abnormal chest imaging without clear cause.

■ Pitfalls

Imaging Findings That Raise Concern of a Complicating Malignancy

With asbestos topping the list, several occupational lung diseases increase the patient's risk for lung cancer, and interpretation of chest imaging for occupational lung disease should consider the possibility of a complicating malignancy. The most likely finding for the presence of bronchogenic carcinoma is a new pulmonary nodule or mass that is out of keeping with the surrounding lung disease, either in appearance or behavior over time (Fig. 20.12). Evidence of cavitation should also raise a red flag for the possibility of complicating malignancy or infection. Other concerning findings include the development of pleural effusion, chest wall invasion, or asymmetric enlargement of adenopathy.

Because occupational lung disease often creates a complicated imaging pattern of nodules, fibrosis, and lymphadenopathy, identification of an early malignancy can be a definite challenge. The asymmetry of an occupational lung disease may mimic malignancy. As stated earlier, PET/CT does offer some benefit in particular situations, such as biopsy planning and atypical round atelectasis. Often, close CT surveillance and/or repeat biopsies provide the only clear evidence to differentiate malignancy from nonmalignant findings.

Identifying and diagnosing mesothelioma in the setting of prior asbestos exposure can also be difficult, particularly because asbestos-related pleural disease can manifest with benign pleural effusion up to 20 years after exposure. Any patient with a new pleural effusion and history or evidence of asbestos exposure should be ruled out for mesothelioma, especially when more than 10 years from exposure (Fig. 20.13). Other imaging appearances of mesothelioma include circumferential pleural thickening, focal pleural-based nodularity thicker than expected pleural plaques, direct invasion of adjacent structures such as the chest wall or mediastinum, new lymphadenopathy, and distant disease.

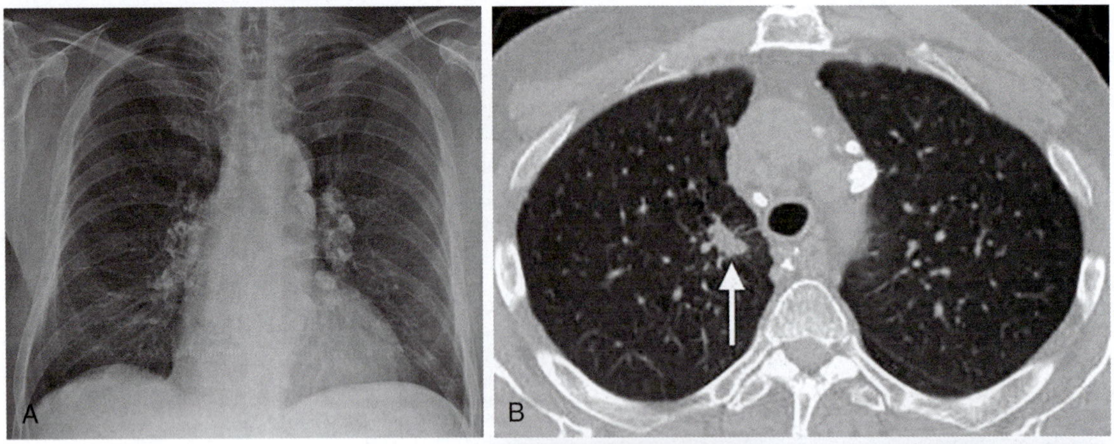

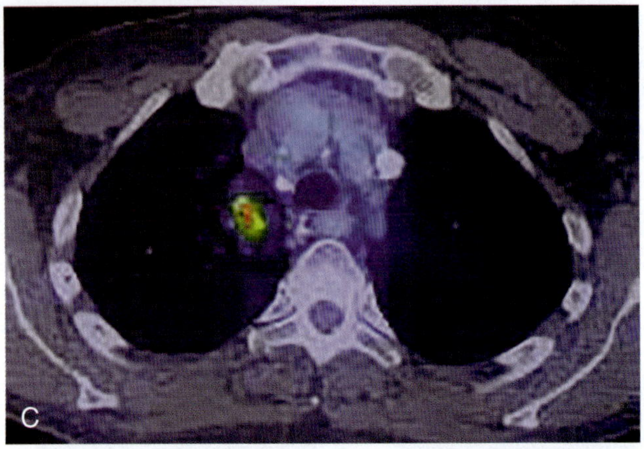

Figure 20.12 Lung cancer in silicosis. (A) Chest radiograph demonstrates the classic appearance of hilar and mediastinal calcified lymphadenopathy with fine upper lobe predominant nodularity. (B) The follow-up chest CT scan reveals a focal nodule in the medial right upper lobe *(arrow)* that also is metabolically active on PET/CT (C).

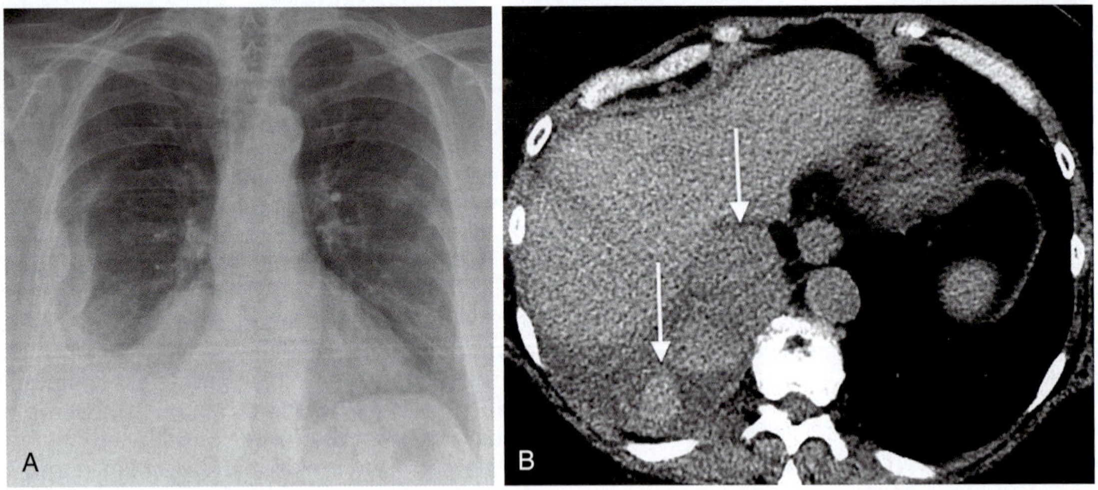

Figure 20.13 Pleural effusion in the setting of asbestos-related pleural disease complicated by mesothelioma. (A) A right pleural effusion is evident on this chest radiograph, with convex contours along the lateral and medial lower lung suggesting a loculation or mass. (B) Noncontrast chest CT in mediastinal window demonstrates pleural masses *(arrows)* associated with the effusion consistent with mesothelioma.

How Smoking Affects the Workup of Occupational and Environmental Lung Diseases

A common coexisting inhalational exposure—smoking—can complicate or cloud the diagnosis of an occupational or environmental lung disease. A smoking history should be elicited as part of every exposure history because smoking may cause or contribute to patient respiratory symptoms and clinical test abnormalities. On imaging, respiratory bronchiolitis produces a poorly defined centrilobular ground-glass nodularity or patchy ground-glass opacities with upper lobe predominance, which happens to overlap with the appearance of early pneumoconiosis and HP on CT. Also, emphysema can be seen in silicosis, asbestosis, and HP when corrected for smoking, so the absence of a smoking history may support the diagnosis of an occupational lung disease when emphysema is present.

It is well known that smoking actually suppresses HP, but this does not exclude the diagnosis. When HP does develop in the setting of smoking, the effect of smoking does not suppress the severity of disease and may even increase the severity.

Finally, smoking further contributes to the risk of lung cancer in the setting of many occupational lung diseases. As stated before, smoking has a synergistic effect with asbestos exposure, increasing the risk of bronchogenic carcinoma by 50 to 100 times. Currently, in the United States, lung cancer screening with chest CT has been exclusively applied to individuals older than 55 years with a smoking history of 30 pack-years, without consideration of other potential occupational or environmental exposures. Perhaps future modifications to lung cancer screening will include risks such as asbestos exposure.

A Normal Chest CT Does Not Exclude an Occupational or Environmental Lung Disease

Several common occupational or environmental lung diseases are known to have potentially normal chest CT findings. Occupational asthma is defined as a temporal relationship between asthma symptoms and a work-related exposure or the development of asthma in the setting of exposure to certain substances known to cause asthma. Asthma may create large and small airway changes on chest CT, such as bronchial wall thickening, bronchiectasis, or air trapping, but may also have a normal chest CT appearance. HP has also been described in the setting of a normal chest CT. In a study of recreation center employees, Lynch et al. have reported that less than 50% of HP biopsy-proven cases revealed CT imaging findings of HP. In addition, a routine inspiratory chest CT can be considered normal but does not exclude the possibility of air trapping found on expiratory CT imaging, which may be the only manifestation of obliterative bronchiolitis or HP.

Finally, deployment-related lung disease (in US Armed Forces recently sent to the Middle East) has demonstrated positive pathologic findings on biopsy, despite normal or near-normal chest CT scans. King et al. found that only 25% of symptomatic postdeployment soldiers with biopsy-proven constrictive bronchiolitis had abnormal findings of small airway disease on chest CT. Subsequent studies and experience have supported the discordance among postdeployment patient symptoms, biopsy results, and medical testing to include chest CT.

■ Conclusion

Whether it is choosing the right study, identifying the characteristic imaging pattern, or managing the complications, radiology plays a pivotal role in the diagnosis and care of those with occupational and environmental lung diseases. With chest radiography reserved primarily for screening and initial evaluation of symptomatic patients, HRCT with inspiratory and expiratory imaging is critical to establish the diagnosis, determine severity, exclude complications, and continue surveillance over time. Some major challenges arise when the following occur: (1) the imaging pattern is atypical or at odds with clinical or pathologic findings; (2) complicating disease such as malignancy or infection overlaps in appearance with the underlying diffuse lung disease; or (3) additional disease processes such as smoking-related lung disease complicate the clinical picture. Considering these challenges reaffirms the need for a multidisciplinary approach to occupational and environmental lung diseases, with active participation of the radiologist.

Bibliography

Agency for Toxic Substances and Disease Registry. Clinical screening guidelines for asbestos-related lung disease. http://www.atsdr.cdc.gov/asbestos/site-kit/docs/clinscrguide_32205_lo.pdf. Accessed June 1, 2015.

Akgun M, Araz O, Ucar EY, et al. Silicosis appears inevitable among former denim sandblasters: a four-year follow up study. *Chest.* 2015;148(3):647–654.

Black B, Szeinuk J, Whitehouse AC, et al. Rapid progression of pleural disease due to exposure to Libby amphibole: "Not your grandfather's asbestos related disease". *Am J Ind Med.* 2014;57(11):1197–1206.

Cox C, Lynch D. Medical imaging in occupational and environmental lung disease. *Curr Opin Pulm Med.* 2015;21:163–170.

Cox C, Rose C, Lynch D. State of the art: imaging of occupational lung disease. *Radiology.* 2014;270(3):281–296.

Das M, Mühlenbruch G, Mahnken AH, et al. Asbestos Surveillance Program Aachen (ASPA): initial results from baseline screening for lung cancer in asbestos-exposed high-risk individuals using low-dose multidetector-row CT. *Eur Radiol.* 2007;17(5):1193–1199.

Gottschall EB. Occupational and environmental thoracic malignancies. *J Thorac Imaging.* 2002;17:189–197.

Hirschmann JV, Pipavath SN, Godwin JD. Hypersensitivity pneumonitis: a historical, clinical and radiologic review. *Radiographics.* 2009;29:1921–1938.

Kim K, Kim C, Lee M, et al. Imaging of occupational lung disease. *Radiographics.* 2001;21:1371–1391.

King MS, Eisenberg R, Newman JH, et al. Constrictive bronchiolitis in soldiers returning from Iraq and Afghanistan. *N Engl J Med.* 2011;365(3):222–230.

Larson TC, Meyer CA, Kapil V, et al. Workers with Libby amphibole exposure: retrospective identification and progression of radiographic changes. *Radiology.* 2010;255(3):924–933.

Lynch DA, Rose CS, Way D, King TE. Hypersensitivity pneumonitis: sensitivity of high-resolution CT in a population-based study. *AJR Am J Roentgenol.* 1992;159:469–472.

Matar LD, McAdams HP, Sporn TA. Pictorial essay: hypersensitivity pneumonitis. *AJR Am J Roentgenol.* 2000;174:1061–1066.

Müller-Quernheim J, Gaede KI, Fireman E, Zissel G. Diagnoses of chronic beryllium disease within cohorts of sarcoidosis patients. *Eur Respir J.* 2006;27(6):1190–1195.

Perez-Alonso A, Cordoba-Dona JA, Millares-Lorenzo JL, et al. Outbreak of silicosis in Spanish quartz conglomerate workers. *Int J Occup Environ Health.* 2014;20(1):26–32.

Podobnik J, Kocijancic I, Kovac V. 3T MRI in evaluation of asbestos-related thoracic diseases—preliminary results. *Radiol Oncol.* 2010;44(2):92–96.

Reichert M, Bensadoun ES. PET imaging in patients with coal workers' pneumoconiosis and suspected malignancy. *J Thorac Oncol.* 2009;4:649–651.

Romero S, Hernandez L, Gil J, et al. Organizing pneumonia in textile printing workers: a clinical description. *Eur Respir J.* 1998;11:265–271.

Sirajuddin A, Kanne JP. Occupational lung disease. *J Thorac Imaging.* 2009;24:310–320.

van Zandwijk N, Clarke C, Henderson D, et al. Guidelines for the diagnosis and treatment of malignant pleural mesothelioma. *J Thorac Dis.* 2013;5:E254–E307.

Webb W, Higgins B. *Pulmonary and Cardiovascular Radiology.* 2nd ed. New York: Lippincott Williams and Wilkins; 2011:504–517.

CHAPTER 21
Hypersensitivity Pneumonitis

Sudhakar Pipavath and Jay Champlin

CHAPTER OUTLINE

■ Introduction

Hypersensitivity pneumonitis is an immunologically mediated lung disease that occurs in susceptible sensitized individuals following inhalational exposure to antigenic organic dust. As such, the antigenic material must be small enough to deposit in the bronchioles and penetrate the alveoli, where it induces an inflammatory response. The vast majority, around 95%, of patients with hypersensitivity pneumonitis are nonsmokers. It is proposed that this may be due to nicotine impairment of T cell function or decreased antibody production following exposure to inhaled antigens in smokers relative to nonsmokers.

Causes of Hypersensitivity Pneumonitis

A multitude of antigenic materials have been implicated as causative agents in hypersensitivity pneumonitis. The two most studied and described types of hypersensitivity pneumonitis are farmer's lung and bird fancier's disease (pigeon breeder's lung). The first of these, farmer's lung, is caused by the inhalation of thermophilic actinomycetes species, including *Saccharopolyspora rectivirgula* (formerly *Micropolyspora faeni*) or *Thermoactinomyces* spp., which grow in moldy hay and grains. Bird fancier's disease (pigeon breeder's lung) typically occurs following exposure to birds and is caused by avian proteins found in feathers and excreta. However, this disease has also been shown to occur following the use of down pillows or laundering a pigeon breeder's clothing. Hypersensitivity pneumonitis has also been described following exposure to air and water systems (Table 21.1) and has been associated with a variety of occupational and recreational exposures (Table 21.2).

Clinical Manifestations

The clinical manifestations of hypersensitivity pneumonitis are highly variable and depend on the frequency, length, and degree of antigenic exposure and on the individual patient's immune response. Hypersensitivity pneumonitis has been subdivided into acute, subacute, and chronic forms. Although this system has been called into question, this chapter will be presented using these subdivisions, as has been the convention.

Acute hypersensitivity pneumonitis typically occurs 4 to 6 hours following the inhalation of a large quantity of antigenic material and is thought to be mediated by a type III hypersensitivity reaction (immune complex deposition). Clinically, acute hypersensitivity pneumonitis presents with severe dyspnea and constitutional or flulike symptoms (e.g., fever, chills, malaise, myalgias, dry or mildly productive cough, chest tightness) mimicking a viral or bacterial infection. Acute hypersensitivity pneumonitis typically resolves over several hours to a few days following termination of exposure to the antigen. However, it may recur following repeat exposure.

Both subacute and chronic hypersensitivity pneumonitis present insidiously following chronic or intermittent low-level exposure to antigenic material and are thought to be mediated by type IV (cell-mediated) hypersensitivity reactions. Clinically, patients present with progressive dyspnea, chronic cough, fatigue, anorexia, and weight

TABLE 21.1 Hypersensitivity Pneumonitis Following Exposure to Air and Water Systems

EXPOSURE	CAUSATIVE AGENT
Humidifiers	*Klebsiella oxytoca*, thermophilic actinomycetes
Air conditioners	Thermophilic actinomycetes
Hot tubs (indoor)	*Mycobacterium avium* complex,[a] *Cladosporium cladosporioides*
Indoor swimming pool	*Pseudomonas* and other gram-negative rods

[a]Whether or not the clinical manifestations of *Mycobacterium avium* complex exposure represents a subset of hypersensitivity pneumonitis or a different but related disease is still a matter of debate.

TABLE 21.2 Hypersensitivity Pneumonitis Associated With Occupational and Recreational Exposures

OCCUPATIONAL OR RECREATIONAL EXPOSURE	CAUSATIVE AGENT[a]
Maple tree bark	*Cryptostroma corticale*
Mushroom workers	Thermophilic actinomycetes, fungal spores
Corn and malt workers	*Aspergillus* spp.
Greenhouse workers and workers with exposure to cheese, dried sausage, cork, or peat moss	*Penicillium* spp.
Automobile industry: painting, parts manufacture or machine operator	Toluene diisocyanate; metal-working fluids (*Mycobacterium avium* complex,[b] *Pseudomonas*, other gram-negative rods)
Foam part production	1,3-bis(isocyanatomethyl) cyclohexane prepolymer
Wood chip boards	Diphenylmethane diisocyanate
Bakers	*Aspergillus fumigatus* and the flour mite *Acarus siro*
Plasterers	Esparto dust
Saxophone player	*Candida, Ulocladium botrytis, Phoma* spp.
Recreational painting	Isocyanate

[a]Low-molecular-weight chemicals may combine with host proteins to form haptens, which then induce hypersensitivity pneumonitis.
[b]Whether or not the clinical manifestations of *Mycobacterium avium* complex exposure represents a subset of hypersensitivity pneumonitis or a different but related disease is still a matter of debate.

loss and may be confused with malignancy. Subacute hypersensitivity pneumonitis typically resolves following a protracted illness. Chronic hypersensitivity pneumonitis, on the other hand, tends to result in irreversible lung damage. Acute exacerbations can occur at any time, even without further antigenic exposure.

Clinical Characteristics That Suggest the Diagnosis

There is currently no consensus regarding the diagnostic criteria for hypersensitivity pneumonitis, and diagnosis is generally only achieved after multidisciplinary collaboration emphasizing the history and physical examination, laboratory findings, imaging, and/or bronchoalveolar lavage (BAL). Although a confident diagnosis of hypersensitivity pneumonitis can be achieved based on the combination of characteristic imaging findings, presence of exposure to a known inciting antigen, BAL results, and/or identification of serum precipitating antibodies (precipitins), histopathologic examination of transbronchial, open, or video-assisted lung biopsy specimen is sometimes required.

History of exposure is a vital component of the workup of suspected hypersensitivity pneumonitis, and it is imperative that common occupational and recreational causes be explored. An important adjunct to this is serum studies for circulating immune complex and precipitins. Despite these measures, the offending agent may never be elucidated.

BAL can lend substantial support to the diagnosis of hypersensitivity pneumonitis. A normal BAL differential includes <10% lymphocytes. In hypersensitivity pneumonitis, BAL tends to demonstrate lymphocytosis (≥20% lymphocytes in current smokers and ≥30% in never-smokers and former smokers), often >50%. A BAL $CD4^+$/$CD8^+$ ratio of <1.8 (often <1) is also typical of hypersensitivity pneumonitis.

Histopathologically, all phases of hypersensitivity pneumonitis demonstrate peribronchiolar inflammation. Given the fleeting nature of acute hypersensitivity pneumonitis, biopsy is rarely required or performed in the acute setting. When biopsied, it typically shows neutrophilic peribronchial and bronchiolocentric (near respiratory or terminal bronchioles) and/or alveolar inflammation. Diffuse alveolar damage and temporally uniform, nonspecific, chronic interstitial pneumonitis may also be seen.

Subacute disease typically shows cellular mononuclear (predominantly lymphocyte and plasma cell) infiltration and bronchiolocentric inflammation (near respiratory or terminal bronchioles), peribronchiolar fibrosis, and poorly formed noncaseating interstitial granulomas. Areas of organizing pneumonia may also be seen. In some cases, antigenic material is visible, or organisms may grow on culture.

As in the acute and subacute forms, lymphocytic peribronchiolar inflammation is also seen in chronic hypersensitivity pneumonitis, but with plasma cell predominance. Like the subacute phase, giant cells or granulomas are also seen, and antigenic material may be visible, or organisms may grow on culture. However, the histologic hallmark of chronic hypersensitivity pneumonitis is fibrosis, which may occur in one of three distinct patterns: homogeneous with linear fibrosis and no architectural distortion (nonspecific interstitial pneumonia [NSIP]-like), peripheral subpleural patchy fibrosis and architectural distortion (usual interstitial pneumonia [UIP]-like), and irregular, predominantly peribronchiolar fibrosis (mixed type).

Imaging Findings

The imaging findings of hypersensitivity pneumonitis are highly variable and dependent on the phase of hypersensitivity pneumonitis.

Conventional Radiographic Findings

Chest radiographs in acute hypersensitivity pneumonitis are usually normal; however, patchy or diffuse homogeneous or heterogeneous opacities may be seen. By contrast, radiographs taken during the subacute phase are generally abnormal and typically demonstrate subtle, poorly defined micronodules, with or without reticulation, in a diffuse or mid and lower lung distribution. There may be small heterogeneous opacities but, unlike the acute phase, diffuse homogenous opacities are generally not seen. Chronic hypersensitivity pneumonitis is characterized radiographically by fibrosis consisting of reticulation, architectural distortion, and volume loss. Nodular or ground-glass opacities are occasionally seen, and radiographs are only rarely normal. The findings in chronic hypersensitivity pneumonitis typically predominate in the mid and upper lungs, with relative sparing of the bases.

High-Resolution CT Findings

High-resolution CT (HRCT) is much more sensitive to the changes seen in hypersensitivity pneumonitis than radiography. Features that may be seen by CT at any stage of disease include ground-glass opacities, poorly defined centrilobular ground-glass nodules, mosaic attenuation, and air trapping. The combination of normal lung interspersed with ground-glass opacities and low-attenuation foci produces a characteristic pattern called the *head cheese sign* (Fig. 21.1). The combination of ground-glass opacity or poorly defined centrilobular nodules and air trapping is suggestive of hypersensitivity pneumonitis, regardless of the stage of disease (other disease conditions such as respiratory bronchiolitis–interstitial lung disease [RB-ILD] may also have this appearance).

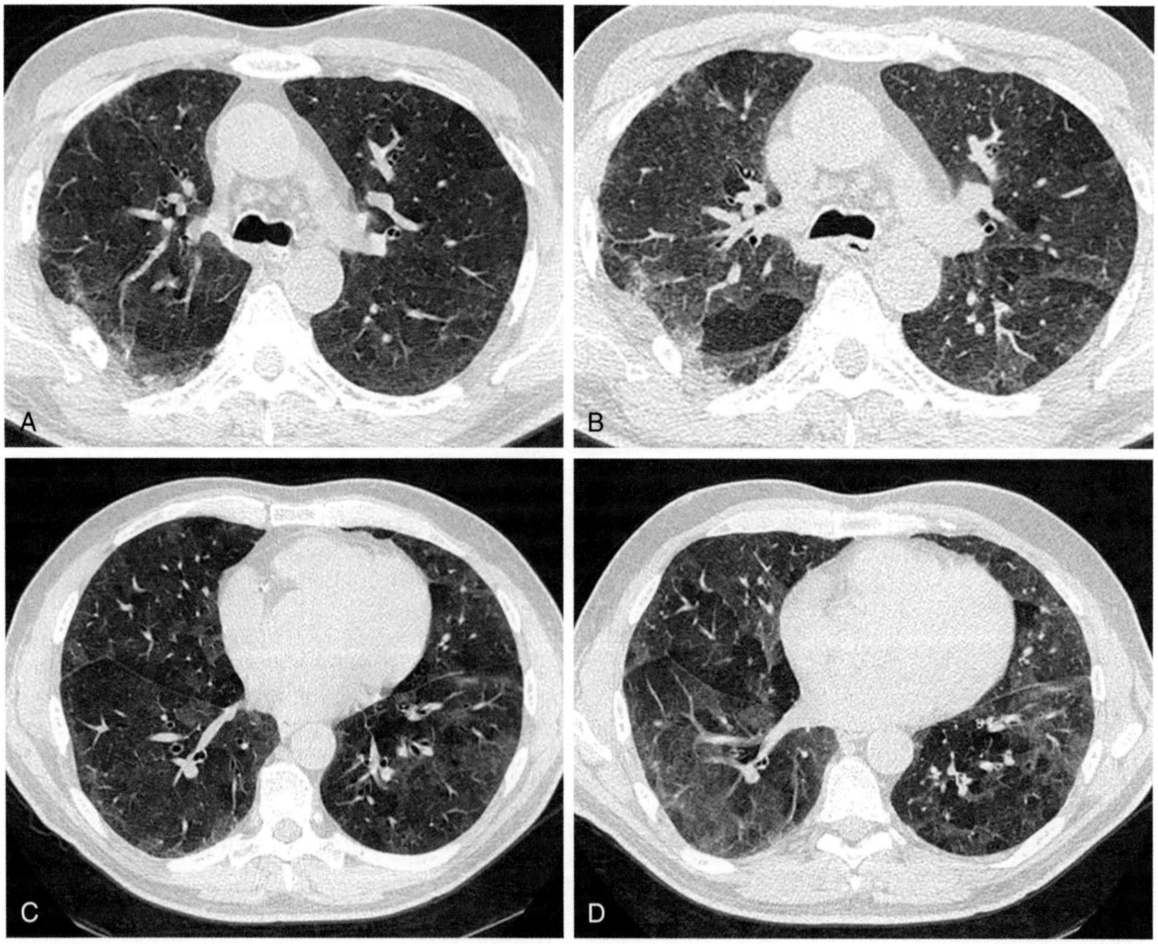

Figure 21.1 Inspiratory (A, C) and expiratory (B, D) CT scans show a combination of ground-glass opacities, normal lung, and air trapping, giving the appearance of the head cheese sign.

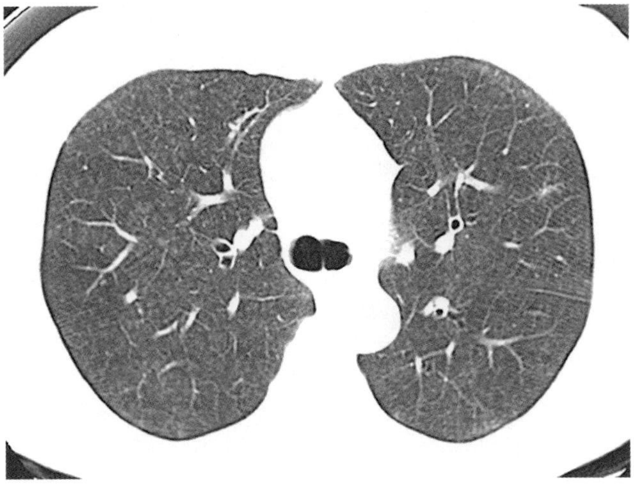

Figure 21.2 Poorly defined centrilobular nodules, uniformly distributed, a finding typically described in subacute hypersensitivity pneumonitis.

Unlike radiographs, HRCT images are usually abnormal in acute hypersensitivity pneumonitis unless the patient is already recovering by the time the study is performed. In the acute phase, HRCT typically demonstrates geographic ground-glass opacities in a mid and lower lung distribution; however, faint, poorly defined, centrilobular ground-glass nodules or diffuse areas of dense consolidation can also be seen. Mosaic attenuation and air trapping are common, as is the head cheese sign.

HRCT findings of subacute hypersensitivity pneumonitis are often the same as those seen in the acute form (diffuse or mid and lower lung predominant, patchy or diffuse geographic, ground-glass opacities and fuzzy, poorly defined centrilobular nodules, mosaic attenuation, air trapping, and head cheese sign). However, poorly defined centrilobular nodules (Fig. 21.2) are seen more often than the acute form, and the degree of ground-glass opacities is usually less than in the acute form. Furthermore, bronchial wall thickening, centrilobular emphysema, and a few thin-walled cysts may rarely be seen.

Chronic hypersensitivity pneumonitis (Fig. 21.3) on HRCT is characterized by fibrosis ranging from interlobular or intralobular interstitial thickening, honeycombing, traction bronchiectasis, and architectural distortion, with upper lobe volume loss. These changes may be superimposed on the findings of subacute hypersensitivity pneumonitis, including geographic ground-glass opacities, small, poorly defined centrilobular nodules, mosaic attenuation, and air trapping. Ground-glass opacities are less prominent in the chronic form than in the acute or subacute form, but are still present.

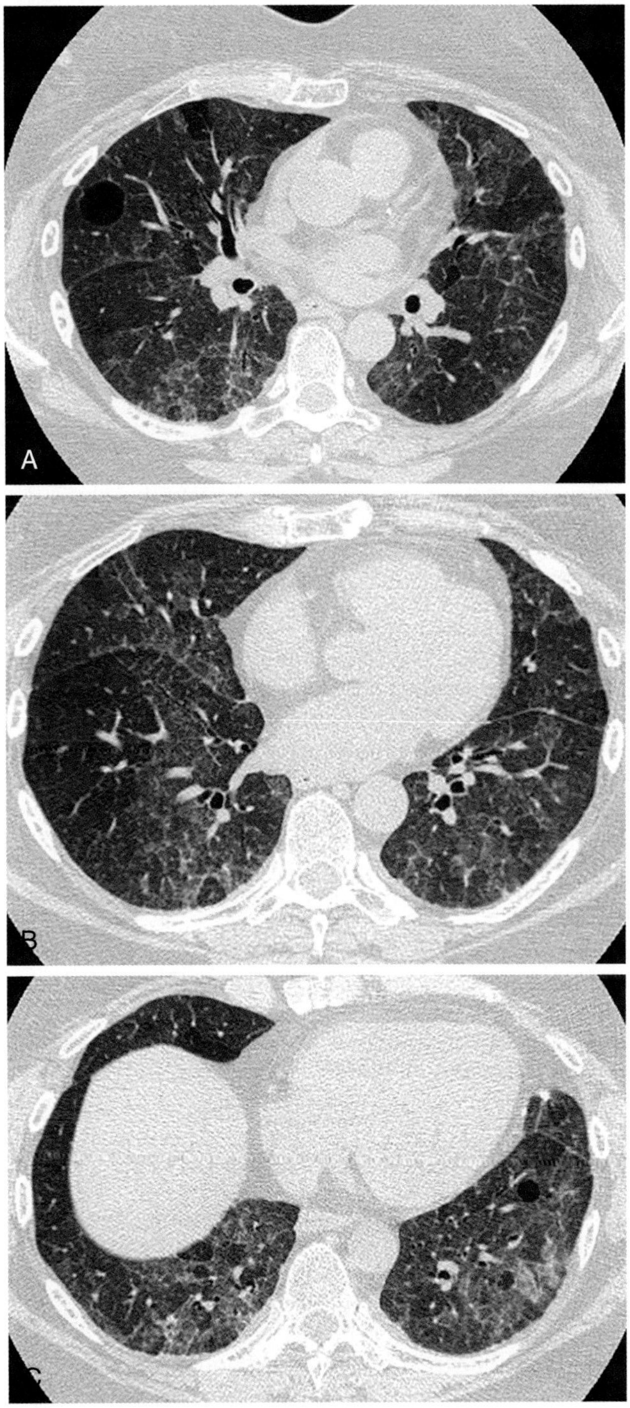

Figure 21.3 (A–C) Reticulation and ground-glass opacity are present, consistent with chronic hypersensitivity pneumonitis.

Imaging Findings Regarding Acuity or Chronicity and Reversibility of the Disease

There is overlap in the different phases of hypersensitivity pneumonitis on HRCT; however, there are specific findings that when present, can often lend support to the diagnosis of subacute or chronic disease. Specifically, findings of fibrosis such as reticulation, traction bronchiectasis, and honeycombing generally indicate chronic hypersensitivity pneumonitis.

The ground-glass opacities, poorly defined centrilobular nodules, mosaic attenuation, and air trapping may be seen at any stage of disease and are generally reversible following removal or avoidance of the offending antigen and corticosteroid therapy. Pulmonary fibrosis, however,

TABLE 21.3 Differential Diagnosis of Hypersensitivity Pneumonitis

PHASE OF ILLNESS	DIFFERENTIAL DIAGNOSIS
Acute (GGO and head cheese sign)	Bacterial or viral infection; pulmonary edema; RB-ILD
Subacute (poorly defined ground-glass attenuation nodules, GGO, with or without air trapping)	Sarcoidosis; chronic beryllium disease; cellular NSIP; RB-ILD
Chronic (reticulation, traction bronchiectasis, with or without air trapping)	Sarcoidosis (atypical pattern with reticulation and honeycombing); IPF; ILD related to connective tissue diseases; fibrotic NSIP

GGO, Ground-glass opacity; *ILD,* interstitial lung disease; *IPF,* interstitial pulmonary fibrosis; *NSIP,* nonspecific interstitial pneumonia; *RB-ILD,* respiratory bronchiolitis–interstitial lung disease.

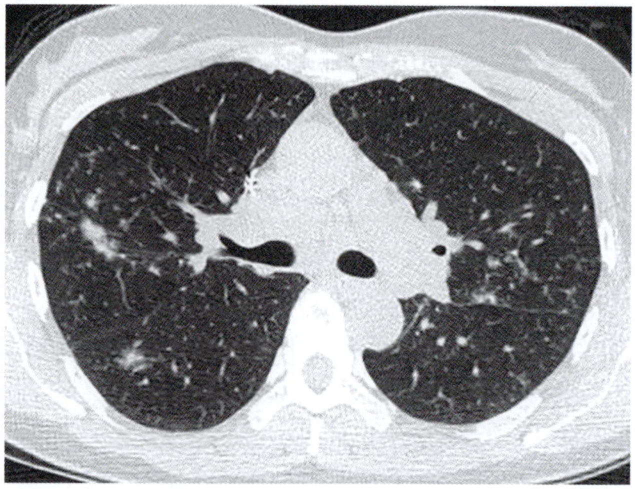

Figure 21.4 Perilymphatic nodules along the fissures, subpleural lung, and bronchovascular tree are highly consistent with sarcoidosis.

is not reversible. Furthermore, it has been shown that the prognosis depends on the presence, extent, and severity of fibrosis, particularly honeycombing and traction bronchiectasis, with more severe fibrosis portending a worse prognosis.

Imaging Findings Suggesting Hypersensitivity Pneumonitis

There are a number imaging findings that when seen, should alert the reader to the possibility of hypersensitivity pneumonitis. These include the following:

- Presence of ground-glass opacities and poorly defined centrilobular nodules with air trapping and/or mosaic attenuation
- Head cheese sign
- NSIP pattern with:
  - Air trapping *or*
  - Poorly defined, centrilobular, ground-glass nodules
- UIP pattern with:
  - Basal sparing
  - Air trapping (mosaic attenuation)
  - Ground-glass opacities
  - Poorly defined centrilobular nodules

■ Differential Diagnosis

The differential diagnosis of hypersensitivity pneumonitis varies, depending on the phase of illness, as noted in Table 21.3.

Narrowing the Differential Diagnosis

It is not always possible to reach a conclusive diagnosis based on imaging findings alone. Clinical information, laboratory studies, BAL, and histology are often required. There are, however, imaging features that when seen, make the diagnosis of hypersensitivity pneumonitis or a competing differential diagnosis more likely.

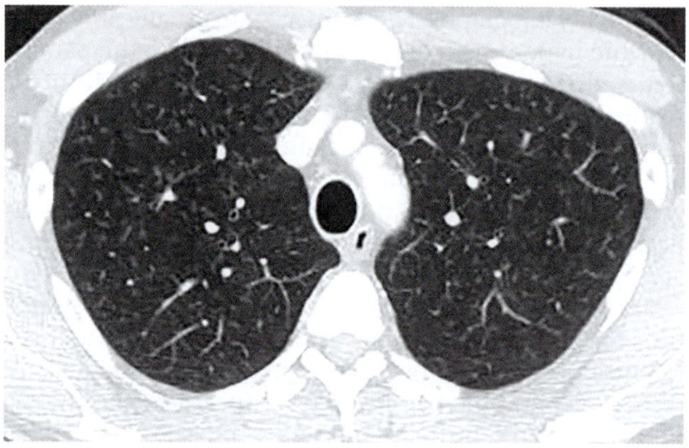

Figure 21.5 Poorly defined centrilobular nodules that are uniformly distributed throughout the lungs are highly suggestive of respiratory bronchiolitis in this smoker.

Sarcoidosis and chronic beryllium disease can mimic both subacute and chronic hypersensitivity pneumonitis. Although these entities are sometimes indistinguishable, differentiation can often be made on the basis of nodule distribution and lymphadenopathy. Sarcoidosis is generally associated with perilymphatic or peribronchovascular nodules and hilar or mediastinal lymphadenopathy (Fig. 21.4). Alternatively, subacute hypersensitivity pneumonitis tends to cause poorly defined, centrilobular nodules in the absence of lymphadenopathy. Similarly, chronic hypersensitivity pneumonitis may present with HRCT findings indistinguishable from sarcoidosis. In this case, lymphadenopathy and the presence of peribronchiolar fibrosis suggest the diagnosis of sarcoidosis. Other causes of poorly defined centrilobular nodules, such as RB-ILD and plexogenic arteriopathy, may also mimic subacute hypersensitivity pneumonitis (Figs. 21.5 and 21.6).

Chronic hypersensitivity pneumonitis may also present with pulmonary fibrosis, which is challenging to

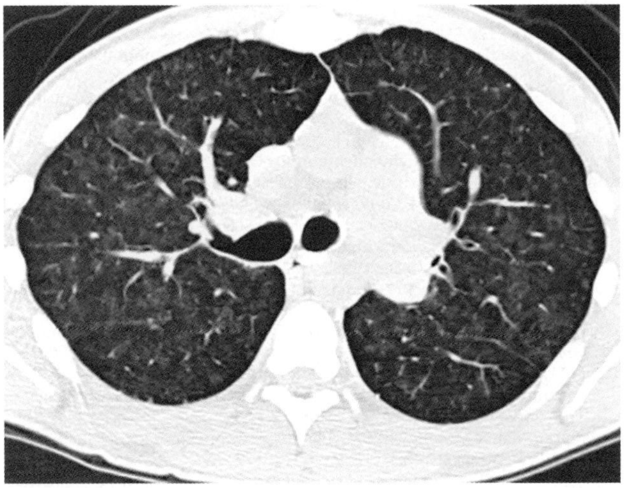

Figure 21.6 Poorly defined centrilobular nodules are present in this patient's lungs, with severe pulmonary arterial hypertension, consistent with cholesterol granulomas and plexogenic arteriopathy.

differentiate from UIP, interstitial pulmonary fibrosis (IPF), or NSIP. In such cases, basal predominant subpleural reticulation with honeycombing in the absence of ground-glass opacities or ground-glass nodules suggests a diagnosis of UIP or IPF. Likewise, either honeycombing or peripheral predominance of disease makes UIP or IPF more likely. By contrast, the presence of ground-glass opacities and poorly defined centrilobular nodules and air trapping and the absence of lower lobe predominance of disease make chronic hypersensitivity pneumonitis more likely. Features favoring NSIP are relative subpleural sparing in the absence of air trapping or honeycombing (Fig. 21.7).

Treatment

The most important aspect of the treatment of hypersensitivity pneumonitis is identification and avoidance of further contact with the offending agent. Although this may sound intuitive, the solution is not always simple. The causative agent is often not identified and, when it is, avoidance may not always be possible. Furthermore, even when it is feasible, patients may elect not to avoid the causative agent. This may be particularly true in bird fancier's disease, in which the source of antigenic material may be considered a member of the patient's family, and there can be significant resistance to parting with the pet, regardless of health consequences. Evading the inciting agent may also pose a challenge in occupational exposures, in which it might be unreasonable or untenable to request that a patient avoid the causative antigen. In such cases, personal protective masks and air purification may be of benefit. Even when the offending agent can be avoided, however, exacerbations have been shown to occur in the absence of reexposure. Pharmacologic options for management have consisted of systemic corticosteroids but, more recently, pentoxifylline and rituximab have been tried.

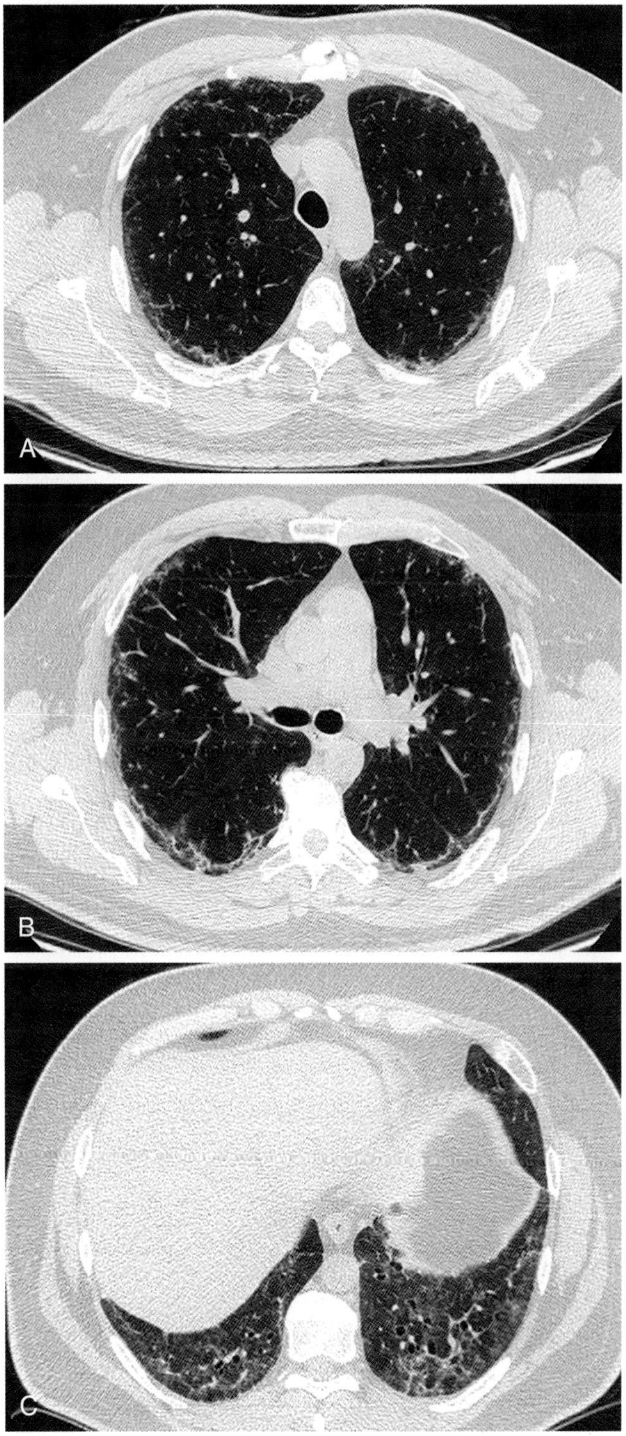

Figure 21.7 (A–C) CT scan shows basilar and peripheral predominant reticulation and ground-glass opacities, with subpleural sparing. Biopsy revealed nonspecific interstitial pneumonia.

Bibliography

Adler BD, Padley SP, Müller NL, Remy-Jardin M, Remy J. Chronic hypersensitivity pneumonitis: high-resolution CT and radiographic features in 16 patients. *Radiology*. 1992;185(1):91–95.

Agostini C, Trentin L, Facco M, Semenzato G. New aspects of hypersensitivity pneumonitis. *Curr Opin Pulm Med*. 2004;10(5):378–382.

Buschman DL, Gamsu G, Waldron JA Jr, Klein JS, King TE Jr. Chronic hypersensitivity pneumonitis: use of CT in diagnosis. *AJR Am J Roentgenol*. 1992;159(5):957–960.

Churg A, Muller NL, Flint J, Wright JL. Chronic hypersensitivity pneumonitis. *Am J Surg Pathol*. 2006;30(2):201–208.

Costabel U, Bonella F, Guzman J. Chronic hypersensitivity pneumonitis. *Clin Chest Med*. 2012;33(1):151–163.

Girard M, Cormier Y. Hypersensitivity pneumonitis. *Curr Opin Allergy Clin Immunol*. 2010;10(2):99–103.

Glazer CS, Rose CS, Lynch DA. Clinical and radiologic manifestations of hypersensitivity pneumonitis. *J Thorac Imaging*. 2002;17(4):261–272.

Gruden JF, Webb WR. CT findings in a proved case of respiratory bronchiolitis. *AJR Am J Roentgenol*. 1993;161(1):44–46.

Grunes D, Beasley MB. Hypersensitivity pneumonitis: a review and update of histologic findings. *J Clin Pathol*. 2013;66(10):888–895.

Hanak V, Golbin JM, Hartman TE, Ryu JH. High-resolution CT findings of parenchymal fibrosis correlate with prognosis in hypersensitivity pneumonitis. *Chest*. 2008;134(1):133–138.

Hanak V, Golbin JM, Ryu JH. Causes and presenting features in 85 consecutive patients with hypersensitivity pneumonitis. *Mayo Clin Proc*. 2007;82(7):812–816.

Hartman TE, Primack SL, Swensen SJ, Hansell D, McGuinness G, Müller NL. Desquamative interstitial pneumonia: thin-section CT findings in 22 patients. *Radiology*. 1993;187(3):787–790.

Hirschmann JV, Pipavath SN, Godwin JD. Hypersensitivity pneumonitis: a historical, clinical, and radiologic review. *Radiographics*. 2009;29(7):1921–1938.

Hodgson MJ, Parkinson DK, Karpf M. Chest x-rays in hypersensitivity pneumonitis: a metaanalysis of secular trend. *Am J Ind Med*. 1989;16(1):45–53.

Holt RM, Schmidt RA, Godwin JD, Raghu G. High resolution CT in respiratory bronchiolitis-associated interstitial lung disease. *J Comput Assist Tomogr*. 1993;17(1):46–50.

Jeong YJ, Lee KS, Chung MP, Han J, Johkoh T, Ichikado K. Chronic hypersensitivity pneumonitis and pulmonary sarcoidosis: differentiation from usual interstitial pneumonia using high-resolution computed tomography. *Semin Ultrasound CT MR*. 2014;35(1):47–58.

Lacasse Y, Cormier Y. Hypersensitivity pneumonitis. *Orphanet J Rare Dis*. 2006;1:25.

Lacasse Y, Girard M, Cormier Y. Recent advances in hypersensitivity pneumonitis. *Chest*. 2012;142(1):208–217.

Lacasse Y, Israël Assayag E, Laviolette M, Cormier Y. Clinical and immunopathological aspects of hypersensitivity pneumonitis. *Rev Mal Respir*. 2004;21(4 Pt 1):769–781.

Lacasse Y, Selman M, Costabel U, et al. Clinical diagnosis of hypersensitivity pneumonitis. *Am J Respir Crit Care Med*. 2003;168(8):952–958.

Lota HK, Keir GJ, Hansell DM, et al. Novel use of rituximab in hypersensitivity pneumonitis refractory to conventional treatment. *Thorax*. 2013;68(8):780–781.

Lynch DA, Newell JD, Logan PM, King TE Jr, Müller NL. Can CT distinguish hypersensitivity pneumonitis from idiopathic pulmonary fibrosis? *AJR Am J Roentgenol*. 1995;165(4):807–811.

Lynch DA, Rose CS, Way D, King TE Jr. Hypersensitivity pneumonitis: sensitivity of high-resolution CT in a population-based study. *AJR Am J Roentgenol*. 1992;159(3):469–472.

Martin SG, Kronek LP, Valeyre D, et al. High-resolution computed tomography to differentiate chronic diffuse interstitial lung diseases with predominant ground-glass pattern using logical analysis of data. *Eur Radiol*. 2010;20(6):1297–1310.

Matar LD, McAdams HP, Sporn TA. Hypersensitivity pneumonitis. *AJR Am J Roentgenol*. 2000;174(4):1061–1066.

Mohr LC. Hypersensitivity pneumonitis. *Curr Opin Pulm Med*. 2004;10(5): 401–411.

Mooney JJ, Elicker BM, Urbania TH, et al. Radiographic fibrosis score predicts survival in hypersensitivity pneumonitis. *Chest*. 2013;144(2):586–592.

Munoz X, Morell F, Cruz MJ. The use of specific inhalation challenge in hypersensitivity pneumonitis. *Curr Opin Allergy Clin Immunol*. 2013;13(2):151–158.

Murayama J, Yoshizawa Y, Ohtsuka M, Hasegawa S. Lung fibrosis in hypersensitivity pneumonitis. Association with CD4+ but not CD8+ cell dominant alveolitis and insidious onset. *Chest*. 1993;104(1):38–43.

Myers JL. Hypersensitivity pneumonia: the role of lung biopsy in diagnosis and management. *Mod Pathol*. 2012;25(suppl 1):S58–S67.

Ohshimo S, Bonella F, Guzman J, Costabel U. Hypersensitivity pneumonitis. *Immunol Allergy Clin North Am*. 2012;32(4):537–556.

Patel RA, Sellami D, Gotway MB, Golden JA, Webb WR. Hypersensitivity pneumonitis: patterns on high-resolution CT. *J Comput Assist Tomogr*. 2000;24(6):965–970.

Paul L, Lehrman SG, Aronow WS. Hypersensitivity pneumonitis: evaluation and management. *Compr Ther*. 2009;35(3–4):177–187.

Sahin H, Brown KK, Curran-Everett D, et al. Chronic hypersensitivity pneumonitis: CT features comparison with pathologic evidence of fibrosis and survival. *Radiology*. 2007;244(2):591–598.

Selman M, Pardo A, King TE Jr. Hypersensitivity pneumonitis: insights in diagnosis and pathobiology. *Am J Respir Crit Care Med*. 2012;186(4):314–324.

Silva CI, Churg A, Müller NL. Hypersensitivity pneumonitis: spectrum of high-resolution CT and pathologic findings. *AJR Am J Roentgenol*. 2007;188(2): 334–344.

Silva CI, Müller NL, Lynch DA, et al. Chronic hypersensitivity pneumonitis: differentiation from idiopathic pulmonary fibrosis and nonspecific interstitial pneumonia by using thin-section CT. *Radiology*. 2008;246(1):288–297.

Silver SF, Müller NL, Miller RR, Lefcoe MS. Hypersensitivity pneumonitis: evaluation with CT. *Radiology*. 1989;173(2):441–445.

Takemura T, Akashi T, Kamiya H, et al. Pathological differentiation of chronic hypersensitivity pneumonitis from idiopathic pulmonary fibrosis/usual interstitial pneumonia. *Histopathology*. 2012;61(6):1026–1035.

Takemura T, Akashi T, Ohtani Y, Inase N, Yoshizawa Y. Pathology of hypersensitivity pneumonitis. *Curr Opin Pulm Med*. 2008;14(5):440–454.

Vourlekis JS, Schwarz MI, Cherniack RM, et al. The effect of pulmonary fibrosis on survival in patients with hypersensitivity pneumonitis. *Am J Med*. 2004;116(10):662–668.

Walsh SL, Sverzellati N, Devaraj A, Wells AU, Hansell DM. Chronic hypersensitivity pneumonitis: high resolution computed tomography patterns and pulmonary function indices as prognostic determinants. *Eur Radiol*. 2012;22(8):1672–1679.

Wild LG, Lopez M. Hypersensitivity pneumonitis: a comprehensive review. *J Investig Allergol Clin Immunol*. 2001;11(1):3–15.

Yi ES. Hypersensitivity pneumonitis. *Crit Rev Clin Lab Sci*. 2002;39(6):581–629.

CHAPTER 22
Eosinophilic Lung Disease

Arlene Sirajuddin and Jeffrey P. Kanne

CHAPTER OUTLINE

■ Introduction

Eosinophilic lung diseases are characterized by the presence of pulmonary opacities and peripheral blood eosinophilia, tissue eosinophilia, or both. Eosinophils are leukocytes that are involved in immune defense and various inflammatory processes. They decrease hypersensitivity reactions by reducing the activity of histamine and leukotriene complexes released by mast cells, as well as by phagocytizing mast cell granules and immune complexes. Eosinophils also release cytotoxic proteins such as major basic protein and eosinophilic cationic protein, which are helpful in destroying parasites, but are also responsible for most of the tissue damage present in eosinophilic lung diseases.

Approach to Diagnosis

Eosinophilic lung diseases can be challenging to diagnose, and a combined clinical, radiologic, and pathologic approach is essential. The clinical history and physical examination are important for determining the extent and duration of signs and symptoms. A diagnosis of asthma, travel history, occupational and environmental exposures, and previous and current medications are also important to identify.

Laboratory studies that aid in the diagnosis of eosinophilic lung disease include a white blood cell count with differential to look for peripheral blood eosinophilia, serum immunoglobulin E (IgE) level, and serum *Aspergillus* precipitins, and stool studies for cysts, ova, and parasites. Peripheral blood eosinophilia is defined as an eosinophil count $>0.4 \times 10^9$/L. Peripheral blood eosinophilia is elevated in most eosinophilic lung diseases.

Diagnostic procedures that can help establish a diagnosis of eosinophilic lung disease include pulmonary function tests and bronchoalveolar lavage (BAL). Pulmonary function tests in patients with eosinophilic lung disease can show different patterns of disease. A restrictive defect usually occurs with acute eosinophilic pneumonia (AEP), chronic eosinophilic pneumonia (CEP), and tropical eosinophilic pneumonia. An obstructive defect usually occurs with allergic bronchopulmonary aspergillosis (ABPA) and Churg-Strauss syndrome (CSS). BAL is an extremely helpful test in diagnosing eosinophilic lung disease. Normal BAL fluid contains <1% eosinophils, whereas eosinophilic lung diseases are associated with BAL fluid with usually >10% eosinophils.

Sputum and tissue analysis can show Charcot-Leyden crystals, which are derived from a protein released by eosinophils. These crystals are present whenever there are large numbers of eosinophils present and thus are typically seen in eosinophilic lung diseases.

Both chest radiography and chest CT can show pulmonary opacities suggestive of eosinophilic lung disease. Transbronchial or surgical lung biopsy may be helpful to confirm the diagnosis in challenging cases.

A diagnosis of eosinophilic lung disease can be made if there is pulmonary opacity present on imaging studies and peripheral blood eosinophilia, biopsy confirmation of tissue eosinophilia, or increased eosinophils in BAL fluid. Additionally, Hodgkin lymphoma, sarcoidosis, infection, and hydatid disease must be excluded before a diagnosis of eosinophilic lung disease can be established.

Available Imaging Modalities to Evaluate Eosinophilic Lung Disease

Imaging procedures available to evaluate pulmonary eosinophilic disease include chest radiography and CT. Chest radiography is useful as a screening examination to detect pulmonary opacities, given its relatively low cost and low patient exposure to ionizing radiation. However, chest radiographic findings are nonspecific and may even be absent in patients with eosinophilic lung disease. In contrast, CT is more sensitive to the presence of lung opacities and sometimes shows a more specific pattern of disease, helping to narrow the differential diagnosis. Furthermore, CT can also be helpful in planning a transbronchial or surgical biopsy. However, compared to chest radiography, CT is more costly and results in higher levels of patient exposure to ionizing radiation.

■ Eosinophilic Lung Diseases

Eosinophilic lung diseases are divided into diseases with known causes and diseases with unknown causes.

- Eosinophilic lung diseases without a known cause:
  1. Simple eosinophilic pneumonia (SEP)
  2. CEP
  3. AEP
  4. Idiopathic hypereosinophilic syndrome
- Eosinophilic diseases with a known cause:
  1. ABPA
  2. Bronchocentric granulomatous inflammation
  3. CSS
  4. Drug reactions
  5. Parasite infection

Diseases Without a Known Cause

Simple Eosinophilic Pneumonia

SEP, also known as Löffler syndrome, is an idiopathic disease characterized by migrating pulmonary consolidation and peripheral blood eosinophilia. Symptoms are often mild and include cough, fever, and dyspnea.

Chest radiographs show migratory foci of consolidation that usually clear spontaneously within 1 month. Foci of consolidation are typically upper lung predominant and peripheral in location. CT shows peripheral ground-glass opacity, consolidation, or both in the mid and upper lungs (Fig. 22.1). Nodules with surrounding ground-glass opacity may also be present. Pleural effusion, cavitation, and lymphadenopathy are absent. Histopathologically, eosinophils are seen infiltrating the alveolar septa and interstitium. The main differential diagnostic considerations include vasculitis and organizing pneumonia. Response to corticosteroids is excellent if treatment is necessary, and the prognosis is excellent.

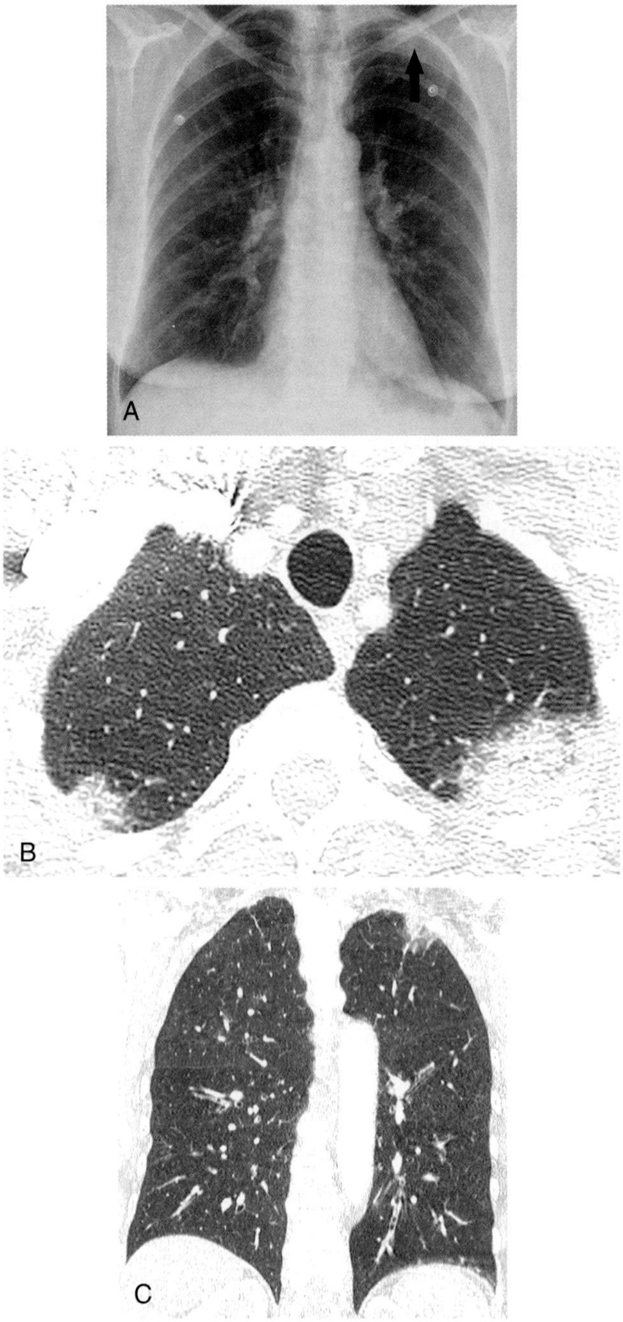

Figure 22.1 Simple eosinophilic pneumonia in a 61-year-old female with asthma. (A) Chest radiograph shows peripheral, ill-defined consolidation within the left apex *(arrow)*. (B) Transverse and coronal (C) CT scans of the lungs show peripheral upper lobe areas of consolidation.

Chronic Eosinophilic Pneumonia

CEP is an idiopathic eosinophilic lung disease with insidious onset. Signs and symptoms are usually present for more than 6 months before the diagnosis is established and include cough, fever, night sweats, dyspnea, and weight loss. Patients usually are middle-age women, and approximately 50% have a history of asthma or atopy.

Patients usually have leukocytosis, an elevated erythrocyte sedimentation rate, and a variable IgE level. Peripheral blood eosinophilia is present in approximately 90% of patients, but may be absent later in the disease process. Pulmonary function tests usually show a restrictive defect, and BAL usually shows >25% eosinophils. Characteristic chest radiographic and CT findings include peripheral areas of upper lung predominant ground-glass

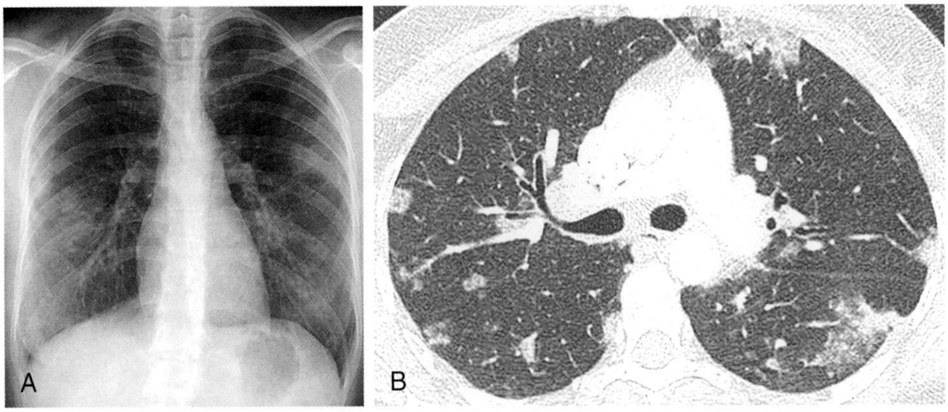

Figure 22.2 Chronic eosinophilic pneumonia in a 38-year-old woman. (A) Chest radiograph and (B) CT scan of the lungs show predominantly peripheral areas of consolidation.

opacity and consolidation, which sometimes contain air bronchograms (Fig. 22.2). However, other patterns of disease, including mixed peripheral and perihilar consolidation and unilateral disease, are also possible. Nodules, reticulation, and pleural effusion are less common findings and usually occur later in the disease course. On histopathology, eosinophils infiltrating into the alveoli and interstitium are present, sometimes forming eosinophilic abscesses.

Treatment of CEP is corticosteroids, often long term because up to 60% of patients relapse. Despite treatment, some patients subsequently develop CSS.

Acute Eosinophilic Pneumonia

AEP is a clinical entity with the following features:

1. Fever <5 days
2. Hypoxemic respiratory failure
3. Opacities on chest radiograph
4. BAL with >25% eosinophils
5. Prompt response to corticosteroids, with no relapse after cessation of therapy
6. Absence of parasitic or fungal infection

AEP can be associated with cigarette smoking and tends to occur with a new onset of smoking, restarting smoking, or significantly increasing the amount of smoking less than 1 month before the onset of symptoms. It can also be seen with exposure to dust. A history of asthma is not very common, and there is no gender predilection. Signs and symptoms include rapid development of nonproductive cough, fever, and dyspnea. Most patients go on to develop respiratory failure necessitating mechanical ventilation.

Peripheral blood eosinophilia may not be present early in the disease course. An abnormally high percentage of eosinophils in BAL fluid is characteristic, even reaching 80%. Chest radiography shows reticular opacities, patchy consolidation, and pleural effusion. Chest CT shows patchy ground-glass opacities, consolidation, pleural effusion, and interlobular septal thickening (Fig. 22.3). Small nodules may also be present. On histopathology, diffuse alveolar damage with eosinophils infiltrating mainly into the interstitium is present. The differential diagnosis of AEP includes lung edema, hemorrhage, infection, and acute respiratory distress syndrome. AEP responds to corticosteroids and does not relapse. Survival is close to 100%.

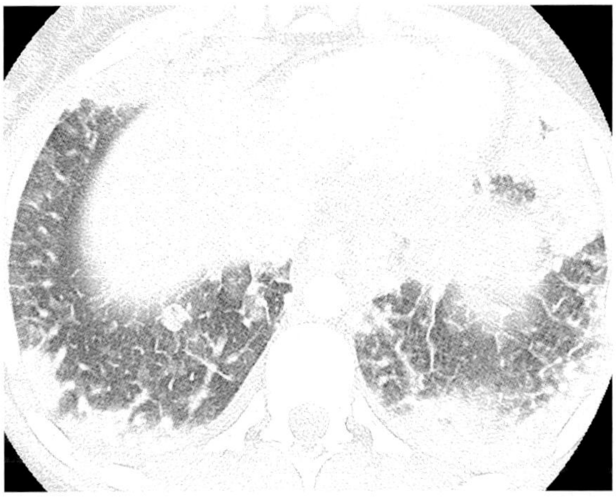

Figure 22.3 Acute eosinophilic pneumonia in an 18-year-old woman who just began smoking. CT scan of the lungs shows septal thickening, patchy consolidation, and pleural effusion.

Idiopathic Hypereosinophilic Syndrome

Idiopathic hypereosinophilic syndrome is characterized by prolonged peripheral blood eosinophilia ($>1.5 \times 10^9$/L) of no recognizable cause, persisting for more than 6 months and resulting in organ dysfunction. It is described as a leukoproliferative disorder because of the presence of monoclonal cell populations found in this disease. Also, cytogenetic analysis sometimes reveals a chromosome 4 deletion resulting in a fusion gene called *FIP1L1–platelet-derived growth factor receptor* α (*FIP1L1-PDGFRA*) fusion gene. Although patients with this *FIP1L1-PDGFRA* fusion gene are included in the group of those with idiopathic hypereosinophilic syndrome, they are considered to have eosinophilic leukemia.

Patients tend to be male and in their third or fourth decade of life. The heart and central nervous system are usually involved. Signs and symptoms include fever, weight loss, neurologic signs and symptoms, including intellectual impairment and neuropathy, and cardiopulmonary signs and symptoms, including cough and dyspnea.

Cardiac complications include endocardial fibrosis, valvular damage, dysrhythmias, restrictive cardiomyopathy, and mural thrombus formation. Lung complications include edema secondary to cardiac failure. Transient patchy consolidation reflecting eosinophilic pneumonia may also be present. BAL fluid shows eosinophilia. On

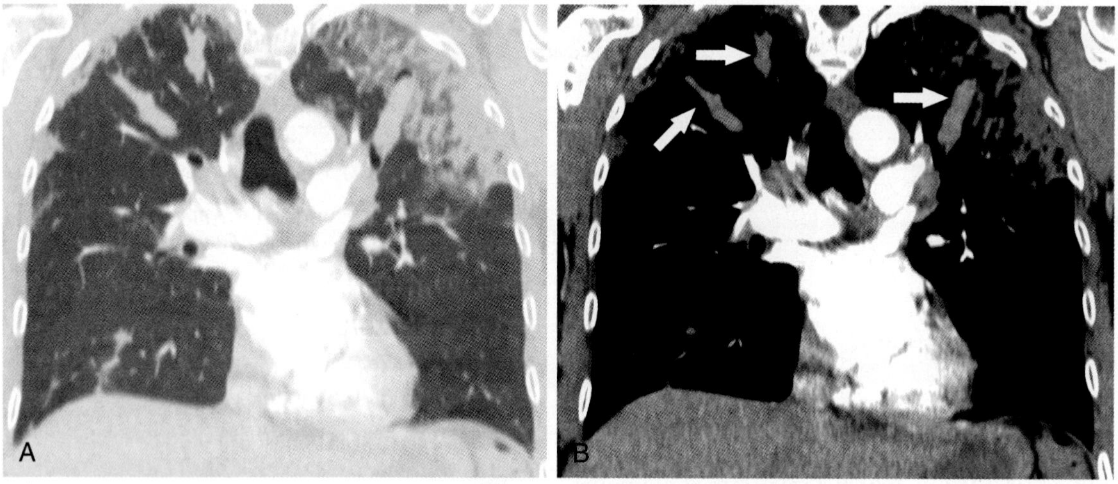

Figure 22.4 A 61-year-old woman with allergic bronchopulmonary aspergillosis and chronic eosinophilic pneumonia. (A) Coronal CT scan of the lungs shows tubular branching structures radiating from the hila, compatible with mucus plugging of dilated bronchi. Left upper lobe peripheral consolidation is compatible with chronic eosinophilic pneumonia. (B) Soft tissue coronal CT scan shows airways plugged with hyperattenuating mucus *(arrows)*.

histopathology, affected organs contain eosinophilic infiltration and areas of necrosis.

Chest radiographs can show focal or diffuse septal lines reflecting mild lung edema or areas of consolidation with more extensive edema. On CT, diffuse septal thickening may be present, as well as other findings, including nodules and focal or diffuse ground-glass opacity, which tends to be peripheral. Pleural effusion is common both on radiographs and CT scans.

Treatment of idiopathic hypereosinophilic syndrome includes corticosteroids, cytotoxic drugs, and monoclonal antibodies. FIP1L1-PDGFRA fusion protein is present in 50% of patients who respond to a protein kinase inhibitor imatinab. Mepolizumab is another available therapy. Improvements in therapy have decreased the 3-year mortality rate to approximately 4%.

Diseases With a Known Cause

Allergic Bronchopulmonary Aspergillosis

ABPA is a hypersensitivity reaction to antigens of *Aspergillus* spp. (*Aspergillus fumigatus* in nearly 90%) and is the most common eosinophilic lung disease, accounting for approximately 75% of patients with pulmonary eosinophilia.

Patients are usually in the second through fourth decades of life and usually have a history of asthma or cystic fibrosis. *Aspergillus* colonizes the airways and forms mycelial plugs in proximal bronchi. Patients subsequently develop an immune response to the fungi, initially an IgE-mediated type I hypersensitivity reaction and subsequently an IgG-mediated type III hypersensitivity reaction. Up to 10% of patients with ABPA also develop allergic fungal sinusitis.

ABPA is usually diagnosed by a combination of clinical and radiographic findings, and biopsy is rarely performed. Diagnostic criteria include asthma, peripheral blood eosinophilia, elevated IgE level, positive skin test for *Aspergillus* antigens, and pulmonary opacity on radiographs. The serum IgE level is extremely useful and corresponds to disease activity. Common signs and symptoms of ABPA included fever, wheezing, and cough. Some patients will expectorate bronchial casts consisting of fungal hyphae and mucus. Five stages of ABPA have been described by Patterson et al.: acute, remission, exacerbation, steroid-dependent asthma, and fibrosis. In the acute phase, patients have peripheral blood eosinophilia, abnormal chest radiographs, immediate positive skin reaction to *Aspergillus* antigen, elevated serum IgE, and usually positive serum precipitins against *Aspergillus*.

In the acute phase, chest radiography and CT show consolidation, bronchial wall thickening, mucoid impaction, centrilobular nodules, and tree-in-bud opacities (Fig. 22.4). The most common finding is mucoid impaction, which appears as a tubular or branching opacity on chest radiographs and has been described as the finger-in-glove sign. On CT, impacted mucus can be water attenuating, soft tissue attenuating, or hyperattenuating. Chronic findings include proximal bronchiectasis and upper lobe volume loss. Aspergillomas can grow in bronchiectatic cavities. Obstructing endobronchial lesions and bronchial atresia should be considered in the differential diagnosis of ABPA.

Histopathologic examination shows bronchocentric granulomas and associated inflammation with histiocytes, lymphocytes, and eosinophils. Fungal hyphae are often present in sputum. Treatment involves managing underlying asthma, corticosteroids, and antifungal medications. One study has shown that relapse occurs in 23% of patients, particularly in those with bronchiectasis and hyperattenuating mucus plugs.

Bronchocentric Granulomatous Inflammation

Bronchocentric granulomatosis is an airway-centered granulomatous histopathologic pattern originally described by Liebow in 1973. The term *bronchocentric*

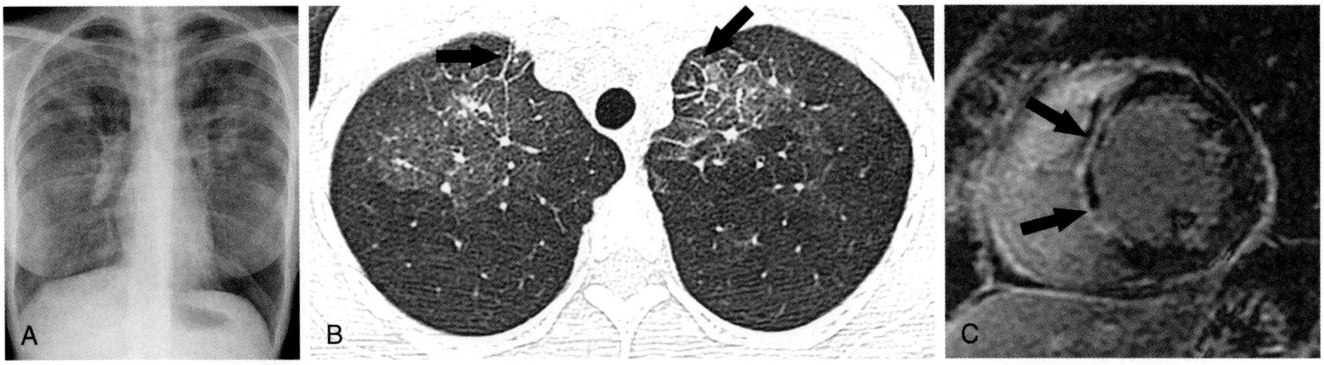

Figure 22.5 Churg-Strauss syndrome in a 29-year-old woman. (A) Chest radiograph shows bilateral patchy consolidation. (B) CT scan of the lung apices shows patchy ground-glass opacity and interlobular septal thickening *(arrows)*. (C) Short-axis postcontrast cardiac MR image shows enhancement of the septal wall *(arrows)* compatible with cardiac involvement by Churg-Strauss syndrome.

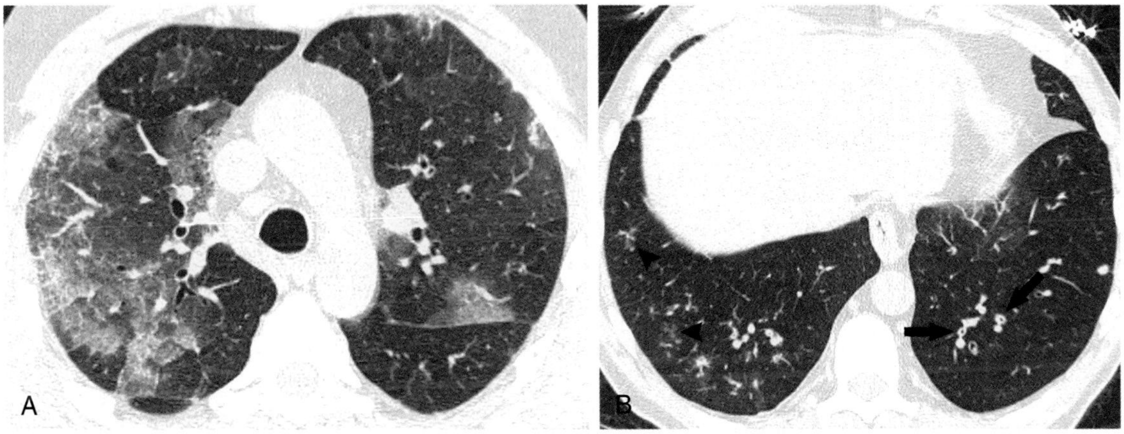

Figure 22.6 Churg-Strauss syndrome in a 60-year-old man. (A) Transverse CT scan of the upper lungs shows scattered areas of ground-glass opacity and consolidation, with some superimposed areas of septal thickening. (B) Transverse CT scan of the lower lungs shows bronchial wall thickening *(arrows)* and nodular areas of ground-glass opacity *(arrowheads)*.

granulomatous inflammation is now preferred and describes a pattern of injury to medium- and small-caliber bronchi, characterized by necrotizing granulomatous inflammation and cellular debris and necrotic granulomas filling the airway lumens. Adjacent pulmonary arteries are unaffected. Most patients with bronchocentric granulomatous inflammation have asthma and ABPA. However, this histopathologic pattern can also occur in nonasthmatic patients, including those with infections such as histoplasmosis, mycobacterial infection, and zygomycosis. Idiopathic bronchocentric granulomatous inflammation is likely the result of an occult infection.

Churg-Strauss Syndrome

CSS, also known as *eosinophilic granulomatosis with polyangiitis,* was first described by Churg and Strauss in 1951. CSS is a necrotizing vasculitis with associated tissue eosinophilia and extravascular granulomas. The cause is unknown but is likely allergic, given its association with asthma and eosinophilia. Patients have symptoms of fever and weight loss.

The diagnosis of CSS requires the presence of four of the following six criteria: (1) asthma; (2) peripheral blood eosinophilia >10%; (3) migratory or transient pulmonary opacities; (4) paranasal sinus abnormality; (5) neuropathy; and (6) tissue or extravascular eosinophils on biopsy. CSS usually involves the lung, but the skin, central nervous system, heart, kidneys, and gastrointestinal tract are also commonly affected.

Other abnormalities include an elevated serum IgE level and elevated levels of BAL fluid eosinophils. The antimyeloperoxidase antineutrophil cytoplasmic antibody (ANCA) test is usually positive. Chest radiography shows bilateral lung consolidation, nodules, and reticulation. Common chest CT findings include peripheral lobular ground-glass opacity and consolidation, centrilobular nodules, septal thickening, and bronchial wall thickening (Figs. 22.5 and 22.6). Less common CT findings include lymphadenopathy and eosinophilic pleural and pericardial effusions. The differential diagnosis includes CEP and other vasculitides. A biopsy, from the lung or elsewhere, is often required for diagnosis.

Histopathologic examination may show tissue eosinophilia, necrotizing granulomatosis, and vasculitis; however, depending on the biopsy size, not all three of these findings may be present together. There is usually transmural inflammation of the vessel wall, with eosinophils and focal areas of necrosis. Vessels may become obliterated

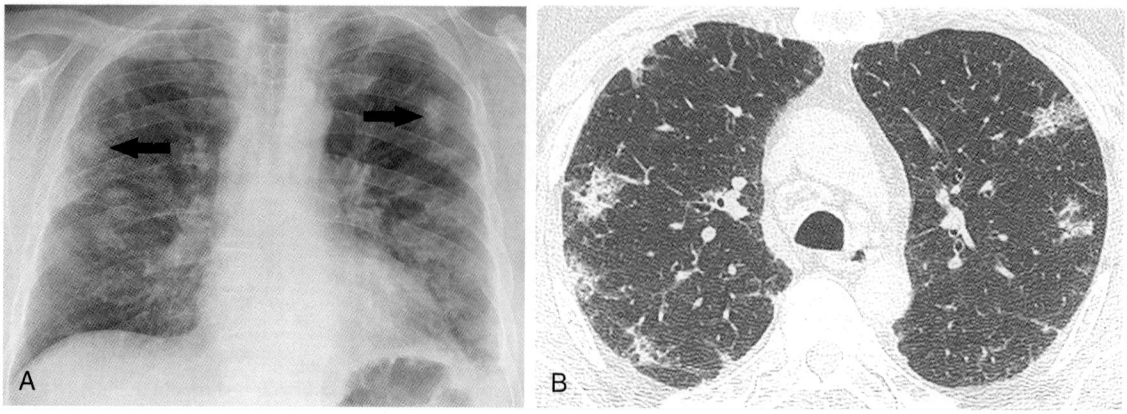

Figure 22.7 Eosinophilic pneumonia in a 47-year-old man secondary to naproxen. (A) Chest radiograph shows multiple nodular areas of opacity bilaterally *(arrows)*. (B) CT scan of the lungs shows patchy peripheral ground-glass opacity and consolidation.

secondary to fibrous tissue. Therapy is corticosteroids, and the long-term prognosis is good.

Drug Reaction–Associated Eosinophilic Lung Disease

Multiple drugs can cause a hypersensitivity reaction associated with pulmonary opacities and peripheral blood eosinophilia, which usually develops days to weeks after starting the new drug. Signs and symptoms can include fever, dyspnea, and skin rash. Multiple causative drugs have been described and include penicillins, sulfonamides, nitrofurantoin, *para*-aminosalicylic acid, chlorpropamide, nonsteroidal antiinflammatory drugs (NSAIDs), gold, hydrochlorothiazide, trimipramine, imipramine, carbamazepine, rapeseed oil, L-tryptophan, and multiple chemotherapeutic agents, most notably methotrexate.

Chest radiographic findings can include ground-glass opacity, consolidation, reticulation, nodules, hilar lymphadenopathy, and occasionally pleural effusion. On chest CT, foci of ground-glass opacity, consolidation, nodules, and septal thickening can be present (Figs. 22.7 and 22.8). Histopathologic examination shows both eosinophils and macrophages within the alveolar spaces, alveolar septa, and adjacent interstitium. Treatment includes corticosteroids and cessation of the causative drug.

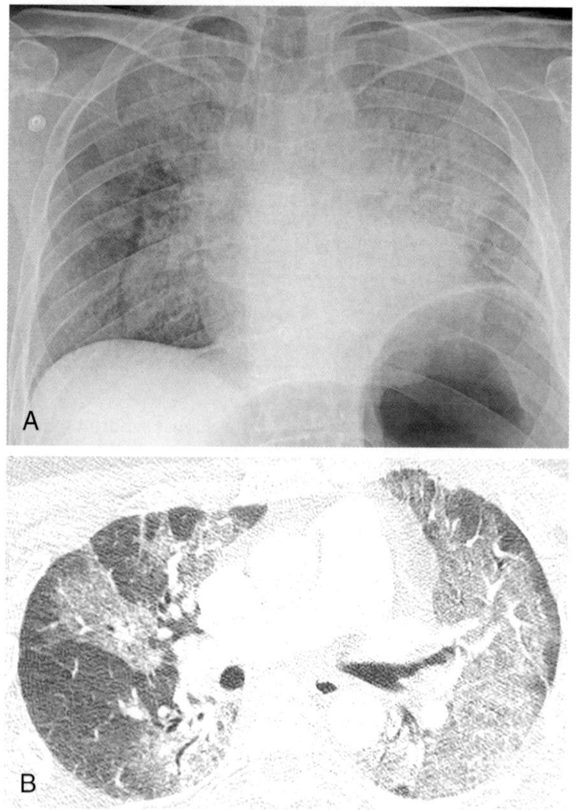

Figure 22.8 Drug-induced eosinophilic pneumonia in a 66-year-old woman secondary to amoxicillin. (A) Chest radiograph and (B) CT scan of the lungs show patchy bilateral ground-glass opacity and consolidation.

Parasite Infection–Associated Eosinophilic Lung Disease

Multiple parasitic infections causing blood and tissue eosinophilia, as well as pulmonary opacities, have been described. Lung involvement can result from direct invasion of the pathogen into the lung or can be secondary to a systemic allergic reaction. Parasitic infections causing eosinophilic lung disease include tropical eosinophilia, worm infestation, schistosomiasis, and pleuropulmonary paragonimiasis (Table 22.1).

Tropical eosinophilia (filariasis) is a systemic disease that results from hypersensitivity to microfilariae, the larva of nematodes. The most common species associated with tropical eosinophilia include *Brugia malayi* and *Wuchereria bancrofti*. Transmission to humans occurs via mosquito bite in endemic areas of India, Southeast Asia, South America, and Northern Africa. Signs and symptoms include weight loss, fatigue, low-grade fever, dyspnea, and chronic cough. Peripheral blood eosinophilia is usually $>3 \times 10^9$/L. Patients usually have elevated serum and BAL IgE levels, positive antifilarial antibody, and BAL fluid consisting of >50% eosinophils. Chest radiographs may be normal or show small nodules and reticulation in a lower lung predominant distribution. CT findings include reticulation, nodules, bronchiectasis, and lobular air trapping. The histopathologic examination shows infiltration

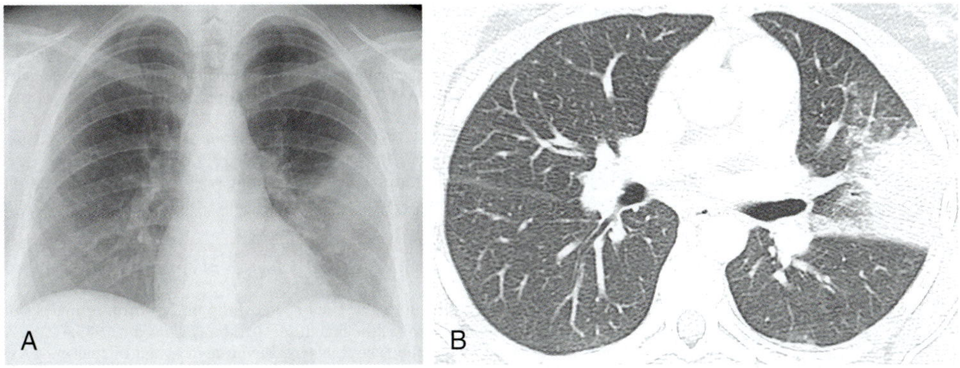

Figure 22.9 Paragonimiasis in a 21-year-old woman who ate undercooked freshwater crab. (A) Chest radiograph shows ill-defined consolidation in the left midlung. (B) CT scan of the lungs shows an area of consolidation within the lingula, abutting the left chest wall. (Courtesy Dr. J. David Godwin, Seattle, WA.)

TABLE 22.1 Common Parasitic Species Causing Eosinophilic Lung Disease

Tropical Eosinophilia	Worm Infestation	Schistosomiasis	Paragonimiasis
Wucheria bancrofti	*Ascaris lumbricoides*	*Schistosoma haematobium*	*Paragonimus westermani*
Brugia malayi	*Strongyloides stercoralis*	*Schistosoma mansoni*	*Paragonimus kellicotti*
Brugia pahangi	*Ancylostoma duodenale*	*Schistosoma japonicum*	
Onchocerca volvulus	*Necator americanus*		
	Toxocara canini		
	Toxocara cati		

of histiocytes and eosinophils into the interstitium and alveoli. Eosinophilic abscesses may also be present. Treatment is with diethylcarbamazine, and there is a 20% relapse rate. If untreated, pulmonary fibrosis eventually develops. Patients with chronic symptoms may not respond well to therapy and can progress to pulmonary fibrosis, despite treatment.

Worm infestation can also result in eosinophilic lung disease. Almost all the worms implicated are nematodes, with the most common species being *Ascaris lumbricoides*. These worms migrate through the lungs during their larval stage, resulting in an allergic reaction, usually SEP. Larvae are present in capillaries, air spaces, and the interstitium. Death of these larvae within the lung incites marked eosinophilic accumulation around the dead larvae.

Almost all patients develop peripheral blood eosinophilia. A skin rash may sometimes be present—for example, with *Strongyloides stercoralis* infection. Although stool studies for ova and parasites are helpful, the diagnosis can be overlooked because some nematodes do not replicate in the digestive system or may not be found in the stool until the female matures. BAL can be useful for diagnosis; larvae are usually identified in BAL fluid, even when absent from the digestive system. Also, serum studies are available for some pathogens, such as *Toxocara*. Chest radiographic findings include miliary nodules, reticulation, and foci of consolidation.

Schistosomiasis is a helminthic infection caused by the human blood fluke. Species include *Schistosoma haematobium, Schistosoma mansoni,* and *Schistosoma japonicum*. Schistosomal cercariae living in fresh water enter the human host via the skin and subsequently enter the blood. They mature in the venous plexus around the bladder, rectum, or mesentery. Lung involvement is less common than at other sites; however, ova are sometimes carried to the pulmonary circulation, where they become lodged in the pulmonary vasculature.

Acute schistosomiasis, also known as Katayama fever, usually occurs in nonimmune travelers and is usually associated with *S. mansoni*. Chronic schistosomiasis occurs in people living in endemic areas. Pulmonary disease is secondary to the presence of schistosome eggs within the pulmonary vasculature. Fibrosis and granuloma formation occur around these eggs and can cause obliteration of pulmonary arterioles, leading to pulmonary hypertension. Chest radiography and CT typically show lung nodules. A peripheral halo of ground-glass opacity may be present around nodules on CT. Enlargement of the pulmonary arteries and right heart chambers suggests pulmonary hypertension.

Pleuropulmonary paragonimiasis is caused by infection with *Paragonimus westermani* or *Paragonimus kellicotti*, usually the result of eating raw or partially cooked infected freshwater crabs and crayfish. The parasite passes through the bowel wall, into the peritoneal cavity, across the diaphragm, and into to the pleural spaces and lungs.

Chest radiographic findings include consolidation and pleural effusion. Some patients may present with spontaneous pneumothorax. CT findings include peripheral low-attenuation nodules, pleural effusion, linear or bandlike areas of consolidation, and foci of ground-glass opacity and consolidation (Fig. 22.9). Bronchiectasis and thin-walled cysts appear later in the disease. The presence of *P. westermani* ova in sputum and BAL fluid confirms the diagnosis. Serologic tests are also available.

■ Some Problem-Solving Issues of Eosinophilic Lung Disease

Development of Eosinophilic Lung Disease in Patients Without a History of Asthma

Although many eosinophilic lung diseases develop in patients with asthma, there are exceptions. A diagnosis of asthma is only established in 50% of patients with

CEP and bronchocentric granulomatous inflammation. Furthermore, the association of asthma and AEP is uncommon. Moreover, idiopathic hypereosinophilic syndrome, drug reactions, and parasite infections are not associated with asthma.

Use of Bronchoalveolar Lavage as Appropriate Workup

BAL can be used as an appropriate workup in those with suspected eosinophilic lung disease in the absence of peripheral blood eosinophilia. Peripheral blood eosinophilia is elevated in most but not all eosinophilic lung diseases. For example, peripheral blood eosinophilia is only elevated in approximately 90% of patients with CEP, and patients with AEP typically do not have peripheral blood eosinophilia in the early course of the disease. The BAL fluid eosinophil count is a much more sensitive examination and tends to be elevated in all eosinophilic lung diseases. If clinical suspicion for eosinophilic lung disease is high, BAL is the preferred diagnostic test.

Distinguishing Eosinophilic Lung Diseases From Disease Mimickers

Overlap between the imaging appearances of several eosinophilic lung diseases and other diseases such as organizing pneumonia and vasculitis can confuse the diagnosis. A combined clinical, radiologic, and pathologic approach is the best method to diagnose eosinophilic lung disease.

Determining the Necessity of Biopsy to Establish a Diagnosis

Biopsy may be necessary to diagnose eosinophilic lung disease when clinical and imaging findings are atypical or nonspecific. This typically occurs in cases of bronchocentric granulomatous inflammation and CSS.

Pitfalls in Diagnosing Pulmonary Eosinophilic Lung Diseases

The major pitfalls in diagnosing pulmonary eosinophilic lung diseases include the absence of peripheral blood eosinophilia, especially initially, as well as nonspecific or atypical findings on imaging. In these cases, further evaluation with BAL and possibly biopsy may be necessary.

Bibliography

Ackerman SJ, Swaminathan GJ, Leonidas DD, et al. Eosinophil proteins: structural biology of Charcot-Leyden crystal protein (galectin-10): new insights into an old protein. *Respir Med.* 2000;94:1014–1016.

Agarwal R, Gupta D, Aggarwal AN, et al. Clinical significance of hyperattenuating mucoid impaction in allergic bronchopulmonary aspergillosis: an analysis of 155 patients. *Chest.* 2007;132:1183–1190.

Al Saieg N, Moammar O, Kartan R. Flavored cigar smoking induces acute eosinophilic pneumonia. *Chest.* 2007;131:1243–1247.

Allen JN, Davis WB, Pacht ER. Diagnostic significance of increased bronchoalveolar lavage fluid eosinophils. *Am Rev Respir Dis.* 1990;142(3):642–647.

Bain BJ. Relationship between idiopathic hypereosinophilic syndrome, eosinophilic leukemia, and systemic mastocytosis. *Am J Hematol.* 2004;77:82–85.

Carrington CB, Addington WW, Goff AM, et al. Chronic eosinophilic pneumonia. *N Engl J Med.* 1969;280:788–798.

Cheever AW, Kamel IA, Elwi AM, et al. *Schistosoma mansoni* and *S. haematobium* infections in Egypt. *Am J Trop Med Hyg.* 1978;27:55–75.

Choi YH, Im JG, Han BK, Kim JH, Lee KY, Myoung NH. Thoracic manifestation of Churg-Strauss syndrome: radiologic and clinical findings. *Chest.* 2000;117(1):117–124.

Chumbley LC, Harrison EG, DeRemee RA. Allergic granulomatosis and angiitis (Churg-Strauss syndrome). Report and analysis of 30 cases. *Mayo Clin Proc.* 1977;52:477–484.

Chusid MJ, Dale DC, West BC, et al. The hypereosinophilic syndrome: analysis of fourteen cases with review of the literature. *Medicine (Baltimore).* 1975;54:1–27.

Cools J, DeAngelo DJ, Gotlib J, et al. A tyrosine kinase created by fusion of the *PDGFRA* and *FIP1L1* genes as a therapeutic target of imatinib in idiopathic hypersosinophilic syndrome. *N Engl J Med.* 2003;348:1201–1214.

Cordier JF. Eosinophilic pneumonias. In: Schwarz M, King T, eds. *Interstitial Lung Disease.* 4th ed. Toronto: Brian C. Decker; 2003:657–700.

Crofton J, Livingstone J, Oswald N, et al. Pulmonary eosinophilia. *Thorax.* 1952;7:1–35.

Ebara H, Ikezoe J, Johkoh T, et al. Chronic eosinophilic pneumonia: evoluation of chest radiograms and CT features. *J Comput Assist Tomogr.* 1994;18(5):737–744.

Epstein DM, Taormina V, Gefter WB, Miller WT. The hypereosinophilic syndrome. *Radiology.* 1981;140(1):59–62.

Franquet T, Muller NL, Gimenez A, Guembe P, de La Torre J, Bague S. Spectrum of pulmonary aspergillosis: histologic, clinical and radiologic findings. *Radiographics.* 2001;21(4):825–837.

Gaensler EA, Carrington CB. Peripheral opacities in chronic eosinophilic pneumonia: the photographic negative of pulmonary edema. *AJR Am J Roentgenol.* 1977;128:1–13.

Gaskin G, Ryan JJ, Rees AJ, et al. Anti-myeloperoxidase antibodies in vasculitis: relationship to ANCA ad clinical diagnosis. *APMIS.* 1990;98:33.

Gonzalez EB, Hayes D, Weedn VW. Chronic eosinophilic pneumonia (Carrington's) with increased serum IgE levels. A distinct subset? *Arch Intern Med.* 1988;148:2622–2624.

Goyal R, White CS, Templeton PA, et al. High attenuation mucous plugs in allergic bronchopulmonary aspergillosis: CT apperance. *J Comput Assist Tomogr.* 1992;16:649–650.

Hueto-Perez-de-Heredia JJ, Dominguez-del-Valle FJ, Garcia E, et al. Chronic eosinophilic pneumonia as a presenting feature of Churg-Strauss syndrome. *Eur Respir J.* 1994;7:1006–1008.

Jederline PJ, Sicilian L, Gaensler EA. Chronic eosinophilic pneumonia. A report of 19 cases and a review of the literature. *Medicine (Baltimore).* 1988;67:154–162.

Jeong YJ, Kim LI, Seo IJ, et al. Eosinophilic lung diseases: a clinical, radiologic, and pathologic overview. *Radiographics.* 2007;27(3):617–637.

Johkoh T, Muller NL, Akira M, et al. Eosinophilic lung diseases: diagnostic accuracy of thin-section CT in 111 patients. *Radiology.* 2000;216(3):773–780.

Katzenstein AL, Liebow AA, Friedman PJ. Bronchocentric granulomatosis, mucoid impaction, and hypersensitivity reactions to fungi. *Am Rev Respir Dis.* 1975;111:497–537.

King MA, Pope-Harman AL, Allen JN, et al. Acute eosinophilic pneumonia: radiologic and clinical features. *Radiology.* 1997;203:715–719.

Koss MN, Robinson RG, Hochholzer L. Bronchocentric granulomatosis. *Hum Pathol.* 1981;12:632–638.

Liebow AA, Carrington CB. The eosinophilic pneumonias. *Medicine (Baltimore).* 1969;48:251–285.

Logan PM, Muller NL. High-attenuation mucous plugging in allergic bronchopulmonary aspergillosis. *Can Assoc Radiol J.* 1996;47:374–377.

Luks AM, Altemeier WA. Typical symptoms and atypical radiographic findings in a case of chronic eosinophilic pneumonia. *Respir Care.* 2006;51:764–767.

Maguire GP, Lee M, Rosen Y, et al. Pulmonary tuberculosis and bronchocentric grnulomatosis. *Chest.* 1986;89:606–608.

Marchand E, Reynaud-Gaubert M, Lauque D, et al. Idiopathic chronic eosinophilic pneumonia. A clinical and follow-up study of 62 cases. The Group d'Etudes et de Recherche sur les Maladies "Orphelines" Pulmonaires (GERM'O'P). *Medicine (Baltimore).* 1998;77:299–312.

Masi AT, Hunder GG, Lie JT, et al. The American College of Rheumatology 1990 criteria for the classification of Churg-Strauss syndrome (allergic granulomatosis and angiitis). *Arthritis Rheum.* 1990;33:1094–1100.

McCarthy DS, Pepys J. Cryptogenic pulmonary eosinophilias. *Clin Allergy.* 1973;3:339–351.

Myers JL, Katzenstein ALA. Granulomatous infection mimicking bronchocentric granulomatosis. *Am J Surg Pathol.* 1986;10:317–322.

Naughton M, Fahy J, FitzGerald MX. Chronic eosinophilic pneumonia. A long-term follow-up of 12 patients. *Chest.* 1993;103:162–165.

Panchal N, Bhagat R, Pant C, et al. Allergic bronchopulmonary aspergillosis: the spectrum of computed tomography appearances. *Respir Med.* 1997;91:213–219.

Parillo JE, Fauci AS, Wolff SM. Therapy of the hypereosinophilic syndrome. *Ann Intern Med.* 1978;89:167–172.

Patterson R, Greenberger PA, Radin RC, Roberts M. Allergic bronchopulmonary aspergillosis: staging as an aid to management. *Ann Intern Med.* 1982;96(3):286–291.

Peters MS, Rodriguez M, Gleich GJ. Localization of human eosinophil granule major basic protein, eosinophil cationic protein, and eosinophil-derived neurotoxin by immunoelectron microscopy. *Lab Invest.* 1986;54:656–662.

Philit F, Etienne-Mastroianni B, Parrot A, et al. Idiopathic acute eosinophilic pneumonia: a study of 22 patients. *Am J Respir Crit Care Med.* 2002;166:1235–1239.

Pope-Harman AL, Davis WB, Allen ED, et al. Acute eosinophilic pneumonia. A summary of 15 cases and review of the literature. *Medicine (Baltimore).* 1996;75:334–342.

Rom WN, Weiden M, Garcia R, et al. Acute eosinophilic pneumonia in a New York City firefighter exposed to World Trade Center dust. *Am J Respir Crit Care Med.* 2002;166(6):797–800.

Rosenberg M, Patterson R, Mintzer R, et al. Clinical and immunologic criteria for the diagnosis of allergic bronchopulmonary aspergillosis. *Ann Intern Med.* 1977;86:405–414.

Rothenberg ME, Klion AD, Roufosse FE, et al. Treatment of patients with hypereosinophilic syndrome with mepolizumab. *N Engl J Med.* 2008;358:1215–1228.

Sandhu M, Mukhopadhyay S, Sharma SK. Tropical pulmonary eosiniophilia: a comparative evaluation of plain chest radiography and computed tomography. *Australas Radiol.* 1996;40:32–37.

Schwartz E, Rozenman J, Perelman M. Pulmonary manifestations of early schistosome infection among nonimmune travelers. *Am J Med.* 2000;109:718–722.

Shintani H, Fujimura M, Yasui M, et al. Acute eosinophilic pneumonia caused by cigarette smoking. *Intern Med.* 2000;39(1):66–68.

Silva CI, Muller NL, Fujimoto K, Johkoh T, Ajzen SA, Churg A. Churg-Strauss syndrome: high resolution CT and pathologic findings. *J Thorac Imaging.* 2005;20(2):74–80.

Souza CA, Muller NL, Johkoh T, Akira M. Drug-induced eosinophilic pneumonia: high-resolution CT findings in 14 patients. *AJR Am J Roentgenol.* 2006;186(2):368–373.

Spry CJF, Davies J, Tai PC, et al. Clinical features of fifteen patients with the hypereosinophilic syndrome. *Q J Med.* 1983;205:1–22.

Sugiyama H, Morishima Y, Kamaeoka Y, et al. Polymerase chain reaction (PCR)-based molecular discrimination between *Paragonimus westermani* and *P. miyazakii* at the metacercarial stage. *Mol Cell Probes.* 2002;16:231–236.

Tazelaar HD, Baird AM, Mill M, et al. Bronchocentric mycosis occurring in lung transplant recipients. *Chest.* 1989;96:92–95.

Tazelaar HD, Linz LJ, Colby TV, et al. Acute eosinophilic pneumonia: histopathologic findings in nine patients. *Am J Respir Crit Care Med.* 1997;155:296–302.

Tillie-Leblond I, Tonnel AB. Allergic bronchopulmonary aspergillosis. *Allergy.* 2005;60:1004–1013.

Turner-Warwick M, Assem ES, Lockwood M. Cryptogenic pulmonary eosinophilia. *Clin Allergy.* 1976;6:135–145.

Uchiyama H, Suda T, Nakamura Y, et al. Alterations in smoking habits are associated with acute eosinophilic pneumonia. *Chest.* 2008;133:1174–1180.

Udwadia FE. Tropical eosinophilia: a review. *Respir Med.* 1993;87:17–21.

Wang JL, Patterson R, Rosenberg M, Roberts M, Cooper BJ. Serum IgE and IgG antibody activity against aspergillus fumigatus as a diagnostic aid in allergic bronchopulmonary aspergillosis. *Am Rev Respir Dis.* 1978;117:917–927.

Ward S, Heyneman LE, Flint JD, Leung AN, Kazerooni EA, Muller NL. Bronchocentric granulomatosis: computed tomographic findings in five patients. *Clin Radiol.* 2000;55(4):296–300.

Weller PF. The immunobiology of eosinophils. *N Engl J Med.* 1991;324(16):1110–1118.

Worthy SA, Muller NL, Hansell DM, Flower CD. Churg-Strauss syndrome: the spectrum of pulmonary CT findings in 17 patients. *AJR Am J Roentgenol.* 1998;170(2):297–300.

CHAPTER 23

Collagen Vascular Diseases and Vasculitis

Julia Capobianco, Bruno Hochhegger, Jeffrey P. Kanne, and Gustavo Meirelles

CHAPTER OUTLINE

Introduction

Collagen vascular diseases (CVDs) are a heterogeneous group of immunologically mediated inflammatory disorders that may involve various organs. They often affect the lungs, mediastinum, and pleura, but the frequency of pulmonary involvement varies according to the specific disease. Additionally, medical treatment may lead to lung infection or drug reaction. Thus imaging is essential in the management of patients with CVD, with early diagnosis and intervention reducing patient morbidity and mortality.

General Aspects of Collagen Vascular Diseases

Collagen Vascular Diseases That Usually Involve the Chest

The defined CVDs that usually involve the lung are rheumatoid arthritis (RA), progressive systemic sclerosis (PSS), systemic lupus erythematosus (SLE), polymyositis (PM), dermatomyositis (DM), mixed connective tissue disease (MCTD), and Sjögren syndrome (SS).

Thoracic Manifestations With Greatest Clinical Impact in Patients With Collagen Vascular Disease

The two thoracic manifestations with the greatest clinical importance in patients with CVD are interstitial lung disease (ILD) and pulmonary arterial hypertension (PAH), which are the major contributors to mortality and morbidity in this patient group.

Best Imaging Techniques and Protocols for Assessing Patients With Collagen Vascular Disease

High-resolution CT (HRCT) is the reference standard technique to image pulmonary diseases in patients with

TABLE 23.1 Frequency of Pulmonary Manifestations of Collagen Vascular Diseases[a]

DISEASE	UIP	NSIP	OP	LIP	DAD	HEMORRHAGE	AIRWAY DISEASE
Rheumatoid arthritis	+++	++	++	+	+	-	+++
Progressive systemic sclerosis	+	+++	+	-	+	-	-
Dermatomyositis/Polymyositis	+	+++	+++	-	++	-	-
Sjögren syndrome	+	++	-	++	+	-	+
Mixed connective tissue disease	+	++	+	-	-	-	-
Systemic lupus erythematosus	+	++	+	+	++	+++	-

[a]Symbols in columns indicate the frequency with which the feature or pattern occurs, with + indicating the lowest, +++ indicating the highest frequency, and - indicating absence of the feature or pattern.
DAD, Diffuse alveolar damage; *LIP,* lymphoid interstitial pneumonia; *NSIP,* nonspecific interstitial pneumonia; *OP,* organizing pneumonia; *UIP,* usual interstitial pneumonia.
Modified from Capobianco J, Grimberg A, Thompson B M, et al. Thoracic manifestations of collagen vascular diseases. *RadioGraphics* 2012;32:33–50.

CVD. Following the development and widespread availability of multidetector CT (MDCT) scanners capable of acquiring near-isotropic data throughout the entire thorax in a single breath-hold, two general approaches are available for performing HRCT. The first and more traditional method entails obtaining axial thin-section (0.625- to 1.5-mm slice thickness) HRCT images spaced at 10- to 20-mm intervals throughout the lungs. The second method uses the ability of MDCT scanners to provide volumetric single breath-hold datasets, allowing spaced, contiguous, and/or overlapping HRCT images to be reconstructed. With MDCT, volumetric data enables multiplanar thin-section HRCT reconstruction, which facilitates the evaluation of the distribution of diffuse lung diseases and the application of postprocessing techniques such as maximum intensity projection, minimum intensity projection, and software that uses volumetric data for quantification of features in the lungs and airways.

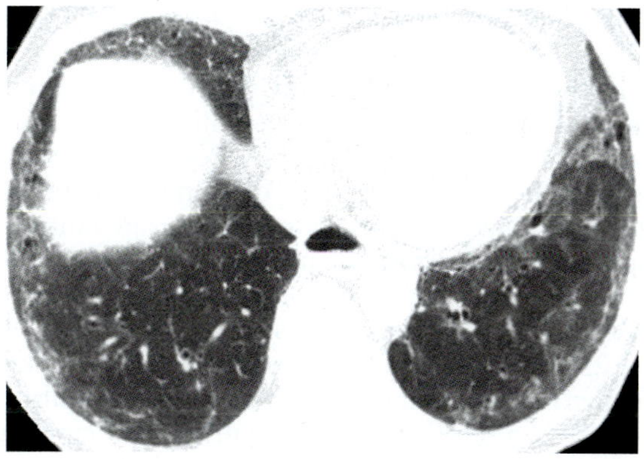

Figure 23.1 A 51-year-old woman with dermatomyositis and a diagnosis of nonspecific interstitial pneumonia on surgical lung biopsy. High-resolution CT demonstrates peripheral ground-glass opacities and reticulation in the lower lobes, with relative subpleural sparing.

Interstitial Pulmonary Diseases in Patients With Collagen Vascular Disease

Most Common Interstitial Pattern

CVD may be associated with various patterns of ILD, and the relative frequency with which these patterns occur varies according to the type of CVD, demographics, and clinical characteristics of those affected (Table 23.1).

Nonspecific interstitial pneumonia (NSIP) is now recognized as a distinct clinicopathologic entity and has been shown to be the most common histologic pattern of ILD in patients with CVD. NSIP encompasses a broad spectrum of histologic features with varying degrees of inflammation and fibrosis, and the temporal uniformity of these pathologic features is the most distinguishing feature from usual interstitial pneumonia (UIP). NSIP is divided into cellular NSIP, which is characterized by inflammation without a substantial fibrotic component, and fibrotic NSIP, in which fibrosis is the dominant finding.

The most common features of NSIP on HRCT are ground-glass opacities, reticulation (usually representing fine fibrosis), and traction bronchiectasis or bronchiolectasis, with a symmetric basal predominant distribution. A lesser degree of involvement of the parenchyma immediately adjacent to the pleura (subpleural relative sparing) can also be seen (Fig. 23.1) and is a distinguishing feature. Other findings include architectural distortion and lower lobe volume loss. Honeycombing is uncommon and occurs primarily in those with advanced fibrosis.

Accurate Detection of Pulmonary Interstitial Disease and Its Importance

Pulmonary alterations (physiologic or anatomic) may be the first manifestations of CVD. Accurate detection of pulmonary involvement in CVD has important therapeutic and prognostic implications because prompt treatment may lead to improved outcomes. Other radiologic findings suggestive of underlying CVD include esophageal dilation, pleural and pericardial effusions and thickening pulmonary arterial enlargement, and osteoarticular disease.

Although the prognosis of NSIP is usually better than that of UIP, NSIP is associated with substantial mortality; nearly 20% of patients die within 5 years after diagnosis.

Patients with cellular NSIP have a more favorable prognosis than those with the fibrotic type. Individuals with CVD-associated ILD usually have a better prognosis than those with idiopathic ILD. Therefore evidence of an underlying CVD should be sought at the initial diagnosis of biopsy-proven NSIP and during the follow-up period, even in the absence of systemic symptoms.

Interstitial Pneumonia With Autoimmune Features and When This Diagnosis Should Be Considered

Some individuals with a diagnosis of idiopathic interstitial pneumonia (IIP) have clinical features that suggest an underlying autoimmune condition but do not meet recognized diagnostic criteria for any CVD. Many terms have already been proposed to describe this process, such as *undifferentiated CVD-associated ILD* (UCVD-ILD), *lung-dominant CVD,* and *autoimmune-featured ILD.*

To achieve consensus about the nomenclature and classification criteria for patients with IIP and features of autoimmunity, the European Respiratory Society/American Thoracic Society Task Force on Undifferentiated Forms of Connective Tissue Disease–Associated Interstitial Lung Disease was formed. The task force agreed on the term *interstitial pneumonia with autoimmune features* (IPAF) for these patients and proposed some classification criteria (Box 23.1), which are centered around three central domains: (1) a clinical domain with specific extrathoracic features; (2) a serologic domain with specific circulating autoantibodies; and (3) a morphologic domain with specific HRCT, histopathologic, and multicompartment features. To be classified as having IPAF, a patient must meet all the a priori requisites and have at least one feature from at least two of the three domains.

Patients with IPAF do not have a classifiable CVD, but are distinct from other individuals diagnosed with IIP. Some of these patients will progress over time to a defined CVD. Prospective studies are still required to validate the proposed classification criteria and assess the natural history and clinical implications of a classification of IPAF.

BOX 23.1 Classification Criteria for Interstitial Pneumonia With Autoimmune Features

1. Presence of an interstitial pneumonia (by HRCT or surgical lung biopsy)
   and
2. Exclusion of alternative causes
   and
3. Absence of criteria for a defined CVD
   and
4. At least one feature from at least two of these domains:
   a. Clinical domain: distal digital fissuring or tip ulceration, inflammatory arthritis or polyarticular morning joint stiffness ≥60 min, palmar telangiectasia, Raynaud phenomenon, unexplained digital edema, unexplained fixed rash on the digital extensor surfaces (Gottron's sign)
   b. Serologic domain: ANA ≥1 : 320, diffuse, speckled, homogeneous patterns or ANA nucleolar pattern or ANA centromere pattern; rheumatoid factor ≥2× upper limit of normal; anti-CCP, anti-dsDNA, anti-Ro (SS-A), anti-La (SS-B), antiribonucleoprotein, anti-Smith, antitopoisomerase (Scl-70), anti-tRNA synthetase, anti-PM-Scl, anti-MDA-5
   c. Morphologic domain:
      1) HRCT patterns: NSIP, OP, NSIP with OP overlap, LIP
      2) Histopathology patterns: NSIP, OP, NSIP with OP overlap, LIP, interstitial lymphoid aggregates with germinal centers, diffuse lymphoplasmacytic infiltration
      3) Multicompartment involvement (in addition to IIP): unexplained pleural effusion or thickening, unexplained pericardial effusion or thickening, unexplained intrinsic airway disease, unexplained pulmonary vasculopathy

ANA, Antinuclear antibody; *CVD,* collagen vascular disease; *HRCT,* high-resolution computed tomography; *IIP,* idiopathic interstitial pneumonia; *LIP,* lymphoid interstitial pneumonia; *NSIP,* nonspecific interstitial pneumonia; *OP,* organizing pneumonia.
Modified from Fischer A, Antoniou KM, Brown KK, et al. An official European Respiratory Society/American Thoracic Society research statement: interstitial pneumonia with autoimmune features. *Eur Respir J.* 2015;46:976–987.

■ Pulmonary Hypertension

Collagen Vascular Diseases Usually Associated With Pulmonary Arterial Hypertension

PAH is defined by a mean resting pulmonary artery pressure ≥25 mm Hg and a pulmonary capillary wedge pressure ≤15 mm Hg. Patients with CVD are considered to have a higher risk for PAH, which may occur in isolation or in combination with ILD. Clinically, and from a therapeutic perspective, the disease in patients with CVD is indistinguishable from its primary form.

PAH is more common in patients with PSS (10%–33%) and MCTD, especially those with predominant scleroderma features. It is less common in SLE (5%–10%) and even more rare in patients with RA, PM/DM, or SS. The limited cutaneous form of systemic sclerosis, also known as CREST syndrome (*c*alcinosis, *R*aynaud disease, *e*sophageal dysfunction, *s*clerodactyly, and *t*elangiectasis), is very often associated with PAH.

Although the pathophysiologic mechanisms of the disease in CVD are not completely understood, its histologic features resemble those seen in primary pulmonary hypertension. Thromboembolic disease may also play a role in patients with SLE and antiphospholipid antibodies.

The most common manifestation of PAH is dyspnea during physical exertion, a nonspecific symptom that makes it difficult to raise the suspicion clinically. For this reason, it is recommended that all patients with PSS and those with MCTD and PSS features undergo noninvasive screening for the early detection of PAH, usually with transthoracic echocardiography. Right heart catheterization is the reference standard for a definitive diagnosis and should be performed when the diagnosis of PAH is suspected.

CT Signs Indicating Pulmonary Arterial Hypertension

Chest CT in patients with PAH may show an increased diameter of the pulmonary arterial trunk (>30 mm), the main pulmonary arteries and their segments, and, in more advanced cases, dilation of the right heart chambers, with contiguous reflux of contrast into the inferior vena cava and hepatic veins. Associated pericardial effusion is a finding that portends a poor prognosis. Pericardial effusion is more common in patients with severe PAH and may be a manifestation of impaired venous and lymphatic drainage resulting from elevated right atrial pressure. CT is also useful for excluding the presence of pulmonary embolism and assessing concomitant ILD.

Cardiac MRI is a complementary method for diagnosing PAH and is currently considered the reference standard for the noninvasive evaluation of right ventricular structure and function. It also provides better evaluation of pulmonary artery flow and compliance as compared with other imaging methods.

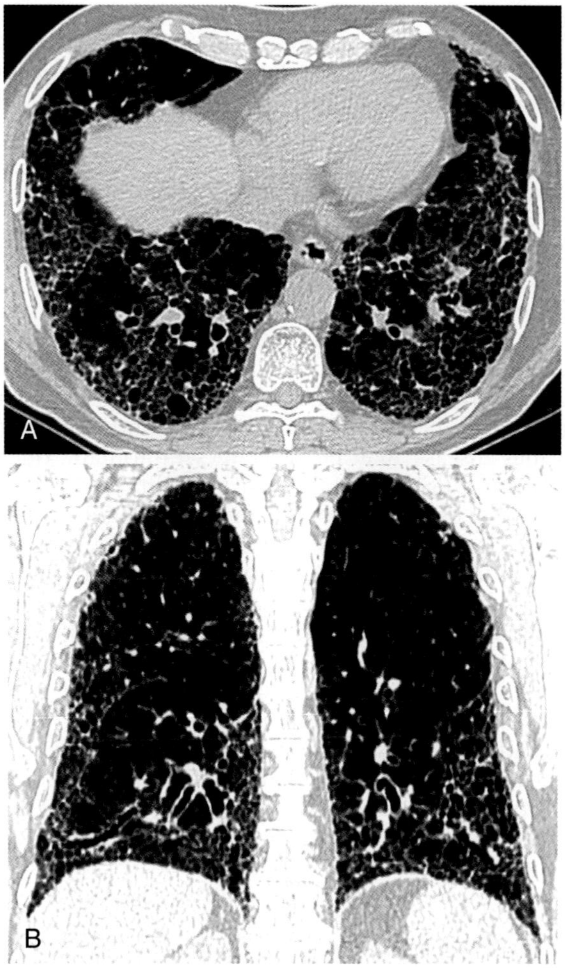

Figure 23.2 A 69-year-old woman with rheumatoid arthritis and chronic dyspnea. (A) Axial and coronal (B) high-resolution CT demonstrates peripheral honeycombing, traction bronchiectasis, and reticular abnormalities in the lower lobes, with subpleural predominance. A surgical lung biopsy showed the usual interstitial pneumonia pattern.

Collagen Vascular Diseases

Rheumatoid Arthritis

RA is a chronic inflammatory disease, typically involving the small joints of the hands and feet in a symmetric fashion. The disease affects mainly women, with peak incidence between 25 and 50 years. Extraarticular manifestations of RA are frequent and may occur in virtually all organ systems. Smoking is associated with a higher risk of developing RA and also with severe forms of the disease.

Main Thoracic Findings

Although RA affects mainly women, pulmonary diseases are more common in men. Respiratory manifestations usually become more prevalent as RA progresses but may present simultaneously with joint symptoms or even predate joint involvement. The prevalence of the different types of RA-associated respiratory diseases is difficult to estimate, but it appears that ILD and pleural disease are most common and ILD, constrictive bronchiolitis, drug reactions, and infections have the greatest impact on patient outcomes.

Most Common Interstitial Findings

The reported prevalence of RA-associated ILD varies significantly, depending on the method of detection and the population examined. ILD had a prevalence initially reported to be around 1.6% to 5%. With the use of HRCT, the prevalence of ILD in unselected RA patients has been found to be as high as 63%. However, clinically significant disease is less common and estimated to occur in approximately 10% of patients.

The main histologic patterns of ILD associated with RA are UIP (Fig. 23.2), NSIP, organizing pneumonia (OP), and diffuse alveolar damage (DAD). Although the radiographic and histologic patterns of NSIP are the most common in the connective tissue disease as a whole, UIP is the most common pattern in RA patients.

Other Thoracic Findings

Pleural involvement is the most common manifestation of thoracic disease in RA, with a frequency of 4% to 75% in postmortem studies. Pleural effusions frequently occur during periods of active arthritis and in patients with subcutaneous nodules, mostly men in their 40s and 50s.

Pulmonary rheumatoid nodules are more common in men than in women and usually result in no symptoms. They are frequently located in the periphery of the right middle lobe or in the upper lobes, ranging from millimeters to several centimeters in diameter. Central cavitation occurs in about 50% of the nodules. Calcification is rare in contrast to silicotic nodules, which commonly calcify. Pulmonary nodules are usually found in patients who have subcutaneous nodules and positive rheumatoid factor.

Progressive Systemic Sclerosis

PSS, or scleroderma, is a chronic multisystem disorder of small vessels and connective tissues characterized by diffuse fibrosis of the skin and internal organs, most frequently the lungs and gastrointestinal tract. The disease has a 3:1 female predilection and typically occurs in the third to fifth decades of life. Almost all patients have skin involvement. Patients with ILD and pulmonary vascular disease may be severely symptomatic due to restrictive lung physiology and low diffusing capacity. Esophageal dysmotility occurs in almost all PSS patients, and gastroesophageal reflux may mimic or overlap with ILD. Cardiac involvement, including right heart dysfunction due to PAH, myocardial fibrosis, and pericardial involvement, may further compound pulmonary symptoms.

Main Thoracic Findings

ILD and PAH are the most common cardiopulmonary findings in PSS. About two-thirds of patients suffering from PSS develop ILD. PAH is present in about 20% of PSS patients and is typically associated with severe pulmonary disease, although it may be an isolated manifestation of PSS. Currently, ILD is the leading cause of death in PSS patients, due to pulmonary fibrosis with or without PAH. The mortality rate from ILD is about 40% within 10 years after the onset of the disease.

Most Common Interstitial Findings

Among interstitial pneumonias, the most frequently seen in PSS patients is NSIP (Fig. 23.3). Typically, the disease affects the posterior regions of the lower lobes, with initially subtle ground-glass opacities, as well as accentuated reticulation that may progress to frank pulmonary fibrosis; this is defined as architectural distortion with reticulation, traction bronchiectasis and bronchiolectasis, and honeycombing.

Other Thoracic Findings

PAH is present in about 20% of PSS patients and is typically associated with severe pulmonary disease, although it may be an isolated manifestation of PSS. Currently, ILD is the leading cause of death in PSS patients, due to pulmonary fibrosis with or without PAH.

Patients with systemic sclerosis have a high prevalence of esophageal (see Fig. 23.3) and pulmonary involvement, but proving a causal relationship is difficult. Few investigators have explored the relationship between esophageal involvement and ILD in PSS. Esophageal dilation is defined by a luminal coronal diameter >9 mm of the infraaortic esophagus. The prevalence of esophageal dilatation varies from 58% to 80% in different series.

This group of patients also has a higher chance of developing malignances during the course of the disease. A recent meta-analysis has found a relative risk of 4.35

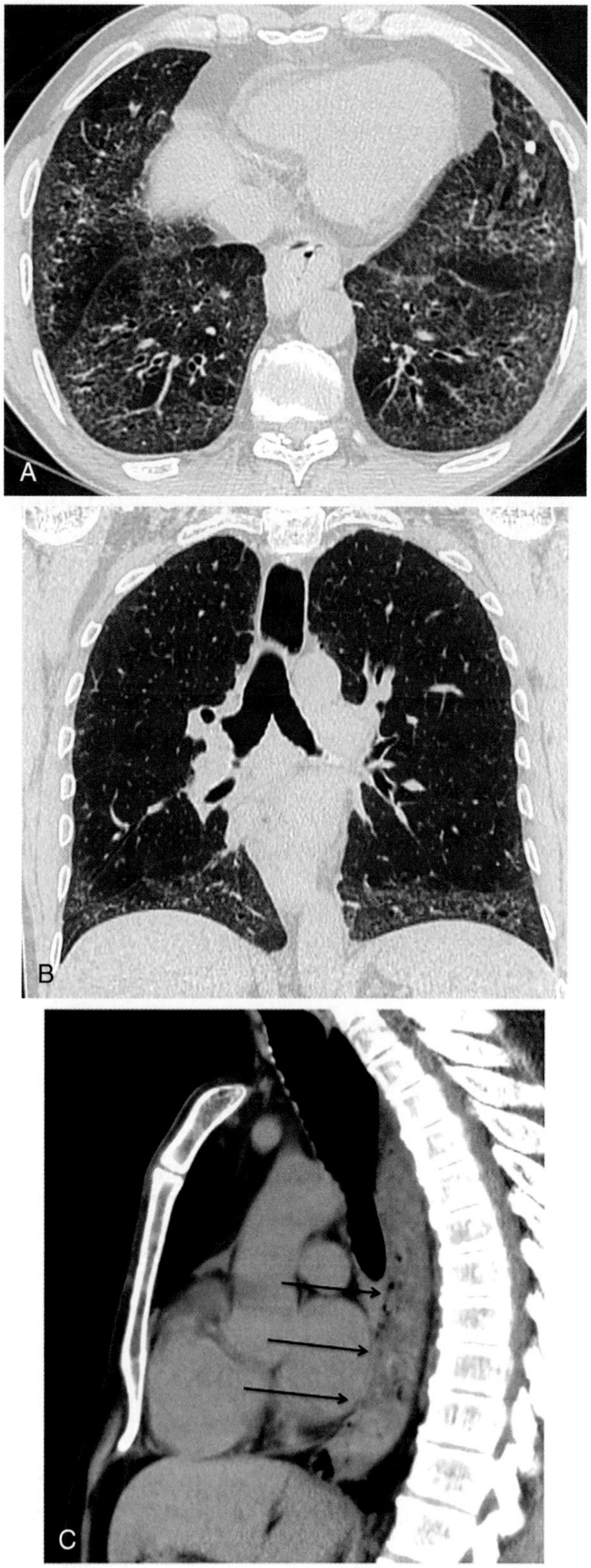

Figure 23.3 A 71-year-old woman with progressive systemic sclerosis, cough, and chronic dyspnea. (A) Axial and coronal (B) high-resolution CT demonstrates peripheral ground-glass opacities and reticular abnormalities in the lower lobes. (C) Sagittal CT reformatted image in soft tissue window demonstrated diffuse esophageal dilation suggesting esophageal disease *(arrows)*. Open lung biopsy demonstrated a nonspecific interstitial pneumonia pattern.

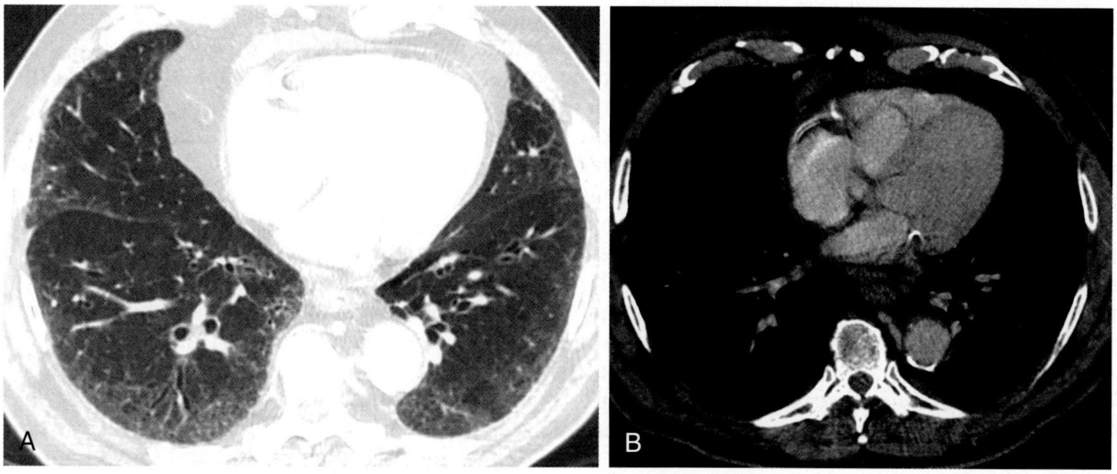

Figure 23.4 A 35-year-old woman with systemic lupus erythematosus, chest pain, and dyspnea. (A) Axial high-resolution CT demonstrates peripheral ground-glass opacities and reticular abnormalities in the lower lobes. Transbronchial lung biopsy demonstrated a nonspecific interstitial pneumonia pattern. (B) CT scan with soft tissue window demonstrates a small pericardial effusion, suggesting pericarditis.

for lung cancer and a relative risk of 2.24 for hematopoietic cancers.

Systemic Lupus Erythematosus

SLE, an autoimmune disorder that primarily affects women (10:1 female-to-male ratio), may affect practically any organ. Predominant manifestations include nondeforming arthritis, serositis, photosensitivity, and renal, hematologic, and central nervous system involvement. Various laboratory abnormalities have been described in SLE, most commonly high-titer antibodies directed against double-stranded DNA, nuclear ribonucleoprotein, Smith (Sm) antigen, Ro/SS-A, and La/SS-B/Ha.

Main Thoracic Findings

The pleuropulmonary manifestations of SLE range in severity from the minor pleuritic pain of serositis to the life-threatening consequences of pulmonary hemorrhage. Many of the abnormalities have nonspecific presentations and require extensive workup to determine the cause. Pleuritis occurs in 17% to 60% of patients at some point in the course of the disease. Although severe parenchymal lung disease is uncommon, pulmonary complications of SLE include acute lupus pneumonitis, diaphragmatic dysfunction and shrinking lung syndrome, cavitating pulmonary nodules, PAH, pulmonary vasculitis, pulmonary embolism (often due to circulating anticardiolipin antibodies), alveolar hemorrhage (reflecting diffuse endothelial injury), chronic interstitial pneumonitis, constrictive bronchiolitis, OP, and opportunistic pulmonary infections or drug toxicity from immunosuppressive therapy.

Most Common Interstitial Findings

Clinically apparent ILD is far less common in SLE than in other CVDs, occurring in 1% to 15% of SLE patients. Although ILD occurs in the setting of SLE, it is often not the direct consequence of the disease. The diagnosis of SLE-ILD relies on a combination of clinical features, chest imaging, histopathology, and abnormalities in lung physiology. A surgical lung biopsy is the gold standard method to diagnose ILD.

The HRCT pattern may be useful in identifying the histologic subtype of ILD, quantifying disease severity, and assessing treatment response. Usually, two (sometimes overlapping) HRCT patterns can be seen in SLE-ILD. One pattern—corresponding to a histologic pattern of NSIP—consists of lower zone, peripherally predominant reticulation often combined with traction bronchiectasis and patchy ground-glass opacities. Areas of consolidation could relate to OP or infection. Another pattern consists of pure ground-glass opacities, with no architectural distortion; this is nonspecific and can be seen in a number of settings, including inflammation, infection, hemorrhage, and edema.

The most common CT pattern of SLE-ILD is that of NSIP (Fig. 23.4); less common patterns include OP, lymphoid interstitial pneumonia (LIP), UIP, desquamative interstitial pneumonia, and DAD.

Other Thoracic Findings

In SLE, other radiographic findings that often occur concomitantly with ILD include pleural and pericardial thickening or effusions (see Fig. 23.4), unilateral diaphragm elevation, cardiomegaly, small lung volumes, and platelike atelectasis. Pleural effusion occurs in 17% to 60% of patients with SLE at some point in the course of the disease.

Inflammatory Myopathies: Dermatomyositis and Polymyositis

DM and PM are the main inflammatory myopathies. These are rare acquired diseases (incidence ≅ 1/100,000 per year) presenting with muscle weakness and inflammation, affecting mainly women, with a peak incidence between 40 and 50 years of age.

Both conditions present with a varying degree of muscle weakness that develops slowly and spares the extraocular muscles (in contrary to myasthenia gravis). Extramuscular manifestations may also be present, such as dysphagia, atrioventricular conduction defects, arrhythmias, heart failure, and pulmonary symptoms. Typical skin manifestations may precede the muscle weakness in DM and include a heliotrope rash (blue-purple discoloration) on the upper eyelids and a raised violaceous rash or papules at the knuckles (Gottron sign). The clinical diagnosis of DM and PM is confirmed by serum muscle enzyme concentrations, electromyography, and muscle biopsy. Skin biopsy may be helpful in certain cases of DM. The antisynthetase syndrome is a related condition that shares many similarities with DM and PM and has a high propensity for pulmonary involvement, involving up to 60% of patients. Lung disease in antisynthetase syndrome is the primary cause of morbidity and may occur without myositis.

Main Thoracic Findings

Thoracic involvement in DM and PM is the main reason for hospital admission in most patients; it is related to worse outcomes and increased mortality. The main thoracic findings in patients with DM and PM are as follows:

- Aspiration secondary to pharyngeal muscle weakness—possibly the most common pulmonary complication in patients with DM or PM, adding significantly to the morbidity and mortality
- ILD, which has a frequency from 5% to 30%
- Hypoventilation and respiratory failure due to respiratory muscles involvement—although an uncommon complication, patients with respiratory failure caused by inflammation of the respiratory muscles usually require intubation and mechanical ventilation.

Other Thoracic Findings

Patients with PM or DM are of increased risk for malignancy. The incidence of cancer association is higher in DM patients, varying from less than 7% to over 30% in some series. Lung cancer is one of the most common neoplasms in these patients (Fig. 23.5), especially in men. Other common cancers are ovarian, breast, gastrointestinal, and non-Hodgkin lymphoma. For PM or DM patients, some factors are associated with an increased risk of malignancy including older age, male gender, dysphagia, cutaneous necrosis, cutaneous vasculitis, rapid onset of myositis (<4 weeks), and elevated serum muscle enzyme levels.

Spontaneous pneumomediastinum and pulmonary hypertension are rare complications of DM and PM but are associated with significant morbidity and mortality.

Most Common Interstitial Findings

The frequency of ILD in DM or PM varies from 5% to 30%, depending on the diagnostic method, and correlates with the presence of anti-Jo1 antibody. The occurrence of ILD may precede the onset of clinical myositis in up to 40% of patients. Four major groups of ILD can be seen: OP, UIP, NSIP, and DAD. The most common pathologic findings are NSIP and OP, often occurring in combination and presenting with the better prognosis among the different groups of ILD that can be seen in DM and PM. The typical imaging features of NSIP have already been discussed; the main imaging findings of OP are bilateral patchy areas of consolidation or ground-glass opacities (Fig. 23.6A), usually in a peripheral, perilobular, or peribronchovascular distribution. These areas of opacities may appear as nodules or masses and often contain air bronchograms. Other CT features are ring-shaped opacities surrounding areas of ground-glass attenuation, also known as the *atoll sign* or *reversed halo sign* (see Fig. 23.6B).

Mixed Connective Tissue Disease

Patients with MCTD exhibit an overlap of features of SLE, PSS, RA, and PM or DM. MCTD affects mostly women (90%), with the highest incidence in the second or third decade of life. The main clinical and laboratory features of MCTD are Raynaud phenomenon, swollen hands, arthritis/arthralgia, acrosclerosis, esophageal dysmotility, myositis, pulmonary hypertension, high-titer fluorescent antinuclear antibody with a speckled pattern, and the presence of antibodies against ribonucleoprotein, at moderate to high levels, in the serum. Most patients with MCTD have a favorable outcome, but thoracic

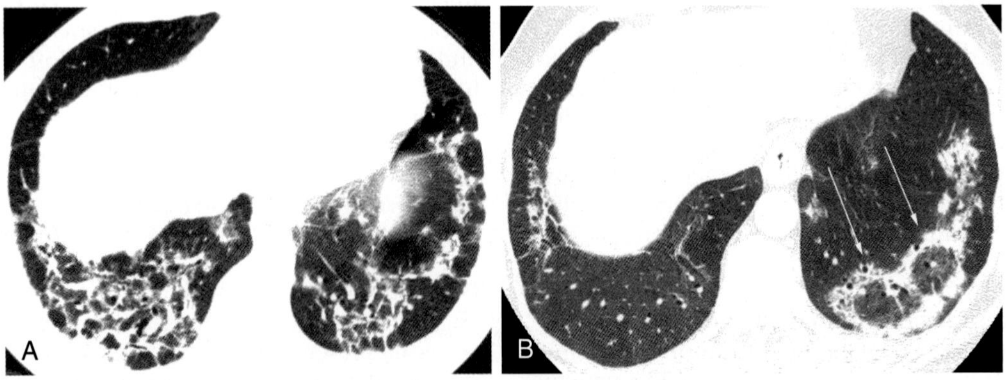

Figure 23.5 (A) A 37-year-old man with dermatomyositis and organizing pneumonia (OP). High-resolution CT (HRCT) shows bilateral areas of consolidation and ground-glass attenuation in a perilobular distribution. (B) A 69-year-old woman with polymyositis and OP. HRCT shows bilateral consolidation and ring-shaped opacities in the left lower lobe and surrounding areas of ground-glass opacity, consistent with the reversed halo sign *(arrow)*.

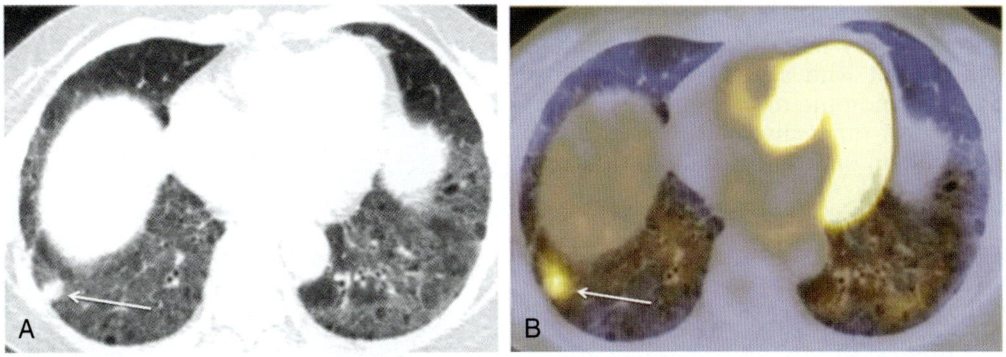

Figure 23.6 A 64-year-old woman with polymyositis, nonspecific interstitial pneumonia (NSIP), and lung cancer. (A) Axial CT image acquired during shallow breathing demonstrates multiple ground-glass opacities in the lower lobes, consistent with the diagnosis of NSIP, and an irregular nodule in the right lower lobe *(arrow)*. (B) Fused PET/CT image shows high metabolic activity in the ground-glass areas and a focal fluorodeoxyglucose (FDG) uptake in the right lower lobe nodule *(arrows)*. The nodule was resected and was consistent with a pulmonary adenocarcinoma.

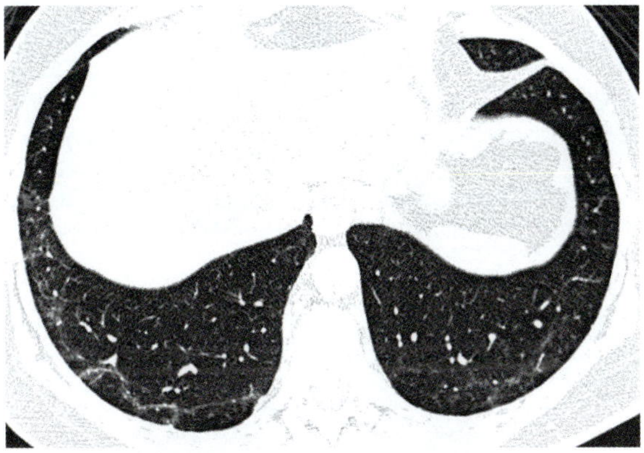

Figure 23.7 A 52-year-old woman with mixed connective tissue disease and nonspecific interstitial pneumonia. High-resolution CT shows peripheral ground-glass opacities, subpleural lines, and reticular abnormalities in the lower lobes, with relative subpleural sparing.

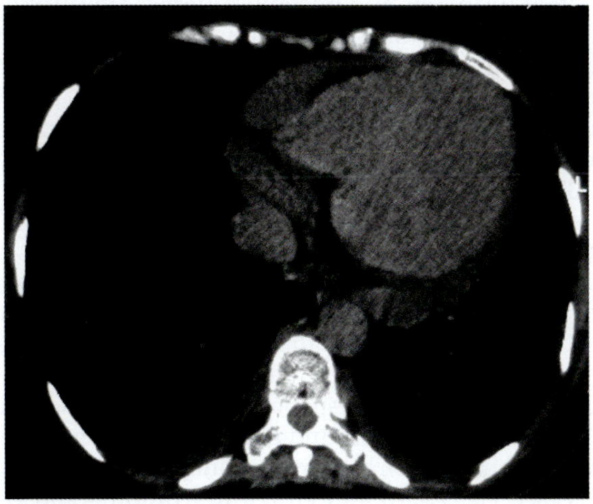

Figure 23.8 A 23-year-old woman with mixed connective tissue disease. This unenhanced CT scan demonstrates small pleural effusions and a pericardial effusion.

involvement, especially PAH, might be a relevant cause of morbidity and mortality.

Main Thoracic Findings

Thoracic involvement is a prevalent feature of MCTD, with a frequency ranging from 20% to 85%. The two most relevant pulmonary complications of the disease are PAH and ILD. PAH has a frequency ranging from 10% to 45% and is not necessarily correlated with the presence of ILD. Pulmonary dysfunction, with a decreasing diffusing capacity for carbon monoxide, is a clue to the development of PAH. PAH is considered a predictor of poor prognosis in MCTD patients; it is the most common disease-associated cause of death.

Most Common Interstitial Findings

ILD is the most common MCTD pulmonary manifestation, with a reported frequency ranging from 21% to 66%. NSIP (Fig. 23.7) is the most common histopathologic and imaging pattern, followed by UIP and LIP. Ground-glass opacity, predominant in the lower and peripheral lungs, is the most common parenchymal abnormality.

Other Thoracic Findings

Esophageal involvement is also a common finding and may be responsible for chronic gastroesophageal reflux, aspiration, and recurrent pulmonary infections. Pleural and pericardial thickening or effusion (Fig. 23.8) may be present in fewer than 10% of patients, mostly in those in whom SLE features predominate. Other thoracic manifestations include thromboembolism, pulmonary vasculitis, infection secondary to aspiration due to esophageal dysmotility, alveolar hemorrhage, and respiratory muscle impairment.

Sjögren Syndrome

SS is an autoimmune disease that affects 0.1% of the population, especially women (female-to-male ratio = 9 : 1) in the fourth or fifth decade of life. The syndrome is characterized by an infiltration of different organs by T lymphocytes, with the lachrymal and salivary glands being the most commonly involved sites.

The main symptoms of SS are xerophthalmia (dry eyes) and xerostomia (dry mouth), and 30% to 40% of patients will present with systemic extraglandular manifestations. The syndrome may be primary, occurring in the absence of other disorders, or secondary, when associated with an underlying condition, such as a CVD.

Main Thoracic Findings

The infiltration of the respiratory tract by T lymphocytes is common in those with SS. Patients with upper respiratory tract involvement often present with dryness and crusting of the nasal mucosa. In more complicated cases, otitis media, epistaxis, and nasal septal perforation may occur. Patients with involvement of the lower airways may present with dry chronic cough, dyspnea on exertion, and recurrent bronchitis.

Patients with SS, especially in the primary form of the disease, may develop ILD, which may present with different histologic and imaging patterns. Airway abnormalities are also a frequent complication of SS. The main imaging findings include bronchial wall thickening, bronchiectasis (Fig. 23.9A), bronchiolectasis, and air trapping. Pleural effusions are rare and almost always occur in patients with secondary SS, more often secondary to SLE and RA.

Most Common Interstitial Findings

The most common presentation of ILD in patients with SS is LIP, but other patterns may be seen, such as NSIP, OP, UIP, bronchiolitis, and diffuse interstitial amyloidosis.

LIP is characterized on the chest radiograph by a reticulonodular pattern, especially in the lower lung zones. HRCT demonstrates ground-glass opacities, thickening of interlobular septa, scattered nodules, and perivascular cysts (see Fig. 23.9B and C). Honeycombing and consolidation are rare. Cysts may also be seen in follicular bronchiolitis due to bronchiolar obstruction secondary to lymphocytic wall infiltration.

Other Thoracic Findings

Patients with SS have an increased risk for lymphoma, usually a B cell, non-Hodgkin type, arising primarily in the salivary glands, but also from mucosa-associated lymphoid tissue from sites such as the lung and stomach. One should suspect a pulmonary lymphoma when a patient with SS develops foci of pulmonary consolidation, large nodules, lymphadenopathy, and/or pleural effusions.

The overall prognosis of SS is good. Morbidity is mainly associated with decreased function of the exocrine organs. Deaths are related to associated diseases (in secondary SS), the development of lymphoproliferative disorders, or acute exacerbation of ILD.

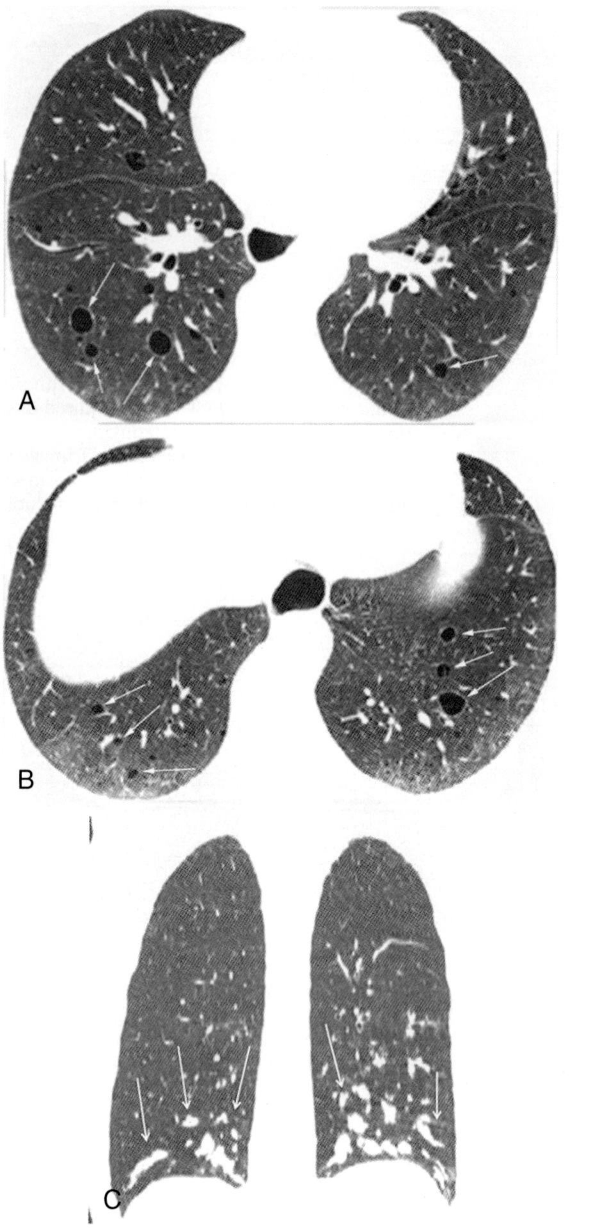

Figure 23.9 (A) A 57-year-old man with Sjögren syndrome (SS). This coronal high-resolution CT (HRCT) image shows multiple bronchiectasis and mucoid impaction *(arrows)* in the lower lobes. (B and C) A 44-year-old woman with SS and lymphoid interstitial pneumonia. Axial HRCT images (B at a higher level than C) show scattered ground-glass opacities, reticulation, and pulmonary cysts *(arrows)*. (From Capobianco J, Grimberg A, Thompson BM, et al. Thoracic manifestations of collagen vascular diseases. *RadioGraphics.* 2012;32:33–50.)

■ Vasculitides

Pulmonary vasculitides comprise a heterogeneous group of rare disorders that share the common feature of inflammation and subsequent destruction of blood vessel walls. Most vasculitides are systemic diseases; the lung can be the primary organ involved or may be one of many. The vasculitides are usually classified by the size of the primary vessels affected or by the pathophysiologic mechanism of disease. The diagnosis of pulmonary vasculitis can be challenging because these diseases are rare and because of the variable clinical manifestations. Diagnosis relies on a combination of clinical, laboratory, imaging, and histopathologic evaluation.

Most Common Vasculitides That Usually Present With Pulmonary Involvement

Most vasculitides that affect the lung belong to the antineutrophil cytoplasmic antibody (ANCA)–associated vasculitis (AAV) group and primarily affect the small vessels. The incidence of pulmonary vasculitis depends on ethnicity; granulomatosis with polyangiitis (GPA) is the most common AAV in North Americans and Europeans, with an incidence of 8 to 10 per million persons per year. In contrast, microscopic polyangiitis (MPA) has been reported to occur more frequently in Japan and China. Eosinophilic granulomatosis with polyangiitis (EGPA; formerly Churg-Strauss syndrome) is the least common of the AAVs, with an incidence of only 1 to 3 per million persons per year. Antiglomerular basement membrane (anti-GBM) antibody disease is an immune complex–mediated small vasculitis that targets the kidneys and lungs and can cause diffuse alveolar hemorrhage (DAH). Takayasu arteritis, a large-vessel vasculitis affecting primarily the aorta, involves the pulmonary arteries in 15% to 60% of patients, although pulmonary involvement may cause little or no clinical manifestations. Pulmonary artery occlusion can occur with long-standing disease. Behçet syndrome affects vessels of all sizes and can involve the pulmonary arteries, leading to aneurysms, thrombosis, or both. Pulmonary involvement occurs almost exclusively in males, and a pulmonary artery aneurysm is associated with high mortality rates. The most common manifestations of pulmonary vasculitides are summarized in Table 23.2.

Most Common Chest CT Findings Suggesting Vasculitis

As with clinical symptoms, the imaging findings of vasculitis are nonspecific and overlap with other disease processes, such as infection, malignancy, and CVD. CT findings of vasculitis range from multifocal ground-glass opacities and consolidation to nodules, masses, and cavities. Tracheobronchial involvement can occur with GPA, and Behçet disease can cause pulmonary artery aneurysms and thrombosis.

Granulomatosis With Polyangiitis

Pulmonary involvement from GPA usually presents with nodules and masses (Fig. 23.10A). Cavitation develops in approximately 50%, particularly as lesions enlarge. The nodules are usually multiple and bilateral and have a predilection for the subpleural and peribronchial regions, with variable craniocaudal distribution. Margins are typically smooth, and some lesions may have a surrounding halo of ground-glass opacity. Central low attenuation is common, reflecting necrosis. With disease progression, lesions usually enlarge and may coalesce into larger inflammatory masses.

The second most common manifestation of GPA in the lung is localized or multifocal consolidation or ground-glass opacity, reflecting areas of hemorrhage, inflammation, or both. Consolidation can be randomly distributed, peribronchial predominant, or subpleural predominant. Approximately 10% of patients will have diffuse ground-glass opacity or consolidation, often with subpleural sparing, reflecting DAH (see Fig. 23.10B). Airway involvement is common with GPA, affecting up to 70% of patients (see Fig. 23.10C). The subglottic trachea is the most common site of disease, but the distal trachea and larger bronchi can also be affected. CT shows single or multiple foci of airway wall thickening and stenosis, usually circumferential. Obstructive atelectasis or infection can develop.

Microscopic Polyangiitis

MPA results in DAH in up to 30% of patients. The appearance of DAH on CT ranges from diffuse bilateral ground-glass opacity to dense consolidation, depending on the extent of alveolar filling (Fig. 23.11A). The

TABLE 23.2 Summary of the Most Common Manifestations of Pulmonary Vasculitides

VASCULITIS	COMMON MANIFESTATIONS	DISTRIBUTION
GPA	• Nodules and masses ± cavitation • Consolidation and ground-glass opacity • Tracheobronchial thickening and narrowing	• Random, peribronchial, subpleural • Focal, patchy, or diffuse • Subglottic most common; usually central airways
MPA	• Consolidation and ground-glass opacity • Poorly defined centrilobular nodules	• Usually bilateral and diffuse • Diffuse or mid and lower lung predominant
EGPA	• Consolidation and ground-glass opacity • Septal thickening	• Nonsegmental, bilateral, and peripheral • Bilateral, dependent
Anti-GBM disease	• Consolidation and ground-glass opacity • Poorly defined centrilobular nodules	• Usually bilateral and diffuse • Diffuse or mid and lower lung predominant
Takayasu arteritis	• Thickening and narrowing of pulmonary arteries	• Focal or multifocal, large pulmonary arteries
Behçet syndrome	• Pulmonary artery aneurysm • Pulmonary artery thrombosis	• Focal or multifocal, large pulmonary arteries • Focal or multifocal

EGPA, Eosinophilic granulomatosis with polyangiitis; *GBM*, glomerular basement membrane; *GPA*, granulomatosis with polyangiitis; *MPA*, microscopic polyangiitis.

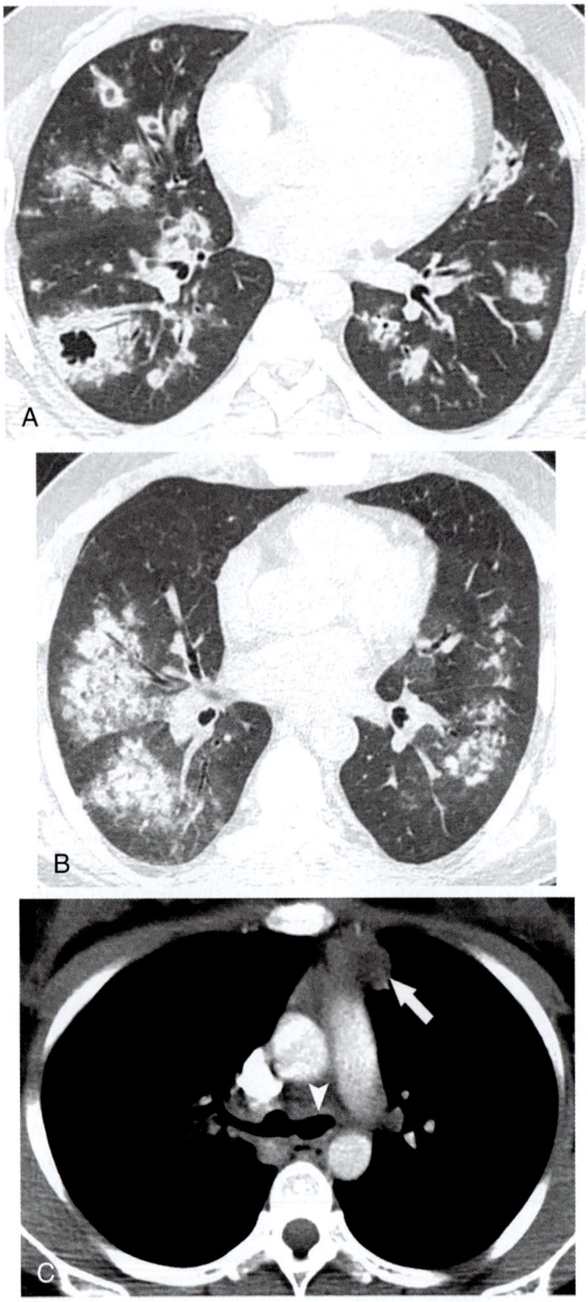

Figure 23.10 (A) A 30-year-old man with granulomatosis with polyangiitis (GPA). This high-resolution CT image shows multiple nodules, some cavitary and some with surrounding ground-glass opacity. (B) A 57-year-old man with GPA and diffuse alveolar hemorrhage (DAH). The image shows bilateral peribronchial consolidation and ground-glass opacity. The relative subpleural sparing is common with DAH. (C) A 15-year-old female with GPA. This contrast-enhanced CT image shows a paramediastinal nodule with central low attenuation *(arrow)* and mild thickening and narrowing of the left main bronchus *(arrowhead)*.

distribution is variable, but a perihilar and mid and basal predominance may occur. Some patients have poorly defined centrilobular nodules on CT. After 24 to 48 hours, as hemorrhage begins to clear, a crazy-paving pattern may be present, defined as ground-glass opacity with superimposed septal lines (see Fig. 23.11B). Recurrent pulmonary hemorrhage can lead to mild fibrosis.

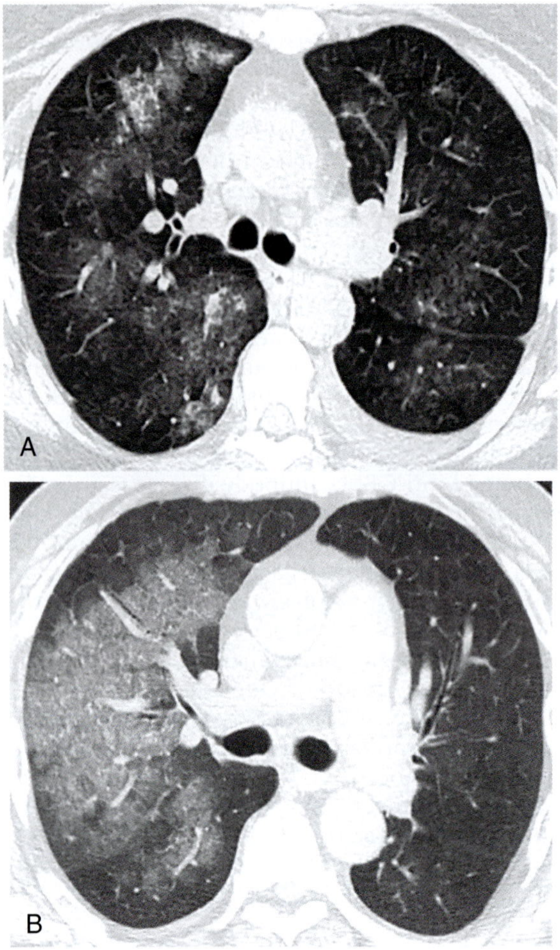

Figure 23.11 (A) A 61-year-old man with microscopic polyangiitis (MPA). This high-resolution (HRCT) image shows bilateral ground-glass opacity and small foci of consolidation in the right lung. Subtle ground-glass attenuation nodules are present in the left upper lobe. (B) A 72-year-old man with subacute diffuse alveolar hemorrhage from MPA. This HRCT image shows a large region of ground-glass opacity in the right lung with subtle superimposed septal lines, creating a crazy-paving appearance.

Eosinophilic Granulomatosis With Polyangiitis

The triad of asthma, hypereosinophilia, and necrotizing vasculitis characterizes EGPA. The lung is the most commonly affected organ. Heart involvement, including myocarditis and coronary arteritis, is the leading cause of death related to EGPA. Bilateral foci of consolidation and ground-glass opacity, typically peripheral, are the most common findings of EGPA on chest CT scans, occurring in up to 90% of patients. This appearance is similar to that of OP or eosinophilic pneumonia (Fig. 23.12A). Approximately 50% of patients with EGPA have smooth septal thickening, reflecting eosinophilic infiltration of the interstitium, edema from heart involvement, or both. Airway manifestations of EGPA on CT include bronchial wall thickening, bronchial dilation, and centrilobular nodules, with or without tree-in-bud opacities, most likely reflecting the effects of asthma (see Fig. 23.12B). Pleural effusions are usually indicative of left heart failure. DAH is rare with EGPA.

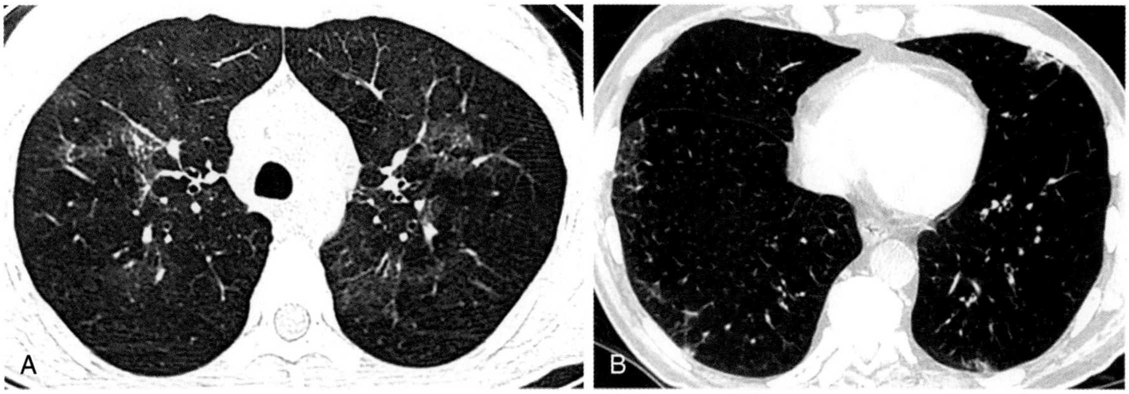

Figure 23.12 (A) A 29-year-old woman with eosinophilic granulomatosis with polyangiitis (EGPA). The high-resolution CT (HRCT) images show patchy ground-glass opacity and mild bronchial wall thickening. (B) A 66-year-old man with EGPA. The HRCT image shows bilateral patchy, peripheral ground-glass opacity and consolidation. Note mild bronchial wall thickening in the left lower lobe.

Distinguishing Vasculitis and Other Diseases

The diagnosis of pulmonary vasculitis is challenging because these diseases are rare, clinical manifestations are variable and nonspecific, and imaging and laboratory findings are also variable and nonspecific. However, the radiologist may suggest the possibility of pulmonary vasculitis when certain imaging features are present. In patients presenting with acute hypoxia and diffuse consolidation or ground-glass opacity on chest imaging, DAH should be considered, especially if the patient has hemoptysis or is anemic. Clinical and laboratory findings of acute glomerulonephritis, in conjunction with lung consolidation and nodules or masses, should also suggest vasculitis. The nodules and masses associated with GPA will change much faster than neoplastic nodules, and many patients with GPA have upper respiratory tract involvement. EGPA should be suspected in patients with adult-onset asthma, other systemic findings such as rash or neuropathy, and areas of increased lung attenuation on CT. Finally, laboratory tests showing elevated serum ANCA levels and, more specifically, anti-myeloperoxidase (anti-MPO) and antiprotease 3 (anti-PR3), are strongly supportive of vasculitis, although the sensitivity and specificity for these autoantibodies vary.

Bibliography

Alibaz-Oner F, Direskeneli H. Update on Takayasu's arteritis. *Presse Med.* 2015;44(6 Pt 2):e259–e265.

Bacon PA. Extra-articular rheumatoid arthritis. In: McCarty DJ, Koopman WJ, eds. *Arthritis and Allied Conditions.* 20th ed. Philadelphia: Lea & Febiger; 1993:811–840.

Bodolay E, Szekanecz Z, Dévényi K, et al. Evaluation of interstitial lung disease in mixed connective tissue disease (MCTD). *Rheumatology.* 2005;44:656–661.

Capobianco J, Grimberg A, Thompson BM, et al. Thoracic manifestations of collagen vascular diseases. *Radiographics.* 2012;32:33–50.

Castañer E, Alguersuari A, Andreu M, et al. Imaging findings in pulmonary vasculitis. *Semin Ultrasound CT MR.* 2012;33(6):567–579.

Dalakas MC, Hohlfeld R. Polymyositis and dermatomyositis. *Lancet.* 2003;362: 971–982.

Eisenberg H, Dubois EL, Sherwin RP. Balchum OJ. Diffuse interstitial lung disease in systemic lupus erythematosus. *Ann Intern Med.* 1973;79(1):37–45.

Epler GR, McLoud TC, Gaensler EA, et al. Normal chest roentgenograms in chronic diffuse infiltrative lung disease. *N Engl J Med.* 1978;298:934.

Fischer A, Antoniou KM, Brown KK, et al. An official European Respiratory Society/American Thoracic Society research statement: interstitial pneumonia with autoimmune features. *Eur Respir J.* 2015;46(4):976–987.

Franquet T. High-resolution CT of lung disease related to collagen vascular disease. *Radiol Clin North Am.* 2001;39(6):1171–1185.

Goldin JG, Lynch DA, Strollo DC, et al. High resolution CT findings in scleroderma-related lung diseases: findings from scleroderma lung study. *Chest.* 2008;134: 358–367.

Hallowell RW, Ascherman DP, Danoff SK, et al. Pulmonary manifestations of polymyositis/dermatomyositis. *Semin Respir Crit Care Med.* 2014;35:239–248.

Hoeper MM. Pulmonary hypertension in collagen vascular disease. *Eur Respir J.* 2002;19(3):571–576.

Honda O, Johkoh T, Ichikado K, et al. Differential diagnosis of lymphocytic interstitial pneumonia and malignant lymphoma on high-resolution CT. *AJR Am J Roentgenol.* 1999;173:71–74.

Joseph J, Sahn SA. Connective tissue diseases and the pleura. *Chest.* 1993;104: 262–270.

Kazerooni EA. High-resolution CT of the lungs. *AJR Am J Roentgenol.* 2001; 177(3):501–519.

Kim EA, Lee KS, Johkoh T, et al. Interstitial lung diseases associated with collagen vascular diseases: radiologic and histopathologic findings. *Radiographics.* 2002;22:S151–S165.

Kligerman SJ, Groshong S, Brown KK, et al. Nonspecific interstitial pneumonia: radiologic, clinical, and pathologic considerations. *Radiographics.* 2009;29(1):73–87.

Kozuka T, Johkoh T, Honda O, et al. Pulmonary involvement in mixed connective tissue disease. *J Thorac Imag.* 2001;16:94–98.

Lally L, Spiera RF. Pulmonary vasculitis. *Rheum Dis Clin North Am.* 2015;41(2): 315–331.

Launay D, Remy-Jardin M, Michon-Pasturel U, et al. High resolution computed tomography in fibrosing alveolitis associated with systemic sclerosis. *J Rheumatol.* 2006;33:1789–1801.

Olson AL, Brown KK, Fischer A. Connective tissue disease-associated lung disease. *Immunol Allergy Clin North Am.* 2012;32(4):513–536.

Orens JB, Martinez FJ, Lynch JPIII. Pleuropulmonary manifestations of systemic lupus erythematosus. *Rheum Dis Clin North Am.* 1994;20:159–193.

Ozerkıs DA, Rubinowitz EA, Homer RJ, et al. Pulmonary manifestations of rheumatoid arthritis. *Clin Chest Med.* 2010;31:451–458.

Prosch H, Schaefer-Prokop CM, Eisenhuber E, et al. CT protocols in interstitial lung diseases—a survey among members of the European Society of Thoracic Imaging and a review of the literature. *Eur Radiol.* 2013;23(6):1553–1563.

Ruano CA, Lucas RN, Leal CI, et al. Thoracic manifestations of connective tissue diseases. *Curr Probl Diagn Radiol.* 2015;44(1):47–59.

Schwarz MI. The lung in polymyositis. *Clin Chest Med.* 1998;19(4):701–712.

Seyahi E, Yazici H. Behçet's syndrome: pulmonary vascular disease. *Curr Opin Rheumatol.* 2015;27(1):18–23.

Silver RM, Miller KS. Lung involvement in systemic sclerosis. *Rheum Dis Clin North Am.* 1990;16:199–216.

Steen VD, Conte C, Owens GR, et al. Severe restrictive lung disease in systemic sclerosis. *Arthritis Rheum.* 1994;37:1283–1289.

Tanaka N, Newell JD, Brown KK, et al. Collagen vascular disease–related lung disease. High-resolution computed tomography findings based on the pathologic classification. *J Comput Assist Tomogr.* 2004;28:351–360.

Tanoue LT. Pulmonary manifestations of rheumatoid arthritis. *Clin Chest Med.* 1998;19:667–685.

Vonk MC, Van Die CE, Snoeren MM, et al. Oesophageal dilatation on high-resolution computed tomography scan of the lungs as a sign of scleroderma. *Ann Rheum Dis.* 2008;67:1317–1321.

CHAPTER 24
Cystic Lung Disease

Rachna Madan and Thanissara Chansakul

CHAPTER OUTLINE

■ Introduction

Cystic lung diseases present a considerable diagnostic challenge mainly because CT findings can be similar in many of these diseases. In addition, a number of pulmonary abnormalities can result in cystic patterns that mimic true lung cysts. However, the combination of characteristic imaging findings, clinical features, and genetic testing, where appropriate, often permits an accurate diagnosis. In this chapter, we review the unique CT features of individual cystic lung diseases and provide a systematic approach to a confident radiologic diagnosis.

■ Spectrum and Prevalence of Cystic Lung Disease

Diffuse cystic lung diseases are rare entities. The most well-known diffuse cystic lung diseases are lymphangioleiomyomatosis (LAM) and pulmonary Langerhans cell histiocytosis (PLCH). The estimated incidence of LAM is from 1 to 2.6 cases/1,000,000 women, although the true incidence is likely higher because LAM is often mistakenly diagnosed for asthma, bronchitis, and chronic obstructive pulmonary disease. PLCH is also uncommon. In a clinical series of 502 patients, the diagnosis of PLCH was made in about 3.4% of individuals undergoing open lung biopsy for chronic diffuse infiltrative lung disease. However, the exact prevalence of PLCH is unknown because a significant number of affected patients may be asymptomatic, and the disorder may undergo spontaneous resolution.

Owing to the recent more widespread use of CT, differential diagnosis of these rare entities becomes more extensive than previously described, including Birt-Hogg-Dubé syndrome (BHD), lymphocytic interstitial pneumonia (LIP), light chain deposition disease (LCDD), and amyloidosis. Infectious processes including *Pneumocystis jiroveci* pneumonia (PJP) and human papillomavirus–associated papillomatosis have also been described to result in cyst formation.

Diffuse cystic lung diseases may be categorized on the basis of CT appearance, clinical history, and serologic evaluation. Many diffuse and focal or multifocal cystic lung diseases demonstrate bronchiolocentric distribution of cysts, as well as abnormal cellular infiltration on histopathology (Table 24.1). Based on their CT appearance, the diseases can be organized based on whether the cysts are sparse or numerous in number and whether there are associated findings, such as nodules or ground-glass opacities. A history of systemic diseases and prior infection is often helpful in narrowing the differential diagnosis (Table 24.2).

■ Demographics, Genetics, and Role of Other Causative Factors

Knowledge about the patient's demographics, family history, medical history, and environmental exposure,

TABLE 24.1 Bronchiolocentric Lesions in Cystic Lung Diseases

CYSTIC LUNG DISEASE	BRONCHIOLOCENTRIC LESION
Pulmonary Langerhans cell histiocytosis (PLCH)	Mixed inflammatory nodule (CD1a-positive Langerhans cells, lymphocytes, macrophages) close to bronchioles
Lymphangioleiomyomatosis (LAM)	Spindle cell proliferation in distal airways
Lymphocytic interstitial pneumonitis (LIP)	Lymphocytic cell proliferation along airways
Desquamative interstitial pneumonitis and respiratory bronchiolitis–interstitial lung disease (RB-ILD)	Pigment-laden macrophages in respiratory bronchioles and alveolar ducts
Amyloid–light chain deposition disease (LCDD)	Peribronchial lymphoplasmacytoid infiltrates and light chain deposition

TABLE 24.2 Cysts Associated With Systemic Disease

SYSTEMIC DISEASE	PATHOLOGY	HIGH-RESOLUTION CT FINDINGS
Primary systemic amyloidosis • Hematologic malignancies • Multiple myeloma, Waldenstrom macroglobulinemia	Amyloid light chain • Deposition in kidneys, heart, lungs	• Calcified nodules and scattered cysts • Lymphadenopathy • Tracheal wall thickening and nodularity
Kappa light chain deposition disease • Hematologic malignancies • Multiple myeloma, Waldenstrom macroglobulinemia	• Non–amyloid kappa light chain • Deposition in kidneys, heart, lungs	• Thin-walled cysts • Nodules, calcifications absent • Progressive abnormality may lead to respiratory failure
Lymphocytic interstitial pneumonitis • Sjögren syndrome, rheumatoid arthritis, HIV, Castleman disease	Lymphocyte proliferation along airways	• Perivascular cysts • Background of patchy ground-glass abnormalities, small nodules

particularly a history of cigarette smoking, is often helpful in narrowing the differential diagnosis.

Lymphangioleiomyomatosis

LAM is almost exclusively a disease of women. Although previously characterized as a disease of women of childbearing age, there has been increasing detection of subclinical disease in postmenopausal women. LAM occurs in two forms, sporadic and in association with tuberous sclerosis complex. The sporadic form accounts for 85% of cases and is generally associated with more severe pulmonary cystic changes. Tuberous sclerosis is an autosomal dominant disease, but 60% of tuberous sclerosis patients have no family history of the disease, and the disease is the result of a new germline mutation. Mutations in the tumor suppressor genes *TSC1* and *TSC2* are associated with the development of LAM. Less than one-third of tuberous sclerosis patients have the classic triad of seizures, adenoma sebaceum, and mental retardation.

Pulmonary Langerhans Cell Histiocytosis and Desquamative Interstitial Pneumonia

PLCH is a disease of smokers, occurring most frequently in young adults with a current or past smoking history. Smoking prevalence has ranged from 80% to 100% in various studies. The diagnosis of PLCH can therefore be confidently excluded in a nonsmoker. Although PLCH was previously reported as more common in men, there is no longer a gender predilection due to increased smoking in women.

Cyst formation has also been described in desquamative interstitial pneumonia (DIP), a smoking-related interstitial lung disease. DIP is a rare disease entity almost exclusively seen in individuals exposed to cigarette smoke. It is characterized by macrophage accumulation within the alveoli. Patients may have dyspnea or cough. Confirmation of the smoking history is mandatory before suggesting a diagnosis of DIP on radiologic grounds.

Birt-Hogg-Dubé Syndrome

BHD is an autosomal dominant disease caused by a mutation in the *BHD* gene, which encodes for the tumor suppressor protein folliculin. Most patients with pulmonary cysts will have facial fibrofolliculomas distributed over the face, neck, and upper trunk. Renal tumors such as oncocytomas and renal cell carcinomas may be seen and are frequently multifocal and bilateral. Hence, identification of subpleural cysts in association with facial fibrofolliculomas should prompt further genetic testing and MRI evaluation of the abdomen to screen for renal neoplasms.

Lymphocytic Interstitial Pneumonia

LIP is a rare entity and may be idiopathic or may be seen more commonly in patients with an underlying immunologic abnormality. In particular, LIP has been associated with Sjögren syndrome, AIDS, primary biliary cirrhosis, Castleman disease, systemic lupus erythematosus, and autoimmune thyroid disease. LIP is more common in women, likely due to the association of LIP with autoimmune disease. It is currently controversial whether LIP represents a benign lymphoproliferative disorder or a form of early lymphoma, and mediastinal and hilar lymph node enlargement is sometimes seen in these patients.

Light Chain Deposition Disease

LCDD occurs in middle-aged patients, with 75% of cases occurring in association with multiple myeloma or macroglobulinemia. LCDD usually involves the kidneys. Although lung involvement is rare, LCDD can result in respiratory failure, necessitating lung transplantation.

Amyloidosis

Pulmonary cysts are rare manifestations of amyloidosis and are usually described with localized amyloidosis in association with Sjögren syndrome. A cystic lung pattern is rarely seen in systemic amyloidosis associated with multiple myeloma, macroglobulinemia, rheumatoid arthritis, tuberculosis, or Crohn disease.

Appropriate Imaging Modalities for the Evaluation of Patients With Cystic Lung Disease

CT is used as a diagnostic study, usually after a standard chest radiograph is obtained or when the chest radiograph result is considered to be abnormal. CT should be performed during deep inspiration at total lung capacity. High-resolution CT (HRCT) using thinner sections of 1 to 1.25 mm is recommended to evaluate the fine details of the pulmonary parenchyma. Contrast material may not be required for routine assessment of cystic lung disease unless there is a concomitant concern for mediastinal, vascular, or pleural abnormalities.

Importance of Ancillary Extrathoracic Findings

Identification of ancillary extrathoracic findings (e.g., renal tumors, skin findings) helps narrow the differential diagnosis and can alert the clinician to the possibility of underlying familial syndrome. Specifically, both tuberous sclerosis and BHD are associated with renal neoplasms.

The most common renal tumor in tuberous sclerosis complex is an angiomyolipoma, which is more common in patients with a *TSC2* gene mutation. The incidence of renal cell carcinoma in tuberous sclerosis is similar to that in the general population but the tumors occur at a younger age, typically in the third decade of life, as compared to the more usual presentation in the fifth decade. Thoracic and/or abdominal chylous effusion is also characteristic of tuberous sclerosis complex. All patients newly diagnosed with LAM should have imaging of the abdomen and pelvis. Annual brain MRI is recommended for all patients with tuberous sclerosis until 21 years of age and then every 2 or 3 years to diagnose and monitor subependymal giant cell astrocytomas.

Imaging of the abdomen and pelvis should also be performed in patients newly diagnosed with BHD. In BHD, renal tumors are often multiple, may be bilateral, and are noted at an earlier age (mean, 50.7 years) than the general population. The tumors include chromophobe oncocytoma, renal cell carcinoma, and clear cell carcinoma.

Pitfalls: How to Differentiate True Cystic Lung Disease From Mimics

On HRCT, the term *lung cysts* refers to a thin-walled (usually <2 mm), well-circumscribed, and well-defined air-containing lesion that is 1 cm or larger in diameter. The mechanism of cyst development is unclear, but in some cases appears to be related to small airway obstruction. Several other pulmonary abnormalities feature a cystic pattern that mimics true cystic lung disease, but do not manifest true lung cysts. These include honeycombing, bronchiectasis, emphysema, and cavitary nodules (Fig. 24.1).

Honeycombing can be differentiated from true cysts because of their thicker walls; they are lined by fibrous tissue. The subpleural location—stacked appearance of cysts—in honeycombing and the presence of other signs of fibrosis also help distinguish honeycombing from true cysts. Bronchiectasis represents dilation and distortion of the airways and hence typically maintains tubular structure or orientation. Coronal and sagittal reformations are helpful in delineating communication with the bronchial tree. Emphysematous bullae and centrilobular emphysema are focal areas of permanent destruction of the bronchiolar walls, with resultant enlargement of the air space distal to the terminal bronchiole. By definition, bullae are 1 cm or more in diameter and have imperceptible walls that are less than 1 mm thick. It is sometimes difficult to distinguish bullae from true lung cysts, although the central location of the vascular structures and other signs of extensive emphysema frequently allow correct diagnosis. Cavitary nodules have much thicker and more irregular walls than true lung cysts.

Problem Solving and Case Scenarios

Diseases Associated With Numerous Cysts (Diffuse Cystic Lung Disease)

Diseases associated with numerous cysts are easy to diagnose due to important differentiating features. The differential diagnosis is short and includes LAM and PLCH; these two disease entities can be differentiated based on demographics, clinical features, and history of smoking, as well as characteristic imaging findings.

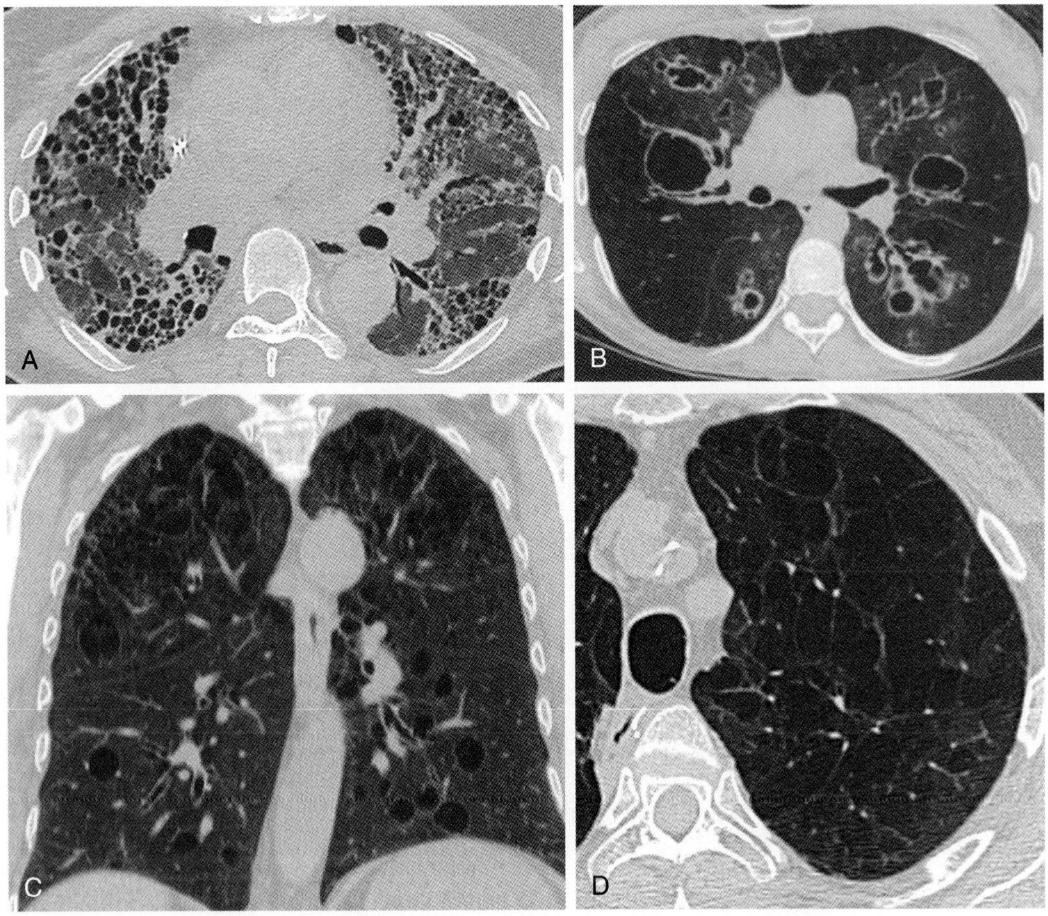

Figure 24.1 Mimics of cystic lung disease. (A) Honeycombing; multiple rows of peripheral stacked cysts with traction bronchiectasis, architectural distortion, and other signs of pulmonary fibrosis. (B) Cystic bronchiectasis. Cysts cluster centrally and communicate with the central airways. (C and D) Centrilobular emphysema and lymphangioleiomyomatosis (LAM) in the same patient. The cysts in the upper lobes have variable polygonal shapes and an imperceptible wall composed of compressed lung tissue and vessels, in keeping with emphysema. The eccentric or central dot is due to perilobular vessels. True cysts in lower lobes are due to LAM and have well-defined thin walls

Clinical Presentation

Patients with numerous cysts frequently present with abnormal pulmonary function test results, airflow obstruction, and low diffusing capacity, given the significant underlying cystic abnormality. The clinical presentation may sometimes be sudden, with acute shortness of breath due to spontaneous pneumothorax from rupture of cysts. Although LAM is considered to be a disease of young women, PLCH is frequently encountered in smokers and is more common in men.

Chest Radiographic and CT Findings

Radiographic abnormalities include increased lung volumes, hyperinflation, linear interstitial opacities, and cystlike lucencies (Fig. 24.2A). Patients with PLCH may also demonstrate a reticulonodular abnormality involving the upper and mid zones of the lungs.

LYMPHANGIOLEIOMYOMATOSIS

On CT images, numerous thin-walled uniform shaped round cysts are seen, frequently >10 in number (see Fig. 24.2B). Extensive cystic abnormality in the vicinity of the fissures may give rise to a beaded appearance of the fissure. The distribution of the cysts is diffuse, including the upper and lower lobes, with no sparing of the lung bases or costophrenic sulci. In addition to the cystic parenchymal abnormality, mediastinal nodal enlargement due to LAM involving the nodes, as well as low-attenuation, free-layering chylous pleural effusions and small pericardial effusions, may also be present (see Fig. 24.2C and D).

PULMONARY LANGERHANS CELL HISTIOCYTOSIS

On CT, a combination of numerous variably shaped cysts and nodules predominates. Irregular stellate-shaped nodules are a feature of early disease, and these can later evolve into thick-walled "Cheerio" cysts and larger, bizarrely shaped cysts due to coalescence. Cysts and nodules frequently demonstrate bronchiolocentric distribution and are most numerous in the upper lobes, with relative sparing of the right middle lobe, lingula, and lung bases. Smoking is strongly associated with PLCH, and end-stage, burnt-out PLCH mimics emphysema due to its upper to mid zone distribution and bizarrely shaped cysts (Fig. 24.3).

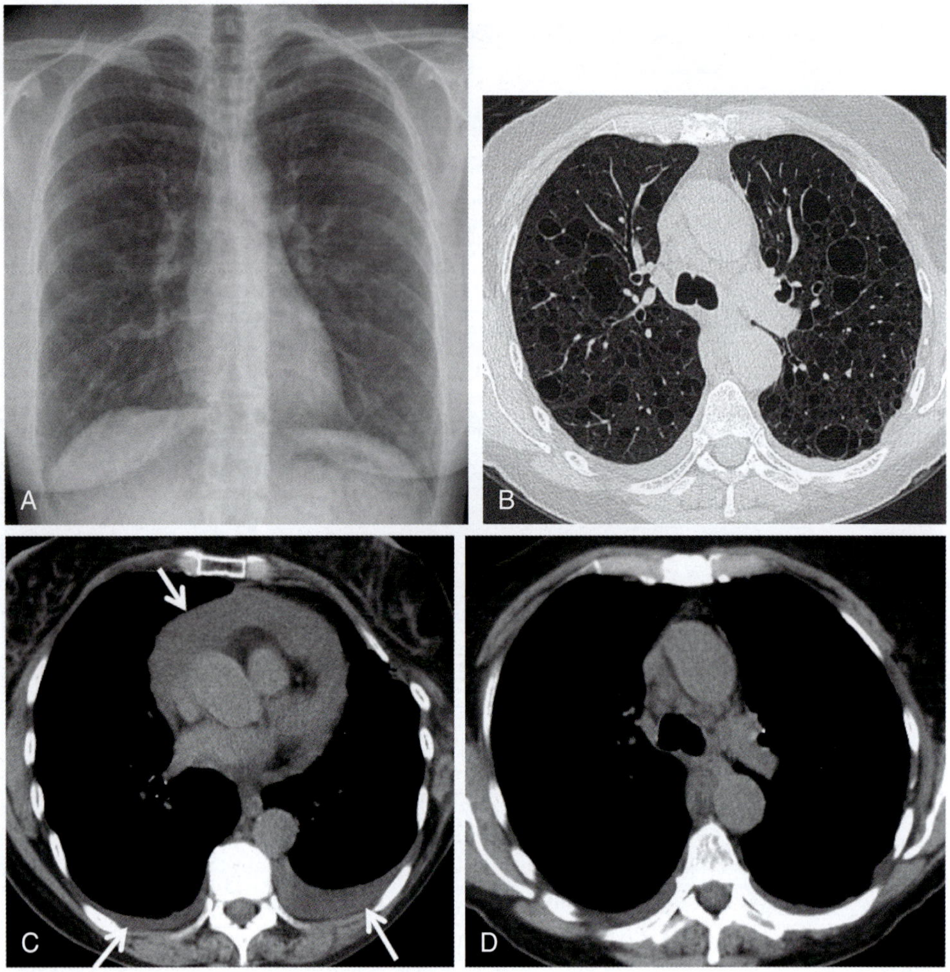

Figure 24.2 Numerous cysts—lymphangioleiomyomatosis. (A) Chest radiograph demonstrates diffuse reticular opacities in both lungs and increased lung volumes. (B) Chest CT scan demonstrates innumerable thin-wall cysts of varying sizes in both lungs. Note normal intervening lung parenchyma. The cysts were seen involving the lungs diffusely. (C and D) CT scans, soft tissue window, demonstrate a moderate-sized pericardial effusion *(arrow)*, as well as small bilateral chylous effusions *(arrows)* and multiple mildly enlarged lymph nodes.

MIMICS AND IMAGING PITFALLS

Entities such as honeycombing and emphysema may mimic cystic lung disease, as described above (see Fig. 24.1).

Diseases Associated With Sparse Cysts (Focal or Multifocal Cystic Lung Disease)

The spectrum of diseases associated with scattered sparse cysts is wider and includes entities such as BHD, LIP, LCDD, and amyloidosis. A confident diagnosis is sometimes not possible because the cysts may be detected incidentally, and underlying systemic disease or an immunologic abnormality may be unknown. In older patients, lung cysts have also been reported in asymptomatic nonsmoking individuals, raising the possibility that they may represent part of the aging process. Hence, scattered cysts are more significant in the younger population.

Clinical Presentation

Patients are usually asymptomatic with respect to the underlying scattered sparse cysts, and the cystic disease is discovered incidentally. Hence, pulmonary function tests are usually normal in these patients. These cases may also be brought to clinical attention due to a spontaneous pneumothorax from a rupture of underlying cysts.

BIRT-HOGG-DUBÉ

Patients have sparse thin-walled cysts, lentiform in shape, mostly seen in a subpleural location in the lower lobes and sometimes close to the pulmonary veins (Fig. 24.4A). A search for ancillary extrathoracic findings, such as facial skin tags, papules, folliculomas, and small renal neoplasms, is crucial in the subsequent management of these patients (see Fig. 24.4B).

LYMPHOCYTIC INTERSTITIAL PNEUMONITIS

Sparse perivascular cysts may be seen in asymptomatic patients with underlying collagen vascular disorders and an immunologic abnormality, such as Sjögren syndrome, HIV infection, or Castleman disease. The cysts may appear pseudoseptated in some cases due to their proximity to adjacent vessels (Fig. 24.5A) and, in some patients, a combination of minimal ground-glass abnormality and nodularity may be seen in the vicinity of the cysts (see Fig. 24.5B).

LIGHT CHAIN DEPOSITION DISEASE AND AMYLOIDOSIS

Cysts with or without nodules may be diagnosed incidentally in patients with plasma cell dyscrasias and may represent kappa light chain deposition disease (κLCDD) or light chain amyloidosis in addition to infection or malignancy.

LCDD is associated with the deposition of a nonamyloid kappa light chain in the kidneys, heart, and lungs,

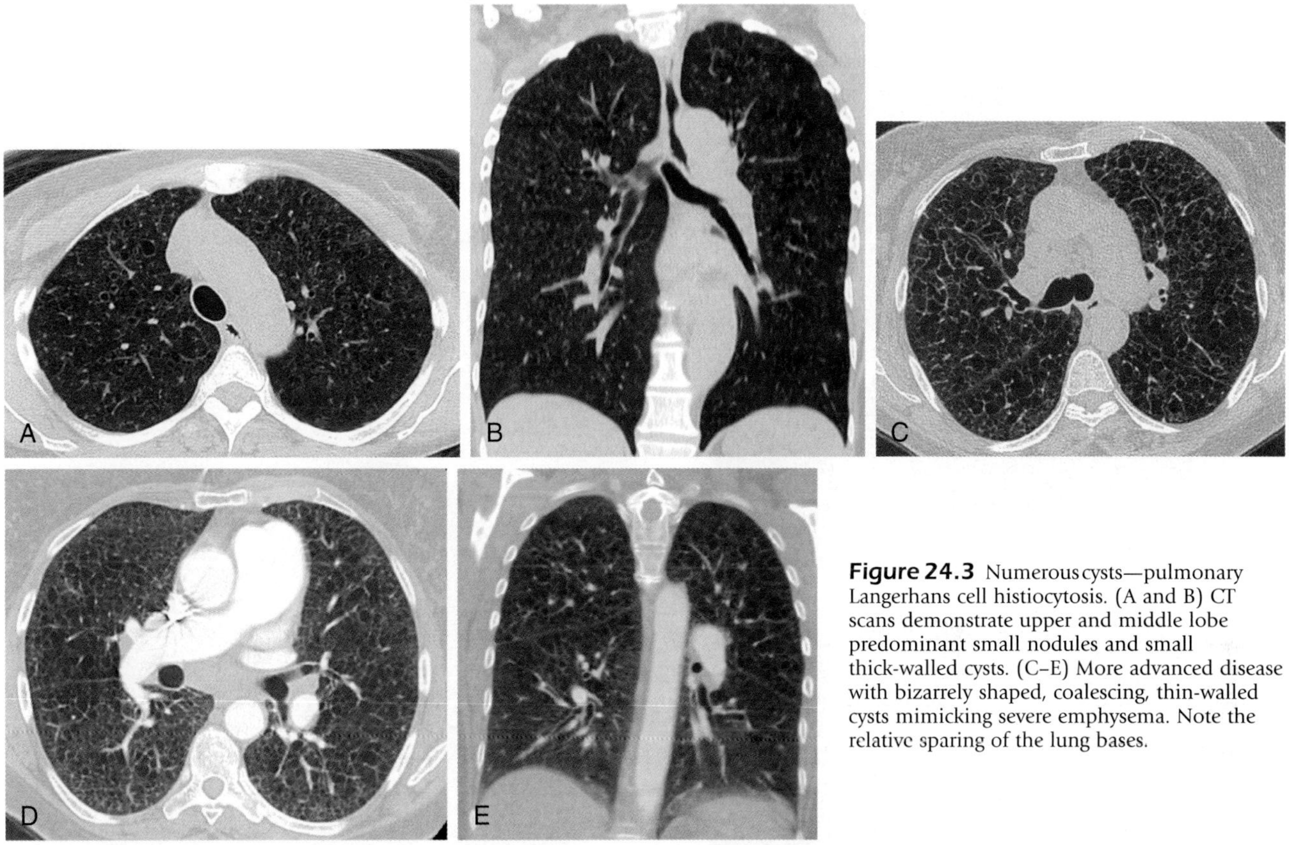

Figure 24.3 Numerous cysts—pulmonary Langerhans cell histiocytosis. (A and B) CT scans demonstrate upper and middle lobe predominant small nodules and small thick-walled cysts. (C–E) More advanced disease with bizarrely shaped, coalescing, thin-walled cysts mimicking severe emphysema. Note the relative sparing of the lung bases.

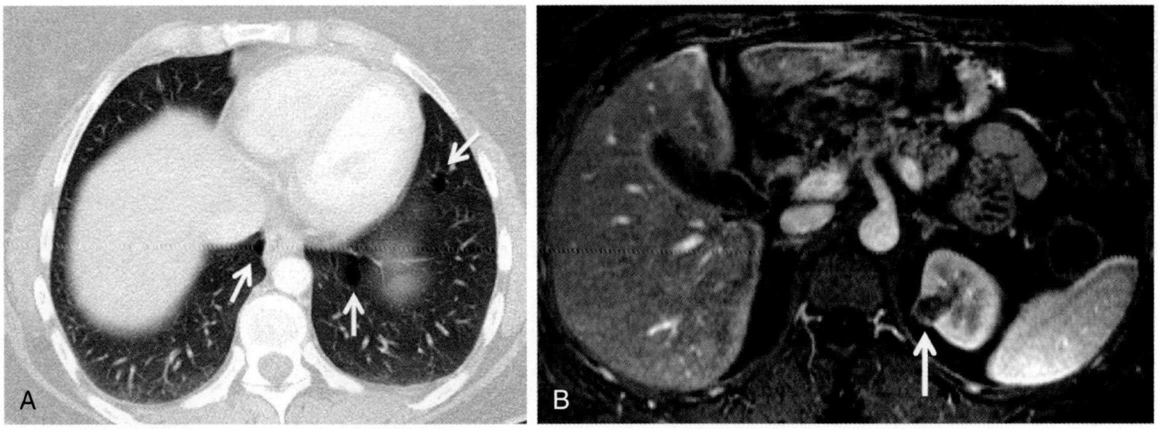

Figure 24.4 Sparse cysts—Birt-Hogg-Dubé syndrome. (A) Axial CT scan demonstrates a few thin-walled cysts in both lower lobes *(arrows)*. (B) Postcontrast axial T1-weighted, fat-suppressed MRI scan demonstrates a hypointense lesion *(arrow)* in the upper pole of the left kidney, representing a clear cell carcinoma.

characterized by multiple, round, thin-walled cysts in the lungs (Fig. 24.6A). Nodules and calcium deposition are generally not seen. In rare cases, the parenchymal abnormalities may be progressive and lead to respiratory failure.

Amyloidosis is frequently associated with calcified nodules besides scattered lung cysts (see Fig. 24.6B and C). Patients may also have adenopathy and nodular tracheal wall thickening. The diagnosis may be suspected in patients with underlying myeloma, macroglobulinemia, or Sjögren syndrome and may subsequently be confirmed on open biopsy of these nodules, which may stain positive for Congo red and show focal ossification.

Diseases Associated With a Combination of Cysts, Nodules, and Thick-Walled Cheerio Cysts

Clinical Presentation

CHEERIO SIGN ON CT

The term *Cheerio sign on CT* refers to a pulmonary nodule with a central lucency, similar to the ring-shaped Cheerios breakfast cereal (Fig. 24.7A). This may arise from the proliferation of neoplastic cells, such as adenocarcinoma, or nonmalignant cells, such as PLCH around a patent airway.

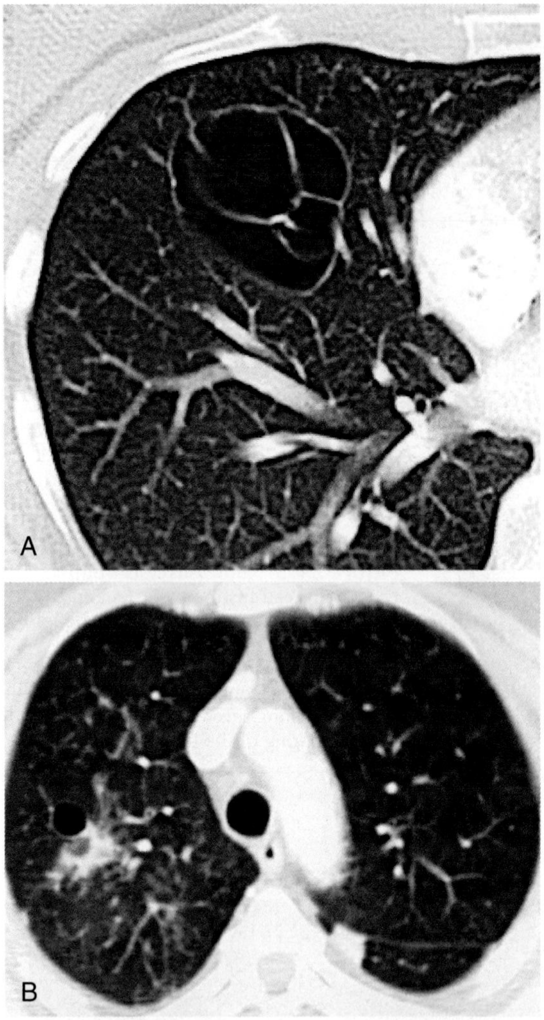

Figure 24.5 Sparse cysts—lymphocytic interstitial pneumonitis. (A) Axial CT scan demonstrates a large thin-walled cyst with a pseudoseptated appearance in the right middle lobe, secondary to proximity to adjacent vessels. (B) Axial CT scan in lung windows in a different patient shows a combination of ground-glass abnormality and nodularity, with superimposed scattered cysts. This represents an earlier phase of disease, and the ground-glass abnormality frequently resolves following treatment with steroids. (Courtesy Dr. Matthew Gilman.)

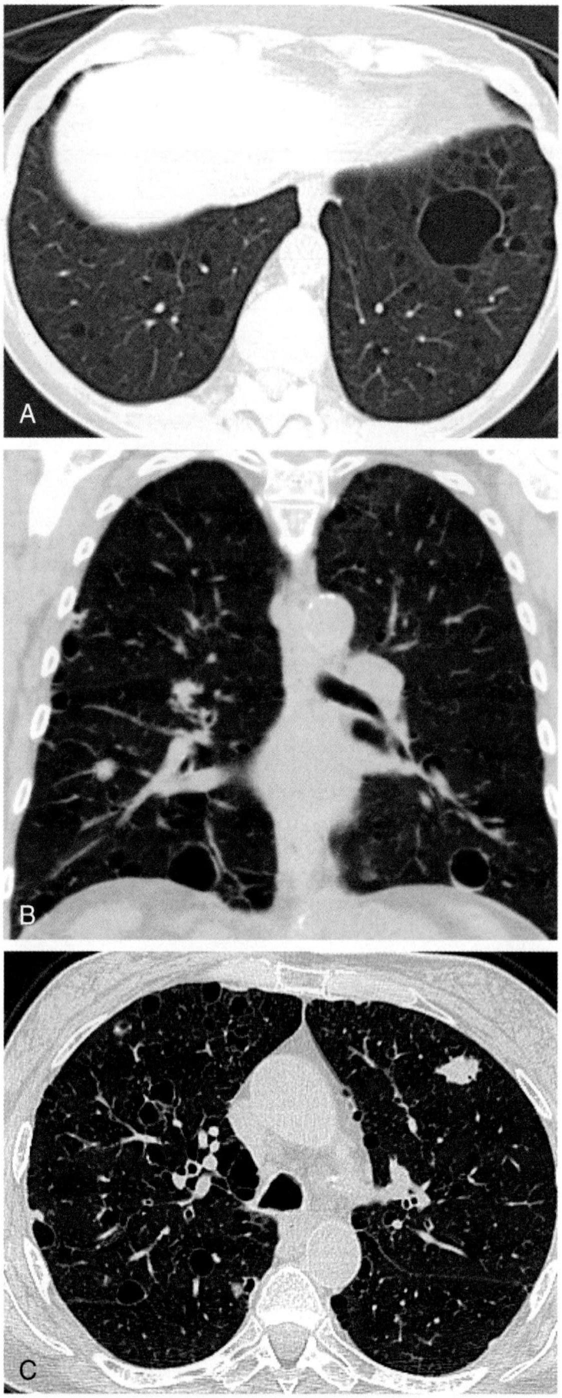

Figure 24.6 Sparse cysts—light chain deposition disease (LCDD) and amyloidosis. (A) Axial CT scan demonstrates a large thin-walled cyst and smaller thin-walled cysts in an asymptomatic patient with multiple myeloma and LCDD. No calcifications or nodules are seen. (B and C) Multiple cysts and a few irregular, partially calcified nodules in a patient with plasmacytoma. Open biopsy of the nodule stained positive with Congo red, confirming amyloidoma, and also revealed plasma cell infiltration.

Cellular proliferation surrounding other types of central radiolucencies, such as pseudocavitation, cavitation, alveoli, or multiple thin-walled cysts, can also produce appearances similar to Cheerios and, as such, this sign may also be seen in metastases, rheumatoid nodules, septic emboli, fungal infection, and vasculitis.

In the early stages of PLCH, small, irregular-shaped bronchiolocentric nodules predominate, which then transform into thick-walled Cheerio cysts (see Fig. 24.7B and C). More advanced disease is characterized by the coalescence of cysts into bizarre shapes. End-stage or burnt-out disease leads to the formation of thin-walled cysts and parenchymal fibrosis and may be difficult to distinguish from advanced emphysema.

Adenocarcinomas may demonstrate the Cheerio sign due to a variety of reasons. In some cases, adenocarcinomas may develop in a bulla or cystic space (Fig. 24.8). Some pathologic entities, including adenocarcinoma in situ, minimally invasive adenocarcinoma, invasive lepidic predominant adenocarcinoma, and invasive mucinous adenocarcinoma, are associated with a lepidic growth pattern with maintained alveolar structure and bronchial patency—hence creating a Cheerios-like appearance on CT.

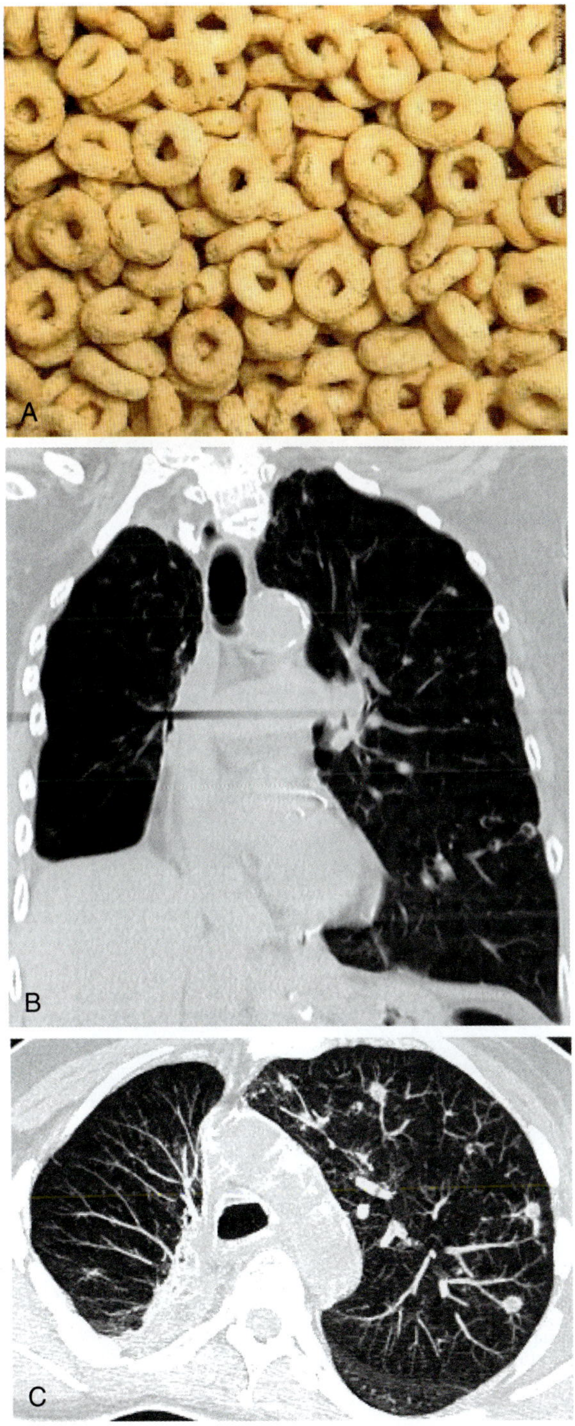

Figure 24.7 Cheerio cysts. (A) Cheerios breakfast cereal. (B and C) Coronal CT scan and axial maximum intensity image in current heavy smoker and prior history of right lung adenocarcinoma demonstrates multiple nodules and thick-walled cysts in the left lung. Open biopsy was done to rule out metastases and confirmed the diagnosis of pulmonary Langerhans cell histiocytosis.

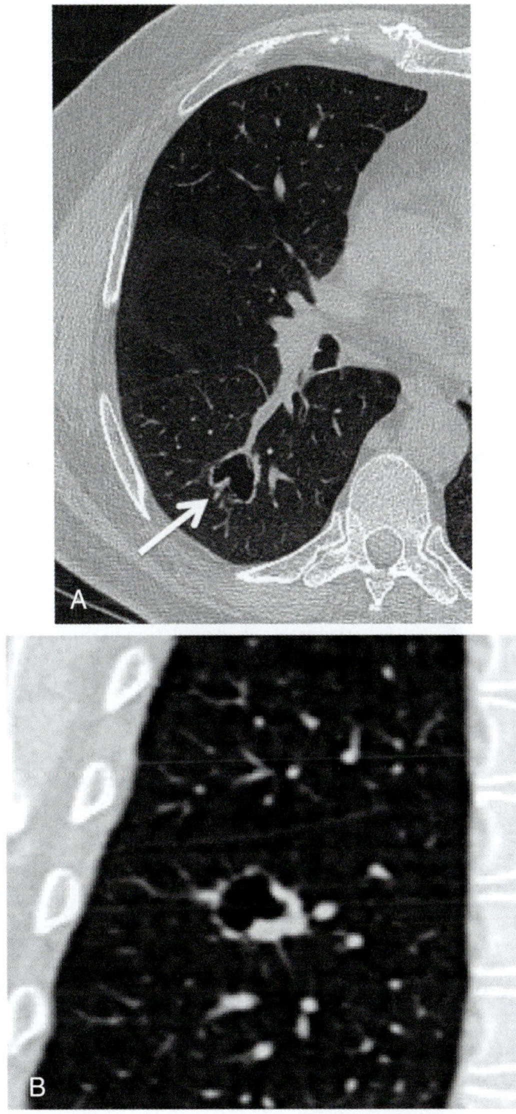

Figure 24.8 Cheerio cysts—adenocarcinoma associated with cystic air space. (A and B) Axial and coronal CT scans reveal an eccentric soft tissue nodularity *(arrow)* along the anterior and medial aspect of the right lower lobe cyst, which had slowly increased in size. Pathology was consistent with adenocarcinoma.

TUMORAL CAVITATION

This may be seen in patients with advanced nonsquamous, non–small cell lung cancer who are receiving chemotherapeutic agents, such as bevacizumab (Avastin, Genentech, San Francisco, CA), which is a humanized monoclonal antibody against vascular endothelial growth factor (VEGF). Cavitation is secondary to central necrosis due to VEGF inhibition and signifies a therapeutic response. Cavitation may develop in the dominant tumor or in the smaller metastatic nodule (Fig. 24.9). Spontaneous pneumothorax has been reported when a responding cavitary lesion communicates with the pleura.

THIN-WALLED CYSTIC METASTASES

These are frequently seen in the setting of underlying sarcoma, squamous cell cancer, transitional cell carcinoma of the bladder, and melanoma. As with other metastatic lesions, cystic metastases tend to have different sizes and a basilar predominance. A potential complication of cystic metastases is the development of a spontaneous pneumothorax (Fig. 24.10).

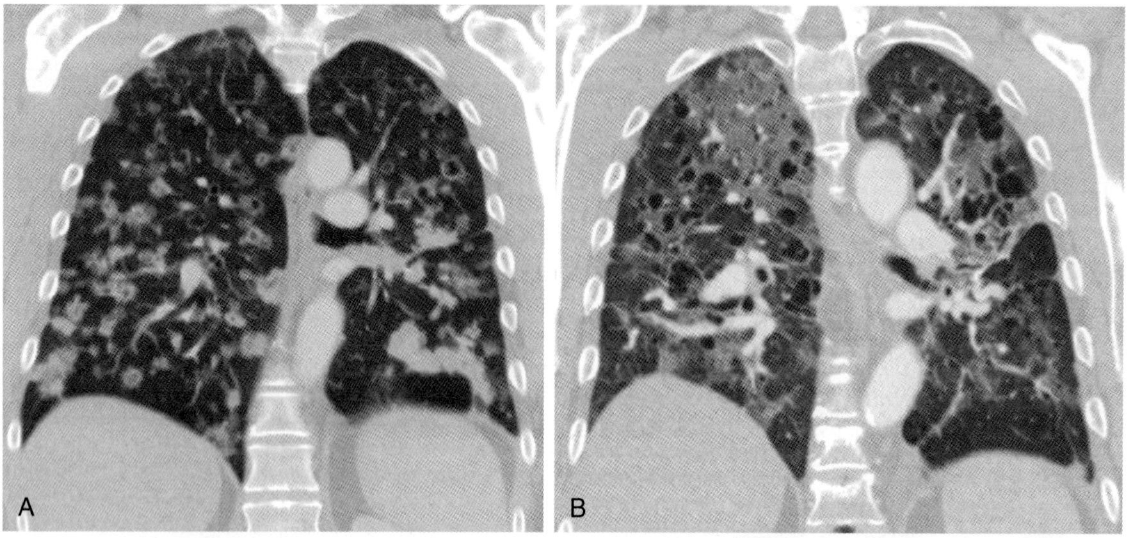

Figure 24.9 Cheerio cysts—cystic changes secondary to bevacizumab. (A and B) Coronal CT scans demonstrates multiple thick-walled cysts in both lungs, representing cavitation of metastatic lesions. Extensive ground-glass abnormality seen in the upper lobes is also considered to be a treatment effect. Bevacizumab causes cavitation in primary and metastatic lung cancers, thought to be secondary to central necrosis due to vascular endothelial growth factor inhibition.

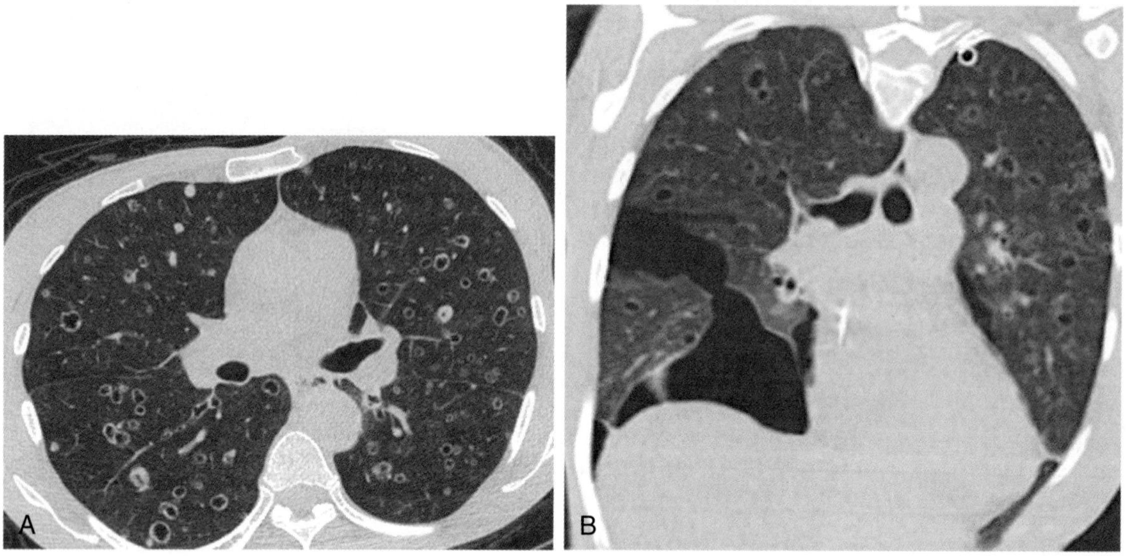

Figure 24.10 Cheerio cysts—cystic metastases presenting acutely with pneumothorax. (A) Axial and (B) coronal CT scans in a patient with müllerian carcinoma being treated with pazopanib. Multiple thick-walled cavitary metastases are seen. Necrosis of subpleural nodules led to bilateral pneumothoraces; this may be a presenting sign of cysts or cystic metastases.

NECROBIOTIC LUNG NODULES

Up to 1% of patients with moderate to severe longstanding rheumatoid arthritis may demonstrate necrobiotic lung nodules (Fig. 24.11). These are frequently subpleural and may cavitate, leading to pneumothorax and bronchopleural fistulae. Because these cavitary nodules mimic infection and malignancy, percutaneous biopsy may be needed.

SEPTIC EMBOLI

These may present as thick-walled cysts with fluid levels and are easily diagnosed due to the history—fever, indwelling catheter, or intravenous drug abuse—and characteristic imaging appearance, including nodules in an angiocentric distribution demonstrating a feeding vessel sign (Fig. 24.12). Septic emboli commonly undergo rapid evolution and cavitation.

The incidence of laryngotracheal papillomatosis and subsequent pulmonary dissemination has significantly decreased due to effective vaccination against human papillomavirus. The radiographic findings include cystic pulmonary lucencies and nodules. On CT, papillomas of the trachea and bronchi are easily visualized. The associated cysts are less numerous than in LAM or

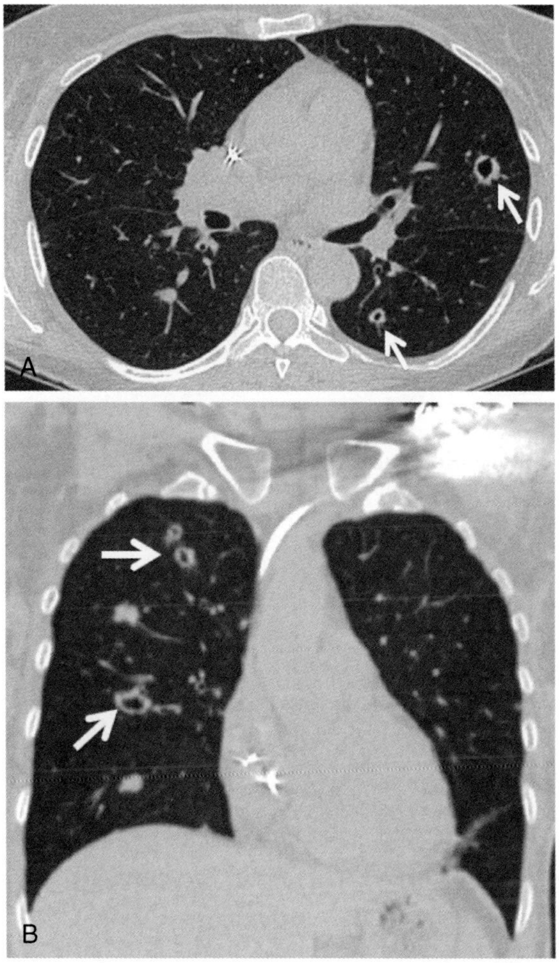

Figure 24.11 Cheerio cysts—rheumatoid arthritis, necrobiotic nodules. (A and B) CT scans demonstrate multiple cavitary lesions in both lungs *(arrows)*, representing cavitated necrobiotic nodules. Biopsy or follow-up imaging is needed for differentiation from malignancy and infection.

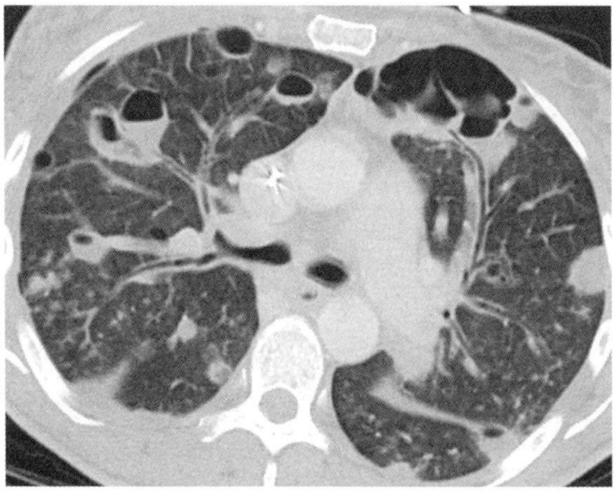

Figure 24.12 Cheerio cysts—septic emboli. Multiple nodules in angiocentric distribution with the feeding vessel sign are characteristic of septic emboli; these undergo rapid evolution and cavitation and demonstrate air-fluid levels.

Langerhans cell histiocytosis and typically have a posterior predominance.

Diseases Characterized by Cysts and Ancillary Findings on Chest CT (e.g., Ground-Glass Abnormalities)

Clinical Presentation

In comparison with LAM or PLCH, other diseases such as LIP, DIP, and some infections are associated with fewer cysts; hence, the distribution of cysts may not aid in refining the differential diagnosis further. Instead, a careful search should be done for features such as ground-glass opacities or nodules because this can assist in suggesting a radiologic differential diagnosis. Although nodules are a well-recognized feature of PLCH, ground-glass opacification is not typically associated with PLCH or LAM.

LIP is characterized by a combination of ground-glass opacification, poorly defined centrilobular nodules, interlobular septal thickening, thickening of the bronchovascular bundles, and scattered perivascular cysts (see Fig. 24.5B). The cysts in LIP are variable in size and sometimes may be large, usually few in number, and peribronchovascular in distribution and may have a pseudoseptated appearance due to proximity to vessels. During the acute phase, ground-glass opacities are seen. In more chronic cases, ground-glass opacities may regress so that cysts are the only residual abnormality (see Fig. 24.5A). The diagnosis of LIP often requires confirmation by transbronchial or open lung biopsy. The usual treatment is steroid therapy, after which ground-glass opacities can resolve. The cysts, however, persist, even after therapy.

In patients with HIV, a combination of findings, including ground-glass opacities and cysts, raises the possibility of LIP or PJP. Clinically, patients with PJP are frequently profoundly hypoxic, with a low diffusing capacity of the lung for carbon monoxide, and the lavage fluid may show elevated levels of 1,3-beta-D-glucan and lactate dehydrogenase and cysts. The extent of ground-glass abnormality is out of proportion to the cystic changes. On CT, PJP often appears as bilateral, multifocal, mainly symmetric ground-glass opacities, and the cysts or pneumatoceles tend to occur mostly after multiple infections; there can be an apical predominance, leading to pneumothoraces, which portend a poor outcome (Fig. 24.13). Cystic changes or pneumatoceles in PJP have been attributed to a combination of factors, such as direct tissue destruction by *Pneumocystis jiroveci*, cytotoxic effect of HIV, release of elastase enzyme by macrophages, and check valve bronchiolar obstruction leading to pneumatocele formation. A cystic abnormality is frequently reversible after the initiation of specific therapy with trimethoprim-sulfamethoxazole, initiation of antiretroviral therapy, and resulting rise in the $CD4^+$ cell count.

DIP is a smoking-related disease, and a diagnosis should be suggested on imaging only after confirming the history of smoking. On HRCT, a characteristic pattern of lower lobe predominant ground-glass opacification, with or without interspersed cysts, may be seen in about one-third of patients (Fig. 24.14).

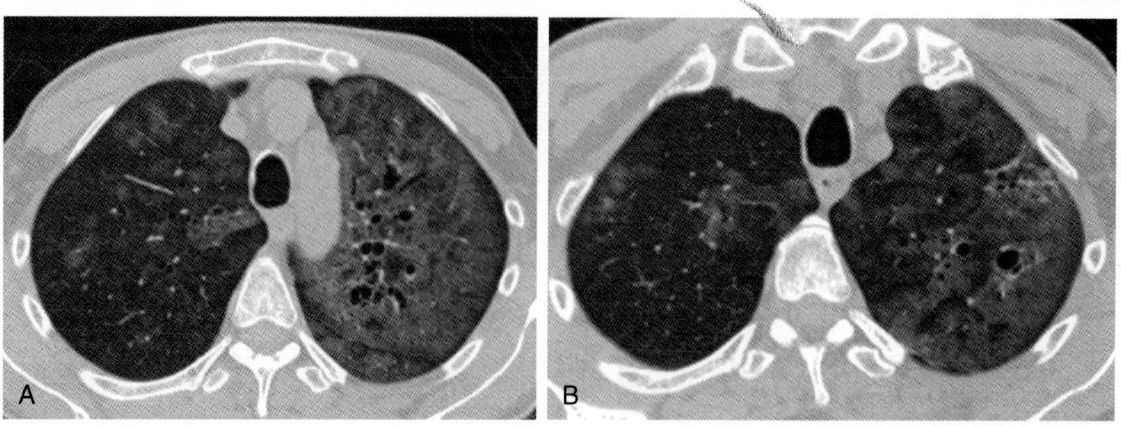

Figure 24.13 *Pneumocystis jiroveci* pneumonia (PJP) with cystic changes. (A and B) Axial chest CT scans demonstrate bilateral ground-glass opacities, greater on the left. Scattered cysts seen in the left upper lobe resolved on subsequent imaging. A reversible cystic change can be seen in up to 30% of patients with PJP.

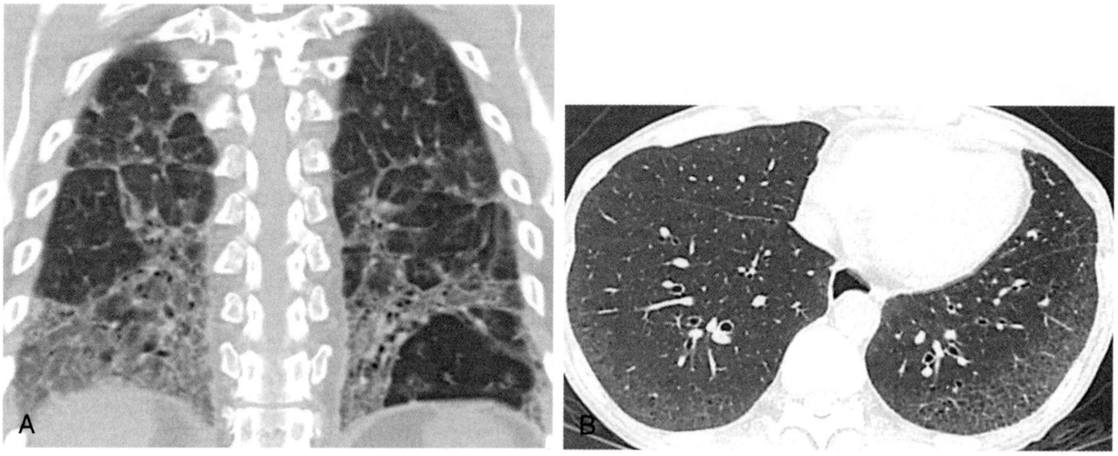

Figure 24.14 Desquamative interstitial pneumonitis. (A) Axial and (B) coronal CT scans in two patients. Extensive ground-glass abnormality with few interspersed cysts is a feature of the disease. The ground-glass abnormality predominates in the peripheral subpleural regions of the middle and lower zones; the distribution is different from other smoking-related diseases, which tend to involve the upper lobes.

■ Conclusion

Lung cysts are not an infrequent finding on HRCT. Further scrutiny with regard to number, distribution, and shape of the pulmonary cysts, as well as for ancillary CT signs, is required to generate a differential diagnosis. A constellation of findings on chest CT may aid in arriving at the correct diagnosis. Although it is easy to diagnose diseases associated with numerous cysts, diseases associated with fewer cysts in asymptomatic patients often pose a diagnostic dilemma. Many cases require correlation with demographics, smoking history, clinical information, family history, and abdominal imaging for a definitive diagnosis. It is also important to recognize that several entities, including cavitary lesions, emphysema, bronchiectasis, and honeycombing, may mimic true cysts. Careful evaluation of the imaging appearances, however, often allows an accurate diagnosis to be established.

Bibliography

Abbott GF, Rosado-de-Christenson ML, Franks TJ, et al. From the archives of the AFIP: pulmonary Langerhans cell histiocytosis. *Radiographics*. 2004;24:821–841.

Abbott GF, Rosado-de-Christenson ML, Frazier AA, et al. From the archives of the AFIP: lymphangioleiomyomatosis: radiologic-pathologic correlation. *Radiographics*. 2005;25:803–828.

Butnor KJ, Guinee DG Jr. Pleuropulmonary pathology of Birt-Hogg-Dubé syndrome. *Am J Surg Pathol*. 2006;30:395–399.

Chorianopoulos D, Stratakos G. Lymphangioleiomyomatosis and tuberous sclerosis complex. *Lung*. 2008;186:197–207.

Hohman DW, Noghrehkar D, Ratnayake S. Lymphangioleiomyomatosis: a review. *Eur J Intern Med*. 2008;19:319–324.

Ryu JH, Swensen SJ. Cystic and cavitary lung diseases: focal and diffuse. *Mayo Clin Proc*. 2003;78:744–752.

Seaman DM, Meyer CA, Gilman MD, et al. Diffuse cystic lung disease at high-resolution CT. *AJR Am J Roentgenol*. 2011;196:1305–1311.

Trotman-Dickenson B. Cystic lung disease: achieving a radiologic diagnosis. *Eur J Radiol*. 2014;83:39–46.

CHAPTER 25

Radiation, Medication, and Illicit Drug–Related Lung Disease

Travis S. Henry

CHAPTER OUTLINE

■ Introduction and Background

Although different in appearances on imaging, radiation and drug-induced lung diseases share several similarities. Both entities may present with a variety of appearances, both in the acute and subacute or chronic settings, and require a high level of suspicion to make the correct diagnosis. Most importantly, these processes share a temporal relationship with the causal event. Furthermore, the two processes may coexist in oncologic patients being treated with radiation and chemotherapy. The imager should always consider both radiation or drug reaction as a cause of otherwise unexplained imaging findings.

■ Radiation-Related Lung Disease

Radiation therapy is a common treatment for many thoracic malignancies and is, therefore, encountered frequently by the thoracic imager, especially in busy oncologic practices. Many of the side effects of radiation are permanent and, because radiation is often administered with intent to cure, imaging abnormalities may be encountered years or decades after treatment. It is important for the imager to understand the basic treatment strategies used and recognize different patterns of radiation pneumonitis and fibrosis so that these entities can be confidently differentiated from infection, tumor recurrence, or another primary tumor.

Purpose of Radiation Treatment

Radiation therapy is an effective treatment option for many intrathoracic malignancies but is most commonly used in the treatment of lung cancer. The purpose of radiation, and the type of radiation used, depends largely on the stage of disease. For example, in stages I and II lung cancers, radiation is potentially curative and may be the only treatment option in patients who are not surgical candidates (e.g., those with severe lung or heart disease). Locally advanced lung cancers with unresectable primary tumors or nodal involvement (stage IIIA) may undergo radiotherapy with the hope of cure or as an adjunct therapy. Patients with metastatic disease may receive radiation as palliation to relieve pain and improve quality of life.

Radiation therapy aims to kill tumor cells by delivering as high a dose as possible to the cancer cell while limiting damage to adjacent normal tissue. Historically, conventional radiation therapy has used parallel radiation beams with opposite orientation (anteroposterior and posteroanterior) to deliver treatment doses of approximately 60 gray (Gy) in daily doses of about 2 Gy each. This technique was limited by the large amount of normal tissue exposed within the radiation fields, including the mediastinum and spinal cord. Oblique beams can be used to boost the dose and reduce exposure to these important structures.

Conventional radiation therapy has largely been replaced by several modern techniques, most notably three-dimensional conformal radiation therapy (3D-CRT) and stereotactic beam radiation therapy (SBRT), that deliver large doses of radiation to a tumor while minimizing adjacent tissue injury. 3D-CRT uses CT images to create a 3D tumor volume, and complex computer algorithms generate multiple oblique radiation fields that deliver the dose to the tumor from many different angles. This technique allows even higher doses of radiation (≥70 Gy) to be delivered to a tumor while limiting the dose to adjacent normal tissues. SBRT is a conformal technique for the treatment of nonoperable stage I lung cancers, with local control rates reported of 80% to 100%. A stereotactic body frame is used to localize the tumor and focus high doses of radiation on a small field.

Many other malignancies are also treated with radiation, and the effects are frequently encountered on thoracic imaging. These include hematologic malignancies such as Hodgkin lymphoma or leukemia, breast cancer, esophageal cancer, and head or neck cancer. The patterns of radiation-related findings in each of these diseases will be discussed later in this chapter.

Pathophysiology and Timeline of Radiation-Related Lung Disease

The lung parenchymal response to radiation is fairly limited and may manifest as one of two patterns—radiation pneumonitis or radiation fibrosis—and there are many factors that contribute to the severity of injury suffered by a particular patient. Technical factors include the volume of lung irradiated, total dose, dose fractionation, and time frame over which the radiation is delivered. Lung injury rarely occurs when total doses are below 20 Gy, but some degree of injury is usually present if more than 40 Gy is administered. Concurrent chemotherapy or withdrawal of steroids may also worsen the lung injury. Individual susceptibility, preexisting lung disease, or prior radiation may also play a role.

The last day of radiation treatment is usually used as a reference point to assess the timeline of radiation pneumonitis and radiation fibrosis. Radiation injury to the lung results in diffuse alveolar damage that evolves through three phases: (1) acute exudative phase, (2) organization and proliferation phase, and (3) chronic fibrotic phase.

Radiation Pneumonitis

The acute exudative phase and organization and proliferation phase correspond to the time frame of radiation pneumonitis and occur within the first 1 to 6 months after completion of therapy. Clinical symptoms include dyspnea, cough, low-grade fever, and/or chest discomfort. The incidence of symptomatic radiation pneumonitis for 3D-CRT is approximately 13% to 37% and much less (4%) for SBRT. Symptoms will usually resolve spontaneously but, in some cases, may require treatment with steroids.

Characteristic imaging findings of radiation pneumonitis on CT include ground-glass opacities (GGOs) and/or consolidation that are almost always confined to the radiation field (Fig. 25.1). The radiation fields

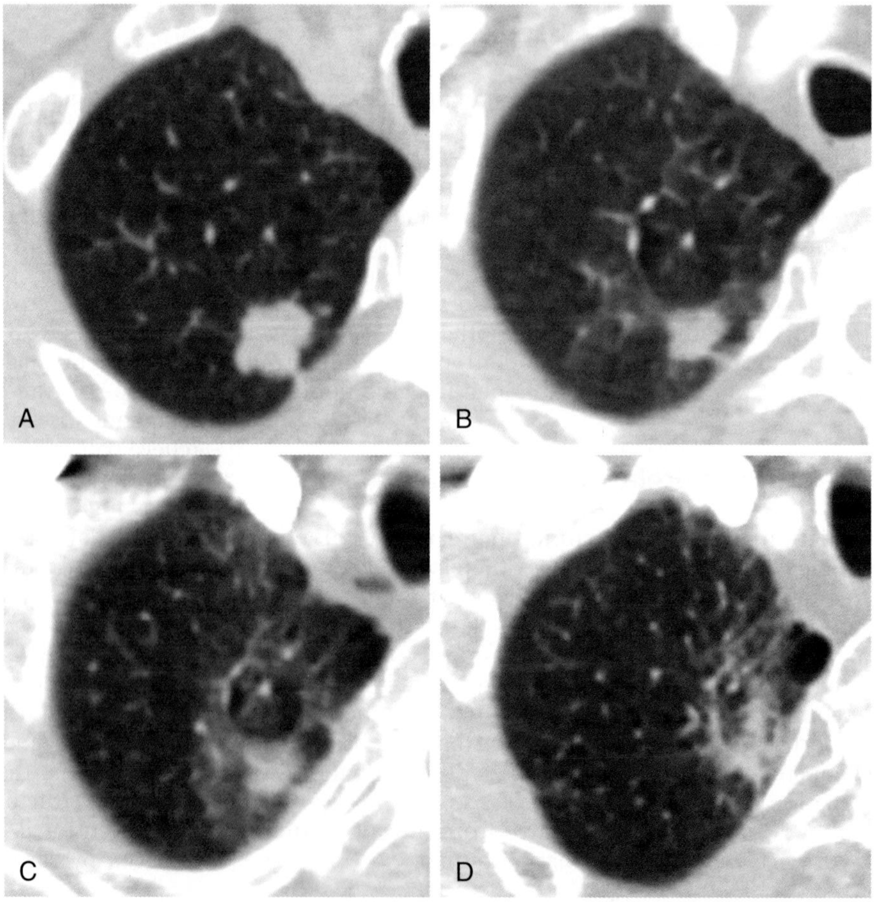

Figure 25.1 A 61-year-old man with stage IA adenocarcinoma of the right upper lobe treated with stereotactic beam radiation therapy. (A) Initial CT scan demonstrates the primary tumor. (B) Follow-up at 3 months shows decrease in tumor size, with subtle surrounding ground-glass opacities (GGOs) representing radiation pneumonitis. (C) At 6 months, the GGOs have increased, and there is now subtle architectural distortion representing the evolution of radiation pneumonitis and fibrosis. (D) Eighteen months after completion of therapy shows resolution of the mass and improvement in the GGOs with progressive fibrosis, including architectural distortion, reticulation, and volume loss.

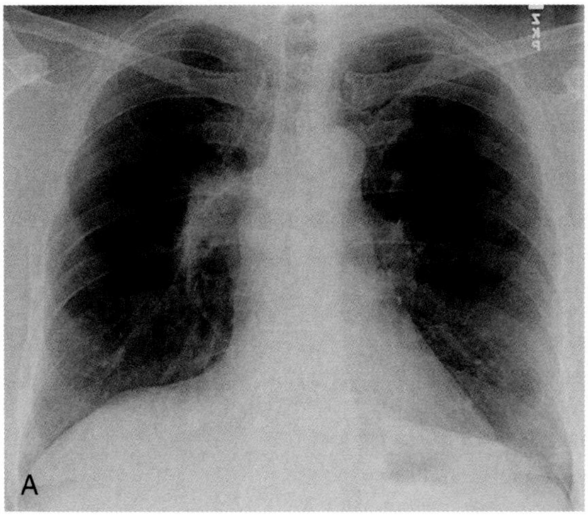

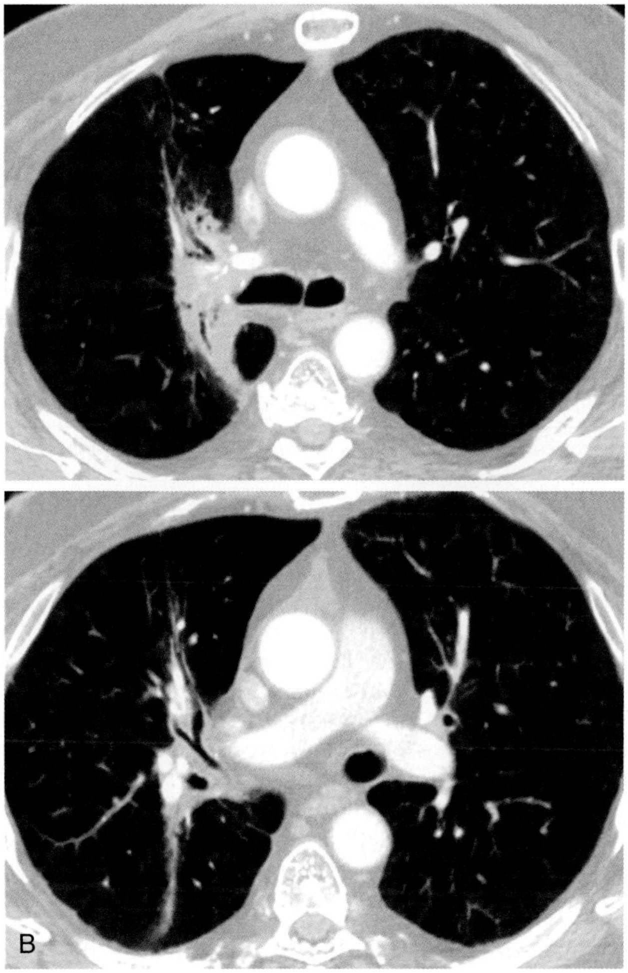

Figure 25.2 A 65-year-old man with radiation fibrosis from treatment of stage IIIA non–small cell lung cancer of the right lung with conventional radiotherapy. (A) Chest radiograph shows characteristic findings of radiation fibrosis, with sharply demarcated consolidation in the right perihilar region and right-sided volume loss. (B) Axial CT images show more fully the sharply marginated fibrosis that crosses fissures and extends anteroposterior along the radiation field. Volume loss with cicatricial atelectasis and traction bronchiectasis are typical findings of radiation fibrosis.

are nonanatomic, so the parenchymal abnormalities often cross fissures and are not confined to a single lobe or segment. In the organization and proliferation phase, imaging findings may evolve as volume loss and bronchiectasis start to develop. Sterile pleural effusions may be present, and pleural thickening in the radiation field may also be observed. These findings may also be visible on chest radiographs, although subtle GGOs may be below the limits of detection.

It is very important to realize that parenchymal abnormalities may develop outside of the radiation field during the radiation pneumonitis time frame; these usually represent an organizing pneumonia (OP), which may be a direct effect of radiation or an immune reaction to radiation injury. This has been reported in up to 20% of patients who have undergone radiation therapy and should not be mistaken for tumor recurrence. Imaging findings of OP outside of the radiation field include GGOs or consolidation that is often migratory and may relapse if steroid therapy ceases.

Radiation Fibrosis

Radiation fibrosis represents the chronic fibrotic phase of lung injury and usually develops 6 to 12 months after the completion of radiation therapy. Symptoms are less frequent than with radiation pneumonitis but, when present, include dyspnea and persistent dry cough. Radiation fibrosis may develop with or without clinically appreciable antecedent pneumonitis.

Histologically, collagen deposition and fibrosis are present in the lung parenchyma. Similar to radiation pneumonitis, the imaging findings may be visible on both radiographs and CT scans, although CT is more sensitive. The main imaging findings include architectural distortion, consolidation with air bronchograms, and traction bronchiectasis with sharp borders that cross fissures and other anatomic landmarks, depending on the radiation field. The fibrosis results in volume loss and corresponding ipsilateral mediastinal shift (Fig. 25.2). Radiation fibrosis should stabilize by 24 months after the completion of therapy. Changes outside this time frame (e.g., especially increased soft tissue, filling in of previously patent bronchi, new nodular borders) should raise suspicion of tumor recurrence, a new tumor, or another process such as infection.

Patterns of Radiation Treatment Seen in the Chest

It is important for the thoracic imager to recognize the different distributions of radiation pneumonitis and

TABLE 25.1 Types of Radiation and Expected Distribution of Abnormalities

EXPECTED DISTRIBUTION OF ABNORMALITIES	TYPES OF RADIATION
Anteroposterior or oblique; extends from one pleural surface to another, may cross fissures	Conventional radiation therapy (usually for lung cancer); 3D-CRT may have a similar distribution but not as severe
Focal, isolated to one region of lung parenchyma	SBRT (possibly 3D-CRT) used to treat a localized lung cancer
Paramediastinal, bilateral	Mantle radiation for Hodgkin disease (or some other types of lymphoma); radiation for thymic tumors
Paramediastinal, unilateral	Radiation for lung cancer nodal disease or esophageal cancer
Unilateral, tangential to chest wall	Radiation for breast cancer
Apical, unilateral	Axillary nodal metastases (usually breast cancer)
Apical, bilateral	Head and neck cancer

SBRT, Stereotactic beam radiation therapy; *3D-CRT,* three-dimensional conformal radiation therapy.

radiation fibrosis that may be encountered. Knowing the type of primary tumor (e.g., lung cancer, esophageal cancer, lymphoma) and time since completion of therapy can improve diagnostic confidence and prevent misinterpretation. Radiation pneumonitis occurs within the first 6 months, whereas radiation fibrosis may develop up to 2 years after completion of therapy (see Fig. 25.1).

Knowing the type of radiation that was administered can help predict where radiation-induced abnormalities occur. Usually, these findings will be seen in the lungs, but any tissues in the radiation field (e.g., skin, soft tissue, bone, vessel, heart) may suffer injury. Conversely, when a pertinent history is not available to the imager, the distribution of abnormalities may allow one to surmise the treatment that was administered. Table 25.1 lists the types of radiation and expected distribution of findings. Examples of different treatment patterns are shown in Fig. 25.3.

If lung parenchymal abnormalities are present, the imager should interrogate the entire radiation field to look for complications, particularly in the setting of lung fibrosis from remote radiation. These findings are discussed in further detail later (see "Long-Term Effects of Radiation").

Differentiating Radiation Pneumonitis and Fibrosis From Other Processes

The primary differential diagnosis for radiation pneumonitis or fibrosis includes tumor recurrence, infection, and a radiation-induced secondary neoplasm. In many cases, the diagnosis may be obvious based on imaging or the clinical presentation alone, but in many cases a multimodality and multidisciplinary approach may be necessary to reach a confident diagnosis. Comparison to prior imaging examinations and knowledge of the treatment regimen are essential.

Tumor Recurrence

Recurrence usually occurs within the first 2 years after completion of therapy, but it can occur after this window. Modern 3D-CRT and SBRT offer lower recurrence rates than conventional treatments because of the higher doses that can be delivered to tumors. Tumors may relapse outside the radiation field and present at imaging as new nodules in the lung, new lymphadenopathy, or lymphangitic carcinomatosis. Tumor recurrence within the radiation field or along the margin of radiation may be more difficult to detect. Clues of recurrence on CT are often subtle and include the following: new soft tissue nodularity or convexity along a radiation field margin; new mass within the radiation field; and secondary signs of soft tissue infiltration, including filling in of previously demonstrated air bronchograms or a new mass effect or compression on vessels and airways (Fig. 25.4). A new pleural effusion long after completion of therapy (months to years) should also raise suspicion of recurrence.

Because recurrence may occur during the first 2 years after completion of therapy, while radiation pneumonitis and fibrosis are evolving, PET-CT may be useful for differentiating the two entities. Although radiation pneumonitis represents a metabolically active response to lung injury, the maximum standard uptake value (SUV_{max}) is usually higher in tumors. However, because of the false-positive potential, PET-CT should generally not be performed in the first 3 months after the completion of radiation therapy. In some cases, tissue biopsy or short-term follow-up imaging is necessary to confirm a diagnosis of recurrence.

Infection

Infection may be particularly difficult to differentiate from radiation pneumonitis because clinical symptoms and imaging findings overlap. Imaging findings that are unusual as a result of radiation pneumonitis, and should prompt evaluation for infection, include tree-in-bud nodules, cavitation, diffuse bilateral abnormalities that extend far beyond the radiation field, or GGOs or consolidation that develop before the completion of radiation therapy. The rapid development of a new abnormality may also be a clue of infection, although steroid withdrawal can incite fairly rapid development of radiation pneumonitis.

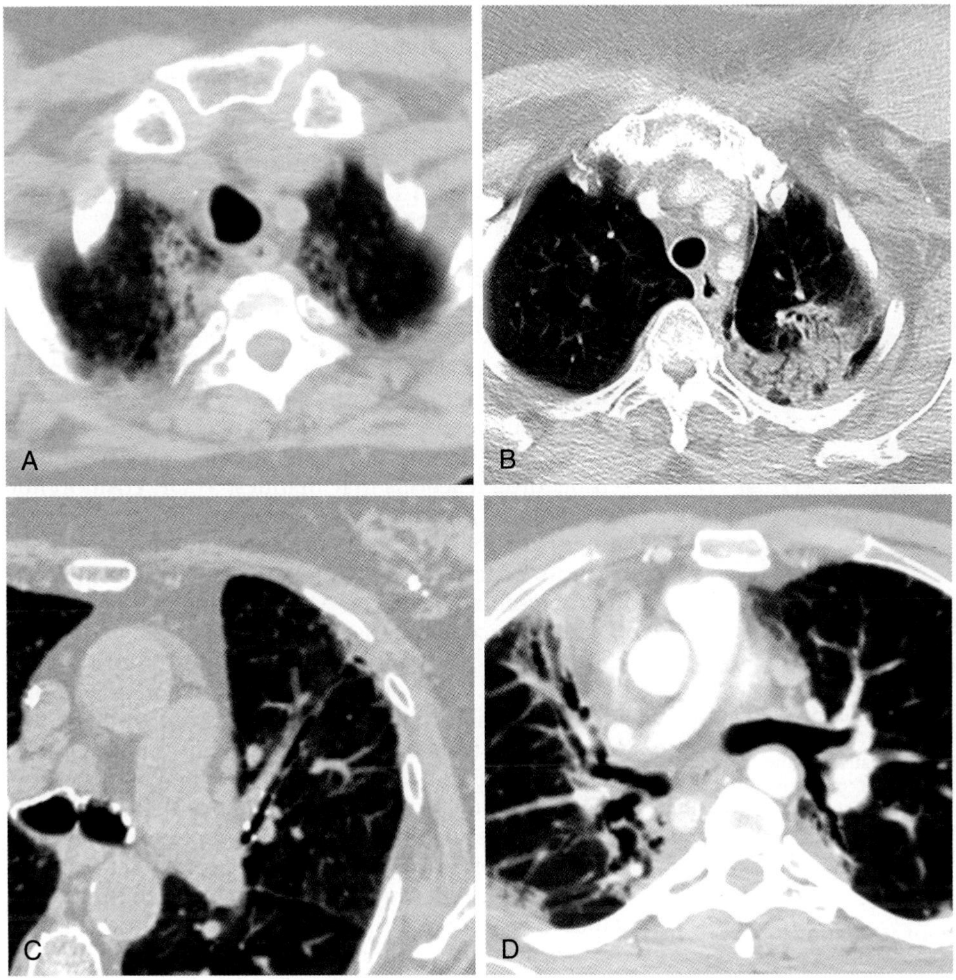

Figure 25.3 Different patterns of radiation fibrosis. (A) Biapical fibrosis in a patient who underwent radiation of the neck for treatment of recurrent papillary thyroid cancer. (B) Unilateral apical fibrosis in a woman with breast cancer with left cervical and axillary nodal metastases treated with radiation. (C) Tangential fibrosis in the anterolateral left lung from breast cancer treated with breast conservation therapy. Also note the metallic tissue marker within the tumor, another clue to the diagnosis. (D) Bilateral paramediastinal radiation for treatment of Hodgkin lymphoma.

Radiation-Induced Tumor

Secondary tumors are a late consequence of radiation therapy (median time, ≈10 years). This should be included on the differential in the appropriate clinical context and is discussed in more detail in the following section.

Long-Term Effects of Radiation

Non-Neoplastic Extrapulmonary Effects

All tissues in the body have varying susceptibilities to radiation-induced damage. In the thorax, this includes the tissues superficial to the lung parenchyma (e.g., subcutaneous tissues, bones, pleura) and mediastinal structures (e.g., vessels, cardiac valves, pericardium, lymph nodes, esophagus, thymus). The most important effects are listed in Table 25.2, and inspection of these structures should be part of a search pattern when they fall within a radiation field.

Radiation-Induced Tumors

A new mass arising in the thorax several years after radiation may represent a second primary tumor developing as a result of the prior radiation therapy. The development of radiation-induced tumors varies according to total dose and technique, but the average latency time is 10 years or longer after radiation therapy. Common tumors such as new lung cancers, lymphoma, acute leukemia, and breast cancers may be the result of radiation, but often the radiation-induced tumors may be unusual, such as various sarcomas (e.g., osteosarcoma, chondrosarcoma, angiosarcoma, undifferentiated soft tissue sarcomas).

■ Medication-Related Lung Disease

More than 1000 different drugs (both prescribed and illicit) have been reported to cause pulmonary toxicity based on numbers from www.pneumotox.com, a useful reference website for researching drug reactions. These pulmonary side effects can result in substantial morbidity and mortality and may be difficult to diagnose because their clinical and radiographic presentation is nonspecific. Often, in practice, biopsy is not performed, and the diagnosis of a drug reaction relies heavily on clinical presentation, imaging findings, and the temporal relationship between drug exposure and onset of symptoms. Prompt recognition of a drug reaction allows the offending agent to be halted, which may result in complete resolution of lung injury or at least halt progression.

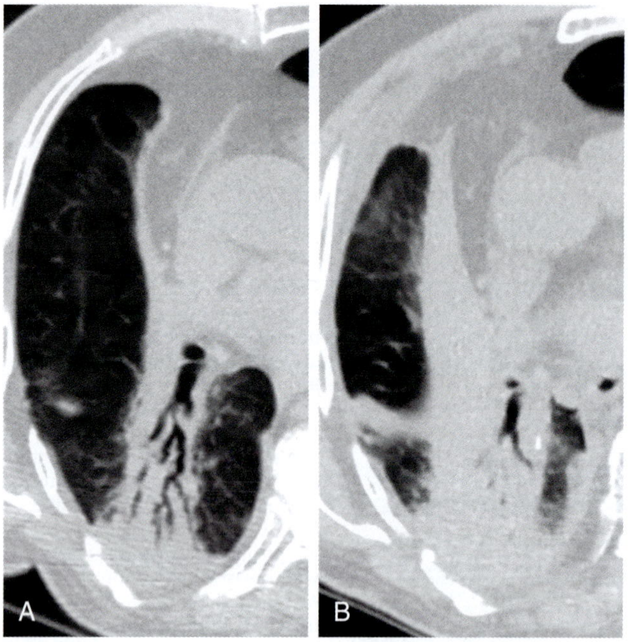

Figure 25.4 A 74-year-old man with unresectable lung cancer and recurrence 4 years after completion of radiation therapy. (A) CT performed 30 months after completion of radiation therapy shows typical findings of radiation fibrosis without recurrence. (B) CT performed 18 months later (48 months after completion of radiation) shows multiple findings of recurrence, including new soft tissue convexity along the lateral radiation margin, opacification of previously dilated bronchi with tumor, and new pleural nodularity.

TABLE 25.2 Long-Term Effects of Radiation

TISSUE OR STRUCTURE AFFECTED	EFFECTS
Bones	Radiation osteonecrosis
Subcutaneous tissues	Edema, fat necrosis
Pleura	Pleural thickening, pleuritis, pleural effusion
Pericardium	Pericardial thickening, pericarditis, pericardial effusion
Vessels (e.g., aorta, arch vessels, coronaries) and valves (e.g., aortic valve)	Accelerated atherosclerotic disease or valvular disease at a young age
Lymph nodes	Calcified lymph nodes—may be sequelae of treated disease
Esophagus	Esophageal strictures—may occur within a radiation field
Thymus	Thymic cysts—may develop after radiation to the mediastinum

Although there are so many drugs that can cause lung injury, most drug reactions tend to fall into one of a few categories that will be the focus of this chapter. It is important to note that many drugs cause more than one pattern of injury, and identification of the exact offending agent may be complicated if a patient is started on multiple drugs that are known to cause a specific reaction at the same time. Illicit drugs can cause many of the following patterns, but additional specific scenarios caused by illicit drugs will also be discussed in the following section.

When a Drug Reaction or Medication-Related Lung Disease Should Be Suspected

Because the clinical presentation and imaging appearance are variable, the simplest answer is that the imager should always consider a drug reaction as a cause of otherwise unexplained pulmonary abnormalities. In the acute setting, drug reactions may present similarly to those of pulmonary edema (hydrostatic or permeability), hemorrhage, or infection. In the subacute to chronic setting, drug reactions may manifest as OP, eosinophilic pneumonia, hypersensitivity reaction, pulmonary vasculitis, pulmonary fibrosis, constrictive bronchiolitis, sarcoid-like reaction, or recurrent pleuritis–pleural effusion. Because these presentations are so variable, definitive diagnosis of drug-induced lung disease depends on the following: (1) temporal relationship between drug exposure and the onset of symptoms and development of imaging abnormalities; (2) radiologic findings compatible with a drug reaction; (3) exclusion of other causes of lung damage, including infection, radiation pneumonitis or fibrosis, or progression of a primary lung disease; and (4) histologic evidence of a lung injury (if biopsy is performed). Early recognition of a drug reaction and prompt cessation of the putative agent are important because findings may stabilize or resolve. Failure to recognize a drug reaction may result in irreversible lung injury or fibrosis.

Different Patterns of Drug-Related Lung Disease

The following sections all represent different patterns of drug reactions. Some of the more common causes of each pattern are listed, where applicable, but the list is ever-growing, especially with the continual introduction of new biologic agents. If one suspects a drug reaction, www.pneumotox.com is an extremely helpful resource. When one of the following patterns is caused by a drug reaction, the findings are almost always indistinguishable from other causes of that pattern. The one major exception is amiodarone, which also affects the attenuation of the lungs and liver secondary to iodine deposition, which will be discussed in its own section.

Diffuse Alveolar Damage

Diffuse alveolar damage (DAD) is a common drug reaction pattern encountered on radiography and CT. Many drugs may cause DAD, including cytotoxic agents (e.g., bleomycin, cyclophosphamide), methotrexate, amiodarone, and illicit drugs, including cocaine and heroin. Patients present with progressively worsening dyspnea, cough, hypoxemia, and possibly fever.

The imaging appearance of DAD from drug reactions is similar to that of DAD from any cause. The imaging findings mirror the pathologic evolution and

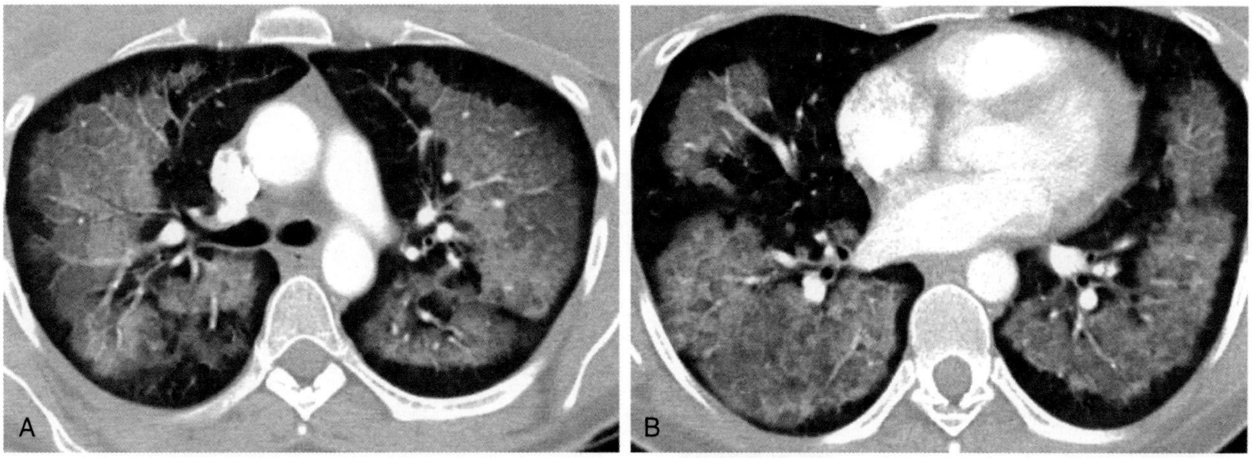

Figure 25.5 A 41-year-old woman with mixed connective tissue disease who developed shortness of breath 2 days following increase of her methotrexate dose. (A and B) Two axial CT images show a typical pattern of permeability edema with bilateral, symmetric, ground-glass opacities and crazy-paving pattern. The absence of peripheral septal thickening and pleural effusions and normal heart size argue against cardiogenic edema. Findings cleared on the chest radiograph 1 week later (not shown) after cessation of methotrexate.

are divided into two phases—exudative and organizing. Pathologically, DAD represents a severe lung injury with pneumocytes and alveolar endothelial cell necrosis and increased permeability. Imaging findings during the acute exudative phase reflect necrosis and permeability edema; these include bilateral parenchymal consolidation that favors the lower lung and midlung zones (Fig. 25.5). Unlike hydrostatic edema, septal thickening and pleural effusions are generally absent, and CT is more accurate than radiography for characterization of these findings.

Progression to the organizing phase of DAD (1–2 weeks after injury) is variable. If the offending agent is removed early, the findings may stabilize and improve. Progression to the organizing stage results from the proliferation of type II pneumocytes and development of fibrosis. This manifests on imaging as architectural distortion and traction bronchiectasis, and, in some cases, honeycombing may be seen.

Organizing Pneumonia

Like DAD, OP is another common drug reaction pattern in the lung. Common causes of OP include amiodarone, bleomycin, interferon, methotrexate, nitrofurantoin, and cyclophosphamide. Imaging findings are typical of other causes of OP and include midlung or lower lung predominant consolidation or GGOs, either in a bronchocentric or peripheral distribution (Fig. 25.6). The reverse halo sign may be present. With the exception of amiodarone, which can cause increased attenuation of lung consolidation (and increased liver attenuation), the findings are indistinguishable from one another.

Patterns of Usual Interstitial Pneumonitis and Nonspecific Interstitial Pneumonitis

Nonspecific interstitial pneumonitis (NSIP) and usual interstitial pneumonitis (UIP) are both recognized patterns of drug reactions, with a long list of causative agents, usually cytotoxic and chemotherapeutic drugs

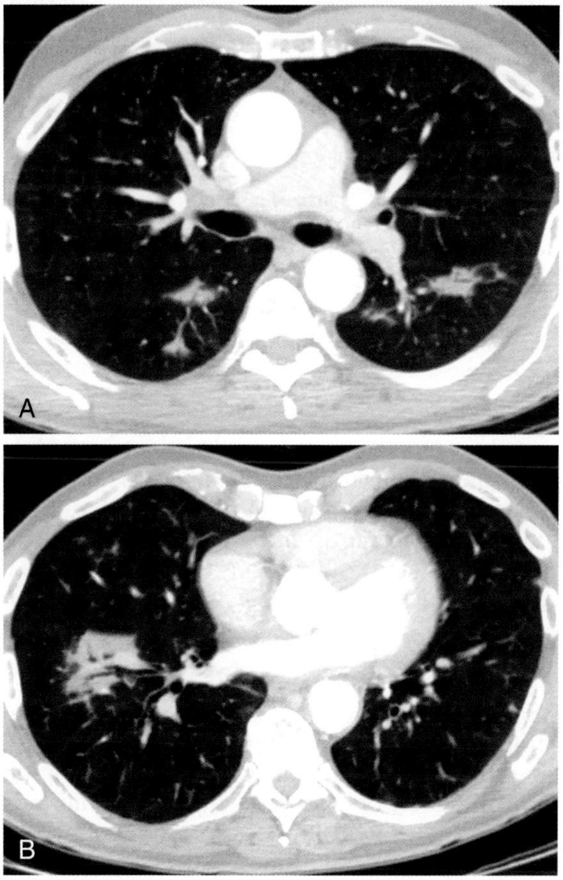

Figure 25.6 A 71-year-old man with melanoma metastatic to bone. He developed respiratory symptoms, including cough and dyspnea, after starting a clinical trial for a monoclonal antibody. CT findings on axial CT images at the level of the carina (A) and in the lower lobes (B) are consistent with organizing pneumonia, including peripheral and peribronchovascular consolidation affecting both lungs. Transbronchial biopsy ruled out infection and metastasis and confirmed the diagnosis. His symptoms and imaging findings resolved after cessation of the clinical trial and administration of steroids.

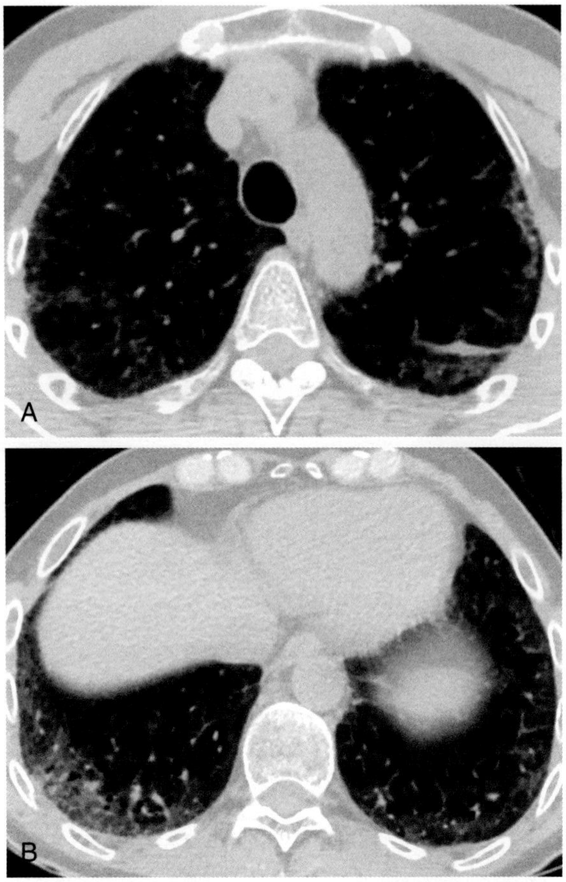

Figure 25.7 A 59-year-old man with bleomycin toxicity for treatment of testicular seminoma and pattern of nonspecific interstitial pneumonitis fibrosis. CT images in the upper lobes (A) and lower lobes (B) show peripheral reticulation, ground-glass opacities, and traction bronchiectasis and bronchiolectasis. On biopsy, a concomitant organizing pneumonia was also present.

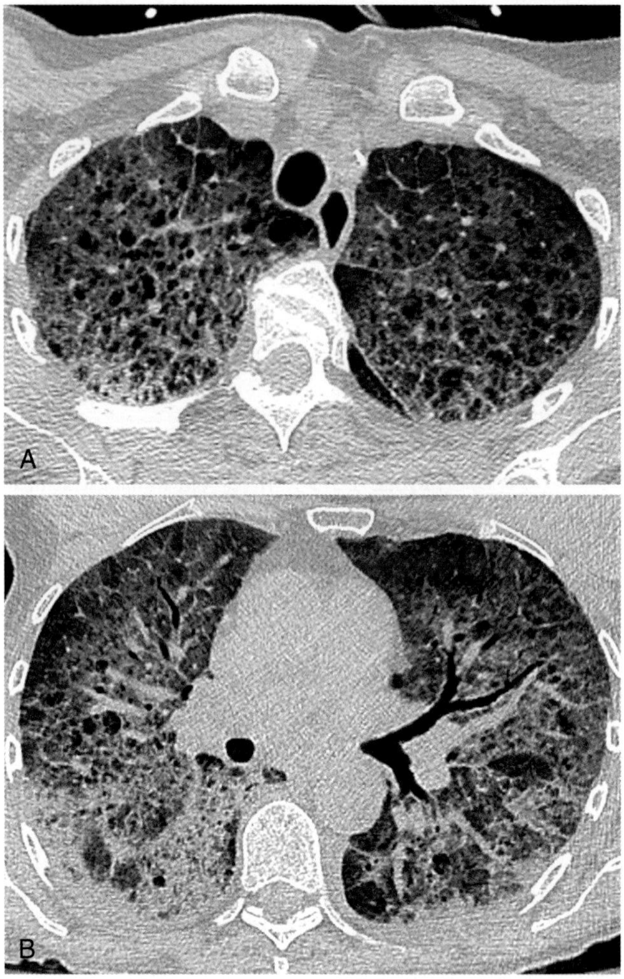

Figure 25.8 A 69-year-old woman with acute hypersensitivity pneumonitis secondary to methotrexate. Axial CT images through the upper lobes (A) and mid-lung zones (B) show upper lobe predominant ground-glass opacities and consolidation. Lung biopsy was consistent with hypersensitivity pneumonitis, and abnormalities resolved after steroid administration and cessation of methotrexate.

(e.g., bleomycin, methotrexate, doxorubicin, carmustine), amiodarone, nitrofurantoin, and penicillamine. Imaging findings are discussed in more detail in the respective sections on UIP and NSIP, but it is important to note that imaging findings of OP and/or DAD may also coexist (Fig. 25.7).

Hypersensitivity Pneumonitis

Hypersensitivity pneumonitis is an uncommon drug reaction. Despite the fact that the causative drugs are ingested, the clinical, pathologic, and radiologic findings are similar to those of hypersensitivity pneumonitis caused by inhaled antigens. CT findings are typical of hypersensitivity pneumonitis and include ill-defined centrilobular ground-glass nodules, more confluent GGOs, consolidation, and variable amounts of lobular air trapping, depending on the chronicity (Fig. 25.8).

Eosinophilic Pneumonia

Drug reactions are a common cause of eosinophilic pneumonia, and the presentation may be acute or insidious. The pathologic diagnosis depends on the presence of peripheral eosinophilia or lung eosinophilia from bronchoalveolar lavage or lung biopsy. Radiographic and CT findings are typical of eosinophilic pneumonia and include peripheral, usually symmetric GGOs, and consolidation, with an upper lobe predominance, although the imaging appearance overlaps with that of OP. Other causes of eosinophilia, including fungal and parasitic infection and systemic disease, must be excluded.

Pulmonary Hemorrhage

Pulmonary hemorrhage may present in the acute or chronic setting; common causes include anticoagulants, amphotericin B, cytotoxic agents, and crack cocaine. Imaging findings include GGOs, with or without septal thickening (crazy-paving pattern), and consolidation. These findings overlap with all other causes of hemoptysis and can appear similar to those of pulmonary edema or pneumonia in the acute setting and are therefore nonspecific. Hemoptysis and pleural effusions are reportedly uncommon.

Sarcoid-Like Reaction

Sarcoid-like reaction is an unusual drug reaction with a relatively short list of offending agents. The most common causes include tumor necrosis factor alpha antagonists, which are used for the treatment of inflammatory arthritis, or interferon therapy, used for malignancies such as melanoma or for nonmalignant conditions such as hepatitis C. Recognition of this pattern is critical, especially in the setting of malignancy, to prevent confusion and misdiagnosis of metastatic disease. Imaging findings of a sarcoid-like reaction include upper lobe predominant nodules in a perilymphatic distribution, with or without mediastinal lymphadenopathy. Steroids may be necessary for the treatment of this reaction, even after cessation of the offending agent.

Pulmonary Hypertension

Several drug classes have been associated with the development of pulmonary arterial hypertension (PAH) and, in many cases, the presentation is indistinguishable from that of idiopathic PAH. Appetite suppressants such as aminorex in the late 1960s, and later fenfluramine and its derivatives, were the first drugs recognized to be risk factors for PAH. Although most of these drugs were banned by 1998, benfluorex (similar to fenfluramine) remained on the market until 2009 in France, and at least 70 cases of PAH have been attributed to benfluorex use.

Other prescribed and illicit drugs have been classified as likely or possible causes of PAH in the most recent updated classification of PAH in 2013. Drugs classified as likely to cause PAH include amphetamines, methamphetamines, and the tyrosine kinase inhibitor dasatinib. Cocaine, amphetamine-like drugs, St. John's wort, interferon-α, and interferon-β have been classified as possible causes of PAH. Injection of crushed tablets (excipient lung) may precipitate pulmonary hypertension (see later).

Amiodarone Toxicity

Amiodarone deserves special attention as a drug for which specific imaging findings may be clues to the diagnosis. Pulmonary toxicity is reported in approximately 5% to 10% of patients on amiodarone and usually begins within months of initiation; the risk is higher with 400-mg or larger daily doses. NSIP and OP are the most common manifestations of amiodarone-associated lung disease, although rare cases of acute lung injury have been reported. Parenchymal opacities may be focal or diffuse but, because the iodine from amiodarone accumulates in type II pneumocytes, these opacities are higher in attenuation than typical consolidation or atelectasis (Fig. 25.9). High attenuation of the liver and

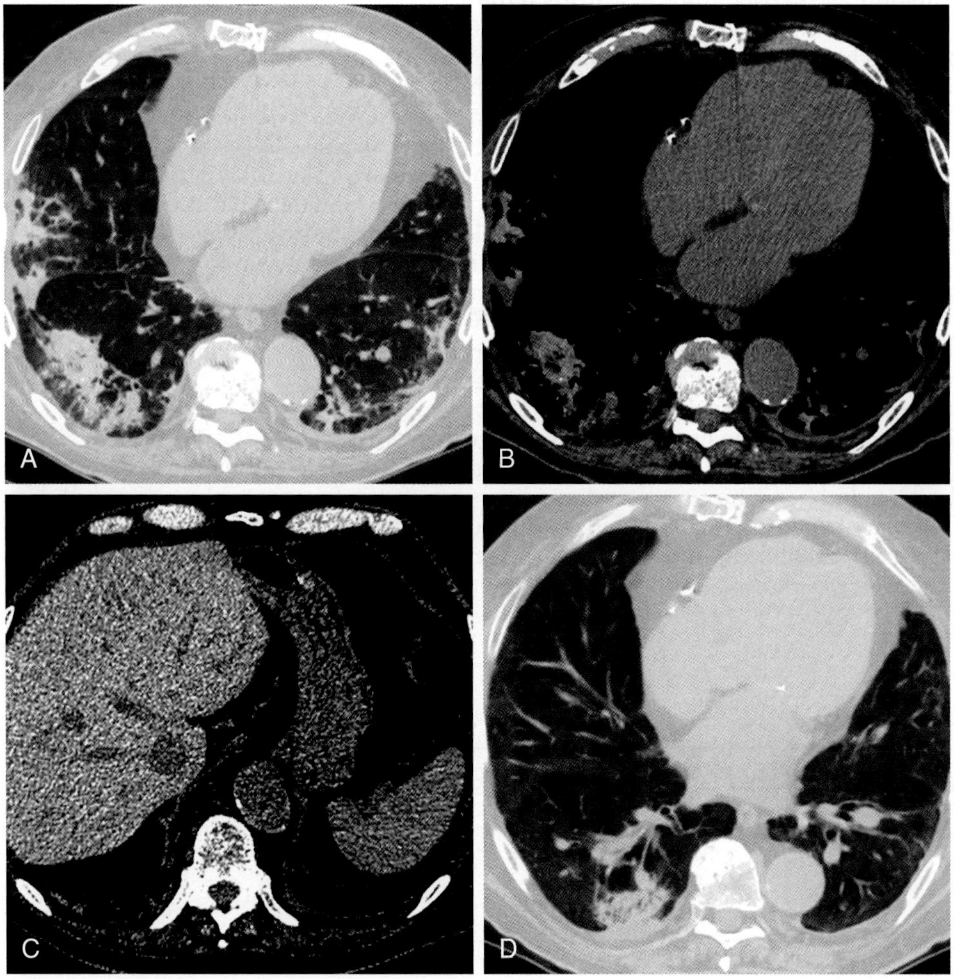

Figure 25.9 A 90-year-old man with amiodarone toxicity. This patient had been on amiodarone for approximately 1 year when he developed worsening dyspnea, cough, and new consolidation on a chest radiograph. (A) Lung windows demonstrate bilateral peripheral areas of consolidation, ground-glass opacities, and reticulation. (B) The consolidation is relatively high attenuation on soft tissue windows, and the liver is also high attenuation on narrow windows (C). (D) Cessation of amiodarone resulted in improvement in symptoms and parenchymal abnormalities on 3-month follow-up CT.

spleen (also due to iodine deposition) are characteristic as well. Ancillary clues of amiodarone use include signs of cardiac dysfunction, such as cardiomegaly or use of a pacemaker.

Drug-Induced Pleural Disease

Pleural reactions are less common than parenchymal drug reactions and therefore may be overlooked. Drug-induced pleural disease may occur in the absence of parenchymal reactions and includes pleural effusions, pleural thickening, and pleuritic chest pain. Exudative effusions, eosinophilic effusions, and chylous effusions have all been reported, and a temporal relationship between the initiation of therapy and development of the effusion is key to the diagnosis. Pleural thickening or pleuritis may occur in the setting of drug-induced systemic lupus erythematosus.

Illicit Drug–Related Diseases

Illicit drug use is associated with many pulmonary and cardiac complications that vary not only by the specific drug that is consumed, but also by the route of administration, presence of impurities or binders used to mix the drug, and sterility (or lack thereof) of the injected substance. The lung is a unique organ in that it can be exposed to inhaled drugs via the airways and injected drugs via the pulmonary circulation. Moreover, the presentation of illicit drug use may be complicated by the drug's effects on other systems including the heart and neurologic system. The myriad of complications from illicit drug use are listed in Table 25.3.

Specific Illicit Drugs

Cocaine

Cocaine can be taken orally, intravenously, or intranasally, whereas crack (cocaine) is the combustible form of the drug that is smoked and is probably the most common illicit drug to cause respiratory symptoms. In the acute setting, symptoms of smoking or inhalation of crack include cough, chest pain, dyspnea, wheezing, and, occasionally, respiratory failure. Chronic or long-term use may cause OP, eosinophilic pneumonia (crack lung), pulmonary fibrosis, talcosis, emphysema, and/or pulmonary hypertension.

Systemic complications of cocaine use result from the sympathomimetic effect of the drug on the cardiovascular system. Effects on the heart include coronary vasospasm and myocardial ischemia or infarction, arrhythmia, and cardiomyopathy. The use of crack cocaine has also been identified as a risk factor for acute aortic syndromes (e.g., dissection, intramural hematoma).

Marijuana

Marijuana causes similar short- and long-term respiratory effects to tobacco use, including chronic cough, sputum production, and wheeze, although patients may develop emphysema at an earlier age than tobacco users. The term *synthetic marijuana* refers to a class of drugs where various chemicals are sprayed onto herbs to mimic the appearance and effects of marijuana. There have been recent case reports of profound respiratory failure from the use of synthetic marijuana, presenting on CT with diffuse centrilobular nodules.

Specific Effects of Illicit Drug Use

Barotrauma

Barotrauma and pneumomediastinum may result from specific smoking practices, regardless of drug, including Valsalva maneuvers during smoking and "shotgunning" (inhaling smoke and then forcefully exhaling it directly into another person's mouth).

Emphysema

Emphysema is a long-term consequence of many illicit drugs, often in distributions that differ from tobacco use, and may be the result of injection or inhalation. Perhaps the most notable cause is IV injection of Ritalin (methylphenidate), which can cause lower lobe–predominant panacinar emphysema similar in appearance to alpha-1-antitrypsin deficiency. Marijuana has been implicated as a cause of bullous emphysema with large paraseptal bullae in young patients who otherwise do not use tobacco, sometimes presenting as giant bullous emphysema. The long-term inhalation of hydrocarbons, including butane, gasoline, glue, and aerosol propellants, may result in panacinar emphysema.

Infective Endocarditis and Septic Emboli

Intravenous drug use is a common cause of infective endocarditis; over 85% of cases involve the right heart, with the tricuspid valve being involved in almost all cases. Damage to the valve from injected particulate matter and injected bacterial load are implicated in the

TABLE 25.3 Complications From Illicit Drug Use

PULMONARY EFFECTS	CARDIOVASCULAR EFFECTS	NEUROLOGIC EFFECTS
Pulmonary edema (hydrostatic or permeability)	Vasospasm	Aspiration
Hemorrhage	Myocardial ischemia, infarct	Neurogenic (permeability) edema
Organizing pneumonia	Dilated cardiomyopathy	
Eosinophilic pneumonia	Acute aortic syndrome	
Hypersensitivity pneumonitis	Excipient lung disease	
Emphysema	Endocarditis, septic emboli	
Pulmonary fibrosis		

development of infective endocarditis, and an altered immune status in the setting of drug use may also predispose patients. Septic emboli represent the pulmonary parenchymal manifestation of right-sided endocarditis in the setting of illicit drug use as the result of the hematogenous dissemination of bacteria.

Imaging findings of septic emboli include peripheral, well-defined spherical nodules (with or without surrounding GGOs) and/or wedge-shaped areas of consolidation in various stages of cavitation (Fig. 25.10). The peripheral distribution of septic emboli reflects the hematogenous spread of infection. A feeding vessel may be seen in some cases but is not necessarily a reliable sign on CT. Septic emboli are rarely macroscopic emboli, as opposed to a bland pulmonary embolism.

When septic emboli are suspected, interrogation of the right heart for the presence of a low-attenuation nodule representing a vegetation (especially along the tricuspid valve) may help confirm the diagnosis. Secondary findings of endocarditis include right-sided chamber dilation and right heart failure from tricuspid (or, less commonly, pulmonic) valve destruction. Other causes of septic emboli and infective endocarditis include infected indwelling catheters, infected pacemakers, and poor dentition.

Excipient Lung Disease

Excipient lung disease (ELD) is the result of the IV injection of crushed oral tablets. Excipients are inert insoluble binders used in the production of the tablets and include talc, cellulose, starch, and crospovidone. When injected, these particles lodge in the pulmonary arterioles and capillaries and incite an angiogranulomatous reaction that may result in arteriolar occlusion and resultant pulmonary hypertension.

Commonly injected medications that cause ELD include analgesics (e.g., methadone, codeine), stimulants, and antihistamines. The most frequent presenting symptom of ELD is dyspnea, which is nonspecific. However, the rapid onset of unexplainable pulmonary hypertension, cor pulmonale, or sudden cardiac death should prompt consideration of ELD. In addition to IV drug users, patients at risk for ELD include those with chronic pain or illness (e.g., malignancy, psychiatric illness, migraine headaches), especially those with an indwelling catheter, or health care workers who have easy access to analgesic tablets.

On CT, ELD has a characteristic appearance of diffuse centrilobular micronodules (often with a vascular tree-in-bud pattern) in combination with pulmonary artery enlargement and findings of right heart strain (Fig. 25.11). The presence of an indwelling catheter is another clue to diagnosis. Many of these excipients are polarizable with histopathology at biopsy or postmortem examination.

Talcosis

Talcosis represents another granulomatous foreign body reaction to excipients in crushed tablets, most notably talc. Respiratory symptoms include progressive dyspnea and symptoms of chronic obstructive pulmonary disease. CT findings of talcosis include innumerable micronodules (~1 mm) and GGOs, with progression to high-attenuation perihilar conglomerate masses that may mimic progressive massive fibrosis of silicosis (Fig. 25.12).

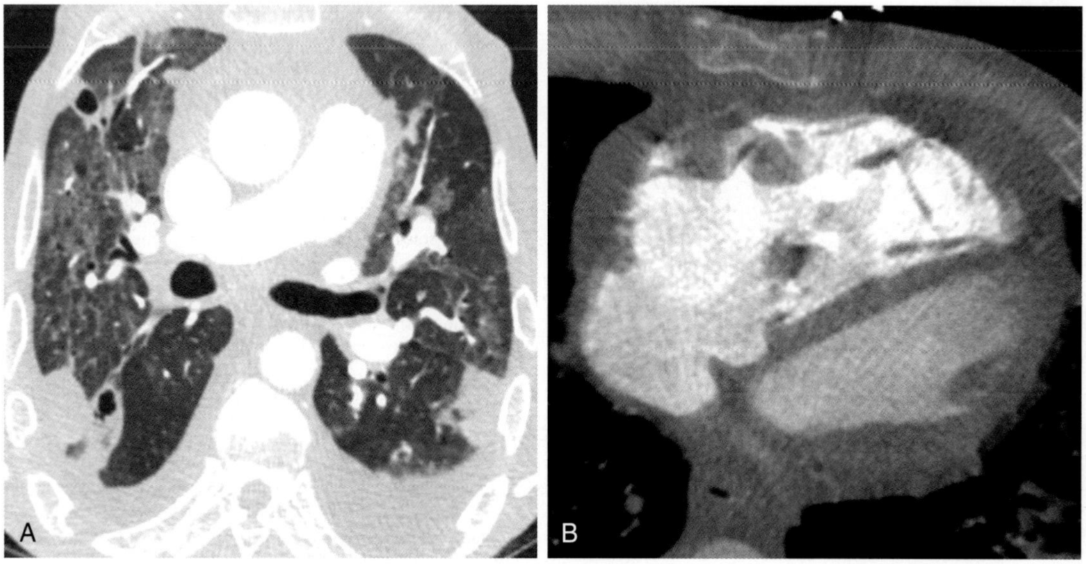

Figure 25.10 A 44-year-old man with methicillin-sensitive *Staphylococcus aureus* tricuspid endocarditis and septic emboli secondary to IV drug use. (A) Axial CT at lung window shows multiple peripheral areas of consolidation and nodules in varying stages of cavitation. (B) Image through the heart at soft tissue window shows a large, multilobulated, low-attenuation vegetation, visible despite cardiac motion. The dilated right atrium and ventricle are secondary clues to severe tricuspid dysfunction.

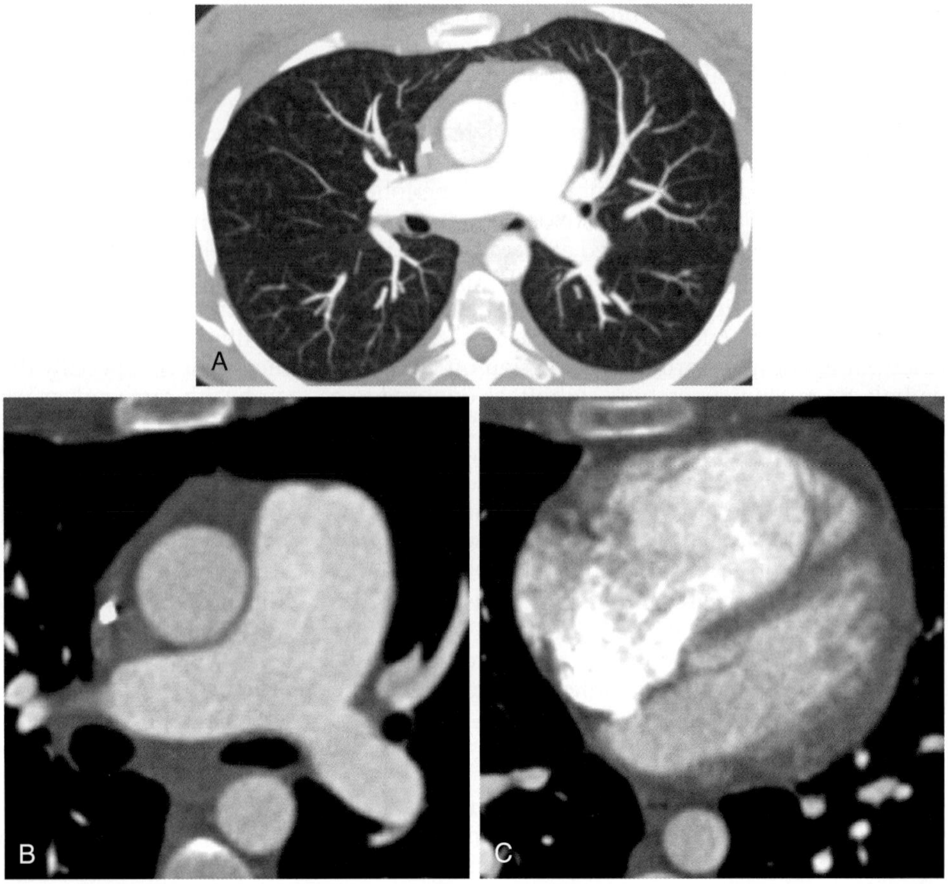

Figure 25.11 A 20-year-old woman with a history of Gardner syndrome, prior colectomy complicated by multiple desmoid tumor resections, and chronic pain killer use. She presented with acute onset of dyspnea and right heart failure. (A) Axial maximum intensity projection image shows diffuse centrilobular nodules in a tree-in-bud configuration. (B and C) Axial images at soft tissue window show profound enlargement of the main pulmonary artery and dilated right heart chambers, indicative of right heart strain. An indwelling catheter is also visible. This constellation of findings was suggestive of excipient lung disease, confirmed when polarizable material was detected on biopsy. Patient admitted to injecting crushed tablets through her central venous catheter.

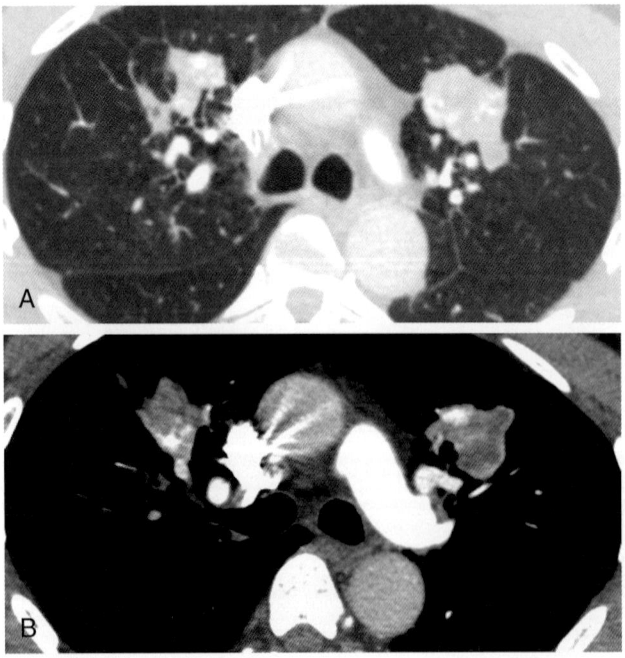

Figure 25.12 Talcosis in a young man with history of intravenous drug use. (A) CT images at lung and soft tissue windows (B) shows bilateral perihilar consolidation with calcification, architectural distortion, and volume loss, resulting in a progressive, massive, fibrosis-like appearance.

Bibliography

Berkowitz EA, Henry TS, Veeraraghavan S, Staton GW Jr, Gal AA. Pulmonary effects of synthetic marijuana: chest radiography and CT findings. *AJR Am J Roentgenol*. 2014;1–8.

Bhargava S, Perlman DM, Allen TL, Ritter JH, Bhargava M. Adalimumab induced pulmonary sarcoid reaction. *Respir Med Case Rep*. 2013;10:53–55.

Biswas S, Badiuddin F. Radiation-induced malignant histiocytoma of the contralateral breast following treatment of breast cancer: a case report and review of the literature. *Cases J*. 2008;1(1):313.

Choi YW, Munden RF, Erasmus JJ, et al. Effects of radiation therapy on the lung: radiologic appearances and differential diagnosis. *Radiographics*. 2004;24(4): 985–997.

Cook RJ, Ashton RW, Aughenbaugh GL, Ryu JH. Septic pulmonary embolism: presenting features and clinical course of 14 patients. *Chest*. 2005;128(1):162–166.

Dodd JD, Souza CA, Müller NL. High-resolution MDCT of pulmonary septic embolism: evaluation of the feeding vessel sign. *AJR Am J Roentgenol*. 2006;187(3):623–629.

Ellis SJ, Cleverley JR, Müller NL. Drug-induced lung disease: high-resolution CT findings. *AJR Am J Roentgenol*. 2000;175(4):1019–1024.

Hsue PY. Acute aortic dissection related to crack cocaine. *Circulation*. 2002;105(13):1592–1595.

Isabela C, Silva S, Müller NL. Drug-induced lung diseases: most common reaction patterns and corresponding high-resolution CT manifestations. *Semin Ultrasound CT MR*. 2006;27(2):111–116.

Karkhanis V, Joshi J. Pleural effusion: diagnosis, treatment, and management. *Open Access Emerg Med*. 2012;4:31–52.

Koenig TR, Munden RF, Erasmus JJ, et al. Radiation injury of the lung after three-dimensional conformal radiation therapy. *AJR Am J Roentgenol*. 2002;178(6):1383–1388.

Kuhlman JE, Teigen C, Ren H, et al. Amiodarone pulmonary toxicity: CT findings in symptomatic patients. *Radiology*. 1990;177(1):121–125.

Larici AR, del Ciello A, Maggi F, et al. Lung abnormalities at multimodality imaging after radiation therapy for non-small cell lung cancer. *Radiographics*. 2011;31(3):771–789.

Matsuno O. Drug-induced interstitial lung disease: mechanisms and best diagnostic approaches. *Respir Res*. 2012;13:39.

Montani D, Seferian A, Savale L, Simonneau G, Humbert M. Drug-induced pulmonary arterial hypertension: a recent outbreak. *Eur Respir Rev.* 2013;22(129):244–250.

Moss R, Munt B. Injection drug use and right-sided endocarditis. *Heart.* 2003;89(5):577–581.

Nguyen ET, Silva CIS, Souza CA, Müller NL. Pulmonary complications of illicit drug use: differential diagnosis based on CT findings. *J Thorac Imaging.* 2007;22(2):199–206.

Nguyen VT, Chan ES, Chou S-HS, et al. Pulmonary effects of IV injection of crushed oral tablets: "excipient lung disease". *AJR Am J Roentgenol.* 2014;203(5):W506–W515.

Oie Y, Saito Y, Kato M, et al. Relationship between radiation pneumonitis and organizing pneumonia after radiotherapy for breast cancer. *Radiat Oncol.* 2013;56.

Park HJ, Kim KJ, Park SH, Kay C-S, Oh JS. Early CT findings of tomotherapy-induced radiation pneumonitis after treatment of lung malignancy. *AJR Am J Roentgenol.* 2009;193(3):W209–W213.

Ravenel JG, McAdams HP, Plankeel JF, Butnor KJ, Sporn TA. Sarcoidosis induced by interferon therapy. *AJR Am J Roentgenol.* 2001;177(1):199–201.

Restrepo CS, Carrillo JA, Martínez S, Ojeda P, Rivera AL, Hatta A. Pulmonary complications from cocaine and cocaine-based substances: imaging manifestations. *Radiographics.* 2007;27(4):941–956.

Rossi SE, Erasmus JJ, McAdams HP, Sporn TA, Goodman PC. Pulmonary drug toxicity: radiologic and pathologic manifestations. *Radiographics.* 2000;20(5):1245–1259.

Sood N, Sood N. A rare case of vanishing lung syndrome. *Case Rep Pulmonol.* 2011;2011(9):1–2.

Stern EJ, Frank MS, Schmutz JF, Glenny RW, Schmidt RA, Godwin JD. Panlobular pulmonary emphysema caused by i.v. injection of methylphenidate (Ritalin): findings on chest radiographs and CT scans. *AJR Am J Roentgenol.* 1994;162(3):555–560.

Ward S, Heyneman LE, Reittner P, Kazerooni EA, Godwin JD, Müller NL. Talcosis associated with IV abuse of oral medications: CT findings. *AJR Am J Roentgenol.* 2000;174(3):789–793.

Wolff AJ, O'Donnell AE. Pulmonary effects of illicit drug use. *Clin Chest Med.* 2004;25(1):203–216.

Yi A, Kim HH, Shin HJ, Huh MO, Ahn SD, Seo BK. Radiation-induced complications after breast cancer radiation therapy: a pictorial review of multimodality imaging findings. *Korean J Radiol.* 2009;10(5):496.

CHAPTER 26

Diffuse Lung Disease With Calcification and Lipid

Hsiang-Jer Tseng and Brent P. Little

CHAPTER OUTLINE

■ Introduction

Certain diffuse lung diseases are associated with high- or low-attenuation lesions. High-attenuation lesions are most often due to calcium deposition from a variety of mechanisms, but can also be due to the accumulation of other radiopaque substances such as iodine (amiodarone lung toxicity) and talc (talcosis). Low-attenuation lesions are predominantly due to the deposition of lipid-containing substances. These diffuse lung diseases can encompass a large range of causes, including infectious, inflammatory, neoplastic, metabolic, occupational exposures, iatrogenic, and idiopathic processes. To make an accurate diagnosis, radiologists need to be cognizant of the morphologies and distribution patterns of these high- or low-attenuation lesions and must be able to assimilate other relevant imaging features and clinical histories. These important distinguishing characteristics, as well as common problem-solving issues and pitfalls, will be discussed in this chapter.

■ Imaging Modalities Used to Assess Diffuse Lung Disease Involving High- or Low-Attenuation Lesions

Radiographs are usually part of the initial workup for diffuse lung disease and can demonstrate large nodules, consolidation, prominent hilar and mediastinal lymphadenopathy, and calcification. Diffuse micronodules and interstitial calcification can present as reticular or reticulonodular opacities on radiographs. However, radiographs have a low sensitivity for detecting smaller lung lesions and often fail to demonstrate fine parenchymal detail and specific attenuation of lung lesions. In addition, diffuse lung disease involving calcification or lipid can mimic pulmonary edema, interstitial lung disease, or atypical infection with radiography. CT with a high-resolution CT (HRCT) technique (thin-slice, high-resolution technique) provides optimal evaluation of diffuse lung disease and is more sensitive and specific in detecting calcification and lipid. On CT, calcified lesions show attenuation similar to that of bone, ranging from 200 to >1000 Hounsfield units (HU). Lesions containing macroscopic fat have negative attenuation values, in general between −50 and −100 HU. Calcification or lipid mixed with other materials, such as soft tissue, will produce intermediate-attenuation values; in addition, volume averaging with adjacent tissue can occur, especially when thicker slices (>1–2 mm) are used for interpretation and when attenuation measurements of very small lesions are attempted. Thin-section CT can also depict the fine parenchymal detail, including patterns of small nodules, that is necessary for the diagnosis of many diffuse lung diseases involving high attenuation or lipid.

Although nuclear medicine examinations such as a technetium-99m methylene diphosphonate (^{99m}Tc-MDP) bone scan and PET can play a role in the evaluation of metastatic disease, they are not the primary modalities for the characterization of diffuse lung disease involving calcification or lipid because uptake of radiotracers can occur in a wide variety of malignant and inflammatory nonmalignant diseases. Chest MRI also has not been traditionally used as a primary method of evaluating these diseases because this modality is inferior to CT in characterizing fine pulmonary parenchymal detail, small nodules, and small foci of fat or calcium.

Diffuse Lung Disease With Calcification or High Attenuation

Diffuse lung disease with calcification or high attenuation can present with nodules, masses, consolidation, or a combination of these. Ancillary findings in some diseases can include calcified lymphadenopathy, septal thickening, and pleural calcification. Nodules and masses can have a wide range of sizes, from tiny nodules <1 mm to masses >10 cm. Diseases can have an upper lung, lower lung, or no particular craniocaudal predominance.

Of the many diseases presenting with nodules, many can be categorized according to the distribution pattern of the calcified lesions relative to the secondary pulmonary lobule. The distribution pattern can be centrilobular, perilymphatic, or random. Centrilobular nodules are located within the central secondary pulmonary lobule and spare pleural surfaces and interlobular septa. Perilymphatic nodules are distributed along the subpleural interstitium, bronchovascular interstitium, and interlobular septa. In a random distribution, nodules are widely distributed without a particular anatomic relation to the secondary lobule; a subset is distributed along the pleural and interlobular septa.

These distribution patterns serve as a good starting point for narrowing the differential diagnosis; additional imaging and clinical features provide further guidance. Certain rare diffuse lung diseases, such as pulmonary alveolar microlithiasis and pulmonary ossification, can have unique calcification patterns that are not typical of the classic distribution pattern discussed above. The list of differential diagnoses for different distribution patterns is summarized in Box 26.1. In the setting of solitary, sparse, multiple calcified nodules or nodules that are large enough to distort the pulmonary lobular architecture, which can be observed in healed granulomatous infection, calcified pulmonary metastasis, and hyalinizing granuloma, the distribution pattern can be difficult to determine, making other diagnostic clues such as clinical histories and other associated imaging features important in problem solving. (See Table 26.2 for a summary of the calcification pattern and associated imaging and clinical features of each disease entity that help differentiate between disease entities that share a similar imaging presentation and identify diseases where the calcification pattern alone provides very limited information.) A disease entity also can have multiple presentations on imaging, adding to the complexity of problem solving.

BOX 26.1 Differential Diagnoses for Diffuse Lung Disease With High-Attenuation Nodules or Masses

Calcified Nodules

Random Distribution
- Healed granulomatous infection
- Healed varicella pneumonia
- Calcified pulmonary metastasis

Perilymphatic Distribution
- Pneumoconioses
- Sarcoidosis
- Amyloidosis (diffuse parenchymal form)

Centrilobular Distribution
- Pulmonary hemosiderosis
- Metastatic pulmonary calcification

Other Patterns of "Calcification"
- Pulmonary ossification
- Pulmonary alveolar microlithiasis

Calcified Masses (>3 cm) or Consolidation
- Progressive massive fibrosis
- Amyloidosis (nodular form)
- Metastatic pulmonary calcification
- Hyalinizing granuloma

High-Attenuation Nodules or Masses Without Visible Calcification
- Talcosis
- Amiodarone lung toxicity
- Pulmonary alveolar microlithiasis

Diseases Causing Calcified Pulmonary Nodules

These can be in a random, perilymphatic, or centrilobular distribution.

Random Distribution

Healed Granulomatous Infections

Healed granulomatous infections are common causes of solitary and multiple calcified nodules in the lung

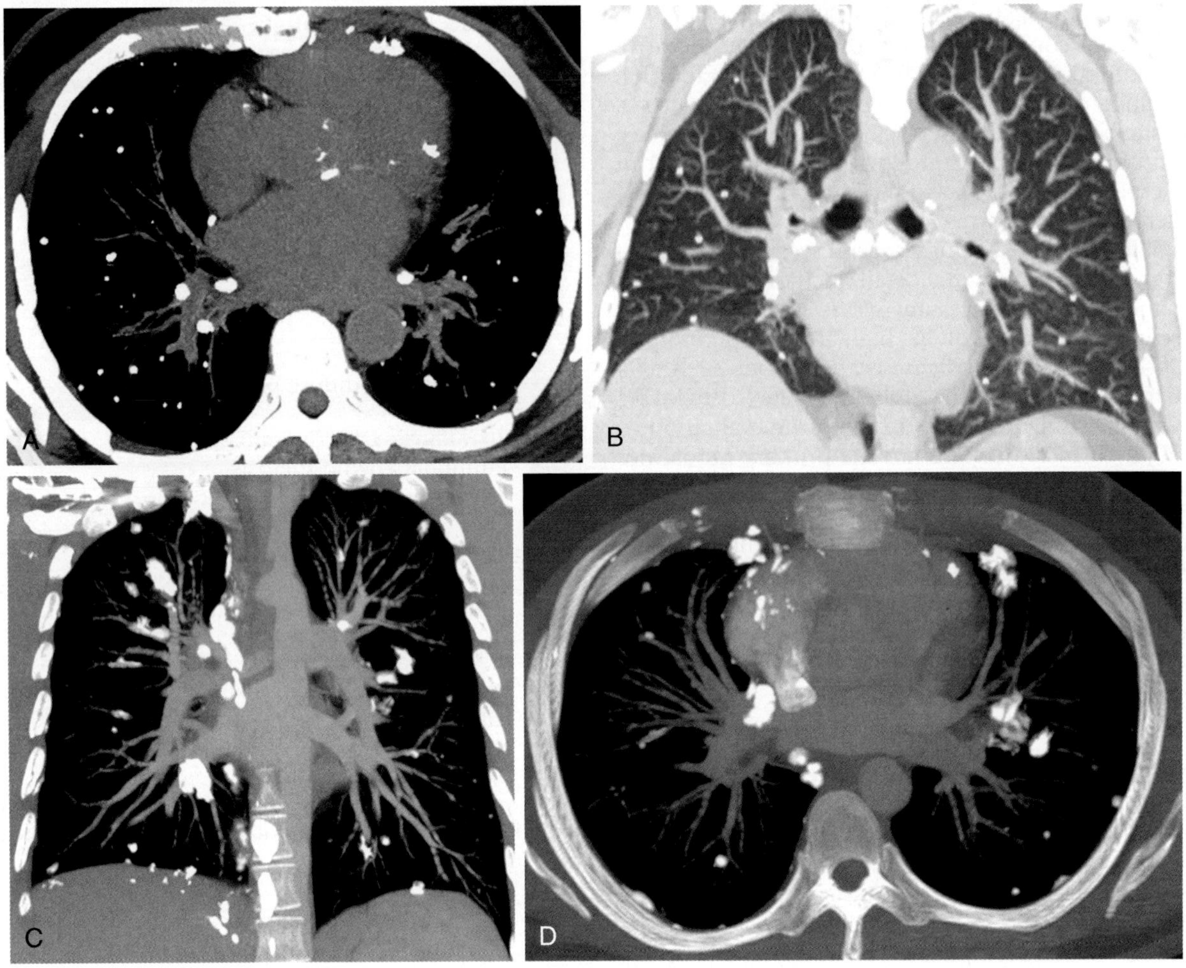

Figure 26.1 (A and B) Remote granulomatous infection in a 70-year-old man from the southern United States with numerous randomly distributed pulmonary nodules in all lobes of the lungs. (A) Axial maximum intensity projection (MIP) reformatted image with lung windows shows numerous completely calcified pulmonary nodules without associated visible soft tissue components. Calcified peribronchial lymph nodes are also present. (B) Coronal CT image with lung windows shows the random distribution of the nodules. No spatial gradient of distribution is seen. Other images showed multiple calcified nodules in the spleen and liver. The appearance is typical for a prior granulomatous infection such as histoplasmosis. (C and D) Osteosarcoma metastases in a 25-year-old man with osteosarcoma of the femur. MIP CT images with bone windows show calcified nodules, lymph nodes, and pleural metastases bilaterally. Although the larger nodules have associated soft tissue, the soft tissue is not visible within many of the smaller nodules, possibly causing confusion with benign patterns of calcification (e.g., as in calcified granulomas).

parenchyma. The nodules usually follow a random distribution or can occur in clusters (Fig. 26.1A and B). In the United States, histoplasmosis is the most common cause of granulomatous infection, whereas tuberculosis is the leading cause worldwide. Other rare causes include coccidioidomycosis and blastomycosis. The pulmonary manifestations of acute primary granulomatous infection vary widely and depend on the amount of exposure, the virulence of the infectious organisms, and the strength of the host's immune system. A granuloma is an area of caseating necrosis that was once a focus of infection, later contained by the host's cell-mediated immune response and subsequently encapsulated by fibrotic tissue. Over the course of months to years, dystrophic calcifications develop with the granulomas. Depending on the size of inoculum, the number of granulomas can vary. Calcification of the diseased lymph nodes and hepatic and splenic granulomas can also be seen with healed granulomatous disease. The imaging appearance of healed histoplasmosis and healed tuberculosis can be indistinguishable. However, multiple splenic calcifications and diffuse nodular calcification patterns are much more commonly seen in histoplasmosis; in addition, significant architectural distortion and/or bronchiectasis with asymmetric, upper lung predominance are more common findings in tuberculosis.

Healed Varicella Pneumonia

Varicella pneumonia is the one of the most common and most severe manifestations of disseminated varicella zoster virus infection in adults, with reported mortality rates of 9% to 50%. Its incidence increases with age, with a peak between the third and fifth decades of life. Some of the risk factors for developing varicella pneumonia include lymphoma, leukemia, immunocompromised status (e.g., as with chronic corticosteroid usage), pregnancy, and a history of smoking. Varicella pneumonia typically develops 3 to 5 days after the classic polymorphic rash (blisters, pustules, and crusty lesions). The predominant histologic finding for acute varicella pneumonia is diffuse alveolar damage. On radiographs, acute varicella pneumonia often presents as multiple ill-defined nodules from 5 to 10 mm, usually without associated mediastinal and hilar lymphadenopathy or pleural effusions. CT reveals multiple noncalcified, coalescent 1- to 10-mm pulmonary nodules with surrounding ground-glass opacity (halo sign) in a centrilobular pattern, with multiple patchy areas of ground-glass opacity. Typical management involves acyclovir and supportive care. Depending on the severity of disease, these pulmonary nodules may resolve within days or up to several weeks following clearing of the skin rash. Some of the nodules can become healed granulomas and gradually evolve into diffuse, calcified, small nodules (1–3 mm). Healed varicella pneumonia can mimic healed histoplasmosis. However, concurrent hepatic and splenic calcified granulomas, if present, favor histoplasmosis as the underlying cause.

Calcified Pulmonary Metastases

Certain malignancies that metastasize to the lungs can manifest as solitary or multiple calcified nodules on imaging. The most commonly encountered example is osteosarcoma, the most common malignant bone tumor in children and young adults (see Fig. 26.1C and D). Up to 90% of patients with osteosarcoma have been found to have pulmonary metastases on autopsy. Tumor cells spread to the lungs hematogenously. A random but overall lower lobe–predominant pattern is observed due to relatively higher perfusion in the lower lobes. Like their primary source, metastatic pulmonary nodules can calcify by heterotopic bone formation within the tumor osteoid matrix. ^{99m}Tc-MDP bone scan can be used to detect metastatic osteosarcoma. However, pulmonary metastatic lesions may not calcify until they grow larger, thereby limiting the sensitivity of bone scanning for detecting small soft tissue metastatic lesions. Therefore, bone scanning is usually used in conjunction with CT. Other primary sarcomas that may show calcified metastases include synovial cell sarcomas, chondrosarcomas (by bone formation within tumor cartilage), and giant cell tumor.

In addition, other nonsarcoma extrapulmonary malignancies have been shown to have calcified lung metastases, including papillary and mucinous adenocarcinoma (of the gastrointestinal tract and ovary) and thyroid medullary carcinoma. In the setting of metastatic mucinous adenocarcinoma, calcium salt can deposit in areas of mucinous degeneration (mucoid calcification), yielding partially calcified nodules with stippled, irregular, or globular eccentric calcification. In the setting of thyroid medullary carcinoma, calcification of metastatic nodules is at least in part due to psammoma body formation. It is also important to note that any treated malignancy in the lung, metastatic or primary, can calcify by dystrophic calcification.

Perilymphatic Distribution

Pneumoconioses

Pneumoconioses are irreversible lung diseases caused by the chronic inhalation of microparticles, such as crystalline silica (silicosis), coal particles (coal workers' pneumoconiosis), beryllium particles (berylliosis), iron oxides (siderosis), tin oxides (stannosis), and barium dust (baritosis). Obtaining the occupational history is essential for the diagnosis of such diseases. Silicosis is associated with mining, sandblasting, stonecutting, quarrying, and manufacture of pottery or glass. Berylliosis is associated with the ceramic, fluorescent light bulb, nuclear weapon, and aerospace industries. Siderosis is associated with iron welding and metal polishing. Stannosis is associated with tin smelting. Baritosis is associated with the chronic inhalation of barium sulfate dusts, which are associated with the manufacture of paint, paper, textile, and numerous other items. Table 26.1 summarizes several important pneumoconioses with their typical associated occupational histories. In general, pneumoconioses have a slow disease progression. Symptoms, including productive cough and progressive dyspnea, as well as radiographic abnormalities, usually follow a latency period of about 10 to 20 years after exposure. However, latency period and disease presentation may change in the setting of high exposure. For example, accelerated silicosis, which can occur in the setting of chronic high exposure, can have a shortened latency of 5 to 10 years with a more severe disease presentation. Acute silicoproteinosis, which is another variant of silicosis caused by high exposure for months to 2 years, can present clinically and pathologically similar to alveolar proteinosis (see below for further discussion). Unlike silicosis, berylliosis has a variable latency period of 2 months to >40 years and can manifest clinically in the setting of minimal exposure. This is largely because its pathogenesis involves activation of adaptive and innate (inflammatory) immune responses.

TABLE 26.1 Pneumoconioses and Associated Occupational Histories

PNEUMOCONIOSES	OCCUPATIONAL HISTORIES
Silicosis	Mining, sandblasting, stonecutting, quarrying, construction, pottery, glass, ceramics manufacture
Coal workers' pneumoconiosis	Coal mining
Beryllium	Ceramics, fluorescent light bulb, nuclear weapons, dental prostheses, alloy machining, automotive and aerospace industries
Siderosis	Iron welding and metal polishing
Stannosis	Tin smelting and bagging
Baritosis	Paint, paper, textile, leather, vinyl, rubber, linoleum, alloy manufacture
Talcosis	Chronic inhalation of baby powder or cosmetic talc; mining, production of paint, rubber, paper, leather, ceramics, and insecticide

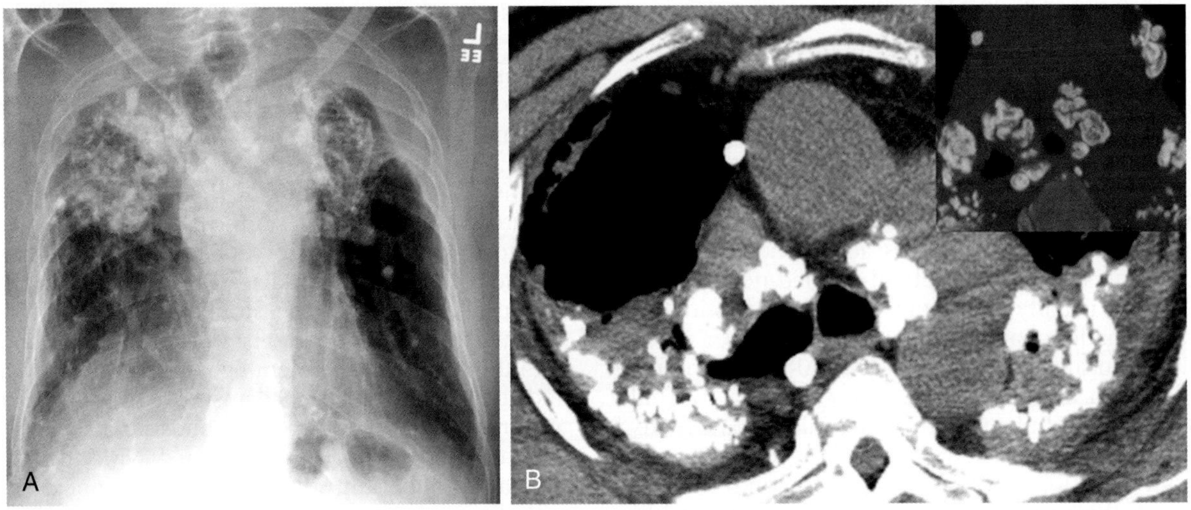

Figure 26.2 Silicosis in a 68-year-old man with occupational exposure to silica dust. (A) Frontal chest radiograph shows bilateral upper lobe volume loss and masslike consolidation in the upper lobes, associated with nodular calcification and calcified hilar and mediastinal lymph nodes. (B) Axial CT scan with soft tissue windows shows coarse nodular calcification of the upper lobe consolidation, with parenchymal distortion and calcified hilar and mediastinal lymph nodes. Coned-down view of the mediastinal lymph nodes at bone windows shows peripheral eggshell calcification.

The typical radiographic findings of chronic simple silicosis and coal workers' pneumoconioses are reticulonodular opacities; calcification may be identified within nodules. On CT, pneumoconioses usually present as numerous small nodules (<10 mm) in a perilymphatic distribution, with or without calcification (Fig. 26.2). These nodules tend to be upper lobe predominant (especially the posterior portions) due to relatively poor lymphatic clearing of the microparticles from the alveoli in the upper lobes; this is a result of lower perfusion and limited respiratory excursion toward the lung apices, with resulting relatively lower lymphatic clearance. Bilateral hilar and mediastinal lymphadenopathy is common, especially in silicosis. Peripherally calcified lymphadenopathy, also known as *eggshell calcification*, can be seen in silicosis, coal workers' pneumoconiosis, and sarcoidosis. In complicated pneumoconioses, the micronodules can grow and form conglomerates (>1 cm) that can gradually migrate toward the hila, a finding known as *progressive massive fibrosis.* When a conglomerate mass grows larger than 4 cm, it can develop central necrosis and punctate calcifications. With similar imaging findings, sarcoidosis can mimic certain pneumoconioses. However, unlike pneumoconioses, sarcoidosis can often present as an isolated lymphadenopathy without parenchymal disease. Typical management involves removal of exposure and supportive care.

Sarcoidosis

Sarcoidosis is an idiopathic chronic inflammatory disease with noncaseating granulomas as the predominant histologic finding. It typically affects young adults with peak age of 20 to 29 years at presentation, with a slight female predominance. In the United States, the age-adjusted annual incidence among African Americans is more than threefold higher than that among whites (35.5 vs. 10.9/100,000 people). African Americans, Swedes, and Danes have the highest prevalence worldwide. Although sarcoidosis in whites tends to be subclinical, the disease presentation in African Americans tends to be more severe and can involve multiple systems, including the heart, nervous system, bone, joints, muscles, skin, eyes, and kidneys, but most commonly the lung. Common symptoms include cough, dyspnea, fatigue, night sweats, weight loss, and erythema nodosum. However, up to 50% of cases remain asymptomatic and are often found incidentally on imaging. Studies have shown that the underlying disease mechanism may be related to a variety of factors, including environmental exposures and genetic, infectious, and immunologic mechanisms.

Pulmonary sarcoidosis usually manifests radiographically as mediastinal and hilar lymphadenopathy (Scadding stage 1) and may develop punctate, amorphous, or eggshell calcification. More advanced disease (stage 2) can have parenchymal and nodal involvement. As the parenchymal disease progresses toward fibrosis, lymphadenopathy can disappear (stage 3). Parenchymal involvement of sarcoidosis can present as reticulonodular opacity with radiography.

On CT, it can present as diffuse, upper lobe–predominant, small nodules in a perilymphatic distribution, nodular septal thickening, and patchy areas of ground-glass opacities. Nodular bronchial and bronchiolar wall thickening can also cause mosaic attenuation of the lung. In complicated disease, nodules can aggregate and form masslike lesions in the upper lobes, with architectural distortion. Although most sarcoidosis cases remain stable or enter remission within a decade after diagnosis, without significant clinical consequences, approximately 20% of patients can progress to end-stage pulmonary sarcoidosis (stage 4; Fig. 26.3), with irreversible, upper lobe–predominant honeycombing, bullae, traction bronchiectasis, and architectural distortion. For many mild cases, symptomatic relief can be achieved by the use of nonsteroidal antiinflammatory drugs. For active

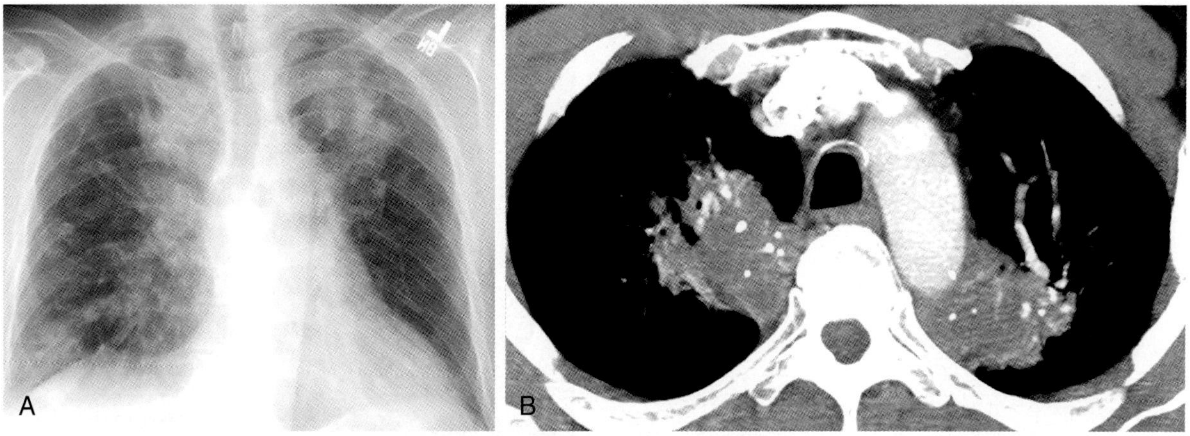

Figure 26.3 Sarcoidosis in a 64-year-old man with sarcoidosis and mass-like fibrosis. (A) Frontal chest radiograph shows bilateral upper lobe volume loss, with upward hilar retraction and symmetric masses in the upper lobes. Smaller masses are also seen in the lower lobes. (B) Axial CT image with soft tissue windows shows upper lobe masses with punctate calcifications, with encasement and retraction of the bronchovascular bundles.

pulmonary sarcoidosis that does not spontaneously resolve in 2 to 3 months, a corticosteroid is often used, despite lack of strong evidence of its efficacy. Severe symptoms often require immunosuppressive agents, such as methotrexate.

Amyloidosis

Amyloidosis has a wide spectrum of imaging presentations in the chest, often mimicking that of other disease entities. Amyloidosis is a multisystem disease in which organ dysfunction is caused by extracellular deposition of insoluble beta-pleated sheets, formed by the overexpression of a range of different proteins. Amyloidosis has a male predominance, with a mean age of 55 to 60 years at the onset of disease. Isolated pulmonary amyloidosis can occur, but up to 80% to 90% of cases of amyloidosis are thought to have systemic involvement. Systemic amyloidosis can be idiopathic (primary) or reactive (secondary) to underlying chronic inflammatory conditions, such as multiple myeloma, rheumatoid arthritis, chronic infections, and familial Mediterranean fever. The clinical presentation depends on the organ involved; the heart and kidney are usually involved in amyloidosis and can manifest as heart failure and nephrotic syndrome.

Two types of pulmonary parenchymal amyloidosis are recognized: nodular and diffuse. The nodular type is typically seen in localized amyloidosis and is usually asymptomatic; the diffuse parenchymal type is usually seen in systemic amyloidosis and carries a poor prognosis, with progressive dyspnea and a mean survival of 16 months. On imaging, the nodular type can manifest as a stable or slow-growing single node or multiple nodules or masses (Fig. 26.4). Nodules range from 0.5 to 15 cm in size. Although some cases have a diffuse distribution of nodules throughout the lung parenchyma, a peripheral and lower lobe predominance occurs in others. Dystrophic calcification can develop within the nodules or masses. The pattern of calcification can be amorphous and sometimes eccentric, at times mimicking either healed granulomatous infection or malignancy. Thin-walled cysts and cavitary nodules may coexist with solid nodules. The diffuse parenchymal form of amyloidosis manifests as an interstitial opacity, interlobular septal thickening, small nodules (<1.5 cm) in a perilymphatic distribution, and, less commonly, traction bronchiectasis and honeycombing. Confluent nodules and consolidation can be seen in a subset of cases.

Mediastinal or hilar lymphadenopathy can occur, at times showing high attenuation or frank calcification. When diffuse small nodules are the dominant features, the differential diagnoses include certain pneumoconioses, granulomatous infection, calcified metastatic disease, and sarcoidosis. When interstitial and septal thickening is the dominant feature, usually peripheral- and basilar-predominant, the imaging findings may mimic a variety of interstitial lung diseases.

Tissue sampling is required to establish a definitive diagnosis. When stained with Congo red, biopsy specimens containing amyloid deposits demonstrate a characteristic positive birefringence with polarized light. Clinical correlation with urine and serum immunoelectrophoresis for multiple myeloma and a history of any known predisposing disease can be helpful. Depending on the specific type of protein deposition involved, treatment options include melphalan (a chemotherapy agent), corticosteroids, stem cell therapy, and treatment of any underlying inflammatory condition(s).

Centrilobular Distribution

Pulmonary Hemosiderosis

Pulmonary hemosiderosis is a rare lung disease characterized by recurrent alveolar hemorrhage and the deposition of hemosiderin in alveoli. Primary pulmonary hemosiderosis can be idiopathic (predominantly affecting infants and young adults, with an incidence of less than two cases per million people) and is thought to be immune-mediated. It can also occur in the setting of Heiner and Goodpasture syndrome, in which the disease mechanisms involve antibodies attacking the basement

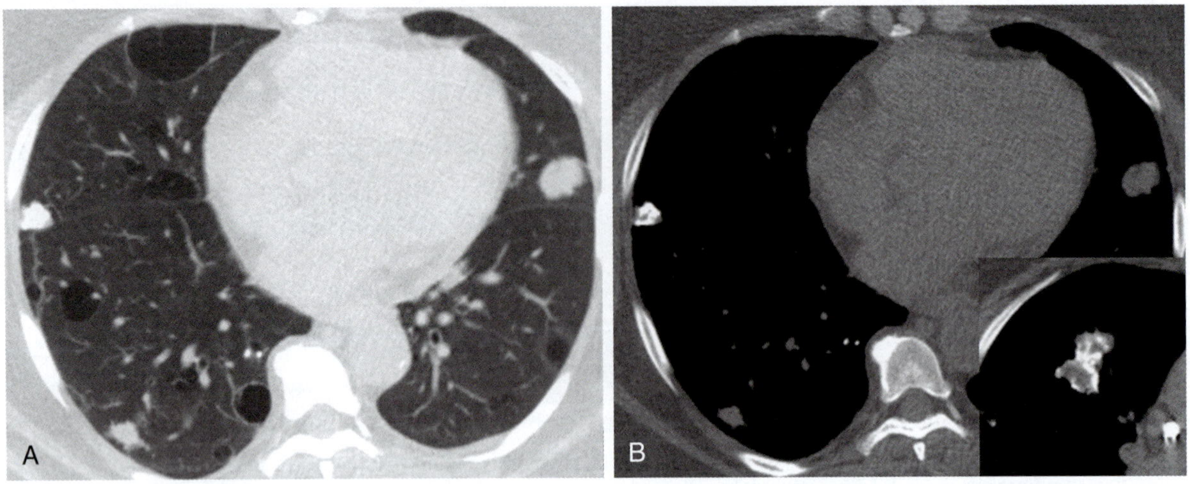

Figure 26.4 Amyloidosis in a 50-year-old woman with pulmonary nodules stable over years of follow-up; the percutaneous biopsy showed amyloidosis. (A) Axial CT image with lung windows shows multiple large nodules and thin-walled cysts. (B) At bone windows, irregular partial calcification is seen in some of the nodules, including the middle lobe and right upper lobe *(inset)*.

membrane of the lung. In the setting of Heiner syndrome, the disease mechanism is triggered by hypersensitivity to cow's milk protein. Secondary pulmonary hemosiderosis is usually due to mitral stenosis, in which recurrent alveolar hemorrhage occurs in the setting of pulmonary capillary hypertension. The classic clinical triad consists of hemoptysis, iron deficiency anemia, and diffuse air space opacities on radiographs. On CT, the condition can present as a profusion of lower lobe–predominant, high-attenuation centrilobular nodules, with or without calcification (Fig. 26.5). Concurrent left atrial enlargement may be observed on imaging in the setting of secondary pulmonary hemosiderosis. The mainstay therapy for primary hemosiderosis is a corticosteroid and other immunosuppressants. Unlike idiopathic pulmonary hemosiderosis, Heiner syndrome carries a good prognosis with the cessation of cow's milk. In the setting of secondary pulmonary hemosiderosis, treatment involves mitral valve repair or replacement. However, nodules can remain, even after valve replacement.

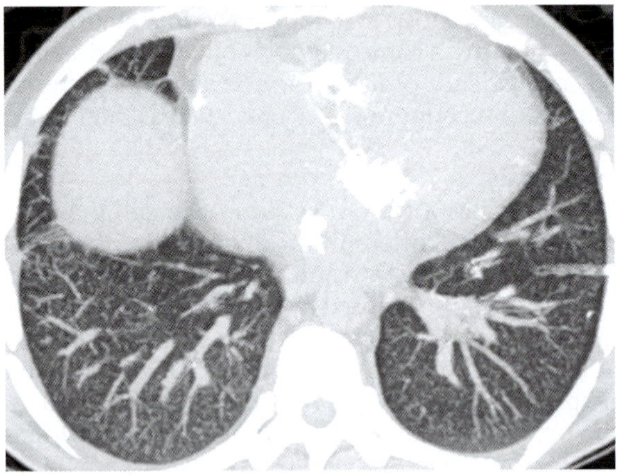

Figure 26.5 Pulmonary hemosiderosis in a 55-year-old man with chronic mitral valve disease and mitral valve replacement. This axial CT scan at lung windows shows innumerable lower lobe–predominant, well-defined centrilobular nodules, most of which are not calcified. One or two 2-mm calcified nodules were also present. Although a biopsy was not done, the patient had no symptoms of infection or other acute process; this appearance is consistent with hemosiderosis secondary to mitral valve disease.

Metastatic Pulmonary Calcification

Metastatic pulmonary calcification is characterized by calcium deposition in normal lung parenchyma as a result of a calcium ion imbalance seen in various disorders, such as primary and secondary hyperparathyroidism (usually chronic renal failure), multiple myeloma, milk-alkali syndrome, hypervitaminosis D, granulomatous disease (e.g., sarcoidosis), IV calcium therapy, and parathyroid hormone–related peptide-secreting malignancies (typically squamous cell carcinoma). The calcium salts are deposited in the alveolar septa and can interfere with gas exchange and cause interstitial fibrosis. Depending on severity, the disease appearance can range from reticular interstitial opacities or diffuse, fluffy, centrilobular ground-glass nodular opacities with punctate calcification to dense consolidation, the most severe form, at times leading to fibrosis (Fig. 26.6). The calcium deposits tend to be upper lobe predominant due to the more alkaline environment from the higher ventilation-to-perfusion ratio in the upper lobes. However, calcium deposits can become more diffuse over time. Concurrent calcification of vessels in the chest wall can occasionally be seen.

■ Diseases Causing Atypical Parenchymal Calcification

These diseases do not conform to classic distribution patterns.

Diffuse Pulmonary Ossification

Diffuse pulmonary ossification is another rare disease characterized by bone formation in the lung. The disorder

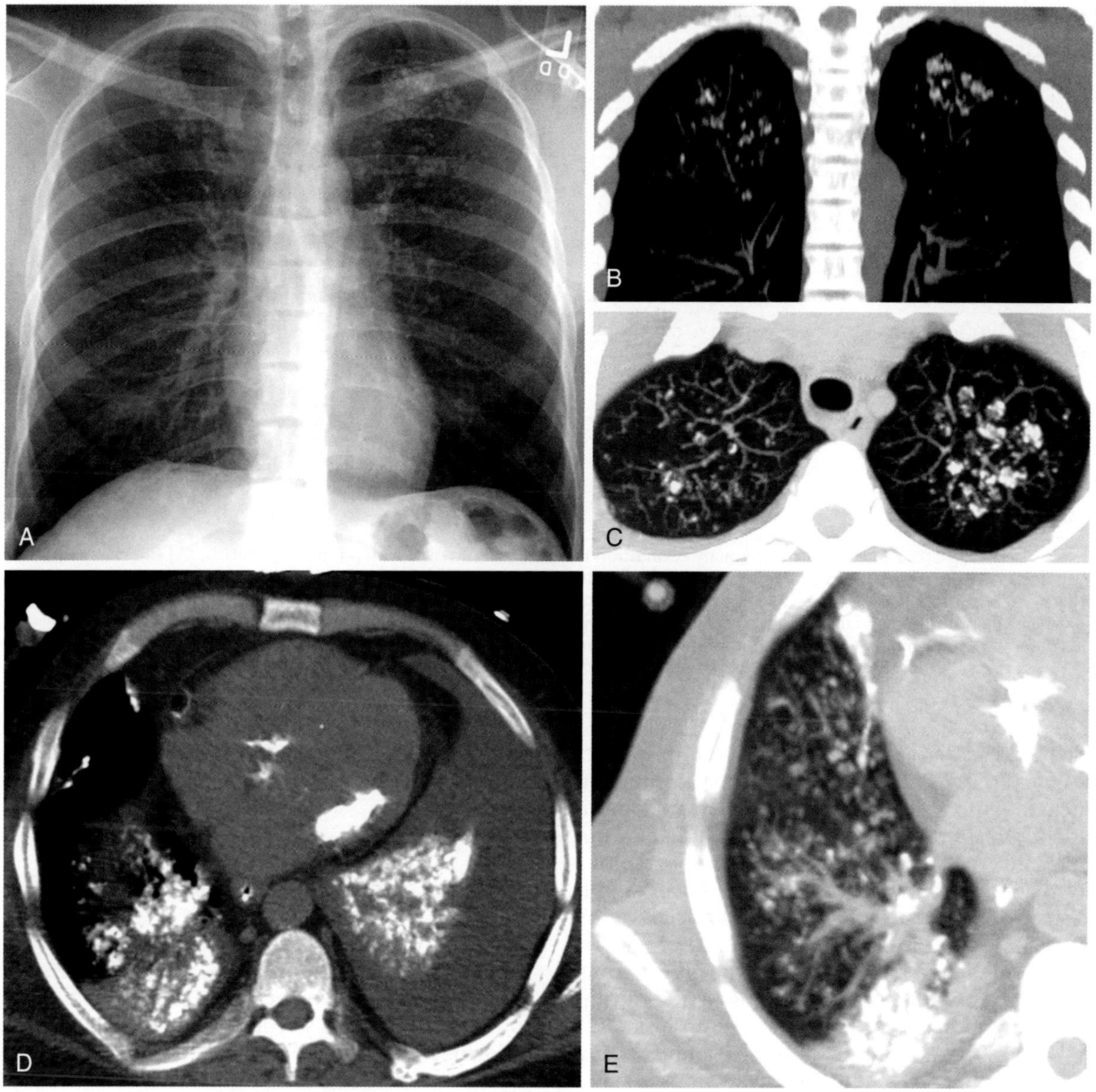

Figure 26.6 (A–C) Metastatic calcification in a 30-year-old man with chronic renal failure with metastatic calcification. (A) The chest radiograph shows clusters of calcified nodules in the upper lobes bilaterally. (B and C) The chest CT images with soft tissue and lung windows show a symmetric distribution of nodules with a centrilobular pattern in the upper lobes. Images of the upper abdomen (not shown) revealed atrophic kidneys with multiple cysts in the setting of chronic dialysis. (D and E) Metastatic calcification in a 52-year-old man with chronic renal failure. (D) This maximum intensity projection CT image with bone windows shows extensive nodular calcification involving the lower lobes; a typical centrilobular predominance is evident at lung windows (E).

can be idiopathic or can occur as a result of repeated diffuse lung injury in the setting of interstitial fibrosis, recurrent bronchopneumonia, chronic aspiration, chronic pulmonary edema, or pulmonary venous hypertension in mitral valve disease. Diffuse ossification has also been reported in cases of pulmonary amyloidosis. Patients are rarely symptomatic due to diffuse pulmonary ossification alone, and the finding is typically made incidentally on imaging or during pathologic analysis for other reasons. Serum calcium and phosphorus levels are normal in the setting of pulmonary ossification. The dendriform type of ossification manifests as branching linear and nodular calcific opacities in regions of architectural distortion and reticulation, usually along the lung periphery, corresponding histologically to branching ossification in areas of septal fibrosis, extending sporadically into alveoli (Fig. 26.7). The nodular type manifests as diffuse round, predominantly subpleural, calcified nodules, corresponding to calcification in the alveolar spaces at histology. Both have lower lobe predominance.

Pulmonary Alveolar Microlithiasis

Pulmonary alveolar microlithiasis is a rare disease characterized by the accumulation of tiny (0.01–3 mm) calcospherites composed of calcium phosphate in the

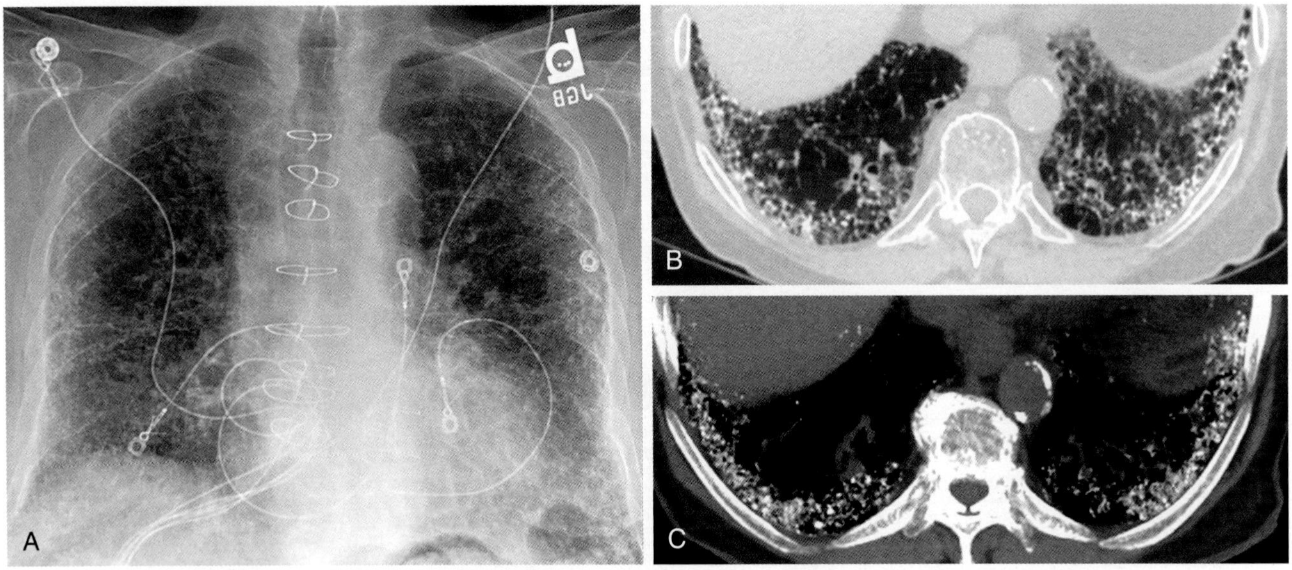

Figure 26.7 Diffuse pulmonary ossification in an 82-year-old man with pulmonary fibrosis. (A) Chest radiograph shows bilateral peripheral reticular opacities and high-density, small nodular opacities following the same distribution. (B) Chest CT scan with lung windows shows peripheral bronchiolectasis, architectural distortion, and mild honeycombing. (C) Maximum intensity projection CT scan with soft tissue windows shows high-attenuation subcentimeter nodular and branching opacities following fibrosis, consistent with dendriform pulmonary ossification.

alveoli. The exact disease mechanism is not fully understood, but studies have suggested a familial component in which mutation of a gene encoding for a sodium-dependent phosphorus transporter in the lung may play an important role. The disease is seen at all ages but is usually diagnosed between birth and 40 years of age. Unlike in cases of metastatic pulmonary calcification, serum calcium and phosphorus levels are normal. The disease is often detected incidentally at imaging because the disease is clinically occult for a long period of time, with very slow progression. The disease can eventually progress to respiratory failure, pulmonary fibrosis, and cor pulmonale. On chest radiographs, it can present as a sandlike pattern of innumerable, middle and lower lung zone–predominant, submillimeter calcified nodules, which can obscure the mediastinal and diaphragmatic borders. On HRCT, the diffuse micronodules are identified in the interlobular septa, interstitium, and pleura of the lower lobes (especially the posterior portions). They appear as calcific peripheral and septal thickening (often without appreciable nodularity), with intervening patchy areas of ground-glass opacity and sometimes striking high-attenuation consolidation, representing a confluence of nodules. A small subset of cases may have high-attenuation nodules without frank calcification at CT or ground-glass opacities with septal thickening.

■ Causes of Calcified Masses or Consolidation

Diffuse lung diseases with calcified masses or consolidation are summarized in Table 26.2. Some disease entities that can present with pulmonary nodules, as discussed in detail previously, such as calcified metastases, metastatic pulmonary calcification, and amyloidosis (nodular form), can also present as calcified masses or consolidation as they progress.

Progressive Massive Fibrosis

Progressive massive fibrosis can form when smaller nodules form a conglomerate >1 cm in the setting of silicosis or coal workers' pneumoconiosis; a similar process can occur in sarcoidosis (see detailed discussions above). Dystrophic calcification can develop within the conglomerate. Progressive massive fibrosis usually has a slow progression and does not cavitate. Rapid changes in size and cavitation should raise the possibility of other diagnoses, such as mycobacterial infection or malignancy.

Hyalinizing Granuloma

Hyalinizing granuloma is a rare cause of multiple calcified nodules or masses. Its disease mechanism is not well understood, but is likely related to a chronic immune response to an endogenous or exogenous antigen or infectious organism, such as *Histoplasma capsulatum* or *Mycobacterium* organisms. Patients often have mild vague respiratory complaints, including dyspnea, cough, chest pain, low-grade fever, and fatigue. Histologically, the disease resembles fibrosing mediastinitis; the center of the lesion consists of a distinctive whorllike pattern of hyaline collagen, with or without focal calcification. On imaging, a hyalinizing granuloma can present as multiple well-marginated nodules or masses (rarely solitary), measuring from a few millimeters to up to 15 cm, and can have central focal irregular calcification (Fig. 26.8).

TABLE 26.2 Summary of Diffuse Lung Diseases With High-Attenuation Lesions

DISEASE	CALCIFICATION PATTERNS	OTHER ASSOCIATED IMAGING FEATURES	CLINICAL FEATURES
Calcified Nodules in a Random Distribution			
Healed granulomatous infection	Solitary or multiple calcified nodules Random distribution or in clusters	±Nodal, splenic and hepatic calcifications Diffuse nodules, splenic and hepatic calcifications more likely due to histoplasmosis Upper lobe predominance, architectural distortion, and/or bronchiectasis can be seen with tuberculosis	Usually due to histoplasmosis and tuberculosis
Healed varicella pneumonia	Multiple subcentimeter calcified nodules (1–3 mm)	No nodal calcification	Polymorphic rash precedes acute varicella pneumonia Lymphoma, leukemia, immunocompromised status, older age, smoking history, pregnancy are risk factors
Calcified pulmonary metastases	Solitary or multiple calcified nodules Lower lobe predominance		Known primary malignancies—sarcomas (especially osteosarcoma), medullary thyroid carcinoma, mucinous and papillary carcinoma
Calcified Nodules in a Perilymphatic Distribution			
Pneumoconioses	Numerous nodules (<1 cm) or consolidation, which may calcify (calcification more common in silicosis) Upper lobe predominance	±Nodal calcification (eggshell pattern) Can form conglomerate nodules and masses (progressive massive fibrosis)	Silicosis and CWP most common Distinctive occupational histories (see Table 26.1), usually with latency period of 10–20 years (can be shortened in setting of high exposure or berylliosis)
Sarcoidosis	Numerous nodules or consolidation, with calcification in a minority of cases Nodules range from 1–2 mm to large nodules and conglomerate masses Upper lobe predominance	±Nodal calcification (eggshell pattern) STAGE 1: Mediastinal and hilar lymphadenopathy STAGE 2: Nodal and parenchymal involvement (small perilymphatic nodules, patchy ground-glass opacities, or masslike lesions) STAGE 3: Parenchymal disease without lymphadenopathy STAGE 4: End-stage fibrosis and honeycombing	Multisystem disorder with noncaseating granulomas as underlying predominant histologic finding; African Americans, Swedes, Danes highest prevalence worldwide Associated with erythema nodosum
Amyloidosis (diffuse parenchymal type)	DIFFUSE PARENCHYMAL TYPE: numerous small calcified or noncalcified nodules (<1.5 cm), and/or consolidation Lower lobe and peripheral predominance	±Nodal calcification or lymphadenopathy Interstitial opacities, septal thickening, smaller nodules (<1.5 cm), consolidation, and, less commonly, traction bronchiectasis and honeycombing	Associated with multiple myeloma and chronic inflammatory states (e.g., rheumatoid arthritis, chronic infections) Systemic amyloidosis often with heart (heart failure) and kidney (nephrotic syndrome) involvement Congo red–stained tissue showing positive birefringence under polarized light
Calcified Nodules in a Centrilobular Distribution			
Pulmonary hemosiderosis	Numerous nodules, with or without calcification Lower lobe predominance	No lymphadenopathy or nodal calcification Atrial enlargement if mitral stenosis is underlying cause	Clinical triad—hemoptysis, iron deficiency anemia, diffuse pulmonary opacities Primary hemosiderosis can be associated with Goodpasture or Heiner syndrome (hypersensitivity to cow milk proteins) Secondary hemosiderosis often associated with mitral stenosis

Continued

TABLE 26.2 Summary of Diffuse Lung Diseases With High-Attenuation Lesions—cont'd

DISEASE	CALCIFICATION PATTERNS	OTHER ASSOCIATED IMAGING FEATURES	CLINICAL FEATURES
Pulmonary metastatic calcification	Numerous centrilobular calcified nodules or dense calcific consolidation In early stages, upper lobe predominance; can become more diffuse over time	Interstitial opacity, diffuse fluffy centrilobular ground-glass nodules, or dense consolidation Concurrent small vessel calcification within the chest wall	Elevated serum calcium and phosphorus levels in primary or secondary hyperparathyroidism (e.g., chronic renal failure), granulomatous disease, multiple myeloma, milk-alkali syndrome, hypervitaminosis D, IV calcium therapy or squamous cell carcinoma
Other Calcification Patterns			
Pulmonary ossification	DENDRIFORM TYPE: numerous tubular calcified opacities along bronchovascular bundles NODULAR TYPE: numerous round subpleural calcified and/or high-attenuation nodules Lower lobe predominance	No lymphadenopathy or nodal calcification	Associated with repeated diffuse lung injuries (e.g., interstitial fibrosis, aspiration, bronchopneumonia, pulmonary edema, pulmonary hypertension in mitral valve disease) Benign and asymptomatic Normal serum calcium and phosphorus levels
Pulmonary alveolar microlithiasis	Calcific interstitial, interlobular septal, and pleural thickening Confluent microcalcification may appear as high-attenuation consolidation Lower lobe predominance	Intervening patching area of ground-glass opacity	Clinically occult with slow progression, despite significant lung involvement on imaging Normal serum calcium and phosphorus levels
Calcified Masses or Consolidation			
Amyloidosis (nodular type)	Calcified or partially calcified nodules	Accompanying thin-walled cysts	
Pulmonary metastatic calcification[a]			
Progressive massive fibrosis	Conglomerate of nodules (>1 cm), with or without calcification in the setting of silicosis and CWP; similar process occurs in sarcoidosis	See "pneumoconioses" and "sarcoidosis" for details	
Hyalinizing granuloma	One or several calcified nodules or masses (several mm to 15 cm)		
High-Attenuation Nodules or Masses or Consolidation Without Calcification			
Talcosis	High attenuation without calcification	EARLY STAGE: diffuse small pulmonary nodules LATE STAGE: nodules can form conglomerates or high-attenuation consolidation (upper lobe predominant) CHRONIC: lower lobe–predominant emphysema	Chronic baby powder exposure, IV delivery of crushed and dissolved oral medications, certain occupational exposures (see Table 26.1)
Amiodarone lung toxicity	High attenuation without calcification	Bibasilar-predominant, high-attenuation consolidation, ground-glass opacity, or, less commonly, nodules Concurrent high attenuation of liver and spleen	Amiodarone usage (especially if daily dose >400 mg or in older adult)
Pulmonary alveolar microlithiasis[b]			

[a]This can also form calcific masses or consolidation as the disease progresses. See "pulmonary metastatic calcification" for details.
[b]This may also present as high-attenuation consolidation as microcalcification accumulates. See "pulmonary alveolar microlithiasis" above for details.
CWP, Coal workers' pneumoconiosis.

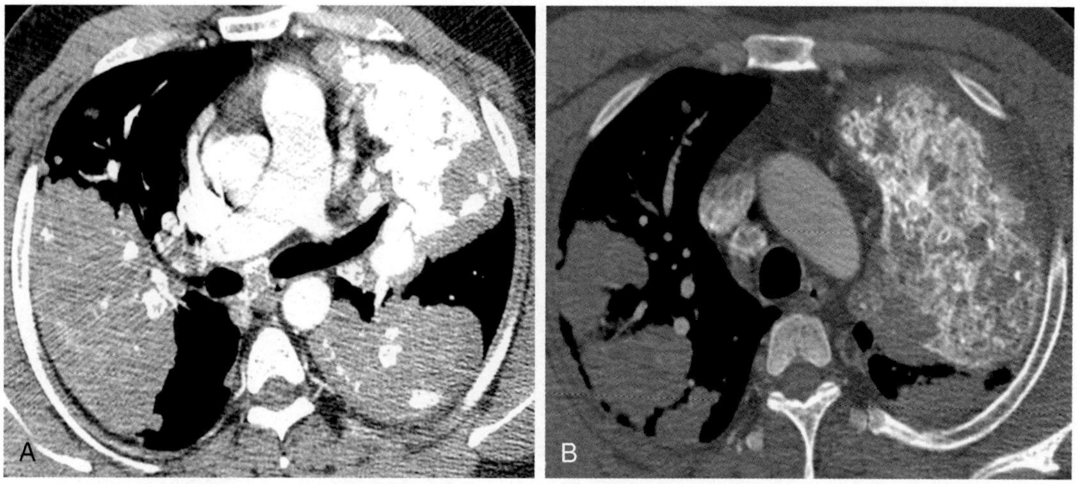

Figure 26.8 Pulmonary hyalinizing granuloma in a 38-year-old man with large, partially calcified masses in all lobes of the lungs; a biopsy revealed the diagnosis. (A) Axial CT image with soft tissue windows shows large masses comprised of both soft tissue and extensive calcification. (B) CT images with soft tissue windows at a different level reveal a lacework of extensive calcification within the soft tissue masses.

Causes of High-Attenuation Nodules, Masses, or Consolidation Without Calcification

Talcosis

Two routes of exposure can lead to pulmonary talcosis. Inhaled talc, usually in the setting of chronic use of older baby powder formulations or occupational exposure (see Table 26.2), can deposit in the alveoli, lymphatics, and interstitium. Talc is also a common filler in oral medications and can cause pulmonary talcosis when IV drug users inject dissolved drug tablets intravenously. The talc particles can embolize to small pulmonary arterioles and eventually migrate into pulmonary interstitium, forming talc-containing granulomas. In the early stages, talcosis can manifest as diffuse small pulmonary nodules. In the late stage, small pulmonary nodules can form upper lobe–predominant, high-attenuation conglomerates, resembling pulmonary massive fibrosis (Fig. 26.9). Lower lobe–predominant, panacinar-like emphysema can sometimes be observed in chronic talcosis. It is unclear whether lower lobe emphysema is caused by talc or the active ingredient (often observed with methylphenidate IV injection). Treatment of acute talcosis generally involves removal of exposure, a corticosteroid, and supportive care.

Amiodarone Lung Toxicity

Amiodarone is a common medication used for refractory ventricular arrhythmias, with a well-known complication of lung toxicity. The risk of developing amiodarone lung toxicity is increased in older adults or with a daily dose >400 mg; however, a long duration of therapy and total cumulative dosage do not appear to confer added risk. On CT, amiodarone lung toxicity can present with any of a range of findings, including ground-glass opacities, consolidation, or, less commonly, nodules or masses. Basilar-predominant, high-attenuation—but not calcified—consolidation is a classic but not universal finding of the disease, attributed to the inherent radiodensity of triiodinated amiodarone incorporated into the type II pneumocytes. Concurrent high attenuation seen in the lung, liver, and spleen is highly suggestive of amiodarone toxicity.

Pulmonary Alveolar Microlithiasis

In patients with long-standing pulmonary alveolar microlithiasis, diffuse innumerable confluent microcalcifications <1 mm can present as high-attenuation or frankly calcified consolidation on HRCT.

Causes of Diffuse Lung Disease With Lipid

Diffuse lung disease containing lipid is uncommon and is caused by a much smaller assortment of diseases than those involving calcification. Lipid-containing lung disease can present as nodules, masses, consolidation, or septal thickening. Lipoid pneumonia and fat-containing pulmonary metastatic disease can present with macroscopic fat on CT, with attenuation values between −60 and −100 HU. The lipoproteinaceous pulmonary contents of pulmonary alveolar proteinosis do not show fat attenuation but have a distinctive CT appearance.

Lipoid Pneumonia

Lipoid pneumonia can occur as an exogenous or endogenous form. Exogenous lipoid pneumonia results from the inhalation or aspiration of animal, vegetable, or mineral oils. The most common causes include aspiration

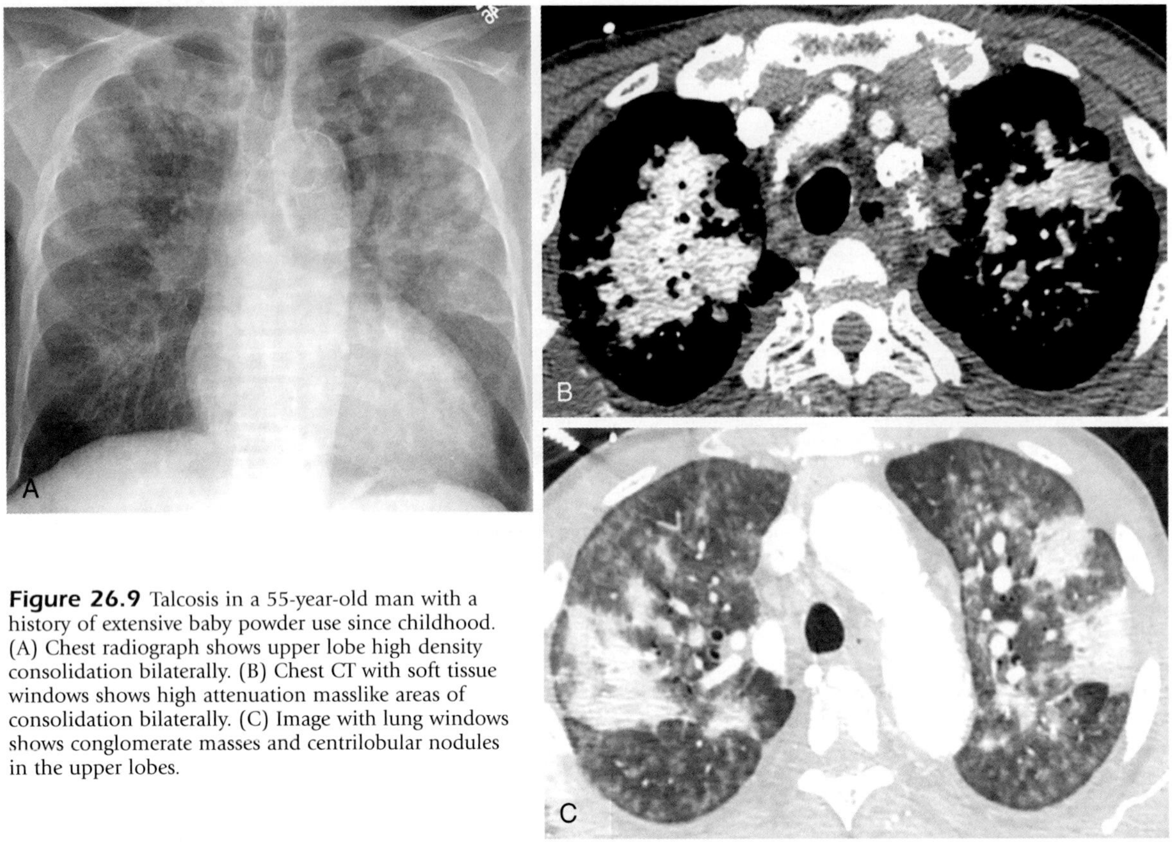

Figure 26.9 Talcosis in a 55-year-old man with a history of extensive baby powder use since childhood. (A) Chest radiograph shows upper lobe high density consolidation bilaterally. (B) Chest CT with soft tissue windows shows high attenuation masslike areas of consolidation bilaterally. (C) Image with lung windows shows conglomerate masses and centrilobular nodules in the upper lobes.

of ingested oils or fats, cod liver oil or other fat-containing laxatives, petroleum jelly, and the nasal application of mineral oils. Even eye drops containing mineral oil have been reported as a cause. Patients at risk of chronic aspiration have a higher incidence of lipoid pneumonia, including the neurologically compromised, those with disordered swallowing mechanisms, at extremes of age, or with gastroesophageal reflux disease. Patients in these categories may have impaired clearance of aspirated substances; in addition, mineral oils fail to elicit the cough reflex common to most other aspirated substances and may impair mucociliary clearance. Endogenous lipoid pneumonia, the less common form, occurs due to the breakdown of alveolar walls and release of cellular lipids in the setting of a primary pulmonary insult. Lung cancer with postobstructive pneumonia, infectious pneumonia, and lipid storage diseases such as Niemann-Pick disease have all been reported as causes.

Acute exogenous lipoid pneumonia usually presents with cough, fever, and dyspnea; leukocytosis and hypoxemia are also common. Clinical presentation in chronic lipoid pneumonia is usually insidious, with about 50% of cases having no symptoms at the time of incidental detection by imaging. When present, symptoms include chronic cough, dyspnea, and, less commonly, fever, weight loss, or hemoptysis. In both acute and chronic lipoid pneumonia, exposure to the inciting agent is often identified after the diagnosis is made through imaging and histologic analysis. Although symptoms usually improve in acute lipoid pneumonia after the exposure ceases, persistent or worsening shortness of breath and other pulmonary symptoms are common in the chronic form.

Characteristic findings at histology include intraalveolar and interstitial lipid-laden macrophages and other associated inflammatory cells. The exogenous form commonly shows extracellular lipids and large, cytoplasmic, fat-containing vacuoles within macrophages, uncommon in the endogenous form. Over time, fibrosis can occur within and adjacent to chronic consolidation. Bronchoalveolar lavage yields lipid-laden macrophages and increased cellularity in many cases; transbronchial biopsy and open lung biopsy are usually diagnostic in the remaining cases.

Radiographs of patients with acute or chronic lipoid pneumonia often show hazy alveolar and interstitial opacities, nodules, consolidation, or masses. Opacities can follow an aspiration pattern of bilateral patchy basilar opacities, but more diffuse bilateral opacities or one or more focal areas of consolidation also can be seen. Pleural effusions can occur in the acute form, but are usually not seen in the chronic setting. Pneumatoceles in regions of air space opacities can develop days or weeks after an episode of acute lipoid pneumonia.

Typical CT findings include fat-containing nodules or consolidation, usually with a dependent distribution. Ground-glass opacities are common, often with superimposed septal thickening in a crazy-paving pattern, corresponding to interstitial and alveolar macrophages and type II pneumocyte infiltration (Fig. 26.10). Masses can occur in the chronic form, presumably due to developing fibrosis, but are uncommon in the acute setting. When

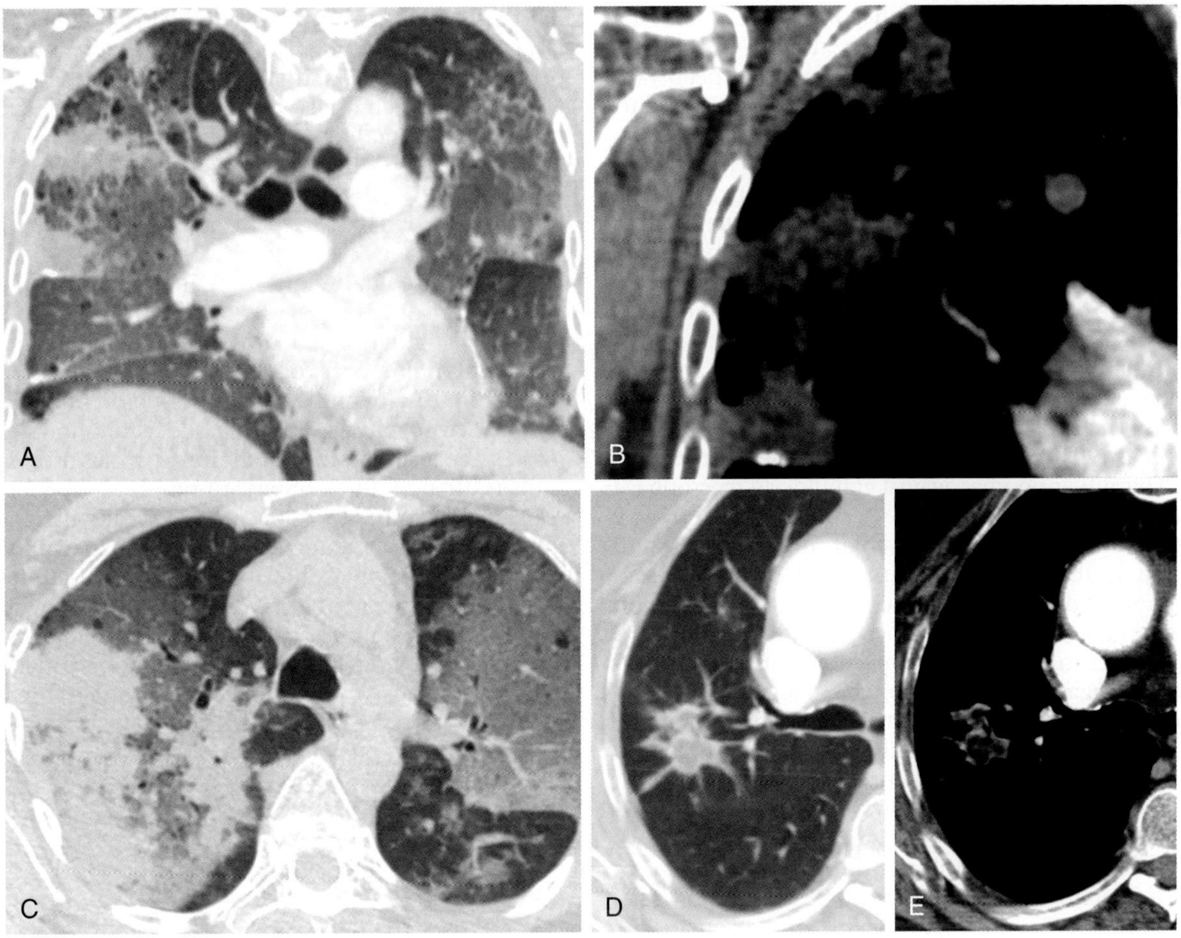

Figure 26.10 Lipoid pneumonia in a 49-year-old woman with biopsy-proven lipoid pneumonia arising from a long history of intranasal petroleum product application during childhood. (A) Coronal CT image with lung windows shows bilateral ground-glass opacities and areas of masslike consolidation. (B) Close-up of right upper lobe with soft tissue windows shows fat attenuation within the masses. (C) Axial CT image with lung windows of the same patient in (A) and (B) shows worsening of ground-glass opacities and extensive consolidation in the right upper lobe. Prompted by worsening shortness of breath and malaise, a biopsy showed *Mycobacterium porcinum* infection. (D) A 75-year-old man with a spiculated nodule in the dependent right upper lobe, resembling a primary lung cancer at lung windows. (E) At soft tissue window, the nodule shows visible fat, in keeping with lipoid pneumonia from chronic mineral oil ingestion.

present, spiculation of nodules and masses can cause confusion with primary lung cancer; such opacities are often FDG-avid on PET, compounding diagnostic difficulty. Although not always present, fat attenuation (less than approximately −70 HU) within nodules or consolidation at CT is highly specific for exogenous lipoid pneumonia; the endogenous form typically does not show fat attenuation.

Complications of lipoid pneumonia potentially seen at imaging include superimposed nontuberculous mycobacterial infection, especially *Mycobacterium fortuitum* and *Mycobacterium chelonei*; free extracellular lipids are thought to enhance the growth of these organisms. New focal areas of consolidation or worsening nodularity in the setting of corresponding symptoms can prompt evaluation for one of these infections. In chronic lipoid pneumonia, interstitial infiltration and fibrosis can rarely lead to pulmonary hypertension and cor pulmonale.

Improvement after elimination of exposure to the offending agent occurs in most patients with acute lipoid pneumonia, with a decrease in associated consolidation, ground-glass opacities, and septal thickening over the course of several weeks to 8 months. However, in chronic disease, many patients may have persistent symptoms and pulmonary opacities for months or years; radiologic findings can remain stable or worsen, developing architectural distortion and fibrosis over time. Serial bronchoalveolar lavage has shown promise, with reductions in lipid-laden macrophages and marked improvement in CT findings in some patients. Steroids, immunoglobulin therapy, and even surgical resection of abnormal portions of lung have been used for therapy, with varying results.

Pulmonary Alveolar Proteinosis

In pulmonary alveolar proteinosis, imbalances in pulmonary surfactant metabolism lead to the abnormal deposition of lipid and protein-containing materials in the alveoli and interstitium. With a prevalence of between 3.7 and 6.2 cases/million per year, alveolar proteinosis is a very rare disease; average age at onset has been variously reported as the fourth, fifth, or sixth decade of life. The clinical course ranges widely, from indolent or asymptomatic disease to severe respiratory failure and death. The most common presenting symptoms are cough and exertional dyspnea. Superimposed infection is a common finding, in part likely resulting from impaired alveolar macrophage function. The most common organisms include *Nocardia*, mycobacteria, and fungal infections such as *Aspergillus*, *Cryptococcus*, and *Histoplasma*.

Pulmonary alveolar proteinosis is classified as acquired or congenital, with the latter comprising a small minority of cases. The most common acquired type, comprising more than 90% of all cases, is the autoimmune type, caused by autoantibodies against granulocyte-macrophage colony-stimulating factor (GM-CSF), a protein necessary for the differentiation of alveolar macrophages and essential for the clearance of pulmonary surfactant from alveoli. Secondary alveolar proteinosis is a less common acquired type, resulting from malfunction of alveolar macrophages in the setting of infection, collagen vascular diseases, drug reaction, hematologic malignancies (most commonly leukemia), and acute inhalational exposures, usually silicosis. The congenital inherited type occurs in less than 2% of cases, due to one or more of several possible mutations that cause surfactant protein production or clearance.

The characteristic histologic finding of alveolar proteinosis is periodic acid–Schiff-positive granular proteinaceous material within the alveoli and bronchioles. Architectural distortion and fibrosis are not typical features. Bronchoalveolar lavage is often sufficient for the diagnosis, revealing frothy milky material with telltale composition at histology. Transbronchial biopsies or even open lung biopsy can be used for the diagnosis of the remaining minority of cases.

At chest radiography, bilateral air space opacities, often with a perihilar distribution mimicking edema or pneumonia, are typical. Found in up to 92% of cases, the characteristic CT appearance consists of bilateral geographic ground-glass opacities with superimposed septal thickening—the crazy-paving appearance (Fig. 26.11). Although crazy-paving pattern is very common in alveolar proteinosis, it is not specific for the disease and, in practice, is seen much more commonly in conditions such as pulmonary edema, diffuse alveolar damage, alveolar hemorrhage, and infection. A sharp demarcation between normal and abnormal lung is often seen in alveolar proteinosis, a finding that can suggest the diagnosis, rather than the more diffuse opacities seen in other diseases. Although lipoid pneumonia can also show a crazy-paving appearance at CT, nodules, masses, and architectural distortion are commonly seen in lipoid pneumonia but are not common in alveolar proteinosis, a potentially useful distinguishing characteristic. In addition, macroscopic fat within a consolidation or nodules is seen in lipoid pneumonia rather than in alveolar proteinosis. Imaging can be valuable to help diagnose superimposed infections, which may present with new areas of consolidation, nodules, or other abnormalities.

The gold standard for alveolar proteinosis is whole-lung lavage, with many patients requiring repeat treatment for persistent symptoms and radiologic findings. Aerosolized GM-CSF has been used, with varying degrees of success. Imaging abnormalities usually improve after lavage.

Fat-Containing Metastatic Disease

A solitary fat-containing nodule in a patient without a primary fat-containing malignancy is nearly pathognomonic of a hamartoma. However, although uncommon, solitary or multiple fat-containing pulmonary metastases can occur, usually in the setting of liposarcoma. CT can show macroscopic fat and soft tissue within nodules and masses; the histology of the pulmonary metastases usually mirrors that of the primary tumor (Fig. 26.12). Fat-containing lymphadenopathy can occur. Although myxoid liposarcoma has a tendency to metastasize to extrapulmonary sites, pleomorphic liposarcoma and dedifferentiated liposarcoma tend to favor the lungs as a metastatic site, and metastatic disease in these subtypes can be isolated to the lungs. The course of pulmonary metastatic disease varies according to histology, ranging from slow growth to more aggressive behavior.

Problem-Solving Issues

Determining if Calcification Is Present at Imaging

In some cases, very high density (similar to bone) at radiography can suggest calcification within nodules or consolidation. In many other cases, CT is required to make the diagnosis. Often, calcification within a lesion is perceived qualitatively at soft tissue and bone windows as being similar in attenuation to bone. Regions of interest drawn within calcification generally show attenuation values of 200 HU or greater within uniformly calcified lesions; volume averaging with soft tissue can occur in partially calcified lesions, leading to attenuation between that of soft tissue and calcification.

Determining if Lipid Is Present at Imaging

Similar to calcification, fat in lung lesions may be detected by qualitative analysis at soft tissue windows. Macroscopic fat appears dark, similar in attenuation to subcutaneous or visceral fat; a corresponding region of interest should show negative attenuation values, generally between −60 and −100 HU. Detection of fat can be central to the diagnosis of a hamartoma or lipoid pneumonia. However, when complexed with other materials, not all lipids can be detected by the analysis of attenuation at CT. For example, the lipoproteinaceous constituents of pulmonary alveolar proteinosis do not show fat attenuation at CT, and diagnosis relies on imaging characteristics, clinical presentation, and histologic correlation.

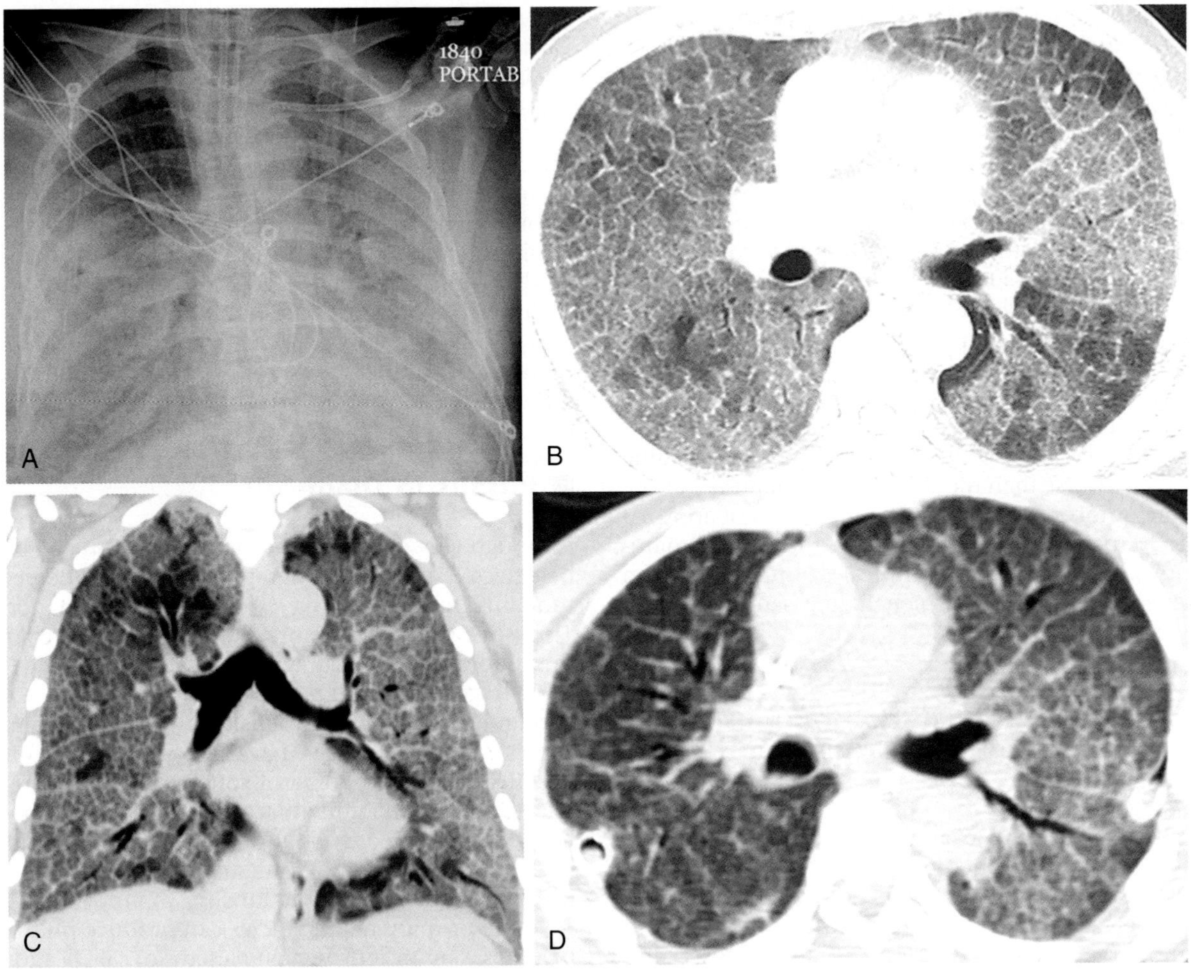

Figure 26.11 Pulmonary alveolar proteinosis in a 64-year-old man with progressive shortness of breath; open lung biopsy showed alveolar proteinosis. (A) Frontal chest radiograph shows bilateral hazy air space opacities in all lobes, with associated air bronchograms. (B) Axial and (C) coronal CT images with lung windows show extensive bilateral ground-glass opacities with accompanying interlobular and intralobular septal thickening, a crazy-paving appearance. (D) One month after whole-lung lavage, ground-glass opacities have improved, and septal thickening is less pronounced.

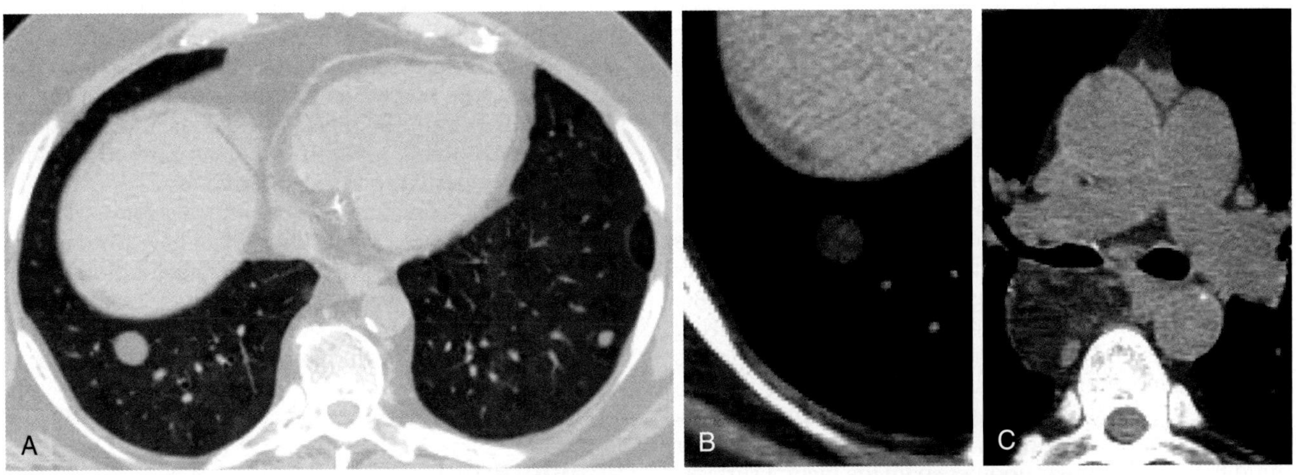

Figure 26.12 Liposarcoma metastasis. Multiple pulmonary nodules containing fat are seen in a patient with metastatic liposarcoma. (A) Right lower lobe and left lower lobe nodules are seen at CT with lung windows. (B) Coned-down view shows macroscopic fat and small soft tissue attenuation foci within the right lower lobe nodule. (C) A fatty mass extending from the right hilum to the right paravertebral space represents an additional metastasis; note small foci of soft tissue attenuation within the mass.

Importance of Acuity of Symptoms in Providing a Rational Differential Diagnosis

The time course of clinical and imaging abnormalities is central to differential diagnosis. For example, although a crazy-paving pattern of lung disease is common in pulmonary alveolar proteinosis and can be seen in chronic lipoid pneumonia, this pattern is far more common in acute lung diseases, such as pulmonary edema, hemorrhage, infection, and diffuse alveolar damage. Healed granulomatous infection, healed varicella pneumonia, and pulmonary ossification are asymptomatic, with stable imaging findings over time. Diseases such as pulmonary alveolar microlithiasis have a very slow disease progression, with the extent of lung involvement on imaging significantly worse than the patient's clinical presentation. Most pneumoconioses have a latency period of approximately 10 to 20 years before imaging and clinical manifestations. However, severe clinical symptoms, with a shortened latency, can be seen in the setting of high exposure.

Importance of Spatial Distributions of Disease in Providing a Differential Diagnosis

Both craniocaudal and axial distributions are important to note. For example, pneumoconioses, sarcoidosis, and metastatic calcification tend to be upper lobe predominant, whereas diffuse pulmonary ossification, lipoid pneumonia, and the diffuse form of amyloidosis tend to be lower lobe predominant. Coronal multiplanar reformatted CT images can be helpful in assessing the craniocaudal distribution of disease. The axial distribution is also important to discern. Perilymphatic diseases such as sarcoidosis have a central peribronchovascular predominance, whereas diseases such as diffuse pulmonary ossification tend to have a peripheral distribution.

Importance of Nodule Distribution Patterns for Diagnosis

Three basic patterns are important for the differential diagnosis of diseases involving small, subcentimeter pulmonary nodules. Random nodules can be seen in diseases with hematogenous spread, including fungal infection leading to calcified granulomas and diseases producing calcified pulmonary metastases. These nodules are widely distributed throughout the lung parenchyma, with a subset of nodules touching but not clustering along fissures and septa. Perilymphatic nodules, such as those seen in sarcoidosis and pneumoconioses, tend to cluster along the peripheral lymphatics (pleural surfaces, fissures, septa) and central lymphatics (bronchovascular bundles). Centrilobular nodules spare the pleural surfaces and tend to occur in clusters, following the regular spacing of secondary pulmonary lobules; they are often detected in metastatic calcification, talcosis, and lipoid pneumonia, among many other diseases.

Importance of Imaging Patterns for Diagnosis of Diffuse Fat-Containing Pulmonary Disease

Regional ground-glass opacities with superimposed interlobular septal thickening—a crazy-paving pattern of lung opacity—can be seen in alveolar proteinosis and lipoid pneumonia. Masses and architectural distortion are more common in chronic lipoid pneumonia than in alveolar proteinosis, and macroscopic fat can be seen in lipoid pneumonia but not in alveolar proteinosis. Multiple fat-containing nodules with smooth or lobulated margins, without a background of diffuse pulmonary disease, can be seen in fat-containing metastases.

■ Pitfalls in Diagnosis

Although very dense calcification in a lesion can usually be detected at chest radiography, CT is the most reliable modality for confirming calcification within nodules. Thin-slice CT is both more sensitive and more specific than radiography for diagnosing calcification.

At larger slice thicknesses (usually >2 mm), volume averaging at CT can cause misleadingly low-attenuation values of a target lesion. For example, a small calcified nodule may appear to be of soft tissue attenuation due to averaging with air in adjacent lung, whereas noncalcified nodules or consolidation may erroneously appear to contain fat. Volume averaging can be minimized by using thin-slice reconstructions (<1–2 mm).

Some primary malignancies can produce pulmonary metastases mimicking benign patterns of calcification. For example, osteosarcoma and (less commonly) chondrosarcoma metastases can show uniform complete calcification. A review of the patient's medical history and symptoms can easily prevent mischaracterization.

Some diffuse lung diseases with calcification and/or high attenuation can produce similar patterns at imaging. For example, upper lobe, high-attenuation nodules can be seen in sarcoidosis, diseases of environmental exposures such as silicosis and talcosis, and metastatic calcification. A thorough exposure history, patient demographics, and medical history may point to the correct diagnosis. In addition, the overall pattern of nodules can provide guidance; for example, metastatic calcification tends to have a centrilobular pattern, whereas sarcoidosis and silicosis have perilymphatic patterns.

The key lipid-containing diffuse lung diseases—alveolar proteinosis and lipoid pneumonia—can have overlapping appearances at radiography and CT. Consolidation, septal thickening, ground-glass opacities, and a crazy-paving appearance can be seen in each. In addition, these two diseases can occur simultaneously or in succession in the same patient.

Bibliography

Baron SE, Haramati LB, Rivera VT. Radiological and clinical findings in acute and chronic exogenous lipoid pneumonia. *J Thorac Imaging*. 2003;18(4): 217–224.

Berk JL, O'Regan A, Skinner M. Pulmonary and tracheobronchial amyloidosis. *Semin Respir Crit Care Med*. 2002;23(2):155–165.

Berteloot L, Taam RA, Emond-Gonsard S, et al. Primary pulmonary alveolar proteinosis: computed tomography features at diagnosis. *Pediatr Radiol.* 2014;44(7):795–802.

Betancourt SL, Martinez-Jimenez S, Rossi SE, Truong MT, Carrillo J, Erasmus JJ. Lipoid pneumonia: spectrum of clinical and radiologic manifestations. *AJR Am J Roentgenol.* 2010;194(1):103–109.

Brown K, Mund DF, Aberle DR, Batra P, Young DA. Intrathoracic calcifications: radiographic features and differential diagnoses. *Radiographics.* 1994;14(6): 1247–1261.

Choi HK, Park CM, Goo JM, Lee HJ. Pulmonary alveolar proteinosis versus exogenous lipoid pneumonia showing crazy-paving pattern: comparison of their clinical features and high-resolution CT findings. *Acta Radiol.* 2010;51(4):407–412.

Criado E, Sanchez M, Ramirez J, et al. Pulmonary sarcoidosis: typical and atypical manifestations at high-resolution CT with pathologic correlation. *Radiographics.* 2010;30(6):1567–1586.

Czeyda-Pommersheim F, Hwang M, Chen SS, Strollo D, Fuhrman C, Bhalla S. Amyloidosis: modern cross-sectional imaging. *Radiographics.* 2015;35(5):1381–1392.

Franquet T, Gimenez A, Bordes R, Rodriguez-Arias JM, Castella J. The crazy-paving pattern in exogenous lipoid pneumonia: CT-pathologic correlation. *AJR Am J Roentgenol.* 1998;170(2):315–317.

Glazer CS, Newman LS. Occupational interstitial lung disease. *Clin Chest Med.* 2004;25(3):467–478.

Gotway MB, Marder SR, Hanks DK, et al. Thoracic complications of illicit drug use: an organ system approach. *Radiographics.* 2002;22(Spec No):S119–S135.

Hadda V, Khilnani GC. Lipoid pneumonia: an overview. *Expert Rev Respir Med.* 2010;4(6):799–807.

Kantarci M, Bayraktutan U, Karabulut N, et al. Alveolar echinococcosis: spectrum of findings at cross-sectional imaging. *Radiographics.* 2012;32(7):2053–2070.

Kashyap S, Mohapatra PR. Pulmonary alveolar microlithiasis. *Lung India.* 2013;30(2):143–147.

Khan A, Agarwal R. Pulmonary alveolar proteinosis. *Respir Care.* 2011;56(7): 1016–1028.

Khan AN, Al-Jahdali HH, Allen CM, Irion KL, Al Ghanem S, Koteyar SS. The calcified lung nodule: what does it mean? *Ann Thorac Med.* 2010;5(2):67–79.

Kim EA, Lee KS, Primack SL, et al. Viral pneumonias in adults: radiologic and pathologic findings. *Radiographics.* 2002;22(Spec No):S137–S149.

Laurent F, Philippe JC, Vergier B, et al. Exogenous lipoid pneumonia: HRCT, MR, and pathologic findings. *Eur Radiol.* 1999;9(6):1190–1196.

Lhote R, Haroche J, Duron L, et al. Pulmonary hyalinizing granuloma: a multicenter study of 5 new cases and review of the 135 cases of the literature. *Immunol Res.* 2017;65(1):375–385.

Maile CW, Rodan BA, Godwin JD, Chen JT, Ravin CE. Calcification in pulmonary metastases. *Br J Radiol.* 1982;55(650):108–113.

Marchiori E, Zanetti G, Mano CM, Hochhegger B. Exogenous lipoid pneumonia. Clinical and radiological manifestations. *Respir Med.* 2011;105(5):659–666.

Nemec SF, Bankier AA, Eisenberg RL. Upper lobe-predominant diseases of the lung. *AJR Am J Roentgenol.* 2013;200(3):W222–W237.

Nicolas M, Moran CA, Suster S. Pulmonary metastasis from liposarcoma: a clinicopathologic and immunohistochemical study of 24 cases. *Am J Clin Pathol.* 2005;123(2):265–275.

Punatar AD, Kusne S, Blair JE, Seville MT, Vikram HR. Opportunistic infections in patients with pulmonary alveolar proteinosis. *J Infect.* 2012;65(2):173–179.

Rossi SE, Erasmus JJ, McAdams HP, Sporn TA, Goodman PC. Pulmonary drug toxicity: radiologic and pathologic manifestations. *Radiographics.* 2000;20(5):1245–1259.

Saeed MM, Woo MS, MacLaughlin EF, Margetis MF, Keens TG. Prognosis in pediatric idiopathic pulmonary hemosiderosis. *Chest.* 1999;116(3):721–725.

Sias SM, Daltro PA, Marchiori E, et al. Clinic and radiological improvement of lipoid pneumonia with multiple bronchoalveolar lavages. *Pediatr Pulmonol.* 2009;44(4):309–315.

Tamura A, Hebisawa A, Fukushima K, Yotsumoto H, Mori M. Lipoid pneumonia in lung cancer: radiographic and pathological features. *Jpn J Clin Oncol.* 1998;28(8):492–496.

Wang T, Lazar CA, Fishbein MC, Lynch JP 3rd. Pulmonary alveolar proteinosis. *Semin Respir Crit Care Med.* 2012;33(5):498–508.

CHAPTER 27
Pulmonary Vascular Diseases

Michael T. Lu, Pedro Vinícius Staziaki, and Evan James Zucker

CHAPTER OUTLINE

Introduction

CT pulmonary angiography (CTPA) to assess for pulmonary embolism (PE) makes up the lion's share of most radiologists' exposure to the pulmonary vascular system and is the focus of this chapter. The pulmonary vascular anatomy is detailed because this can be the crucial determinant to differentiate embolism from artifact. Other modalities for pulmonary vascular assessment, including radiography, MRI, and catheter angiography, are briefly discussed. Finally, select congenital and other pulmonary vascular pathologies are described.

Pulmonary Vascular Anatomy

The adult pulmonary circulation consists of the pulmonary arteries (PAs), pulmonary veins, and bronchial arteries. In anatomically normal individuals, the main pulmonary artery (MPA) or pulmonary trunk arises from the right ventricular (RV) outflow tract distal to the pulmonic valve and then divides into the right and left pulmonary arteries (RPA and LPA, respectively). This bifurcation is readily visible on axial CT slices and is usually conveniently located near the carina, which makes this a popular location to place a bolus-tracking region of interest for CTPA. The LPA arches over the left main stem bronchus and gives rise to the left upper and lower lobar PA branches. The RPA is longer, arches over the right main stem bronchus, and gives rise to upper, middle, and lower lobar PAs. This anatomic relationship between the RPA and LPA and their associated bronchi is critical for determining situs in congenital heart disease, although this is of limited usefulness in most adult patients. The right upper lobe PA divides into apical, posterior, and anterior segmental PAs. The right middle lobe PA divides into lateral and medial segmental arteries. The right lower lobe PA divides into superior, anterior, posterior, medial, and lateral segmental arteries. On the left side, the upper lobe artery divides into apicoposterior, anterior, and lingular arteries, which further divide into superior and inferior segmental arteries. The lower lobe artery divides into superior, anteromedial, lateral, and posterior basal segmental arteries. The word *central* is also often used to refer to the main, left, and right PAs. PAs travel next to bronchi, whereas pulmonary veins travel separately from the bronchi (Fig. 27.1)—a useful pearl to differentiate arteries from veins when they cannot be followed back to the heart.

PAs should be of similar caliber as adjacent bronchi; a substantial disparity in size should raise suspicion for pathology. PAs narrow as they branch (Fig. 27.2); this anatomic feature can be helpful when differentiating an embolus from an artifact because emboli should catch at these branch points.

Pulmonary venous anatomy is more variable than pulmonary arterial anatomy. In most patients, there are two left and two right pulmonary veins that drain to the left atrium, but many normal variations have been described. The distal veins parallel to the course of the PAs until the proximal segmental regions; thereafter, each

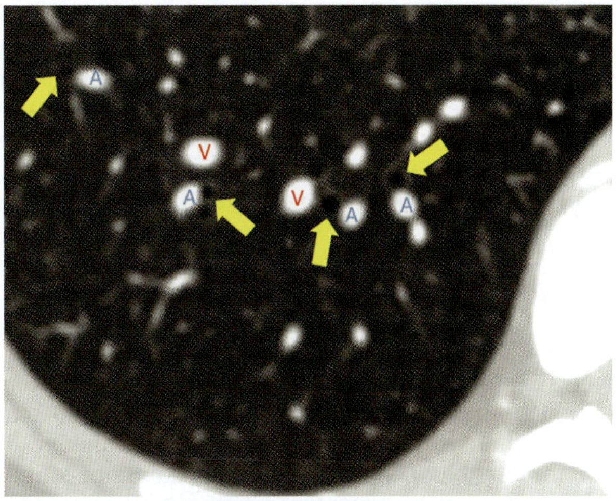

Figure 27.1 Normal right lung base pulmonary vascular anatomy on CT. Pulmonary arteries *(blue A)* travel in parallel with bronchi *(arrows)*. Pulmonary veins *(red V)* travel separately from the arteries and bronchi. These anatomic relationships help distinguish arteries from veins when they cannot be followed back to the heart—for example, when there is a potential filling defect on the top slices of an abdominal CT.

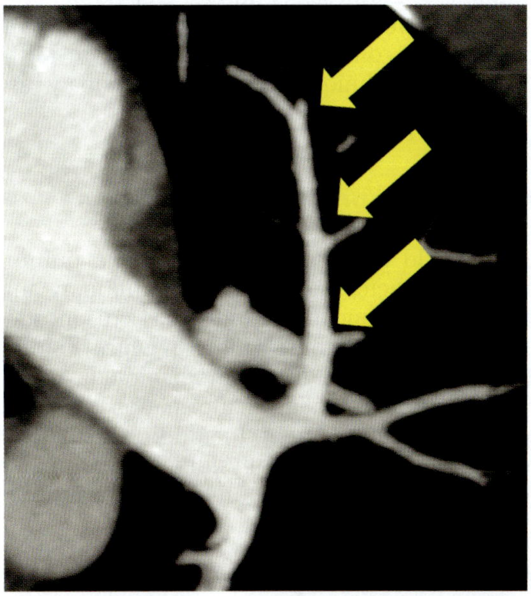

Figure 27.2 Axial maximum intensity projection image of normal left upper lobe pulmonary artery branches. Note how the artery narrows as it branches *(arrows)*; emboli commonly lodge at these branch points.

takes a distinct course. Usually, the right upper lobe veins course adjacent and lateral to the superior vena cava (SVC). The right middle lobe vein combines with the upper lobe vein to form a common confluence and then drains into the left atrium. The right inferior lobe pulmonary vein drains posteriorly and medially into the left atrium as a separate ostium. On the left, the upper lobe pulmonary vein takes a posterior and medial course after the convergence of the superior segment and lingular veins, draining into the left atrium. The left lower lobe vein has a long posterior and medial course; the descending thoracic aorta often indents the vein, but this is typically of no clinical significance.

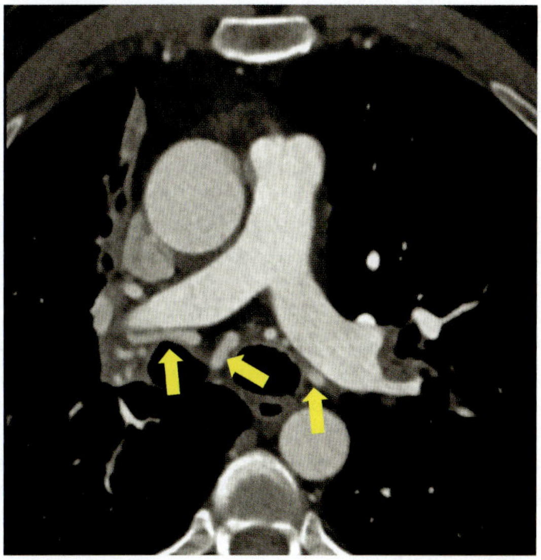

Figure 27.3 Axial CT pulmonary angiography demonstrating dilated, tortuous bronchial arteries *(arrows)*.

Bronchial arteries are the final component of the pulmonary vasculature. There are typically two left bronchial arteries that arise from the descending thoracic aorta. There is usually a single right bronchial artery that arises from the first aortic intercostal artery or by a trunk with the left upper bronchial artery. In the adult, the bronchial arteries usually contribute little to the pulmonary circulation. However, in pathologic states that cause diminished pulmonary arterial circulation (e.g., due to tetralogy of Fallot or PA stenosis), the bronchial arteries serve as an important collateral pathway (Fig. 27.3).

■ Imaging Modalities

Chest Radiography

Chest radiographs remain the first-line modality in the evaluation of pulmonary vascular disease and are especially useful for excluding nonvascular disease such as pneumonia or effusion. Although radiographic findings have been described in many of the pulmonary vascular diseases discussed in this chapter, as a whole they lack both sensitivity and specificity and have been superseded by other techniques.

Ventilation-Perfusion Scintigraphy

The ventilation-perfusion (V/Q) scan is a nuclear medicine technique introduced in the 1960s for the assessment of pulmonary ventilation and blood flow. Perfusion scintigraphy is performed with intravenous (IV) injection of technetium-99m (^{99m}Tc)-labeled macroaggregated albumin, which ranges in size from 10 to 40 μm and localizes in precapillary arterioles. Ventilation scanning is performed typically with inhaled xenon-133 or

^{99m}Tc-labeled aerosols. Prior to the early to mid-2000s, V/Q scanning was the first-line diagnostic test for PE, along with compression sonography of the lower extremities for deep venous thrombosis (DVT). The major limitation of V/Q for PE was its probabilistic nature, with a large proportion of inconclusive results, particularly in patients who had abnormal chest radiographs. In the United States, V/Q has since been largely replaced by CTPA, which allows for direct visualization of the PAs and pulmonary emboli. However, it is worth remembering the advantages of V/Q for select patient populations. V/Q delivers substantially less radiation dose to the breasts, and for this reason the 2012 American Thoracic Society/Society of Thoracic Radiology guidelines favored V/Q over CTPA for young or pregnant women with a normal chest radiograph and no lower extremity DVT on compression sonography. V/Q also does not require iodinated contrast and thus is useful for patients with renal insufficiency or contrast allergy.

Multidetector CT

CTPA performed with multidetector CT (MDCT) has revolutionized the assessment of the pulmonary vasculature and has in practice replaced invasive pulmonary angiography as the gold standard for diagnosis. With modern scanners, the entire thorax can be imaged in a single breath-hold. CT offers exquisite spatial, contrast, and temporal resolution and can demonstrate even small subsegmental pulmonary arterial branches. At the same time, disease processes affecting the lungs and other portions of the chest beyond the pulmonary vasculature can be assessed.

A typical CTPA protocol uses a test bolus or bolus tracking technique to determine the appropriate scan delay after contrast injection at which the attenuation of the PAs is maximized. Some prefer a caudocranial CTPA acquisition based on reports of a lower rate of artifacts, but other studies have found no substantial difference between caudocranial and standard craniocaudad techniques. For the diagnostic scan, a bolus of 70 to 140 mL of contrast at a concentration of 300 to 375 mg iodine/mL is injected preferentially via an 18- to 20-gauge IV placed in an antecubital vein at a typical rate of 3 to 5 mL/s, followed by a saline flush. Radiation doses may be decreased by lowering the peak kilovoltage (kVP) while increasing the product of tube current and exposure time (mAs) to maintain image quality. Iterative reconstruction algorithms also allow dose reduction without sacrificing image quality compared to standard filtered backprojection algorithms. Because the subsegmental PAs are quite small, the image reformats should be generated to maximize spatial resolution. The axial slice thickness should be ≤1.25 mm. The reconstructed field of view should be limited to the lungs (ribs to ribs) to maximize xy plane spatial resolution. Coronal and sagittal reformations are often helpful for problem solving.

There has been considerable recent interest in the potential added value of dual-energy CT in evaluating pulmonary vascular disease, such as PE. Dual-energy CTPA is obtained using two different photon spectra—for example, at 140 and 80 kV. In addition to the standard grayscale CT images, an iodine distribution map is generated, which correlates with perfusion to the lung. This allows assessment of the extent and severity of perfusion deficits to the lung caused by various pulmonary vascular insults (e.g., arterial obstruction by emboli), which may be correlated with prognosis or alter management.

MRI/Magnetic Resonance Angiography

MRI/magnetic resonance angiography (MRI/MRA) is a promising tool for assessing the pulmonary vasculature. Unlike competing modalities, such as CT or V/Q scintigraphy, there is no ionizing radiation. Although evaluation for PE is best performed with IV gadolinium contrast agent, MRA can be performed without IV contrast, a welcome alternative in patients with renal impairment. Both anatomic and perfusion imaging can also be simultaneously acquired. Nevertheless, a number of challenges limit the more widespread use of pulmonary vascular MRA. These include long examination times, which may be difficult for dyspneic patients, lower spatial resolution (≈1–2 mm vs. <1 mm for CT), poorer sensitivity for small pulmonary emboli, and high technical difficulty. With continuing improvements in MRI and familiarity with techniques, the use of pulmonary vascular MRA may become more common.

Invasive Pulmonary Angiography

Once the gold standard for imaging the pulmonary vasculature, catheter-based invasive pulmonary angiography is now infrequently performed as a diagnostic test. It is generally reserved for situations in which an intervention is planned, such as drug or mechanical thrombolysis, embolization of aneurysms, malformations, or collateral vessels, and stent placement. In addition, catheter angiography can provide direct physiologic measurement of the degree of shunting and pulmonary pressures.

■ Acute Pulmonary Embolism

Currently, most PA imaging is performed for the evaluation of PE. A PE is a clot that has migrated, or embolized, from a distant source, usually the deep veins of the lower extremities, and becomes lodged within the PAs. It is the third leading cause of cardiovascular disease after myocardial infarction and stroke, affecting 600,000 people annually and accounting for more than 10% of in-hospital deaths, with an untreated mortality rate as high as 30%. PE is notoriously difficult to diagnose clinically. Presenting symptoms such as chest pain, tachycardia, and tachypnea are nonspecific. Clinical prediction rules such as the modified Wells criteria and use of the serum D-dimer have low specificity. The PIOPED II (Prospective Investigation of Pulmonary Embolism Diagnosis II) established CTPA as the de facto gold standard for the diagnosis of PE, with subsequent studies finding a sensitivity and specificity approaching 100% and 97%, respectively.

Alternative modalities include V/Q scintigraphy (V/Q scan), MRA, and invasive pulmonary angiography. In following sections, the distinguishing imaging features of PE in its varied forms are discussed, with an emphasis on MDCT and an attention to diagnostic pitfalls.

Practical Approach to Interpreting CT Pulmonary Angiography for Pulmonary Embolism

Quality

The quality of the CTPA should first be assessed to determine whether PE can be confidently excluded and to what level. This usually hinges on the contrast bolus and respiratory motion. It has been reported that a mean attenuation of 250 Hounsfield units (HU) in the MPA is necessary to exclude PE; in actual practice, main, lobar, and even segmental pulmonary emboli can sometimes be excluded with worse opacification. If the study is limited, this uncertainty and to what level (main, lobar, segmental, subsegmental) PE can be confidently excluded should be reported so that the health care provider can decide whether additional testing is necessary.

Search Pattern

There is no one correct way to read a CTPA for PE, but for the sake of instruction, we present our search pattern. Start with a gestalt pass (i.e., look at the entire image) through the stack of thin (≤1.25-mm) axial images and then focus on individual quadrants (upper left, lower left, upper right, lower right) while scrolling through the axial images. Finally again take a last gestalt pass through a set of coronal multiplanar reformatted images (MPRs). Coronal (or sagittal) MPRs can be very helpful to identify pulmonary emboli oriented in the axial plane and for completely occluded segmental or subsegmental PAs that would be difficult to perceive on axial images. Standard mediastinal window and level settings could wash out emboli by making the PAs appear too bright, so a PE-specific window width/level setting of 700/100 has been proposed. In practice, we find that the best window varies substantially based on the contrast bolus. RV trabeculations should be visible on PE windows because they have a similar to slightly higher attenuation than clot (Fig. 27.4).

CT Pulmonary Angiography Findings of Acute Pulmonary Embolism

Pulmonary emboli should have a serpentine shape because they were originally casts of deep veins. The embolus should be longer than it is wide and oriented down the barrel (long axis) of the artery (Fig. 27.5). PAs narrow as they branch (see Fig. 27.2), so emboli should catch at these branch points. The embolus should have a sharp, well-defined border (Fig. 27.6). Any filling defect that does not fit these criteria should be scrutinized as a possible artifact.

Artifacts

At most centers, only 5% to 7% of CTPA findings are positive for PE. Treatment of PE, in most cases 3 months to a lifetime of anticoagulation, carries substantial cost and inconvenience. Furthermore anticoagulation carries an approximately 0.5% annual risk of major hemorrhage, with a substantially higher rate during the first 3 months of treatment and in patients with bleeding risk factors. Thus the misdiagnosis of PE has the potential to cause substantial harm.

When a possible filling defect is detected on CT, the first step is to confirm that it lies within a PA and not a vein. The pulmonary veins enhance heterogeneously and can mimic pulmonary emboli (Fig. 27.7); pulmonary vein thrombus is very rare and is usually seen in the setting of direct malignant invasion or as a postprocedural complication. On chest CT, this is easily accomplished

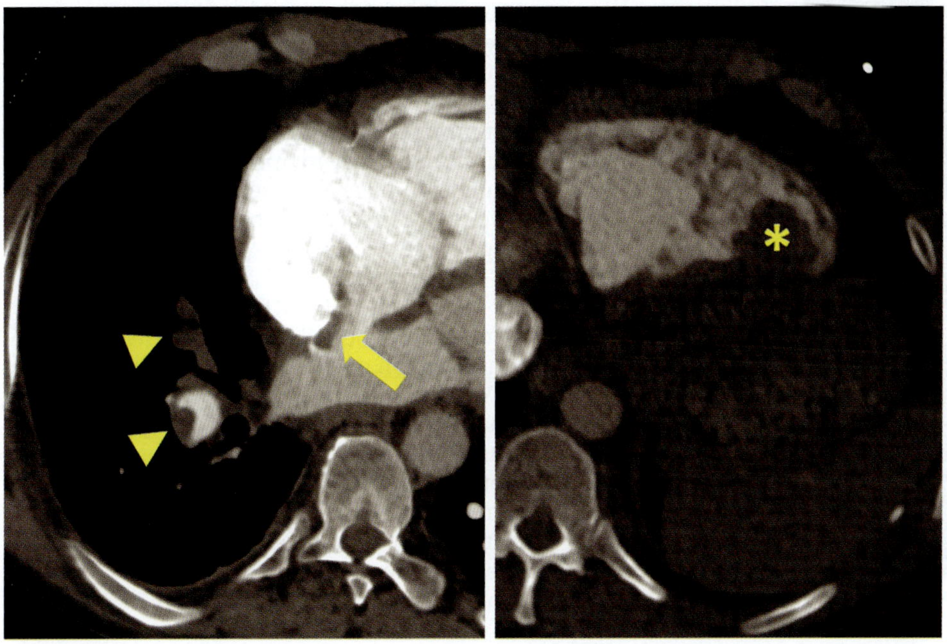

Figure 27.4 Embolus in transit, with clot caught in an interatrial septal aneurysm *(arrow)* and in the right ventricular apex *(asterisk)*. In addition to a pulmonary embolism *(arrowheads)*, this patient suffered a stroke due to an embolism traversing a patent foramen ovale.

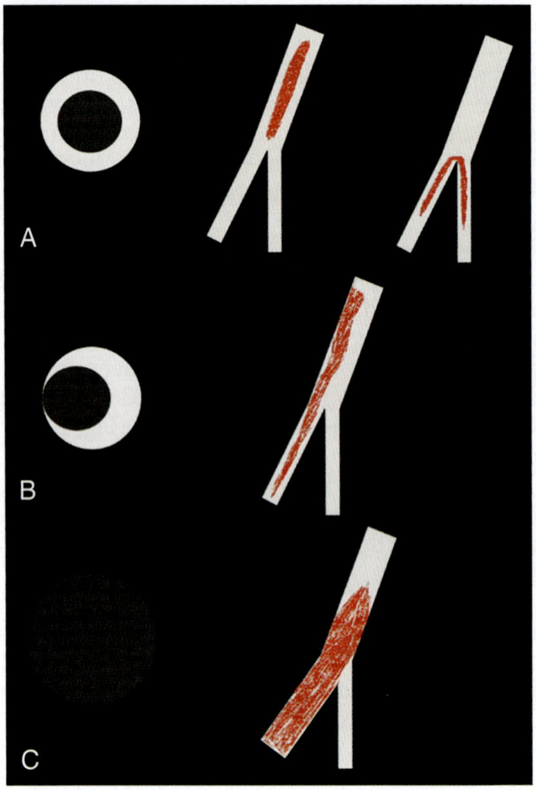

Figure 27.5 Three classic appearances of acute pulmonary embolism have been described. (A) A central filling defect with the polo mint short axis and tram track longitudinal appearance. Pulmonary arteries (PAs) narrow as they branch, so emboli tend to catch at branch points. (B) Eccentric embolus lies against the vessel wall. Note the acute angle between the embolus and wall on the axial cross section. In contrast, chronic emboli have obtuse angles. (C) A completely impacted and engorged PA is larger than uninvolved neighbors.

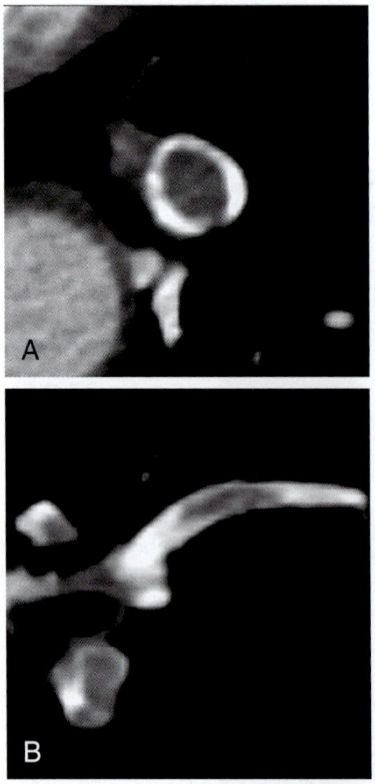

Figure 27.6 (A) Polo mint and (B) tram track signs of pulmonary embolism.

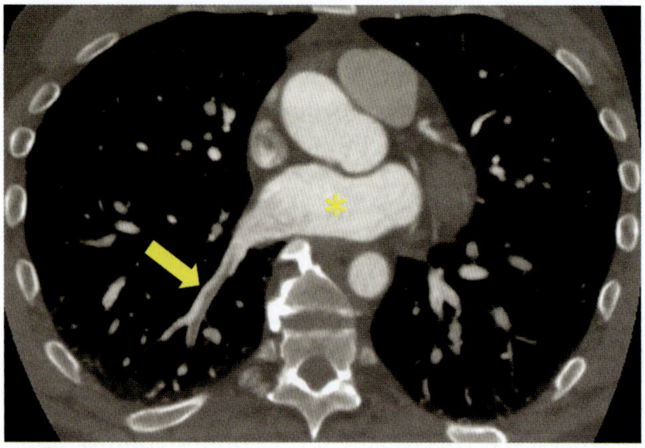

Figure 27.7 Pseudo-filling defect in a pulmonary vein *(arrow)* emptying into the left atrium *(asterisk)*. Pulmonary venous opacification is often heterogeneous and can mimic a pulmonary embolism.

by following the vessel back to the right ventricle (PA) or left atrium (pulmonary vein). On abdominal CT, the heart is often not included, so the fact that the PAs travel in parallel with the bronchi should be used as described in Fig. 27.1. When there is uncertainty about whether a finding is a PE, a practical approach is to look first for additional emboli. Pulmonary emboli often occur in multiples, and if a second definite PE is present, there is no need to perseverate over a difficult finding.

RESPIRATORY MOTION ARTIFACT

This is the most common cause of indeterminate CTPA. When the patient breathes during the CT acquisition, portions of the lung, bronchi, and PAs can overlap, and this volume averaging can mimic PE (Figs. 27.8 and 27.9). This is usually easily detected by switching to lung windows, which will demonstrate blurring of the lung parenchyma and occasionally what is known as a characteristic *seagull sign*.

IMAGE NOISE OR QUANTUM MOTTLE

This degrades image quality and is particularly detrimental for the evaluation of small segmental and subsegmental PAs. Image noise is usually an issue in obese patients who cannot raise their arms and have large pleural effusions or an elevated hemidiaphragm. Higher contrast flow rates, higher kVp and mAs settings, and thicker slice and iterative image reconstruction algorithms can help reduce image noise.

MIXING OR FLOW-RELATED ARTIFACTS

These are among the most difficult to resolve on CTPA. Transient interruption of contrast can occur if the patient performs a Valsalva maneuver or deep inspiration during the contrast injection, resulting in a transient increase in the proportion of unopacified inferior vena cava (IVC) blood emptying into the right side of the heart. This results in a portion of the PA having lower attenuation than its proximal and distal neighbors. Similarly, locally increased pulmonary vascular resistance can occur upstream of parenchymal changes, such as atelectasis or pneumonia. Flow artifacts often have ill-defined borders or demonstrate a density gradient, which can be very helpful for distinguishing from PE (Fig. 27.10; see Fig. 27.8). When the morphologic features fail, attenuation can be helpful for differentiating flow artifact from PE. Although attenuation can vary substantially based on the scan protocol, it has been reported that small acute pulmonary emboli have a mean attenuation around 35 HU (range, 5–65 HU); chronic emboli are more dense, with a mean attenuation of 90 HU (range, 50–160 HU; Fig. 27.11). In general, attenuation is much less helpful than morphology for differentiating acute versus chronic PE, but it is useful for flow artifacts. The closer the attenuation is to 35 HU, the more likely is a PE. On the other hand, ill-defined margins and an attenuation near or above 90 HU favors flow artifact. Because attenuation can vary with the CTPA protocol, it is better to rely on the morphology of the filling defect first and use attenuation as supporting evidence only. When there is diagnostic uncertainty, it is reasonable to repeat CTPA.

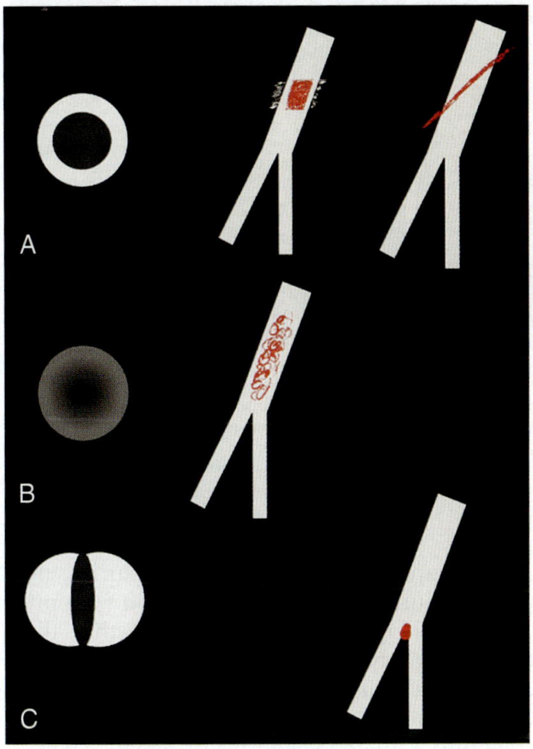

Figure 27.8 Unlike pulmonary emboli, artifacts do not have a serpentine appearance, may not be oriented down the barrel of the vessel, do not catch at branch points, and may have hazy, ill-defined borders. (A) Filling defects that are globular, not oriented along the long axis of the vessel, or do not catch at a vessel branch point suggest artifact. Volume averaging with adjacent lung or bronchus due to respiratory motion often looks like a filling defect and is easily identified on lung windows. (B) Hazy intermediate attenuation without a sharp border suggests flow or mixing artifact. (C) Volume averaging with normal lymphoid tissue at vessel bifurcations is best identified on coronal or sagittal images.

EDGE ENHANCEMENT ARTIFACT

This results from the use of high spatial frequency reconstruction kernels (lung and bone algorithm). These so-called hard kernels improve visualization of such structures as the airways and pulmonary interstitium, but they also tend to create artifacts at the periphery of the PAs that mimic PE. Therefore, PE should be assessed using standard soft tissue reconstruction kernels.

LOW-DENSITY MUCUS PLUGS

Occluding bronchi surrounded by a relatively high density bronchial wall can be misinterpreted as PE. This artifact is easily resolved by following the filling defect back to the heart or trachea.

Prognosis and Treatment

Once the diagnosis of acute PE has been made, attention should shift to prognostic findings that can help guide patient management. Death from PE occurs due to RV dysfunction and failure. The best-studied and most reliable measure of RV dysfunction on CT is a dilated right ventricle (Fig. 27.12). Normally, the left ventricle should have a greater diameter than the right; when the RV/left ventricular (LV) diameter ratio is >1, the right ventricle

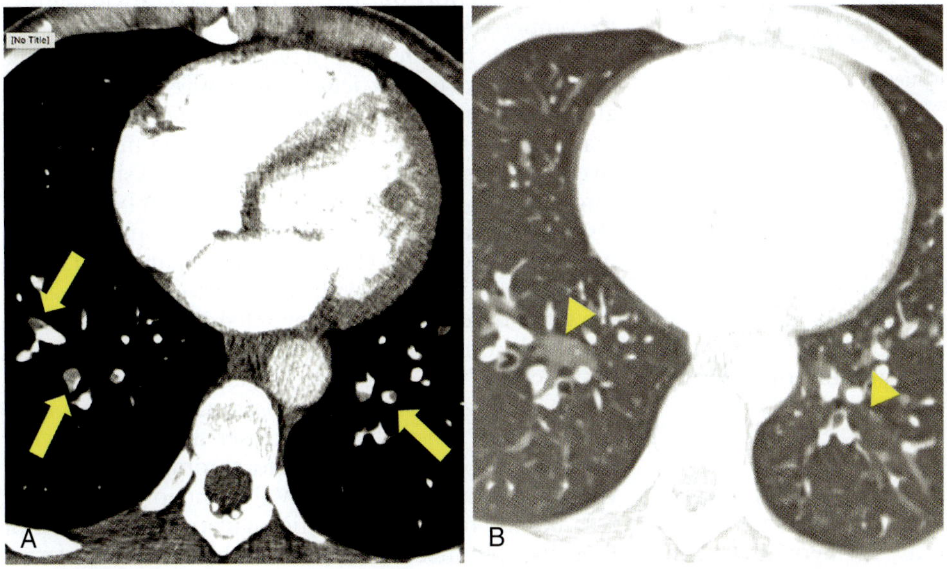

Figure 27.9 Apparent filling defects (A; *arrows*) identified as respiratory motion artifacts (B; *arrowheads*) by switching to lung windows.

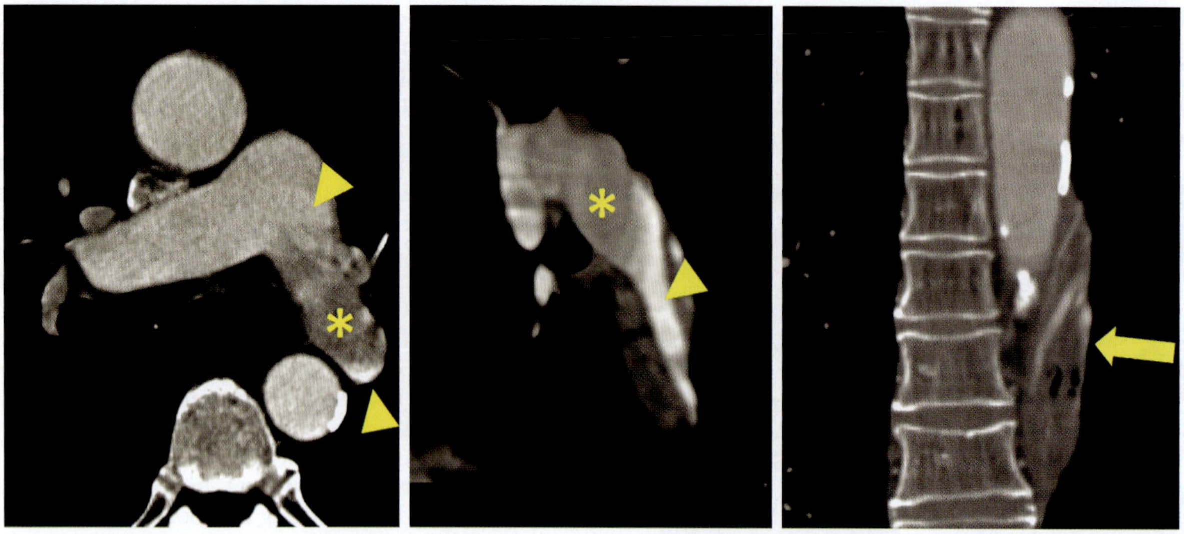

Figure 27.10 Hazy flow artifact *(asterisk)* in the left main and lower lobar pulmonary arteries in a patient with increased pulmonary vascular resistance due to collapse of the left lower lobe *(arrow)*. In this case, there is dense contrast both before and after the flow artifact *(arrowheads)*, indicating transient interruption of the contrast bolus by inferior vena cava blood.

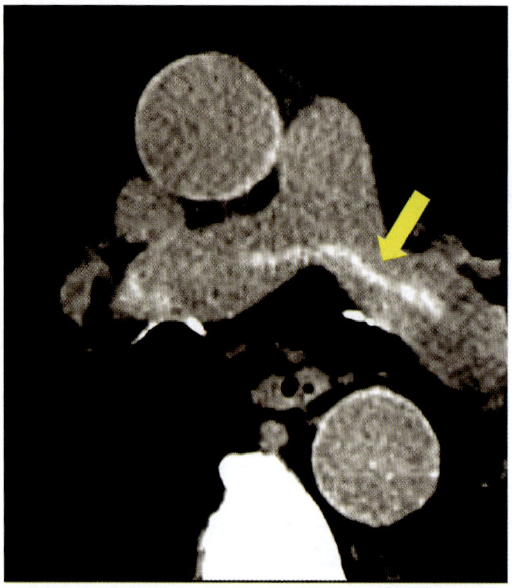

Figure 27.11 Unusual case of a high-attenuation saddle pulmonary embolism (PE; *arrow*) visible on noncontrast CT. A PE usually has similar attenuation to blood and is only rarely visible without intravenous contrast.

is enlarged (see Fig. 27.2). A meta-analysis of 49 studies in over 13,000 patients found that an increased RV/LV diameter ratio conferred a 2.5-fold risk of all-cause mortality and a 5-fold increased risk of PE-related mortality compared to persons without an abnormal RV/LV ratio. Approximately 50% of patients with PE will have an RV/LV diameter ratio >1, and up to 25% of patients with no PE on CTPA will also have an enlarged right ventricle by this criterion. Thus RV enlargement is not a specific sign of RV dysfunction and should be interpreted in the context of clinical stability, RV hypokinesis on echocardiography, and serum biomarkers such as troponin or brain natriuretic peptide. Comparison with prior CTs can be very helpful to determine whether the right ventricle is acutely enlarged and increases specificity.

Supportive CT signs of RV dysfunction include leftward bowing of the interventricular septum and reflux of contrast into a dilated vena cava or hepatic veins. These findings are less reliable because septal bowing is difficult to evaluate accurately on non–ECG-gated axial images, and power injection can cause reflux of contrast into the IVC in the absence of elevated right heart pressure. Of note, PA clot burden is not a reliable predictor of risk after adjusting for RV enlargement. Anecdotally, many young patients with large central emboli have minimal symptoms, whereas patients with diminished cardiopulmonary reserve can have profound symptoms from small peripheral emboli. The best measure of risk is not the quantity of clot but the right ventricle's ability to compensate.

The single best predictor of risk after acute PE is systemic hypotension, which is defined as *massive PE* and trumps all prognostic imaging findings. Untreated patients with massive PE have a poor prognosis, so the most aggressive therapies such as systemic thrombolysis, catheter thrombolysis, and surgical or catheter thrombectomy are reserved for these patients. It is worth emphasizing that massive PE refers to clinical hemodynamic instability and is often discordant with clot burden. For this reason, the word *massive* should be avoided in the CTPA report to avoid confusion. Normotensive patients with RV dysfunction on CT, echocardiography, or by biomarkers are defined as having *submassive PE*. Patients with submassive PE usually merit closer monitoring; select patients may also be candidates for thrombolysis. Patients with PE and no evidence of RV dysfunction are at lower risk and are treated with anticoagulation. Treatment of PE is in rapid flux due to the introduction of oral factor

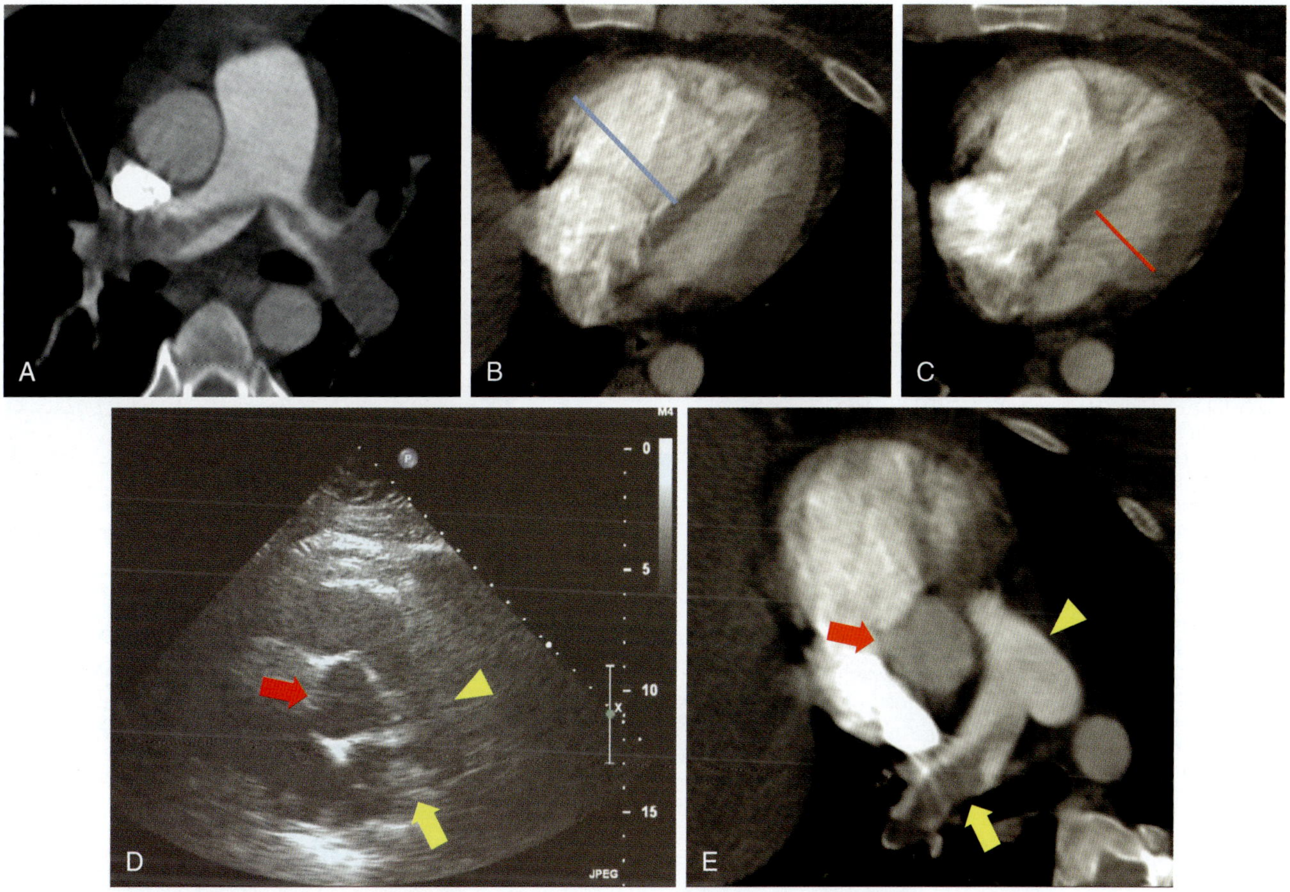

Figure 27.12 (A) A saddle pulmonary embolism (PE) straddling the pulmonary artery (PA) bifurcation extends into the right, left, lobar, and segmental branches. (B and C) Right ventricular (RV) dilation suggests RV dysfunction (also known as *right heart strain*). The right ventricle is enlarged when it is greater in diameter than the left ventricle. The RV and left ventricular (LV) diameters should be measured at the level at which they are largest and are often on different axial images. (D and E) RV dysfunction can be confirmed with echocardiography. Echocardiographic signs of RV dysfunction include an RV/LV diameter ratio >1, RV end-diastolic diameter >3 cm, or RV hypokinesis. Paradoxic interventricular septal motion and tricuspid regurgitation may also be present. McConnell's sign, defined as RV hypokinesis with sparing of the RV apex, has been described as a specific sign for PE. In this unusual case, a mobile echogenic clot was visible in the proximal right PA *(yellow arrow)* on the echocardiogram. Note the adjacent aortic root *(red arrow)* and main PA *(arrowhead)*, with correlation to an oblique multiplanar reconstruction image from CT pulmonary angiography.

Xa inhibitors (e.g., rivaroxaban, apixaban) and direct thrombin inhibitors (e.g., dabigatran). Until recently, initial treatment was dominated by IV unfractionated and subcutaneous low-molecular-weight heparin, followed by long-term treatment with warfarin or subcutaneous low-molecular-weight heparin. However, the new factor Xa and direct thrombin inhibitors are increasingly used as an oral alternative, with more consistent dosing than warfarin. The duration of treatment is usually between 3 and 6 months for those with provoked thromboembolism (e.g., recent surgery) and indefinite for those without modifiable risk factors (e.g., malignancy). IVC filter placement should be considered when anticoagulation is contraindicated. IVC filters may also be placed in carefully selected patients with low cardiopulmonary reserve and a high risk for additional emboli.

Secondary Signs of Pulmonary Embolism on CT Pulmonary Angiography

A variety of ancillary parenchymal abnormalities may be observed on CT. These include atelectasis, pleural effusion, mosaic attenuation representing regional oligemia, peripheral consolidation with central ground-glass opacity representing pulmonary infarction, and focal ground-glass opacity representing pulmonary hemorrhage (Fig. 27.13). However, none of these findings are specific for the diagnosis of PE.

Pulmonary infarction represents coagulative ischemic necrosis in a portion of the lung, which is normally supplied by the pulmonary and bronchial arteries as well as the pulmonary veins. Initial stages involve localized alveolar hemorrhage due to ischemia and reperfusion,

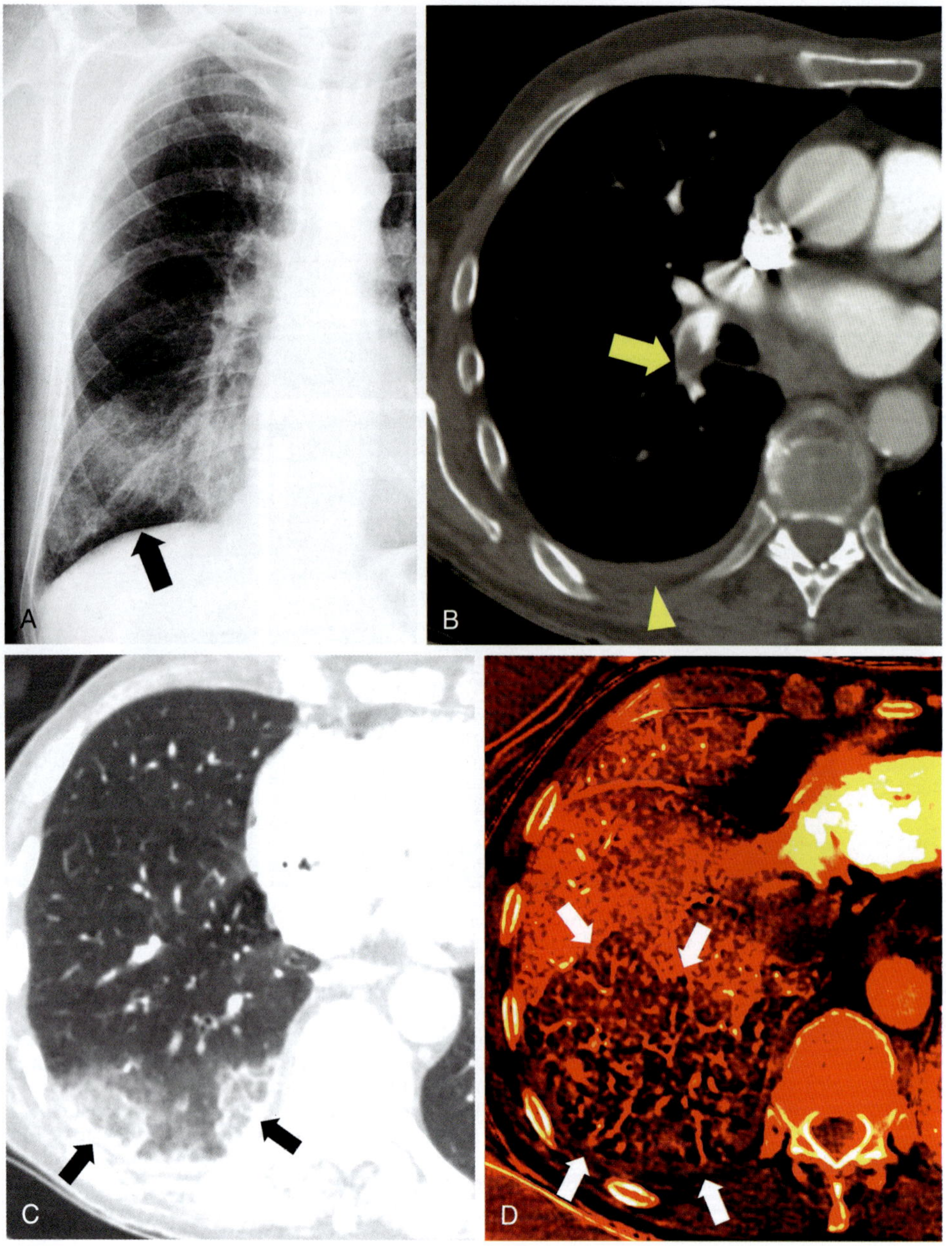

Figure 27.13 (A) Frontal chest radiograph demonstrates right lower lobe opacity *(black arrow)*. (B) A right interlobar pulmonary embolism (PE; *yellow arrow*) and small right pleural effusion *(yellow arrowhead)* are visible on CT pulmonary angiography. (C) Wedge-shaped opacities *(black arrows)* at the periphery of the right lower lobe are compatible with infarcts. A central bubbly lucency is characteristic of an early infarct that will progress to homogeneous consolidation. (D) A dual-energy iodine map of the right lower lobe demonstrates diminished perfusion *(white arrows)* in a polygonal region that follows the lobular anatomy and is substantially larger than lung opacities, both features of PE and infarct.

with later progression to an irreversible fibrotic scar. PE is the most common cause of pulmonary infarction. The risk is highest when emboli involve distal small to medium-sized pulmonary arterial branches ≤3 mm, with insufficient compensatory bronchial collateralization. Pleuritic chest pain is a common presenting symptom.

The most characteristic finding of pulmonary infarction is Hampton's hump, a wedge-shaped, broad, pleural-based opacity with a truncated apex and convex border, originally described on chest radiographs (Fig. 27.14). On CT, additional supportive although less common features of pulmonary infarction include internal central lucencies within the peripheral area of consolidation (bubbly consolidation), thickened vessels leading to the apex of the opacity, and linear stranding from hilum to apex. Cavitation occurs in less than 1 in 10 infarctions. Decreased enhancement within the consolidated lung is present in 95% of cases, but this is a nonspecific finding that can also be observed in pneumonia and tumor. Unilateral pleural effusion is another supportive feature. CT is also useful for delineating infarct-related complications such as sterile or purulent effusions. The advent of dual-energy CT may assist in the diagnosis; a segmental perfusion defect is seen on the iodine map corresponding to the area of opacified and infarcted lung. Pulmonary infarctions may also be visualized on a variety of other (although not first-line) imaging modalities. Ultrasound demonstrates a wedge-shaped hypoechoic structure with a hyperechoic center caused by reverberation artifact. MRI shows a peripheral, wedge-shaped signal

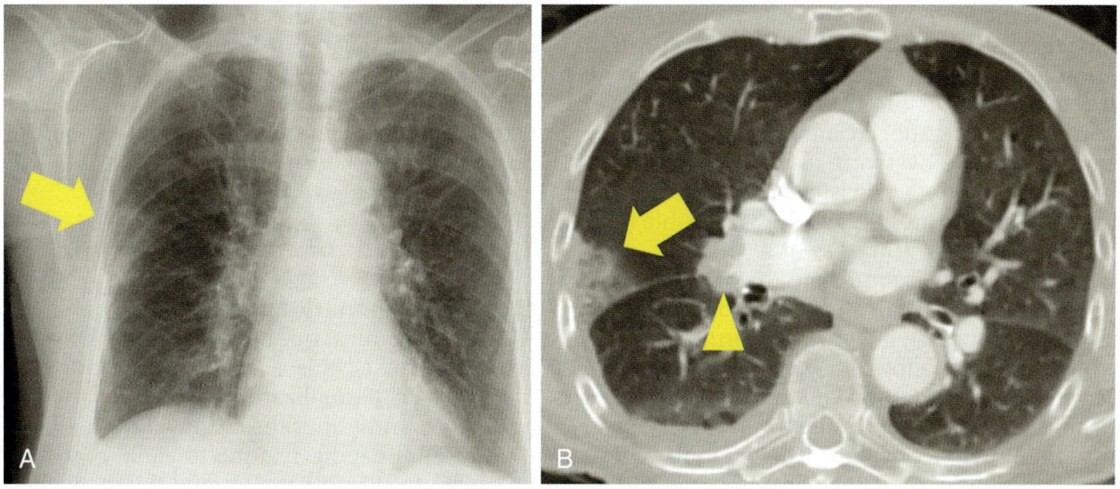

Figure 27.14 Hampton's hump on a chest radiograph (A; *arrow*) corresponding to a pulmonary infarct on CT pulmonary angiography. Note right-sided pulmonary emboli on the CT scan (B; *arrowhead*).

abnormality that is T2-hyperintense and becomes increasingly T1-hypertense with increasing age of the infarction. On V/Q scans, a triple-match pattern is observed, with an area of radiographic parenchymal opacity corresponding to both ventilation and perfusion defects. PET using ^{18}F-fluorodeoxyglucose (FDG) may show peripheral radiotracer avidity along the infarct periphery with central photopenia or, alternatively, diffuse uptake within the infarct.

Other Imaging Modalities for Pulmonary Embolism

Chest radiographs are usually not helpful beyond excluding another cause for chest pain. When present, the most common radiographic findings include atelectasis, focal parenchymal opacity, and pleural effusion. Less common findings include diaphragmatic elevation, oligemia, and central PA enlargement. Two eponyms associated with PE, the Westermark sign and Hampton's hump, are commonly mentioned but infrequently seen on chest radiographs. The Westermark sign is characterized by focal peripheral radiolucency representing decreased vascularity beyond an occluded PA, accompanied by mild central pulmonary arterial dilation. Hampton's hump is a peripheral wedge-shaped, pleural-based opacity, typically representing a pulmonary infarct. A normal chest radiograph does not exclude PE, but can be helpful for the interpretation of V/Q scanning as the next imaging test.

V/Q scintigraphy should be considered as an alternative to CTPA for patients with renal insufficiency, iodinated contrast allergy, or pregnancy. Based on ventilation (V) and perfusion (Q) images with correlation with chest radiographs, the probability of acute PE is estimated. Perfusion defects are small, moderate, or large if they affect <25%, 25% to 75%, or >75% of an anatomic lung segment, respectively. A V/Q mismatch is defined as a perfusion defect with no corresponding ventilation abnormality. Scans are commonly evaluated according to the modified PIOPED II criteria. Results are categorized as a normal or very low (<10%), low (≤20%), intermediate (20%–79%), or high (≥80%) probability of PE. Very low probability scans consist of one to three small perfusion defects with a normal chest radiograph (original PIOPED criteria). Large, moderate, and small defects are defined as >75%, 26% to 75%, and <25% of a lung segment, respectively. Low-probability scans may include nonsegmental perfusion defects, perfusion defects with much larger radiographic abnormalities, matched V/Q defects with a normal radiograph and some areas of normal perfusion, or small perfusion defects with normal radiographs. Intermediate probability scans may demonstrate one matched V/Q defect with a normal radiograph, one moderate to two large (or equivalent) V/Q mismatches, or a V/Q abnormality not otherwise classifiable. A high probability scan includes two or more large or an equivalent combination of moderate and large V/Q mismatches.

Most PE arises from DVT of the lower extremities. Ultrasound is the first-line modality for the assessment of DVT, with an accuracy approaching 100% for the lower extremities and 95% for the upper extremities. Veins are typically imaged in the transverse and sagittal planes using grayscale imaging, supplemented by color and spectral Doppler, using at least a 5-MHz linear probe. Lack of venous compression with gentle transducer pressure is the primary diagnostic criterion for DVT; other findings are less sensitive and less specific. Acute DVT characteristically causes venous distention but is often anechoic and otherwise indistinguishable from a normal vessel on static grayscale imaging. Doppler flow may be absent. With only partially obstructive acute DVT, there is typically loss of respiratory phasicity in the venous waveform, with a dampened response to calf augmentation (squeezing maneuver). In later stages, DVT becomes more echoic but can mimic slow flow; thus, an echogenic filling defect is not specific for the diagnosis. Chronic, unresolved DVT appears as thickening and increased echogenicity of the vein walls, which are resistant to compression. In the lower extremity, it is also important to assess for the presence of a monophasic waveform in the common femoral vein, a reliable predictor of more proximal venous obstruction. In the upper extremity, it is noteworthy that the subclavian vein is not readily compressed due to the overlying clavicle, and the brachiocephalic veins are not well visualized by ultrasound; thus only secondary features of DVT may be visible (e.g., abnormal color Doppler flow, loss of respiratory variation). Treatment of DVT is similar to that of PE.

CT venography (CTV) is an alternative to ultrasound. CTV is convenient because it can be performed concurrently with CTPA; it also allows for better visualization of the pelvic veins and IVC. However, there is a substantial associated radiation dose. Acute DVT appears on CTV as an intraluminal filling defect, often involving multiple venous segments and possibly accompanied by venous distention. Chronic DVT manifests as calcified thrombi, small thick-walled veins with heterogeneous enhancement, and the presence of multiple collaterals veins. MR venography, performed with or without IV gadolinium contrast, can show findings similar to CTV without ionizing radiation. Although both CT and MR are accurate for the evaluation of DVT, they should be considered second-line therapy compared to compression sonography.

MRI/MRA is another alternative to MDCT and can demonstrate similar anatomic findings, as well as perfusion deficits, when local experience is sufficient. However, the PIOPED III trial of MR pulmonary angiography to exclude PE found that 25% of pulmonary MR angiograms were technically inadequate to exclude PE. Although some expert sites had better (and others worse) results, this speaks to the fact that MRA cannot supersede CTPA for the evaluation of PE; rather, it should be considered as a problem-solving tool when CTPA or V/Q are not possible or yield indeterminate results. Invasive pulmonary angiography is now a last resort when other diagnostic modalities are insufficient or intervention is planned.

Incidental Pulmonary Embolism, Isolated Subsegmental Pulmonary Embolism, and Overdiagnosis

On oncology and postoperative contrast chest CT scans, incidental pulmonary emboli are common. Up to 5% of routine staging contrast chest CT scans have an incidental PE. Recall that only 5% to 7% of CTPAs performed expressly for suspected PE are positive, and so PE is nearly as common on routine staging contrast chest CT as on CTPA. For this reason, the PAs should be included in the search pattern for all contrast-enhanced CT of the chest and abdomen.

The clinical significance of incidental pulmonary emboli is controversial. At our practice, most oncology patients with small and asymptomatic incidental PEs are treated as outpatients. Some consider isolated subsegmental pulmonary emboli (ISSPE) as a separate category. Small observational studies suggest that asymptomatic ISSPE in patients with normal cardiopulmonary reserve and no DVT have good outcomes, even without anticoagulation. Registry data have suggested that mortality due to PE has remained constant, despite a substantial increase in PE diagnosis during the CTPA era, suggesting that some patients are overdiagnosed and may not need treatment. Prospective randomized controlled trials are necessary to determine whether patients with ISSPE should be treated more conservatively.

Types of Embolisms

Chronic Pulmonary Embolism

A common clinical question is whether PE is chronic or acute. In practice, this is a difficult question because the first signs of recanalization can occur anywhere from hours to months after the event. Chronic PE has several unique CT imaging features that, like acute PE, may be categorized into vascular and parenchymal findings (Fig. 27.15). Pulmonary arterial involvement in chronic PE has one of four forms: (1) complete occlusion of an artery that is smaller than adjacent patent arteries and forms a concave contrast cutoff known as a *pouch deformity* (Fig. 27.16); (2) a nonobstructive, peripheral (eccentric, mural) intraluminal filling defect that has a crescent shape, forms obtuse angles with the vessel wall, and

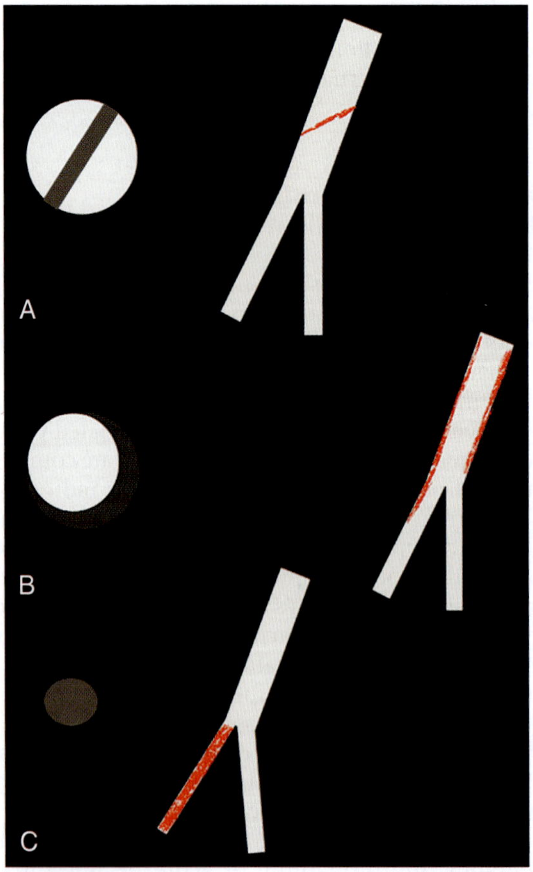

Figure 27.15 Common appearance of a chronic pulmonary embolism (PE). (A) Band or web across the pulmonary artery (PA). (B) Recanalized thrombus forms a convex angle against the vessel wall and may not stop at branch points. In contrast, acute PE forms acute angles with the vessel wall. (C) Small, chronically occluded PA. In contrast, acutely occluded PAs are normal or enlarged in diameter.

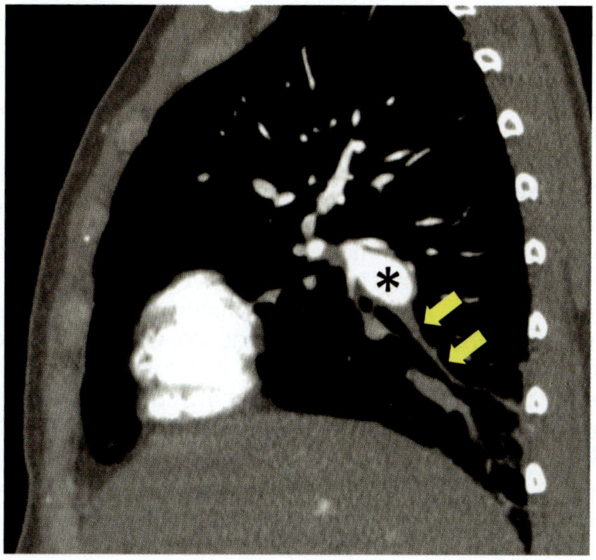

Figure 27.16 Sagittal CT pulmonary angiography scan of right lower lobar pulmonary artery (PA) mycotic aneurysm *(asterisk)* and small, chronically occluded PA *(arrows)* in an intravenous drug user.

sometimes calcifies; (3) contrast material traversing through thickened and commonly smaller arteries; or (4) a band or web in a contrast-filled artery. A band describes a thin ribbon-like structure that is attached to the vessel wall at two ends, whereas a web is a complex band with branches. Calcification within eccentric vessel wall thickening may also be observed in the absence of a visible intraluminal thrombus. Other vascular findings include vascular stenosis or beading and bronchial or systemic artery collateralization. Bronchial artery enlargement >2 mm is more typical of chronic PE than of acute PE and is an indicator of a more central clot burden. Secondary pulmonary arterial hypertension (as detailed later in this chapter) may result in enlargement of the central PAs, including MPA dilation >29 mm.

The most characteristic CT pulmonary parenchymal finding in chronic PE is a mosaic attenuation pattern in the lungs, consisting of geographic areas of higher and lower attenuation on lung window settings. The vessels in areas of hyperlucency are often diminutive in caliber. Other findings may include peripheral parenchymal opacities, scarring, and pleural thickening, which may represent sequela of prior lung infarction. Bronchiectasis may also occur.

Chronic thromboembolic pulmonary hypertension (CTEPH) is a feared long-term complication occurring in 0.5% to 4% of PE cases. CTEPH is defined by a mean pulmonary arterial pressure >25 mm Hg persisting 6 months after an acute PE, with a pulmonary vascular resistance ≥3 Wood units (240 dyne s/cm^5) with unresolving pulmonary arterial obstruction, despite 3 months or more of uninterrupted anticoagulation. Although the exact mechanism remains unclear, it is thought that persistent thromboemboli become incorporated into vessel walls, leading to vessel luminal narrowing, occlusion, and elevation in pulmonary vascular resistance. Risk factors for CTEPH include chronic inflammatory conditions such as inflammatory bowel disease and chronic osteomyelitis, myeloproliferative disorders, prior splenectomy, and ventriculoarterial shunts. Symptoms are nonspecific, such as exertional dyspnea, and may be mistaken for more common conditions, such as ischemic heart disease or interstitial lung disease.

Pulmonary Embolism: Beyond Bland Clot

Pulmonary emboli are usually bland (thrombotic). However, a variety of substances may embolize, including infected material (septic emboli), cement, tumor, amniotic fluid, and fat.

Septic Embolism

Septic pulmonary emboli are thrombi-containing microorganisms that become lodged in the PAs. They usually arise in the setting of tricuspid valve endocarditis. Other risk factors include infected central venous catheters, septic peripheral thrombophlebitis, and immunocompromised states, such as organ transplantation. Symptoms may include fever, cough, and hemoptysis in patients with a known active extrapulmonary infectious source. Septic emboli are characteristic of Lemierre syndrome, characterized by oropharyngeal infection in young adults, with subsequent thrombophlebitis of the internal jugular vein.

Radiographic findings include variably sized (1–3 cm) peripheral lung nodules with ill-defined borders that often cavitate. Analogously, CT shows spherical and potentially cavitary subpleural nodules with a dependent distribution in addition to wedge-shaped heterogeneous opacities with peripheral rim enhancement. Air bronchograms may be present. A feeding vessel leading to the nodules (feeding vessel sign) is classic but not specific. Similarly, the halo sign, consisting of a central nodule surrounded by a ground-glass halo due to adjacent hemorrhagic infarction, may be present but is not specific. Associated findings may include mediastinal lymphadenopathy and pleural effusions. The SVC and heart should also be screened for thrombi and vegetations.

Cement Embolism

Cement (polymethylmethacrylate) embolism is an uncommon complication of percutaneous vertebroplasty, arising in 3.5% to 23% of procedures. Cement leaks into the vertebral venous plexuses and IVC and then travels to the PAs. Patients are usually asymptomatic but may develop dyspnea. Rare deaths have been reported. Early imaging should be considered, particularly in patients in whom this complication is suspected during intraprocedural fluoroscopy. Chest radiographs may demonstrate bilateral, branching, linear radiopaque structures just after vertebroplasty, corresponding to the embolized cement. CT shows multiple tubular areas of high attenuation in the PAs. Paravertebral high-attenuation cement may also be evident. Management is controversial. In symptomatic patients, anticoagulation and supportive care are recommended. Surgical removal of the cement is not commonly pursued but has been reported.

Tumor Embolism

Tumor embolism refers to the movement of distant primary neoplastic cells to the lumen of the PAs, where the cells become lodged. Breast, hepatocellular, renal cell, gastric, prostate, and choriocarcinoma are the most common underlying extrapulmonary malignancies. The exact incidence is not known, but tumor embolism has been reported in 3% to 26% of autopsies. Clinically, tumor emboli may be suspected in patients with a known malignancy who experience subacute dyspnea and signs of right heart failure or pulmonary hypertension.

Macroscopic (large) tumor emboli are best seen by CTA and appear as filling defects in the PAs. These features mimic bland pulmonary emboli, which also occur in cancer patients, thus making precise diagnosis challenging. Features that should raise suspicion for tumoral rather than bland emboli include enhancing filling defects on delayed CT imaging and persistence, despite a long course of anticoagulation. Other clues are the presence of dilated and beaded peripheral arteries or an identifiable tumoral component. Microscopic tumor emboli are sufficiently small that imaging findings may be nonexistent or minimal and nonspecific. V/Q scans may demonstrate multiple subsegmental perfusion defects. Subtle CT findings may include the presence of mildly enlarged small arteries with a beaded appearance and smooth or nodular septal thickening. A tree-in-bud pattern may also be observed and is caused by tumor involvement of centrilobular arterioles, combined with a thrombotic microangiopathy. Supportive but nonspecific findings in a tumor embolism include the presence of subpleural wedge-shaped consolidations representing areas of pulmonary infarction and peripheral ground-glass opacities suggesting pulmonary hemorrhage. Widespread tumor emboli may lead to secondary imaging features of pulmonary arterial hypertension and right heart strain.

When tumor emboli are disseminated, the prognosis is grim. Few treatment options are available. However, early targeted chemotherapy may lead to clinically significant improvement for some tumors, such as choriocarcinoma and Wilms tumor.

Amniotic Fluid Embolism

Amniotic fluid embolism is characterized by the transit of fetal squamous cells, mucin, meconium, lanugo hairs, or vernix caseosa into the mother's pulmonary vasculature. It results from forced passage of amniotic fluid into the maternal blood due to tearing of uterine veins during normal labor in 70% of cases. In the remainder, amniotic fluid embolism is caused by placental disruption related to surgery or trauma. Clinical symptoms are dire, with abrupt onset dyspnea and cyanosis progressing rapidly to widespread pulmonary edema, shock, and cardiopulmonary collapse. Maternal and fetal mortality rates are estimated at 80% and 40%, respectively.

Radiographs show diffuse bilateral air space opacities that cannot be distinguished from fulminant pulmonary edema and other cause of acute respiratory distress, such as hemorrhage and aspiration. Areas of consolidation may resolve within several days but can persist. Cardiomegaly may occur due to developing pulmonary hypertension and RV failure (cor pulmonale). CT may show diffuse bilateral ground-glass opacities but its use is limited in practice due to the severity of the disease.

The prognosis in amniotic fluid embolism is ominous. Mortality rates as high as 50% within the first hour of onset have been reported. Treatment options are limited; emergency cesarean section is recommended for the best chances of fetal survival.

Fat Embolism

Fat embolism refers to the migration of fat, usually originating in bone marrow, into the systemic or pulmonary circulation. This causes both obstruction of the vessel and a localized inflammatory response. Fat embolism arises in up to 3% of patients with an isolated long bone fracture, increasing to 33% of patients with severe pelvic trauma. Other causes include major burns, pancreatitis, hemoglobinopathy, and liposuction. A triad of symptoms known as fat embolism syndrome occurs within 12 to 48 hours of the event, consisting of petechial rash, mental status changes, and respiratory distress.

Chest radiographs show bilateral patchy or diffuse air space opacities with a predilection for the lower peripheral lungs, resembling the findings in acute respiratory distress syndrome. The absence of cardiomegaly, pleural effusion, septal lines, and pulmonary venous hypertension allows differentiation from cardiogenic pulmonary edema. Moreover, the radiographic findings in fat embolism are typically delayed by 1 to 2 days from the inciting event. These features help distinguish fat embolism from lung contusion, whose radiographic abnormalities are present immediately, are generally unilateral and asymmetric, and tend to resolve within 1 day. CT demonstrates confluent areas of consolidation, ground-glass opacities, and ill-defined centrilobular and subpleural nodules that can be subtle, and a crazy-paving pattern is also seen. Late in the presentation, diffuse calcifications along the course of peripheral PAs may be present. Visible fat or bone marrow deposits appearing as low-attenuation filling defects may also rarely be observed in the PAs on CT.

No specific treatment exists for fat embolism. Supportive care is essentially the only option. The mortality rate is estimated at 10% to 20%.

Other Pulmonary Vascular Findings

Pulmonary Artery Sarcoma

PA sarcoma is a rare malignancy arising from the PAs, with only several hundred cases reported in the literature. Nevertheless, it is an important entity to consider because it mimics PE. More than 50% of PA sarcomas are initially mistaken for chronic PE. Presenting symptoms such as dyspnea, chest pain, cough, and hemoptysis are nonspecific.

Distinguishing PA sarcoma from embolism by imaging can be challenging. However, several findings should raise suspicion for the diagnosis. On CT, PA sarcoma tends to occupy and expand the entire lumen of the main or proximal right and left PAs, an unusual pattern for PE (Fig. 27.17). This has been termed the *wall eclipsing sign*. Attenuation of the mass can be heterogeneous due to necrosis or hemorrhage, unlike bland thrombus. Patchy

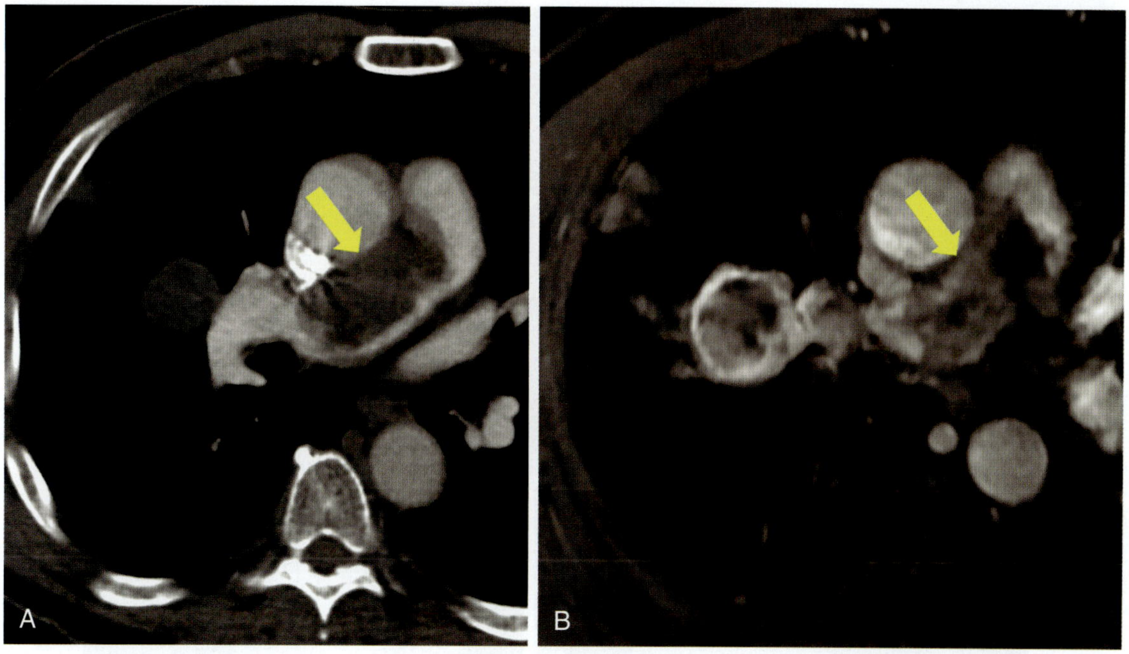

Figure 27.17 Pulmonary artery (PA) sarcoma. (A) CT pulmonary angiography demonstrates a filling defect nearly occluding the right PA *(arrow)*. (B) MRI demonstrates that it enhances heterogeneously, which is characteristic for PA sarcoma. Also note heterogeneously enhancing right lung masses.

and delayed enhancement of the mass may be seen, best visualized on a venous phase. Occasionally, the sarcoma may ossify, although this finding can be confused with calcification in chronic PE. Finally, the degree of arterial obstruction is often out of proportion to symptoms because there has been time to develop collaterals.

In a small pilot study using dual-energy CT, PA sarcoma was associated with significantly higher iodine concentration and iodine-related HU attenuation compared to PE, but this technique is not widely used. On MRI, sarcoma is T1-hyperintense and enhances with IV gadolinium contrast, findings that are not present in chronic PE. Finally, sarcoma, unlike PE, may be FDG-avid on PET. Extension beyond the lumen of the PA and metastatic disease to the lung or mediastinum are definitive features of sarcoma but usually present only late in the course of the disease. An extrathoracic malignancy with a propensity for venous invasion and tumor embolism such as hepatocellular, renal, or adrenal carcinoma should also be excluded.

In situ Pulmonary Artery Thrombus

Clot that arises primarily within the PAs is termed *in situ thrombosis*. This should be distinguished from pulmonary arterial embolism, which originates from a distant source. In situ thrombus is rare but may form when pulmonary arterial pressure approaches that of the systemic arterial system or when there is turbulent pulmonary arterial blood flow, promoting endothelial damage and activating the clotting cascade. In situ thrombus is most commonly seen with significant congenital shunts and resulting severe pulmonary hypertension (Fig. 27.18). It can also be seen with primary pulmonary hypertension, right heart failure, obstructive lung disease, nephrotic syndrome, or as a complication of right heart cauterization. Thrombus at the stump of a pneumonectomy can also be seen but is thought to be of little clinical consequence.

Although distinguishing in situ thrombosis from PE by imaging can be challenging, several features support the diagnosis. In situ thrombus tends to be peripheral and adherent to the arterial wall, in contrast to acute pulmonary emboli, which are usually centrally located. Layering calcifications may also be observed, similar to the calcifications seen with atherosclerotic disease in the systemic arterial system. Treatment focuses on resolving the underlying cause of thrombosis. In contrast to PE, anticoagulation is often not used because it increases the risk of bleeding and often does not resolve the clot.

Pulmonary Hypertension

Pulmonary hypertension (PH) is defined by a mean PA pressure (based on right heart catheterization) >25 mm Hg at rest or >30 mm Hg with exercise. It may be idiopathic but also has a variety of secondary causes, including CTEPH, pulmonary venous hypertension (e.g., from left heart disease), obstructive sleep apnea, lung disease or hypoxemia, and pulmonary vasculature disorders such as the rare pulmonary capillary hemangiomatosis and pulmonary venoocclusive disease. Presenting symptoms such as fatigue and dyspnea are nonspecific and often insidious, resulting in delayed diagnosis.

MDCT is useful in both diagnosing PH and establishing secondary and potentially treatable causes. It has been reported that an MPA transverse diameter ≥29 mm has

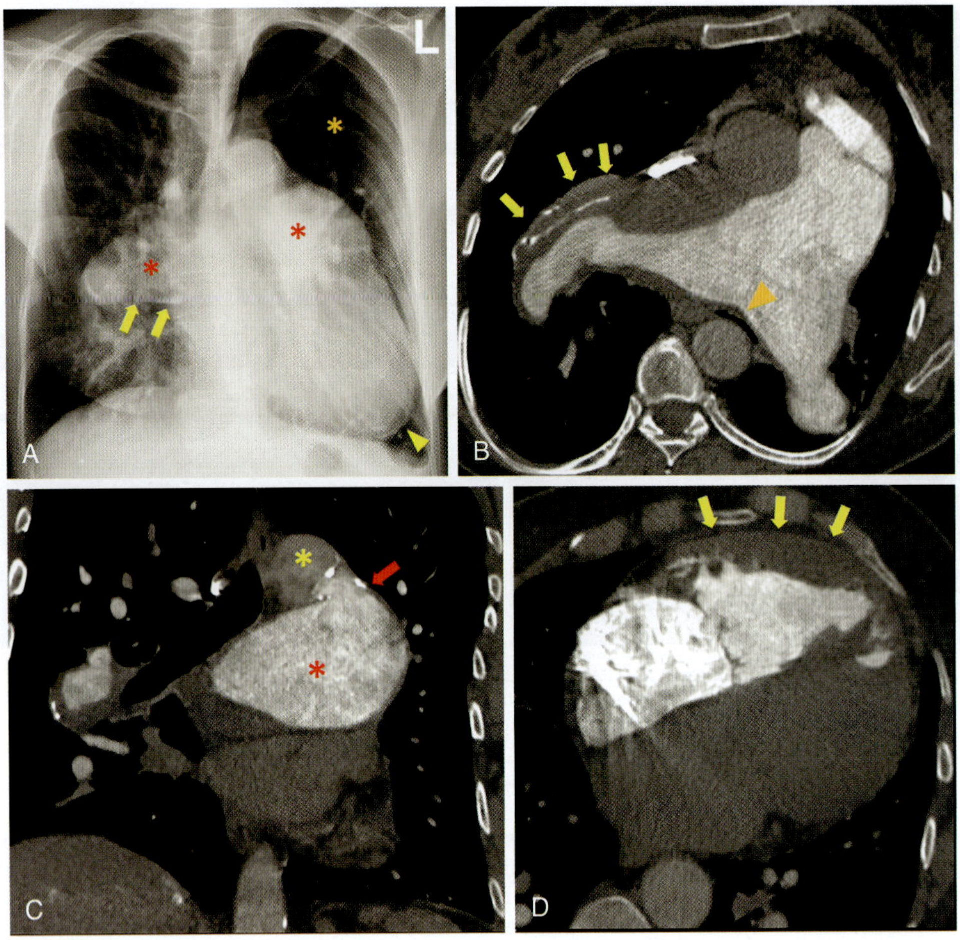

Figure 27.18 (A) Frontal chest radiograph with marked dilation of the pulmonary arteries (PAs; *red asterisks*). Calcified in situ thrombus is seen in the right PA (RPA; *yellow arrows*). There is an upturned cardiac apex *(yellow arrowhead)*, characteristic of right ventricular (RV) dilation. (B) Hyperinflated left lung *(orange asterisk in A)* is due to left bronchus compression by the PAs *(orange arrowhead)* visible on axial CT pulmonary angiography scan. Layering, partially calcified thrombus in the RPA *(yellow arrows)* characteristic of in situ thrombus, is caused by chronic endothelial damage due to severely elevated pulmonary arterial pressures and has similar imaging features to atherosclerotic atheroma in the systemic arteries. Note also the thickened wall of the PA *(arrowhead)*. (C) This degree of PA dilation is usually seen in the setting of a congenital shunt, in this case a patent ductus arteriosus that reopened after a failed repair *(red arrow)*. Blush of contrast from the PA *(red asterisk)* into the aorta *(yellow asterisk)* suggests that pulmonary arterial pressure exceeds systemic arterial pressure, leading to a right-to-left shunt (Eisenmenger syndrome). (D) RV hypertrophy *(yellow arrows)* has developed in response to severe pulmonary hypertension.

an 87% sensitivity and 89% specificity for PH. However many sites use thresholds of ≥33 mm for higher specificity. An MPA-to-ascending aorta diameter ratio >1 also demonstrates a specificity >90% and positive predictive value of 95% for the diagnosis. The right and left PAs are considered enlarged if they are more than 18 to 20 mm at 1 cm from their origin. The lobar arteries are considered dilated if they are larger than their accompanying bronchi. Peripheral vessels may appear tapered due to vasoconstriction.

Secondary cardiac signs include right atrial and RV enlargement, defined by transverse diameters >35 mm and >45 mm, respectively. There may be inversion or bowing of the interventricular septum toward the left ventricle. Reflux of high-attenuation contrast may also be seen into a dilated IVC and hepatic veins. Pericardial effusion or thickening is a feature of more advanced PH. In addition, secondary lung parenchymal findings may be observed, including a mosaic pulmonary parenchymal attenuation pattern, centrilobular ground-glass opacities, septal lines, and small pleural effusions.

Pulmonary Artery Aneurysm

Pulmonary vasculature aneurysms and pseudoaneurysms are rare. They usually arise in the PAs but can affect the pulmonary veins or bronchial arteries. True aneurysms involve all three layers of the vessel wall, whereas false (pseudo) aneurysms do not and, in fact, represent contained ruptures. As in other body regions, an aneurysm is defined as ≥50% focal increase in the diameter of a vessel compared with the adjacent normal vessel. Trauma and infection are two of the most common causes of PA aneurysms. PA aneurysms are also a classic manifestation of the rare vasculitis, Behçet disease.

Traumatic Pseudoaneurysms

Traumatic PA pseudoaneurysms are usually iatrogenic, related to PA catheter (e.g., Swan-Ganz) placement, chest tube insertion, or biopsy, and rarely caused by penetrating or nonpenetrating chest trauma. Presenting symptoms include chest pain, hypoxia, and hemoptysis. Chest radiographs may reveal hilar enlargement, nonspecific consolidation, or an apparent lung nodule or mass. CTA is the imaging test of choice and allows precise characterization of the size, number, location, and extent of pseudoaneurysms. Although pseudoaneurysms vary in shape and dimensions, they usually enhance similarly to the nearby PAs. Central PA injury may result in irregularity of the vessel wall, with associated mediastinal hematoma. Morbidity and mortality rates from ruptured pseudoaneurysms resulting in hemoptysis are high, and thus early recognition and treatment are crucial. Pulmonary arterial coil or balloon embolization is preferred. Second-line management options include surgical ligation, wedge resection, lobectomy, and endovascular stent graft insertion.

Infectious Pseudoaneurysms

Prior to the advent of antibiotics, infectious (mycotic) PA pseudoaneurysms were usually caused by tuberculosis and syphilis. They now typically occur in the setting of infective endocarditis, invasive fungal infection, or IV drug abuse. Mycotic pseudoaneurysms result from bacteremia, with subsequent vasa vasorum embolization, vascular occlusion by septic emboli, or vessel erosion due to adjacent pulmonary infection or lymphatic invasion. Massive hemoptysis is the most feared complication, with a mortality rate exceeding 50%.

Radiographs may show single or multiple rounded nodules, characteristically with lower lung predominance. CT is most useful for precise diagnosis and preprocedural planning. Acutely, mycotic pseudoaneurysms appear as enhancing nodules similar to the attenuation of vessels associated with a cavity or necrotizing pneumonia and may mimic tumor. In subacute and chronic settings, the dilated vessel is the primary imaging finding, with resolution in the surrounding pulmonary parenchymal changes. Rapid change in size of a vascular masslike lesion should raise concern for infection rather than neoplasm. Rasmussen aneurysms are a type of PA pseudoaneurysm caused by tuberculosis. They are typically singular, small (<1 cm), and surrounded by parenchymal consolidation or a lung cavity. However, they may be massive or multiple.

Definitive treatment is surgical, including aneurysmectomy or aneurysmorrhaphy, lobectomy, or banding. Less invasive alternatives include aneurysm occlusion with coils or detachable balloons. Antibiotics are typically administered for at least 6 weeks and are continued until blood cultures are negative and inflammatory markers have normalized.

Behçet Disease

Behçet disease is a chronic relapsing vasculitis with multiorgan involvement. It usually affects Mediterranean, Middle Eastern, and Japanese men in the third decade of life. The classic presentation is uveitis combined with recurrent oral and genital ulcers. Pulmonary involvement occurs in only 5% of patients, usually with late-stage disease. However, PA pseudo aneurysms are among the most common findings in Behçet patients with pulmonary involvement. In fact, the PA is the most frequently involved vessel after the aorta. Multiple bilateral aneurysms ranging from 1 to 7 cm in size is the classic pattern, with a predilection for the right lower lobar PA followed by the right and left PAs. PA pseudoaneurysms in Behçet disease portend a poor prognosis and are associated with massive hemoptysis and a mortality rate of 30% to 50% within 2 years.

On chest radiographs, the most frequent finding is a parahilar nodular or masslike structure that may be bilateral or unilateral. Rarely, the apparent nodule may be located in the lung periphery or large enough to involve the pleural surface. Associated pulmonary parenchymal findings may include wedge-shaped, rounded, irregular, or linear lung opacities representing areas of atelectasis, hemorrhage, or infarction. CT is the preferred modality for diagnosis, showing a contrast-enhancing fusiform or saccular vascular dilation with variable intraluminal thrombus. The PAs distal to the aneurysm also tend to thrombose. Associated features may include venous system involvement, including SVC or brachiocephalic vein occlusion or aneurysmal dilation. Prominent collaterals, including enlarged bronchial arteries and arteriovenous shunts, may also develop. CT also allows more accurate assessment of associated pulmonary parenchymal findings, as well as the pleura (effusions) and mediastinum (pericardial effusion, mediastinitis). A concomitant abdominal aortic aneurysm or occlusion is not uncommon and may be assessed at the same time.

Behçet PA pseudoaneurysms may regress with medical treatments such as corticosteroids and cytostatic agents. However, progressively enlarging pseudoaneurysms or recurrent hemoptysis may necessitate more invasive management. Selective transcatheter embolization using coils or acrylic glue has gained traction over surgery when feasible. If hemoptysis persists despite embolization, bronchial artery embolization may also be considered.

Congenital Abnormalities

A variety of congenital processes may affect the pulmonary vasculature. Two entities with distinct imaging features encountered not uncommonly in radiology practice are pulmonary arteriovenous malformations (AVMs) and partial anomalous pulmonary venous return (PAPVR).

Arteriovenous Malformations

Pulmonary AVMs are direct abnormal communications between PAs and veins. They are highly associated with hereditary hemorrhagic telangiectasia (HHT), or Osler-Weber-Rendu syndrome, an autosomal dominant genetic condition with variable penetrance. As many as 80% of pulmonary AVMs arise in patients with HHT, and up to 35% of HHT patients have pulmonary AVMs. When small, AVMs may be asymptomatic. However, they can enlarge and lead to clinically significant right-to-left shunting, leading to dyspnea on exertion, hypoxia, cyanosis, and clubbing. Shunting also poses a risk of transient ischemic attack or stroke and brain abscess. Hemoptysis or hemothorax may occur in severe cases.

Radiographs are not sensitive but may show opacities corresponding to the AVMs, tend to arise in the peripheral subpleural lower lungs, and characteristically demonstrate at least two branching vessels. MDCT is the preferred test, with a sensitivity of 98%, surpassing even invasive pulmonary angiography. On CT, AVMs appear as serpentine masses with dilated feeding arteries and draining veins. Multiple draining arteries and veins are seen in approximately 20% of cases, and multiple lesions occur more frequently in HHT. Measurement of the arterial feeder diameter is most important; if ≥3 mm, embolization treatment is indicated. Although precise guidelines have not been established, the measurement should be made as close to the AVM nidus as possible and beyond any parenchymal branches. MRA has been show to perform similarly to CT for lesions ≥3 mm and thus is an alternative for AVM follow-up and screening of HHT patients. Concurrent hepatic AVMs are not uncommon, so imaging may be extended to the abdomen.

Coil embolization is now considered the safest and most effective treatment for pulmonary AVMs and is preferred to surgery. Repeated intervention may be needed. If left untouched, AVMs with arterial feeders ≥3 mm pose a 50% risk of stroke, brain abscess, or other complication.

Partial Anomalous Pulmonary Venous Return

PAPVR is a congenital anomaly characterized by abnormal drainage of one to three pulmonary veins into systemic veins or the right atrium rather than the left atrium, creating a left-to-right shunt. Its prevalence is estimated at 0.7% of the general population. The disorder is associated with Turner syndrome and atrial septal defects. Most commonly, the left upper pulmonary vein drains into the left brachiocephalic vein. Bilateral PAPVR is seen in 4% of cases. Direct drainage to the right atrium is rare. Scimitar syndrome is a specific type of PAPVR in which an anomalous, crescent-shaped pulmonary vein (resembling the Turkish scimitar sword on imaging) usually drains the entire right lung; common concurrent abnormalities include cardiac dextroposition, right lung hypoplasia, and systemic arterial supply to the right lower lung from the abdominal aorta. Although PAPVR is usually incidental and asymptomatic, a significant shunt can lead to symptoms of dyspnea, fatigue, palpitations, and chest pain.

Radiographic findings depend on the PAPVR anatomy and degree of shunt but include an abnormal left mediastinal contour representing a so-called vertical vein, a thickened right paratracheal stripe corresponding to a dilated SVC, cardiomegaly with right atrial and ventricular enlargement, pulmonary edema, and dilated central PAs. CT or MRI is the preferred imaging test, with a sensitivity approaching 100% for the diagnosis of PAPVR. CT allows precise delineation of the aberrant veins and any associated cardiovascular or lung anomalies. Alternatively, MRI has the added benefit of allowing quantification of the degree of left-to-right shunting via the Qp:Qs ratio, with a Qp:Qs >1.5 as a commonly referenced threshold for pursuing surgical correction. Many patients with PAPVR will also have a sinus venosus atrial septal defect, which is best visualized on cardiac MRI.

Bibliography

Bhalla S, Raptis CA. Vascular chest emergencies. In: Mirvis SE, Kubal WS, Shanmuganathan K, Soto JA, Yu JS, eds. *Problem Solving in Emergency Radiology*. 1st ed. Elsevier; 2013:231–242.

Carter BW, Abbott GF. Pulmonary arteries. In: Abbara S, Kalva SP, eds. *Problem Solving in Cardiovascular Imaging*. 1st ed. Elsevier; 2013:668–684.

Ceylan N, Bayraktaroglu S, Erturk SM, Savas R, Alper H. Pulmonary and vascular manifestations of Behcet disease: imaging findings. *AJR Am J Roentgenol*. 2010;194(2):W158–W164.

Chen MM, Coakley FV, Kaimal A, Laros RK Jr. Guidelines for computed tomography and magnetic resonance imaging use during pregnancy and lactation. *Obstet Gynecol*. 2008;112(2 Pt 1):333–340.

D'Avila A, Scanavacca M, Sosa E, Ruskin JN, Reddy VY. Pericardial anatomy for the interventional electrophysiologist. *J Cardiovasc Electrophysiol*. 2003;14(4):422–430.

Ghaye B, Ghuysen A, Bruyere PJ, D'Orio V, Dondelinger RF. Can CT pulmonary angiography allow assessment of severity and prognosis in patients presenting with pulmonary embolism? What the radiologist needs to know. *Radiographics*. 2006;26(1):23–39.

Gilman MD, Kazerooni EA Standardized reporting of CT pulmonary angiography for acute pulmonary embolism; 2014. https://www.rsna.org/uploadedFiles/RSNA/Content/Science_and_Education/Quality/Standardized%20Reporting%20of%20CT%20Pulmonary%20Angiography%20for%20Acute%20Pulmonary%20Embolism.pdf. Accessed August 10, 2015.

Hunsaker AR, Lu MT, Goldhaber SZ, Rybicki FJ. Imaging in acute pulmonary embolism with special clinical scenarios. *Circ Cardiovasc Imaging*. 2010;3(4):491–500.

Kwak MK, Kim WY, Lee CW, et al. The impact of saddle embolism on the major adverse event rate of patients with non-high-risk pulmonary embolism. *Br J Radiol*. 2013;86(1032):20130273.

Lacomis JM, Wigginton W, Fuhrman C, Schwartzman D, Armfield DR, Pealer KM. Multi-detector row CT of the left atrium and pulmonary veins before radio-frequency catheter ablation for atrial fibrillation. *Radiographics*. 2003;23 Spec No:S35–S48, discussion S48–S50.

Leung AN, Bull TM, Jaeschke R, et al. American Thoracic Society documents: an official American Thoracic Society/Society of Thoracic Radiology clinical practice guideline—evaluation of suspected pulmonary embolism in pregnancy. *Radiology*. 2012;262(2):635–646.

Lu MT, Cai T, Ersoy H, et al. Interval increase in right-left ventricular diameter ratios at CT as a predictor of 30-day mortality after acute pulmonary embolism: initial experience. *Radiology*. 2008;246(1):281–287.

Lu MT, Demehri S, Cai T, et al. Axial and reformatted 4-chamber RV/LV diameter ratios on CT pulmonary angiography as predictors of death after acute pulmonary embolism. *AJR Am J Roentgenol*. 2012;198(6):1353–1360.

Meinel FG, Nance JW, Schoepf UJ, et al. Predictive value of computed tomography in acute pulmonary embolism: systematic review and meta-analysis. *Am J Med*. 2015;128(7):747–759.

Nguyen ET, Silva CI, Seely JM, Chong S, Lee KS, Muller NL. Pulmonary artery aneurysms and pseudoaneurysms in adults: findings at CT and radiography. *AJR Am J Roentgenol*. 2007;188(2):W126–W134.

Pahade JK, Litmanovich D, Pedrosa I, Romero J, Bankier AA, Boiselle PM. Quality initiatives: imaging pregnant patients with suspected pulmonary embolism: what the radiologist needs to know. *Radiographics*. 2009;29(3):639–654.

Porres DV, Morenza OP, Pallisa E, Roque A, Andreu J, Martinez M. Learning from the pulmonary veins. *Radiographics*. 2013;33(4):999–1022.

Rajiah P, Desai MY. Pulmonary veins, atria, and atrial appendage. In: Abbara S, Kalva SP, eds. *Problem Solving in Cardiovascular Imaging*. 1st ed. Elsevier; 2013:643–656.

Stein PD, Chenevert TL, Fowler SE, et al. Gadolinium-enhanced magnetic resonance angiography for pulmonary embolism: a multicenter prospective study (PIOPED III). *Ann Intern Med*. 2010;152(7):434–443, w142–w143.

Stein PD, Yaekoub AY, Matta F, et al. Resolution of pulmonary embolism on CT pulmonary angiography. *AJR Am J Roentgenol*. 2010;194(5):1263–1268.

Wieseler KM, Bhargava P, Kanal KM, Vaidya S, Stewart BK, Dighe MK. Imaging in pregnant patients: examination appropriateness. *Radiographics*. 2010;30(5):1215–1229, discussion 1230–1233.

Wittram C. How I do it: CT pulmonary angiography. *AJR Am J Roentgenol*. 2007;188(5):1255–1261.

Wittram C, Kalra MK, Maher MM, Greenfield A, McLoud TC, Shepard JA. Acute and chronic pulmonary emboli: angiography-CT correlation. *AJR Am J Roentgenol*. 2006;186(6 suppl 2):S421–S429.

Wittram C, Maher MM, Halpern EF, Shepard JA. Attenuation of acute and chronic pulmonary emboli. *Radiology*. 2005;235(3):1050–1054.

Wittram C, Maher MM, Yoo AJ, Kalra MK, Shepard JO, McLoud TC. CT angiography of pulmonary embolism: diagnostic criteria and causes of misdiagnosis. *Radiographics*. 2004;24:1219–1238.

CHAPTER 28
Congenital Heart and Vascular Disease

Carlos A. Rojas and Tony Hany Fattouch

CHAPTER OUTLINE

Introduction

Congenital heart and vascular diseases are relatively uncommon malformations of the heart or great vessels that occur during embryologic development. With advances in medical and surgical treatments, most patients survive into adulthood, and it is imperative for the chest radiologist to be familiar with the imaging findings of common malformations and their postoperative appearance. Although echocardiography remains the first step in the assessment of these patients, these imaging modalities, with technical advances in CT and MRI, have become key elements in the evaluation of the anatomy and detection of the defects and functional assessment of patients with congenital heart and vascular abnormalities.

Imaging Techniques

Both electrocardiographic (ECG)-gated CT and MRI play important roles in the detection of congenital anomalies of the heart and great vessels.

Electrocardiographic-Gated CT

This is an imaging modality with great spatial resolution and is therefore a useful tool to assess congenital anatomic defects, associated abnormalities, postoperative anatomy, and complications in the postoperative patient. Each examination should be tailored to answer the clinical question posed. Unenhanced, low-dose images are typically useful to identify high-density postoperative changes and avoid misinterpretation of the contrast-enhanced images. The contrast injection protocol, contrast volume, and/or contrast mix should be determined specifically for each patient. With the use of ECG gating, coronary artery analysis can be performed. Although cardiac MRI is more accurate in the evaluation of ventricular volumes and function, ventricular volumes and function can also be quantified using dedicated postprocessing software with the use of retrospective gating CT imaging. The use of delayed imaging can be helpful when trying to assess patency of baffles and/or conduits, especially in patients with Fontan morphology, due to their delayed filling.

Cardiac MRI

Cardiac MRI allows evaluation of the anatomy and functionality of the heart. It is the gold standard for the evaluation of ventricular volumes and function. Every cardiac MRI examination is tailored to answer the clinical question presented. The use of noncine, black blood, and bright blood sequences through the chest are useful in the assessment of the mediastinum and great vessels. The use of bright blood cine images is useful in the assessment of the anatomy and functionality of the heart.

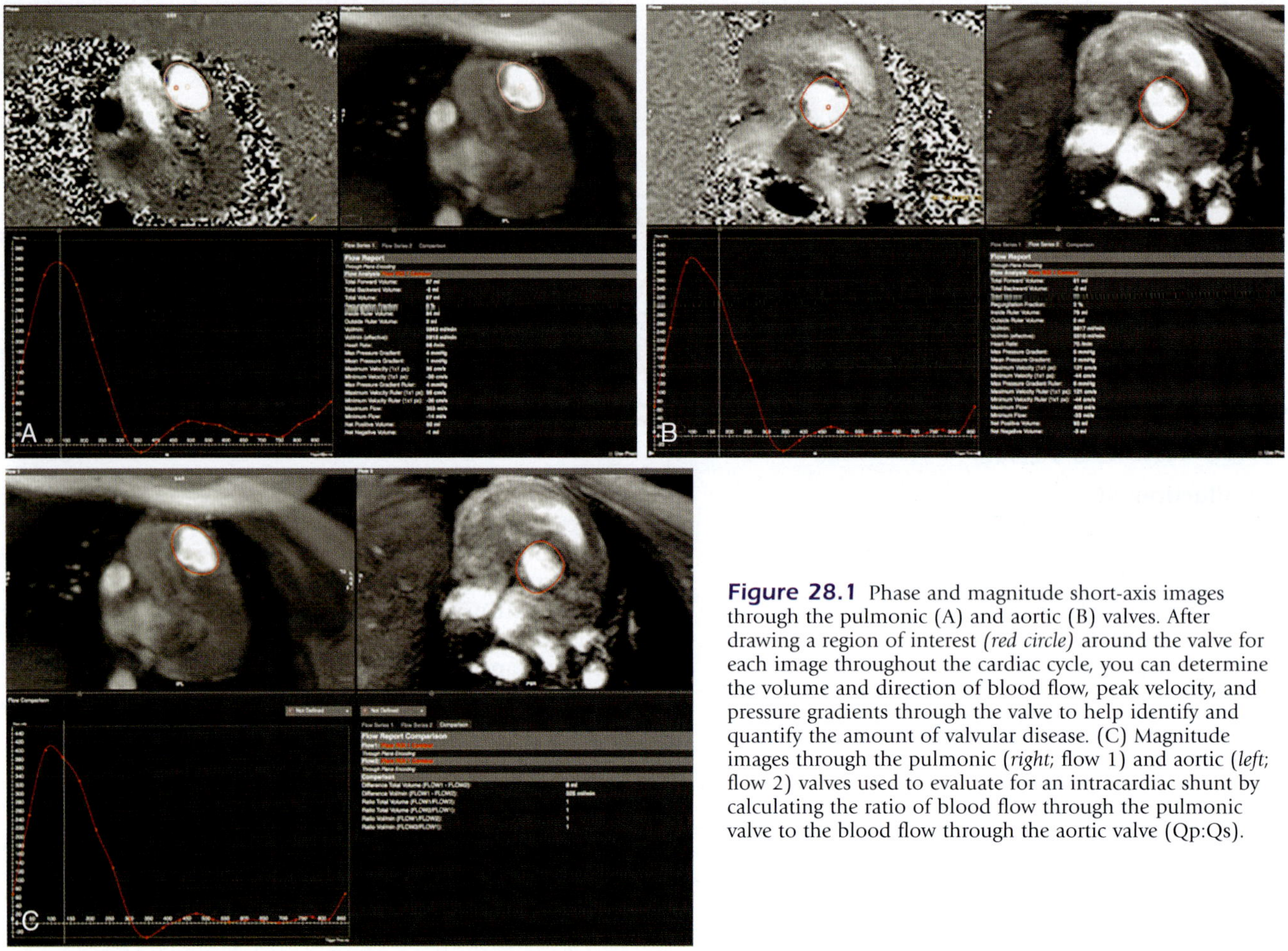

Figure 28.1 Phase and magnitude short-axis images through the pulmonic (A) and aortic (B) valves. After drawing a region of interest *(red circle)* around the valve for each image throughout the cardiac cycle, you can determine the volume and direction of blood flow, peak velocity, and pressure gradients through the valve to help identify and quantify the amount of valvular disease. (C) Magnitude images through the pulmonic (*right*; flow 1) and aortic (*left*; flow 2) valves used to evaluate for an intracardiac shunt by calculating the ratio of blood flow through the pulmonic valve to the blood flow through the aortic valve (Qp:Qs).

Phase contrast images are performed to quantify flow and velocities through a particular imaging plane. Phase contrast images are prescribed orthogonal to the blood flow being assessed to obtain the most accurate evaluation. Phase contrast images allow reproducible flow and velocity quantification and are commonly used during valvular assessment (Fig. 28.1). In patients with congenital heart disease, this imaging technique becomes paramount for the evaluation of intracardiac shunts by quantifying Qp:Qs and by quantifying valvular function. MRI angiography is often used in the assessment of vascular anatomy and associated abnormalities.

■ General Approach

It is important to have a systematic review of patients with complex congenital heart disease to ensure that all relevant abnormalities are detected and the report is complete. Analysis of the chest should start with assessment of the aortic arch (left or right) and branching pattern. The most common anomalies of the arch are a right-sided arch with mirror image branching pattern (highly associated with congenital heart defects) and a right-sided aortic arch with an aberrant left subclavian artery. It is also important to evaluate the aorta caliber to exclude aneurysm formation as well as detect areas of narrowing, in particular at the aortic isthmus, as can be seen in coarctation. Evaluation of the pulmonary arteries should follow to assess for enlargement of the main pulmonary artery (PA), which is commonly seen in patients with elevated pulmonary arterial pressures. Evaluation of the pulmonary branch arteries can reveal areas of stenosis. Venous connections should be assessed for normal drainage patterns. The most common venous anomaly is a persistent left superior vena cava (SVC). This vein normally courses to the left of the aortic arch and drains into the coronary sinus. Rarely, this vein drains into the left atrium, creating a right-to-left shunt. It is important to review the connections of the pulmonary veins into the left atrium to exclude anomalous pulmonary venous return. When evaluating the heart, it is important to remember the segmental approach developed by Van Praagh et al. based on embryologic development. It consists of three steps. The first is to determine the visceroatrial situs; the second consists of determining the morphologic right versus left ventricle and their relation to each other; and the third consists of defining the ventriculoarterial (VA) connections and their relation to each other.

The orientation of the base-apex of the heart should be described separately—dextrocardia, mesocardia, and levocardia. The position of the heart within the chest should also be described separately (levoposition, dextroposition, mesoposition). Situs ambiguous, situs inversus with levocardia, and situs solitus with dextrocardia are usually associated with congenital heart defects.

The first step is to determine the visceroatrial situs, which is defined as the relationship between the atria and thoracoabdominal organs. To determine which of the two atria is the morphologic left or right atrium, look at the shape of the atrial appendage. The left atrial appendage has an elongated, finger-like shape; the right atrial appendage has a broad base attachment and triangular shape (Fig. 28.2). Another clue in deciding the left versus the right atrium is the venoatrial concordance. The right atrium is the chamber receiving the inferior vena cava (IVC). When neither of these two methods works to determine the morphologic left versus right atrium, the right atrium should be considered the atrium on the side of the trilobed lung. Once you have determined the left versus right atrium, you now have to determine the position of the liver, spleen, and stomach. There are three types of situs—situs solitus, which is the normal arrangement, situs inversus, which the opposite of the normal arrangement, and situs ambiguous, which is the in-between arrangement. The situs ambiguous is also known as the *heterotaxy syndrome* and can be further classified into bilateral right sidedness (asplenia) and bilateral left sidedness (polysplenia).

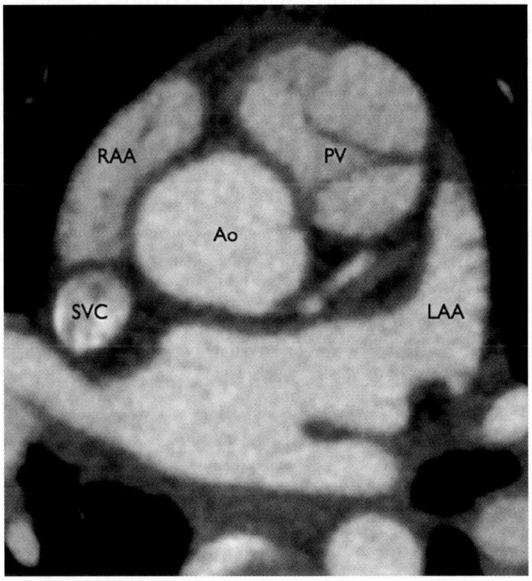

Figure 28.2 Axial oblique image at the level of the atrial appendages from cardiac CT demonstrates the typical broad-based attachment and triangular shape of the right atrial appendage *(RAA)* and the typical, elongated finger-like shape of the left atrial appendage *(LAA)*. *Ao*, Aorta; *PV*, pulmonary valve; *SVC*, superior vena cava.

The second step consists of determining the ventricular loop orientation. To determine the rotation of the ventricle, you first have to identify the morphologic right ventricle. The most helpful way to recognize the right ventricle is to identify a muscular infundibulum and resultant muscular separation between the atrioventricular (AV) and semilunar valves (Fig. 28.3). Other important characteristics of the morphologic right ventricle include the presence of a septal leaflet in the AV valve, the presence of a moderator band, papillary muscles that attach to the septum and free wall, and interventricular septal trabeculation. A D-looped right ventricle is the normal looping of the heart, with the right ventricle located on the right position and the aortic valve located to the left of the pulmonic valve. An L-looped right ventricle will have the morphologic right ventricle in the left position and the aortic valve to the left of the pulmonic valve.

The third step includes identifying the position and origin of the great vessels. The normal position of the great vessels is with the PA origin located anterior and to the left of the ascending aorta. Situs inversus in the opposite. In D-transposition, the aorta is located anteriorly and arises from the right ventricle. In L-transposition, there is an anteriorly located aorta arising from the morphologic right ventricle, which is located on the left and is connected

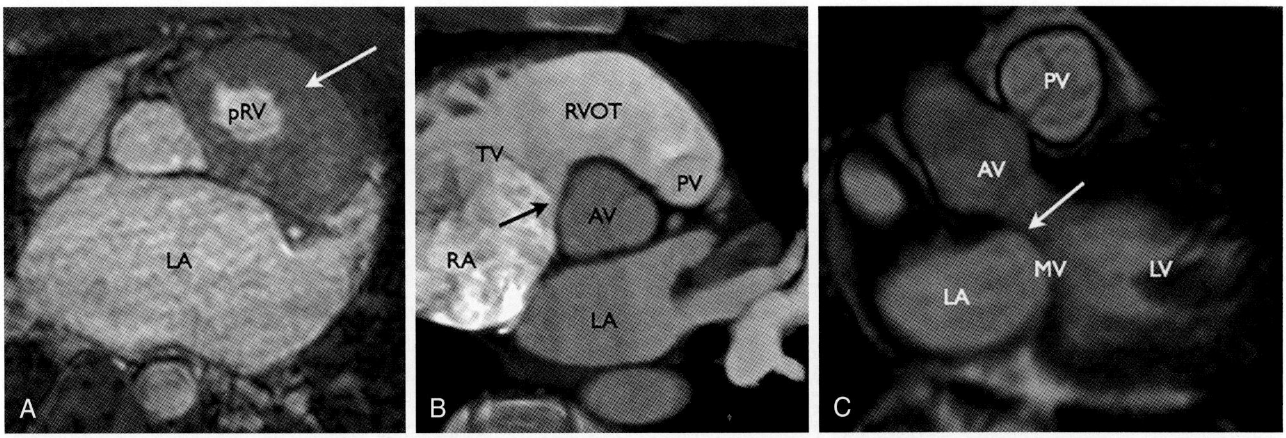

Figure 28.3 (A) Axial image from a contrast-enhanced ECG-gated, respiratory-navigated MR angiography of the chest demonstrates the muscular infundibulum *(white arrow)* of the right ventricle in this patient with a congenitally corrected L-transposition of the great arteries. (B) Short-axis view of the aortic valve *(AV)* from cardiac CT demonstrates the muscular separation between the atrioventricular and semilunar valves *(black arrow)*, which is characteristic of the right ventricle. (C) Steady-state free precession cine image of the pulmonic valve *(PV)* demonstrates the lack of a muscular separation between the atrioventricular and semilunar valves *(white arrow)*, characteristic for the left ventricle *(LV)*. *LA*, Left atrium; *MV*, mitral valve; *pRV*, pulmonic right ventricle; *RVOT*, right ventricular outflow tract; *TV*, tricuspid valve.

to the left atrium. This results in the morphologic right ventricle to the left of the pulmonic valve. The term *D and L malposition* refers to a normal origin but abnormal position of the great vessels in the chest.

■ Bicuspid Aortic Valve

A bicuspid aortic valve is one of the most common types of congenital heart disease, with an estimated incidence of 0.9% to 2%. It is more common in males than in females, with a 2 to 3 : 1 ratio. It is inherited as an autosomal dominant trait with incomplete penetrance and results in incomplete separation of the valve leaflets during development. The most common leaflets to demonstrate the incomplete separation are the left and right cusps (70%–86%), followed by the right and noncoronary cusp (12%). It is imperative to assess the aortic valve morphology during systole because a raphe (fibrous ridge at the site of fusion of the conjoined cusps) can simulate a trileaflet valve during diastole. Bicuspid aortic valves can be associated with aortic coarctation, supravalvular aortic stenosis, subvalvular aortic stenosis, ventricular septal defects (VSDs), patent ductus arteriosus (PDA), and sinus of Valsalva aneurysms (Fig. 28.4). Patients with a bicuspid aortic valve develop aortic stenosis more commonly than patients with a trileaflet valve. To a lesser degree, these patients can also develop aortic regurgitation. Bicuspid aortic valve is considered a risk for infective endocarditis and is often associated with aortic root or ascending aortic dilation. Associated syndromes include Loeys-Dietz and Turner syndromes.

Echocardiography is the most common imaging modality to assess and follow up patients with a bicuspid aortic valve. Its high temporal and spatial resolution, ability to quantify velocities, gradients, and valve areas, as well as the lack of use of ionizing radiation and nephrotoxic contrast agents, make it the imaging modality of choice.

The use of CT and MRI has been growing, in particular in the preoperative evaluation of the aorta and in the follow-up of a thoracic aortic aneurysm. CT, with the use of multiplanar reformats, is a very accurate and reproducible method of measuring the aorta. The use of a retrospective ECG-gated acquisition allows for the morphologic assessment of the valve and planimetry of the valve opening area and/or regurgitant orifice. Cardiac MRI allows for anatomic assessment similar to CT and, with the use of phase contrast images, allows quantification of peak velocities to determine the peak systolic gradient (using the modified Bernoulli equation: gradient $= 4v^2$, where $v =$ velocity) to determine the severity of aortic stenosis and flow quantification and the degree of aortic regurgitation.

The type of surgical procedure in a patient with a bicuspid aortic valve depends on whether the patient needs aortic valve intervention, aortic repair, or both. Aortic valve intervention without repair of the aorta can be performed by aortic valvuloplasty, surgical aortic valve replacement, or the Ross procedure. Transcatheter aortic valve replacement has an uncertain role in patients with a bicuspid aortic valve due to the lack of experience. Aortic valvuloplasty or balloon valvotomy is not recommended in older patients with calcified leaflets. It has a role in adolescents and young adults with aortic stenosis without significant calcification. Surgical intervention in adolescents or young adults with symptomatic bicuspid aortic valve is usually accomplished with a bioprosthetic valve. The use of a pulmonary autograft and right-sided reconstruction with a pulmonary homograft (Ross procedure) is limited due to its technical complexity and complications in the aortic autograft, the pulmonic homograft, and the availability of simpler and more effective alternatives (e.g., mechanical and bioprostheses, including stentless bioprosthetic valves).

Combined aortic valve replacement and ascending aorta repair can be done with a prosthetic aortic valve and supracoronary aortic graft. In patients who need aortic valve replacement and have a dilated aortic root and ascending aorta, a composite graft that includes the aortic valve, aortic root, and ascending aorta can be used (Bentall procedure). Re-implantation of the coronaries is needed in this type of procedure. Surgery to replace the aortic root or ascending aorta in patients with a bicuspid aortic valve is performed when the aortic root or ascending aorta measures 5.5 cm or greater. If there is a family history of aortic dissection or rapid growth

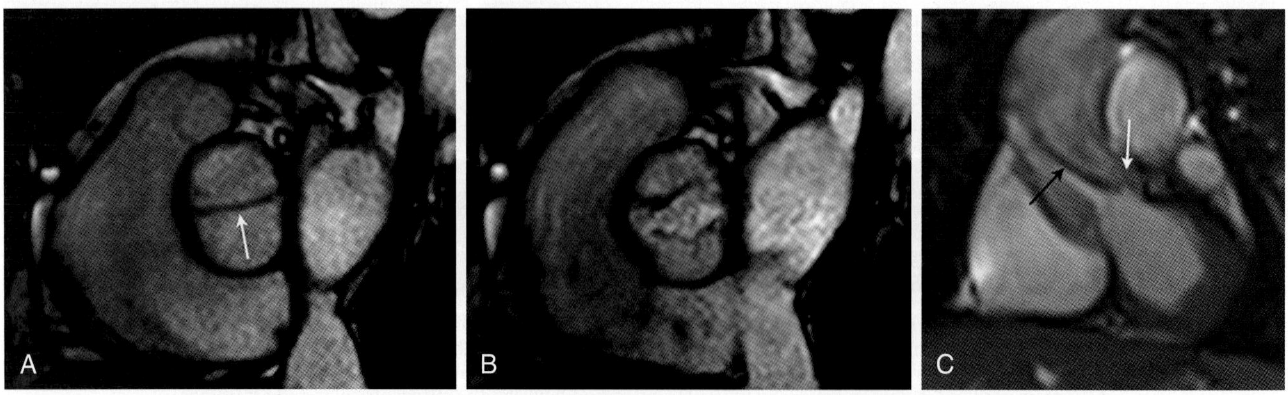

Figure 28.4 Oblique axial steady-state free precession (SSFP) images in both diastole (A) and systole (B) demonstrate a bicuspid morphology of the aortic valve with a fishmouth opening. Note the presence of only a single commissure. (C) Oblique coronal SSFP image during systole demonstrates the typical doming of the aortic valve leaflets *(white arrow)* with a dephasing jet of associated aortic stenosis *(black arrow)*.

(>5 mm/year), surgery is suggested at 5.1 to 5.5 cm. If the patient is undergoing aortic valve surgery due to severe stenosis or regurgitation, the aorta should be repaired if larger than 4.5 cm. Repair of the aortic bicuspid valve depends on the patient's symptoms.

■ Aortic Coarctation

Aortic coarctation is a congenital narrowing of the descending thoracic aorta, typically at the level of the ductus arteriosus (DA). It accounts for approximately 4% to 6% of all congenital heart defects and occurs more in males than in females. The cause is unknown, but underdevelopment of the aortic arch secondary to decreased anterograde flow and extension of ductal tissue into the wall of the aorta are the two leading theories. A genetic predisposition is present, given the association with Turner syndrome.

Aortic coarctation is usually seen in conjunction with other congenital abnormalities, including bicuspid aortic valve, single-ventricle variants, endocardial cushion defects, D-transposition, VSDs, atrial septal defects (ASDs), PDA, and aortic or subaortic stenosis (Fig. 28.5). Close association with an aortic aneurysm is also common.

The clinical presentation varies depending on the severity of the narrowing. In cases of severe narrowing, patients present in the neonatal age with heart failure due to increased left ventricular (LV) afterload once the PDA closes. In cases of mild narrowing, patients can go unrecognized until they are adults. In these patients, systolic hypertension recorded in the upper extremities, with low blood pressure in the lower extremities and diminished or delayed femoral pulses, is the classic clinical presentation.

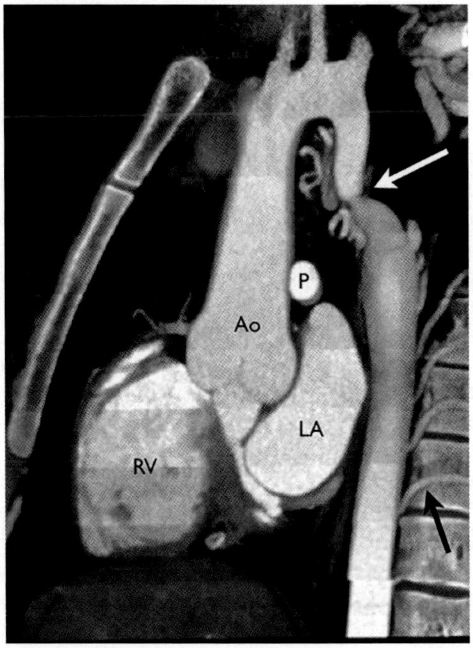

Figure 28.5 Sagittal volume-rendered image from a chest CT scan demonstrates an aortic coarctation *(white arrow)* occurring within the aortic isthmus. Note how there are multiple thoracic collaterals *(black arrow)*. *Ao*, Aorta; *LA*, left atrium; *P*, pulmonary artery; *RV*, right ventricle.

There is a spectrum of anatomic variants, from the classic short-segment coarctation that includes long segmental narrowing, tubular hypoplasia, and pseudocoarctation. ECG-gated CT is a helpful imaging tool for the anatomic assessment of aortic coarctation before and after treatment. With CT's great spatial resolution, the area of narrowing can be accurately measured. Furthermore, with the visualization of the entire chest during the same image acquisition, you can assess for the presence of collateral vascularity. CT is commonly used as a diagnostic tool and for the follow-up of patients after surgical correction. Cardiac MRI and MR angiography (MRA) are also helpful for the evaluation of these patients and do not use ionizing radiation. With the use of phase contrast images, prescribed at and a few centimeters distal to the coarctation, flow and velocity across the coarctation can be quantified. Using the peak velocity and modified Bernoulli equation (gradient = $4v^2$), the peak gradient across the coarctation can be estimated. Furthermore, with the prescription of phase contrast images of the distal thoracic aorta (at the level of the diaphragm), you can assess for recruitment of blood flow through collateral vascularity. Any increase in blood flow in the distal descending thoracic aorta relative to the flow at or just distal to the coarctation is considered abnormal and is suggestive of collateral vascularity.

Treatment of aortic coarctation should be performed as early as possible. The type of treatment used (balloon angioplasty ± stenting vs. surgery) depends on the expertise of the treating team and associated malformations.

Problem Solving

Trying to differentiate between coarctation and pseudocoarctation can be difficult. The imaging characteristics that can differentiate them are as follows.

An elongated aorta anchored at the ligament arteriosus is compatible with a pseudocoarctation. It is also called *kinking or buckling of the aorta*. No significant narrowing is noted in pseudocoarctation with gradients less than 20 mm Hg on MRI phase contrast images. No collateral vascularity is present with pseudocoarctation.

■ Atrial Septal Defects

ASDs account for approximately 13% of congenital heart disorders. ASDs can be classified as defects resulting from abnormal development of the interatrial septum (e.g., in ostium secundum and ostium primum defects) and defects resulting in interatrial communication with a normally developed interatrial septum (e.g., sinus venosus and unroofed coronary sinus defects).

It is important to discuss the embryologic development of the interatrial septum briefly to understand ASDs and their imaging appearance better. The normal septation of the atria begins in the fifth week of gestation, with the septum primum growing from the superior aspect of the common atria down toward the endocardial cushions. The gap between the free end of the septum primum and the endocardial cushions is called the *ostium primum*. The fusion between the septum primum and the endocardial cushions closes the ostium primum. Multiple small fenestrations (that later coalesce) occur in the septum primum, called the *ostium secundum*. The septum secundum forms as an invagination of the atrial wall to the right of the septum primum. As the septum secundum continues to grow caudally, it eventually covers the ostium secundum. It is important to know that the septum secundum does not completely divide the two atria, leaving an oval-shaped hole called the *fossa ovalis*. The fossa ovalis is covered solely by the overlapping septum primum. At birth, with the expansion of the lungs, the right-sided pressures drop, causing a left-to-right gradient, which results in permanent opposition of the septum primum against the septum secundum. In two-thirds of the population, the septum primum fuses permanently with the septum secundum and, in the remaining population, there is a probe-patent fossa ovalis (patent foramen ovale [PFO]; Fig. 28.6).

An ostium primum ASD corresponds to 15% to 20% of all ASDs. It results from an abnormal fusion between the septum primum and endocardial cushions, resulting in a persistent ostium primum defect. It is considered the mildest form of an endocardial cushion defect. This type of defect is uncommon and usually is seen as part of an endocardial cushion defect, with an associated VSD and mitral and/or tricuspid valve clefts (Fig. 28.7A and B).

An ostium secundum ASD corresponds to 70% of all ASDs. It results from excessive apoptosis of the septum primum or incomplete development of the septum secundum, resulting in a defect in the fossa ovalis region. These defects are more common in females than in males. Although most of these defects occur sporadically, there are rare familial cases. Single or multiple defects can be present. The defects can vary in size and shape. These defects can associate with other septal defects (e.g., primum or sinus venosus) and/or extracardiac abnormalities as in Holt-Oram syndrome (autosomal dominant; limb defects and septal defects; see Fig. 28.7C and D).

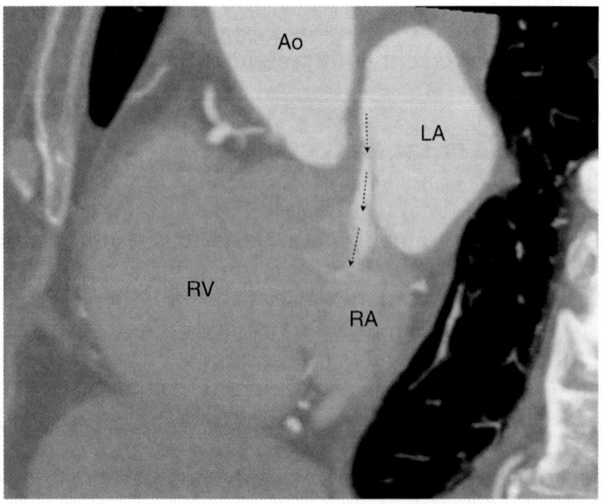

Figure 28.6 Sagittal oblique image from a cardiac CT scan in a 42-year-old man with atypical chest pain. Incidentally noted is a high-attenuation jet directed from the left atrium to the right atrium *(black dashed arrows)* through a patent foramen ovale. *Ao*, Aorta; *LA*, left atrium; *RA*, right atrium; *RV*, right ventricle.

Sinus venosus ASDs are defects located between the venous inflow of the SVC or IVC and left atrium. These account for 5% to 10% of all ASDs. The superior sinus venosus defects are more common than inferior defects. Both types of defects are associated with partial anomalous pulmonary venous return. These defects result in left-to-right shunting at the level of the atria, with an intact interatrial septum. They are thought to result from lack of septation between the right superior pulmonary vein and SVC (superior sinus venosus) or right inferior pulmonary vein and IVC (inferior sinus venosus; Fig. 28.8).

Coronary sinus defects (also called *unroofed coronary sinuses*) are the least common type of ASDs, accounting for less than 1%. They result from lack of separation between the atrial wall and coronary sinus. A large percentage of these patients also have a persistent left SVC (Fig. 28.9).

The treatment options of ASDs vary, depending on the type of defect, size of the defect, number of defects, and associated abnormalities. It is performed in patients with significant left-to-right shunting (Qp:Qs >1.5). It is important to know that large defects can result in significant dilation of the right-sided chambers and elevation of right heart pressures. When elevation of the pulmonary arterial pressure surpasses the systemic pressure shunt, reversal occurs. At this point, these patients are dependent on the high PA pressures to force blood across the capillary bed, and therefore surgical correction is contraindicated. Usually, ASDs are repaired surgically. Percutaneous closure of secundum ASDs can be performed safely in patients with single small defects.

Problem Solving

Sinus venosus defects with anomalous pulmonary venous return are difficult to recognize with transthoracic echocardiography due to their location. In patients with a suspected intracardiac shunt and normal appearance of the interatrial septum on echocardiography, further evaluation with CT or MRA should be performed. Think of sinus venosus defects in a patient with a positive bubble study, enlarged right-sided chambers in which the septal defect cannot be clearly seen by transthoracic echocardiography. These patients typically present with a dilated right heart and pulmonary hypertension from chronic right-sided volume overload. On CT or MR images these defects are seen as an abnormal communication between the SVC or IVC and left atrium. They are associated with a partial anomalous pulmonary venous return into the SVC, IVC, or right atrium.

Differentiating between a secundum-type ASD and PFO can be challenging. A PFO is not considered an ASD, given that there is normal development of the atrial septal structures. It is the lack of fusion between the septum primum and septum secundum that results in a potential communication between these two chambers, a PFO. A PFO is present in one-third of the population. The flow through a PFO can be continuous or intermittent. A secundum defect results from an abnormal development of the septum primum and/or septum secundum, resulting in

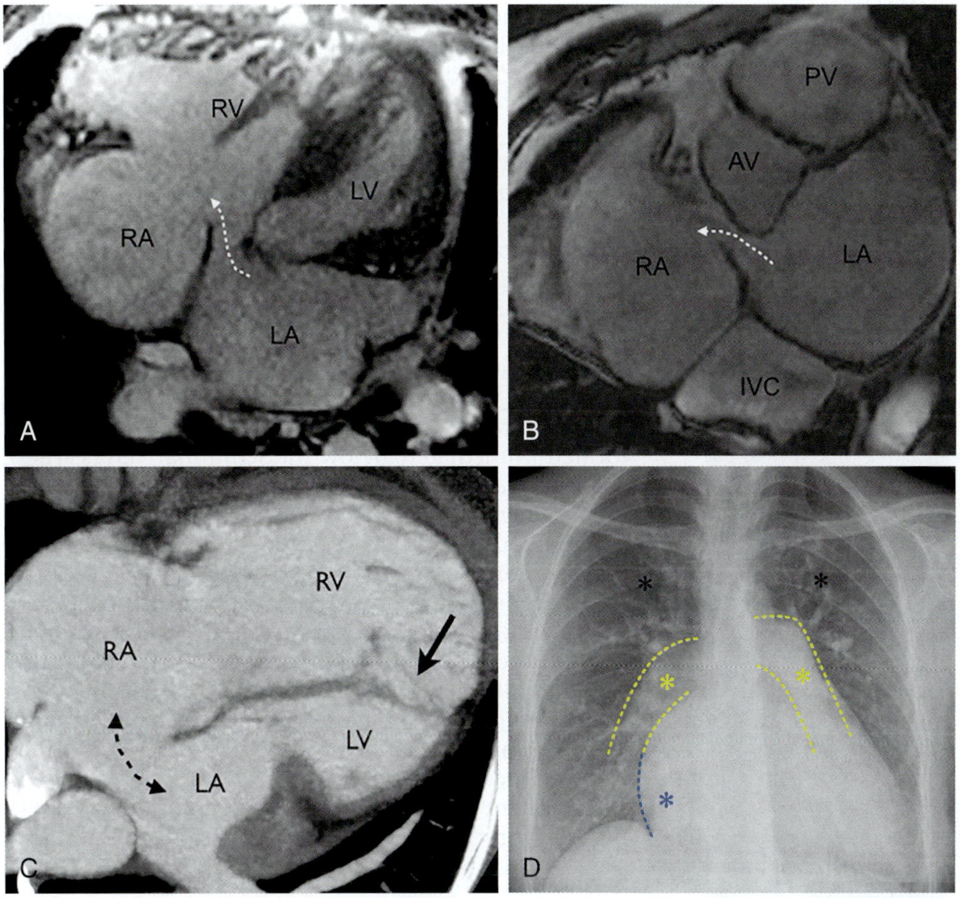

Figure 28.7 (A and B) Four-chamber (B) and short-axis (C) steady-state free precession images demonstrate an ostium primum atrial septal defect *(white dashed arrow)*. Note the secondary right ventricular enlargement. (C) Four-chamber image from cardiac CT demonstrates a large ostium secundum atrial septal defect with free interatrial communication *(black dashed arrow)*. Note the typical appearance of a left-to-right shunted heart with increased right-sided pressures, evidenced by massive dilation of the right-sided heart chambers and leftward bowing of the interventricular septum *(black arrow)*. (D) Frontal PA chest radiograph demonstrates the typical appearance of a left-to-right shunted heart. Note how the right atrium *(blue dashed line)* is dilated *(blue asterisk)*. The pulmonary arteries *(yellow dashed lines)* are also enlarged *(yellow asterisks)*, and there is resulting increased pulmonary vasculature throughout both lungs *(black asterisks)*. *AV*, Aortic valve; *IVC*, inferior vena cava; *LA*, left atrium; *LV*, left ventricle; *PV*, pulmonic valve; *RA*, right atrium; *RV*, right ventricle.

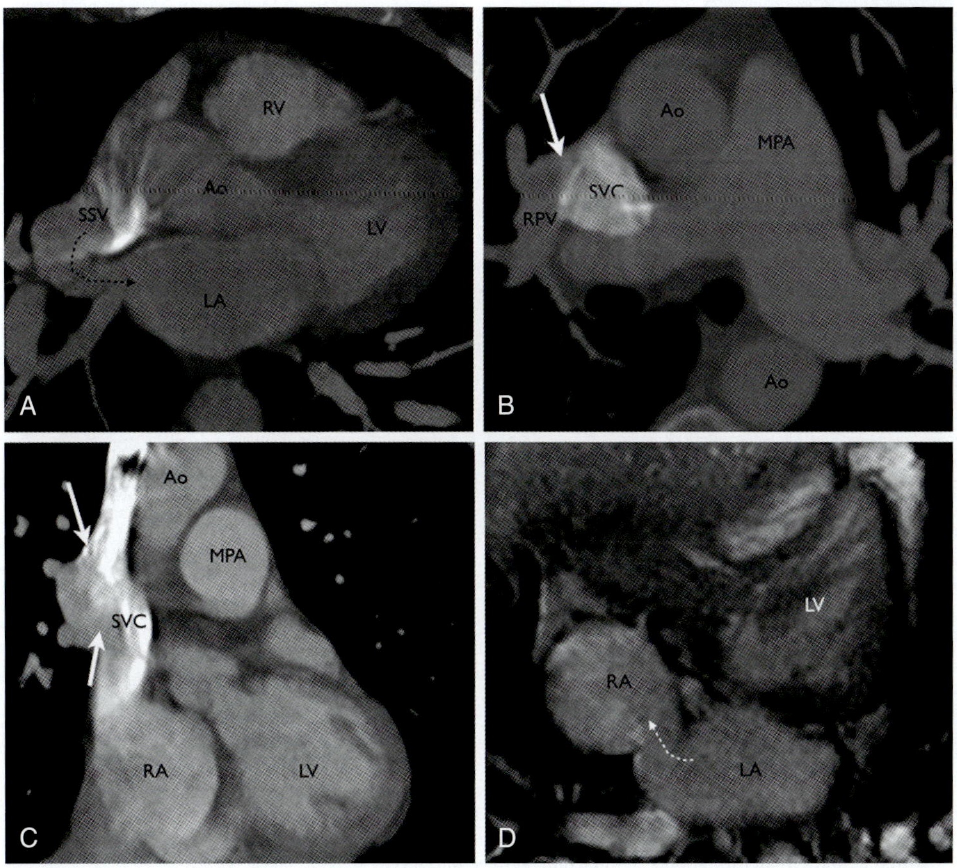

Figure 28.8 (A and B) Axial images from a chest CT angiography demonstrate a superior sinus venosus atrial septal defect *(SSV)*, which connects the inferiormost portion of the superior vena cava *(SVC)* to the left atrium *(LA)*. Additionally, there is partial anomalous pulmonary venous return of several right-sided branches into the SVC *(white arrows)*. (C) Coronal image from the same patient again demonstrating partial anomalous pulmonary venous return of several right-sided branches into the SVC *(white arrows)*. (D) Four-chamber steady-state free precession image demonstrates an inferior sinus venosus atrial septal defect *(white dashed arrow)* located near the junction with the inferior vena cava. *Ao*, Aorta; *LV*, left ventricle; *MPA*, main pulmonary artery; *RA*, right atrium; *RPV*, right pulmonary vein; *RV*, right ventricle.

a permanent interatrial communication. Morphologically, the PFO has a tunnel shape, whereas the ASD is a hole.

■ Ventricular Septal Defects

VSDs are the most common congenital lesion of the heart. It is present in nearly 50% of all patients with a congenital heart malformation. They occur isolated or in conjunction with other defects. There are multiple classifications of these types of defects in the literature, which complicates the subject. Similar to ASDs, VSDs can be classified as four different types—membranous, subarterial, muscular, and inlet. An important anatomic landmark in the classification of VSDs is the crista supraventricularis, which is a muscular protrusion that divides the right ventricular (RV) body and RV outflow tract (RVOT) and separates membranous VSDs (below the crista supraventricularis) from the subarterial VSDs (above the crista supraventricularis).

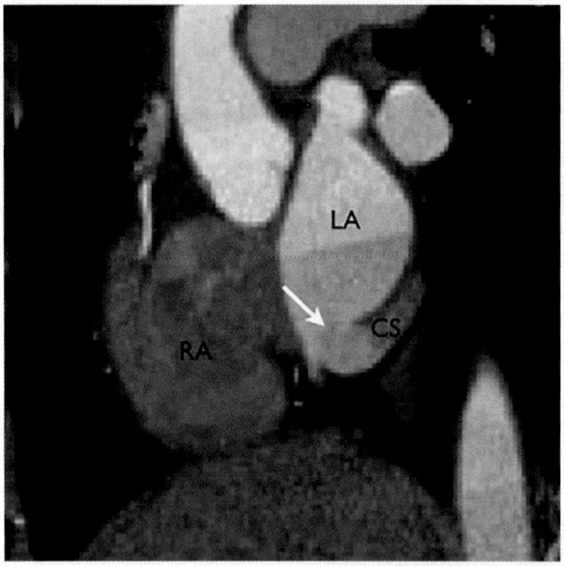

Figure 28.9 Oblique sagittal image from cardiac CT demonstrates an unroofed coronary sinus atrial septal defect *(arrow)* with communication of the coronary sinus *(CS)* with the left atrium *(LA)*. *RA*, Right atrium. (Courtesy Dr. Juan Carlos Batlle, Baptist Health South Florida, Radiology Associates of South Florida.)

Membranous VSDs are the most common type of VSDs, accounting for approximately 75% of VSDs. These defects are also known as *perimembranous, infracristal,* or *paramembranous VSDs*. They are located immediately below the aortic valve and anterior to the septal leaflet of the tricuspid valve (Fig. 28.10A). They can close spontaneously by apposition and scarring of the septal leaflet of the tricuspid valve or by prolapse of the aortic cusp.

Subarterial VSDs account for 5% of VSDs. They are located immediately below the semilunar valves. These defects are also known as *outlet, subpulmonic, infundibular, doubly committed,* or *conoseptal VSDs*. They rarely close spontaneously.

Muscular VSDs account for 20% of VSDs. They can be single or multiple and small or large. Approximately two-thirds of these defects are located in the apical segment. Most of them close spontaneously (see Fig. 28.10B).

Ventricular septal defects are usually seen in patients with complex congenital heart disease. Isolated cases of VSDs are rare. Evaluation of VSDs is typically performed using echocardiography.

Treatment of VSDs is usually surgical for defects resulting in significant left-to-right shunting (Qp:Qs >1.5).

■ Coronary Anomalies

Coronary anomalies can be difficult to classify due to the numerous variations of normal coronary anatomy. They can be grouped into four main categories:

1. Absent left main trunk (separate origin of the left circumflex and left anterior descending arteries [LADs] from the left sinus of Valsalva)

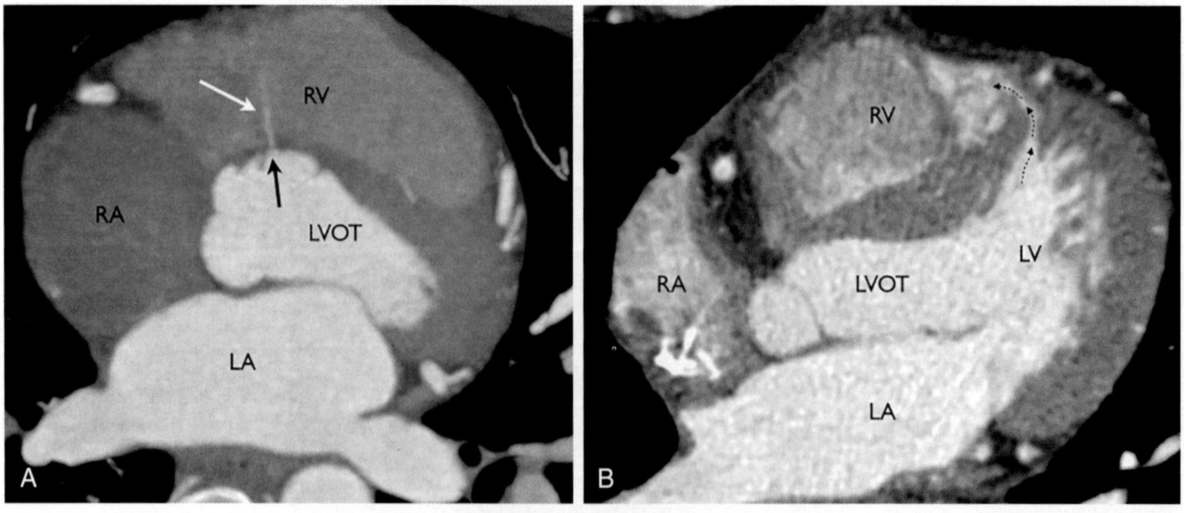

Figure 28.10 (A) Axial image from cardiac CT demonstrates a perimembranous ventricular septal defect *(black arrow)* with thin jet iodinated contrast extending from the left ventricular outflow tract *(LVOT)*, immediately below the level of the aortic valve, into the right ventricle *(RV; white arrow)*. (B) Axial image from a different patient demonstrates a muscular ventricular septal defect *(black dashed arrows)*. *LA*, Left atrium; *LV*, left ventricle; *RA*, right atrium.

2. Anomalous location of coronary ostium in the aortic root or near the proper aortic sinus of Valsalva for each coronary artery
3. Anomalous location of the coronary ostium outside the normal coronary aortic sinuses (e.g., noncoronary sinus, ascending aorta, left ventricle, right ventricle, PA, aortic arch)
4. Anomalous location of the coronary ostium at the improper sinus or single coronary pattern—right coronary artery (RCA) arising from the left sinus, LAD arising from the right sinus, left circumflex artery arising from the right sinus, and left main coronary artery arising from the right sinus—with an anomalous course (e.g., retroaortic, prepulmonic, septal, interarterial)

Most coronary anomalies have no clinical relevance and are incidental imaging findings. The coronary anomalies that have been linked to angina and major adverse cardiac events are the anomalous origin of the LAD or left main from the right sinus with an interarterial course and, to a lesser degree, the anomalous origin of the RCA from the left sinus with an interarterial course. The proposed mechanisms of myocardial ischemia are coronary compression during systole, narrow intramural course, slitlike ostium, and acute angle of takeoff. The anomalous origin of the RCA from the left sinus with an interarterial course can be further divided into a high interarterial course (above the pulmonic valve level) and low interarterial course (below the pulmonic valve level). The high interarterial course has a higher association with angina and major adverse cardiac events than the low interarterial course, which is thought to be due to systolic compression of the anomalous vessel between the expanding aortic root and PA (Fig. 28.11).

Many patients with coronary anomalies are treated on a case-by-case basis. Surgical treatment depends on the type of anomaly and the patient's symptomatology. Surgical intervention consists of coronary artery bypass grafting or unroofing of the intramural coronary artery segment.

An anomalous origin of the coronary arteries from the PA is a hemodynamically significant abnormality that results in myocardial ischemia. The anomalous coronary artery (arising from the PA) perfuses the myocardium

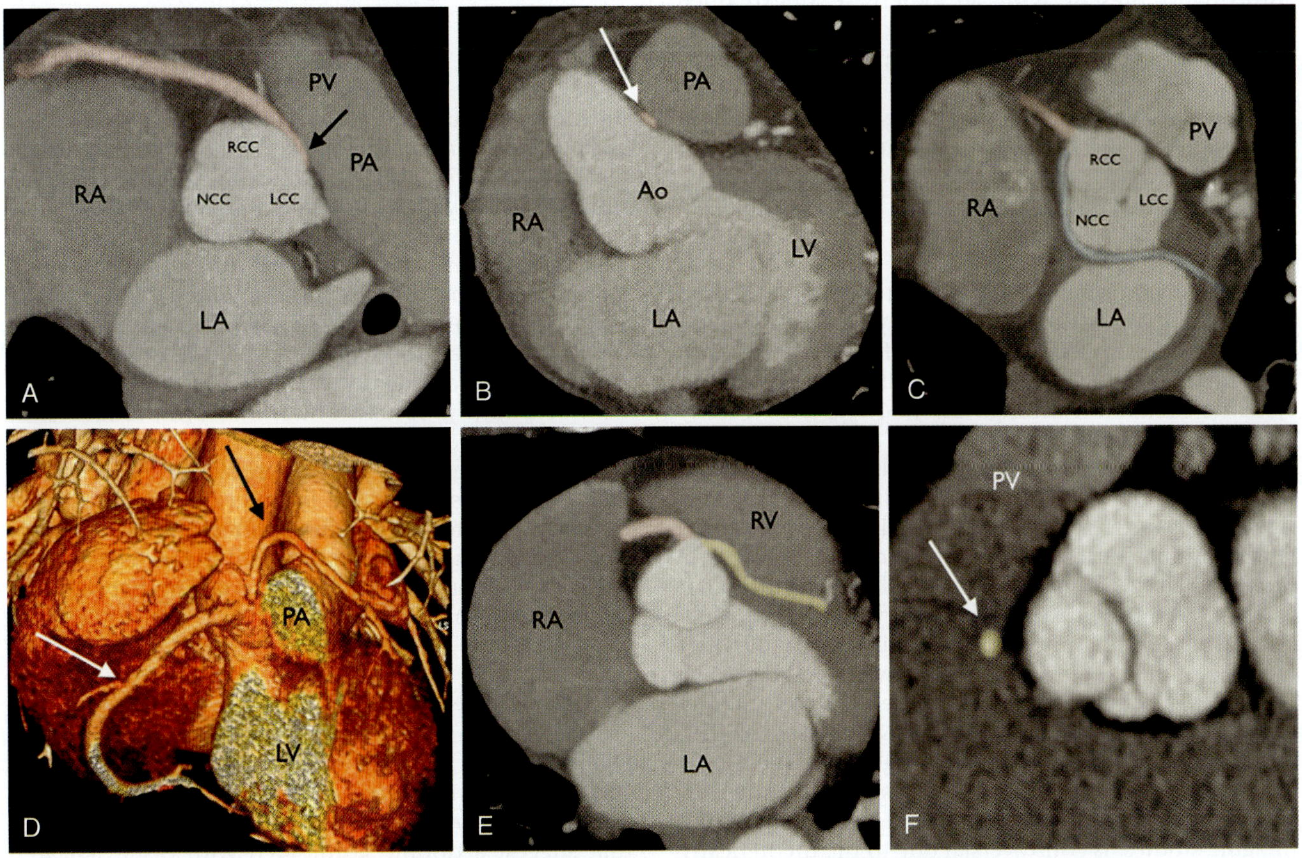

Figure 28.11 (A and B) Axial and coronal oblique images from cardiac CT demonstrates an anomalous right coronary artery (RCA), outlined in pink, arising from the left coronary cusp *(LCC)*, with an interarterial course. Note the slitlike ostium and acute angle of takeoff *(black arrow in A)*, as well as the slitlike appearance of the RCA in between the aorta *(Ao)* and pulmonary artery *(PA; white arrow in B)*. (C) Axial oblique image from cardiac CT demonstrates an anomalous left circumflex coronary artery, outlined in blue, arising from the right coronary cusp *(RCC)*, with a retroaortic course. (D) Three-dimensional volume-rendered image from cardiac CT demonstrates an anomalous left anterior descending coronary artery (LAD; *black arrow*) arising from the LCC, with a prepulmonic course. (E and F) Axial and sagittal oblique images from cardiac CT demonstrate an anomalous LAD *(outlined in yellow)* arising from the RCA *(white arrow in F)* with a septal course. Note how the LAD is surrounded by myocardium *(white arrow)*. *LA*, Left atrium; *LV*, left ventricle; *NCC* noncoronary cusp; *PV*, pulmonic valve; *RA*, right atrium; *RV*, right ventricle.

with a low- pressure, low-oxygen system that results in myocardial ischemia and can lead to ischemic cardiomyopathy. Furthermore, this type of anomaly results in collateral vessel formation that creates a steal phenomenon from the normal origin of the coronary artery to the anomalous coronary, resulting in a left-to-right shunt. The most common variant of this anomaly is the anomalous left coronary artery arising from the PA (ALCAPA), also known as *Bland-White-Garland syndrome*. The anomalous origin of the RCA arising from the PA (ARCAPA) is far less common and is related to fewer symptoms. Both these anomalies are repaired surgically when discovered.

Problem Solving

One commonly encountered diagnostic and clinical dilemma is myocardial bridging. Myocardial bridging is defined as an intramyocardial, rather than epicardial, segment of a coronary artery. Its incidence on CT angiography (CTA) has been reported as high as 58%, suggesting that this is an incidental imaging finding, without clinical relevance. The one caveat to this are teenagers or young adults who present with an otherwise unexplained exertional angina and the presence of a myocardial bridge. In these patients, use of a physiologic test (e.g., with nuclear myocardial perfusion) can be helpful to confirm or exclude myocardial bridging as the cause of the symptoms and to guide treatment options.

■ Patent Ductus Arteriosus

The DA derives from the left sixth aortic arch. It is needed during fetal circulation and typically closes spontaneously 10 to 15 hours after delivery. The high-resistance pulmonary circulation empties into the lower resistance systemic circulation through the DA. The DA typically extends from the distal aortic arch (at the level of the takeoff of the left subclavian) and the junction of the left PA and main PA (Fig. 28.12). In the setting of a right-sided aortic arch, the DA usually arises from the left innominate artery and inserts into the region of the proximal left PA. In the setting of a right-sided aortic arch with an aberrant left subclavian artery, the DA typically arises from the aberrant left subclavian artery and inserts into the proximal left PA, creating a vascular ring.

Surgical closure of a clinically evident PDA is typically performed in the newborn through video-assisted thoracoscopic surgical ligation. Pharmacologic therapy is used exclusively in premature infants. The treatment of silent PDAs (nonaudible), encountered incidentally during imaging studies, is controversial due to the theoretically small risk of bacterial endocarditis.

■ Vascular Rings and Slings

A vascular ring is an aortic arch anomaly in which the trachea and esophagus are completely surrounded by arterial vascular structures. This results in compression of the tracheobronchial tree and/or esophagus. Vascular rings are the most important vascular cause of tracheal obstruction. The two most common complete vascular rings are a double aortic arch and right-sided aortic arch, with an aberrant left subclavian artery and left ligamentum arteriosus.

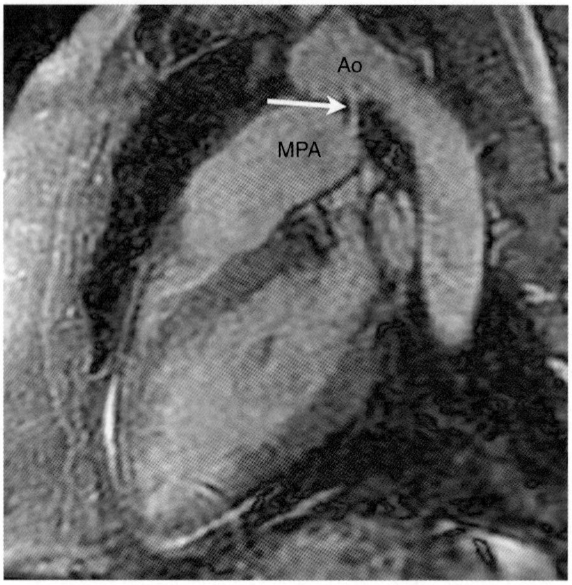

Figure 28.12 Sagittal image from a three-dimensional, balanced, steady-state gradient echo sequence from cardiac MRI demonstrates a patent ductus arteriosus *(arrow)* connecting the descending thoracic aorta *(Ao)* and the main pulmonary artery *(MPA)*.

Other less common variants include a left aortic arch with an aberrant right subclavian with right ligamentum arteriosus, left aortic arch with a right descending aorta and right DA, and right aortic arch with a left descending aorta (circumflex aortic arch) and left DA (Fig. 28.13).

Incomplete vascular rings are less likely to be associated with respiratory or gastrointestinal symptoms. These include a pulmonary sling, aberrant left or right subclavian, and innominate artery compression. The innominate artery compression results in anterior compression of the trachea due to the innominate artery arising posteriorly along the arch. A pulmonary sling results from an anomalous origin of the left PA coursing between the trachea and esophagus (Fig. 28.14).

Problem Solving

Distinguishing between a right-sided aortic arch with mirror branching pattern and a double aortic arch with distal left arch atresia is difficult. Imaging characteristics that suggest a double aortic arch with distal left arch atresia include inferior and posterior tethering of the left subclavian from the atretic fibrous cord and ligamentus arteriosus and the symmetric branching pattern of the carotid and subclavian arteries on axial imaging. The presence of an aortic diverticulum in the proximal aspect of the descending thoracic aorta can also be present, aiding in the diagnosis (Fig. 28.15).

A right-sided aortic arch with mirror image branching pattern is highly associated with congenital heart disease.

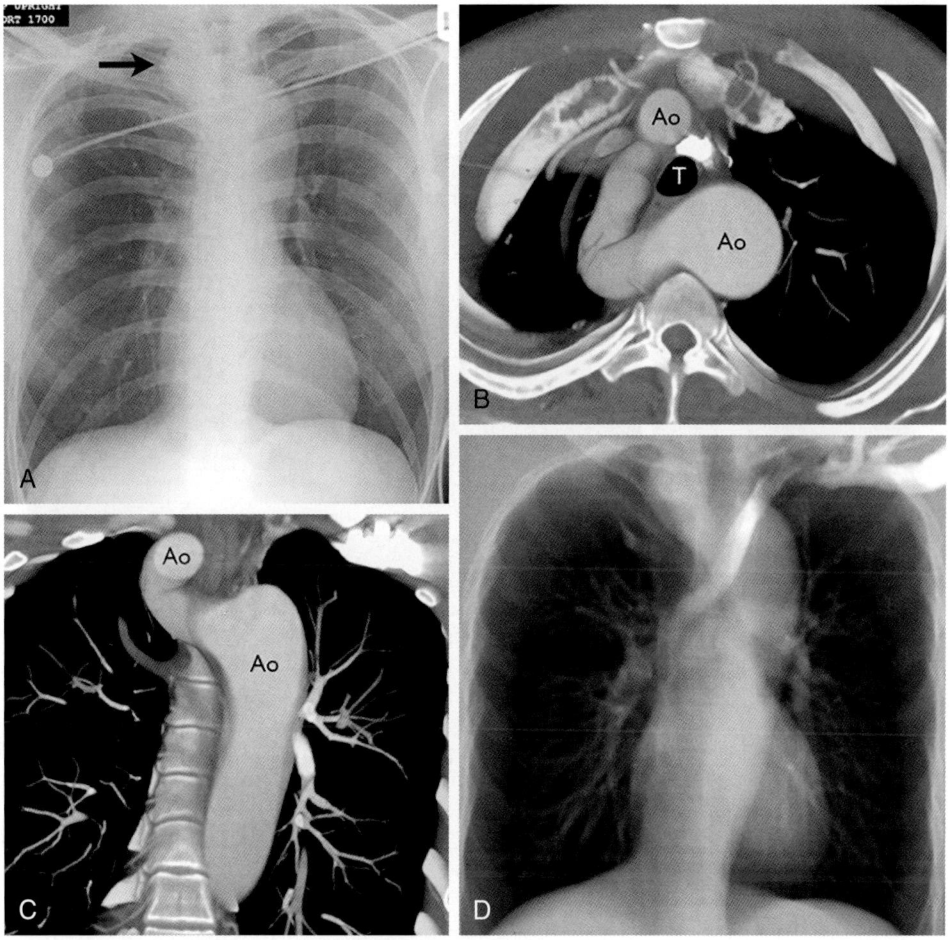

Figure 28.13 A 41-year-old man with a circumflex aorta *(Ao)*. (A) Posteroanterior frontal chest radiograph demonstrates a right paratracheal opacity *(black arrow)* with mass effect on the adjacent trachea. (B and C) Oblique axial and coronal volume-rendered images from CT in the same patient demonstrates a circumflex aorta. Note how there is a right aortic arch; however, the aorta crosses the midline and descends in the normal position just left of midline. (D) Mean projection image from the same CT scan demonstrates the circumflex aorta and helps correlate the findings on the chest radiograph. *T*, Trachea.

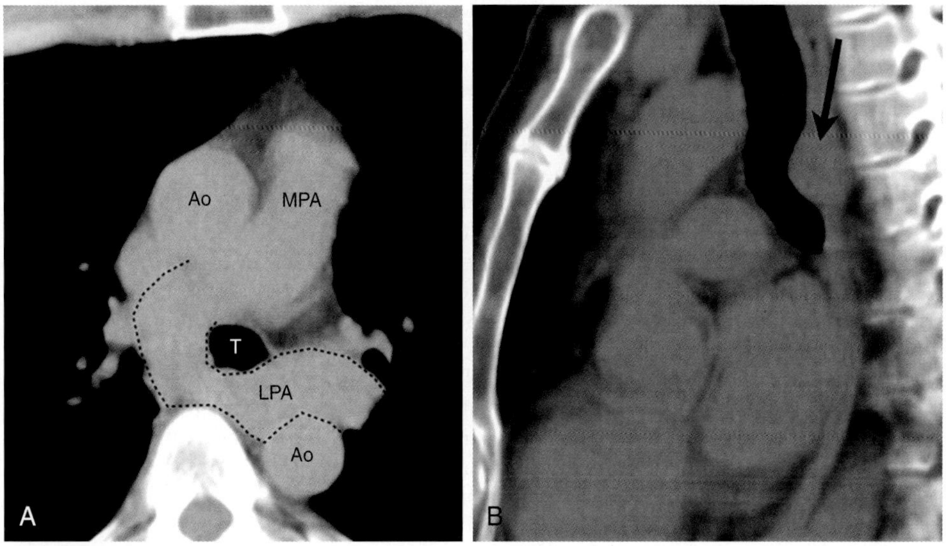

Figure 28.14 Axial (A) and sagittal (B) images from chest CT demonstrates a pulmonary sling where the left pulmonary artery *(LPA; outlined in dashed black lines)* wraps around the trachea *(T)*. (B) Sagittal image from chest CT demonstrates the characteristic location of the LPA *(arrow)* between the esophagus and trachea. *Ao*, Aorta; *MPA*, main pulmonary artery.

Tetralogy of Fallot

First described in 1888 by the French physician Etienne-Louis Arthur Fallot, tetralogy of Fallot (TOF) consists of pulmonic stenosis, overriding aorta, VSD, and RV hypertrophy. It accounts for 7% to 10% of all cases of congenital heart disease. It is thought to be related to anterior displacement of the interventricular septum during embryogenesis. This results in narrowing of the RVOT and secondary RV hypertrophy. The anterior location of the interventricular septum results in an overriding aorta and incomplete fusion of the interventricular

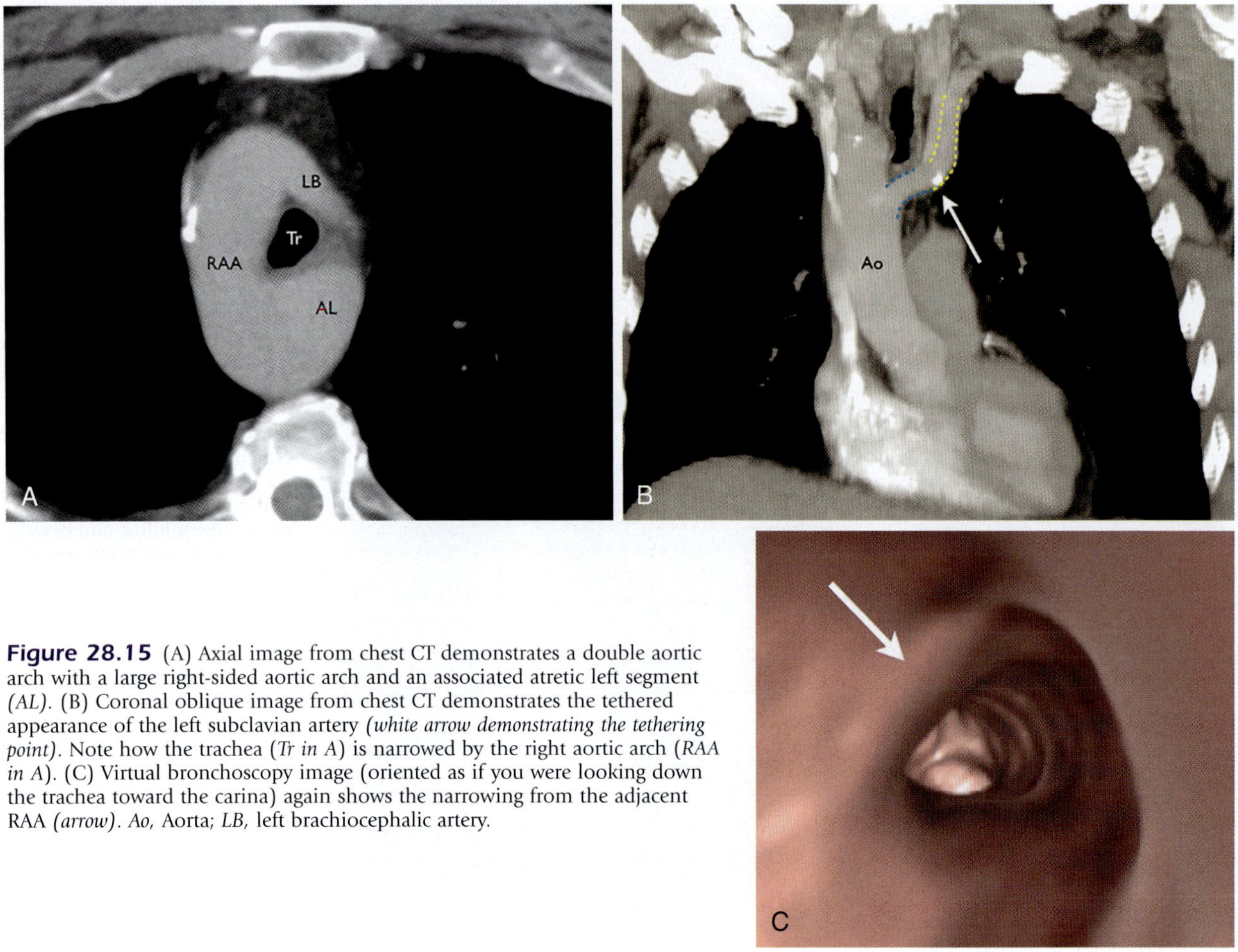

Figure 28.15 (A) Axial image from chest CT demonstrates a double aortic arch with a large right-sided aortic arch and an associated atretic left segment *(AL)*. (B) Coronal oblique image from chest CT demonstrates the tethered appearance of the left subclavian artery *(white arrow demonstrating the tethering point)*. Note how the trachea (*Tr in A*) is narrowed by the right aortic arch (*RAA in A*). (C) Virtual bronchoscopy image (oriented as if you were looking down the trachea toward the carina) again shows the narrowing from the adjacent RAA *(arrow)*. *Ao,* Aorta; *LB,* left brachiocephalic artery.

septum. It can be associated with many other congenital abnormalities, including but not limited to a right-sided aortic arch, coronary artery anomalies, and dilation of the aorta. A PDA is present in two-thirds of patients with TOF. Surgical repair of TOF patients is typically performed in the first year of life and aims to achieve VSD closure and augmentation of the RVOT. Creation of shunts to increase pulmonary arterial flow is not currently used.

The three most common surgical procedures to correct TOF are an infundibulectomy, transannular patch repair, and right ventricle to PA conduit placement, depending on the severity of the RVOT stenosis. The preferred surgical procedure in cases of mild to moderate RVOT stenosis with a normal pulmonic valve is an infundibulectomy, which consists of resection of the hypertrophied myocardium. In most patients with marked stenosis of the RVOT or pulmonary annulus, a transannular patch repair with VSD closure is the treatment of choice. In patients with a severe variant of TOF, in which atresia of the pulmonic valve or PA is present, a right ventricle to PA conduit is performed. Pulmonary insufficiency is the most common complication in patients who have undergone repair of TOF, in particular patients who have had transannular patch repair. Although most conduits used to repair severe TOF are valved, it is frequent to have valvular degeneration, resulting in insufficiency. Conduit stenosis also results from chronic degeneration. It ranges from mild to severe and can result in RV dilation, arrhythmias, and contractile dysfunction. Aneurysm formation at the site of patch repair is another common complication, seen in up to 50% of these patients. Recurrent or persistent RVOT obstruction is the most common complication related to isolated infundibulectomy.

The role of advanced cardiac imaging, in particular cardiac MRI, in patients with repaired TOF is paramount. Steady-state free precession (SSFP) images are used to assess ventricular volumes and systolic function accurately, whereas velocity-encoded cine (VEC) is used for flow quantification. Accurate assessment of the ventricular end-diastolic volumes indexed to body surface area is used to guide the timing of valvular replacement in the setting of moderate to severe pulmonary regurgitation, as delineated below. The use of VEC images can accurately quantify the degree of pulmonary valvular regurgitation or stenosis and detect a shunt (Qp:Qs) in the setting of persistent or recurrent VSD. MRA is routinely performed in all new patients with TOF repair to assess for pulmonary branch stenosis and additional morphologic assessment.

Indications for pulmonary valve replacement in patients with repaired TOF or similar physiology with moderate or severe pulmonary regurgitation (regurgitation fraction ≥25%) are as follows:

1. Asymptomatic patient with two or more of the following criteria:
   a. RV end-diastolic volume index >150 mL/m^2 or z-score >4; patients whose body surface area falls outside published normal data: RV/LV end-diastolic volume ratio >2
   b. RV end-systolic volume index >80 mL/m^2
   c. RV ejection fraction <47%
   d. LV ejection fraction <55%
   e. Large RVOT aneurysm
   f. QRS duration >140 ms
   g. Sustained tachyarrhythmia related to right heart volume load
   h. Other hemodynamically significant abnormalities:
      (1) RVOT obstruction with RV systolic pressure ≥ two-thirds systemic
      (2) Severe branch PA stenosis (<30% flow to affected lung) not amenable to transcatheter therapy.
      (3) At least moderate tricuspid regurgitation
      (4) Left-to-right shunt from residual ASDs or VSDs with pulmonary-to-systemic flow ratio ≥1.5
      (5) Severe aortic regurgitation
      (6) Severe aortic dilation (diameter ≥5 cm)
2. Symptomatic patients: Symptoms and signs attributable to severe RV volume load documented by cardiac magnetic resonance or alternative imaging modality, fulfilling one or more of the quantitative criteria detailed above; examples of symptoms and signs include the following:
   a. Exercise intolerance not explained by extracardiac causes (e.g., lung disease, musculoskeletal anomalies, genetic anomalies, obesity), with documentation by exercise testing with metabolic cart (≤70% predicted peak VO_2 for age and gender not explained by chronotropic incompetence)
   b. Signs and symptoms of heart failure (e.g., dyspnea with mild effort or at rest not explained by extracardiac causes, peripheral edema)
   c. Syncope attributable to arrhythmia

■ Transposition of the Great Arteries

Dextrotransposition of the Great Arteries

Dextrotransposition of the great arteries (D-TGA) results from abnormal conotruncal rotation resulting in an abnormal position and connection of the great vessels with the ventricles (VA discordance). The atria and ventricles are normally positioned and connected (AV concordance). This results in closed loop parallel circuits that are incompatible with life. To survive after delivery, there has to be communication between the two circuits, such as a PDA, ASD, or VSD. It is more common in infants of diabetic mothers. There are many associated cardiovascular anomalies, such as VSD, coarctation, pulmonary outflow obstruction, and mitral and tricuspid stenosis and atresia. Coronary anomalies are frequent, with the most common variant being an anteriorly located noncoronary cusp.

Surgical correction of this defect can be performed at the atrial level (Mustard and Senning procedures) or at the arterial level with an arterial switch. The arterial switch (Jatene procedure) has replaced the atrial switch. It is performed by cutting the aorta off the right ventricle above the coronary arteries and cutting the PA off the left ventricle above the pulmonic valve, then the aorta is reattached to the left ventricle and the PA reattached to the right ventricle. Reimplantation of the aorta to the PA root and of the PA to the aortic root is performed. The coronaries are excised off the aortic root with a surrounding button and re-implanted into the neoaorta. The Lecompte maneuver places the main PA anterior to the aorta, with the left and right main PAs to the sides of the aorta (Fig. 28.16). The Jatene arterial switch has a more favorable outcome compared to the atrial level switch because the morphologic ventricles are correctly paired with their workload. Dilation of the neoaorta is common, reported in up to 50% of patients. The main complication of this procedure is stenosis of the PA at the anastomosis.

Levotransposition of the Great Arteries

Levotransposition of the great arteries (L-TGA) is abnormal conotruncal rotation resulting in the aortic root located anterior and to the left of the PA. The great vessels run parallel to each other in the sagittal plane, as in patients with D-TGA. Contrary to D-TGA, in L-TGA patients have abnormally connected atria and ventricles (AV discordance), as well as abnormally connected ventricles and arteries (VA discordance), resulting in a congenitally corrected transposition. It is important to know that the valves follow their ventricles so that the morphologic left ventricle will always have a mitral valve, and the morphologic right ventricle will always have a tricuspid valve. The same applies for the semilunar valves in the sense that the aorta will always have an aortic valve and the PA will always have a pulmonic valve. The AV and VA discordance results in a morphologic right ventricle located on the left, handling the workload of a morphologic left ventricle and vice versa. This can ultimately lead to heart failure. Associated anomalies include VSDs, pulmonic stenosis, apical displacement of the tricuspid valve, and ventricular noncompaction. Until recently, surgical correction was focused on correcting the associated anomalies, but with the increased recognition of the long-term complications of uncorrected L-TGA, a double-switch operation is now performed. In this procedure, atrial and arterial level switches are performed.

■ Univentricular Conditions

Numerous conditions result in a functionally single ventricle for which the surgical treatment is usually similar. The goal

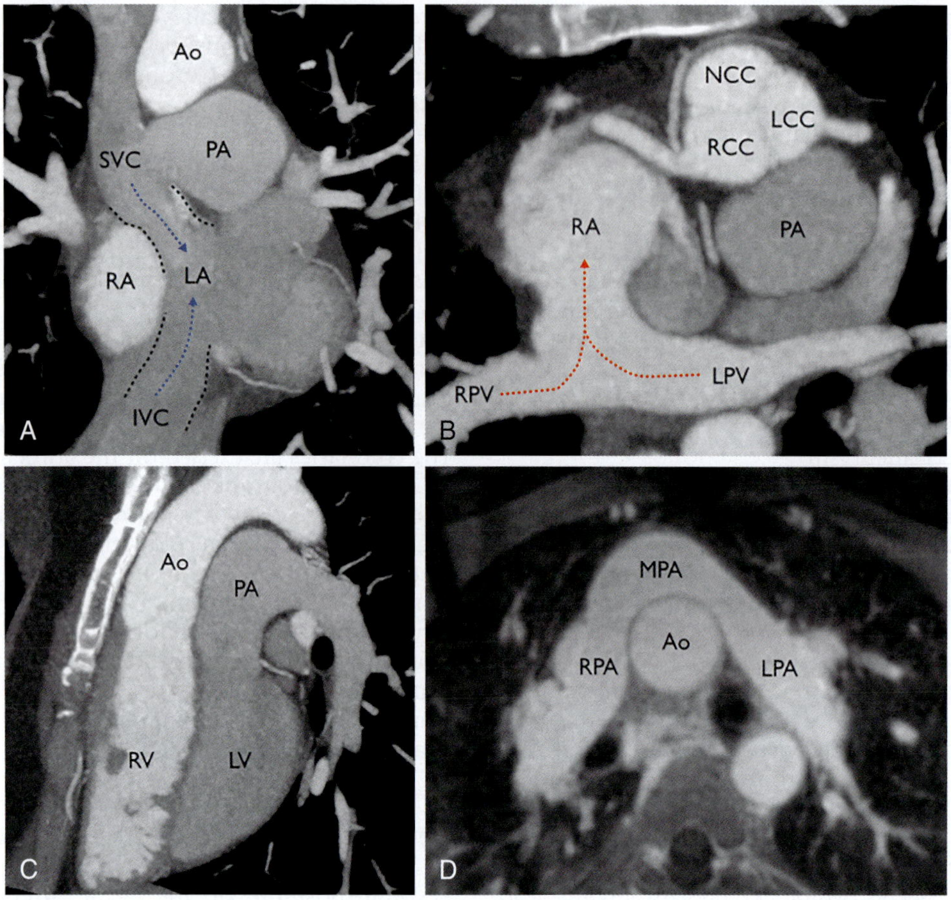

Figure 28.16 D-transposition of the great arteries in a 30-year-old woman status post–Mustard procedure. (A) Oblique coronal cardiac CT image demonstrates patent superior and inferior limbs of systemic baffles *(black dashed lines)* directing venous blood from the superior vena cava *(SVC)* and inferior vena cava *(IVC)* into the left atrium *(LA; blue dashed lines)*. (B) Axial cardiac CT image demonstrates pulmonary veins draining into the right atrium *(RA; red dashed arrows)*. Also note that the aorta lies anterior to the pulmonary artery *(PA)*, with an expected configuration of the sinus of Valsalva following surgical correction with the noncoronary cusp *(NCC)* positioned anterior to both the right and left coronary cusps (*RCC* and *LCC*). (C) Oblique sagittal cardiac CT image demonstrates the aorta *(Ao)* arising from the right ventricle *(RV)* and the PA arising from the left ventricle *(LV)*. (D) D-transposition of the great arteries in a 20-year-old man status post–Jatene procedure with a Lecompte maneuver. Axial image from a contrast-enhanced, ECG-gated, respiratory-navigated MR angiography of the chest demonstrates the location of the main pulmonary artery *(MPA)* anterior to the ascending aorta with draping of the right and left pulmonary arteries (*RPA* and *LPA*) around the ascending aorta *(Ao)*. *LPV*, Left pulmonary vein; *RPV*, right pulmonary vein.

of surgical treatment is to separate the pulmonary and systemic circulations and allow the single ventricle to work on the systemic circulation. This is accomplished by connecting the deoxygenated blood returned from the body directly into the PA. Surgical correction is done in stages.

The first stage focuses on establishing reliable blood flow to the pulmonary arterial system to allow for normal development. This was accomplished in the past by performing a Blalock-Taussig shunt (subclavian artery to ipsilateral PA). Other surgical possibilities used in the past include a Potts shunt (anastomosis between the left PA and descending thoracic aorta) and the Waterston shunt (anastomosis between the right PA and ascending aorta). However, these are no longer performed due to many complications. Currently, a modified Blalock-Taussig (B-T) shunt is preferred due to fewer complications. The modified B-T shunt uses a synthetic graft that connects the subclavian artery to the PA. The Sano procedure is a modification of this first-stage surgery, in which a right ventricle to PA conduit is created.

The second-stage operation establishes a superior cavopulmonary connection, and the systemic to PA shunt is removed. This was accomplished in the past by a Glenn connection, which involved isolating the right PA from the main PA and connecting it to the SVC. Currently, a bidirectional Glenn is used, in which the main PA is isolated from the single ventricle, and the SVC is connected to the right PA. In this setting, the venous return of the upper body fills the left and right PAs passively. A hemi-Fontan procedure is the preceding step toward an intracardiac Fontan, whereas a bidirectional Glenn is the preceding step for an extracardiac Fontan conduit.

In the third stage, the systemic and pulmonary circulations are completely isolated. This is accomplished by routing the blood return of the IVC into the PA. In patients who have had a bidirectional Glenn anastomosis, an

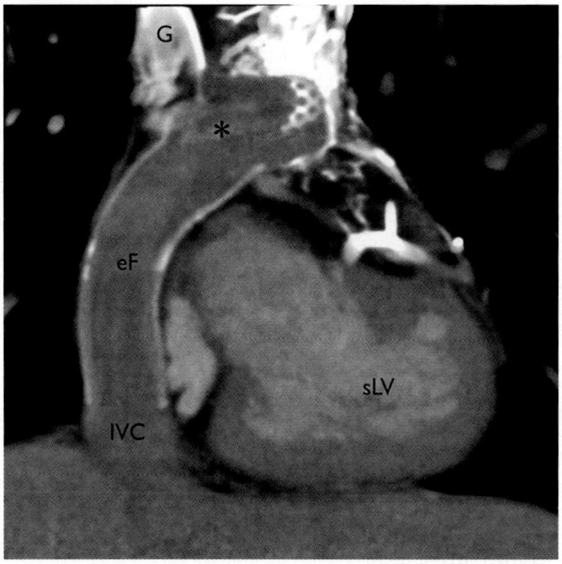

Figure 28.17 Tricuspid atresia, status post-Fontan and bidirectional Glenn anastomosis. Oblique coronal image from cardiac CT in a 19-year-old man demonstrates a patent extracardiac Fontan *(eF)*, which directs blood from the inferior vena cava *(IVC)* to the confluence of the pulmonary arteries *(asterisk)*. There is also a patent bidirectional Glenn *(G)*, which directs blood from the superior vena cava to the confluence of the pulmonary arteries. *sLV*, Systemic left ventricle.

extracardiac conduit is placed connecting the IVC with the PA. In patients with a hemi-Fontan, an intracardiac baffle is performed (Fig. 28.17).

Imaging of patients with Fontan procedures using MRI is crucial for the evaluation of ventricular size and function using SSFP images. VEC images are used for the evaluation of the Fontan conduit or baffle and Glenn shunt for their patency. MRA is used to detect venovenous collaterals and pulmonary arteriovenous malformations, seen in up to 25% of patients with an isolated superior cavopulmonary anastomosis.

Problem Solving

Evaluation for pulmonary embolism is difficult in patients with the Fontan procedure due to artifacts related to a mix of contrast and poor opacification of the left pulmonary arterial branches. The best method to determine the presence of pulmonary embolism in these patients is through CT pulmonary angiography performed during simultaneous injections of contrast in the lower and upper extremity veins, using bolus tracking to trigger when optimal enhancement is achieved. Obtaining an additional second delay phase imaging can be beneficial. Other limited imaging modalities that can be useful are MRA and a split injection VQ scan.

Evaluation of the patency of the Fontan graft and Glenn connections using CT can be difficult due to the inability to opacify the IVC PA conduit using an upper extremity injection. In these cases, the intravenous administration of contrast can be performed with two different protocols to answer this question. The first protocol includes performing two separate simultaneous injections through the upper and lower extremities to obtain simultaneous opacification of the Fontan and Glenn connections while opacifying the right and left chambers. To obtain this, a long contrast injection with a low injection rate is preferred. The second protocol involves a delayed scan (60–90 s after the administration of contrast) to allow for venous opacification.

■ Conclusion

Congenital abnormalities of the heart and great vessels are rare, but have been increasingly seen in adults patients who have undergone successful surgical correction. It is important for the radiologist to be familiar with common surgical procedures and their imaging appearance to recognize complications and guide patient care.

Bibliography

Angelini P. Congenital heart disease for the adult cardiologist: coronary artery anomalies—an entity in search for an identity. *Circulation*. 2007;115:1296–1305.

Attenhofer Jost CH, Schaff HV, Connolly HM, et al. Spectrum of reoperations after repair of aortic coarctation: importance of an individualized approach because of coexistent cardiovascular disease. *Mayo Clin Proc*. 2002;77:646–653.

Brickner ME, Hillis LD, Lange RA. Congenital heart disease in adults. Second of two parts. *N Engl J Med*. 2000;342:334–342.

Brown ML, Burkhart HM, Connolly HM, et al. Coarctation of the aorta: lifelong surveillance is mandatory following surgical repair. *J Am Coll Cardiol*. 2013;62:1020–1025.

Eckart RE, Scoville SL, Campbell CL, et al. Sudden death in young adults: a 25-year review of autopsies in military recruits. *Ann Intern Med*. 2004;141:829–834.

Engelfriet P, Boersma E, Oechslin E, et al. The spectrum of adult congenital heart disease in Europe: morbidity and mortality in a 5 year follow-up period. The Euro Heart Survey on adult congenital heart disease. *Eur Heart J*. 2005;26:2325–2333.

Geva T. Repaired tetralogy of Fallot: the roles of cardiovascular magnetic resonance in evaluating pathophysiology and for pulmonary valve replacement decision support. *J Cardiovasc Magn Reson*. 2011;13(1):9.

Jacobs JP, Burke RP, Quintessenza JA, et al. Congenital heart surgery nomenclature and database project: ventricular septal defect. *Ann Thorac Surg*. 2000;69(suppl 4):S25–S35.

Johri AM, Rojas CA, El-Sherief A, et al. Imaging of atrial septal defects: echocardiography and CT correlation. *Heart*. 2011;97(17):1441–1453.

Lapierre C, Déry J, Guérin R, Viremouneix L, Dubois J, Garel L. Segmental approach to imaging of congenital heart disease. *Radiographics*. 2010;30(2):397–411.

Lee HJ, Hong YJ, Kim HY, et al. Anomalous origin of the right coronary artery from the left coronary sinus with an inerarterial course: subtypes and clinical importance. *Radiology*. 2012;262:101–108.

Ordovas KG, Muzzarelli S, Hope MD, et al. Cardiovascular MR imaging after surgical correction of tetralogy of Fallot: approach based on understanding of surgical procedures. *Radiographics*. 2013;33(4):1037–1052.

Parikh SR, Hurwitz RA, Hubbard JE, et al. Preoperative and postoperative "aneurysm" associated with coarctation of the aorta. *J Am Coll Cardiol*. 1991;17:1367–1372.

Ringel RE, Gauvreau K, Moses H, Jenkins KJ. Coarctation of the aorta stent trial (COAST): study design and rationale. *Am Heart J*. 2012;164:7–13.

Rojas CA, El-Sherief A, Medina HM, et al. Embryology and developmental defects of the interatrial septum. *AJR Am J Roentgenol*. 2010;195(5):1100–1104.

Rojas CA, Jaimes C, Abbara S. Ventricular septal defects: embryology and imaging findings. *J Thorac Imaging*. 2013;28(2):W28–W34.

Silversides CK, Kiess M, Beauchesne L, et al. Canadian Cardiovascular Society 2009 consensus conference on the management of adults with congenital heart disease: outflow tract obstruction, coarctation of the aorta, tetralogy of Fallot, Ebstein anomaly and Marfan's syndrome. *Can J Cardiol*. 2010;26:e80–e97.

Van Praagh S, Carrera ME, Sanders SP, et al. Sinus venosus defects: unroofing of the right pulmonary veins—anatomic and echocardiographic findings and surgical treatment. *Am Heart J*. 1994;128:365–379.

Verheugt CL, Uiterwaal CS, Grobbee DE, Mulder BJ. Long-term prognosis of congenital heart defects: a systematic review. *Int J Cardiol*. 2008;131:25–32.

Warnes CA, Williams RG, Bashore TM, et al. ACC/AHA 2008 guidelines for the management of adults with congenital heart disease: a report of the American College of Cardiology/American Heart Association Task Force on Practice Guidelines (writing committee to develop guidelines on the management of adults with congenital heart disease). *Circulation*. 2008;118:e714–e833.

CHAPTER 29
Acquired Diseases of the Aorta

Jonathan H. Chung, Suhny Abbara, and Tami J. Bang

CHAPTER OUTLINE

Introduction

The aorta is the largest artery in the body, arising from the left ventricular outflow tract and branching throughout the body. The spectrum of thoracic aortic disease is wide, with causes that may be chronic or acute, congenital or acquired, and symptomatic or asymptomatic.

The clinical presentation of acquired thoracic aortic disease ranges from asymptomatic (as in the case of an ascending thoracic aortic aneurysm) to severe acute chest pain (in the case of aortic dissection). Technologic advances in multidetector computed tomography (MDCT), as well as increasing availability of advanced imaging, has increased clinical awareness of aortic diseases and has largely replaced direct catheter angiography as the method of aortic imaging.

Determining Who Needs Imaging

In the setting of acute chest pain, basic imaging is often performed, and cross-sectional advanced imaging may be pursued, depending on the degree of clinical suspicion for aortic disease. Imaging is also often performed in the setting of acute trauma (blunt or penetrating thoracic trauma); imaging modalities may be chosen based on the mechanism of trauma and/or degree of clinical suspicion for vascular injury.

Additionally, chronic aortic diseases may be followed with serial examinations. These imaging studies are often performed for surveillance of diseases (e.g., a thoracic aortic aneurysm), in which changes or increases in size may prompt more aggressive or surgical management.

Imaging Techniques

Radiography

Chest radiographs are often the first radiologic examination performed in the setting of acute or chronic thoracic aortic disease. The main utility of chest radiography resides in the frontal projection, and it is often used as a screening tool for the exclusion of acute aortic disease. However, radiography plays a limited role in the detailed workup of thoracic aortic diseases, mainly because of the limited anatomic detail and poor contrast resolution.

Advantages of Radiography

Chest radiography has the distinct advantage of being quick, readily available, and portable. Radiography plays a central role in the initial evaluation of an unstable patient or in a patient who cannot be easily positioned or moved. Frontal chest radiography may serve as a useful screening tool because a normal chest radiograph has a 98% negative predictive value in the setting of blunt trauma.

Although radiography uses ionizing radiation, the dose is relatively low. In cases when aortic disease has already been characterized, radiography may be a useful tool for surveillance by detecting change over time. Plain film radiography is useful for the detection of calcifications (particularly atherosclerotic calcifications), especially in the aorta and in valve leaflets or annuli. It is also helpful in the surveillance of support devices and localization of prosthetic devices (e.g., prosthetic valves, vascular endografts, pacemaker leads).

Disadvantages and Limitations of Radiography

Radiography has many limitations, mostly owing to the two-dimensional acquisition of images and low contrast resolution. This limits accurate and reproducible measurements of the mediastinum.

Although radiography may demonstrate the outward contours of the mediastinum, abnormalities of the intima are not apparent. As such, acute abnormalities such as dissection, penetrating aortic ulcer (PAU), and intramural hematoma (IMH) are usually not apparent radiographically.

Radiography also has the disadvantage of artifacts secondary to positioning, inspiratory effort, and projection. As an example, anterior-posterior imaging magnifies the size of the mediastinum more than a posterior-anterior image. Additionally, supine positioning or hypoinflation can artificially make the cardiomediastinal contours appear larger. Consequently, measurements and comparisons may be inaccurate owing to the lack of reproducible images.

Problem Solving With Radiography

Radiography of the chest is typically performed with the patient in an upright position, with posterior-anterior and lateral projections. This minimizes distortion of the mediastinal contours and artifacts related to positioning. However, in the emergent setting (e.g., spinal trauma, acute chest pain, hemodynamic instability), this may not be possible. In these cases, anterior-posterior projection radiography may be substituted.

Although relatively insensitive, the chest radiograph may display signs of acute aortic pathology. For example, mediastinal widening or obscuration of the normal aortic contours may suggest an aortic abnormality. And, although rare, inward displacement of atherosclerotic calcifications is virtually diagnostic of acute aortic dissection. Although these cases almost always proceed to cross-sectional imaging for further characterization, abnormal findings on the radiograph may be the first warning sign of serious aortic pathology.

Computed Tomography

CT was introduced in the early 1990s, providing a noninvasive alternative to catheter-directed angiography. Early iterations of CT used single detectors, requiring extended acquisition times and prohibitively long breath-holds. Additionally, the first iodinated contrast agents were hyperosmolar and associated with high rates of adverse reactions.

Since the advent of MDCT, acquisition times have significantly decreased, allowing for imaging to be obtained in a single breath-hold. Furthermore, thin slices and reconstruction software have allowed for isovolumetric multiplanar reconstruction at the radiologist's workstation. Newer contrast agents are low osmolar and associated with lower rates of allergic reactions and renal injury.

Advantages of CT

CT is a relatively quick examination that allows for accurate and reproducible three-dimensional (3D) images of the aorta. With modern MDCT, multiplanar reconstructions can be made to evaluate and characterize the aorta accurately.

Actual image acquisition for a CT of the thoracic aorta can be performed in a matter of seconds, particularly with the advent of newer technology, such as dual-source scanners. However, overall, CT is more time consuming than radiography because it requires patient preparation (securing intravenous access), scanner setup, and time for image postprocessing. Nevertheless, the complete process of CT imaging from start to finish can be completed in a matter of minutes. This allows for noninvasive imaging of critically ill patients and can expedite management and treatment decision making. A secondary advantage to the fast acquisition of CT pertains to pediatric patients or patients in pain—short acquisition times are easier to tolerate and avoid motion artifacts from patient discomfort.

Disadvantages and Limitations of CT

An inherent disadvantage of CT imaging is the ionizing radiation associated with image acquisition. The radiation dose is of particular concern when imaging is performed in pediatric patients or when serial examinations are performed for disease surveillance.

Additionally, diagnostic imaging of the aortic lumen requires administration of IV contrast. However, IV contrast is contraindicated in the case of severe chronic renal insufficiency (glomerular filtration rate <30); in these cases, contrast-enhanced CT imaging cannot be performed. It should be mentioned, however, that patients with end-stage renal disease may receive iodinated contrast if hemodialysis is performed after contrast administration.

Furthermore, allergies to iodinated contrast are not uncommon, and the use of iodinated contrast may be contraindicated (e.g., in the case of anaphylaxis). Even in cases of mild allergy, premedication takes between 7 and 13 hours, which is usually not feasible in the assessment of traumatic injury or acute chest pain.

Although CT has a relatively short acquisition time, motion artifacts, including cardiac motion and breathing, may result in an artifact that degrades images. However, newer scanners with dual-source technology and more detectors may reduce artifacts and decrease scan times.

Problem Solving With Noncontrast CT

The noncontrast phase is an essential part of every examination of the aorta. Noncontrast evaluation allows for the characterization of intimal atherosclerotic calcifications, which may be obscured by contrast in an angiographic phase. Similarly, surgical material such as sutures or pledgets are intrinsically dense on CT; without a precontrast image, these can be mistaken for contrast leak or pseudoaneurysm.

Importantly, an acute IMH is most evident on noncontrast CT. This is seen as a crescentic hyperdensity tracking along the vessel wall. However, this may be obscured on the angiographic phase or may be mistaken for atheromatous plaque or mural thrombus instead of acute pathology.

The radiation dose may be reduced by a number of methods. Automated tube current modulation should always be used, when available. In the case of thin or pediatric patients, lower tube kVp may also be used. Newer scanners with dual-source technology can have faster image acquisition at lower radiation doses. Dual-source technology has also been used in virtual noncontrast imaging, eliminating the dose from an additional CT sequence. However, this technology is relatively new and is not universally available. Newer software using iterative reconstruction (as opposed to filtered backprojection) can reduce image noise, allowing for diagnostic images with lower radiation doses.

Problem Solving With Contrast-Enhanced CT

Contrast-enhanced CT angiography (CTA) is the mainstay for the emergent evaluation of acute aortic diseases. Contrast is used for the opacification of the vessel lumen, which allows for targeted evaluation of the intima.

Contrast is injected intravenously at a rate of 3 to 5 mL/s, usually followed by a saline chaser that allows contrast advancement through the circulatory system while decreasing contrast volume. Bolus-tracking strategy is generally used, with a region of interest set over the blood pool (typically the ascending aorta). When the density of the ascending aorta has reached a threshold, scanning begins.

In some cases, a delayed scan may be performed 2 minutes after injection of contrast. Delayed scans may assess for late contrast opacification of a false lumen (in the case of aortic dissection) or delayed opacification of an endoleak in the case of endograft repair. Additionally, delayed images may demonstrate contrast extravasation that is not apparent on angiographic phase.

Nearly all examinations are subject to postprocessing, including multiplanar (axial, sagittal, and coronal) reformats and maximum intensity projection images. The additional use of interactive reformatting software can allow for oblique reformats (e.g., candy cane view of the thoracic aorta). Three-dimensional surface rendering of the aorta can aid in the additional characterization of thoracic disease and treatment planning.

Magnetic Resonance Imaging

MRI is an imaging method that does not use ionizing radiation and provides an alternative to the use of CT in cross-sectional thoracic imaging. MRI uses a combination of a strong magnetic field and radiofrequency pulses to create cross-sectional images. In contrast to CT, this requires multiple sequences (image acquisitions). The most useful tool in aortic imaging by MRI is usually contrast-enhanced (using gadolinium-based contrast agents) magnetic resonance angiography (MRA). However, some MRA sequences may also be obtained using noncontrast protocols, which are useful in cases where gadolinium contrast is contraindicated.

Advantages of MRI

Magnetic resonance imaging has the distinct advantage of providing cross-sectional images without the use of ionizing radiation. This is ideal for many situations, particularly in the case of young patients or patients who need serial studies for surveillance. MR images provide multiplanar reformatted images, which may be adjusted to any plane that is tailored to any patient's individual anatomy. In addition to anatomic information, MRI can provide functional imaging through the use of cinematic and phase contrast sequences.

Another advantage of MR over CT is the use of contrast agents. When iodine allergy precludes a contrast-enhanced CT examination, gadolinium may be administered without cross-reactivity. Additionally, when all IV contrast agents are contraindicated (see below), noncontrast MRA may also provide useful and diagnostic information.

Disadvantages and Limitations of MRI

A major disadvantage to MR is its long acquisition time. A full MR study may take from 30 to 60 minutes. This is not ideal in the cases of acute aortic syndromes, when decisions for intervention are made in a matter of minutes, not hours. Moreover, the long acquisition times may require sedation, particularly in pediatric patients.

In the case of obese patients, the size of the magnet may preclude its use. Magnet size varies by manufacturer and model but, overall, MRI bores are typically narrower than those of CT and may not permit the imaging of obese patients.

Due to the high magnetic fields and tissue heating associated with MR, certain devices are contraindicated. Examples include pacemakers, automated implantable cardiac defibrillators, spinal stimulators, and deep brain stimulators. Metallic fragments in the orbits, brain, or spinal canal may also preclude the use of MRI because fragment heating or motion may result in adjacent tissue damage.

Contrast agents in MRI (gadolinium-based) are excreted through the renal system. Due to the risk of nephrogenic systemic fibrosis, gadolinium agents are contraindicated in those with renal failure. Unlike iodinated contrast, gadolinium remains contraindicated in all cases of renal failure, even when the patient is on hemodialysis.

Problem Solving With Noncontrast MRI

Multiple techniques are used in noncontrast MRI evaluation of the aorta. Black blood sequences (traditionally spin echo sequences) yield high-contrast images of the aortic wall-lumen interface and mediastinal structures. Bright blood (gradient echo) sequences can use both static and cinematic techniques and can yield anatomic and functional data. Also, with the use of velocity-encoded cine sequences, quantitative vascular flow data can be acquired. 3D time-of-flight images can be used for noncontrast angiography. However, time-of-flight images are prone to artifacts (particularly in the setting of slow or turbulent flow) and are less useful when IV contrast can be used.

Problem Solving With Contrast-Enhanced MRI
Following a noncontrast MRI sequence, contrast-enhanced MR images are obtained after the IV administration of gadolinium-based contrast agents. The timing of contrast bolus is critical in the acquisition of MRA sequences because the intravascular phase of contrast enhancement is short.

Contrast-enhanced MRA exploits the T1-shortening characteristics of gadolinium. A postcontrast T1-weighted sequence of the aorta can be obtained using single–breath-hold techniques. Images are obtained in any number of projections and can be reformatted into maximum intensity projection or surface rendered images.

Similar to CT, a noncontrast series of images must first be obtained. In addition to providing a baseline to evaluate relative enhancement, this allows for subtraction images to be calculated from the added information.

■ Aortic Anatomy

Normal Thoracic Aortic Anatomy

The thoracic aorta arises from the left ventricular outflow tract at the aortic valve and extends to the level of the diaphragm (Fig. 29.1). Like all arteries, the aorta is comprised of three layers. The intima is the innermost layer. Aortic media has smooth muscle cells and comprises the middle layer of the aorta. The adventitia is the outermost layer. The adventitia has its own aortic supply, known as the *vasa vasorum,* which is a network of feeding arteries that encase the aorta. The vasa vasorum can play a role in the development of aortic disease.

The thoracic aorta is divided into three anatomic sections—ascending aorta, aortic arch, and descending aorta. The aortic root is the first portion of the thoracic aorta, between the aortic annulus and the sinotubular junction. The sinuses of Valsalva are considered part of the aortic root and give rise to the coronary arteries. It is important to remember that the first 3 cm of the ascending aorta are within the reflections of the pericardium, an important consideration in the evaluation of ascending aortic disease.

The arch of the aorta starts at the origin of the brachiocephalic artery and extends to the origin of the left subclavian artery (Fig. 29.2). The aortic arch has three branches—brachiocephalic artery, left common carotid artery, and left subclavian artery. The end of the left subclavian artery is at the aortic isthmus, where the left subclavian artery extends to the ligamentum arteriosum.

The descending aorta extends from the isthmus to the diaphragm. Multiple branches arise from the descending aorta, including the bronchial arteries, spinal arteries, intercostal branches, and superior phrenic branches.

Normal Variants of Aortic Anatomy

In 7% of the asymptomatic population, the left vertebral artery arises directly from the aortic arch. This is usually of little clinical significance, but is helpful to know prior to catheter-directed angiography or surgery.

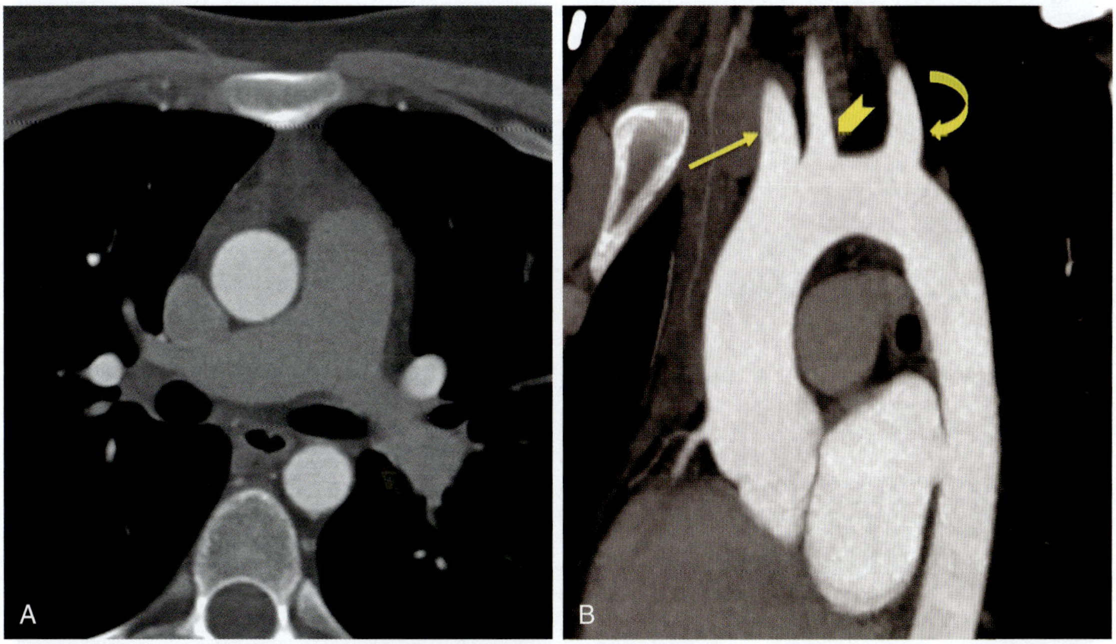

Figure 29.1 Normal aortic anatomy on CT angiogram. (A) Axial CT angiogram image of a normal ascending and descending aorta. The normal thoracic aorta measures less than 4 cm. (B) Sagittal oblique maximum intensity projection of a normal thoracic aorta demonstrates its extension from the aortic root to the diaphragm. It has conventional three-vessel branching. The great vessels typically arise from the aortic arch in the following order: right brachiocephalic *(straight arrow)*, left common carotid *(arrowhead)*, and left subclavian *(curved arrow)* arteries.

Another common variant to the aortic arch branching is the two-vessel arch, which is characterized by a common origin of the brachiocephalic and left common carotid artery, occurring in up to 25% of the normal population (Fig. 29.3). This anatomic variant has been termed the *bovine arch*, which is actually a misnomer—a cow's aortic arch actually has a single brachiocephalic trunk from which the subclavian arteries and a bicarotid trunk arise.

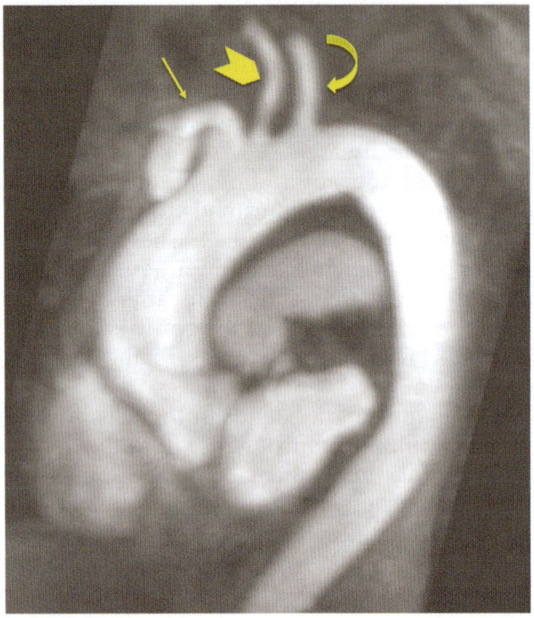

Figure 29.2 Sagittal oblique maximum intensity projection reformat of a contrast-enhanced MR angiogram, demonstrating normal contours of the thoracic aortic arch and branching to the right brachiocephalic *(straight arrow)*, left common carotid *(arrowhead)*, and left subclavian *(curved arrow)* arteries.

In approximately 0.5% of the population, the right subclavian artery arises directly from the aorta. However, in these cases, the subclavian artery arises distal to the left subclavian origin, taking an aberrant retroesophageal course across the mediastinum.

A ductus diverticulum is also a common aortic arch variant, which occurs at the aortic isthmus. This focal contour abnormality may be complicated by aneurysmal dilation of the diverticulum.

Pseudocoarctation occurs in the setting of an elongated, redundant thoracic aorta. In this case, the redundant portions of the vessel become kinked on themselves. These redundant folds in the aorta can mimic focal narrowing or congenital coarctation of the aorta. Pseudocoarctation is common in patients with Turner syndrome as a result of an elongated transverse portion of the aortic arch.

A cervical aortic arch occurs when the aortic arch extends superiorly beyond the clavicles, into the thoracic inlet. This may be an isolated finding or may occur in the setting of congenital heart and/or thoracic disease.

Pitfalls in the Evaluation of Aortic Anatomy

Pseudocoarctation Versus Coarctation

A true coarctation is a congenital narrowing of the aorta, which occurs at the aortic isthmus (at the level of the ductus arteriosus). Thus a true coarctation results in

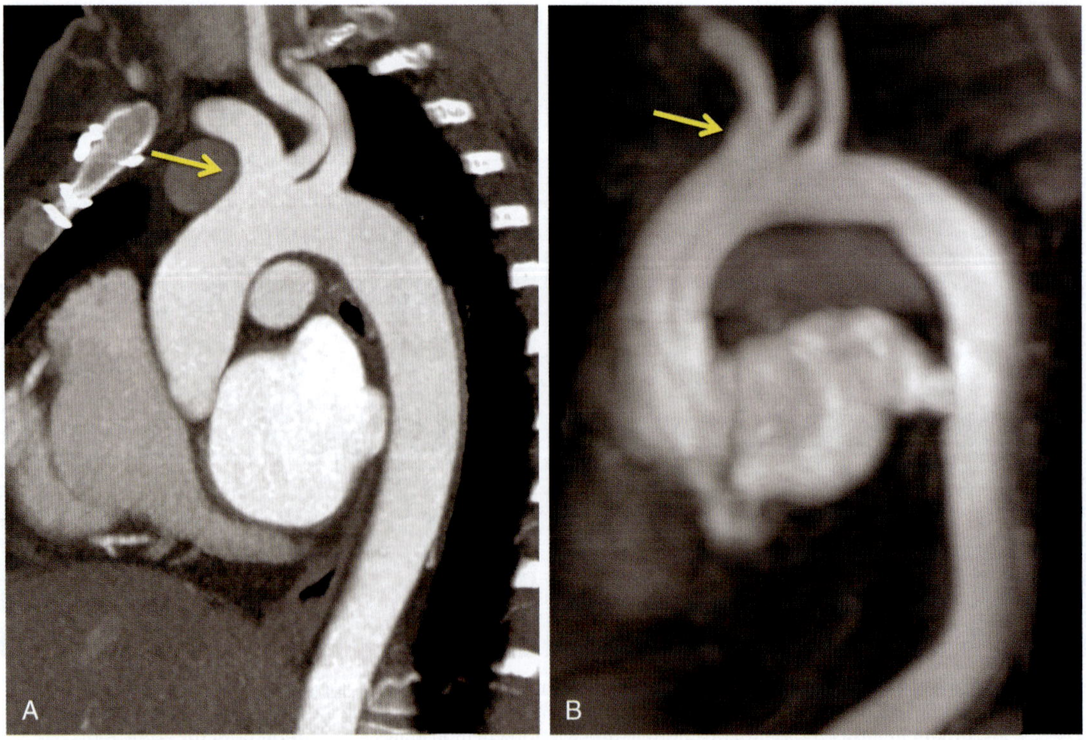

Figure 29.3 Two-vessel arch. (A) Sagittal oblique maximum intensity projection reformatted images of a CT angiogram and (B) contrast-enhanced MR angiogram in two patients with a bovine aortic arch. Note the two-vessel configuration resulting from a common origin of the right brachiocephalic and left common carotid arteries *(arrows)*.

obstruction of flow. Secondary signs of coarctation include left ventricular hypertrophy or enlarged collateral vessels, such as the intercostal and internal mammary arteries.

In contrast, pseudocoarctation results from redundancy of an ectatic aorta. Redundant folds in the aorta can give the appearance of luminal narrowing, although the overall flow in the aorta is not actually obstructed. As such, there should be no collateral vessels and normal flow on phase contrast MRI.

Chronic Diseases of the Aorta

Atherosclerosis

Causes of Atherosclerosis

Atherosclerosis is the result of chronic inflammation in an artery secondary to long-standing hypertension. Lipids are deposited into the vessel wall, and inflammatory cytokines and cells infiltrate the vessel wall. A contained atheromatous plaque has a fibrous cap, which protects the lipid core from exposure to the vessel lumen. A plaque may be calcified or noncalcified.

Appearance of Atherosclerosis

Radiographs are relatively insensitive for the detection of noncalcified atheromatous plaque. However, calcified atherosclerosis may be visible in the aortic arch (on a frontal projection) or in the aortic wall (on lateral views). Noncontrast CT is very sensitive for the detection of calcified atherosclerosis; however, noncalcified plaque may not be visible. In contrast, CTA is very sensitive for the detection of noncalcified plaque, whereas calcifications may occasionally be obscured.

MRA is very sensitive for the detection of atherosclerosis, namely as an irregularity along the aortic vessel wall. Calcifications, on the other hand, may be difficult to detect on MRI.

Thoracic Aortic Aneurysm

Normal Dimensions of the Aorta

PROBLEM SOLVING: MEASURING THE AORTA

The normal aorta is a curved 3D structure. Thus measurement of the aortic lumen in standard axial, sagittal, and coronal planes may underestimate or overestimate the actual dimensions of the vessel. Thin-section data and interactive reformatting software are essential for the accurate and reproducible measurement of the aorta. Interactive software allows for true reconstruction in the plane of the aorta as it turns and results in accurate cross-sectional analysis of the aorta. This is important not only in the evaluation of acute aortic disease, but also in the surveillance of aortic disease (e.g., evaluating an aortic aneurysm for increasing size). By convention, aortic size is measured from the outermost portion of the aortic wall (outer diameter).

Appearance of a Thoracic Aortic Aneurysm

By definition, an aortic aneurysm occurs when all three layers of the aorta (intima, media, and adventitia) become dilated. Although size criteria have been debated, the generally accepted cutoff for normal aortic size is 4 cm (Fig. 29.4).

On a radiograph, this manifests as a large, ectatic, and tortuous aorta. However, artifacts related to projection and multiple overlapping mediastinal structures make measurements of the aorta unreliable by radiographic appearance only. This is better evaluated with multiplanar reformats on cross-sectional imaging, such as contrast-enhanced CT or MRI.

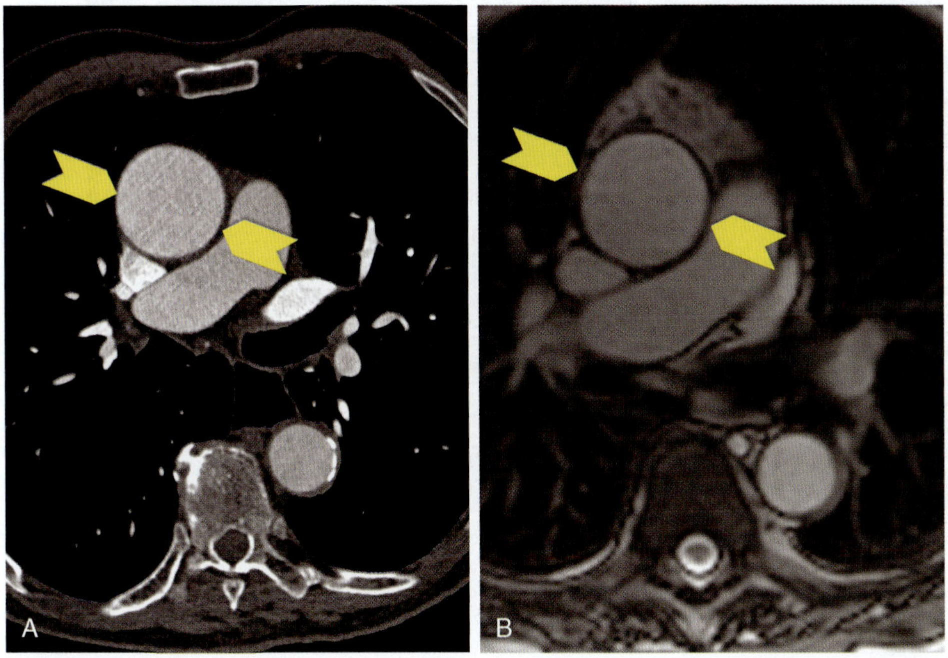

Figure 29.4 Ascending aortic aneurysm. (A) Axial images of a CT angiogram and axial contrast-enhanced MR angiogram (B) demonstrating dilation of the ascending thoracic aorta, up to 4.7 cm in diameter *(arrowheads)*. Note the caliber of the ascending aorta relative to the descending aorta.

Most thoracic aortic aneurysms (60%) occur in the ascending aorta. The descending thoracic aorta is affected in 40% of cases.

Clinical Significance of a Thoracic Aortic Aneurysm

Due to altered hemodynamics and decreased tensile strength of the aorta, the aneurysmal aorta is inherently weak. The aneurysmal aorta has a higher likelihood of aortic dissection and/or rupture. The risk factors predicting aneurysm rupture are overall size and rate of enlargement. As the aortic size increases, the tensile strength of the aorta decreases, thus increasing the likelihood of rupture.

■ Acute Aortic Syndromes

Intramural Hematoma

Causes of Intramural Hematoma

An IMH is an acute aortic syndrome characterized by acute hemorrhage into the aortic media. It is thought to result from rupture of the vasa vasorum into the vessel wall. An IMH may have an intact intima, although complicated cases may have focal aortic dissection or intimal interruption.

The most common predisposing factor for IMH is hypertension. IMH may also occur because of trauma or a PAU.

Appearance of Intramural Hematoma

IMH is best characterized on noncontrast CT. On axial images, IMH appears as a crescentic density in the wall of the aorta (Fig. 29.5). The IMH is hyperdense and has different MRI signal characteristics relative to aortic blood pool as the hematoma organizes and becomes thrombosed (Fig. 29.6).

Noncontrast CT is essential for the characterization of the IMH. Otherwise, contrast in the vessel lumen may obscure the hyperdensity of the IMH.

IMH is classified similarly to an aortic dissection. IMH involving the ascending aorta is classified as type Stanford A, and IMH distal to the left subclavian artery is classified as type Stanford B.

Management of Intramural Hematoma

IMH is treated similarly to aortic dissection, based on the Stanford A and B classification. IMH has a variable clinical course and may resolve over time or lead to aneurysmal dilation or frank dissection. Stanford type A IMH is usually treated as a surgical emergency, and Stanford type B IMH is usually treated medically.

Problem Solving: How to Differentiate Intramural Hematoma From Vasculitis

From an imaging standpoint, differentiating IMH and vasculitis can be difficult. Both are associated with aortic wall thickening on cross-sectional imaging.

Clinical and demographic information may be helpful in differentiating vasculitis from IMH. Takayasu arteritis (the most common vasculitis to affect the aorta) usually affects young women of Asian descent. In contrast, IMH is more often associated with hypertension and usually affects older individuals.

Additionally, vasculitis is an inflammatory condition affecting the aorta. In the case of active inflammation, the aorta may enhance following administration of IV

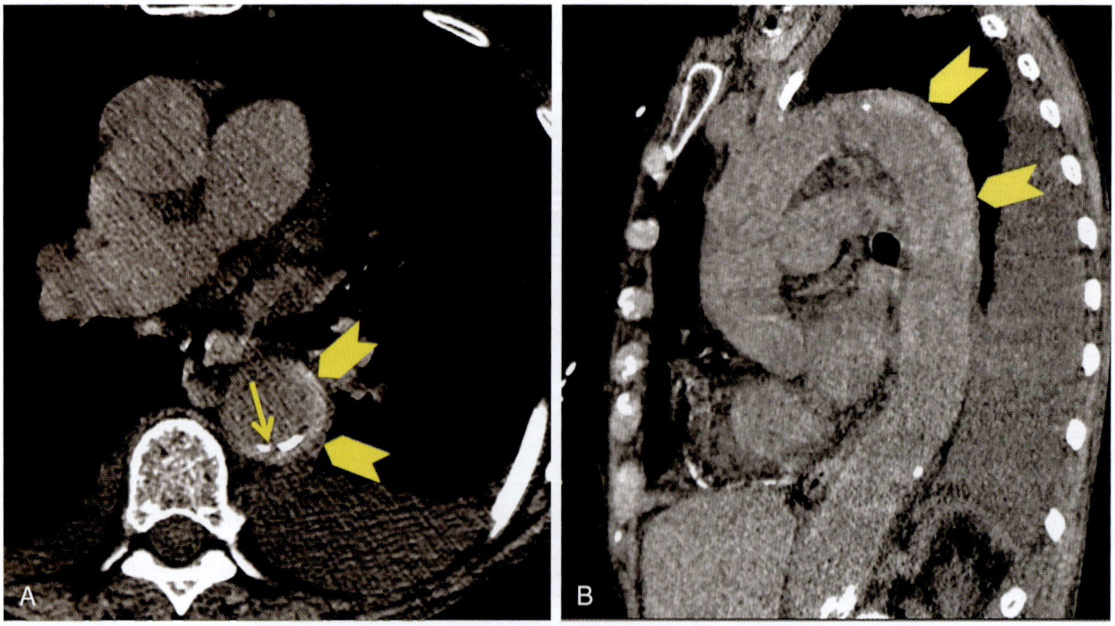

Figure 29.5 Acute intramural hematoma (IMH) on noncontrast CT. (A) Noncontrast axial and sagittal oblique (B) noncontrast views of the aorta with a crescentic, hyperdense IMH *(arrowheads)*. Note background atherosclerosis and the relation of the hematoma to the intimal calcifications *(arrow)*, which clearly demonstrates the intramural location of the hyperdense hematoma.

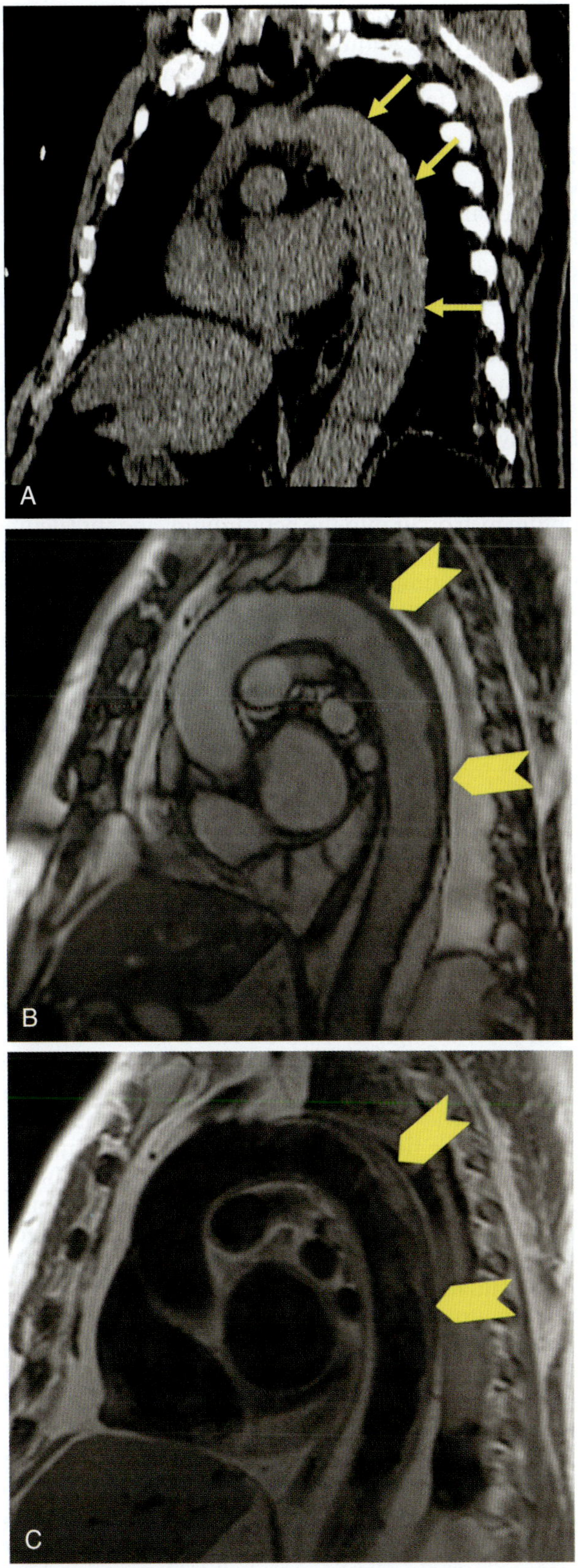

Figure 29.6 Sagittal oblique views of acute intramural hematoma (IMH). (A) Sagittal oblique noncontrast CT demonstrates an eccentric curvilinear hyperdensity in the descending aorta *(arrows)*, compatible with an acute IMH. (B) Noncontrast sagittal oblique balanced steady-state free precession and (C) T2 black blood images show irregular abnormal signal *(arrowheads)* in the aortic vessel wall corresponding to the IMH.

contrast and result in a so-called double-ring configuration of enhancement. In contrast, IMH does not enhance.

Penetrating Aortic Ulcer

Causes of a Penetrating Aortic Ulcer

PAU is an acute aortic syndrome that occurs in the setting of atheromatous aortic plaque. PAU develops when the ulcerated plaque disrupts the aortic intima. This leads to disruption of the elastic lamina and may extend into the aortic media.

The most common predisposing factor for PAU is hypertension. PAU occurs in the setting of extensive atherosclerosis in the aorta. Patients with PAU may present with acute chest pain. In some cases, patients are asymptomatic, and the finding may be incidental when imaging is performed for other reasons.

Appearance of a Penetrating Aortic Ulcer

PAU is best detected on contrast-enhanced CT. It is characterized by a contrast-filled outpouching beyond the normal contours of the aorta.

In the setting of PAU, the ulceration of plaque disrupts the vessel wall. In the mildest of cases, this only affects the aortic intima. However, a PAU may also extend beyond the aortic intima and may lead to an IMH or aortic dissection.

Problem Solving: How to Differentiate a Penetrating Aortic Ulcer From Plaque

Even with cross-sectional imaging, PAU can be difficult to differentiate from ulcerated plaque along the aortic intima. Multiplanar reformatting may be helpful in outlining the contours of the aortic wall and the relationship of plaque relative to the aorta. By definition, a PAU must show contrast opacification beyond the confines of the aortic wall (Fig. 29.7).

Aortic Dissection

Causes of Aortic Dissection

Aortic dissection occurs from tearing of the aortic intima; blood fills the space between the intimal flap and the media, which is otherwise only a potential space. Spontaneous dissections usually occur secondary to hypertension. However, other causes of luminal disruption (e.g., PAU, trauma) may also result in the propagation of a dissection flap.

Appearance of a Dissection

Aortic dissection is characterized by an intimal flap that becomes displaced into the aortic lumen. Downstream of the intimal defect, the potential space of the media becomes filled by blood or contrast and is termed the *false lumen.* Pressure from the blood flow forces the intimal flap to extend downstream. On cross-sectional imaging, an aortic dissection has an intimal flap separating the true and false lumens.

Classification of Aortic Dissections

Aortic dissections are classified by the Stanford classification system. Dissections that involve the ascending aorta

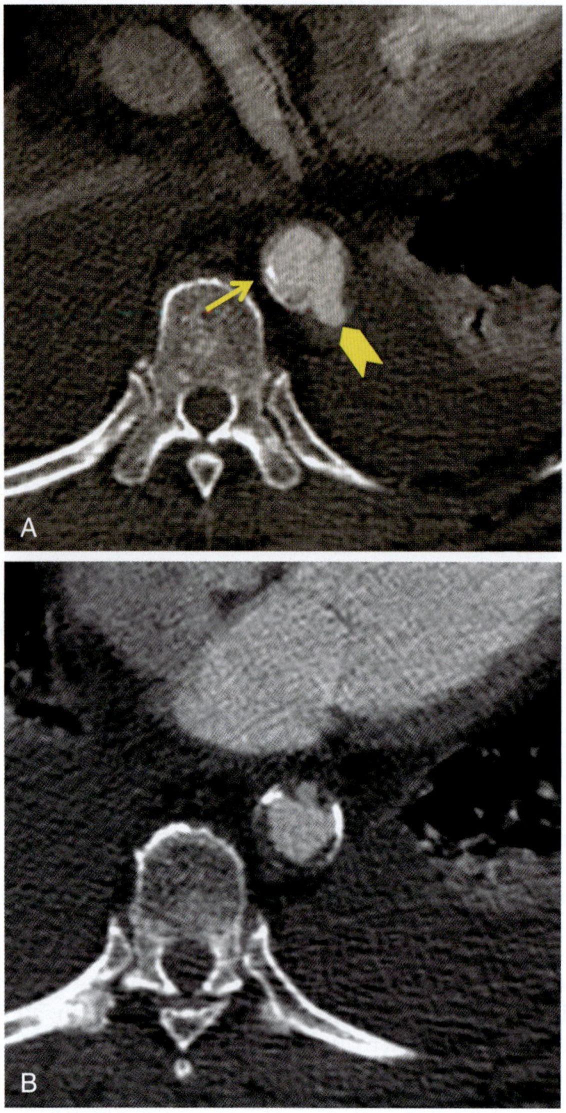

Figure 29.7 Penetrating aortic ulcer (PAU). (A) Contrast-enhanced CT image of a PAU. Note the intimal calcifications *(arrow)* denoting the margin of the aortic intima. Iodinated contrast in the PAU clearly extends beyond the normal vessel wall *(arrowhead)*. (B) In comparison, a different axial slice in the same patient demonstrates ulcerated plaque. Note the relation of the contrast relative to the atherosclerotic calcifications and how the IV contrast does not extend beyond the aortic wall.

are classified as Stanford class A in the radiology literature (Fig. 29.8). Dissections that start distal to the origin of the left subclavian artery are classified as Stanford class B by the radiology literature; the innominate artery is the transition point in the surgical literature (Fig. 29.9). The most important point is that the morphology of the aortic dissection be clearly communicated to the surgical team at the local medical center. Stanford type A dissections are usually managed as surgical emergencies. Stanford type B dissections are typically managed medically with blood pressure control.

In the case of Stanford type B dissection, the aorta is usually followed with serial examinations to evaluate for extension of the intimal flap or for signs of enlarging aortic aneurysm. Chronic aortic dissections may have features that are not present in acute aortic dissections. As an example, a long-standing false lumen may thrombose and calcify over time. Additionally, chronic aortic dissections may develop fenestrations or communication between the true and false lumens through the intimal flap.

Complications of Aortic Dissection

Acutely, an aortic dissection flap separates the aorta into true and false lumens. The false lumen is typically larger than the true lumen and may even narrow the true lumen to a flow-limiting state. In the aortic arch, exclusion by a dissection flap may compromise flow to the left subclavian artery, resulting in differential blood pressure in the upper extremities. In the abdominal aorta, this phenomenon may lead to bowel ischemia or renal injury.

Additionally, aortic dissections may propagate into the downstream branches (see Fig. 29.8B and C). In a Stanford type A dissection, the flap may propagate into the aortic root or coronary arteries; in these cases, vessel rupture may occur into the pericardium, and threatening cardiac tamponade may result (Fig. 29.10). Additional branches, including the subclavian, carotid, mesenteric, and iliac arteries, may also be involved.

Chronically, aortic dissection results in an inherent weakening of the aorta, and aneurysmal dilation may result. Also secondary to slow flow, the false lumen may thrombose; the thrombus may break off, resulting in downstream infarcts.

Role of Imaging in Aortic Dissection

Although often obtained in the initial evaluation of acute chest pain, plain film radiographs are not sensitive or specific for the detection of aortic dissection. However, in some cases, intimal atherosclerotic calcifications may be inwardly displaced secondary to blood in the aortic media. Although this is a very rare finding in plain film radiography, it is virtually diagnostic of aortic dissection when present (Figs. 29.11 and 29.12).

Owing largely to its short acquisition times and ready availability, CT has become the mainstay in the evaluation of acute aortic dissection. CT is highly sensitive and specific for the detection of aortic dissection, but does require the use of ionizing radiation and iodinated contrast. In contrast, MRI does not use ionizing radiation and can be performed with or without contrast. As such, MRI is ideal for the surveillance of chronic aortic dissection (evaluating for propagation of the dissection flap or for aneurysm enlargement) and for the evaluation of dissection in the setting of chronic renal disease. However, the long acquisition times associated with MRI make it less useful in the evaluation of acutely ill or hemodynamically unstable patients.

Cross-sectional imaging (including CT or MRI) plays a key role in the evaluation for complications of aortic dissection. Specifically, CT can be useful when evaluating for the extent of dissection flap propagation, as well as for immediate complications, including hemopericardium, ischemia, and vessel rupture.

Problem Solving: Differentiating True Lumen Versus False Lumen

In the case of a thrombosed false lumen, differentiating the true and false lumens is usually not difficult. However,

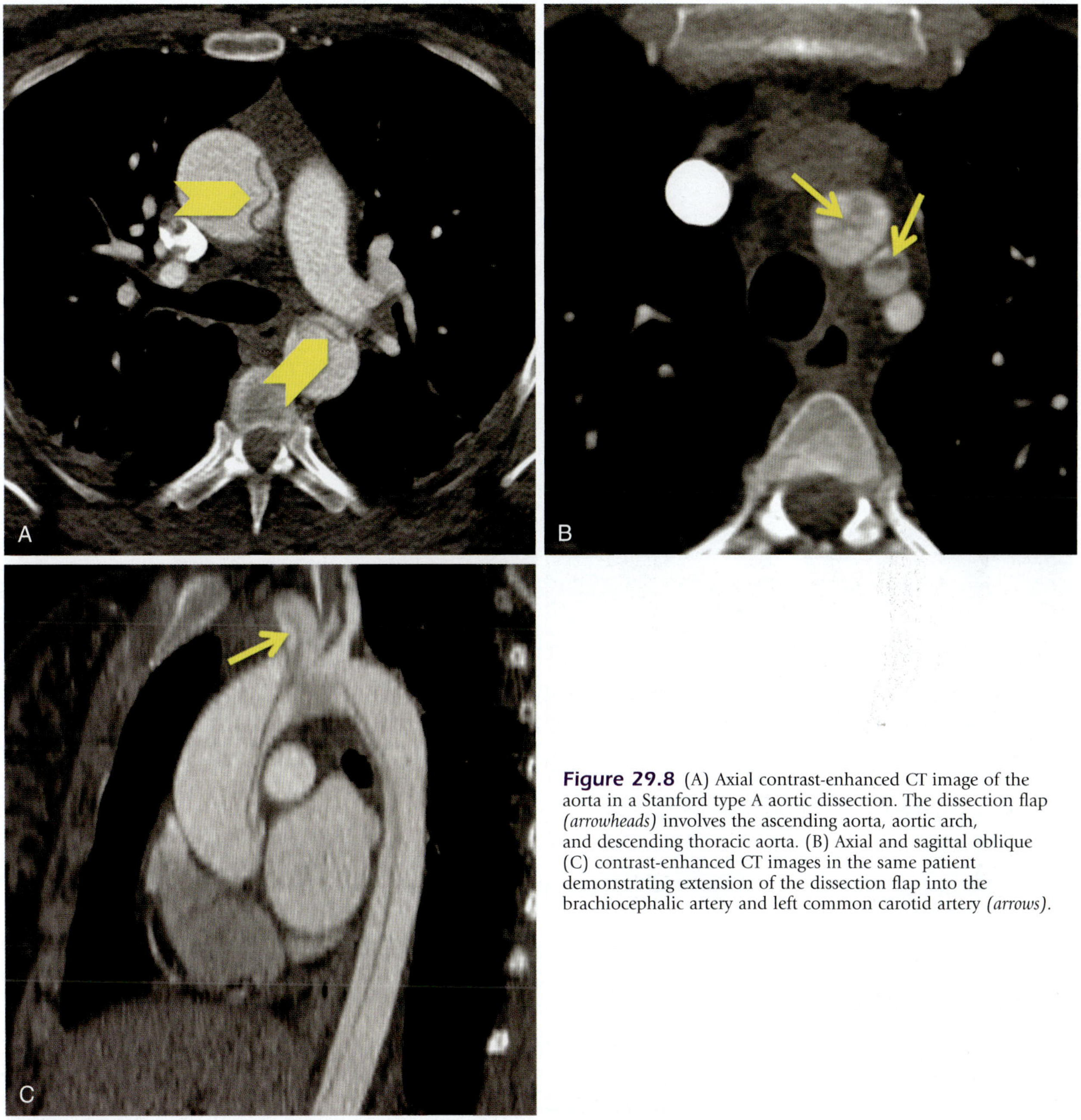

Figure 29.8 (A) Axial contrast-enhanced CT image of the aorta in a Stanford type A aortic dissection. The dissection flap *(arrowheads)* involves the ascending aorta, aortic arch, and descending thoracic aorta. (B) Axial and sagittal oblique (C) contrast-enhanced CT images in the same patient demonstrating extension of the dissection flap into the brachiocephalic artery and left common carotid artery *(arrows)*.

in the setting of acute aortic dissection, differentiation can be difficult.

The true lumen should be continuous with the normal parts of the aorta, both upstream and downstream of the dissection flap. Additionally, the true lumen usually spirals along the posterior aspect of the aortic arch and along the anterior aspect of the descending aorta.

Due to differential filling, the false lumen should exhibit delayed filling relative to the true lumen. Changing the viewing windows of a CT image may aid in differentiating lumens.

A reliable differentiating feature between the true and false lumens of an aortic dissection is the so-called beak sign, which occurs when the false lumen has an acute angle at the end of the dissection, created by the intimal flap and normal vessel media or adventitia. Multiplanar and oblique reformatting can be very useful in identifying this feature (Fig. 29.13).

Although not a reliable indicator, the false lumen is usually larger than the true lumen. Additionally, the cobweb sign—thin strandlike filling defects from residual media fibers—can help identify the false lumen (although only present in a minority of cases).

Pitfalls in the Evaluation of Acute Aortic Syndromes

Motion Artifacts

Longer acquisition times are associated with a higher likelihood of motion artifact. The most common motion artifacts result from patient breathing and cardiac motion.

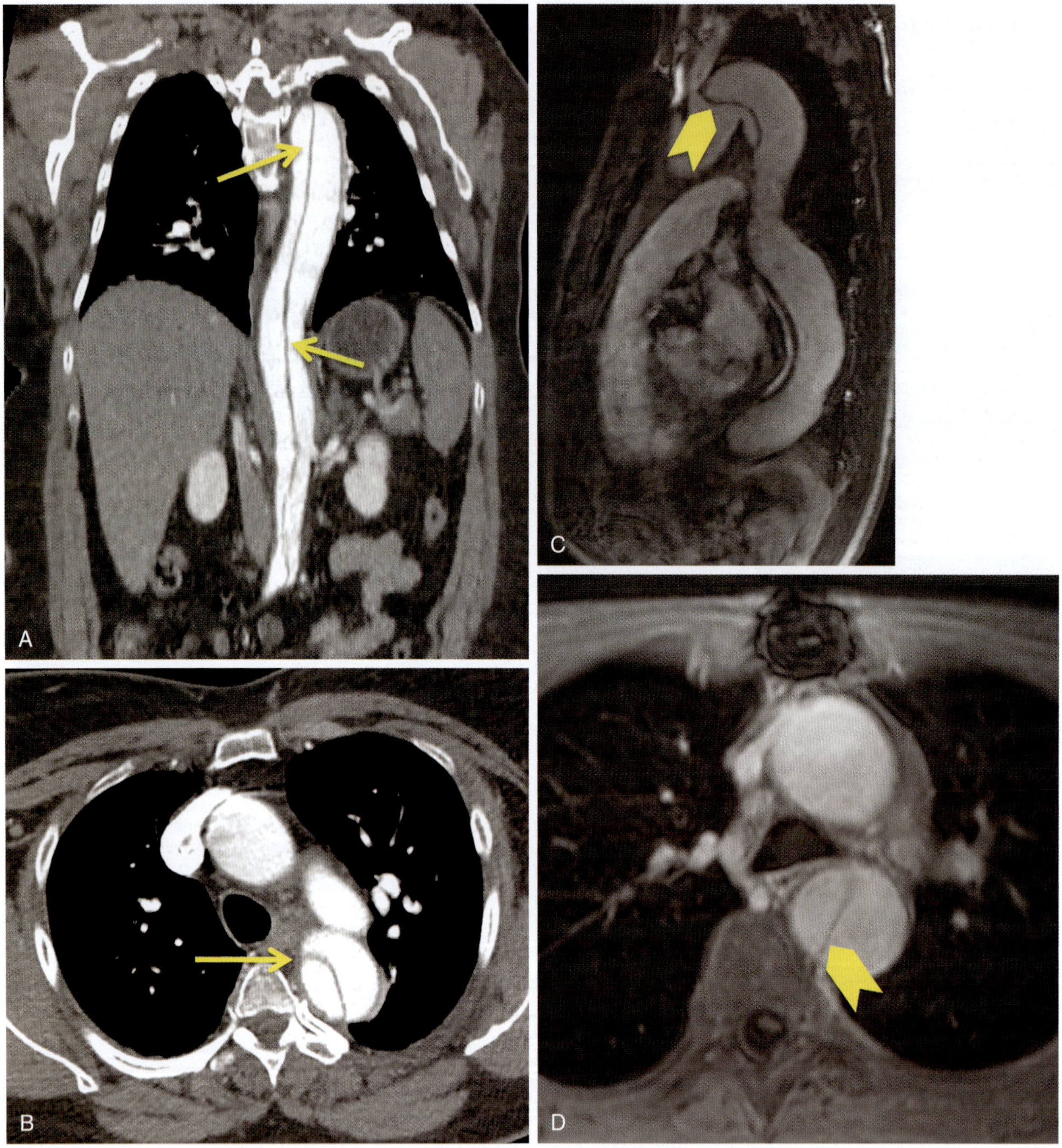

Figure 29.9 Stanford type B aortic dissection. (A) Coronal and axial (B) contrast-enhanced CT angiogram image of a Stanford type B aortic dissection. The dissection flap *(arrows)* initiates beyond the origin of the left subclavian artery. The dissection flap propagates downstream to the level of the aortic bifurcation. (C) Sagittal and axial (D) postcontrast MR angiogram images of a different patient with a Stanford type B aortic dissection. The dissection flap *(arrowhead)* begins downstream of the left subclavian artery. There is no involvement of the ascending aorta.

Other factors such as patient agitation, altered mental status, extreme shortness of breath, or young patient age may also increase motion artifact.

Motion may result in bandlike artifacts along the vessel wall, which can mimic a dissection flap. Additionally, motion can complicate accurate measurement of the aorta.

With the use of MDCT, acquisition times have substantially decreased. Using newer technologies (e.g., Flash scanning [Siemens] or dual-source CT), the entire aorta may be imaged in a single breath-hold, thus reducing breathing artifact. Cardiac electrocardiographic (ECG) gating, in which images are obtained in diastole, can

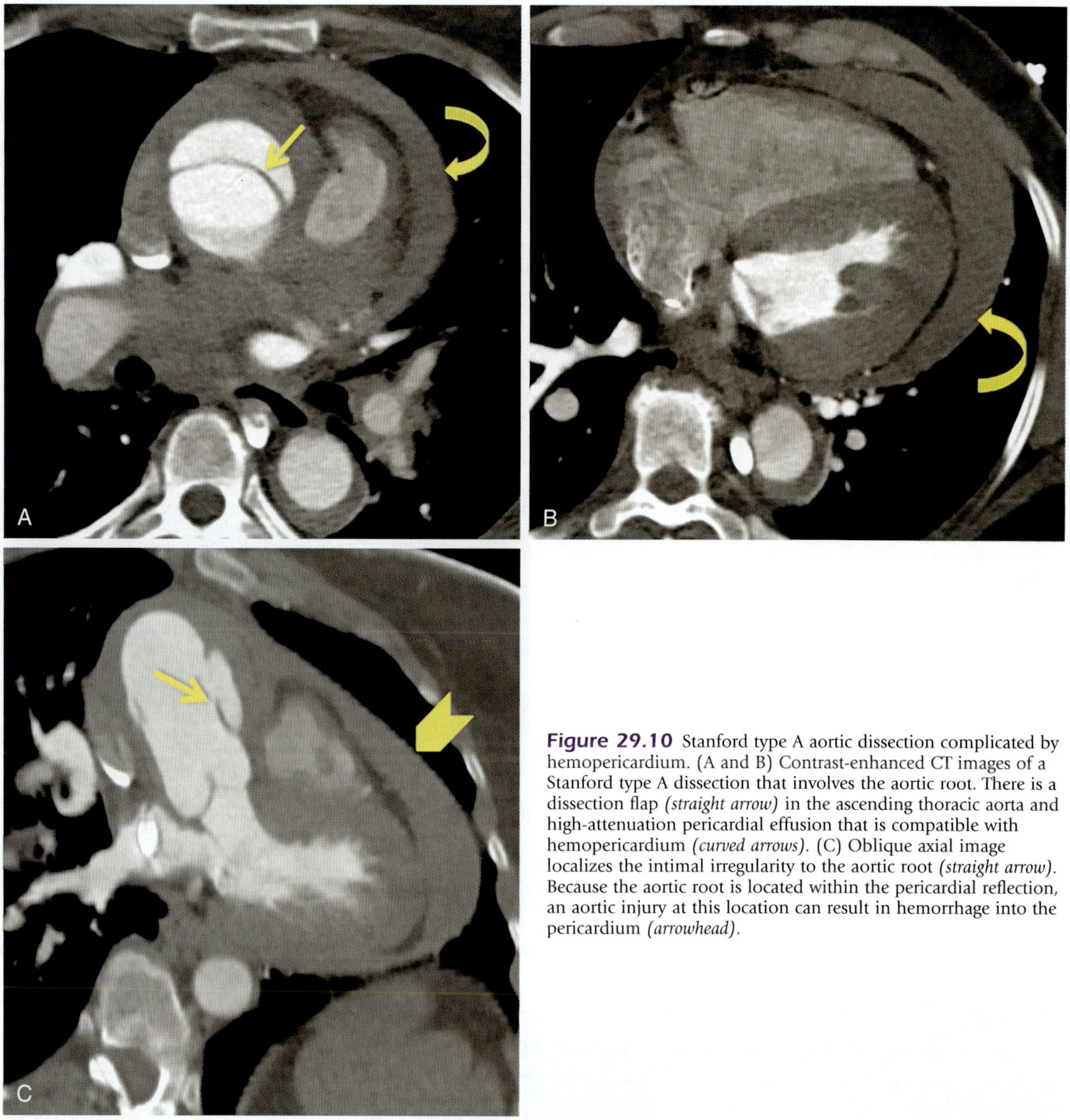

Figure 29.10 Stanford type A aortic dissection complicated by hemopericardium. (A and B) Contrast-enhanced CT images of a Stanford type A dissection that involves the aortic root. There is a dissection flap *(straight arrow)* in the ascending thoracic aorta and high-attenuation pericardial effusion that is compatible with hemopericardium *(curved arrows)*. (C) Oblique axial image localizes the intimal irregularity to the aortic root *(straight arrow)*. Because the aortic root is located within the pericardial reflection, an aortic injury at this location can result in hemorrhage into the pericardium *(arrowhead)*.

eliminate cardiac motion artifact. In other cases, sedation or anesthesia may be useful in decreasing patient agitation or motion.

Inclusion of Noncontrast Images

As mentioned before, MDCT has become the mainstay in the evaluation of acute aortic syndromes. CTA has become essential for evaluating syndromes such as PAU and aortic dissection. However, the high density of contrast in the aortic lumen may obscure abnormalities in the aortic wall, and certain abnormalities (e.g., IMH) may be not be readily apparent on postcontrast images. As such, it is imperative that every CT examination of the aorta include a noncontrast phase to evaluate the density of the aortic wall relative to the blood pool.

Aortic Trauma

Because it is the largest artery in the body, injuries to the aorta can have devastating results. Shear injuries to the aorta occur from blunt thoracic trauma or sudden deceleration. However, complete aortic injuries (through all three layers of the aorta) result in rapid exsanguination, and patients often do not survive long enough to undergo imaging.

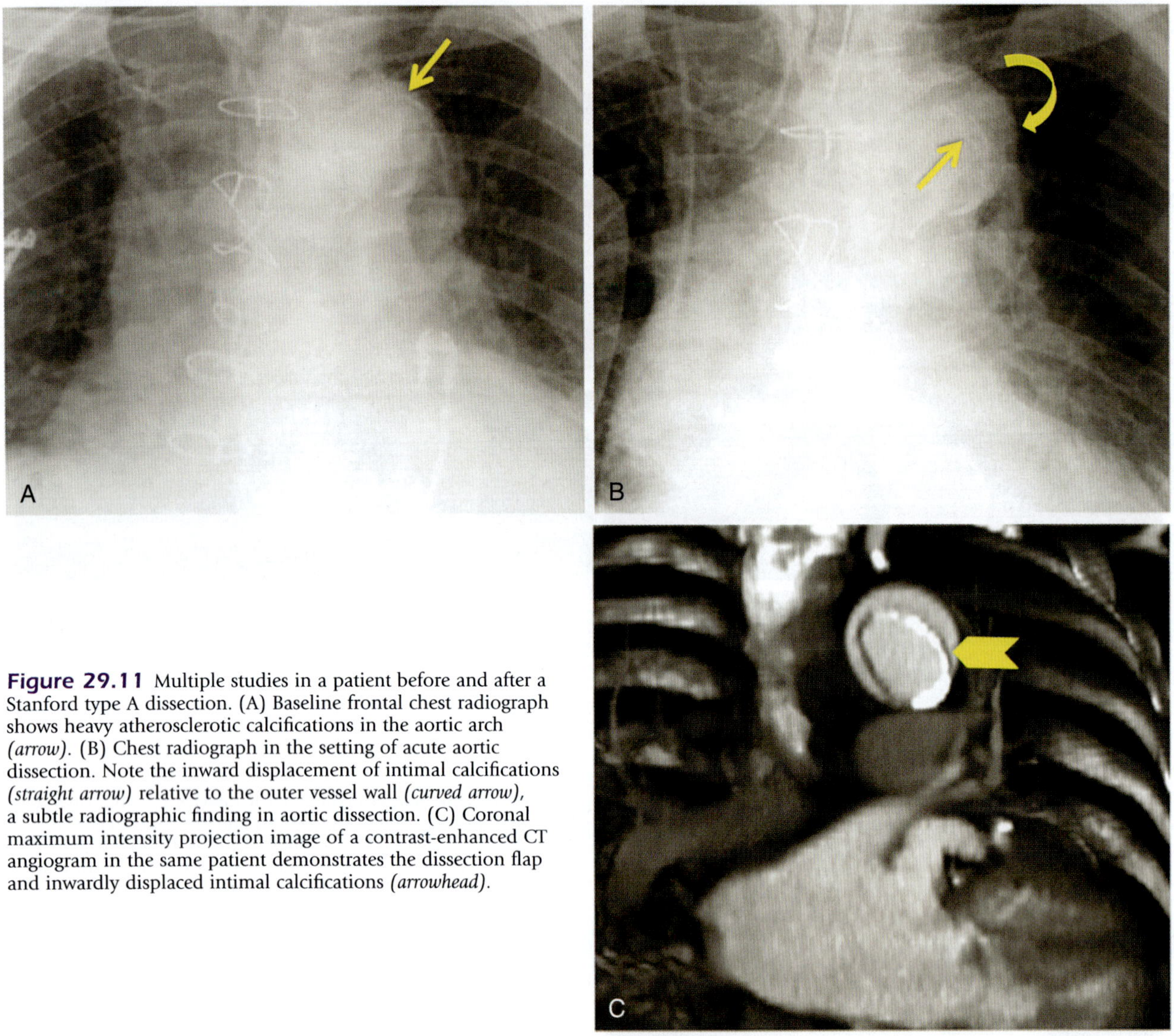

Figure 29.11 Multiple studies in a patient before and after a Stanford type A dissection. (A) Baseline frontal chest radiograph shows heavy atherosclerotic calcifications in the aortic arch *(arrow)*. (B) Chest radiograph in the setting of acute aortic dissection. Note the inward displacement of intimal calcifications *(straight arrow)* relative to the outer vessel wall *(curved arrow)*, a subtle radiographic finding in aortic dissection. (C) Coronal maximum intensity projection image of a contrast-enhanced CT angiogram in the same patient demonstrates the dissection flap and inwardly displaced intimal calcifications *(arrowhead)*.

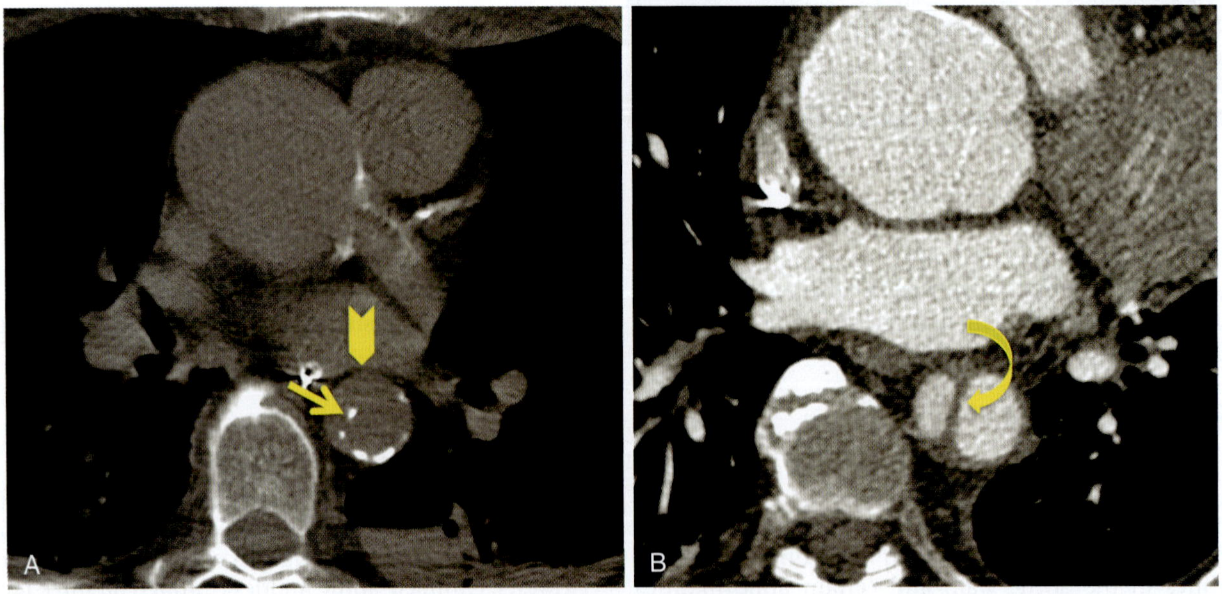

Figure 29.12 Intimal disruption in aortic dissection. (A) Noncontrast chest CT scan demonstrates inward displacement of atherosclerotic calcifications *(arrow)* relative to the outer contour of the descending thoracic aorta *(arrowhead)*. (B) Contrast-enhanced examination in the same patient demonstrates an intimal flap *(curved arrow)*.

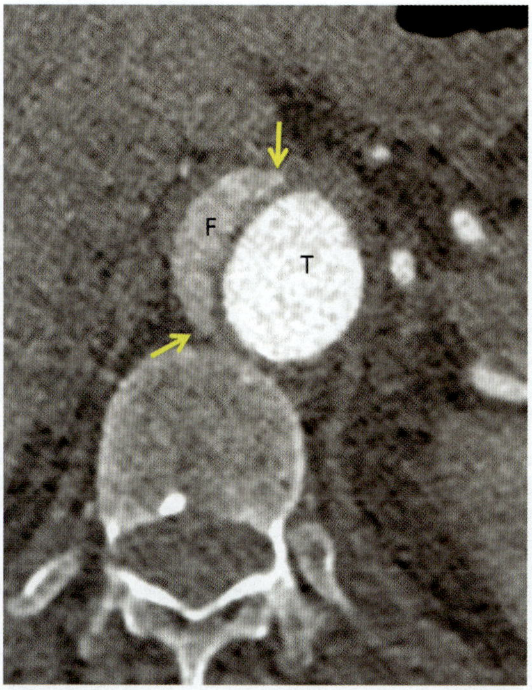

Figure 29.13 Axial contrast-enhanced CT scan demonstrates a dissection flap in the descending thoracic aorta/abdominal aorta. Differential perfusion allows for identification of the true lumen *(T)* and false lumen *(F)*. The beak sign *(arrows)* refers to acute angles of the dissection flap relative to the outer aortic contours, which helps identify the false lumen (in addition to the differential perfusion).

Imaging Modalities Useful in Trauma

Although limited, the first step in evaluation of blunt or penetrating thoracic trauma is usually frontal chest radiography. This is almost always performed with the patient in a supine position with anterior-posterior projection because concerns for spinal injury usually preclude upright positioning.

As previously described, radiography is not useful in the evaluation of aortic intimal injury. However, it may be useful in detecting secondary signs of aortic injury, namely mediastinal hematoma. A hematoma may result in mediastinal widening, thickening of the right paratracheal stripe, or loss of the normal aortopulmonary window. Other radiographic clues such as hemothorax, high rib fractures, sternal fractures, and scapular fracture suggest a high-mechanism injury that increases likelihood of aortic injury.

MDCT is the most commonly used modality in the evaluation of acute aortic trauma, owing largely to its availability and fast acquisition times. Contrast-enhanced CT is highly sensitive for the detection of acute aortic injury, as well as for associated injuries, including fractures, pulmonary contusions, pneumothorax, and pericardial effusion.

MRI is of limited use in the setting of trauma. The time required for an examination would delay clinical decision making, when minutes can affect survival.

Location of Acute Traumatic Aortic Injuries

Shear injuries of the aorta result from blunt aortic trauma or sudden deceleration. Injuries occur where the aorta is tethered to the chest wall or other structures. Therefore, the most common sites of injury are the aortic root, aortic isthmus (where the aorta is tethered by the ligamentum arteriosum), or diaphragmatic hiatus. However, it is important to remember that multiple sites of injury are possible along the aorta.

Pseudoaneurysm

A pseudoaneurysm (or false aneurysm) is best described as a contained aortic rupture. In contrast to an aneurysm, where all three layers of the vessel are dilated, a pseudoaneurysm results in a focal outpouching of only one or two of the layers. In these cases, the traumatic injury disrupts the aortic intima and aortic media, with the adventitia remaining intact. The distensible adventitia becomes dilated, secondary to the intraluminal blood pressure.

APPEARANCE OF A PSEUDOANEURYSM

A pseudoaneurysm results in a focal contour abnormality at the site of injury. This usually occurs at the aortic isthmus, where the ligamentum arteriosum renders the aorta prone to deceleration injury. However, because pseudoaneurysm occurs with a high mechanism of trauma, it is usually associated with other mediastinal abnormalities, including mediastinal hematoma.

Traumatic Aortic Dissection or Transection: Typical Imaging Appearance of Aortic Trauma

In the case of severe injury and hemodynamic instability, imaging may not be pursued to expedite emergent surgical intervention. However, as CT becomes increasingly available with decreasing acquisition times, aortic injuries are being increasingly imaged.

Imaging appearance changes based on the degree of injury. When only the innermost layer of the aorta is injured, a mild intimal irregularity or small intimal flap may be the only finding (Fig. 29.14). Deeper aortic wall injury may result in focal weakening of the aortic wall, resulting in a pseudoaneurysm (Fig. 29.15). In the most extreme cases of full-thickness aortic injury, frank extravasation of contrast into the mediastinum may be visible. Low-grade injuries (e.g., limited injuries to the aortic intima) may be managed medically and with follow-up examination. However, high-grade injuries or those that increase in size over serial examinations require surgical or endovascular intervention.

Pitfalls in the Imaging of Aortic Trauma

Motion

Again, motion can confound the evaluation of the aorta in the setting of trauma. In the era of MDCT, most studies can be performed in a single breath-hold, reducing respiratory motion artifacts. However, cardiac motion may be problematic and may result in artifactual irregularity of

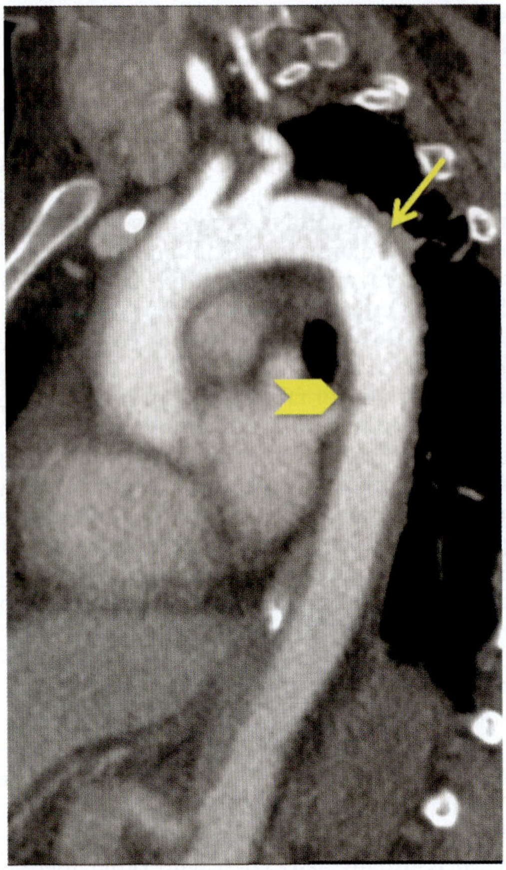

Figure 29.14 Aortic trauma. Sagittal oblique reformat of a contrast-enhanced CT scan after high-velocity traumatic injury. Intimal injury occurs in the region of the aortic isthmus *(arrow)* and extends downstream *(arrowhead)*.

the aortic wall. This can result in normal aortic contours being mistaken for a pseudoaneurysm or a true aortic trauma being mistaken for artifact.

As for the evaluation of acute aortic syndromes, ECG cardiac gating may prove useful in the detection of acute aortic trauma. However, this technology is not available in all locations or at all times of day, and urgency of the patient's injuries may not allow for this additional step.

Secondary signs of trauma may be helpful in the differentiation between true trauma and artifact. Aortic injury usually occurs in the setting of high-velocity or high-mechanism trauma. Concomitant high-mechanism injuries such as sternal or scapular fractures are more likely in the setting of aortic trauma. Also, associated mediastinal hematoma, mediastinal fat stranding, or adjacent pulmonary contusions can also suggest the presence of acute aortic injury.

Normal Variants in Aortic Anatomy

PROBLEM SOLVING: AORTIC SPINDLE VS. AORTIC INJURY

The aortic spindle is a variant in normal aortic anatomy whereby a short segment of the descending aorta (just distal to the isthmus) increases in caliber. This fusiform dilation is thought to be a remnant of fetal anatomy and is typically an incidental finding when imaging is pursued for other reasons. This change in aortic caliber may be mistaken for acute injury in the setting of trauma; however, smooth margins and the lack of surrounding hematoma may help the observer differentiate this variant from true aortic injury.

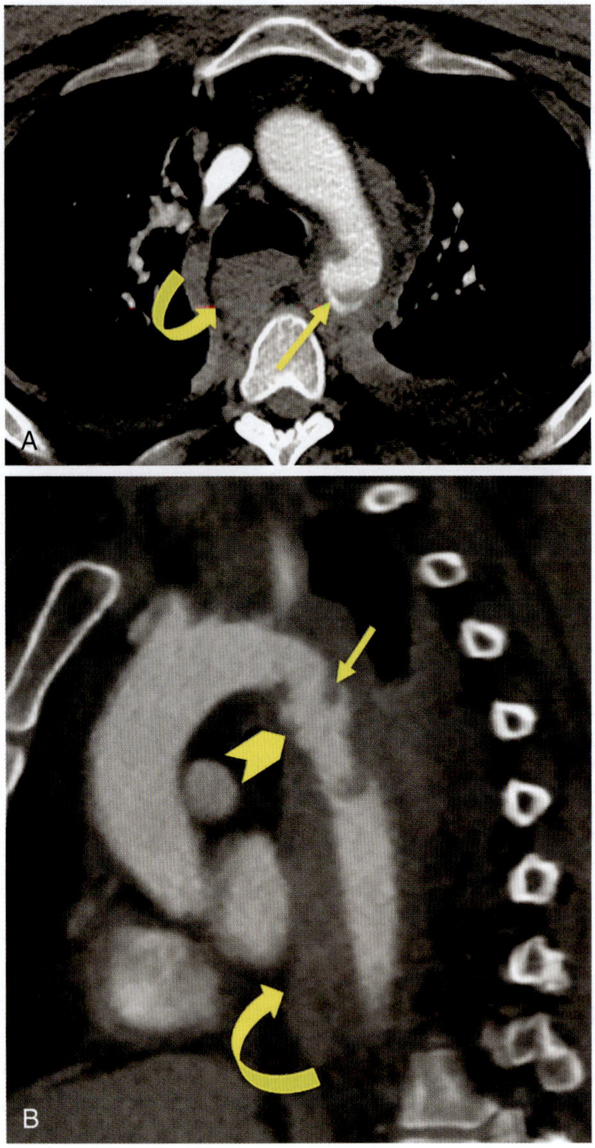

Figure 29.15 Contained aortic rupture and pseudoaneurysm formation. Axial (A) and sagittal oblique (B) images from a CT angiogram demonstrate a focal irregularity of the intima at the level of the isthmus *(straight arrows)*. Additionally, there is focal irregularity and outpouching of the aorta at this level *(arrowhead)*, compatible with pseudoaneurysm formation in the setting of a contained aortic rupture. Note surrounding mediastinal blood *(curved arrows)*.

PROBLEM SOLVING: PSEUDOANEURYSM VS. DUCTUS DIVERTICULUM

Ductus diverticulum is a focal outpouching along the inferior aspect of the aorta that occurs at the previous site of ductus arteriosus attachment. Both ductus diverticulum and traumatic aortic injury occur at the isthmus. A ductus diverticulum may be seen in up to one-third

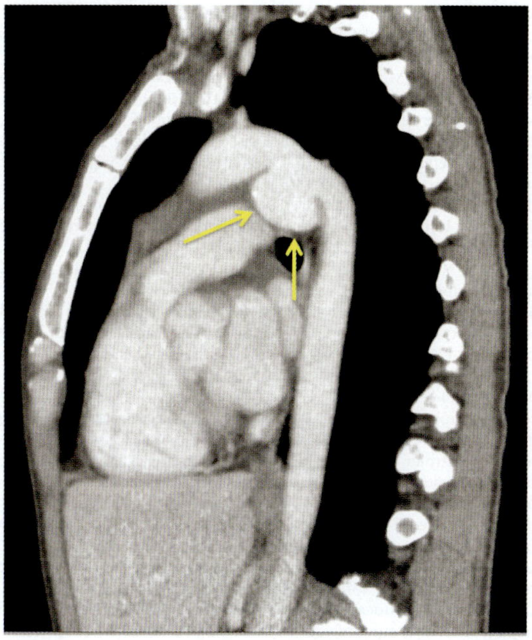

Figure 29.16 Sagittal oblique contrast-enhanced CT image of the aorta in a patient with ductus diverticulum aneurysm *(arrows)*. This anatomic variant occurs at the isthmus, which is also a common location for trauma. Understanding the typical location of a ductus diverticulum is important in differentiating this variant from true pathology. Also, the focal intimal calcifications are compatible with a chronic process, arguing against an acute injury.

of the asymptomatic population. However, this focal aortic contour abnormality may mimic a pseudoaneurysm or some other focal traumatic injury.

A typical ductus diverticulum has smooth contours and obtuse angles to the aorta. In contrast, aortic trauma is usually more irregular, may have acute angles to the aorta, and can project in any direction. However, it is import to note that atypical aortic diverticula in unexpected locations and projections do exist. Also, aneurysmal dilation of the diverticulum may result in acute angles relative to the aorta, further confounding imaging findings (Fig. 29.16).

Most importantly, secondary findings of trauma can support the diagnosis of traumatic aortic injury over a benign variant. Traumatic aortic injury rarely occurs in the absence of a mediastinal hematoma. Additional findings of high mechanism trauma (e.g., multiple fractures, pulmonary contusions, abdominal solid organ injury) favor trauma over a normal variant.

Conclusion

The spectrum of acquired aortic diseases includes a variety of abnormalities, such as acute diseases that require prompt intervention as well as slowly progressive abnormalities that may be followed or managed medically. A detailed understanding of their radiologic appearance and knowledge of common imaging pitfalls may aid the radiologist in promptly and correctly identifying diseases of the aorta and directing further management.

Bibliography

Abbara S, Kalva S, Cury RC, Isselbacher E. Thoracic aortic disease: spectrum of multidetector computed tomography imaging findings. *J Cardiovasc Comput Tomogr*. 2007;1(1):40–54.

Alfson DB, Ham SW. Type B Aortic dissections: current guidelines for treatment. *Cardiol Clin*. 2017;35(3):387–410.

Armerding MD, Rubin GD, Beaulieu CF, et al. Aortic aneurysmal disease: assessment of stent-graft treatment-CT versus conventional angiography. *Radiology*. 2000;215(1):138–146.

Attenhofer Jost CH, Schaff HV, Connolly HM, et al. Spectrum of operations after repair of aortic coarctation: importance of an individualized approach because of coexistent cardiovascular disease. *Mayo Clin Proc*. 2002;77(7):646–653.

Batra P, Bigoni B, Manning J, et al. Pitfalls in the diagnosis of thoracic aortic dissection at CT angiography. *Radiographics*. 2000;20(2):309–320.

Berko NS, Jain VR, Godelman A, et al. Variants and anomalies of thoracic vasculature on computed tomographic angiography in adults. *J Comput Assist Tomogr*. 2009;33(4):523–528.

Bonaca MP, O'Gara PT. Diagnosis and management of acute aortic syndromes: dissection, intramural hematoma, and penetrating aortic ulcer. *Curr Cardiol Rep*. 2014;16(10):536.

Bosner RS, Pagano D, Lewis ME, et al. Clinical and patho-anatomical factors affecting expansion of thoracic aortic aneurysms. *Heart*. 2000;84(3):277–283.

Burkhart HM, Gomez GA, Jacobson LE, et al. Fatal blunt aortic injuries: a review of 242 autopsy cases. *J Trauma*. 2001;50(1):113–115.

Chung JH, Ghoshhajra BB, Rojas CA, et al. CT angiography of the thoracic aorta. *Radiol Clin N Am*. 2010;48(2):249–264.

Clouse WD, Hallett JW, Schaff HV, et al. Improved prognosis of thoracic aortic aneurysms: a population-based study. *JAMA*. 1998;280(22):1926–1929.

Coady MA, Davies RR, Roberts M, et al. Familial patterns of thoracic aortic aneurysms. *Arch Surg*. 1999;134(4):361–367.

Coady MA, Rizzo JA, Hammond GL, et al. Surgical intervention criteria for thoracic aortic aneurysms: a study of growth rates and complications. *Ann Thorac Surg*. 1999;67(6):1922–1926, discussion 1953–1958.

Davies RR, Gallo A, Coady MA, et al. Novel measurement of relative aortic size predicts rupture of thoracic aortic aneurysms. *Ann Thorac Surg*. 2006;81(1):169–177.

Davies RR, Goldstein LJ, Coady MA, et al. Yearly rupture or dissection rates for thoracic aortic aneurysms: simple prediction based on size. *Ann Thorac Surg*. 2002;73(1):17–27, discussion 27–28.

Fan ZM, Zhang ZQ, Ma XH, et al. Acute aortic dissection with intimal intussusception: MRI appearances. *AJR Am J Roentgenol*. 2006;186(3):841–843.

Feczko JD, Lynch L, Pless JE, et al. An autopsy case review of 142 nonpenetrating (blunt) injuries of the aorta. *J Trauma*. 1992;33(6):846–849.

Geyer LL, Schoepf UJ, Meinel FG, et al. State of the art: iterative CT reconstruction techniques. *Radiology*. 2015;276(2):339–357.

Gomes AS, Bettmann MA, Boxt LM, et al. Acute chest pain—suspected aortic dissection. American College of Radiology. ACR appropriateness criteria. *Radiology*. 2000;215(suppl):1–5.

Greenberg RK, Secor JL, Painter T. Computed tomography assessment of thoracic aortic pathology. *Semin Vasc Surg*. 2004;17(2):166–172.

Hagan PG, Nienaber CA, Isselbacher EM, et al. The International Registry of Acute Aortic Dissection (IRAD): new insights into an old disease. *JAMA*. 2000;283(7):897–903.

Hayashi H, Matsuoka Y, Sakamoto I, et al. Penetrating atherosclerotic ulcer of the aorta: imaging features and disease concept. *Radiographics*. 2000;20(4):995–1005.

Heinemann M, Laas J, Karck M, et al. Thoracic aortic aneurysms after acute type A aortic dissection: necessity for follow-up. *Ann Thorac Surg*. 1990;49(4):580–584.

Husainy MA, Sayyed F, Puppala S. Acute aortic syndrome—pitfalls on gated and non-gated CT scan. *Emerg Radiol*. 2016;23(4):397–403.

Isselbacher EM. Thoracic and abdominal aortic aneurysms. *Circulation*. 2005;111(6):816–828.

Johnson PT, Chen JK, Loeys BL, et al. Loeys-Dietz syndrome: MDCT angiography findings. *AJR Am J Roentgenol*. 2007;189(1):W29–W35.

Kaatee R, Van Leeuwen MS, De Lange EE, et al. Spiral CT angiography of the renal arteries: should a scan delay based on a test bolus injection or a fixed scan delay be used to obtain maximum enhancement of the vessels? *J Comput Assist Tomogr*. 1998;22(4):541–547.

Kaji S, Nishigami K, Akasaka T, et al. Prediction of progression or regression of type A aortic intramural hematoma by computed tomography. *Circulation*. 1999;100(19 suppl II):II281–II286.

Kazerooni EA, Bree RL, Williams DM. Penetrating atherosclerotic ulcers of the descending thoracic aorta: evaluation with CT and distinction from aortic dissection. *Radiology*. 1992;183(3):759–765.

Kuzmik GA, Sang AX, Elefteriades JA. Natural history of thoracic aortic aneurysms. *J Vasc Surg*. 2012;56(2):565–571.

Layton KF, Kallmes DF, Cloft HJ, et al. Bovine aortic arch variant in humans: clarification of a common misnomer. *AJNR Am J Neuroradiol*. 2006;27(7):1541–1542.

Lee CH, Goo JM, Ye HJ, et al. Radiation dose modulation techniques in the multidetector CT era: from basics to practice. *Radiographics*. 2008;28(5):1451–1459.

LePage MA, Quint LE, Sonnad SS, et al. Aortic dissection: CT features that distinguish true lumen from false lumen. *AJR Am J Roentgenol*. 2001;177(1):207–211.

Lin FY, Devereaux RB, Roman MJ, et al. Assessment of the thoracic aorta by multidetector computed tomography: age- and sex-specific reference values in adults without evident cardiovascular disease. *J Cardiovasc Comput Tomogr*. 2008;2(5):298–308.

Lobato AC, Puech-Leao P. Predictive factors for rupture of thoracoabdominal aortic aneurysm. *J Vasc Surg*. 1998;27(3):446–453.

Lu TL, Huber CH, Rizzo E, et al. Ascending aorta measurements as assessed by ECG-gated multi-detector computed tomography: a pilot study to establish normative values for transcatheter therapies. *Eur Radiol*. 2009;19(3):664–669.

Maksimowicz-McKinnon K, Hoffman GS. Takayasu arteritis: what is the long-term prognosis? *Rheum Dis Clin North Am*. 2007;33(4):777–786, vi.

Mao SS, Ahmadi N, Shah B, et al. Normal thoracic aorta diameter on cardiac computed tomography in healthy asymptomatic adults; impact of age and gender. *Acad Radiol*. 2008;15(7):827–834.

Meszaros J, Morocz J, Szlavi J, et al. Epidemiology and clinicopathology of aortic dissection. *Chest*. 2000;117:1271–1278.

Moore AG, Eagle KA, Bruckman D, et al. Choice of computed tomography, transesophageal echocardiography, magnetic resonance imaging, and aortography in acute aortic dissection: international registry of acute aortic dissection (IRAD). *Am J Cardiol*. 2002;89(10):1235–1238.

Morgan-Hughes GJ, Marshall AJ, Roobottom CA. Refined computed tomography of the thoracic aorta: the impact of electrocardiographic assistance. *Clin Radiol*. 2003;58(8):581–588.

Morris JH, Mix D, Cameron SJ. Acute aortic syndromes: update in current medical management. *Curr Treat Options Cardiovasc Med*. 2017;19(4):29.

Nelsen KM, Spizarny DL, Kastan DJ. Intimointimal intussusception in aortic dissection: CT diagnosis. *AJR Am J Roentgenol*. 1994;162(4):813–814.

Nienaber CA, von Kodolitsch Y, Nicholas V, et al. The diagnosis of thoracic aortic dissection by noninvasive imaging procedures. *N Engl J Med*. 1993; 328(1):1–9.

Nienaber CA, von Kodolitsch Y, Petersen B, et al. Intramural hemorrhage of the thoracic aorta: diagnostic and therapeutic implications. *Circulation*. 1995;92(6): 1465–1472.

Nistri S, Sorbo MD, Marin M, et al. Aortic root dilatation in young men with normally functioning bicuspid aortic valves. *Heart*. 1999;82(1):19–22.

Nuenninghoff DM, Hunder GG, Christianson TJ, et al. Incidence and predictors of large-artery complication (aortic aneurysm, aortic dissection, and/or large-artery stenosis) in patients with giant-cell arteritis: a population based study over 50 years. *Arthritis Rheum*. 2003;48(12):3522–3531.

Ocak I, Lacomis JM, Deible CR, et al. The aortic root: comparison of measurements from ECG-gated CT angiography with transthoracic echocardiography. *J Thorac Imaging*. 2009;24(3):223–226.

Pagni S, Denatale RW, Boltax RS. Takayasu's arteritis: the middle aortic syndrome. *Am Surg*. 1996;62(5):409–412.

Parikh SR, Hurwitz RA, Hubbard JE, et al. Preoperative and postoperative "aneurysm" associated with coarctation of the aorta. *J Am Coll Cardiol*. 1991;17(6):1367–1372.

Quint LE, Francis IR, Williams DM, et al. Evaluation of thoracic aortic disease with the use of helical CT and multiplanar reconstructions: a comparison with surgical findings. *Radiology*. 1996;201(1):37–41.

Quint LE, Williams DM, Francis IR, et al. Ulcerlike lesions of the aorta: imaging features and natural history. *Radiology*. 2001;218(3):719–723.

Raptis CA, Hammer MM, Raman KG, et al. Acute traumatic aortic injury: practical considerations for the diagnostic radiologist. *J Thorac Imaging*. 2015;30(3):202–213.

Rojas CA, Restrepo CS. Mediastinal hematomas: aortic injury and beyond. *J Comput Assist Tomogr*. 2009;33(2):218–224.

Roos JE, Willmann JK, Weishaupt D, et al. Thoracic aorta: motion artifact reduction with retrospective and prospective electrocardiography-assisted multi-detector row CT. *Radiology*. 2002;222(1):271–277.

Rubin GD. MDCT imaging of the aorta and peripheral vessels. *Eur J Radiol*. 2003;45(suppl 1):S42–S49.

Safir J, Kerr A, Morehouse H, et al. Magnetic resonance imaging of dissection in pseudocoarctation of the aorta. *Cardiovasc Intervent Radiol*. 1993;16(3):180–182.

Schoenhoff FS, Zanchin C, Czerny M, et al. Aorta related and all-cause mortality in patients with aortic intramural hematoma. *Eur J Vasc Endovasc Surg*. 2017;54(4):447–453.

Sebastia C, Quiroga S, Boye R, et al. Aortic stenosis: spectrum of diseases depicted at multisection CT. *Radiographics*. 2003;23:S79–S91.

Stanson AW, Kazmier FJ, Hollier LH, et al. Penetrating atherosclerotic ulcers of the thoracic aorta: natural history and clinicopathologic correlations. *Ann Vasc Surg*. 1986;1(1):15–23.

Steenburg SD, Ravenel JG, Ikonomidis JS, et al. Acute traumatic aortic injury: imaging evaluation and management. *Radiology*. 2008;248(3):748–762.

Svensson LG, Crawford ES, Hess KR, et al. Experience with 1509 patients undergoing thoracoabdomial aortic operations. *J Vasc Surg*. 1993;17(2):357–368.

Takach TJ, Reul GJ, Duncan JM, et al. Sinus of valsalva aneurysm or fistula: management and outcome. *Ann Thorac Surg*. 1999;68(5):1573–1577.

Therrien J, Thorne SA, Wright A, et al. Repaired coarctation: a "cost-effective" approach to identify complications in adults. *J Am Coll Cardiol*. 2000;35(4):997–1002.

Tops LF, Wood DA, Delgado V, et al. Noninvasive evaluation of the aortic root with multislice computed tomography implications for transcatheter aortic valve replacement. *JACC Cardiovasc Imaging*. 2008;1(3):321–330.

Valente T, Rossi G, Lassandro F, et al. MDCT evaluation of acute aortic syndrome (AAS). *Br J Radiol*. 2016;89(1061):20150825.

Von Kodolitsch Y, Aydin MA, Koschyk DH, et al. Predictors of aneurysmal formation after surgical correction of aortic coarctation. *J Am Coll Cardiol*. 2002;39(4): 617–624.

Von Kodolitsch Y, Csosz SK, Koschyk DH, et al. Intramural hematoma of the aorta: predictors of progression to dissection and rupture. *Circulation*. 2003;107(8): 1158–1163.

Wang GX, Hedgire SS, Le TQ, et al. MR angiography can guide ED management of suspected acute aortic dissection. *Am J Emerg Med*. 2017;35(4):527–530.

Williams MP, Farrow R. Atypical patterns in the CT diagnosis of aortic dissection. *Clin Radiol*. 1994;49(10):686–689.

Zhao DL, Liu XD, Zhao CL, et al. Multislice spiral CT angiography for evaluation of acute aortic syndrome. *Echocardiography*. 2017;34(10):1495–1499.

CHAPTER 30

Ischemic Cardiac Disease

Julian L. Wichmann, Akos Varga-Szemes, Pal Spruill Suranyi, and U. Joseph Schoepf

CHAPTER OUTLINE

■ Introduction: Using Cardiovascular Imaging

Cardiovascular diseases remain one of the most common causes of death in industrialized nations. Over the last decade, substantial technical advances in cardiovascular imaging have been made and have helped mature such modalities from research techniques into clinical applications. Ischemic cardiac disease is defined as an efficiency loss of the myocardium due to inadequate oxygen supply, which is mostly caused by obstructive coronary artery disease (CAD). Several parameters that can be obtained through cardiovascular imaging have been shown to allow for more precise risk stratification and management in patients with ischemic heart disease.

Indications for Imaging

Risk assessment remains the main indication for cardiovascular imaging in clinical routine. Coronary computed tomography angiography (CCTA) has been incorporated into most major guidelines as a first-choice standard examination to detect CAD, assess coronary artery bypass graft (CABG) lumen patency, and visualize congenital heart disease. A number of multicenter studies have demonstrated high sensitivity and specificity for CCTA in comparison with invasive coronary angiography (ICA). Although the severity of coronary stenosis may be overestimated with CCTA, its high negative predictive value has established it as a modality to rule out CAD reliably. The use of CCTA in the emergency department to triage patients with acute chest pain and suspected CAD has also been recommended by multiple studies.

Although CCTA is per definition an anatomic examination, other functional imaging modalities generally need to be used to assess the hemodynamic significance of detected coronary stenosis. Such myocardial perfusion imaging (MPI) is mostly performed using single-photon emission CT (SPECT) or magnetic resonance imaging (MRI), although other modalities can also be used (e.g., positron emission tomography, stress echocardiography, fractional flow reserve CT [CT-FFR]). This explains why a comprehensive workup in patients with ischemic cardiac disease is commonly based on multimodality imaging. However, multiple factors and patient characteristics influence the selection of an appropriate imaging modality and protocol (Box 30.1).

Determining the Appropriate Imaging Modality

X-Ray (Chest X-Ray, Invasive Coronary Angiography)

In most patients presenting to the emergency department, an initial chest x-ray is obtained. Although not routinely used to detect ischemic cardiac disease, it can provide certain indicators of CAD because extensive coronary

BOX 30.1 Parameters Influencing Cardiac Imaging Protocol Selection

Technical Parameters
CT detector design and arrays
Available CT radiation and contrast dose reduction techniques
Postprocessing algorithms (3D, 4D, and CT-FFR)
MR field strength and bore width

Patient Factors
Age
Gender
Body weight and habitus
Heart rate
Heart rhythm
Blood pressure
Medical and surgical history
Renal function
Ability to follow breathing commands
Presence of devices and implants
Claustrophobia

Clinical Parameters
Indications for imaging
Appropriateness for imaging
Specific clinical questions
Impact on further clinical pathway

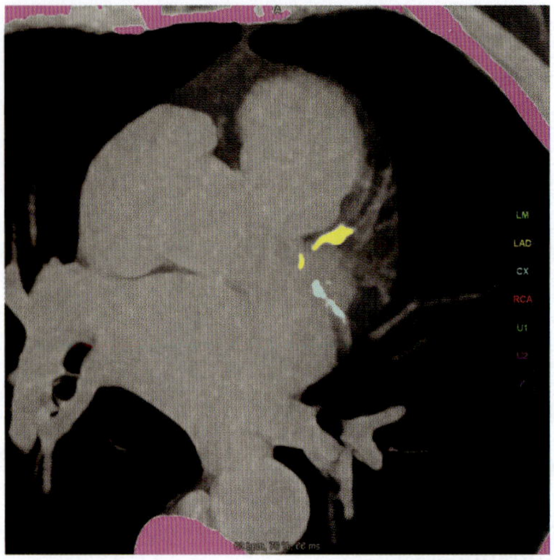

Figure 30.1 Evaluation of calcium scoring and Agatston score in a 77-year-old male patient. Material with a high density (threshold, 130 Hounsfield units) is automatically identified by the software and rendered in pink. Manual allocation of focal coronary calcium spots has been performed and extensive calcifications in the left anterior descending *(yellow)* and circumflex *(turquoise)* coronary artery segments are visualized on maximum-intensity projections. The total Agatston score in this patient was 387.8.

calcification may be visible or characteristic enlargement of certain cardiac chambers may indicate valvular disease and heart failure.

In routine clinical practice assessment of ischemic cardiac disease, x-ray technology is usually used more during ICA. This invasive approach remains the gold standard to assess CAD, especially because FFR measurements also allow for an accurate evaluation of the hemodynamic significance of coronary stenosis. CAD detected on CCTA may be reaffirmed using ICA, the severity can be quantified using FFR, and it can be simultaneously treated with balloon angioplasty and stent placement when appropriate.

Computed Tomography (Coronary CT Angiography, CT Myocardial Perfusion Imaging)

Due to several major technical improvements over the last decades, CT has evolved into a routinely used modality to detect multiple cardiac pathologies. Currently, it is still mostly used to detect or rule out CAD. For an initial evaluation, a low-dose, unenhanced calcium scoring scan is usually performed to detect calcified coronary plaques (Fig. 30.1). The resulting Agatston score based on this dataset can be used for risk stratification based on an extensive body of research regarding the prognostic value of this calcium score. Nevertheless, especially in younger patients, noncalcified coronary soft plaque or, in the acute setting, a clot or embolus may be present, which would remain undetected on a noncontrast scan. Therefore, a contrast-enhanced CCTA study may be necessary to assess coronary artery patency and high-risk coronary anomalies (e.g., interarterial or intramural course). CCTA is also used to evaluate CABG patency, and newer scanner generations allow for the detection of in-stent thrombosis due to higher spatial and temporal resolution and improved metal artifact reduction algorithms. The combination of recently introduced dose-saving technologies has allowed for a substantial dose reduction, down to submillisievert levels in clinical practice. Thus CCTA has been established as an adequate first-line, rule-out test in patients with suspected CAD, with low to intermediate probability.

In an effort to provide comprehensive cardiac assessment, static and dynamic MPI using CT (CTMPI) has been made feasible (Fig. 30.2). A growing body of evidence demonstrates that additional CTMPI may be helpful to identify patients with hemodynamically relevant coronary artery stenosis. An advantage of CTMPI over other established myocardial viability imaging modalities is the opportunity for a comprehensive, single-modality cardiac assessment. By performing both examinations in the same time slot, without additional patient positioning, this may ultimately prove to be a more time-efficient and cost-effective imaging solution.

Cardiac Magnetic Resonance

Due to several major technical improvements over the last decades, cardiac magnetic resonance (CMR) has evolved into the gold standard for the assessment of left and right ventricular function and myocardial viability without the use of ionizing radiation. There is growing evidence that stress myocardial perfusion CMR is a superior alternative to SPECT for the detection of perfusion deficits. Some have even suggested that this modality may also be particularly useful in women, whose epicardial coronary arteries show no obstruction but who have suspected coronary microvascular dysfunction. An increasing number of pacemakers and intravascular stents are MR-compatible, and several single-shot, free-breathing protocols and motion

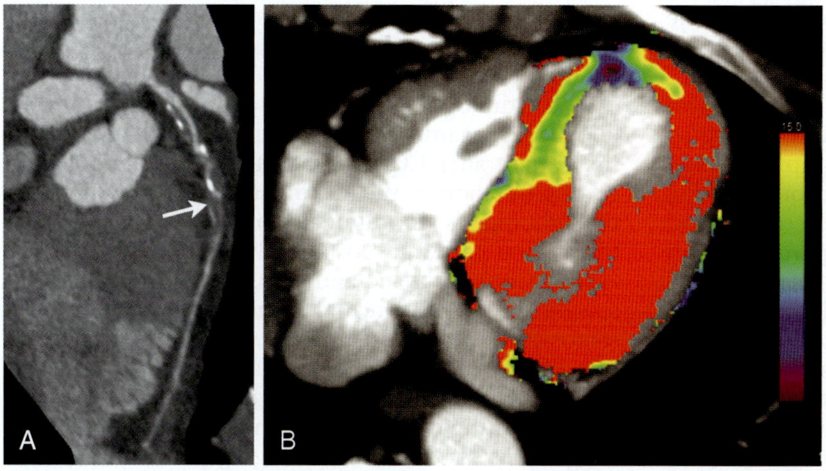

Figure 30.2 Correlation of coronary stenosis and myocardial perfusion deficit. (A) Coronary CT angiography demonstrates multiple mixed plaques of the left anterior descending coronary artery *(arrow)*. (B) Color-coded CT myocardial perfusion imaging shows a focal anteroseptal perfusion deficit in the corresponding vessel territory. Red indicates peak values for myocardial blood volume; purple indicates lowest values.

correction algorithms are available for most imaging indications. In addition, CMR late gadolinium enhancement (LGE) imaging remains the examination of choice for the visualization of myocardial necrosis and scar, as well as the myocardial involvement in a variety of other structural diseases (e.g., cardiac amyloidosis, sarcoidosis, myocarditis). Furthermore, stress dobutamine CMR is a viable alternative to stress dobutamine echocardiography.

Nevertheless, CMR still tends to be more time-consuming than cardiac CT, and some patients still refuse or abort MR examinations due to severe claustrophobia. Thus some of the concepts of CMR, including late-enhancement imaging, have been transferred to CT to allow for similar examination characteristics in selected patients, although such techniques are still under development.

Nuclear Studies

SPECT remains an established MPI technique to detect myocardial ischemia due to the substantial body of research regarding its value as a prognostic indicator. Nevertheless, its relatively high radiation exposure, requirement for a radionuclide tracer, and rather low specificity have led to the development of the other aforementioned MPI techniques. Although cardiac positron emission tomography using ^{82}Rb or ^{13}N-ammonia is also feasible, it is only used by a minority in clinical routine, primarily due to the logistical difficulties in obtaining these radiotracers.

■ CT Imaging Algorithms

Examining Patients With Suspected Coronary Artery Disease

When a patient is referred for cardiac imaging, the radiologist should tailor an appropriate imaging protocol determined by indication, the patient's clinical parameters, and the technical capabilities of the scanner used. Coronary artery imaging currently remains mainly a CT domain. First, it should be determined whether the clinical question can be answered with purely anatomic data of the coronary arteries or whether it requires functional data and possibly even additional myocardial perfusion assessment. In addition, in the emergency room setting, an emergent triple rule-out CTA of the entire chest may be warranted, instead of standard CCTA.

Patients with a low to intermediate pretest likelihood for CAD are the ideal candidates for CCTA. Some patients with known CAD may benefit from a CCTA—for example, to assess for coronary stent or bypass graft patency. Patients with a prior CABG require a larger field of view to visualize the internal mammary arteries fully.

A noncontrast, low-dose, calcium scoring scan is usually performed for initial risk assessment, for an initial overview of cardiac anatomy, and for optimal protocol selection, but can be omitted in patients with implanted coronary stents, prior infarct, or a CABG.

Image quality is mainly determined by the used acquisition protocol and the patient's heart rate and body habitus. Most cardiac CT examinations require electrocardiogram (ECG) synchronization, even though newer scan technologies may provide exemptions. A widely accepted guideline is to scan patients with a heart rate <80 beats/min with prospectively ECG-triggered protocols to reduce radiation exposure, whereas patients with a heart rate of >80 beats/min are scanned with retrospectively ECG-gated protocols to ensure diagnostic image quality.

To achieve a lower heart rate, some patients may require oral or IV beta blockers unless contraindicated (e.g., in severe asthma). Many patients referred for cardiac CT also have a history of hypertension or arrhythmia and are already medicated with beta blockers. Sublingual application of nitroglycerin provides coronary artery dilation, which may improve visualization. It should be administered 3 to 5 minutes prior to the scan but is contraindicated in patients currently medicated with other vasodilators (e.g., sildenafil) because severe hypotension is a possible complication.

Both bolus tracking and test bolus techniques can be used for CCTA to ensure optimal scan timing. Depending on the scanner generation, functional analysis requires retrospectively ECG-gated protocols or can be performed using newer padding techniques for prospectively triggered acquisition modes. Late-enhancement imaging 7 to 15 minutes after the angiographic phase to detect myocardial scarring can be optionally performed, depending on the patient's clinical history and indications for imaging.

Image reconstruction and three-dimensional postprocessing plays a crucial role in cardiac CT. Patients with severe calcifications or stents may benefit from reconstructions with sharper kernels, which could improve vessel conspicuity. Curved multiplanar reconstructions (cMPRs) are helpful for the visualization of plaque geometry and for the assessment of stenosis severity, particularly in complex cases. Alternatively, where available, CT-derived FFR values could be assessed and included in the clinical decision making process. Three-dimensional volume rendering is especially useful for visualization of CABG anatomy and cardiac malformations. Snapshot images should be made available for colleagues from other subspecialties for intervention planning. It should be noted, however, that the severity of coronary artery stenosis is usually slightly overestimated on CCTA compared to ICA.

Reporting the Findings

Each cardiac CT report should begin with describing the scanning technique and image reconstruction parameters. If available, the resulting Agatston score from the calcium scoring scan should be stated with the corresponding MESA (Multi-Ethnic Study of Atherosclerosis) percentile adjusted for age, race, and gender (http://www.mesa-nhlbi.org/calcium/input.aspx). For analysis of CCTA images, it is usually helpful to provide a brief description for each major coronary artery (right, left main, left anterior descending, left circumflex coronary arteries, and, if present, the ramus intermedius) describing vessel course, plaque presence, and distribution. Due to our inability to quantify stenosis severity accurately, coronary stenosis should be described qualitatively as mild (<30%), moderate (30%–70%), or severe (>70%). Coronary anomalies, especially those with malignant potential, should also be described here.

Even if normal, cardiac anatomy should be mentioned at least briefly, and anatomy of the greater vessels should be assessed. Special attention should be paid to the myocardium because perfusion defects (acute or chronic) may be visible as segments with hypoattenuation. Chronic changes, including myocardial thinning, fatty metaplasia, calcifications, and aneurysm, should also be reported. If functional imaging was performed, quantitative results (e.g., ejection fraction, end-diastolic and end-systolic volumes) should be reported, and regional wall motion abnormalities should be mentioned, when present.

It is imperative to evaluate all provided image series for extracardiac findings because CCTA may be the first cross-sectional imaging modality performed in patients with suspected CAD without any prior history of hospitalization. The lungs should be examined in a separate image series reconstructed with a wide field of view and sharper lung kernel to avoid missing smaller pulmonary nodules. Acute or chronic pulmonary disease (e.g., pneumonia, emphysema, fibrosis) and pleural effusion should also be described. A separate image series of the thorax reconstructed with a dedicated soft tissue kernel should be reviewed to detect masses or lymphadenopathy. Finally, the chest wall, osseous structures, and partially visualized abdomen (and, in some cases, the lower neck) should be examined.

The radiologist, unfortunately, often has only little knowledge regarding the scheduled clinical workflow of the patient after CCTA. In addition, the interpretation of a CCTA report by the treating physician may vary from the radiologist's report but also has the potential to alter the clinical pathway substantially. CCTA is an excellent examination for triage and to rule out CAD, but lacks specificity to predict actual hemodynamic relevance of stenosis. Therefore it is advisable to give a broad description of the coronary status and to highlight potentially significant stenosis, which may represent culprit lesions without stating the actual percentage of stenosis values. Suggestions for additional imaging procedures (CMR, SPECT) may be appreciated by the treating physician but are not mandatory. In conclusion, as with all reports, the main clinical question should be answered, instead of reusing the same report template for all cases.

Reducing Radiation and Contrast Dose

Several recent technologic innovations have helped substantially lower radiation exposure from CCTA and required contrast material dose in routine clinical practice and can be applied in most patients. Conventionally, CCTA has been performed using retrospectively ECG-gated protocols with continuous radiation and relatively high tube voltages for sufficient tissue penetration, with effective doses of 10 to 18 mSv. Prospectively ECG-gated protocols result in intermittent radiation and consequently lower radiation exposure substantially. Depending on the patient's heart rate and scanner generation, patients can be examined using these prospectively-gated protocols in sequential (<80 beats/min) or high-pitch (<65 beats/min) acquisition. High-pitch scanning has made CCTA with <1 mSv feasible, but remains restricted to specific patient populations.

Newer scanner generations provide an automated in-scan adaptation of tube voltage and tube current modulation, which can substantially reduce radiation exposure without impacting image quality. Although older scanners were operated with a tube voltage of 120 kVp, newer scanners allow for a reference tube voltage of as low as 70 kVp due to improvements in detector technology (Fig. 30.3). Low tube voltage acquisition during contrast-enhanced CT allows for a significant dose reduction and may also result in a superior contrast-to-noise ratio due to a far stronger iodine attenuation compared to standard acquisition, with only a moderate increase in image noise. In addition, postprocessing using iterative reconstruction algorithms can mitigate such distinct image noise, further improving image quality with low tube voltage acquisition.

Most of these techniques for the reduction of radiation exposure can be simultaneously applied for reducing contrast material volume. Due to the increased iodine attenuation with low tube voltage acquisition, less contrast material is required. In addition, high-pitch CCTA protocols usually require less contrast material also due to rapid image acquisition.

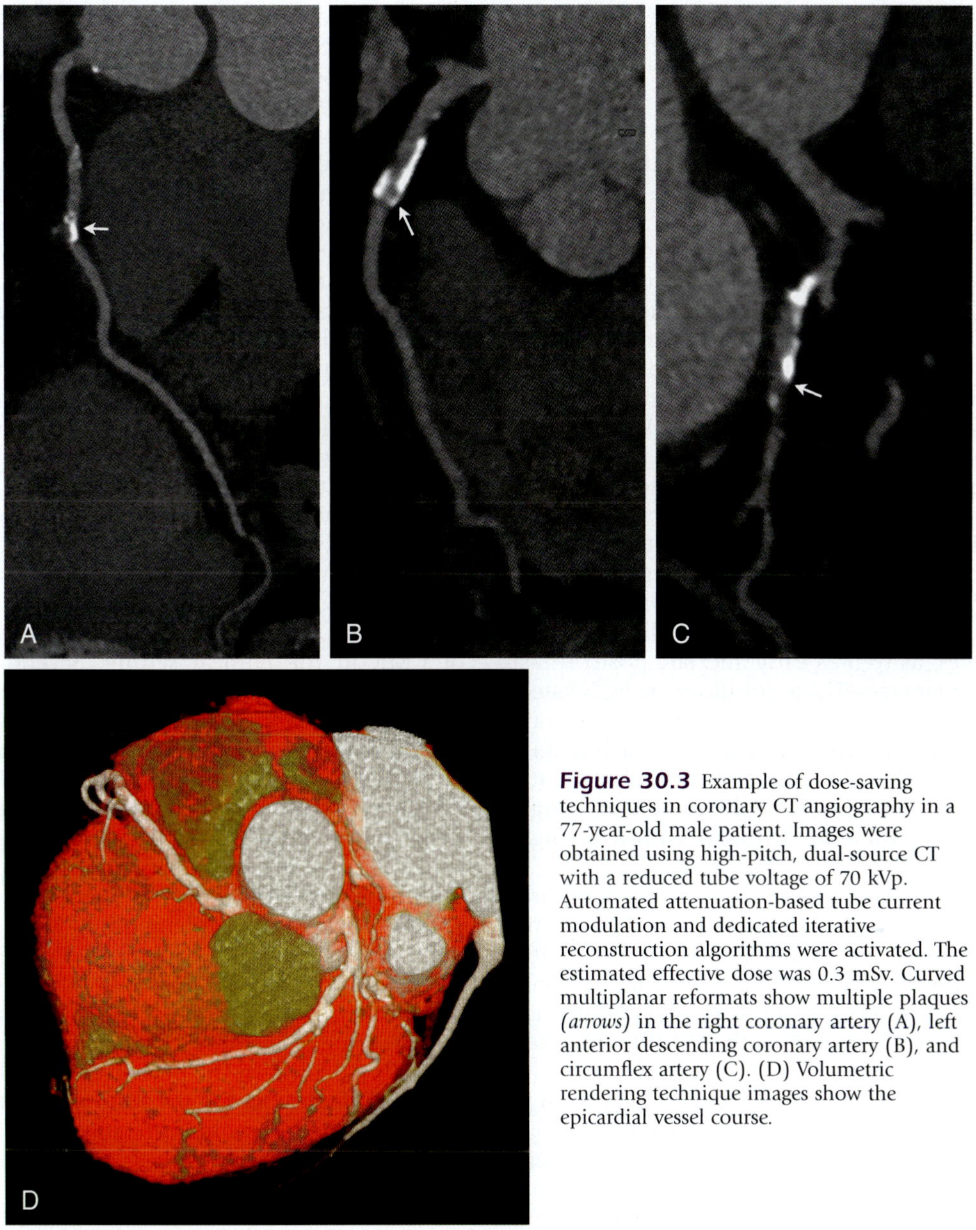

Figure 30.3 Example of dose-saving techniques in coronary CT angiography in a 77-year-old male patient. Images were obtained using high-pitch, dual-source CT with a reduced tube voltage of 70 kVp. Automated attenuation-based tube current modulation and dedicated iterative reconstruction algorithms were activated. The estimated effective dose was 0.3 mSv. Curved multiplanar reformats show multiple plaques *(arrows)* in the right coronary artery (A), left anterior descending coronary artery (B), and circumflex artery (C). (D) Volumetric rendering technique images show the epicardial vessel course.

Cardiac Magnetic Resonance Imaging Algorithms

Contraindications to the Use of Cardiac Magnetic Resonance

Due to the strong magnetic field used to operate the MR scanner, there are certain safety provisions for which every patient undergoing CMR must be screened. Unknown active devices, ferromagnetic implants, unknown aneurysm clips, metallic fragments in the eye, implantable cardioverter-defibrillators (ICDs), and any implant known to be MR-unsafe are absolute contraindications for CMR. There are relative contraindications when the CMR study can possibly be performed after a thorough risk-benefit assessment. Such conditions include severe claustrophobia, large metal wires, and active devices that have not been tested for MR safety. Most pacemakers belong to the latter group; pacemakers, however, can be programmed to MR mode before the CMR examination after consultation with the treating cardiologist. When scanning these patients, the imaging parameters have to be adjusted using more conventional gradient echo sequences to reduce energy deposition and metal-induced susceptibility artifacts.

The presence of newer stents, heart valves, coils, and occluder devices represents relative contraindications. Patients with such implants can usually be imaged after a certain time specified by the manufacturer. Novel MR-conditional implantable pacemakers are now available, and new generations of ICDs have been tested for MR use. Although an increasing number of devices and implants released from year to year are MR-safe, the artifacts caused by the presence of these implants still represent a challenge in image interpretation. However, because most pacemaker and ICD leads are anchored in the right heart, the visualization of the left ventricle is only minimally affected in most cases.

Examining Patients With Suspected Coronary Artery Disease

Although CT is the current noninvasive standard of care for the evaluation of coronary artery morphology, and there are efforts to develop CT techniques for the assessment of functional parameters, the evaluation of myocardial function and perfusion remains within the domain of CMR, mainly due to its significantly higher temporal resolution. When a patient with CAD is referred for CMR, a variety of diagnostic questions may arise to determine the imaging protocol suitable for the given clinical scenario.

Patients with heart failure of unknown cause and patients with known CAD typically undergo a routine protocol, sometimes referred to as a *viability protocol,* which includes localizers, T2-weighted, cine, and rest perfusion images, as well as early and late postcontrast inversion recovery images. The acquisitions are ECG-gated. Most of these images are segmented—that is, they are collected in several consecutive heartbeats, which require 7- to 20-s long breath-holds to keep the diaphragm at a relatively constant level. Some of the images are single shot, meaning that they are acquired within a single heartbeat.

Cine loops are acquired with 20- to 40-ms temporal resolution in three standard long-axis (two-, three-, and four-chamber views) and multislice short-axis orientations, allowing for the assessment of global and regional cardiac function and valves. Rest myocardial perfusion is assessed after the administration of the gadolinium-based contrast agent, which facilitates the evaluation of the myocardial first-pass contrast uptake. Rest perfusion is especially beneficial in cases of a suspected intracardiac thrombus or mass. Early gadolinium enhancement images are collected 2 minutes postcontrast to assess for thrombus or microvascular perfusion defects, and LGE imaging is performed 10 to 20 minutes after contrast administration to evaluate myocardial contrast accumulation.

In patients with symptoms suggesting stress-inducible ischemia, a stress protocol can be added to the above-described routine protocol. Dobutamine stress CMR can be performed to detect stress-induced wall motion abnormalities. However, the administration of dobutamine is contraindicated in several cardiac conditions, such as severe arterial hypertension, unstable angina, acute myocardial infarction, severe aortic stenosis, and hypertrophic obstructive cardiomyopathy. A more frequently performed protocol is vasodilator stress perfusion imaging, designed to detect stress-induced ischemia in the myocardium. This approach is based on the considerably slower first-pass kinetics of the contrast agents in the myocardial territories affected by ischemia. Adenosine (0.14 mg/kg/min for 3 minutes) and regadenoson (0.4-mg bolus) are the most frequently used pharmacologic stressors. One day before the administration of the stressor, food and beverages containing caffeine must be suspended. The use of these stressors is contraindicated in several conditions such as hypersensitivity to the medication, second- or third-degree atrioventricular block, long QT syndrome, sick sinus syndrome, active wheezing in chronic obstructive pulmonary disease, severe hypotension, and unstable angina. Heart rate, oxygen saturation, and blood pressure should be monitored before, during, and after the stress protocol.

CAD is often associated with valvular disease (e.g., aortic valve calcification and stenosis, mitral insufficiency due to papillary muscle infarction). In such cases, CMR offers the opportunity to evaluate not only valve anatomy and motion, but also the blood flow through the valve. Phase contrast velocity mapping sequences are used to map blood velocity, similarly to Doppler echocardiography. Using the phase contrast acquisition, peak velocities as well as the forward and regurgitant volumes can be quantitatively assessed. Novel phase contrast CMR sequences can even be applied in a free-breathing fashion and in four dimensions.

Coronary MR angiography is a relatively new domain of CMR in the clinical setting. Several experimental studies have been conducted to investigate the feasibility of CMR for the visualization of the coronary arteries. Although CMR outperforms CT in temporal resolution, its spatial resolution is still inferior to CT. In addition, the collection of a three-dimensional dataset requires imaging during several heartbeats, resulting in alignment issues between images acquired at different heartbeats and multiple breath-holds. There are some prototype sequences available implementing combined ECG and respiratory gating or various motion correction algorithms to provide good image quality and also patient comfort by eliminating breath-holds. Using such sequences, the proximal and mid courses of the coronary arteries can be visualized. However, the presence of calcification in the coronary arteries (and in the aortic valve) leads to further challenges in image interpretation due to significant dephasing artifacts.

Administering a Gadolinium Agent

Gadolinium-based contrast agents are relatively safe. The number of hypersensitivity reactions reported is significantly less than for iodinated contrast media. A major concern regarding these agents arose several years ago, when cases with nephrogenic systemic fibrosis (NSF) were associated with the administration of certain gadolinium agents. However, the causal relationship between gadolinium administration and the development of NSF has not been clarified so far. Newer concerns have been recently voiced over the long-term permanent accumulation of gadolinium in the body, but the exact clinical significance is yet unknown. Novel contrast agents with a cyclic structure exhibit significantly higher molecular stability, providing increased patient safety. According to the current guidelines, a gadolinium agent must not be used in patients with severe kidney problems (glomerular filtration rate [GFR] <30 mL/min per 1.73 m^2) and in newborns younger than 4 weeks of age.

Reporting the Findings

The report should be started with the description of the CMR protocol and the contrast medium and amount used, followed by the findings in a structured order. A general description of the calibers of the atria and ventricles, interatrial and interventricular septal discontinuity, and pericardial status should be provided.

Further assessment of the CMR images requires a complex overview of the various acquisitions. It is particularly important to match the findings of the T2-weighted, cine, perfusion, and early and late enhancement images. For example, a signal increase in a certain myocardial territory in T2-weighted images may correspond to hypokinesis of the same segment in cine, a hypointense region on rest perfusion and early gadolinium enhancement images, and hyperintensity in the delayed phase, consistent with acute myocardial infarction. Thus the findings in each image set should be separately reported, matched, and summarized as an impression.

The presence of myocardial edema in T2-weighted images should be discussed. T2 hyperintensity may indicate myocardial edema (Fig. 30.4), whereas T2 hypointensity may represent the presence of heme-containing blood degradation products due to intramyocardial hemorrhage. Edema may indicate acute infarction or inflammation. Hemorrhage may be caused by the revascularization of an occluded coronary artery.

Global and regional cardiac function can be qualitatively evaluated using long- and short-axis cine images (Fig. 30.5). Quantitative assessment of global left ventricular function is usually based on the short-axis cine image set. As part of the global functional assessment, the end-diastolic and end-systolic volumes, stroke volume, ejection fraction, cardiac output, and myocardial mass can be calculated for the left and right ventricles. These values are usually indexed to the body surface area. Qualitative and quantitative regional cardiac function is based on segmental wall thickening. The evaluation is usually performed using the American Heart Association

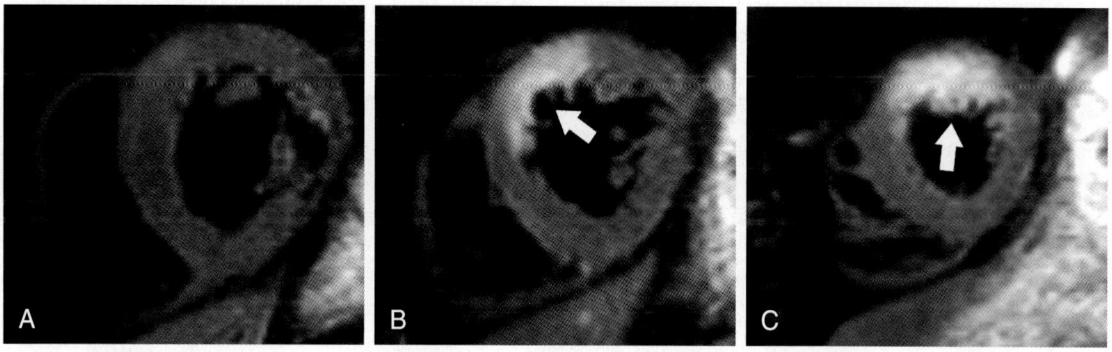

Figure 30.4 Basal (A), midventricular (B), and apical (C) short-axis T2-weighted images from a patient with acute myocardial infarction. The elevated signal intensity *(arrows)* in the anteroseptal and anterior segments of the mid and apical sections of the ventricle corresponds to acute myocardial edema.

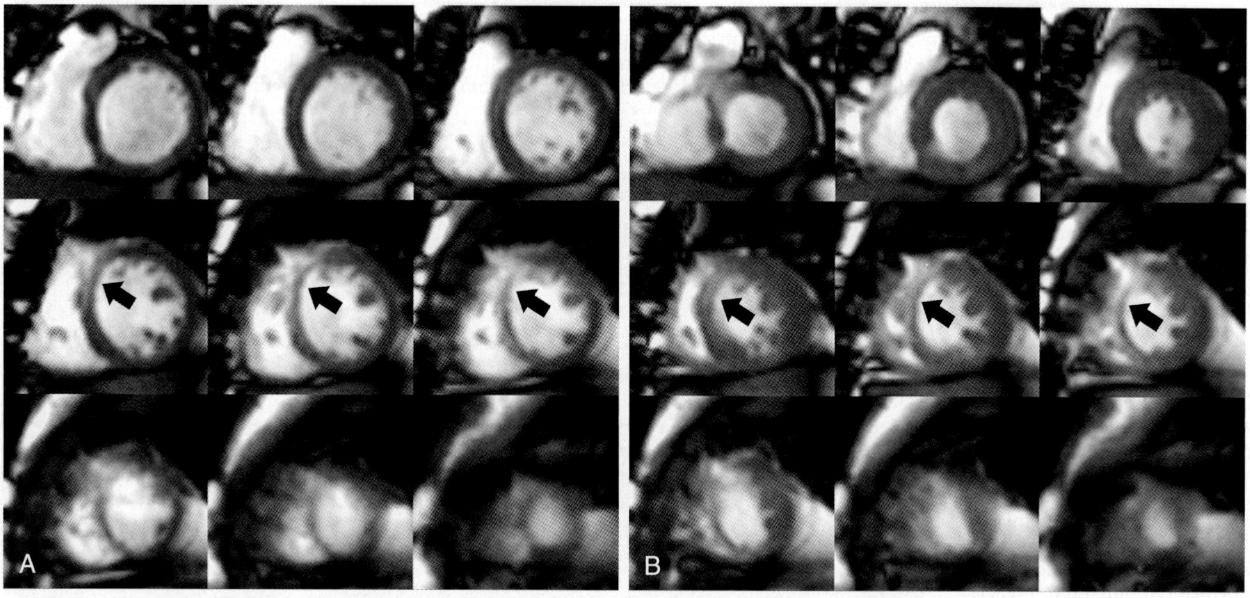

Figure 30.5 Short-axis–oriented multislice cine images at end-diastole (A) and end-systole (B). Substantial myocardial thinning and hypokinesis can be observed in the midventricular anteroseptal segments *(arrows)*.

17-segment, left ventricular model. Visual assessment is used for qualitative interpretation (normokinetic, hypokinetic, akinetic, or dyskinetic); absolute and fractional wall thickening or wall motion (i.e., endocardial displacement) values are calculated for quantitative evaluation.

The evaluation of the stress perfusion studies is more complex. First, only true perfusion defects should be reported. A perfusion defect is defined as a hypointense region including at least two adjacent myocardial segments, according to the 17-segment model, and visible over several consecutive heartbeats. Because only three or four different slice positions can be imaged within one cardiac cycle, perfusion imaging does not provide full left ventricular coverage. Usually, three short-axis (apical, mid, and basal) and one long-axis image series are collected. To report perfusion deficits, one should specify which section and which segments are affected and also provide the percentage of wall thickness involved. Perfusion defects observed during rest usually correspond to permanent myocardial damage, such as prior myocardial infarction. Stress-only perfusion defects are considered reversible (Fig. 30.6). Novel software algorithms also allow for the quantitative perfusion analysis and calculation of absolute myocardial blood flow.

Finally, gadolinium enhancement should be evaluated. Early gadolinium enhancement images are used to detect hypointense microvascular obstruction (no-reflow) and intracardiac thrombus. LGE images highlight both acute and subacute myocardial necrosis and chronic scar (Fig. 30.7). These image sets usually provide full left ventricular coverage. The enhancement observed in the myocardium should be reported based on the 17-segment model. One should specify the myocardial section (apical, mid, or basal) and segments in which the enhancement was detected. The pattern of myocardial necrosis and scar of ischemic origin should always respect the myocardial territory of the involved coronary artery based on the 17-segment model, whereas the extent of the lesion should affect at least two adjacent myocardial segments. It is paramount to confirm that the pattern is suggesting ischemic cause—that is, primarily subendocardial. Other patterns (e.g., patchy, subepicardial, midmyocardial) typically suggest a nonischemic cause.

Several approaches have been reported for the classification of the extent of the hyperenhancing (nonviable) areas, such as the number of segments affected, percentage of wall thickness affected (transmurality described as involving 0%–25%, 25%–50%, 50%–75%, or 75%–100%

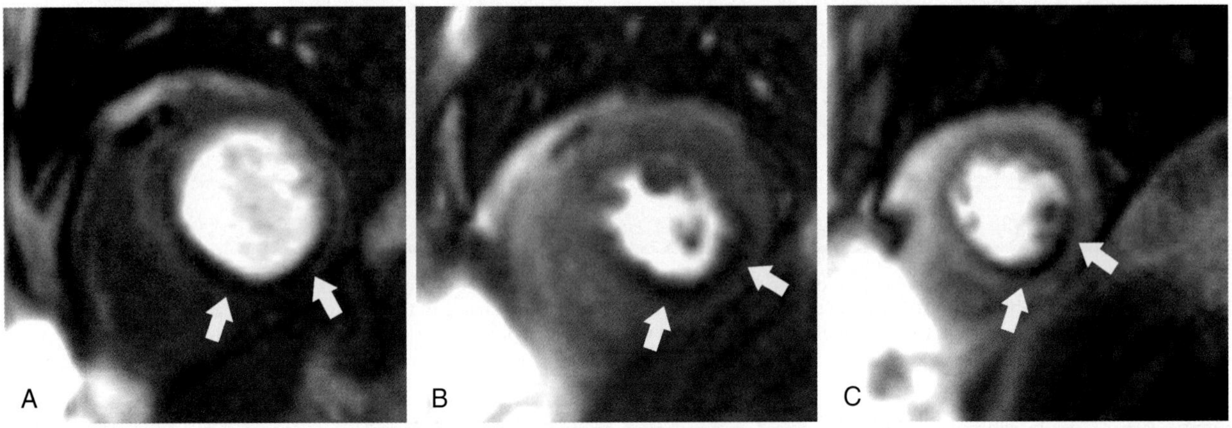

Figure 30.6 Stress myocardial perfusion study in a patient with acute chest pain. Basal (A), midventricular (B), and apical (C) short-axis slices are shown. A stress perfusion defect was detected in the inferoseptal and inferolateral segments of the basal and midventricular myocardium, as well as in the inferior segment of the apical section *(arrows)*.

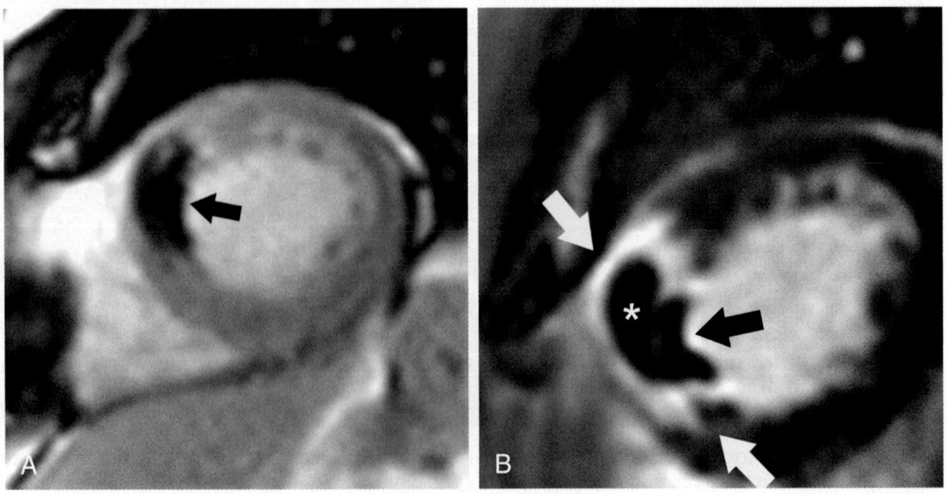

Figure 30.7 Early and late gadolinium enhancement study in a patient with acute myocardial infarction and adjacent mural thrombus. (A) Early enhancement image shows an unenhanced region in the myocardium consistent with microvascular obstruction and a mural thrombus *(arrow)* in the anteroseptal segment. (B) Late enhancement image depicts a bright region *(white arrows)* surrounding a dark area consistent with acute infarct with central microvascular obstruction *(asterisk)*. The nonenhanced mural thrombus is also shown *(black arrow)*.

of the wall thickness), and purely quantitative methods used. Quantification is usually based on a certain thresholding algorithm, which can discriminate the normal myocardium from the lesion. The actual infarct size can be reported as absolute volume or percentage of the total myocardium.

■ Problem Solving

High or Arrhythmic Heart Rate

Image quality of cardiac CT is highly influenced by artifacts caused by movement of the myocardium and adjacent vascular structures. When the heart contracts in a regular rhythm, electrocardiographic synchronization detects this pattern and provides optimal radiation exposure during intervals of the cardiac cycle with little movement. This concept is the foundation for dose-saving protocols with electrocardiographic synchronization. A high or arrhythmic heart rate may potentially interfere with such algorithms. Thus older scanner generations generally used retrospectively ECG-gated protocols in these patients, with consequently high ionizing radiation doses. Newer scanner generations provide far better algorithms for imaging under these conditions.

Ectopy is relatively common and may be present in patients with and without a history of cardiac disease. It is therefore crucial to assess the ECG during scan preparation with the patient on the table because it is usually intermittent and infrequent. Additional administration of beta blockers may suppress some but not all ectopic activity. Nevertheless, current scanner generations are also able to detect ectopy in real time during a scan and adjust for it. Several studies have demonstrated that prospectively ECG-triggered protocols can be used in patients with ectopy and other forms of arrhythmia without compromising image quality. Even high-pitch protocols with radiation exposure <1 mSv can be applied. With current scanner generations, full helical acquisition with consequently far higher radiation exposure should not be necessary for the assessment of coronary artery patency and CAD.

Atrial fibrillation used to be a contraindication for dose-saving protocols or even cardiac CT in general. Due to faster scanning with newer scanner generations, multiple recent studies have demonstrated that most dose-saving techniques can be applied, even in these patients. In addition, atrial fibrillation patients referred for cardiac CT often actually require visualization of the left atrium, left atrial appendage, and pulmonary veins, instead of high-resolution imaging of the coronary arteries. This has a direct impact on the optimal imaging protocol and resulting radiation exposure. Thus depending on the indication, which should be discussed with the referring physician, high-pitch acquisition with a reduced tube voltage and automated dose modulation software may be performed in these patients.

CMR image quality is similarly sensitive for arrhythmia. The best-quality images require segmented acquisition—that is, the acquisition of a single image is distributed over several heartbeats—and the equal length of the cardiac cycles involved in the data collection is particularly important. Most cine CMR sequences are implemented in a retrospectively ECG-gated approach. In patients with frequent ectopic activity, a more time-consuming technique, prospective ECG gating, can be used, which can skip ectopic cardiac cycles. Alternatively, real-time cine sequences can be used, although the temporal resolution in these sequences is suboptimal. First-pass perfusion imaging, early- and late-enhancement (viability) imaging, however, can be performed with single-shot imaging, which is an advantage in patients with arrhythmia.

Obesity

Image quality is directly influenced by the photon count and therefore by tissue penetration and passage through the patient's body. Overweight patients still pose a challenge to cross-sectional imaging modalities. However, recent innovations regarding x-ray generators, photon shields, and detector technology have substantially improved the image quality of CT examinations in obese patients. Nevertheless, the basic principle for CT in obese patients remains an increase of the emitted energy by adjusting the x-ray tube voltage and current. The type of examination and indication for imaging should also be taken into account. Contrast-enhanced examinations, and especially CT angiography studies, can usually be performed with lower tube voltage settings that result in increased intravascular attenuation.

Due to the anatomic properties of the lungs, the image contrast of chest CT in obese patients can be expected to be superior compared to imaging of the abdomen. In general, most chest CT examinations can be safely performed at 100 kVp if automated tube current modulation is activated. The newest scanner generations have made contrast-enhanced cardiac CT examinations at 70 to 80 kVp feasible, but usually require the use of dedicated postprocessing. In addition, newer scanner generations provide improved photon emission at low tube voltages to provide diagnostic image quality, with coincidental dose reduction (Fig. 30.8). Nevertheless, even with a higher tube voltage, the existing solutions for reduced radiation exposure can be used, such as selection of a prospectively ECG-gated protocol. Even high-pitch acquisition can be performed in obese patients with sinus rhythm and bradycardia (<65 beats/min). Particularly in patients with a low likelihood for CAD, cardiac CT, even at lower tube voltages, will provide sufficient image quality to rule out coronary stenosis. In patients with known CAD, previously implanted stents, or a CABG, a standard tube voltage of 100 kVp or higher should be selected.

In CMR, obesity is a less significant issue in terms of image quality or imaging protocols. The main limiting factor in imaging of obese patients is the bore size. Most scanners have a bore diameter of 60 cm. At the beginning of the cardiac scan, localizers are used to place the heart in the isocenter of the magnet. If the region of the heart is moved to the isocenter, at least the upper abdomen must also fit into the bore due to its relatively long size. This means that the abdominal girth plus the coil together

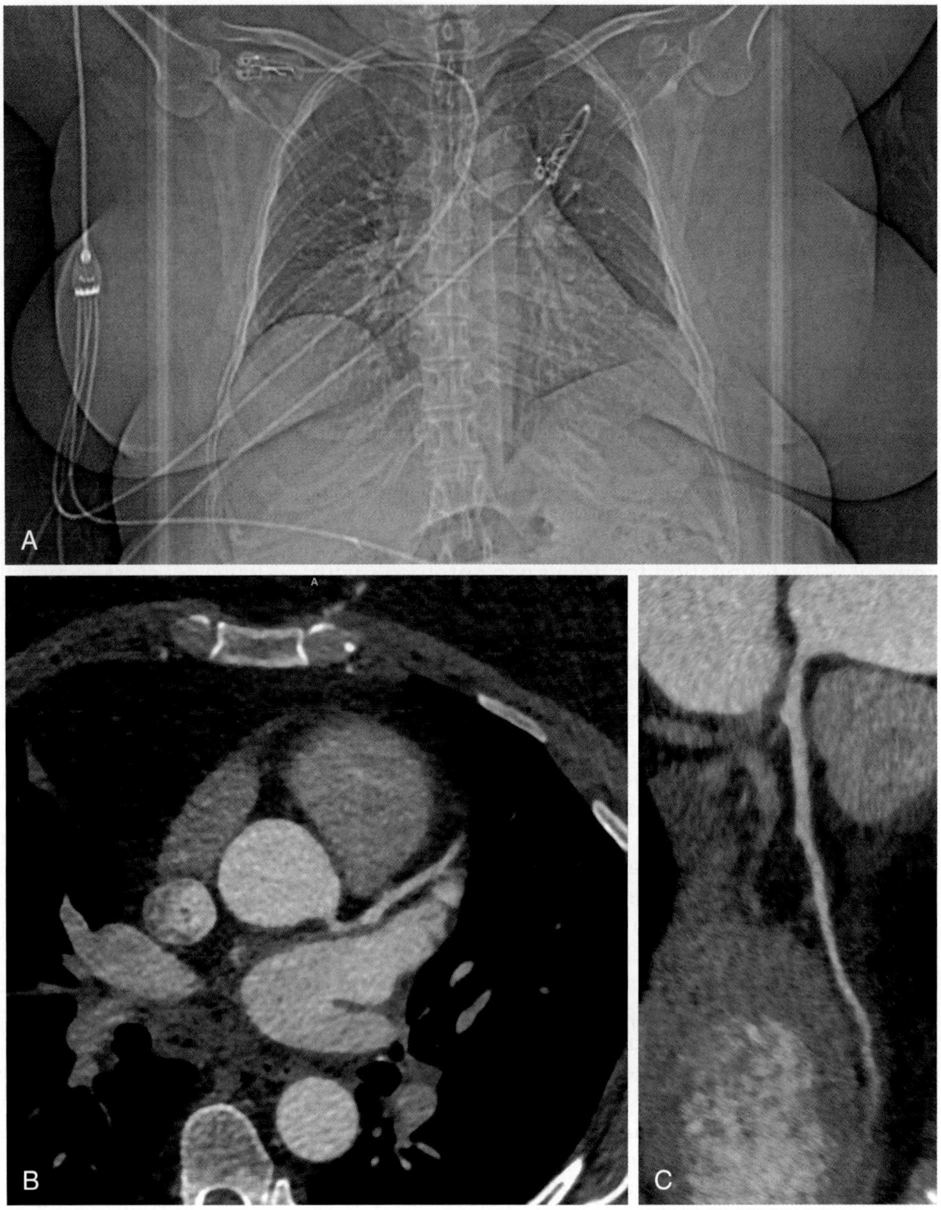

Figure 30.8 Example case of coronary CT angiography (CCTA) in a 50-year-old obese female patient with a body mass index of 41.5 kg/m^2. (A) Scout images demonstrate a large thoracic diameter. CCTA was performed with a prospectively ECG-gated sequential protocol on third-generation dual-source CT. (B) Axial images and curved multiplanar reformats (C) of the left anterior descending coronary artery demonstrate diagnostic image quality.

(if the coil partially covers the upper abdomen) should be less than the bore diameter. Usually, though, the limiting factor is the patient circumference with hands by the side, measured at the widest point in the chest, including the shoulders and upper arms. When a patient does not fit into a regular size magnet, a large-bore 3-T MR scanner (70 cm), if available, may be used to perform the cardiac scan, or alternative imaging modalities should be taken into consideration.

High-Density Elements

Although CT technology provides high image resolution and soft tissue contrast at fast acquisition times, it may still be impaired by beam-hardening artifacts and scatter caused by high-density elements, such as surgical clips, coronary stents, pacemaker wires, and valve prostheses in cardiac patients. In addition, extensive coronary calcium and contrast material inflow can cause these artifacts, which may drastically limit assessment of the heart and coronary arteries.

A first step to approach this problem is to evaluate the scout images and coronary calcium scans (if performed). On these, any elements that may cause such artifacts will be clearly visible, and scan protocols for the actual CT angiography can be promptly adjusted. In the past, image acquisition protocols with high tube voltage (120–140 kVp) and current were used to reduce such artifacts. However, this also results in a substantial increase in radiation exposure. With current scanner generations, two different approaches are available. Most CT vendors provide dedicated iterative metal artifact reduction algorithms, which are able to decrease such artifacts substantially. When using these algorithms, imaging can be performed at a standard tube voltage of

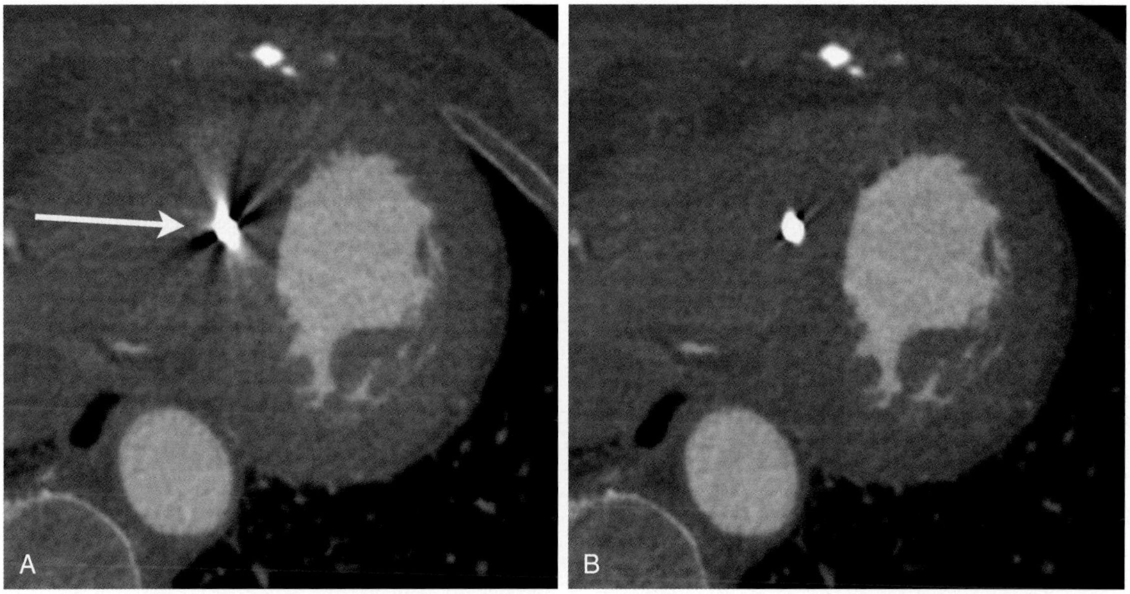

Figure 30.9 Effects of a dedicated iterative metal artifact reduction algorithm in a 70-kVp cardiac scan. (A) Beam-hardening artifacts arising from the tip of a pacemaker wire *(arrow)* superimpose the septal myocardium. (B) Metal artifact reduction eliminates most streak artifacts and improves evaluation of the myocardium.

100 kVp in most patients (Fig. 30.9). Such algorithms usually require raw data and therefore need to be activated on the scanner interface. In addition, the resulting image series should be reconstructed with a sharper kernel to reduce artifacts further.

Dual-energy CT has been established as a different approach to this problem. In addition to various post-processing possibilities, monoenergetic reconstructions have been shown to obliterate beam-hardening effects effectively from high-density elements.

The corresponding MR safety issues of high-density elements (e.g., metallic implants, implantable devices) are discussed in the section titled "Cardiac Magnetic Resonance Imaging Algorithms." The MR compatibility of an implant should always be confirmed with the manufacturer before placing the patient into the scanner. Even if the implant is MR-compatible, the presence of a metallic structure in the magnetic field close to the region imaged may cause significant susceptibility artifacts, depending on the sequence used. Sternal wires and pacemaker leads, the most common metallic parts close to the heart, do not cause major artifacts that affect the diagnostic value of a CMR scan. Artificial valve replacements may result in substantial signal loss at the level of the valve, limiting the evaluation of the valve itself, but it is still possible to perform flow assessment of the valve and visualize the effects of valvular abnormality and complications.

Vascular and valve calcification, another common finding in patients with ischemic heart disease, may also cause spin dephasing and consequent signal loss in the areas of the calcium deposits. This signal loss may affect valve assessment (diameter and area measurements) and influence the evaluation of the vascular components (e.g., ostia of the coronary arteries).

In case of significant artifacts yielding nondiagnostic studies, the referring physician should be informed, and alternative imaging approaches to answer the diagnostic questions should be suggested.

In-Stent Lumen Assessment

Coronary artery stents pose a special challenge for cardiac imaging due to beam-hardening effects, which may overlay the coronary lumen. However, in-stent lumen assessment is a relatively common task for cardiac imaging due to the risk of in-stent thrombosis, especially within the first year after stent implantation. In general, most of the techniques already presented for coping with beam-hardening artifacts from high-density elements also apply to in-stent imaging: low tube voltage acquisition should be used less frequently, sharper kernels should be used for reconstruction, and iterative reconstruction algorithms should be used. Most new-generation CT scanners are able to provide adequate image quality for in-stent lumen assessment in larger stents.

In addition, novel techniques specifically developed for the evaluation of in-stent lumen patency have been developed. By measuring the attenuation values in the coronary lumen proximal and distal to stents, the coronary opacification gradient can be assessed. This simple approach has been shown to help detect in-stent thrombosis, although it seems to work particularly well in smaller stents. Software-based digital subtraction angiography is an established technique in neurovascular imaging, but remains a research topic in cardiac CT. Nevertheless, most stents can be examined with good image quality in clinical routine by adjusting scan and image reconstruction parameters and meticulously evaluating cMPR datasets.

Claustrophobia

Due to the small diameter of the MR bore, many patients complain about claustrophobia after a certain time during the examination. Different strategies have been tested to increase patient comfort. Wider bore magnets are available, which also fit patients with a higher body mass index, and special constructions with mirrors have been developed that allow the patient to look out from the bore. Listening to music during the MR examination may also have a beneficial effect. In severe cases, sedation may be used. In outpatients, 5 to 10 mg of orally administered diazepam may relieve the patient's symptoms. In rare cases, even general anesthesia can be considered.

Difficulty With Breath-Holding

Cardiac patients frequently have difficulties with long breath-holds necessary for most of the CMR acquisitions. In such cases, the length of the acquisition time (the length of the breath-hold) can be reduced, or free-breathing protocols can be used. The length of the acquisition is influenced by several parameters; however, the most effective way to decrease the acquisition time is reducing the number of segments imaged and/or lowering spatial resolution. These modifications will consequently result in a reduction of image quality. In severe cases, the use of free-breathing protocols might be necessary, such as real-time cine imaging (with low temporal and spatial resolution) and single-shot acquisitions (the whole image is collected in a single cardiac cycle).

■ Pearls and Pitfalls

CT Imaging

- Preimaging evaluation of patients scheduled for cardiac CT is crucial to determine factors influencing the optimal imaging protocol with diagnostic image quality and low radiation exposure.
- Radiation dose from cardiac CT is mainly influenced by protocol selection based on heart rhythm and frequency.
- Further radiation dose reduction can be achieved by lowering tube voltage and current. Iterative reconstruction algorithms should be additionally applied to improve image quality.
- Special attention should be paid to material which may potentially cause beam-hardening artifacts as imaging protocols have to be modified and additional post-processing should be used.
- New-generation scanners allow for cardiac CT with diagnostic image quality even in patients with arrhythmia or atrial fibrillation without exposing the patient to high radiation exposure.
- Dedicated post-processing in cardiac CT is also particularly helpful for image interpretation. cMPRs should be routinely created and assessed.

Cardiac Magnetic Resonance Imaging

- Appropriate patient screening is essential to identify possible contraindications, such as metallic implants and implanted devices.
- The majority of newer implants are MR compatible. Special attention is necessary regarding ICDs.
- Kidney function must be assessed in patients undergoing contrast-enhanced CMR if a reliable GFR value from the past 30 days is not available.
- In patients with arrhythmias, prospective ECG gating can be used.
- In patients with difficulty holding their breath, free-breathing single shot and respiratory navigator-gated sequences may be employed.

■ Conclusion

Patients with ischemic cardiac disease represent a unique and demanding population for CT and CMR imaging in clinical routine. Radiologists are expected to use the latest technologies to reduce radiation exposure in CT and achieve high image quality and diagnostic accuracy. Recent technological innovations have introduced suitable solutions for most problems for both modalities. Comprehensive patient evaluation before imaging remains key and protocols must be specifically tailored during the examination. Thus, cardiac imaging remains one of the few examinations in radiology with a high patient-physician interaction and adjustment of scan parameters. Nevertheless, cutting-edge technologies should be routinely applied to emphasize the crucial clinical role of CT and MRI for cardiac imaging next to established methods, especially invasive techniques (i.e., ICA).

Bibliography

Achenbach S, Marwan M, Ropers D, et al. Coronary computed tomography angiography with a consistent dose below 1 mSv using prospectively electrocardiogram-triggered high-pitch spiral acquisition. *Eur Heart J*. 2010;31(3): 340–346.

Al Sayari S, Kopp S, Bremerich J. Stress cardiac MR imaging: the role of stress functional assessment and perfusion imaging in the evaluation of ischemic heart disease. *Radiol Clin North Am*. 2015;53(2):355–367.

Anderson KM, Odell PM, Wilson PW, Kannel WB. Cardiovascular disease risk profiles. *Am Heart J*. 1991;121(1 Pt 2):293–298.

Bamberg F, Becker A, Schwarz F, et al. Detection of hemodynamically significant coronary artery stenosis: incremental diagnostic value of dynamic CT-based myocardial perfusion imaging. *Radiology*. 2011;260(3):689–698.

Baumann S, Wang R, Schoepf UJ, et al. Coronary CT angiography-derived fractional flow reserve correlated with invasive fractional flow reserve measurements — initial experience with a novel physician-driven algorithm. *Eur Radiol*. 2015;25(4):1201–1207.

Cerqueira MD, Weissman NJ, Dilsizian V, et al. Standardized myocardial segmentation and nomenclature for tomographic imaging of the heart. A statement for healthcare professionals from the cardiac imaging committee of the Council on Clinical Cardiology of the American Heart Association. *Circulation*. 2002;105(4):539–542.

Choi JH, Min JK, Labounty TM, et al. Intracoronary transluminal attenuation gradient in coronary CT angiography for determining coronary artery stenosis. *JACC Cardiovasc Imaging*. 2011;4(11):1149–1157.

Cury RC, Abbara S, Achenbach S, et al. CAD-RADS™: Coronary Artery Disease — Reporting and Data System: An Expert Consensus Document of the Society of Cardiovascular Computed Tomography (SCCT), the American College of Radiology (ACR) and the North American Society for Cardiovascular Imaging (NASCI). Endorsed by the American College of Cardiology. *J Am Coll Radiol*. 2016;13(12 Pt A):1458–1466.e9.

De Cecco CN, Varga-Szemes A, Meinel FG, Renker M, Schoepf UJ. Beyond stenosis detection: computed tomography approaches for determining the functional relevance of coronary artery disease. *Radiol Clin North Am.* 2015;53(2): 317–334.

Douglas PS, Hoffmann U, Patel MR, et al. Outcomes of anatomical versus functional testing for coronary artery disease. *N Engl J Med.* 2015.

Ebersberger U, Makowski MR, Schoepf UJ, et al. Magnetic resonance myocardial perfusion imaging at 3.0 tesla for the identification of myocardial ischaemia: comparison with coronary catheter angiography and fractional flow reserve measurements. *Eur Heart J Cardiovasc Imaging.* 2013;14(12):1174–1180.

Expert Panel on MRS, Kanal E, Barkovich AJ, et al. ACR guidance document on MR safe practices: 2013. *J Magn Reson Imaging.* 2013;37(3):501–530.

Flohr TG, De Cecco CN, Schmidt B, Wang R, Schoepf UJ, Meinel FG. Computed tomographic assessment of coronary artery disease: state-of-the-art imaging techniques. *Radiol Clin North Am.* 2015;53(2):271–285.

Geyer LL, Glenn GR, De Cecco CN, et al. CT evaluation of small-diameter coronary artery stents: effect of an integrated circuit detector with iterative reconstruction. *Radiology.* 2015;140427.

Hao D, Ai T, Goerner F, Hu X, Runge VM, Tweedle M. MRI contrast agents: basic chemistry and safety. *J Magn Reson Imaging.* 2012;36(5):1060–1071.

Hendel RC, Patel MR, Kramer CM, et al. ACCF/ACR/SCCT/SCMR/ASNC/NASCI/SCAI/SIR 2006 appropriateness criteria for cardiac computed tomography and cardiac magnetic resonance imaging: a report of the American College of Cardiology Foundation Quality Strategic Directions Committee Appropriateness Criteria Working Group, American College of Radiology, Society of Cardiovascular Computed Tomography, Society for Cardiovascular Magnetic Resonance, American Society of Nuclear Cardiology, North American Society for Cardiac Imaging, Society for Cardiovascular Angiography and Interventions, and Society of Interventional Radiology. *J Am Coll Cardiol.* 2006;48(7):1475–1497.

Hoffmann U, Truong QA, Schoenfeld DA, et al. Coronary CT angiography versus standard evaluation in acute chest pain. *N Engl J Med.* 2012;367(4):299–308.

Lin K, Carr JC. MR imaging of the coronary vasculature: imaging the lumen, wall, and beyond. *Radiol Clin North Am.* 2015;53(2):345–353.

Meyer M, Haubenreisser H, Schoepf UJ, et al. Closing in on the K edge: coronary CT angiography at 100, 80, and 70 kv-initial comparison of a second- versus a third-generation dual-source CT system. *Radiology.* 2014;273(2):373–382.

Nordbeck P, Ertl G, Ritter O. Magnetic resonance imaging safety in pacemaker and implantable cardioverter defibrillator patients: how far have we come? *Eur Heart J.* 2015;36(24):1505–1511.

Piccini D, Monney P, Sierro C, et al. Respiratory self-navigated postcontrast whole-heart coronary MR angiography: initial experience in patients. *Radiology.* 2014;270(2):378–386.

Pletcher MJ, Tice JA, Pignone M, Browner WS. Using the coronary artery calcium score to predict coronary heart disease events: a systematic review and meta-analysis. *Arch Intern Med.* 2004;164(12):1285–1292.

Renker M, Nance JW Jr, Schoepf UJ, et al. Evaluation of heavily calcified vessels with coronary CT angiography: comparison of iterative and filtered back projection image reconstruction. *Radiology.* 2011;260(2):390–399.

Renker M, Schoepf UJ, Wang R, et al. Comparison of diagnostic value of a novel noninvasive coronary computed tomography angiography method versus standard coronary angiography for assessing fractional flow reserve. *Am J Cardiol.* 2014;114(9):1303–1308.

Schoepf UJ, Becker CR, Ohnesorge BM, Yucel EK. CT of coronary artery disease. *Radiology.* 2004;232(1):18–37.

Schoepf UJ, Zwerner PL, Savino G, Herzog C, Kerl JM, Costello P. Coronary CT angiography. *Radiology.* 2007;244(1):48–63.

Schwitter J, Wacker CM, Wilke N, et al. MR-IMPACT II: magnetic resonance imaging for myocardial perfusion assessment in coronary artery disease trial: perfusion-cardiac magnetic resonance vs. single-photon emission computed tomography for the detection of coronary artery disease: a comparative multicentre, multivendor trial. *Eur Heart J.* 2013;34(10):775–781.

Secchi F, De Cecco CN, Spearman JV, et al. Monoenergetic extrapolation of cardiac dual energy CT for artifact reduction. *Acta Radiol.* 2014.

Srichai MB, Barreto M, Lim RP, Donnino R, Babb JS, Jacobs JE. Prospective-triggered sequential dual-source end-systolic coronary CT angiography for patients with atrial fibrillation: a feasibility study. *J Cardiovasc Comput Tomogr.* 2013;7(2):102–109.

Takx RA, Blomberg BA, El Aidi H, et al. Diagnostic accuracy of stress myocardial perfusion imaging compared to invasive coronary angiography with fractional flow reserve meta-analysis. *Circ Cardiovasc Imaging.* 2015;8(1).

Taylor AJ, Cerqueira M, Hodgson JM, et al. ACCF/SCCT/ACR/AHA/ASE/ASNC/NASCI/SCAI/SCMR 2010 appropriate use criteria for cardiac computed tomography. A report of the American College of Cardiology Foundation Appropriate Use Criteria Task Force, the Society of Cardiovascular Computed Tomography, the American College of Radiology, the American Heart Association, the American Society of Echocardiography, the American Society of Nuclear Cardiology, the North American Society for Cardiovascular Imaging, the Society for Cardiovascular Angiography and Interventions, and the Society for Cardiovascular Magnetic Resonance. *J Am Coll Cardiol.* 2010;56(22): 1864–1894.

Thomson LE, Wei J, Agarwal M, et al. Cardiac magnetic resonance myocardial perfusion reserve index is reduced in women with coronary microvascular dysfunction. A National Heart, Lung, and Blood Institute-sponsored study from the women's ischemia syndrome evaluation. *Circ Cardiovasc Imaging.* 2015;8(4):e002481.

Wichmann JL, Bauer RW, Doss M, et al. Diagnostic accuracy of late iodine-enhancement dual-energy computed tomography for the detection of chronic myocardial infarction compared with late gadolinium-enhancement 3-T magnetic resonance imaging. *Invest Radiol.* 2013;48(12):851–856.

CHAPTER 31
Imaging of Cardiomyopathy and Myocarditis

Brian B. Ghoshhajra, Pedro Vinícius Staziaki, and Marie-Helene Levesque

CHAPTER OUTLINE

■ Introduction

Cardiomyopathies and myocarditis are disorders frequently encountered in clinical practice, and imaging plays a major role in the diagnosis, management, and follow-up of these diseases. This chapter will describe imaging of the cardiomyopathies that have characteristic imaging features and that are most commonly imaged in clinical practice.

■ Imaging: What, Why, and How

Definition of a Cardiomyopathy

Cardiomyopathies are diseases of the heart muscle that may eventually lead to cardiac dysfunction or arrhythmias. They encompass a heterogeneous group of several myocardial disorders that manifest with various structural and functional phenotypes. Despite the common clinical use of the terms *ischemic* and *hypertensive cardiomyopathies,* cardiomyopathy does not include impaired cardiac function caused by cardiovascular disorders, such as atherosclerotic coronary artery disease (CAD), cardiac valve disease, systemic hypertension, or congenital heart disease, as defined by the 2006 American Heart Association (AHA) and 2008 European Society of Cardiology statements. The AHA classification divides the cardiomyopathies into primary and secondary cardiomyopathies, based on the predominant organ of involvement. Primary cardiomyopathies are confined to heart muscle and may be genetic, acquired, or mixed genetic and acquired (Table 31.1). Secondary cardiomyopathies represent pathologic involvement of the myocardium in the context of a generalized systemic disorder (Table 31.2).

Reasons for Imaging Cardiomyopathy

An important role of imaging patients with cardiomyopathy is to differentiate the ischemic from nonischemic pattern of disease because heart failure is usually caused by myocardial ischemia and infarction. Ischemic disease is important to diagnose with coronary angiography, coronary CT angiography (CTA), or cardiac magnetic resonance imaging (CMR) because left ventricular (LV) function can improve following coronary revascularization in the presence of substantial viable myocardium. On CMR, abnormal late gadolinium enhancement (LGE) involving the subendocardium with a variable degree of transmurality and distributed in the vascular myocardial territory of a coronary artery is compatible with ischemic disease. CMR is a validated tool to differentiate viable from scarred myocardium with decreased potential of recuperation (nonviable) based on abnormal LGE involving less (viable) or more (nonviable) than 50% of the wall thickness.

Imaging is essential to assess the phenotypic expression of nonischemic cardiomyopathy and degree of cardiac dysfunction. CMR can identify infarcted or scarred myocardium by the presence of abnormal LGE, which has prognostic value and may influence clinical management—for example, deciding on the implantation of an automatic implantable cardioverter-defibrillator. Finally, the lack of ionizing radiation makes echocardiography and CMR important tools for screening relatives of patients with hypertrophic cardiomyopathy (HCM) or arrhythmogenic right ventricular cardiomyopathy or dysplasia (ARVC/D) and for the serial assessment of treatment response and complications of various cardiomyopathies.

Procedural Considerations

Problem Solving With Echocardiography

Transthoracic echocardiography is usually the first-line imaging modality to identify various cardiomyopathy phenotypes, assess for wall motion abnormalities, and measure chamber volume, ventricular ejection fraction, and wall thickness. Doppler echocardiography is helpful to evaluate cardiac valves and diastolic dysfunction. However, echocardiography is limited by substantial interstudy and interobserver variability. It may be inconclusive because of suboptimal acoustic window (e.g., obese patients) or because some areas (e.g., cardiac apex and the right ventricular [RV] free wall) are poorly visualized by transthoracic echocardiography. Transesophageal echocardiography improves visualization, but it is an invasive procedure requiring intubation of the esophagus, with a small risk of esophageal perforation, bleeding, and aspiration.

TABLE 31.1 American Heart Association Classification of Primary Cardiomyopathies

TYPE	EXAMPLES
Genetic	HCM, ARVC/D, LVNC
Acquired	Myocarditis, stress, and PPCM
Mixed	DCM, restrictive cardiomyopathy

ARVC/D, Arrhythmogenic right ventricular cardiomyopathy or dysplasia; *DCM*, dilated cardiomyopathy; *HCM*, hypertrophic cardiomyopathy; *LVNC*, left ventricular noncompaction; *PPCM*, peripartum cardiomyopathy.

Problem Solving With Coronary CT Angiography

In newly diagnosed cardiomyopathy, it is important to ensure that the cardiac dysfunction is not caused by CAD-related ischemia or infarction. Although catheter angiography is the gold standard test, coronary CTA is a validated noninvasive alternative in patients with a low pretest probability of CAD (e.g., young patients with no risk factors for CAD). Functional data can be acquired to assess for wall motion abnormalities and measure the chamber volume, ventricular ejection fraction, and myocardial wall thickness. Delayed imaging after injection of iodinated contrast may also be performed to detect myocardial fibrosis, a technique similar to the LGE sequence in CMR. Although the contrast resolution, accuracy, and reproducibility of CMR to assess cardiac function and myocardial fibrosis are superior, coronary CTA is a helpful alternative in patients with contraindications to CMR (e.g., pacemaker). Incidental CT findings in the lung or mediastinum may suggest the cause of a cardiomyopathy. For example, abnormal LGE in the myocardium in the presence of mediastinal and hilar lymphadenopathy with lung nodules is suspicious for sarcoidosis. Signs of congestive heart failure may be seen on CT, including interlobular septal thickening, ground-glass opacity, pleural effusion, and borderline enlarged bilateral hilar lymph nodes.

Problem Solving With Cardiac Magnetic Resonance Imaging

CMR has become the most valuable modality to image cardiomyopathies and will be the focus of this chapter. It is complementary to other imaging modalities to assess for cardiac and pericardial morphology and cardiac and valve function, as well as myocardial perfusion. It also provides uniquely distinct data on the characterization of myocardial tissue. The imaging technique and protocols need to be tailored to the suspected pathology; therefore proper clinical information should be obtained prior to scanning time, and acquisition of the CMR images should be closely monitored.

TABLE 31.2 American Heart Association Classification of Secondary Cardiomyopathies

TYPE	EXAMPLES
Infiltrative	Amyloidosis; Gaucher, Hurler, and Hunter disease
Storage	Hemochromatosis, glycogen storage, Anderson-Fabry and Niemann-Pick diseases
Toxicity	Drugs, heavy metals, chemical agents
Endomyocardial	Tropical endomyocardial fibrosis, hypereosinophilic syndrome
Granulomatous	Sarcoidosis
Endocrine	Diabetes mellitus, hyperthyroidism, hypothyroidism, hyperparathyroidism, pheochromocytoma, acromegaly
Cardiofacial	Noonan syndrome, lentiginosis
Neuromuscular, neurologic	Friedreich ataxia, Duchenne-Becker muscular dystrophy, Emery-Dreifuss muscular dystrophy, myotonic dystrophy, neurofibromatosis, tuberous sclerosis
Nutritional deficiencies	Thiamine, vitamin C (scurvy), carnitine
Autoimmune, collagen	Systemic lupus erythematosus, dermatomyositis, rheumatoid arthritis, scleroderma, polyarteritis nodosa
Consequence of cancer therapy	Anthracyclines, cyclophosphamides, radiation

ASSESSING MYOCARDIAL MORPHOLOGY

Black blood imaging, using a fast spin-echo sequence with blood suppression performed through a double-inversion recovery pulse technique, is used to acquire static images with high in-plane spatial resolution of the morphology of the heart, pericardium, and great vessels. This sequence produces images in which the myocardium has intermediate signal intensity (SI) contrasting with the adjacent dark blood and bright epicardial fat.

Bright blood imaging, using a balanced steady-state free precession (SSFP) sequence acquired in multiple planes (vertical and horizontal long axis, three chamber, and short axis), provides cine images of high temporal resolution in which the blood pool is bright relative to the adjacent intermediate SI of the myocardium.

ASSESSING MYOCARDIAL FUNCTION

Bright blood imaging, using an ECG-segmented balanced SSFP sequence, yields dynamic functional imaging of the heart and can be acquired in any plane. The presence of regional wall motion abnormality can be depicted on SSFP sequence, with or without myocardial tagging technique. A stack of 20 to 30 consecutive, breath-hold, short-axis SSFP images, each acquired during a different cardiac cycle, from the base to the apex, can be interrogated with dedicated viewing software. It is the most accurate and reproducible method for the quantitative assessment of biventricular end-diastolic volumes, end-systolic volumes, ejection fractions, and myocardial mass. Quantitative assessment of the LV volume, ejection fraction, and mass of comparable accuracy can be achieved using a series of long-axis views radially acquired around the anatomic axis of the left ventricle. When CMR is performed to evaluate for ARVC/D, additional SSFP sequences are usually acquired in the right ventricular outflow tract (RVOT), as well as in the long-axis view of the right ventricle and axial plane for a better depiction of the motion of the RVOT and RV free walls.

CHARACTERIZING MYOCARDIAL TISSUE

MYOCARDIAL EDEMA. T2-weighted imaging, using a dual-echo, double-inversion recovery, fast spin-echo sequence in the short-axis plane, is used to detect fluid accumulation in the myocardium caused by focal myocardial edema and/or necrosis. It is depicted by abnormally high T2-weighted SI compared to the adjacent intermediate SI of the normal myocardium. However, diffuse myocardial edema with a homogeneous increase in the T2-weighted SI is more difficult to detect than focal edema. To improve detection of diffuse myocardial edema, the T2 ratio can be calculated to normalize the SI of the myocardium to that of the skeletal muscle. Myocardial T2 mapping, generated by acquiring multiple T2-weighted images repeated with different T2 preparation times, provides both visual and quantitative analyses of the myocardial edema and is a promising tool to diagnose diffuse myocarditis.

MYOCARDIAL IRON DEPOSITION. Iron is a paramagnetic element that alters the local magnetic field and results in a significant decrease in T2*-weighted SI of the affected myocardium. Levels of cardiac iron deposition can be quantified on T2*-weighted images, which is helpful to monitor patients with primary hemochromatosis or secondary hemosiderosis.

MYOCARDIAL FAT. T1-weighted spin-echo imaging is helpful to depict fatty myocardial replacement associated with cardiomyopathies. Focal fatty replacement of the myocardium exhibits high SI on T1-weighted images and can be confirmed with fat saturation showing a loss of SI. Although ARVC/D is characterized by fibrofatty replacement of the myocytes on histology, the presence of fat in the RV wall on imaging is not a diagnostic criterion of ARVC/D due to lack of specificity for this common finding. It usually represents a physiologic change related to age. The presence of subendocardial fatty metaplasia of the LV myocardium in the territory of a coronary artery is indicative of prior myocardial infarction. The presence of myocardial fat has also been described in cardiomyopathy associated with tuberous sclerosis complex or muscular dystrophy and in dilated cardiomyopathy (DCM).

MYOCARDIAL FIBROSIS. LGE imaging, performed with an inversion recovery, gradient echo T1-weighted sequence, is an extremely powerful tool to characterize cardiomyopathies based on the pattern of myocardial fibrosis. Images are acquired 10 to 20 minutes after the injection of gadolinium, with the trigger delay set for systole or diastole. Images are usually acquired in the short-axis view, but additional orthogonal views are often useful to confirm the presence of an abnormality and better visualize the apex. The inversion time is set to null the normal (RV or LV) myocardium that should appear dark, whereas the pathologic myocardium appears bright due to necrosis (acute disease) or fibrosis (chronic disease) expanding the extracellular space and accumulating gadolinium. The pattern of abnormal LGE can be diffuse, patchy, nodular, or linear in appearance, and its distribution is divided into subendocardial, midmyocardial, and subepicardial regions. The subendocardium is the innermost portion of the myocardium and is the most sensitive to ischemia and infarction. The subepicardium refers to the outermost portion of the myocardium. The midmyocardium (or mesocardium) is the myocardium lying between the subendocardium and subepicardium. The localization of abnormal LGE in the LV myocardium is described using the 17-segments model of the AHA with six basal segments, six midventricular segments, four apical segments, and the apex. The pattern of abnormal LGE not only enables differentiation between ischemic and nonischemic cardiomyopathy but also provides a differential diagnosis to establish the cause of the nonischemic cardiomyopathy (Table 31.3).

The LGE imaging technique is designed to optimize discrimination between the enhancement of focal myocardial fibrosis (abnormal LGE) and enhancement of normal myocardium nulled by the selected inversion recovery time. As a result, it fails to demonstrate diffuse myocardial fibrosis because its signal is diffusely suppressed by the selected inversion recovery time. Different CMR techniques have been developed to detect diffuse myocardial fibrosis, such as the T1-weighted early global enhancement ratio, which compares the early uptake of gadolinium in the myocardium to the uptake in skeletal muscle. The T1-weighted early global enhancement ratio is increased in diffuse myocardial

TABLE 31.3 Pattern of Abnormal LGE of Different Cardiomyopathies

PATTERN OF LGE	DIFFERENTIAL DIAGNOSIS
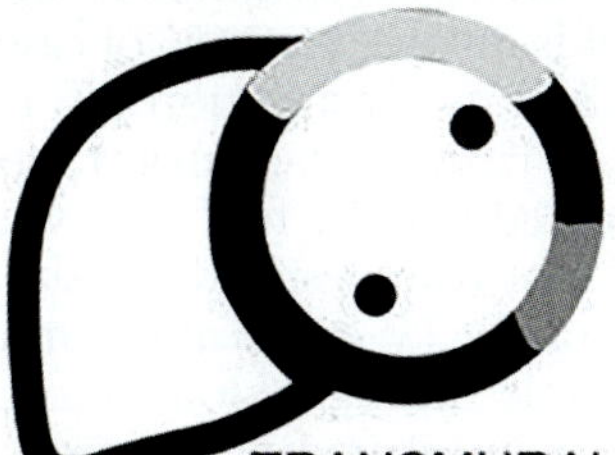 TRANSMURAL	Vascular territory (light gray) • Transmural myocardial infarct Potentially nonvascular territory (dark gray) • Myocarditis • Sarcoidosis
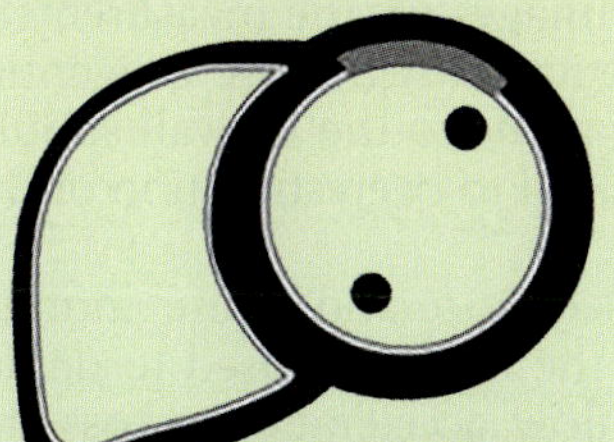 ENDOCARDIAL	Vascular territory (dark gray) • Multivessel myocardial infarcts (light gray) • Amyloidosis • Hypereosinophilic syndrome • Endocardial fibrosis
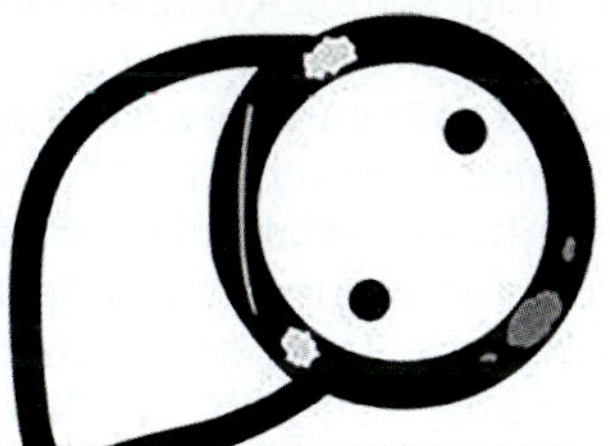 MESOCARDIAL	Linear (light gray) • Idiopathic DCM • Myocarditis RV insertion points (white) • HCM • RV pressure overload Patchy and/or nodular (dark gray) • Myocarditis • Sarcoidosis • HCM • Amyloidosis • Chagas disease • Anderson-Fabry disease
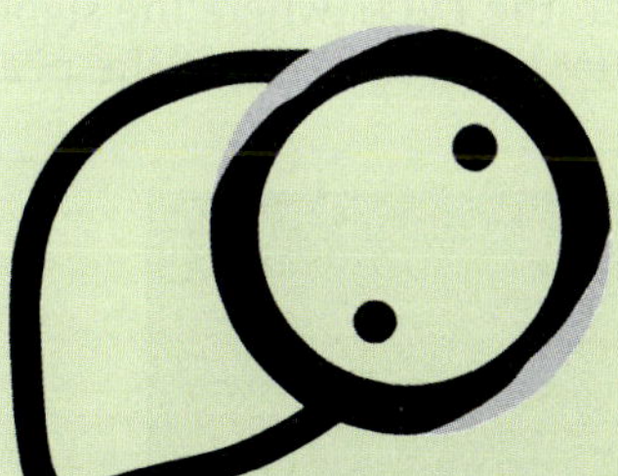 EPICARDIAL	Myocarditis Sarcoidosis Chagas disease Anderson-Fabry disease

DCM, Dilated cardiomyopathy; *HCM*, hypertrophic cardiomyopathy; *LGE*, late gadolinium enhancement.

fibrosis, as well as in myocarditis. This can be measured via multiple T1-weighted acquisitions before and after contrast, in correlation with the hematocrit level, via a technique known as extracellular volume ratio calculation, which is a marker of diffuse abnormalities, most often fibrosis. Another technique, called *T1 mapping*, can visualize and quantify changes in T1 signal due to diffuse myocardial fibrosis, often occurring before any other imaging findings. T1 mapping is performed using fast gradient echo sequences with multiple increasing inversion times (50–1000 ms), without and/or after injection of gadolinium. Precontrast T1 mapping measures intrinsic myocardial contrast. T1 is higher when the extracellular compartment is increased due to fibrosis, edema, or amyloidosis. T1 is lower in lipid (seen in Anderson-Fabry disease) and iron accumulation. Postcontrast T1 mapping quantifies the expansion of the extracellular volume (interstitium) due to fibrosis, amyloidosis, or edema.

ASSESSING MYOCARDIAL PERFUSION

A T1-weighted perfusion sequence performed at rest after the injection of gadolinium can demonstrate a defect of myocardial perfusion in the region of myocardial scarring, and this can be helpful to differentiate scarring from myocardial edema, which has normal to increased perfusion when both myocardial scarring and edema show an abnormal LGE.

ASSESSING FOR BLOOD FLOW ACCELERATION

Intracardiac or transvalvular blood flow acceleration resulting from stenosis or regurgitation may be visualized on SSFP or gradient-recalled echo sequences (e.g., an acceleration jet in the left ventricular outflow tract [LVOT] in obstructive HCM). However, phase contrast imaging is more sensitive and provides an accurate quantification of flow velocities and volumes. It is used to assess for valve stenosis or regurgitation, to measure the degree of obstruction in obstructive HCM, and to assess diastolic dysfunction in restrictive cardiomyopathy.

■ Primary Cardiomyopathies

Genetic Cardiomyopathies

Imaging Hypertrophic Cardiomyopathy

HCM is characterized by inappropriate LV hypertrophy with nondilated ventricular chambers and unexplained by any other cardiac or systemic disease, such as aortic stenosis or systemic hypertension. HCM is caused by mutation in one of the genes encoding sarcomeric proteins and is characterized on histology by disorganization of the myofibrils with myocardial hypertrophy and fibrosis. HCM is the most common primary genetic cardiomyopathy, with an estimated prevalence of 0.2% in the general population; 60% of cases are genetically transmitted, and familial clustering of HCM is frequent. The clinical presentation and natural history of HCM are highly variable. Some individuals remain asymptomatic and undiagnosed, whereas others may present with symptoms of intraventricular obstruction (usually occurring at the level of the LVOT), myocardial ischemia, diastolic dysfunction, heart failure, or ventricular arrhythmia. HCM is the most common cause of sudden cardiac death (SCD) caused by ventricular arrhythmias in young individuals and apparently healthy athletes, with a mortality rate of about 0.5% to 1.0% per year.

An increased end-diastolic wall thickness of the LV myocardium of 15 mm or greater in adults (or the equivalent threshold relative to body surface area in children) is the hallmark of HCM. Patients with hypertension or who practice regular and intensive physical training (so-called athlete's heart) may have ventricular hypertrophy due to remodelling, but the LV wall thickening is usually symmetric (concentric) and borderline increased (12–15 mm; normal LV wall thickness <12 mm), and an athlete's heart often presents with concomitant mild LV dilation proportional to the LV wall thickening.

There are several morphologic variants of HCM according to the distribution of the wall thickening. Asymmetric septal hypertrophy is the most common variant, predominating in the anterior and anteroseptal walls of the basal LV. A spiral pattern of LV wall thickening is common, starting in the anterobasal wall and moving in a counterclockwise spiral toward the LV apex to involve the inferoseptal wall (Fig. 31.1). The apical variant of HCM is a nonobstructive form, with thickening of the LV apex and/or loss of the normal tapering of the LV wall thickness from the base toward the apex. There is obliteration of the apical cavity, sometimes with a spadelike appearance of the LV cavity (Fig. 31.2A). Apical HCM has a high prevalence in Japan, and the diagnosis is suspected in the presence of T-wave inversion in the anterolateral leads on the electrocardiogram (ECG). Another variant of HCM is the midventricular form (see Fig. 31.2B). It often induces an intracavitary gradient between the LV apex and base, causing a noncontractile apical aneurysm (2% of HCM patients) at risk for apical thrombus formation. Symmetric (concentric) HCM is a less common variant (5%). RV involvement is seen in 18% of HCM patients. In a minority of patients with HCM (5%–10%), there is progressive adverse ventricular remodelling, leading to end-stage dilated HCM.

On echocardiography, the diagnosis of HCM relies on the demonstration of LV wall thickness >15 mm and/or an increased ratio (>1.5:1) of septal to opposed posterior LV wall thickness. Doppler echocardiography can evaluate for diastolic dysfunction that is often present in HCM due to increased chamber stiffness and impaired ventricular relaxation. Nevertheless, about 6% to 12% of HCM cases are undetected by echocardiography, likely because some areas (e.g., LV anterolateral wall, cardiac apex, RV free wall) are not well visualized by echocardiography. The measurement of precise wall thicknesses by ultrasound has been shown to be discrepant with gold-standard MRI in roughly half of patients, most often due to overestimation, with clinically significant thresholds involved in 16% of cases.

The primary role of CMR is clarification of the diagnosis and phenotype of HCM. Cine images typically show normal or increased systolic function, with normal to decreased ventricular volumes, and can show near-complete obliteration of the LV cavity at the midventricular and/or apical levels during systole. The LV end-diastolic wall thickness is measured perpendicular to the myocardial wall on short-axis SSFP images, combined with long-axis SSFP images for the measurement of the wall thickness of the apical segments. Tangential orientation of the imaging plane to the LV wall should be avoided because it may lead to overestimation of the wall thickness.

A three-chamber SSFP sequence and phase contrast imaging performed across the LVOT are used to depict and quantify the systolic flow acceleration across the LVOT, adjacent to the upper septal hypertrophy in the asymmetric septal variant of HCM. A three-chamber view is the best to assess for systolic anterior motion of the anterior mitral valve leaflet that may further exacerbate the LVOT obstruction and cause a posteriorly directed jet of mitral regurgitation, with left atrial enlargement (see Fig. 31.2C) A phase contrast sequence is used to measure peak velocities across the LVOT that can be translated into a pressure gradient using the modified Bernoulli equation (mm Hg = 4 × [peak velocity, in m/s^2]). A gradient >55 mm Hg is considered obstructive and may be present at rest or provoked by exercise, Valsalva maneuver, or administration of amyl nitrite. The imaging plane of the phase contrast sequence should be positioned perpendicular to the LVOT where the signal void is best visible to ensure measurement of the peak

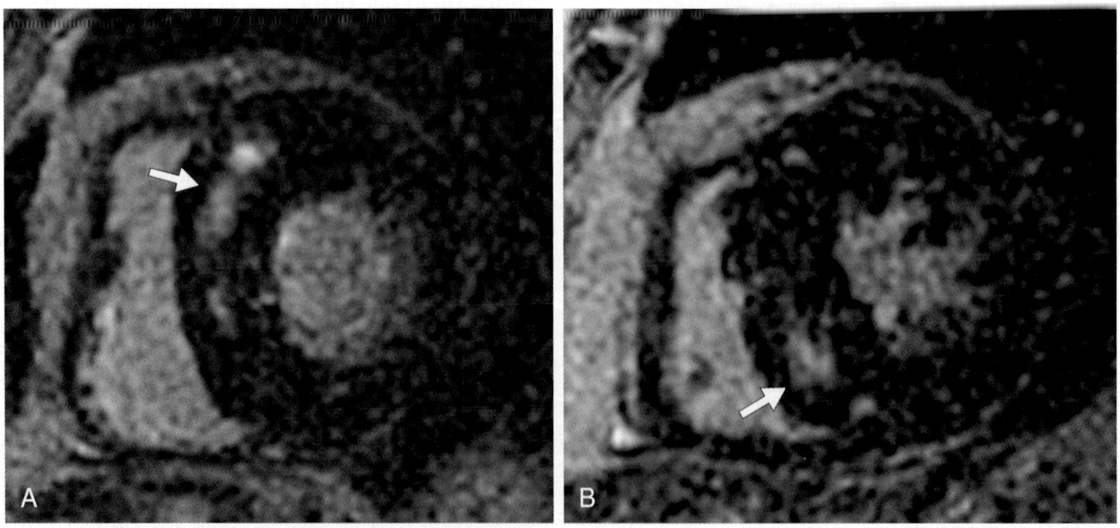

Figure 31.1 (A and B) Asymmetric septal hypertrophic cardiomyopathy (HCM). This short-axis late gadolinium enhancement (LGE) sequence shows the typical patchy midwall LGE in HCM *(arrows)* affecting the segments that are the most thickened. It also demonstrates the spiral pattern of myocardial hypertrophy in HCM, starting in the anteroseptal wall at the base (A) and moving in a counterclockwise spiral toward the LGE apex, thereby involving the inferoseptal wall at the midventricular level (B).

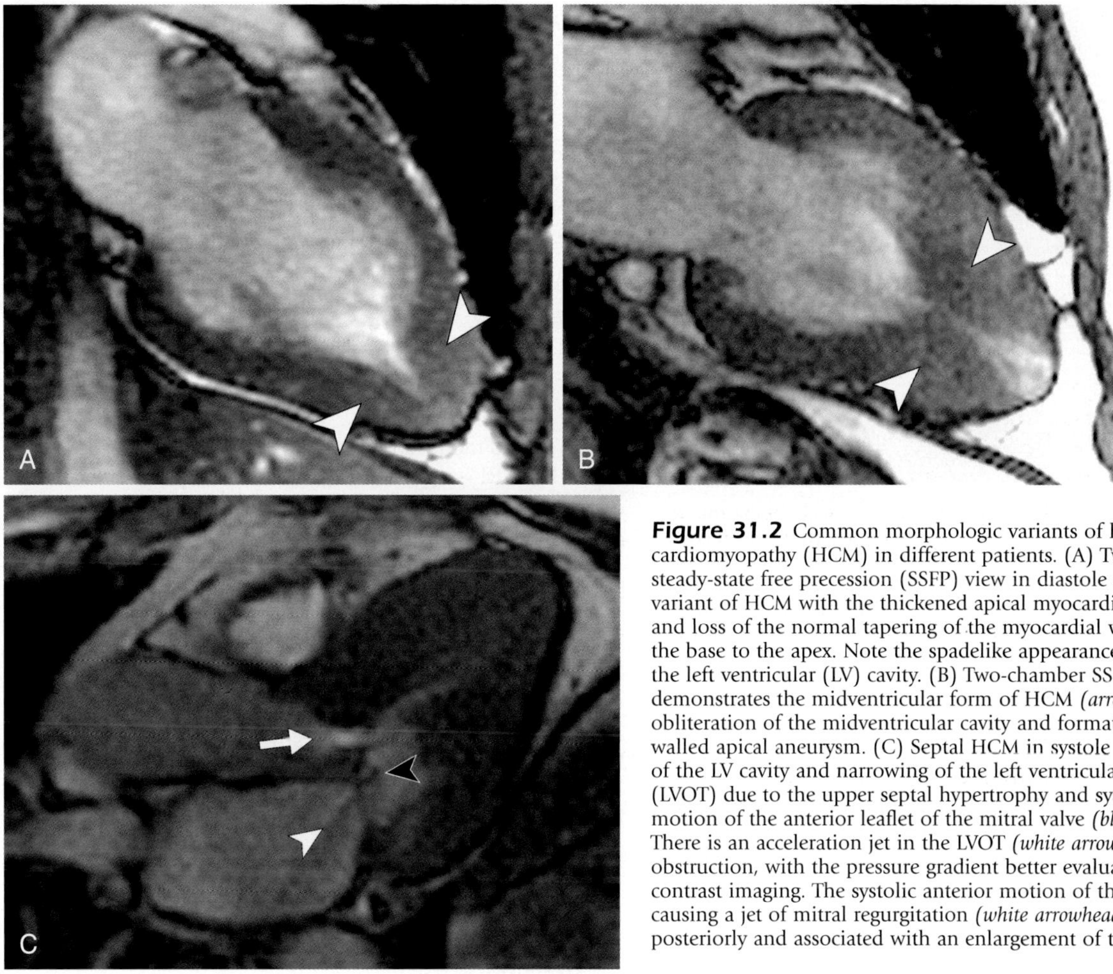

Figure 31.2 Common morphologic variants of hypertrophic cardiomyopathy (HCM) in different patients. (A) Two-chamber steady-state free precession (SSFP) view in diastole shows the apical variant of HCM with the thickened apical myocardium *(arrowheads)* and loss of the normal tapering of the myocardial wall thickness from the base to the apex. Note the spadelike appearance of the shape of the left ventricular (LV) cavity. (B) Two-chamber SSFP image in systole demonstrates the midventricular form of HCM *(arrowheads)* with obliteration of the midventricular cavity and formation of a thin-walled apical aneurysm. (C) Septal HCM in systole with obliteration of the LV cavity and narrowing of the left ventricular outflow tract (LVOT) due to the upper septal hypertrophy and systolic anterior motion of the anterior leaflet of the mitral valve *(black arrowhead)*. There is an acceleration jet in the LVOT *(white arrow)* suggestive of obstruction, with the pressure gradient better evaluated with phase contrast imaging. The systolic anterior motion of the mitral valve is causing a jet of mitral regurgitation *(white arrowhead)* directed posteriorly and associated with an enlargement of the left atrium.

velocity encountered in the LVOT. Phase contrast imaging is also used to quantify mitral regurgitation or measure the pressure gradient between the base and apex in the midventricular form of HCM.

LGE sequences should be obtained to assess for myocardial fibrosis in the areas of ventricular hypertrophy. The typical pattern of abnormal LGE in HCM is patchy, located in the midmyocardium of the hypertrophied segments or adjacent to the RV insertion points at the midventricular level. The presence and extent of abnormal LGE is an independent predictor of an adverse outcome, such as ventricular arrhythmias, SCD, and heart failure.

CMR is helpful to evaluate treatment response in HCM. The effects of medical treatment on the degree of LVOT obstruction can be monitored with phase contrast imaging. The success of surgical septal myomectomy, septal alcohol ablation, or septal coiling can be assessed with cine images, phase contrast imaging, and LGE imaging to locate and evaluate the extent of the site of septal reduction, detect if this area is too small or located outside the target area, and monitor the pressure gradients across the LVOT. Reduction of LVOT obstruction in symptomatic patients is associated with improved systolic function and a significant reduction in the myocardial mass.

On coronary CTA, deep myocardial bridging of the left anterior descending coronary artery occurs more frequently in HCM than in other cardiac disorders, with or without LV hypertrophy. Deep muscular clefts (or crypts) in the basal inferoseptal wall of the LV can be present in normal subjects, but is now recognized as a morphologic expression of HCM that is sometimes present in HCM mutation carriers who have not yet developed the disease (Fig. 31.3).

Imaging Arrhythmogenic Right Ventricular Cardiomyopathy

ARVC/D is a rare inherited autosomal dominant disorder characterized by genetic mutations in the cardiac desmosomes, which provides structural links between myocytes. It results in progressive loss of myocytes in the right ventricle and, less commonly, in the left ventricle, with inflammation, repair, and fibrofatty replacement of myocardial tissue. It predominantly affects the inferior, apical, and infundibular part of the thin RV wall (so-called triangle of dysplasia) and the inferolateral wall of the LV, leading to focal areas of RV wall thinning, aneurysm formation, dyskinesis, and eventually evolving to global RV dilation and dysfunction. The estimated prevalence of ARVC/D in the general population ranges from 1 in 1000 to 5000, with an increased prevalence in Italy. Its clinical manifestations are variable and include ventricular arrhythmias with a substantial risk of SCD, particularly in young people and athletes. This disorder is progressive, and early detection is important in patients

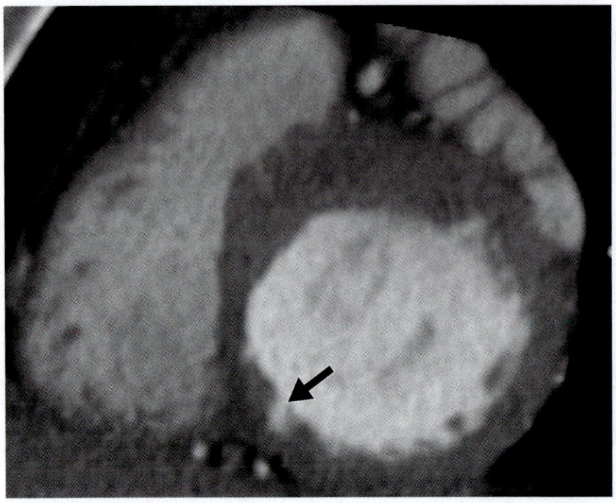

Figure 31.3 Myocardial crypt—short-axis CT image in diastole in a 39-year-old man presenting to the emergency department with chest pain. CT angiography shows the absence of coronary artery disease, but there is an incidental finding of a muscular crypt in the basal inferoseptal wall *(arrow)*, with normal left ventricular wall thickness. Although this can be present in normal subjects, it is sometimes present in hypertrophic cardiomyopathy mutation carriers who have not yet developed the disease.

with ventricular arrhythmias or positive family history of ARVC/D to prevent SCD by implantation of an automatic implantable cardioverter-defibrillator.

RV endomyocardial biopsy is an invasive procedure with low diagnostic yield in ARVC/D because of the patchy and predominantly epicardial distribution of the fibrofatty replacement. Diagnostic criteria for ARVC/D were established by the Arrhythmogenic Right Ventricular Dysplasia Task Force in 1994 and include major and minor criteria for structural, histologic, electrocardiographic, arrhythmic, and genetic features. Revised criteria were proposed in 2010 to increase the diagnostic sensitivity and to include specific imaging criteria for two-dimensional echocardiography, CMR, and angiography (Box 31.1). Either two major criteria, one major plus two minor criteria, or four minor criteria have to be present to diagnose ARVC/D. Because imaging findings can only account for one major or one minor criterion, the diagnosis of ARVC/D does not rely solely on imaging and requires additional criteria based on family history, electrocardiographic changes, and/or endomyocardial biopsy. Diagnosis of ARVC/D is challenging, and imaging findings may be normal in the early stage, although patients are still at risk for SCD.

On echocardiography, the major task force criteria for ARVC/D are regional RV wall motion abnormality with enlargement of the RVOT or decreased RV systolic function. Other echographic findings are trabecular derangement and a hyperreflective moderator band. On CMR, SSFP sequences performed with the patient in a prone position with axial, sagittal, and short-axis views yield excellent depiction of the thin RV free wall. Findings of ARVC/D include wall thinning and regional wall motion abnormalities of the RV free wall, with dyskinesia and saccular outpouchings/aneurysms in systole. The term *accordion sign* refers to an extended area of multiple focal

BOX 31.1 2010 Revised Task Force Major Criteria for the Diagnosis of Arrhythmogenic Right Ventricular Cardiomyopathy or Dysplasia[a]

Global or regional dysfunction and structural alterations
- By two-dimensional echocardiography—regional RV akinesia, dyskinesia, or aneurysm, plus one of the following (end-diastole):
  - PLAX RVOT ≥32 mm (corrected for body size [PLAX/BSA] ≥19 mm/m^2)
  - PSAX RVOT ≥36 mm (corrected for body size [PLAX/BSA] ≥21 mm/m^2)

    or
  - Fractional area change ≤33%
- By MRI—regional RV akinesia or dyskinesia or dyssynchronous RV contraction, plus one of the following:
  - Ratio of RV end-diastolic volume to BSA ≥110 mL/m^2 (male) or ≥100 mL/m^2 (female)

    or
  - RV ejection fraction ≤40%
- By RV angiography—regional RV akinesia, dyskinesia, or aneurysm

Endomyocardial biopsy
- Decreased myocytes, with fibrous replacement of RV free wall

ECG repolarization abnormalities
- Inverted T waves in right precordial leads

ECG depolarization and conduction abnormalities
- Epsilon wave

Arrhythmias

Familial history

BSA, Body surface area; *ECG*, electrocardiogram; *PLAX*, parasternal long-axis view; *PSAX*, parasternal short-axis view; *RV*, right ventricular; *RVOT*, right ventricular outflow tract.
[a]The minor criteria are not detailed in this box.

bulgings of the RV free wall in systole (Fig. 31.4). RV wall motion abnormalities solely confined to the area of the RV wall surrounding the insertion site of the moderator band should be interpreted with caution because it may be a normal variant in healthy subjects. RV dilation, enlargement of the RVOT, RV dysfunction, and dysplastic RV trabeculations are present in more advanced stages of ARVC/D. Even if fatty myocardial infiltration is the hallmark of ARVC/D on histology, the presence of fat on imaging is not included in the revised task force criteria because it usually represents physiologic changes related to aging. Nevertheless, high-resolution, T1-weighted, spin-echo images continue to be routinely performed in some institutions to assess for fatty infiltration of the RV wall, which may be confirmed with fat saturation. Abnormal LGE is seen in up to 70% of ARVC/D cases, but is not a component of the revised task force criteria.

Imaging Left Ventricular Noncompaction

Left ventricular noncompaction (LVNC) cardiomyopathy (also called *spongy myocardium* or *LV hypertrabeculation*)

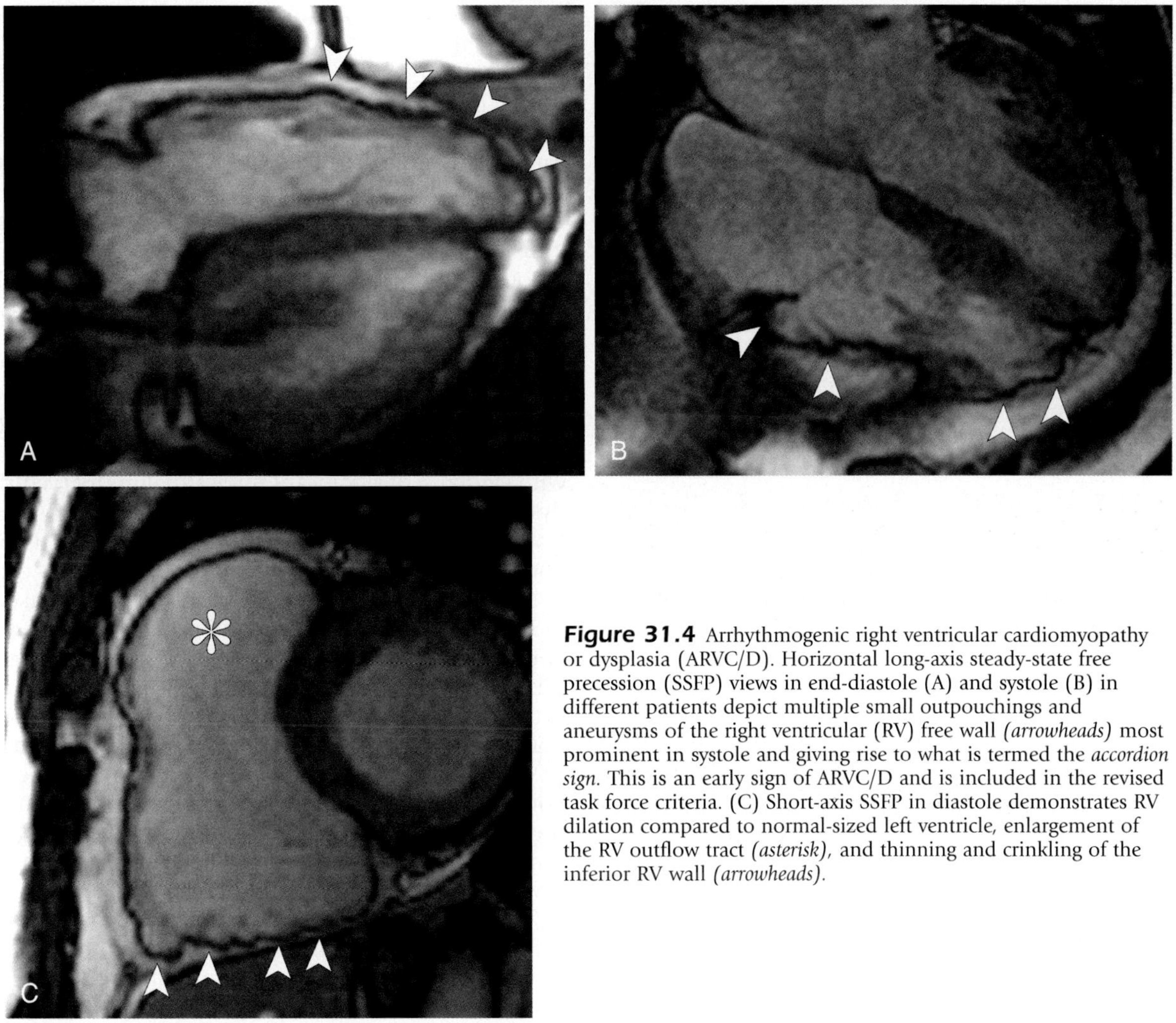

Figure 31.4 Arrhythmogenic right ventricular cardiomyopathy or dysplasia (ARVC/D). Horizontal long-axis steady-state free precession (SSFP) views in end-diastole (A) and systole (B) in different patients depict multiple small outpouchings and aneurysms of the right ventricular (RV) free wall *(arrowheads)* most prominent in systole and giving rise to what is termed the *accordion sign*. This is an early sign of ARVC/D and is included in the revised task force criteria. (C) Short-axis SSFP in diastole demonstrates RV dilation compared to normal-sized left ventricle, enlargement of the RV outflow tract *(asterisk)*, and thinning and crinkling of the inferior RV wall *(arrowheads)*.

is characterized by an extensive layer of noncompacted myocardium lining the LV cavity. LV dilation, regional or global LV hypokinesis, and impaired LV systolic function may eventually develop. LVNC is found in pediatric and adult patients and may be isolated or associated with congenital heart abnormalities. Complications include systolic dysfunction, thromboembolic disease, ischemia, ventricular arrhythmia, and SCD. The exact pathogenesis of LVNC is uncertain, but the most accepted hypothesis is that it is caused by an intrauterine arrest of the process of compaction of the loosely interwoven meshwork of myocardial fibers, which normally progresses from epicardium to endocardium, beginning at the base and septum and proceeding toward the apex and lateral wall. This would explain why the apex and lateral and inferior walls at the midventricular level are the most commonly affected segments. Involvement of the right ventricle may be seen but is not a reliable marker because the right ventricle is more trabeculated than the left ventricle in normal individuals.

Morphologic diagnostic criteria have been established on echocardiography and CMR to enable the differentiation of LVNC from normal subjects and other diseases mimicking LVNC, such as hypertrabeculation due to HCM, DCM, and LV hypertrophy from hypertension. On echocardiography, LVNC is diagnosed in the presence of four major diagnostic criteria: (1) absence of coexisting cardiac abnormality; (2) ratio of noncompacted to compacted myocardium of more than 2:1 measured at end-systole; (3) segmental distribution predominantly involving the apex, midlateral, and/or midinferior wall; and (4) color Doppler evidence of flow within the deep trabecular recesses. On CMR, the diameter ratio of noncompacted to compacted myocardium is measured at end-diastole, as opposed to end-systole on echocardiography on an SSFP sequence acquired perpendicular to the wall. Tangential orientation of the imaging plane to the LV wall should be avoided because it may lead to overestimation of the relative extent of the noncompacted layer. A ratio of noncompacted to compacted myocardium of 2.3:1 or greater in more than one segment of the LV wall is considered specific for the diagnosis of LVNC (Fig. 31.5). However, more recent data in normal individuals without cardiac disease or hypertension have demonstrated that a ratio of more than 2.3:1 is present in at least one region in 43% and two regions in 6% of normal individuals, suggesting that reevaluation of the current CMR criteria for LVNC may be necessary. LGE imaging

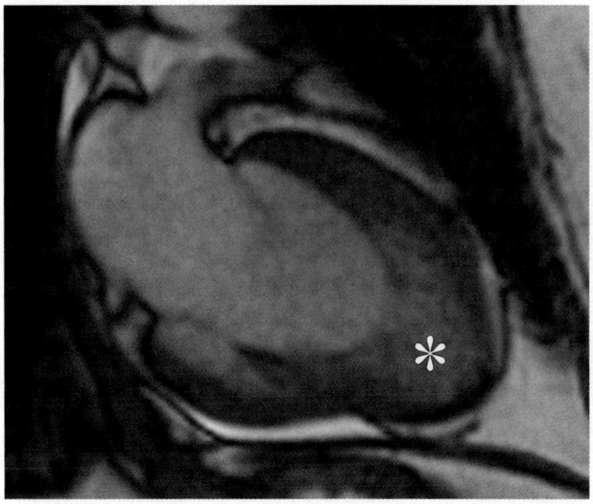

Figure 31.5 Left ventricular noncompaction (LVNC). This two-chamber steady-state free precession sequence at end-diastole shows an increase in subendocardial LV trabeculation in the apical segment *(asterisk)*. The ratio of noncompacted to compacted myocardium is greater than 2.3:1. This was seen in more than one segment of the LV wall on additional views; therefore this is consistent with LVNC.

is helpful to assess for LV thrombi forming within the noncompacted myocardium. Myocardial fibrosis may be seen predominating in the subendocardium, adjacent to the noncompacted myocardium, and correlating with the degree of LV systolic dysfunction.

Acquired Cardiomyopathies

Imaging Myocarditis

Myocarditis is an acquired cardiomyopathy characterized by acute or chronic inflammation of the myocardium, with edema, necrosis, and possibly fibrotic scars. Viral infections (e.g., parvovirus, human herpesvirus, adenovirus, coxsackievirus) account for most cases in previously healthy patients, but any infectious agent may cause myocarditis. Other possible triggers of myocardial inflammation are drug hypersensitivity reaction, toxin, or systemic immunologic disorder (e.g., inflammatory bowel disease, giant cell myocarditis, systemic lupus erythematosus, thyrotoxicosis, Wegener granulomatosis). The clinical presentation of acute myocarditis is variable, and early recognition is often difficult due to nonspecific symptoms and findings on the ECG, echocardiogram, and laboratory tests at initial presentation. The diagnosis of acute myocarditis should be considered for the following clinical presentations: (1) in patients presenting with symptoms resembling acute coronary syndrome with increased level of cardiac serum biomarkers but no obstructive CAD; (2) flulike syndrome, fever, malaise, and arthralgia; or (3) unexplained new onset of congestive heart failure, especially when younger than 40 years. Prognosis is usually good, but some patients will progress toward dilated cardiomyopathy, eventually requiring cardiac transplantation. Although endomyocardial biopsy is still considered the gold standard test for definitive diagnosis of myocarditis and viral genome detection, it is an invasive procedure prone to sampling error and low sensitivity.

CMR has become a valuable alternative to endomyocardial biopsy for suspected myocarditis. The role of CMR is to exclude other ischemic and nonischemic causes of cardiomyopathies, evaluate and monitor myocardial tissue injury and systolic function, differentiate acute from healed myocarditis, and detect concomitant pericardial effusion and pericarditis. Although nonspecific for myocarditis, SSFP images may reveal regional or global wall motion abnormalities, increased LV volume, and depressed LV ejection fraction.

The international consensus group on CMR in myocarditis has proposed diagnostic CMR criteria, also known as the Lake Louise criteria, that can be applied in patients with recent onset or persisting symptoms of myocarditis, with evidence of significant myocardial injury (ventricular dysfunction, new electrocardiographic changes, or elevated troponin levels), and without significant obstructive CAD. There are three criteria for assessing inflammatory changes of the myocardium on CMR, including myocardial edema (T2 ratio), hyperemia or capillary leak (early global enhancement ratio), and myocardial fibrosis or necrosis (abnormal LGE). In the presence of two or more of the three criteria, myocarditis can be diagnosed with a diagnostic accuracy of 78%, compared to an accuracy of 68% if only LGE is performed. An update to the "Lake Louse" consensus criteria is expected in 2018 and may incorporate newer sequences like T1 and T2 mapping as a replacement for the more antiquated ratio methods invoked in the original criteria.

To assess for myocardial edema, T2-weighted triple-inversion recovery images, with inversion pulses for fat and blood suppression acquired in the short axis of the left ventricle, provide good contrast between the high SI of edema and the intermediate SI of the normal myocardium (Fig. 31.6A). A body coil is used to prevent signal inhomogeneity. The distribution of myocardial edema may be regional or diffuse. Because diffuse edema is difficult to detect by visual assessment, the T2 ratio is a quantitative analysis normalizing the SI of the myocardium to that of the skeletal muscle (erector spinae or latissimus dorsi). It is measured by manually tracing endocardial and epicardial contours of the myocardium and a region of interest (ROI) in the skeletal muscle of the same slice: T2 ratio = (SI myocardium)/(SI skeletal muscle). A T2 ratio of 1.9:1 or greater or visualization of regional myocardial edema is one of the three Lake Louise consensus criteria for the diagnosis of myocarditis.

Myocardial hyperemia reflects reversible myocardial inflammatory changes, with greater accumulation of gadolinium in regions of myocardial inflammation due to acute cell damage, that allow gadolinium to accumulate in the intracellular space. It is detected by contrast-enhanced, T1-weighted, fast spin-echo techniques, with image acquisition before and during the first 3 minutes after gadolinium injection. Images are acquired with a body coil, during free breathing, in short-axis or axial views and with a saturation band across the atria. ROIs are traced over the entire LV myocardium and a skeletal muscle on the same slice of the precontrast T1-weighted image and are copied to the corresponding contrast-enhanced images.

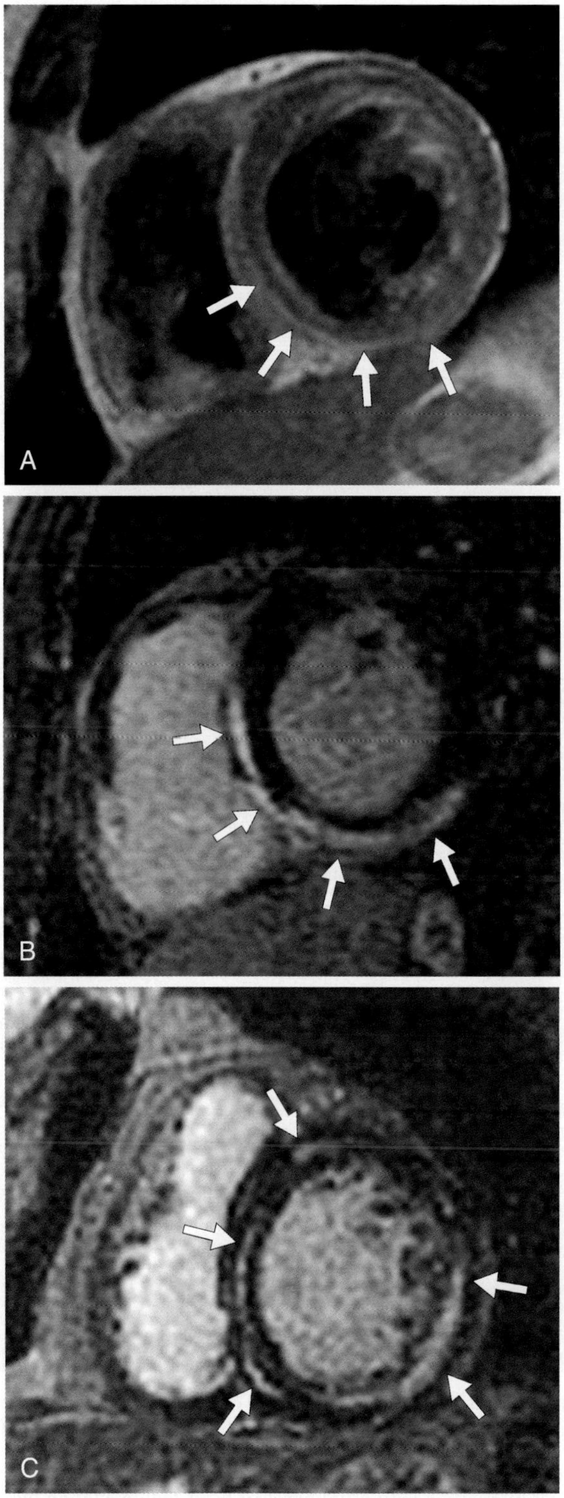

Figure 31.6 Myocarditis. Short-axis T2-weighted (A) and late gadolinium enhancement (LGE) images (B) show myocardial edema. This is depicted by increased signal intensity on T2-weighted images in a subepicardial distribution in the septal, inferoseptal, and inferior walls at the midventricular level (A; *arrows*), with corresponding abnormal LGE (B; *arrows*) in a 19-year-old man with viral myocarditis. (C) Short-axis LGE sequence in a 29-year-old woman with myocarditis in the setting of systemic lupus erythematosus (SLE) shows diffuse abnormal LGE, predominantly involving the midwall *(arrows)*. Myocarditis is clinically evident in 10% of patients with SLE, but the incidence at autopsy approaches 40%.

The early global enhancement ratio can be calculated by the following:

$$\text{Early global enhancement ratio} = ([SI_{postmyo} - SI_{premyo})/SI_{premyo})/([SI_{postskm} - SI_{preskm}])/SI_{preskm})$$

where $SI_{postmyo}$ and SI_{premyo} are the myocardial SI after and before gadolinium, and $SI_{postskm}$ and SI_{preskm} are the skeletal muscle SI after and before gadolinium. An early global enhancement ratio of 4:1 or more (1.5-T scanner from one vendor), 5:1 or more (1.5-T scanner from a different vendor), or an absolute increase of myocardial enhancement ($[SI_{postmyo} - SI_{premyo}]/SI_{premyo}$) of 45% or more reflects myocardial inflammation and satisfies one of the three Lake Louise consensus criteria.

The presence of abnormal LGE is the third CMR criterion for myocarditis. The pattern of abnormal LGE is variable and usually involves the subepicardium or mesocardium, typically in the inferolateral wall. Abnormal LGE may be focally transmural, but usually does not follow a vascular distribution and does not solely involve the subendocardium (see Fig. 31.6B).

Although the Lake Louise consensus criteria are commonly used in clinical practice to assess for myocarditis, there are significant limitations altering the value of these criteria. For example, the ROIs in the skeletal muscle used to calculate the T2 ratio and early global enhancement ratio may be nearly impossible to obtain due to muscular atrophy or may be altered by field homogeneity or active myositis. T1 and T2 mapping may improve the assessment of myocardial edema and fibrosis, respectively.

Imaging Chagas Cardiomyopathy

Chagas heart disease is caused by *Trypanosoma cruzi*. It is a leading cause of morbidity and mortality in Latin America and should be considered in patients with such an epidemiologic history. It can be confirmed by positive serologic antibody (immunoglobulin G) for *T. cruzi*. The disease has an acute phase and a chronic phase. Acute Chagas infection is usually acquired during childhood and occurs most often unnoticed, rarely presenting with pericardial effusion, tamponade, or, less commonly, myocarditis. Chronic Chagas cardiomyopathy evolves for several decades after acute infection, and patients present with dilated cardiomyopathy and a variable degree of myocardial fibrosis, and 50% of cases have an apical aneurysm in the left ventricle or right ventricle (Fig. 31.7). The pattern of abnormal LGE is nonischemic, involving the mesocardium and subepicardium, usually in the apical and basal inferolateral segments of the LV wall.

Imaging Stress Cardiomyopathy

Stress cardiomyopathy (also known as *Takotsubo cardiomyopathy, broken heart syndrome,* or *apical ballooning syndrome*) is an acquired reversible cause of LV systolic dysfunction, with transient ST-segment elevation on the ECG and minimal myocardial serum biomarker release in the absence of obstructive CAD. It represents 1% to 2% of acute coronary syndromes and preferentially affects postmenopausal women. It is precipitated by

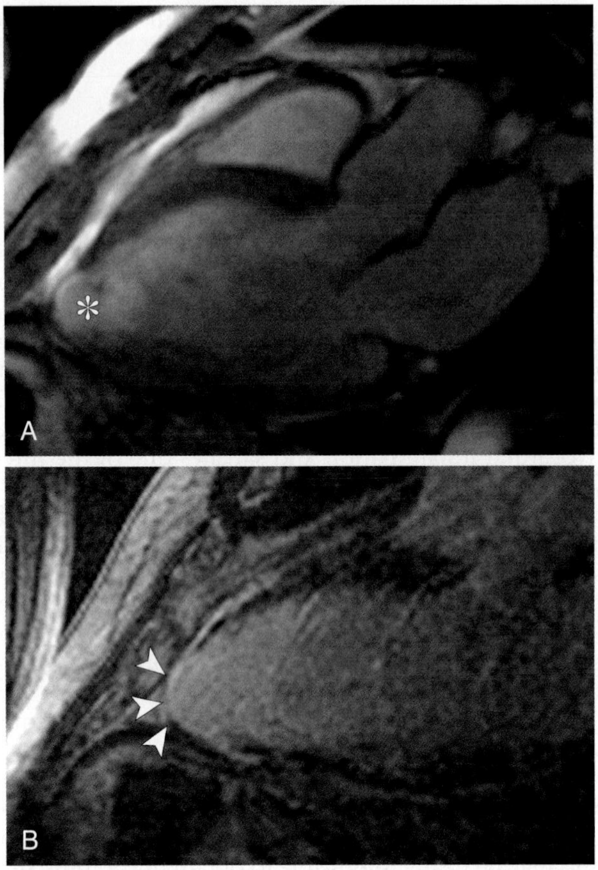

Figure 31.7 Chagas cardiomyopathy. (A) Three-chamber steady-state free precession and two-chamber late gadolinium enhancement (LGE) (B) sequences in a 74-year-old presenting with heart failure. There is moderate dilation of the left ventricle, with moderately decreased left ventricular systolic function. There is an apical aneurysm of the left ventricle (A; *asterisk*) with abnormal LGE of the thin aneurysmal wall (B; *arrows*). The patient was found to have positive serologic antibody for *Trypanosoma cruzi*.

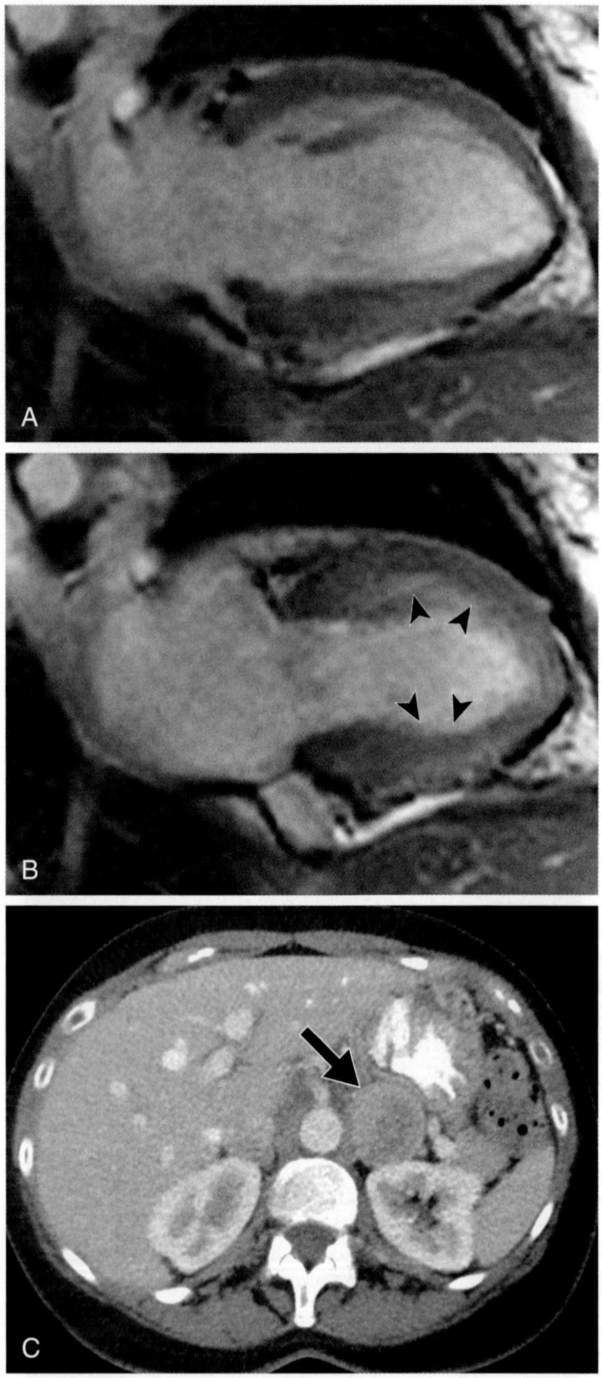

Figure 31.8 Catecholamine-induced cardiomyopathy. Two-chamber steady-state free precession images at end-diastole (A) and end-systole (B) demonstrate hypokinesis restricted to the midventricular left ventricle *(arrowheads)*, with relative sparing of the base and apex in a 46-year-old woman presenting with acute onset of heart failure after an elective cosmetic surgery. (C) She was later found to have a pheochromocytoma of the left adrenal gland *(arrow)*.

emotional or physical stressors, such as the death of a relative or recent surgery. The pathophysiology of stress cardiomyopathy is not fully understood, but a similar cardiac disorder has been described in patients with pheochromocytoma-producing catecholamines. The prognosis is excellent because supportive treatment leads to spontaneous complete recovery in nearly all patients.

The typical form of stress cardiomyopathy (82% of cases) is akinesia of the LV apex, with apical ballooning of the LV cavity in systole and preserved myocardial function of the basal segments. Wall motion abnormalities extend beyond the territory of a single epicardial coronary artery. There is apical ballooning of both ventricles in a minority of cases. On ventriculography performed during cardiac catheterization, the apical ballooning resembles an octopus fishing pot with a round bottom and a narrow neck, which is called *Tako-Tsubo* in Japanese. Other variants of stress cardiomyopathy are the midventricular form (17%), with hypokinesis restricted to the midventricle and relative sparing of the apex, and the reverse form (1%), with hypokinesis of the base and sparing of the midventricle and apex. On CMR, radial long-axis cine SSFP images are useful to demonstrate the wall motion abnormalities and ventricular dysfunction (mean LV ejection fraction of 47.7%; Fig. 31.8). Myocardial edema may be observed on T2-weighted images; myocardial scarring on an LGE sequence may be seen but is usually absent and it is not a predominant feature. Localizer images should be scrutinized to exclude adrenal or extraadrenal pheochromocytoma as the cause of the stress cardiomyopathy.

Imaging Peripartum Cardiomyopathy

Peripartum cardiomyopathy (PPCM) is defined as heart failure developing between the last month of pregnancy and up to 5 months postpartum in the absence of preexisting heart disease. It is characterized by myocardial inflammation, with or without concomitant pericarditis. The cause of PPCM remains uncertain, but hypotheses include viral myocarditis, abnormal immune response to pregnancy, abnormal response to altered hemodynamics of pregnancy, and abnormal metabolism of prolactin. Its incidence is approximately 1 in 3000 to 4000 in the United States and even higher in African Americans. The diagnosis may be delayed because patients present with signs of heart failure that may resemble normal physiologic changes of pregnancy (e.g., pedal edema, fatigue, dyspnea). Patients may also present with complications, such as systemic or pulmonary emboli from ventricular thrombi, arrhythmia, or SCD. Approximately 50% of cases recover completely without complications, but the prognosis is poor in PPCM lasting longer than 6 months.

Imaging findings in PPCM are similar to other causes of dilated cardiomyopathy, and PPCM is a diagnosis of exclusion. The role of imaging is to quantify the severity of myocardial dysfunction and exclude other causes of cardiac dysfunction in pregnancy (e.g., myocardial infarction, underlying valve heart disease, congenital heart disease exacerbated by the altered hemodynamics of pregnancy). Due to the issues of CT radiation and gadolinium exposure of the fetus, echocardiography plays an important role in the pregnant patient. CMR without gadolinium may be performed to assess ventricular function and valves, but gadolinium is a class C drug that should be avoided during pregnancy. In the postpartum patient, gadolinium can be used but is not very helpful because there is no specific pattern of abnormal LGE to characterize PPCM. Multimodality imaging findings in PPCM are enlarged cardiac chambers that should be carefully assessed for the presence of an intracavitary thrombus because these patients are at high risk for cardiac thrombus formation due to the peripartum hypercoagulable state and the cardiac dysfunction, with blood stasis.

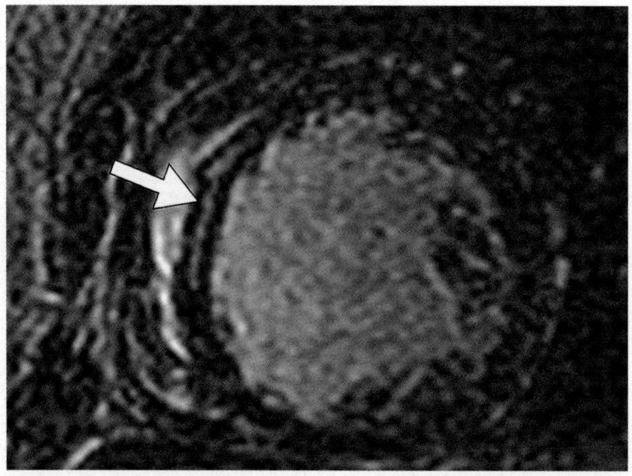

Figure 31.9 Idiopathic dilated cardiomyopathy. This short-axis late gadolinium enhancement (LGE) image shows dilation of the left ventricle with linear LGE in the midwall of the interventricular septum *(arrow)*, which is characteristic of midwall fibrosis of idiopathic dilated cardiomyopathy.

Mixed Cardiomyopathies

Imaging Dilated Cardiomyopathy

DCM is the most common acquired cardiomyopathy worldwide and is characterized by dilation and decreased contractility of the left, right, or both ventricles, occurring in the absence or out of proportion to CAD or abnormal loading conditions (e.g., hypertension, valve disease). DCM has a wide range of causes. The genetic (familial) form of DCM may be responsible for 20% to 48% of cases, and numerous associated genetic mutations have been identified. DCM can also be secondary to myocarditis, toxins exposure (e.g., chronic alcohol intake, cocaine, anthracyclines, heavy metals), systemic disorders (e.g., autoimmune, collagen vascular disease, sarcoidosis, end-stage renal disease), endocrine disorders (thyroid dysfunction), metabolic disorders (nutritional deficiencies), or may be idiopathic.

Multimodality imaging of DCM demonstrates dilated ventricles and globally depressed systolic function. The role of imaging is to differentiate the ischemic from the nonischemic form of DCM. The ischemic form of DCM has a poorer prognosis and different treatment options, including possible coronary revascularization. Invasive coronary catheter angiography used to be performed to exclude CAD-related disease in patients with DCM, but coronary CTA and LGE sequence on CMR are now increasingly used as an alternative. In DCM, there is usually no abnormal LGE. Less commonly, there is linear abnormal LGE in the midwall, particularly in the interventricular septum, reflecting midwall segmental fibrosis seen in idiopathic DCM and associated to an increased risk of arrhythmias (Fig. 31.9). Patchy LGE may also be seen. LGE imaging and an additional LGE sequence with a long inversion recovery time (e.g., inversion time of 600 ms) are helpful to assess for intracavitary LV thrombus that may form in a poorly contractile ventricle. A phase contrast sequence can assess valve dysfunction secondary to DCM.

Imaging Restrictive Cardiomyopathy

Restrictive cardiomyopathy is the least common form of cardiomyopathy. It is characterized by increased stiffness of the myocardium causing impaired ventricular filling, diastolic dysfunction, and heart failure. Restrictive cardiomyopathy encompasses a wide range of pathologies involving the myocardium and/or endocardium and presenting with restrictive physiology. This includes primary idiopathic restrictive cardiomyopathy, myocardial fibrosis, myocardial infiltrative diseases (e.g., amyloidosis, sarcoidosis), myocardial storage diseases (e.g., hemochromatosis, Anderson-Fabry disease), and endomyocardial diseases (e.g., hypereosinophilic syndrome).

On imaging, ventricular volumes are normal or reduced, and the myocardial wall thickness is normal. There is increased ventricular filling pressure, with biatrial

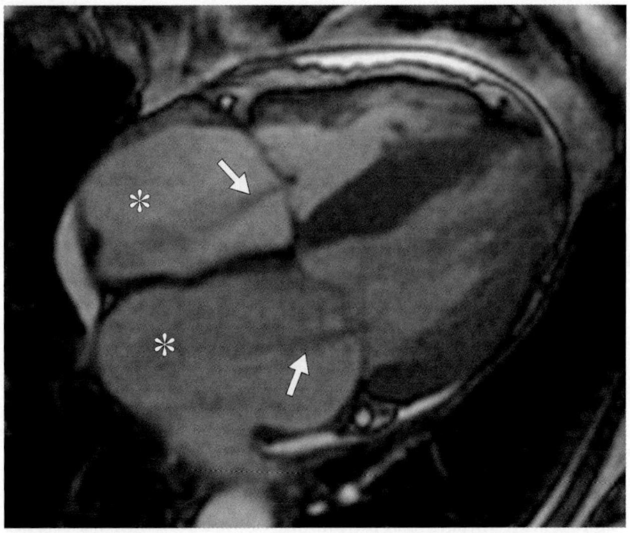

Figure 31.10 Restrictive cardiomyopathy—four-chamber steady-state free precession MR image in a patient with diastolic heart failure and restrictive cardiomyopathy secondary to amyloidosis. There is concentric wall thickening of nondilated ventricles and biatrial dilation *(asterisks)*, with jets *(arrows)* of regurgitation of the atrioventricular valves. The findings are characteristic of restrictive physiology.

enlargement and atrioventricular valve regurgitation (Fig. 31.10). Atrial thrombi may occur. The main differential diagnosis is constrictive pericarditis, because impaired ventricular filling and diastolic dysfunction are hallmarks of both disorders. Differentiation with CMR is important because restrictive cardiomyopathy is treated medically, whereas constrictive pericarditis is treated with a pericardiectomy. Pericardial thickening (>4 mm) and septal bounce are findings suggestive of constrictive pericarditis. Septal bounce is a paradoxic bouncing motion of the interventricular septum occurring during early diastole, initially directed toward and then away from the left ventricle and accentuated by inspiration. T2* and LGE sequences are helpful to assess for an underlying cause of restrictive cardiomyopathy, such as hemochromatosis or amyloidosis.

■ Secondary Cardiomyopathies

Imaging Endomyocardial Diseases

Endomyocardial diseases are secondary restrictive cardiomyopathies categorized in two different forms according to geographic distribution and clinical presentation, even though there is significant overlap between both forms—hypereosinophilic syndrome and tropical endomyocardial fibrosis. Hypereosinophilic syndrome is a systemic disorder characterized by increased peripheral eosinophilia for more than 6 months resulting in end-organ damage, including cardiac involvement known as Loeffler endomyocarditis. Hypereosinophilic syndrome occurs in temperate countries, is more rapidly progressive, and is seen in different clinical scenarios associated with hypereosinophilia—neoplasm (eosinophilic leukemia), infections (parasites), allergic agents, or idiopathic. Tropical endomyocardial fibrosis is primarily a disease of the young (bimodal peak incidence at ages 10 and 30 years) occurring in Africa, south India, and Brazil. Its pathogenesis is largely unknown, but several theories have been proposed, including hypereosinophilia, infections (e.g., toxoplasmosis, rheumatoid fever, malaria, parasites), environmental exposure (e.g., cerium in the soil), and immunologic and genetic causes.

Loeffler endomyocarditis predominantly affects the apex and subvalvular regions of one or both ventricles. It is caused by the infiltration of eosinophils in the myocardial wall, with subsequent degranulation and necrosis, causing endomyocarditis, with progressive wall thickening in the first stage of the disease. The second stage of the disease is characterized by frequent mural and apical thrombus formation, and in the third stage it is characterized by extensive subendocardial fibrosis in the cardiac apex. Severe tricuspid and mitral regurgitation is a common finding due to scarring and deformation of the chordae tendinae, with tethering of the papillary muscles.

On echocardiography and CMR, there is concentric wall thickening of the mid to apical left ventricle and/or right ventricle (Fig. 31.11). There is significant reduction of the end-diastolic ventricular volumes, severe atrioventricular valve dysfunction, and biatrial enlargement. Obliteration of the ventricular apex may resemble the apical variant of HCM, but the restrictive filling pattern with biatrial enlargement is more consistent with hypereosinophilic syndrome. There is abnormal LGE in the subendocardium of the left ventricle and/or right ventricle at the apex or diffuse, but extending beyond the territory of a single epicardial coronary artery. The major differential diagnosis of this abnormal LGE is amyloidosis, but the blood pool is bright in endomyocardial disease, whereas the blood pool is dark in patients with amyloidosis due to the abnormal kinetics of gadolinium. Mural thrombus is a common complication, even with preserved systolic function, and this should be assessed on an LGE sequence. Accessory findings on CT and CMR include peripheral consolidation in the lungs caused by pulmonary eosinophilia.

Imaging Cardiac Sarcoidosis

Cardiac involvement is clinically evident in 5% of patients with sarcoidosis, but is likely underdiagnosed because myocardial lesions are found in 20% to 60% of cases on autopsy. In these patients, with a subclinical asymptomatic course, there is still substantial increased risk of ventricular arrhythmias, conduction block, and SCD. Early diagnosis of cardiac involvement is important to prevent complications. The clinical course is variable, from spontaneous regression to progression with DCM and heart failure.

Imaging findings are variable, depending on the histologic stages of sarcoidosis, and are better depicted by CMR. In the acute stage, noncaseating granulomatous infiltration of the myocardium causes inflammation with a regional increase in T2 signal, early gadolinium enhancement on perfusion imaging, and enhancement on LGE sequence. Focal myocardial thickening is often

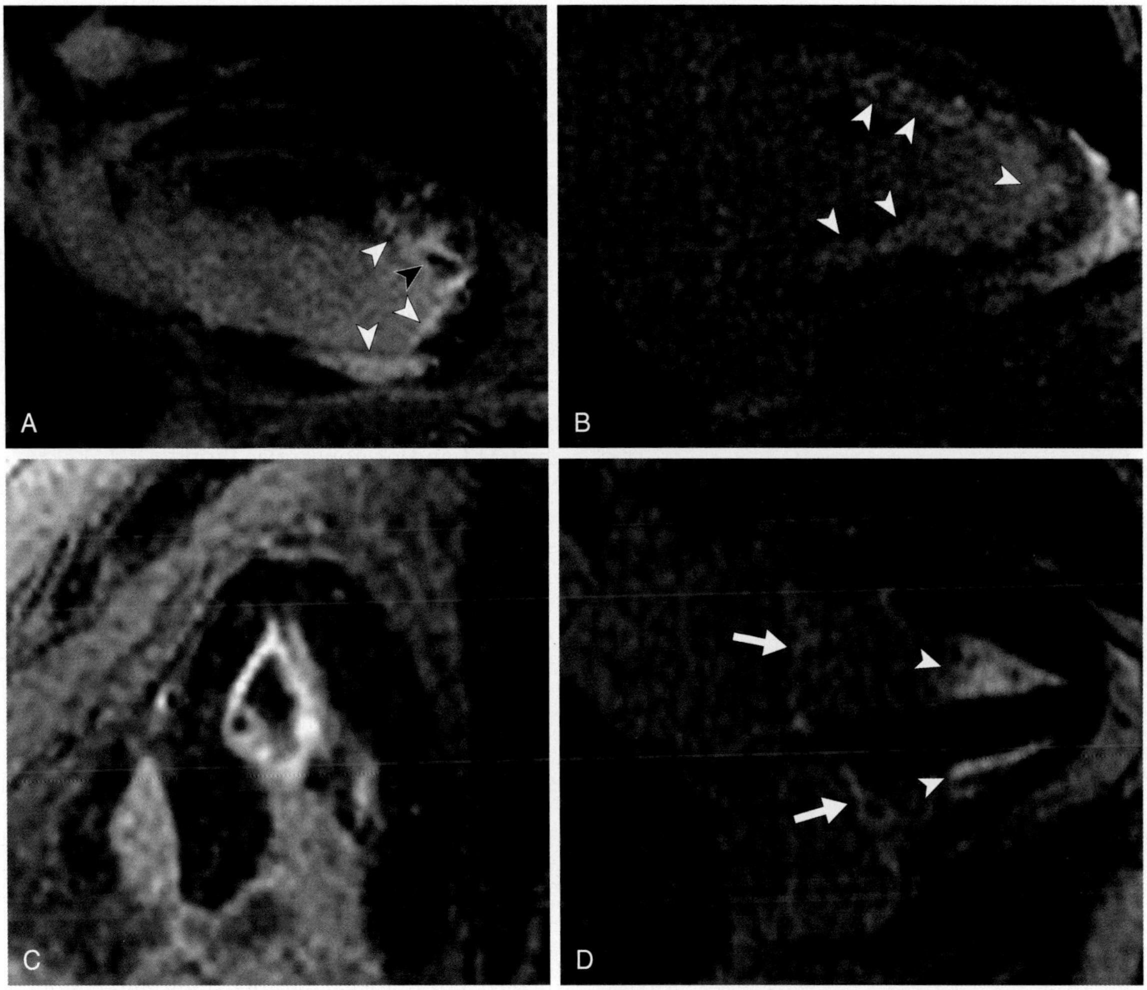

Figure 31.11 Various clinical scenarios of endomyocardial disease. (A) Hypereosinophilic syndrome in a 56-year-old man. This two-chamber late gadolinium enhancement (LGE) image shows abnormal subendocardial LGE in a nonvascular distribution, predominating at the ventricular apex *(white arrowheads)* with mural thrombus *(black arrowhead)*. The patient suffered from embolic stroke. (B) Eosinophilic endocarditis due to eosinophilic leukemia in a 76-year-old woman. This two-chamber LGE view shows diffuse abnormal subendocardial LGE of the left ventricle. (C) Loeffler syndrome. There is diffuse abnormal LGE of the left ventricular subendocardium with an intracavitary thrombus, which commonly occurs in the second stage of the disease after the inflammatory phase. (D) There is resolution of the thrombus in the third stage of the disease, characterized by extensive subendocardial fibrosis in the apex of both ventricles *(arrowheads)* and in the subvalvular regions *(arrows)*.

seen because of the edema. In the more advanced postinflammatory stage, abnormal LGE reflecting replacement fibrosis may develop, sometimes with myocardial wall thinning. Segmental contraction abnormalities may be present in all stages. Cardiac sarcoidosis occurs in a variety of patterns on T2-weighted images and an LGE sequence, but is typically patchy or nodular in appearance, involving the mesocardium and subepicardium, or is focally transmural. It is usually located in the basal segment of the interventricular septum (Fig. 31.12). Cardiac sarcoidosis may resemble myocarditis; the diagnosis is challenging when cardiac dysfunction is the first manifestation of sarcoidosis. Localization of imaging findings in the basal portion of the septal wall and the nodular pattern suggest sarcoidosis over myocarditis. Abnormal LGE in a patient with known extracardiac disease is also strongly suspicious for cardiac sarcoidosis. In doubtful cases, CMR findings are helpful to guide the endomyocardial biopsy toward pathologic regions, because sensitivity of the biopsy is as low as 20% due to focal myocardial involvement in most cases. Diffuse severe cardiac sarcoidosis affects a minority of patients and is depicted by diffuse myocardial thickening, edema, and global hypokinesis, evolving to DCM in the advanced stage. Another role of CMR is to monitor the response of cardiac sarcoidosis to therapy reflected by resolving myocardial inflammation on T2-weighted images and perfusion imaging and possible decrease of abnormal LGE. Finally, CT and CMR findings of extracardiac sarcoidosis should be assessed, including lung nodules, mediastinal and hilar lymphadenopathy, and signs of pulmonary hypertension, such as enlargement of the pulmonary artery, RV hypertrophy, and dilation.

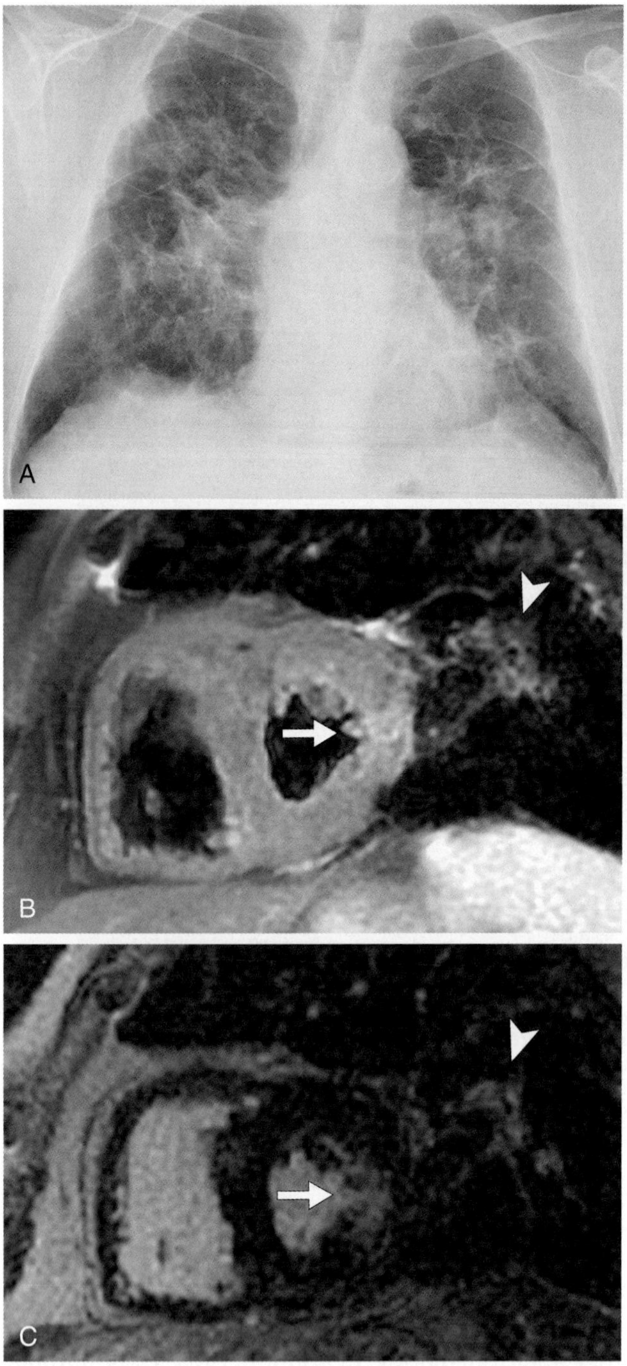

Figure 31.12 Sarcoidosis. (A) Chest radiograph shows paratracheal and hilar enlargement, with fibrotic changes predominating in the midzone of the lungs, consistent with sarcoidosis. (B) T2-weighted and late gadolinium enhancement (LGE; C) images depict cardiac involvement of sarcoidosis, with a nodular focus of myocardial edema (B; *arrow*) and corresponding abnormal LGE (C; *arrow*) involving the midwall of the inferolateral wall at the midventricular level. The pulmonary opacities are seen by cardiac magnetic resonance imaging *(arrowheads)*.

Imaging Amyloidosis

Cardiac amyloidosis is a secondary infiltrative cardiomyopathy resulting from the extracellular deposition of insoluble fibrillary amyloid proteins throughout the myocardium, atrium, and valves. It can be the first and only manifestation of amyloidosis or may be discovered while investigating a patient with systemic amyloidosis. Cardiac involvement is present in 50% of cases of systemic amyloidosis, leading to the prognosis of the disease because this restrictive cardiomyopathy progresses to diastolic heart failure. Light chain amyloidosis is the most common form affecting the heart and has a particularly poor prognosis; median survival <6 months if untreated. Many other forms of amyloidosis are recognized, including hereditary (ATTRm), senile (ATTRwt), and dialysis-related amyloidosis. The gold standard test for the diagnosis of cardiac amyloidosis is endomyocardial biopsy with Congo red staining, but this procedure is invasive. In clinical practice, the diagnosis of cardiac amyloidosis is usually suggested by echocardiography and supported by CMR and/or noncardiac biopsy.

Echocardiography findings include concentric hypertrophy of both ventricles (wall thickness >12 mm), increased echogenicity of the myocardium, and prominent valves from amyloid infiltration. Doppler echocardiography shows a restrictive pattern, with progressive diastolic dysfunction over serial examinations. The ejection fraction is usually preserved until late in the disease. However, other diseases such as HCM and hemochromatosis may mimic these echocardiography findings.

CMR has the advantage of tissue characterization and has good sensitivity (80%) and high specificity (94%) compared to endomyocardial biopsy. On CMR, cardiac amyloidosis typically causes concentric ventricular wall thickening (>12 mm) with nondilated ventricles. Thickening (>6 mm) of the interatrial septum and posterior right atrial wall is a common feature (Fig. 31.13). The LV ejection fraction is normal or decreased, with restrictive physiology depicted by restricted diastolic filling and biatrial enlargement. In cardiac amyloidosis, there is expansion of the extracellular space by amyloid deposition and associated endomyocardial fibrosis. On CMR, this results in a characteristic pattern of abnormal myocardial and blood-pool gadolinium kinetics (see Fig. 31.13). Expansion of the myocardial extracellular space creates an environment in which gadolinium is retained, with abnormal LGE seen in 79% to 97% of patients. The pattern of abnormal LGE in the myocardium may be diffusely transmural, diffusely subendocardial, or focal and patchy. However, abnormal LGE may be difficult to assess because of the rapid washout of gadolinium from the myocardium. The delay to perform an LGE sequence after gadolinium injection is therefore shorter than that for other cardiomyopathies—5 minutes after gadolinium injection compared to 10 to 20 minutes. Abnormal LGE may also be difficult to depict because there is incomplete nulling of the myocardial signal on the inversion recovery sequence caused by the alteration in T1 signal by amyloid deposition, resulting in difficulty to determine the optimal inversion time to null normal myocardium. In general, if difficulty with myocardial suppression is noted, cardiac amyloidosis should strongly be considered as the cause. Phase-sensitive inversion recovery sequences, which are less sensitive to the selection of a specific inversion time for myocardial nulling, are often useful in this setting. Systemic expansion of the extracellular space is also believed to explain the absence of residual gadolinium within the blood pool on LGE images, resulting

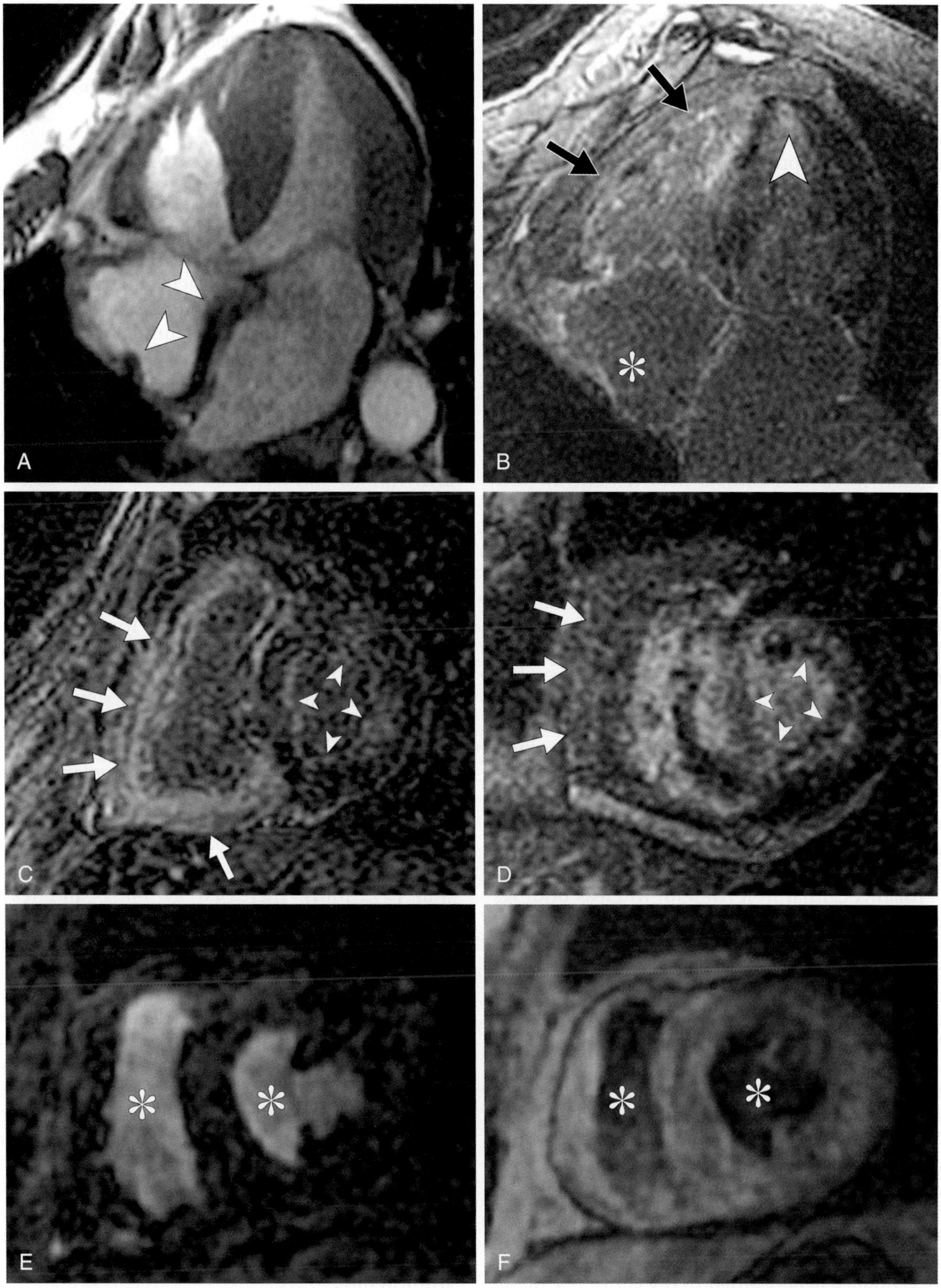

Figure 31.13 Amyloidosis in different patients. (A) This four-chamber steady-state free precession view shows concentric ventricular wall thickening of nondilated ventricles and thickening of the interatrial septum and posterior right atrial wall *(arrowheads)*. Four-chamber (B) and short-axis late gadolinium enhancement (LGE; C) views show diffuse subendocardial LGE of the left ventricle *(white arrowheads)* and transmural LGE of the right ventricular (RV) wall *(black and white arrows in B and C, respectively)*. There is diffuse LGE of both atria *(asterisk)* and atrioventricular valves in (B). (D) Short-axis LGE demonstrates more important LGE of the left ventricle *(white arrowheads)* and severe thickening of the RV wall due to amyloid deposition *(white arrows)*. Short-axis cine inversion recovery at 155 ms (E) and 255 ms (F) demonstrates the abnormal kinetics of gadolinium in amyloidosis, with nulling of the myocardium (becoming dark) at 155 ms before nulling of the blood pool *(asterisks)* at 255 ms.

in the characteristic dark blood pool with a myocardium that remains bright using the normal range of inversions times due to suboptimal myocardial nulling. This abnormal kinetics of gadolinium in amyloidosis can also be depicted with short-axis images acquired at multiple inversion times (cine inversion recovery) showing abnormal nulling of the myocardium occurring prior to nulling of the blood pool.

Imaging Cardiac Hemochromatosis and Siderotic Cardiomyopathy

Iron overload cardiomyopathy is defined as systolic or diastolic dysfunction secondary to the increased deposition of iron in the heart caused by primary hemochromatosis or secondary hemosiderosis. Primary hemochromatosis is an autosomal recessive disorder affecting iron metabolism, usually presenting in middle-aged patients with increased skin pigmentation, abnormal liver function tests, elevated serum ferritin level, and cardiac involvement in one-third of cases. Secondary hemosiderosis is a form of iron overload resulting from repeated blood transfusions in patients with chronic anemia (e.g., β-thalassemia major, sickle cell disease, myelodysplasia). Secondary hemosiderosis tends to manifest at an early age, typically in adolescence. Both forms have similar imaging findings on CMR. They can sometimes be differentiated based on organ distribution because both affect the liver, but primary hemochromatosis involves the pancreas whereas secondary hemosiderosis also involves the spleen and bone marrow. Because iron deposition in the myocardium is not related to iron deposition in other organs, cardiac-specific measurements of the iron overload are necessary. Early recognition of the disease in asymptomatic patients is important to prevent heart failure and dilated cardiomyopathy. CMR provides a safe and noninvasive method to assess for myocardial iron content, whereas findings on echocardiography are nonspecific; endomyocardial biopsy is an invasive procedure of limited sensitivity because iron deposition tends to be patchy.

On echocardiography and CMR, there is a normal to mildly increased wall thickness with diastolic dysfunction and restrictive physiology. Systolic dysfunction and DCM usually do not appear until the iron concentration reaches a critical level. CMR can identify and quantify the iron deposition load in the myocardium based on changes in the T2* signal characteristics of the myocardium. Iron causes local alterations in the magnetic field, with a resultant shorter relaxation time and darker SI of the myocardium compared to skeletal muscles on T2-weighted and T2*-weighted images. A specific T2*-weighted sequence is used for quantification of myocardial iron load. The sequence is performed in the short-axis plane of the left ventricle at the midventricular level using a breath-hold gradient-echo sequence acquired at multiple echo times. A ROI is traced in the interventricular septum, away from the blood pool and epicardial veins. The SI within the ROI is measured for each image and plotted against echo time to form an exponential decay curve, a phenomenon called *T2* decay* (Fig. 31.14). To obtain the mean T2*, an exponential trend line is fitted with the equation: $y = K_e^{\ TE/T2^*}$ (where K_e is a constant, TE indicates echo time, and y is the SI). In myocardial iron overload, T2* values are typically lower than 20 ms. This technique may also be used to monitor the effectiveness of iron chelation therapy because a myocardial T2* increase also correlates with the recovery of LV function.

Imaging Cardiac Involvement in Anderson-Fabry Disease

Anderson-Fabry disease is one the various metabolic storage diseases (e.g., type I or II glycogenosis, Gaucher, Neimann-Pick diseases, galactosialidosis, mucopolysaccharidosis) that may induce an infiltrative cardiomyopathy caused by the abnormal accumulation of a substance. Cardiac involvement in these diseases is common and represents an important cause of morbidity and mortality. Deposition leads to LV hypertrophy and diastolic dysfunction that eventually progresses to systolic dysfunction and heart failure if left untreated. Complications include arrhythmias and ischemia due to small-vessel disease. Anderson-Fabry disease is an autosomal recessive lysosome mutation that causes increased glycosphingolipid accumulation in the myocardium. Anderson-Fabry disease is usually diagnosed during childhood or adolescence, but cardiac involvement appears in the third or fourth decade. It is of particular interest for imagers because it causes LV wall thickening in a pattern that mimics the concentric form of HCM. About 6% to 12% of patients who present with late-onset HCM are subsequently found to have Anderson-Fabry disease. It is critical to distinguish both entities because early detection of Anderson-Fabry disease and the initiation of enzyme replacement therapy can significantly reduce the myocardial mass and improve myocardial function.

On echocardiography and CMR, Anderson-Fabry cardiomyopathy shows diffuse thickening of the LV wall (>12 mm), increased LV mass, and features of diastolic dysfunction, with preserved systolic function in the earlier stage. Glycosphingolipid deposition in the subendocardium may result in a characteristic binary appearance on echocardiography, characterized by increased echogenicity of the endocardium separated from the hyperechoic myocardium by a hypoechoic space and optimally visible along the interventricular septum. On CMR, approximately 50% of cases have abnormal LGE in a nonischemic pattern usually involving the midmyocardium and subepicardium, sparing of the subendocardium, and predominating in the basal inferolateral LV wall, contrasting with HCM, which does not commonly involve only this segment of the left ventricle (Fig. 31.15). In the terminal stage, the basal inferolateral LV wall may show marked thinning and severe regional wall motion abnormality.

■ Conclusion

Cardiac imaging, particularly CMR, offers valuable information for diagnosing and monitoring cardiomyopathies. A comprehensive CMR study, adapted to the specific clinical question, is an excellent noninvasive imaging technique that can differentiate ischemic from nonischemic cardiomyopathies and recognize patterns of disease

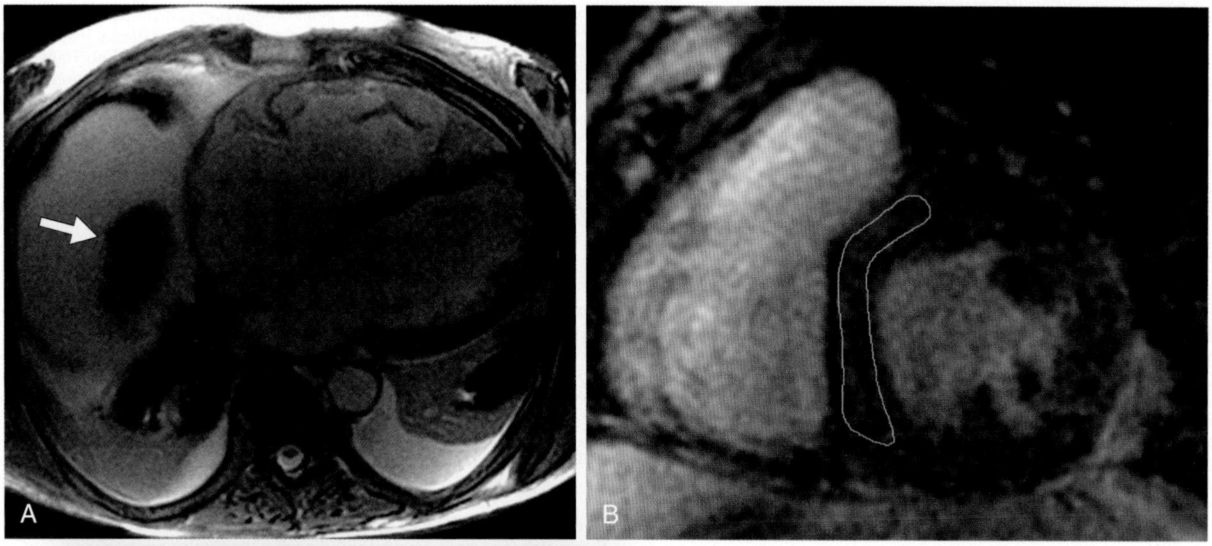

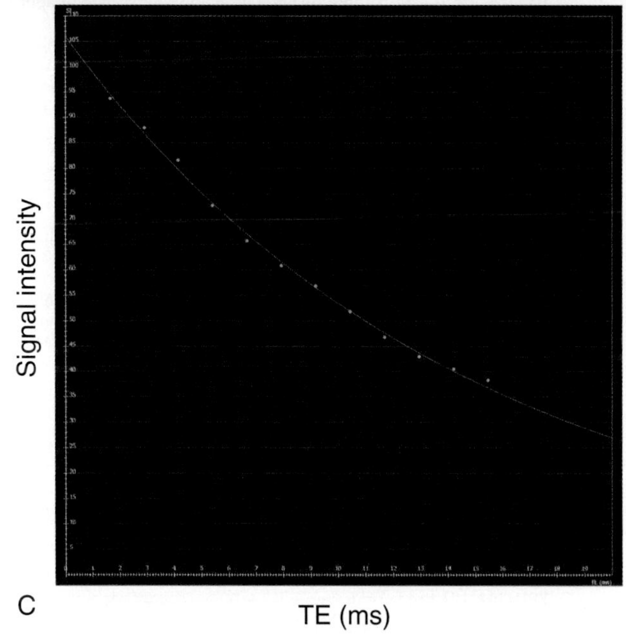

Figure 31.14 Secondary hemosiderosis in an alcoholic patient with cirrhosis, chronic anemia, and esophageal varices requiring multiple blood transfusions. (A) Axial localizer shows decreased signal intensity (SI) of the liver *(arrow)*, bone marrow in the spine, and left ventricular myocardium, with dilation of the cardiac chambers. (B) and (C) depict the myocardial iron quantification process in this patient. A region of interest is traced in the interventricular septum *(orange contour)* of multiple gradient echo T2* images acquired at the same level with a variable echo time *(TE)*. Acquired data of variable myocardial SI according to different echo times are plotted on a graph to calculate the T2* decay time, which was 16 ms in this patient (a value of <20 ms is abnormal and is consistent with increased iron deposition).

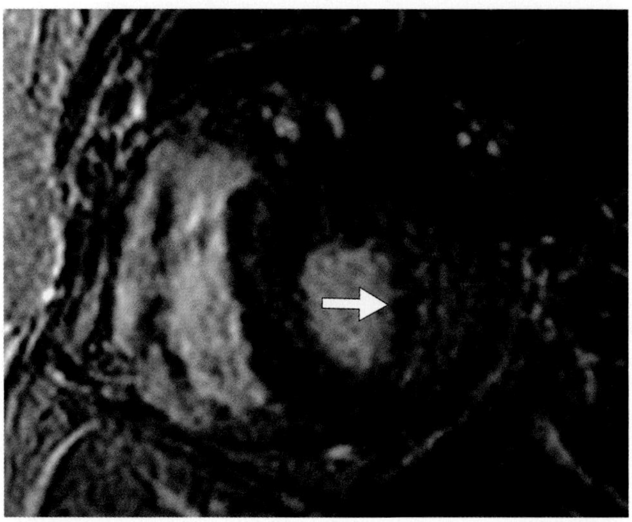

Figure 31.15 Anderson-Fabry disease. This short-axis late gadolinium enhancement (LGE) image shows myocardial thickening and hazy midwall LGE predominating in the basal inferolateral left ventricular wall *(arrow)*.

that can narrow the differential diagnosis in patients with nonischemic disease. It has become a valuable alternative to endomyocardial biopsy in many clinical scenarios. CMR not only provides valuable information regarding cardiac morphology, function, and myocardial tissue, but it can also detect the presence of fibrotic myocardial replacement, which is appealing for the risk stratification of potential harmful complications, such as cardiac arrhythmias, heart failure, and SCD. However, imaging of cardiomyopathies can be challenging because there is overlap of the imaging features between different cardiomyopathies; some cardiomyopathies do not have specific imaging features or may have normal imaging findings, despite the presence of myocardial pathology on histology.

Bibliography

Abdel-Aty H, Boye P, Zagrosek A, et al. Diagnostic performance of cardiovascular magnetic resonance in patients with suspected acute myocarditis: comparison of different approaches. *J Am Coll Cardiol.* 2005;45(11):1815–1822.

Acquatella H. Echocardiography in Chagas heart disease. *Circulation*. 2007;115(9): 1124–1131.

Anderson LJ, Holden S, Davis B, et al. Cardiovascular T2-star (T2*) magnetic resonance for the early diagnosis of myocardial iron overload. *Eur Heart J*. 2001;22(23):2171–2179.

Baessler B, Luecke C, Lurz J, et al. Cardiac MRI texture analysis of T1 and T2 maps in patients with infarctlike acute myocarditis. *Radiology*. 2018;289(2):357–365.

Bogaert J, Taylor AM. Heart muscle diseases. In: Bogaert J, Dymarkowski S, Taylor AM, Muthurangu V, eds. *Clinical Cardiac MRI*. 2nd ed. Springer; 2012:275–353.

Chan AK, Somarouthu B, Ghoshhajra B. Magnetic resonance imaging for hypertrophic cardiomyopathy update. *Top Magn Reson Imaging*. 2014;23(1): 33–41.

Deva DP, Williams LK, Care M, et al. Deep basal inferoseptal crypts occur more commonly in patients with hypertrophic cardiomyopathy due to disease-causing myofilament mutations. *Radiology*. 2013;269(1):68–76.

Eitel I, von Knobelsdorff-Brenkenhoff F, Bernhardt P, et al. Clinical characteristics and cardiovascular magnetic resonance findings in stress (Takotsubo) cardiomyopathy. *JAMA*. 2011;306(3):277–286.

Friedrich MG. Cardiomyopathies. In: Manning WJ, Pennell D, eds. *Cardiovascular Magnetic Resonance*. 2nd ed. Philadelphia: Churchill Livingstone; 2010:515–531.

Friedrich MG, Sechtem U, Schulz-Menger J, et al. Cardiovascular magnetic resonance in myocarditis: A JACC white paper. *J Am Coll Cardiol*. 2009;53(17): 1475–1487.

Henry TS, Cummings KW. Myocardial nonischemic cardiomyopathies. In: Abbara S, Kalva SP, eds. *Problem-Solving in Cardiovascular Imaging*. Elsevier; 2013: 505–521.

Hindieh W, Weissler-Snir A, Hammer H, et al. Discrepant measurements of maximal left ventricular wall thickness between cardiac magnetic resonance imaging and echocardiography in patients with hypertrophic cardiomyopathy. *Circ Cardiovasc Imaging*. 2017;10(8):e006309.

Hundley WG, Bluemke DA, Finn JP, et al. ACCF/ACR/AHA/NASCI/SCMR 2010 expert consensus document on cardiovascular magnetic resonance: a report of the American College of Cardiology Foundation Task Force on expert consensus documents. *Circulation*. 2010;121(22):2462–2508.

Kawel N, Nacif M, Arai AE, et al. Trabeculated (noncompacted) and compact myocardium in adults: the multi-ethnic study of atherosclerosis. *Circ Cardiovasc Imaging*. 2012;5(3):357–366.

Kimura F, Matsuo Y, Nakajima T, et al. Myocardial fat at cardiac imaging: how can we differentiate pathologic from physiologic fatty infiltration? *Radiographics*. 2010;30(6):1587–1602.

Kwong RY, Falk RH. Cardiovascular magnetic resonance in cardiac amyloidosis. *Circulation*. 2005;111(2):122–124.

Marcus FI, McKenna WJ, Sherrill D, et al. Diagnosis of arrhythmogenic right ventricular cardiomyopathy/dysplasia: proposed modification of the task force criteria. *Circulation*. 2010;121(13):1533–1541.

Marcus FI, McKenna WJ, Sherrill D, et al. Diagnosis of arrhythmogenic right ventricular cardiomyopathy/dysplasia: proposed modification of the task force criteria. *Eur Heart J*. 2010;31(7):806–814.

Maron BJ, McKenna WJ, Danielson GK, et al. American College of Cardiology/ European Society of Cardiology clinical expert consensus document on hypertrophic cardiomyopathy. A report of the American College of Cardiology Foundation Task Force on Clinical Expert Consensus Documents and the European Society of Cardiology Committee for Practice Guidelines. *J Am Coll Cardiol*. 2003;42(9):1687–1713.

Maron BJ, Towbin JA, Thiene G, et al. Contemporary definitions and classification of the cardiomyopathies: an American Heart Association scientific statement from the Council on Clinical Cardiology, Heart Failure and Transplantation Committee; Quality of Care and Outcomes Research and Functional Genomics and Translational Biology Interdisciplinary Working Groups; and Council on Epidemiology and Prevention. *Circulation*. 2006;113(14):1807–1816.

McCrohon JA, Moon JC, Prasad SK, et al. Differentiation of heart failure related to dilated cardiomyopathy and coronary artery disease using gadolinium-enhanced cardiovascular magnetic resonance. *Circulation*. 2003;108(1):54–59.

McKenna WJ, Thiene G, Nava A, et al. Diagnosis of arrhythmogenic right ventricular dysplasia/cardiomyopathy. Task force of the working group myocardial and pericardial disease of the European Society of Cardiology and of the Scientific Council on Cardiomyopathies of the International Society and Federation of Cardiology. *Br Heart J*. 1994;71(3):215–218.

Moon JC, McKenna WJ, McCrohon JA, Elliott PM, Smith GC, Pennell DJ. Toward clinical risk assessment in hypertrophic cardiomyopathy with gadolinium cardiovascular magnetic resonance. *J Am Coll Cardiol*. 2003;41(9):1561–1567.

Moon JC, Messroghli DR, Kellman P, et al. Myocardial T1 mapping and extracellular volume quantification: a Society for Cardiovascular Magnetic Resonance (SCMR) and CMR Working Group of the European Society of Cardiology consensus statement. *J Cardiovasc Magn Reson*. 2013;15:92.

Mouquet F, Lions C, de Groote P, et al. Characterisation of peripartum cardiomyopathy by cardiac magnetic resonance imaging. *Eur Radiol*. 2008;18(12): 2765–2769.

O'Donnell DH, Abbara S, Chaithiraphan V, et al. Cardiac MR imaging of nonischemic cardiomyopathies: imaging protocols and spectra of appearances. *Radiology*. 2012;262(2):403–422.

O'Hanlon R, Grasso A, Roughton M, et al. Prognostic significance of myocardial fibrosis in hypertrophic cardiomyopathy. *J Am Coll Cardiol*. 2010;56(11):867–874.

Petersen SE, Selvanayagam JB, Wiesmann F, et al. Left ventricular noncompaction: insights from cardiovascular magnetic resonance imaging. *J Am Coll Cardiol*. 2005;46(1):101–105.

Richardson P, McKenna W, Bristow M, et al. Report of the 1995 World Health Organization/International Society and Federation of Cardiology Task Force on the definition and classification of cardiomyopathies. *Circulation*. 1996;93(5):841–842.

Sharkey SW, Lesser JR, Zenovich AG, et al. Acute and reversible cardiomyopathy provoked by stress in women from the United States. *Circulation*. 2005;111(4): 472–479.

Sievers B, Addo M, Franken U, Trappe HJ. Right ventricular wall motion abnormalities found in healthy subjects by cardiovascular magnetic resonance imaging and characterized with a new segmental model. *J Cardiovasc Magn Reson*. 2004;6(3):601–608.

Sparrow PJ, Merchant N, Provost YL, Doyle DJ, Nguyen ET, Paul NS. CT and MR imaging findings in patients with acquired heart disease at risk for sudden cardiac death. *Radiographics*. 2009;29(3):805–823.

Vermes E, Friedrich MG. Current role of magnetic resonance imaging for suspected myocarditis. In: Abbara S, Kalva SP, eds. *Problem Solving in Cardiovascular Imaging*. Elsevier; 2013:423–430.

Vignaux O. Cardiac sarcoidosis: spectrum of MRI features. *AJR Am J Roentgenol*. 2005;184(1):249–254.

Walker CM, Chung JH, Reddy GP. Septal bounce. *J Thorac Imaging*. 2012;27(1):W1.

Watkins H, Ashrafian H, Redwood C. Inherited cardiomyopathies. *N Engl J Med*. 2011;364(17):1643–1656.

CHAPTER 32

Cardiac and Vascular Tumors

Nagina Malguria, Attila Tóth, and Suhny Abbara

CHAPTER OUTLINE

Introduction

Cardiac tumors, benign and malignant types, are uncommon, with an incidence of 0.002% to 0.3% on autopsy series. However, even benign cardiac tumors may present with significant obstructive symptoms or be a substrate for arrhythmias. Tumors in the left side of the heart have the potential to cause systemic or neurologic embolic phenomena. The goals of imaging in cardiac masses are as follows:

1. Anatomic localization of the mass, which may sometimes provide a clue to the specific diagnosis
2. Tissue characterization
3. Distinction from thrombi, other non-neoplastic benign entities, and anatomic variants

Conventional radiographs are rarely useful in evaluating cardiac masses, unless the lesions are big or lead to cardiomegaly. Imaging evaluation of cardiac masses usually begins with echocardiography and, because it is so widely used, cardiac masses are often discovered incidentally on echocardiography. However echocardiography has its limitations; it is operator dependent and may be limited by acoustic windows—for example, in large patients and those with chronic obstructive pulmonary disease.

Computed tomography (CT) has a significant role in evaluating cardiac masses in view of high spatial acquisition and the ability to acquire multiplanar data rapidly. Its ability to characterize fat and calcium accurately may help narrow the differential diagnosis in some cases. MRI, with its high tissue contrast resolution and multiplanar imaging, is often the modality of choice for evaluating cardiac masses. The MRI planes may need to be tailored to a specific mass location. A standard protocol for the evaluation of cardiac masses begins with scout images, followed by steady-state free precession (SSFP) images in standard planes (paraseptal or vertical long-axis, horizontal long-axis, short-axis stack, three-chamber views). T1 axial fast spin-echo images, without—and, if needed, with—fat suppression should be performed in planes best suited to evaluate the mass in question. T2-weighted images are obtained to evaluate edema or T2 characteristics of the mass. Tagging may be useful in masses that infiltrate the myocardium or involve the pericardium. First-pass perfusion images, acquired during gadolinium administration, are useful to evaluate vascularity of the mass. Delayed gadolinium images at 8 to 15 minutes are acquired in a short-axis view to cover the left ventricle and in any additional planes that may be necessary to show the mass. In between the perfusion images and delayed gadolinium images, fast spin-echo, postcontrast T1 images may be obtained in optimal planes, which are determined by the location of the mass.

Benign Tumors of the Heart

Myxoma

Among primary cardiac tumors, 90% are benign and, of these, the most common are myxomas (50%–80%). They are three times more common in females than males and

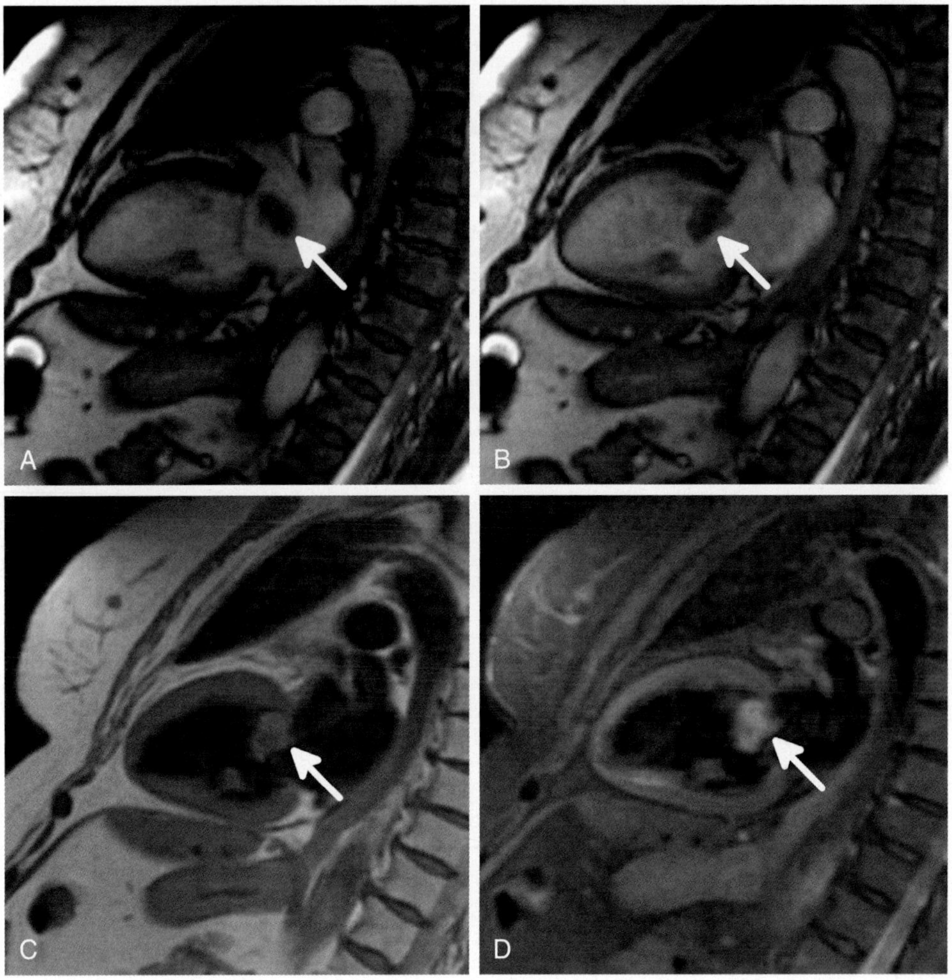

Figure 32.1 Mobile left atrial myxoma *(arrows)*. (A) Early systolic image from steady-state free precession (SSFP) cine sequence in two-chamber (2CH) or vertical long-axis view shows left atrial mass. (B) Late diastolic image taken from a 2CH SSFP cine. The left atrial mass enters the left ventricle during the cardiac cycle. (C) Black blood T1 image showing heterogenous T1-weighted signal in the lesion, slightly lower compared to the myocardium. (D) Triple-inversion recovery (dark blood, fat-suppressed) demonstrating nonhomogeneously increased T2-weighted signal of the mass.

usually present in the fourth to sixth decades of life. In 60% to 80% of cases, myxomas are seen in the left atrium (Fig. 32.1), in the region of the interatrial septum and fossa ovalis, followed by the right atrium (15%–28%), right ventricle (8%; Fig. 32.2), left ventricle (3%–5%), and, rarely, the valves. About 10% of these are biatrial, often extending via the fossa ovalis from the left atrium to the right.

Most myxomas occur sporadically, but approximately 7% occur syndromically, with the Carney complex, an X-linked autosomal dominant syndrome consisting of cardiac and extracardiac myxomas, spotty skin pigmentation, endocrine overactivity, and schwannomas. Myxomas associated with the Carney complex occur in younger patients, who are more likely to be male, and tend to recur after resection. Recent studies have shown that both sporadic myxomas and those associated with the Carney complex may have a mutation in the *PRKAR1A* gene, suggesting a plausible genetic origin for at least some of these tumors.

Clinically, approximately, 10% to 15% of myxomas are asymptomatic at the time of diagnosis. Alternatively, they may present with systemic constitutional symptoms due to interleukin production or obstructive symptoms related to left and right heart failure. A large, mobile, left atrial myxoma may prolapse through the mitral valve, causing functional mitral obstruction, or a so-called wrecking ball effect due to back and forth prolapse of the tumor through the mitral valve. Embolic manifestations are seen in 30% to 50% of myxomas and usually involve the cerebral and retinal circulations.

Pathologically, myxomas are rounded lobular masses, with a bosselated surface. Cystic forms of myxoma have been reported. One-third of myxomas are calcified, and some may demonstrate hemorrhage. On gross pathology, one-third of myxomas are papillary, and the remaining are polypoidal. The papillary myxomas are the ones more likely to present with neurologic and systemic embolic events due to detached fragments, whereas the polypoidal types are more likely to present with obstructive symptoms. Right atrial myxomas are more likely to be calcified than left atrial myxomas.

Imaging

Myxomas are heterogeneously low attenuating on CT, usually demonstrating lower or, less frequently, equal enhancement to that of the surrounding myocardium. Calcification, if present, is well seen on CT, usually visualized as a coarse or punctate calcification, and is more common in right atrial myxomas but uncommon in left atrial myxomas. Atrial myxomas have a narrow attachment to the interatrial septum.

On MRI, myxomas are typically isointense on T1-weighted images and hyperintense on T2-weighted sequences.

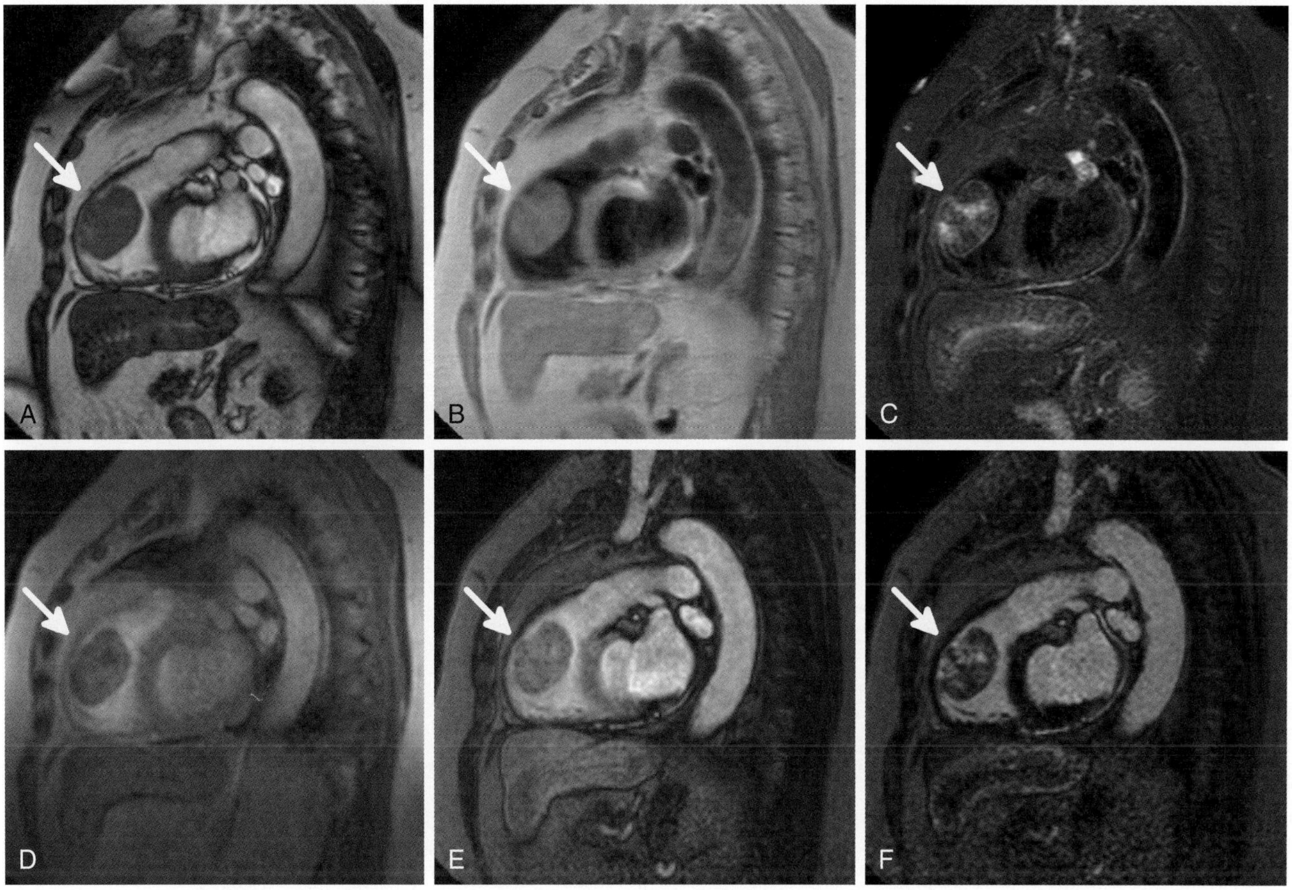

Figure 32.2 Myxoma *(arrows)* of the right ventricular outflow tract. (A) Steady-state free precession image of the right ventricle. The slightly nonhomogeneous T2-/T1-weighted signal is mostly similar to the myocardium. (B) Black blood, T1-weighted turbo spin-echo (TSE) image in the same view; nonhomogeneous, intermediate signal intensity. (C) T2-weighted TSE image. Nonhomogeneous signal characteristics show areas of increased and decreased signal intensity. Myxomatous components and some blood degradation products can cause a signal increase, whereas calcification and hemosiderin (or, to a lesser extent) fibrotic components result in decreased signal. (D) First-pass perfusion image showing nonhomogeneous contrast uptake during administration of extracellular IV contrast material (Gd-DO3A-butrol). (E) Early enhancement inversion recovery turbo field-echo image taken 2 to 7 minutes after contrast administration using intentionally long inversion times, demonstrating mildly nonhomogeneous contrast enhancement. (F) Delayed enhancement inversion recovery turbo field-echo image taken 10 to 20 minutes after contrast administration using inversion times to null the myocardium. The mass shows nonhomogeneous contrast enhancement as a sign of a heterogenous histologic structure.

Balanced SSFP images demonstrate the mobility of atrial myxomas (see Fig. 32.1), which may prolapse through the atrioventricular valves, causing temporary obstruction. On the balanced SSFP images, myxomas are generally hypointense compared to the blood pool and hyperintense to the normal myocardium. On early first-pass images, they may show no or mild enhancement; demonstrating a greater degree of heterogenous enhancement on late gadolinium enhancement sequences, performed 10 to 15 minutes after contrast enhancement. Heterogeneity on postcontrast images is related to areas of necrosis, hemorrhage, fibrosis, and calcification (see Fig. 32.2).

Lipoma

Description

Cardiac lipomas are the second most common primary tumors of the heart. They may occur anywhere and usually present at a young age. They are well-encapsulated lesions, made up of mature adipocytes; about 50% are subepicardial and midmyocardial in origin, and the remaining 50% are subendocardial in location. Lipomas may occur sporadically in the heart or in association with tuberous sclerosis. Lipomas are usually discovered incidentally and are asymptomatic but, depending on their size, may grow large enough to cause coronary artery or pericardial compression (subepicardial), arrhythmias (intramyocardial), or outflow obstruction (subendocardial).

Imaging

On CT and MRI, they follow the typical appearance of fat-containing tissues—that is, low density on CT and bright on T1 MRI sequences—and are suppressed with the application of fat saturation (or suppression) pulses. A useful additional clue is the similar signal intensity of the surrounding mediastinal or chest wall fat on CT, as well as T1- and T2-weighted sequences.

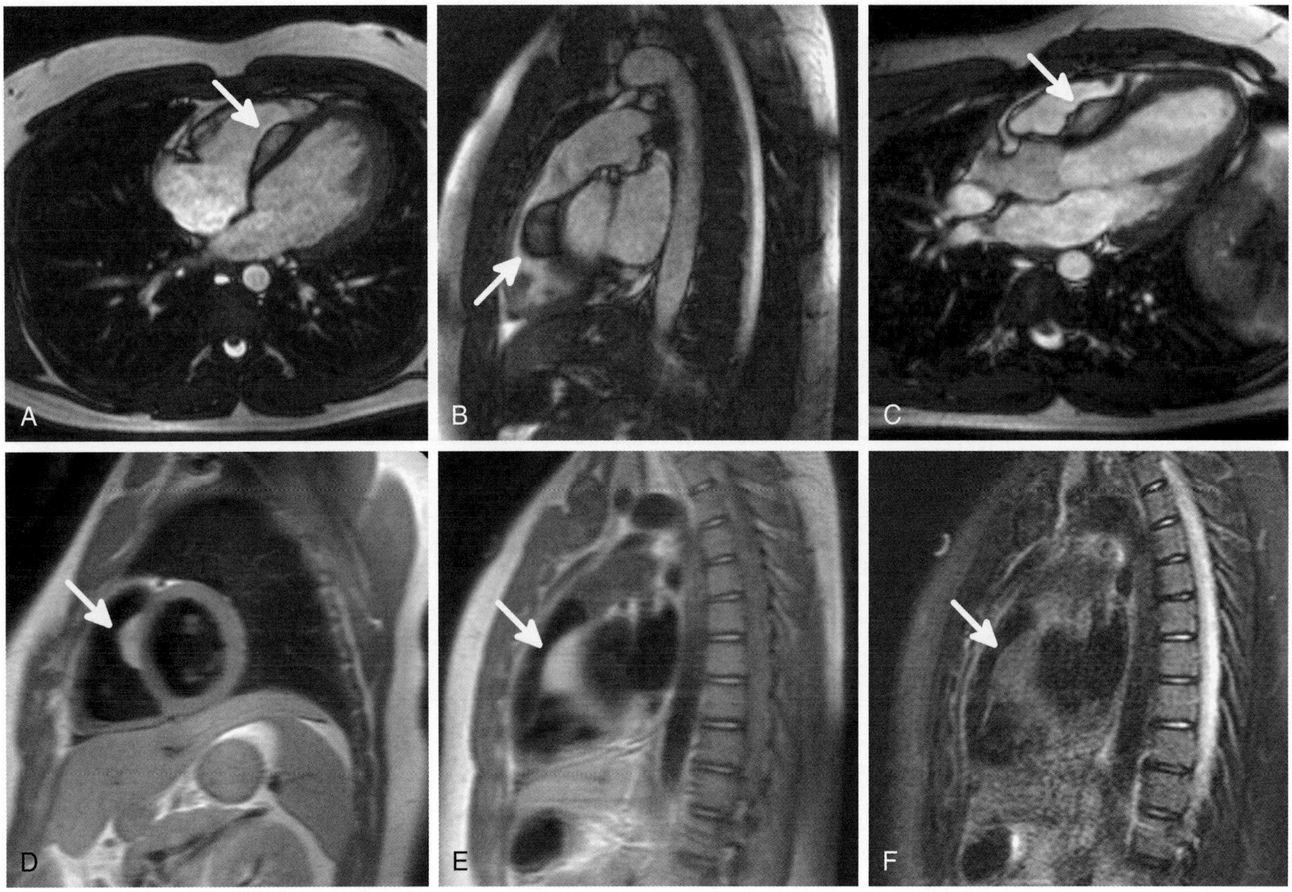

Figure 32.3 Lipoma *(arrows)* of the interventricular septum. (A) Steady-state free precession (SSFP) axial image demonstrates a lesion with a dark rim in the interventricular septum projecting into the right ventricle. (B) SSFP right ventricular outflow tract image of the lesion. (C) SSFP three-chamber view of the same lesion. (D) T1-weighted fast spin-echo (FSE), black blood, short-axis image. The lesion matches subcutaneous fat in its signal characteristics. (E) T1-weighted FSE right ventricular outflow tract image demonstrates the lesion in another plane. (F) Signal dropout of the lesion on the fat-suppressed, T2-weighted, triple inversion recovery FSE image.

Lipomas are avascular and do not enhance with contrast (Fig. 32.3).

Cardiac lipomas need to be distinguished from lipomatous hypertrophy of the interatrial septum, which is often seen in older and overweight patients. In contrast to lipomas, these typically involve the interatrial septum, with sparing of the fossa ovalis, creating a typical dumbbell appearance (Fig. 32.4). The presence of metabolically active brown fat in this entity may cause it to be metabolically active on positron emission tomography scans.

Fibroma

Description

Cardiac fibromas are the second most common congenital tumor and usually present in pediatric or young adult life. They have a propensity to involve the ventricles, left more often than the right. They are typically well circumscribed and may be centrally calcified. It is the most common resected cardiac neoplasm in children and the second most common benign primary tumor found at autopsy in children. Prevalence among males and females is equal. Syndromic cardiac fibromas occur in association with Gorlin syndrome, an autosomal dominant condition associated with multiple basal cell carcinomas, jaw cysts, skeletal anomalies, and a tendency to develop neoplasms in several organ systems.

Imaging

Most of the cardiac fibromas are solitary and usually occur in the interventricular septum or ventricular free wall. Central dystrophic calcification is best identified by CT. On MRI, these lesions are isointense to hyperintense on T1-weighted sequences and slightly hypointense on T2-weighted images. On delayed postgadolinium images, they may either demonstrate intense enhancement or a central hypointense area with a well-demarcated, isointense surrounding shell (Figs. 32.5 and 32.6).

Rhabdomyoma

Description

Rhabdomyomas are the most common primary tumors in children. They usually present in the first year of life.

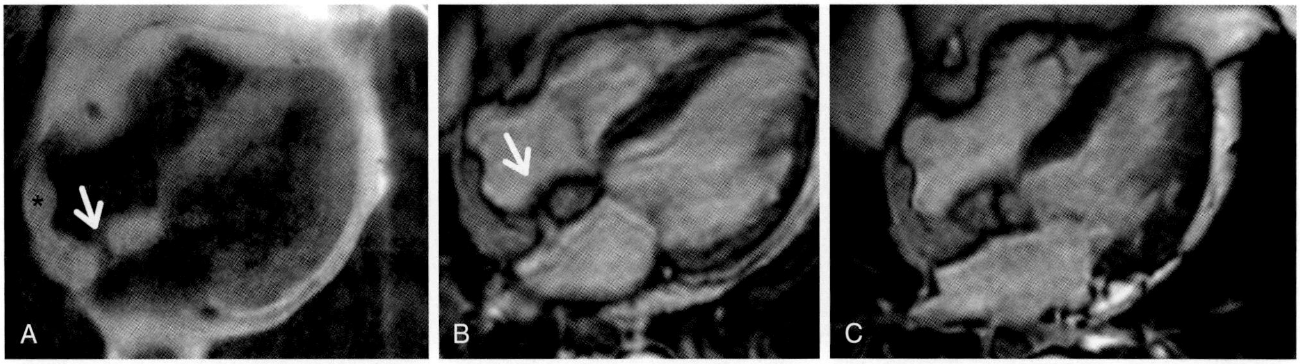

Figure 32.4 Lipomatous hypertrophy of the interatrial septum. (A) Axial double-inversion recovery image, high signal in the interatrial septum, in a dumbbell shape, with sparing of the interatrial septum *(arrow)*. Note the signal in the interatrial septum matches that of the epicardial fat. In this case, fatty infiltration is also seen along the posterior wall of the right atrium, continuing into the crista terminalis. Still diastolic images from axial (B) and four-chamber (C) steady-state free precession sequences demonstrate etching artifact due to a fat-fluid interface in the interatrial septum, with sparing of the fossa ovalis (*arrow*, B) through the process.

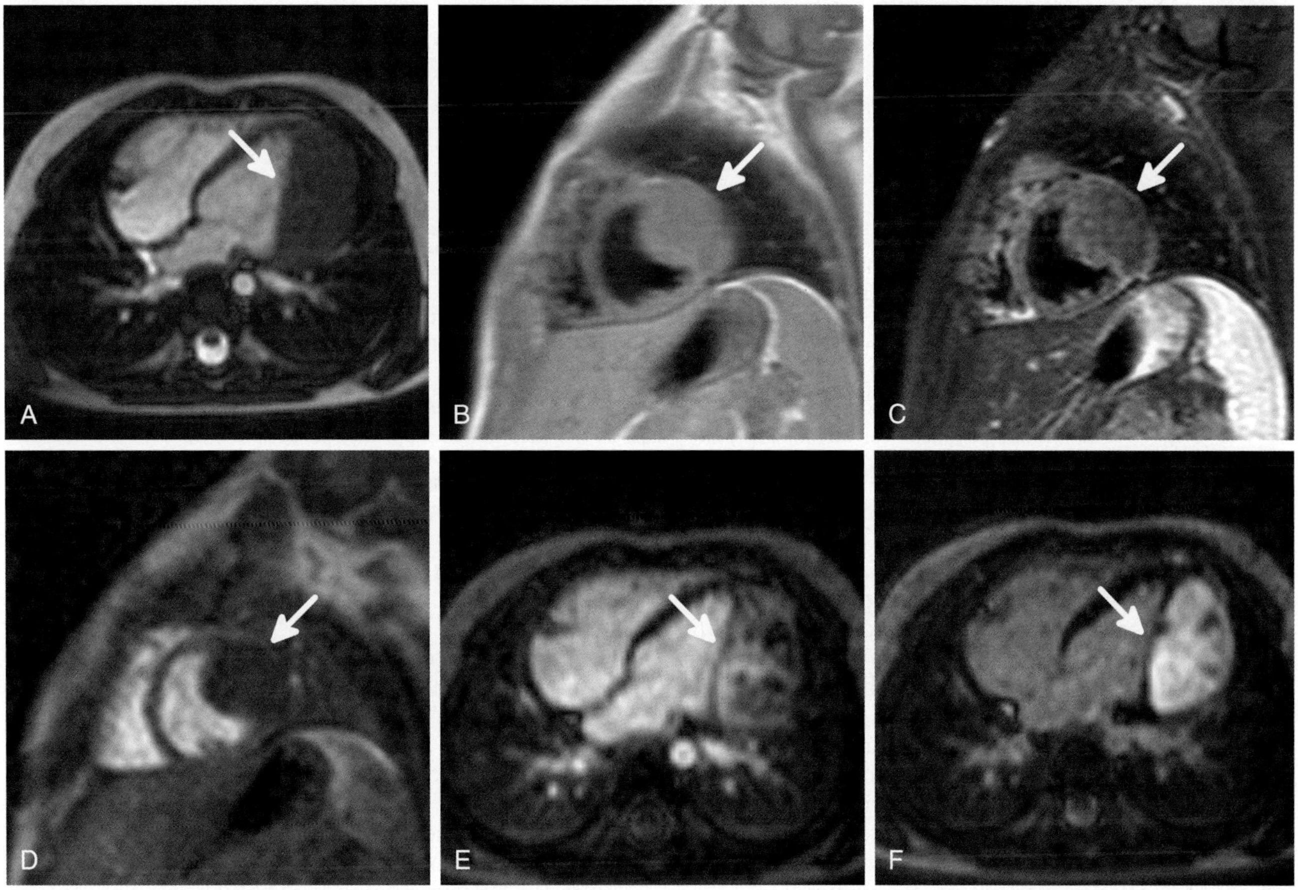

Figure 32.5 Fibroma *(arrows)* of the left ventricle in a 4-year-old boy causing ventricular arrhythmias. The patient underwent implantable cardioverter-defibrillator placement. (A) Steady-state free precession four-chamber image demonstrates an isoattenuating mass in the lateral wall of the left ventricle. (B) Short-axis (SA) T1-weighted, blood-suppressed turbo spin-echo image. The mass shows intermediate signal intensity. (C) SA fat-saturated T2-weighted image. The fibroma is slightly darker compared to the myocardium. (D) SA first-pass perfusion image during extracellular contrast material application. The tumor does not take up contrast. (E) Four-chamber early postcontrast image taken 2 to 3 minutes after gadolinium administration, nulled to the myocardium. The mass shows heterogenous contrast enhancement. (F) Four-chamber inversion recovery delayed hyperenhancement image taken 20 minutes after contrast material injection. The tumor demonstrates marked late enhancement. The borders are well defined.

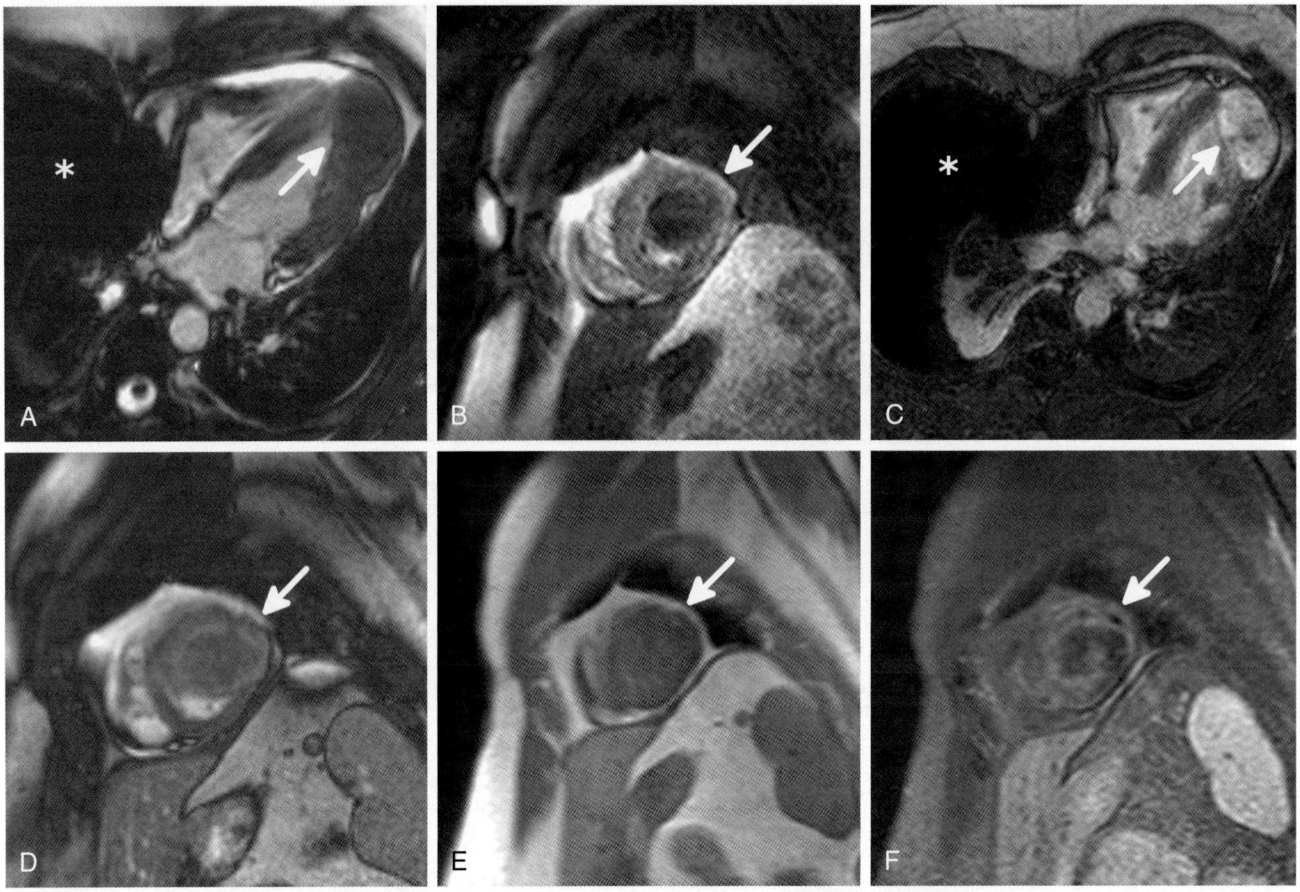

Figure 32.6 Left ventricular fibroma *(arrows)*. An unsuspected finding is spontaneous pneumothorax (PTX). (A) Four-chamber (4CH) balanced steady-state free precession (b-SSFP) frame. The tumor is isointense compared to the myocardium (*asterisk,* PTX). (B) Short-axis first-pass perfusion image. The mass shows low vascularization during extracellular gadolinium contrast material administration. (C) 4CH delayed enhancement (inversion recovery turbo field-echo) image. The fibroma demonstrates marked enhancement 10 minutes after injection (*asterisk,* PTX). The collapsed right lung can be seen ventrolateral to the spinal column, behind the asterisk. (D) Short-axis b-SSFP frame after contrast administration demonstrates peripheral enhancement. (E) Short-axis, T1-weighted, blood-suppressed turbo spin-echo image. The mass has slightly heterogenous signal intensity. (F) Short-axis, T2-weighted, blood-suppressed spectral inversion recovery image. The fibroma has a central nonhomogeneous decreased signal.

Rhabdomyomas demonstrate a high association with tuberous sclerosis, with about 60% to 80% of cardiac rhabdomyomas associated with tuberous sclerosis, and over 50% of patients with tuberous sclerosis having rhabdomyomas. Multiplicity of lesions has an even higher association with tuberous sclerosis. They are well-circumscribed lesions, ranging from a few millimeters to a few centimeters in size. Histologically, they are hamartomas. They arise intramurally in the ventricular myocardium. Most rhabdomyomas regress spontaneously by the age of 4 years, and surgical removal is reserved for symptomatic lesions causing obstruction.

Imaging

Rhabdomyomas are often diagnosed on antenatal ultrasound, where they are hyperechoic. They are generally isointense to the surrounding myocardium on T1-weighted images and hyperintense on T2-weighted sequences (unlike fibromas). They typically show no significant or only minimal early gadolinium enhancement and are isointense on delayed enhanced sequences.

Hemangioma

Description

Hemangiomas are vascular tumors that account for 5% to 10% of all cardiac tumors. Histologically they may be cavernous, capillary, arteriovenous, or usually mixed.

Imaging

On cardiac MR images, hemangiomas are typically heterogeneous and hyperintense on T1- and T2-weighted images due to slow blood flow and show intense post-contrast enhancement due to their high vascular content, but there may be regions of inhomogeneity due to calcification and fibrous septa (Figs. 32.7 and 32.8).

Paraganglioma

Description

Paragangliomas are neuroendocrine tumors. Within the heart, they usually originate from the sympathetic nervous

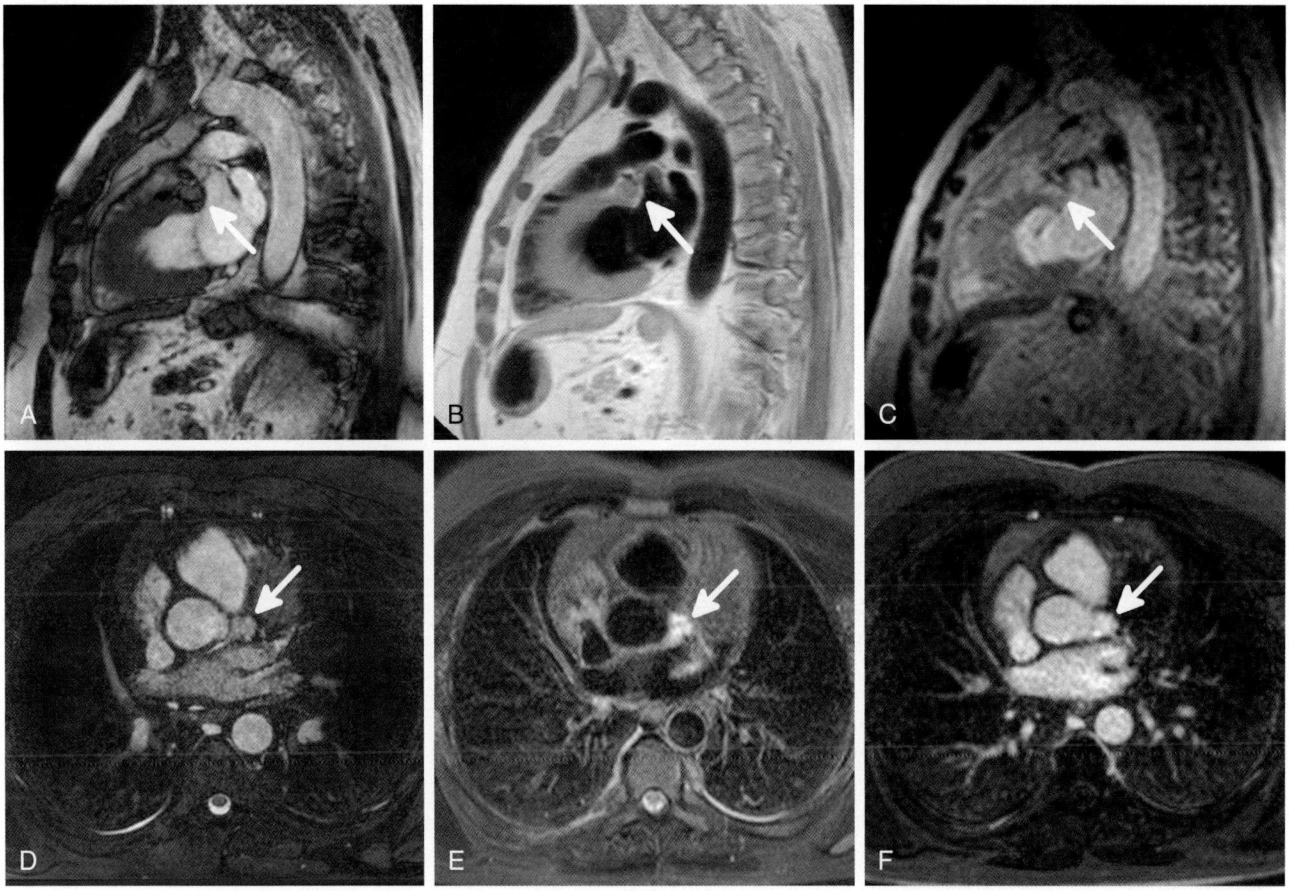

Figure 32.7 Hemangioma. Coronary CT angiography performed for chest complaints revealed no coronary lesions, but showed a mass located under the left main coronary artery bifurcation, adjacent to the aortic root *(arrows)*. This is a relatively common location of a paracardiac hemangioma. Cardiac MRI was performed for further characterization. (A) Sagittal balanced steady-state free precession end-diastolic frame. This well-circumscribed abnormality has a higher T2-/T1-weighted signal compared to the myocardium. (B) Sagittal T1-weighted black blood turbo spin-echo (TSE) image. The tumor shows intermediate signal, similar to the myocardium. (C) Sagittal first-pass image. Marked first-pass contrast uptake suggests a highly vascularized tumor. (D) Axial reconstruction of an isotropic three-dimensional, high-resolution, navigator-driven, T2-prepped, fat-suppressed, balanced fast field echo sequence. No signs of involvement of the adjacent structures. (E) Axial T2-weighted black blood TSE image. The tumor shows increased signal intensity compared to the myocardium. (F) Axial delayed enhancement image after gadolinium contrast administration. The enhancement resembles that of the blood pool.

system and may display catecholamine-related symptoms. These lesions may occasionally occur as a part of multiple endocrine neoplasia syndromes and may be associated with similar lesions elsewhere in the body. These lesions usually have a predilection to arise from the epicardium—including the interatrial groove and atrioventricular groove—or the root of the great vessels and project intrapericardially. Genetic testing may reveal succinate dehydrogenase-related mutations. Their natural life history is variable; some tend to regress, some persist unchanged, and some may enlarge. On imaging, these tumors may be positive on nuclear medicine metaiodobenzylguanidine scans. They show avid enhancement on CT and MRI (Fig. 32.9).

Papillary Fibroelastoma

Description

Papillary fibroelastomas are benign tumors, which predominantly affect the valves, accounting for 75% of all valvular neoplasms. Grossly, they have a papillary frondlike structure; the shape varies—some tumors have a well-developed head and others have elongated stalklike projections. Microscopically, these lesions are comprised of avascular connective tissue lined by endothelium. The most common location is the aortic valve, followed by the mitral valve, tricuspid valve, and pulmonic valve. These tumors may be asymptomatic, or left-sided lesions may present with stroke or other systemic embolic phenomena.

Imaging

These lesions are often incidentally discovered on echocardiography. On MRI, they appear as small, highly mobile homogenous valvular masses, with hypointense signal intensity and surrounding turbulent flow on cine images. Visualizing the tumor may pose difficulties because of its mobile nature (Fig. 32.10). They enhance on post-contrast images, allowing distinction from thrombi. They occasionally may calcify, and CT is the best modality to identify the presence of calcification.

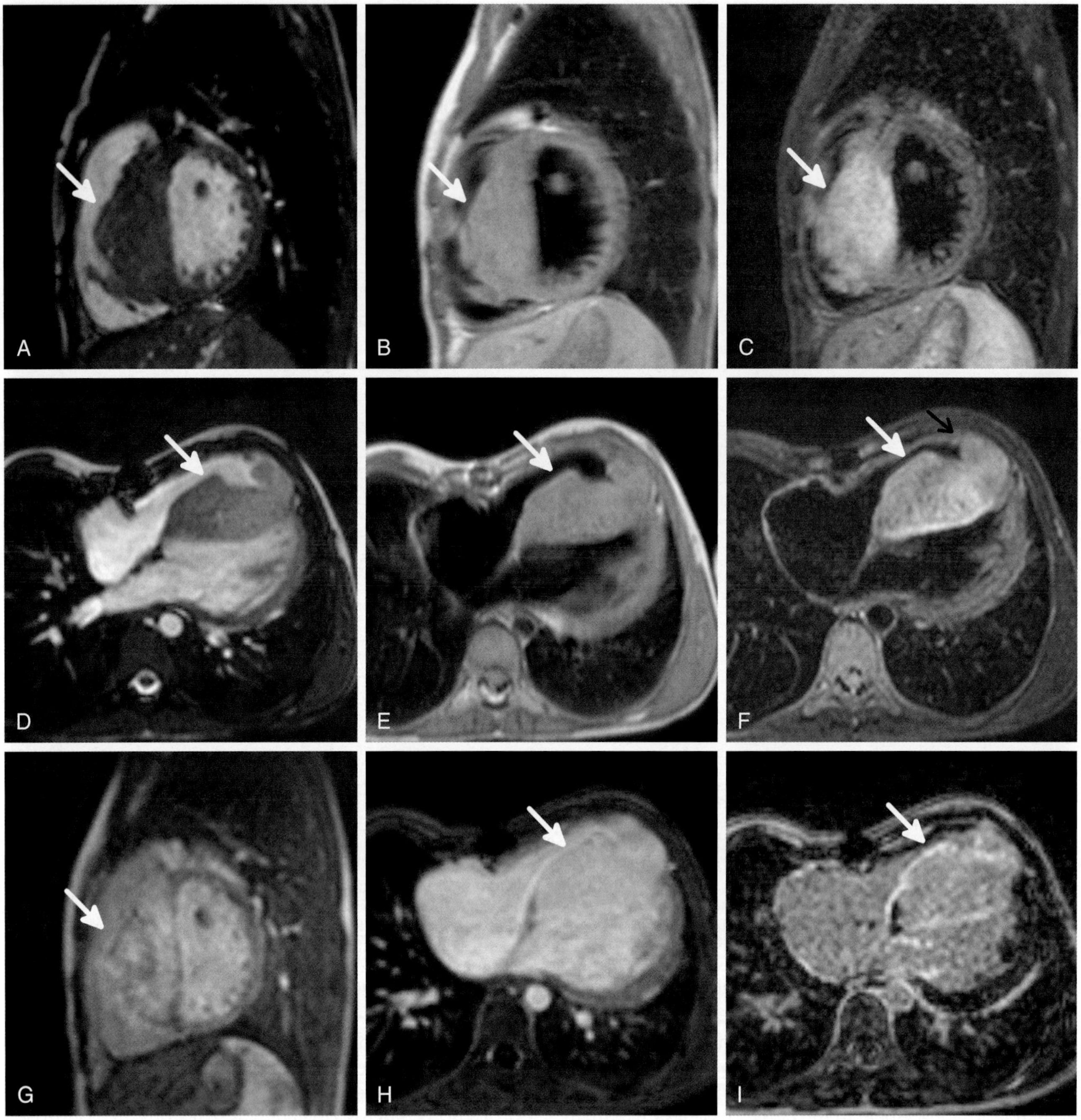

Figure 32.8 Hemangioma. The patient's hemangioma was discovered in early childhood while open heart surgery was performed to close her atrial septal defect. After several years of follow-up, the patient developed ventricular arrhythmias. Cardiac MRI was requested for further workup of the hemangioma *(white arrows)*. (A) Sagittal balanced steady-state free precession (b-SSFP) end-diastolic frame. The thickened interventricular septum and right ventricular trabeculae can be visualized. T2-/T1-weighted signal intensity is approximately equal to the myocardium. (B) Sagittal T1-weighted black blood turbo spin-echo (TSE) image. The tumor shows intermediate signal, similar to the myocardium. (C) Sagittal T2-weighted black blood TSE image. The hemangioma spans the interventricular septum and spreads into several right ventricular trabeculae. (D) Axial b-SSFP end-diastolic frame after contrast administration. The tumor developed higher T2-/T1-weighted signal intensity compared to the myocardium. (E) Axial T1-weighted black blood TSE image. The tumor shows an intermediate signal, similar to the myocardium. (F) Axial T2-weighted black blood TSE image. The hemangioma spans all along the interventricular septum and spreads into several right ventricular trabeculae and a portion of the right ventricular apex *(black arrow)*. (G) Sagittal early enhancement magnitude image after extracellular gadolinium contrast administration. The contrast uptake is nonhomogeneous, but roughly similar to the blood pool. (H) Axial early enhancement image. The enhancement resembles the blood pool. (I) Axial delayed enhancement image. The outer rim of the tumor shows hyperenhancement, whereas the vast majority of the lesion is homogeneous with that of the blood pool.

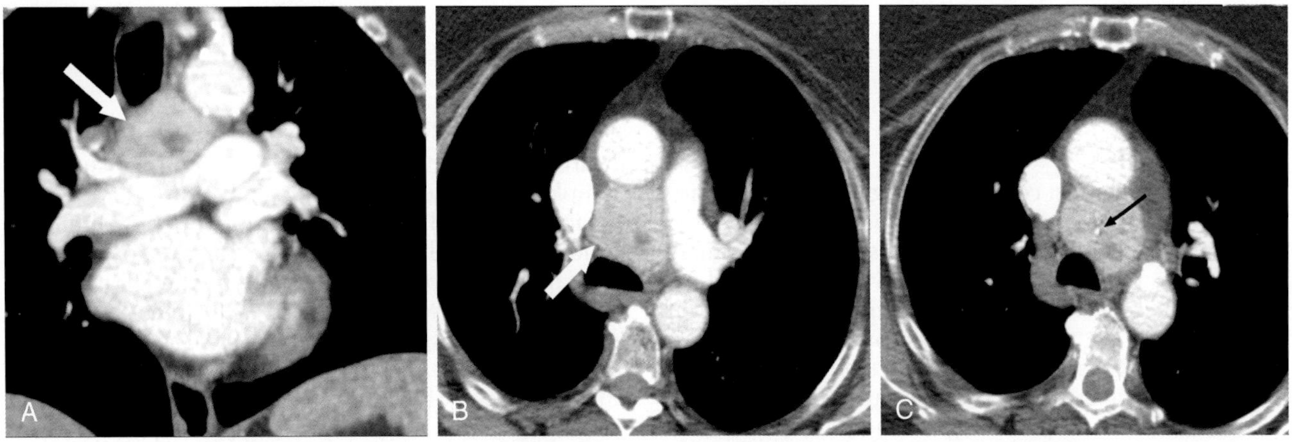

Figure 32.9 Coronal (A) and axial (B) reconstructions from a cardiac CT demonstrate an enhancing heterogenous mass *(white arrow)* between the base of the pulmonary artery and the aorta, typical location for a paraganglioma. (C) Axial reconstruction (at a level higher than B) demonstrates punctate calcification within the tumor *(black arrow)*.

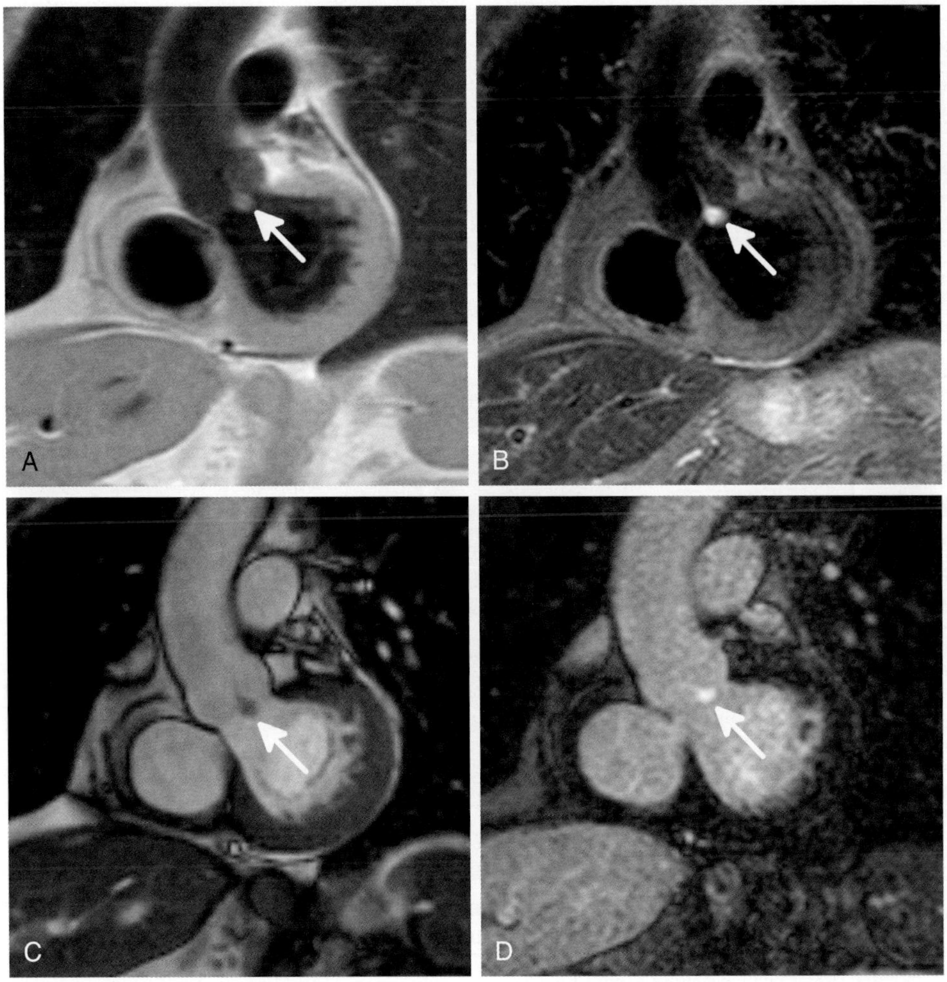

Figure 32.10 Papillary fibroelastoma of the aortic valve *(arrows)*. This may be hard to spot and depict properly on cardiac MR images due to its highly mobile nature. Unless the attaching stalk is short, the small mass can move in and out of the slice or become blurred. (A) T1-weighted, blood-suppressed, left ventricular outflow tract (LVOT) image. The mass shows intermediate signal intensity. (B) T2-weighted, blood-suppressed spectral inversion recovery, LVOT image. The tumor demonstrates high signal. (C) Balanced steady-state free precession frame in the LVOT view. The signal intensity is similar to other soft tissues. (D) Delayed enhancement image 10 to 20 minutes after extracellular gadolinium contrast material (Gd-BOPTA) administration. The mass demonstrates marked contrast accumulation, distinguishing it from thrombus.

Malignant Tumors of the Heart

Metastasis

Description

Metastasis is the most common malignancy of the heart, being approximately 30 to 40 times more common than primary lesions. Lung cancer is the most common primary malignancy to metastasize to the heart, followed by lymphoma, leukemia, breast cancer, and esophageal cancer (Figs. 32.11 to 32.14). Melanoma has the highest frequency of metastasis to the heart but, being a less common malignancy than lung and breast cancer, accounts for a lower percentage of metastatic tumors in the heart. Metastatic spread can occur via direct invasion (e.g., lung, breast, esophagus), hematogenous spread (e.g., melanoma, leukemia, lymphoma), transvenous spread via the great vessels (e.g., renal, hepatoma, adrenal cortical cancers, retroperitoneal tumors), and via mediastinal lymphatics.

Imaging

The most common site of metastatic involvement in the heart is the pericardium, usually from direct spread or lymphatic invasion. The imaging manifestations are nodular or masslike thickening of the pericardium and exudative pericardial effusion. If hemorrhagic or exudative, pericardial effusion may be hyperdense on CT and bright on T1-weighted MRI sequences. In general, most metastatic lesions to the heart are dark on T1-weighted sequences and bright on T2-weighted sequences, with the exception of melanoma, which is bright on T1 sequences. In the case of the transvenous spread of right-sided renal cancers and hepatocellular carcinomas, the inferior vena cava (IVC) may demonstrate enhancing filling defects on contrast-enhanced CT and multiphase MRI, extending into the right atrium.

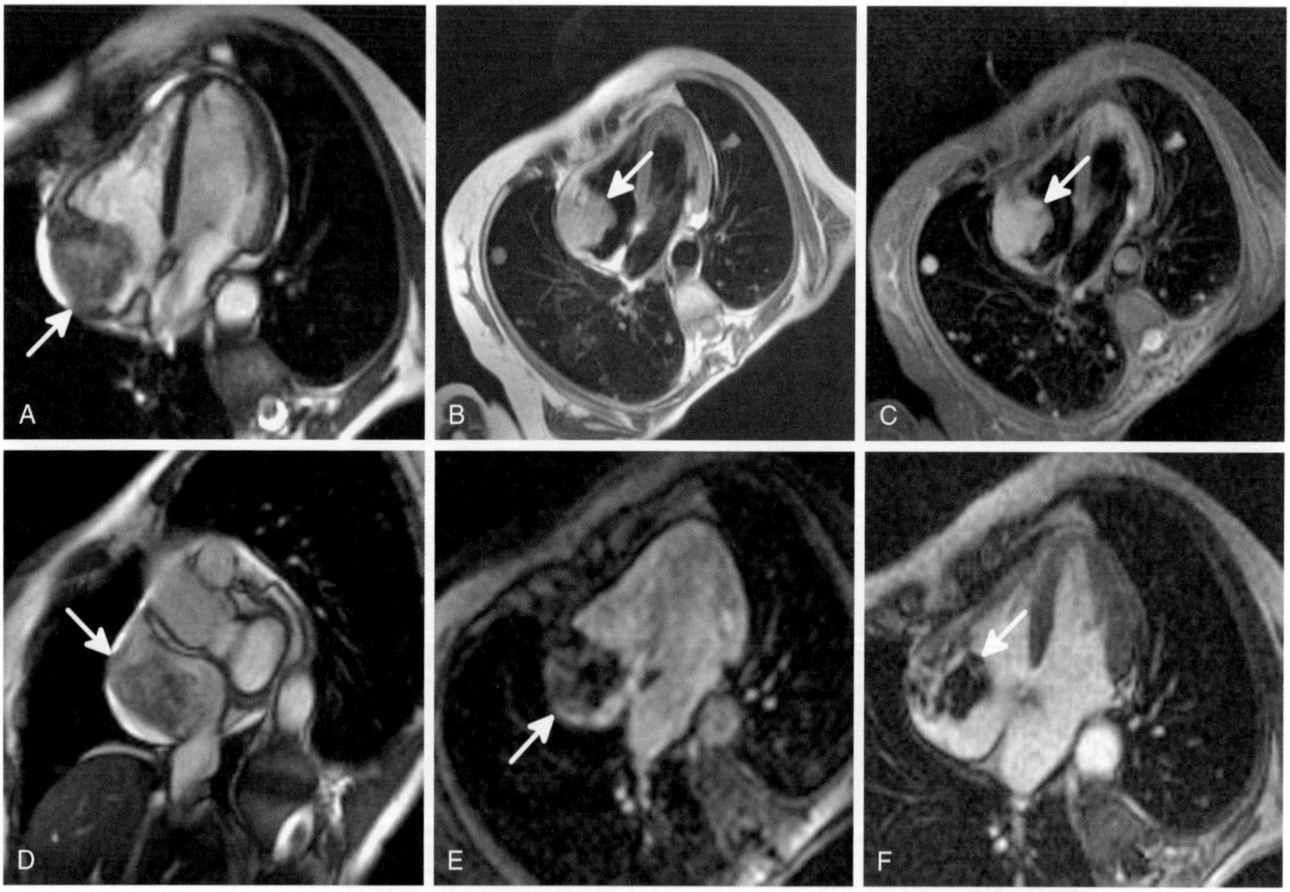

Figure 32.11 Patient with known prior breast cancer. The echocardiogram raised the suspicion of atrial metastasis. An arrow points to the tumor. (A) Four-chamber (4CH) steady-state free precession (SSFP) end-diastolic frame—nonhomogeneous tumor involving the right atrial wall, extending to the right atrioventricular groove. (B) 4CH T1-weighted black blood fast spin-echo image. The T1-weighted signal is a little brighter than the myocardium. Various metastatic nodules are seen in the lungs. (C) 4CH, T2-weighted, black blood, fat-suppressed (triple) image. Heterogeneously increased signal intensity is seen. Multiple pulmonary metastatic nodules are more obvious. (D) Short-axis SSFP end-diastolic frame after contrast material administration demonstrates heterogenous enhancement in the lesion. (E) 4CH first-pass perfusion image, nonhomogeneous early uptake, suggests that the lesion is a vascular tumor rather than a thrombus. (F) 4CH delayed enhancement image, nonhomogeneous enhancement, of the intracardiac metastatic lesion. Pulmonary nodules cannot be visualized on these images.

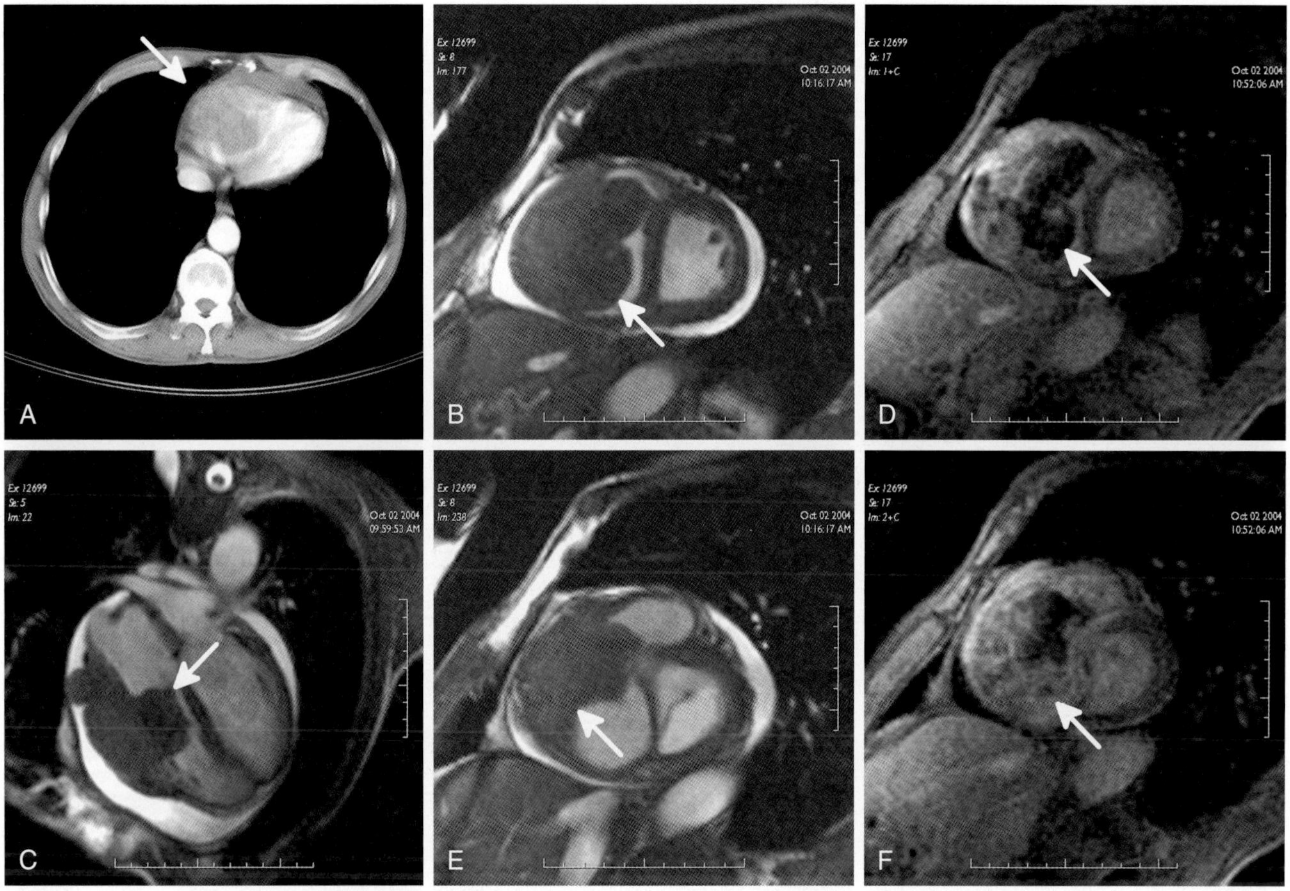

Figure 32.12 History of rectal cancer. Chest CT raised the suspicion of a metastasis in the right ventricle. An arrow points at the tumor. (A) Axial chest CT image after iodinated contrast administration demonstrates a right ventricular mass. Note pericardial effusion. (B) Short-axis (SA) steady-state free precession (SSFP) image, end-diastolic frame. The T2-/T1-weighted signal of the metastatic lesion is similar to the myocardium. There is overlying pericardial effusion. (C) SA delayed enhancement image, with nonhomogeneous contrast uptake in the metastatic lesion. (D) Four-chamber fast imaging using steady-state acquisition end-diastolic frame. The metastasis *(arrow)* crosses the border between the right atrium and ventricle, infiltrating the right atrioventricular groove, usually a sign of malignancy. (E) SA SSFP end-diastolic frame toward the base of the heart. The metastasis reaches the aortic root. (F) SA late enhancement image. Nonhomogeneous contrast uptake in the metastasis.

Primary Malignancies of the Heart

Sarcomas are the most common primary malignant neoplasm of the heart, of which angiosarcoma is the common. Primary cardiac lymphoma confined to the heart is rare, but is the second most common primary malignancy of the heart. On immunophenotyping, malignant angiosarcoma is positive for vascular markers such as CD31 and CD34; malignant lymphomas are reactive for leukocyte common antigen and pan–B cell markers such as CD20 or pan–T cell markers such as CD3. In contrast, metastatic carcinoma is generally positive for cytokeratin, and metastatic melanoma is positive for S100.

Sarcomas

Description

Sarcomas are the most common primary malignant tumors of the heart and occur mainly in adulthood, usually between the second and third decades. Overall, these tumors have a poor prognosis, with an expected mean survival rate of 25 months. Of the cardiac sarcomas, angiosarcoma is the most common, accounting for about 37% of all cases. A sarcoma with no distinct histologic pattern is considered undifferentiated sarcoma and is the second most common primary cardiac malignancy. Other rare types include synovial sarcoma, malignant fibrous histiocytoma, intimal sarcoma, osteosarcoma, and leiomyosarcoma.

Rhabdomyosarcomas are the most common primary malignancy of the heart in childhood. Angiosarcomas are more common on the right side and usually arise from the lateral wall of the right atrium; as they grow, they may grow through the epicardial fat, across the atrioventricular valve plane into the right ventricle (Fig. 32.15). According to at least one recent series, other sarcomas are equally distributed between the left and right sides of the heart. Sarcomas arising from the left side tend to be better circumscribed and less infiltrative, metastasize later, and have overall better survival.

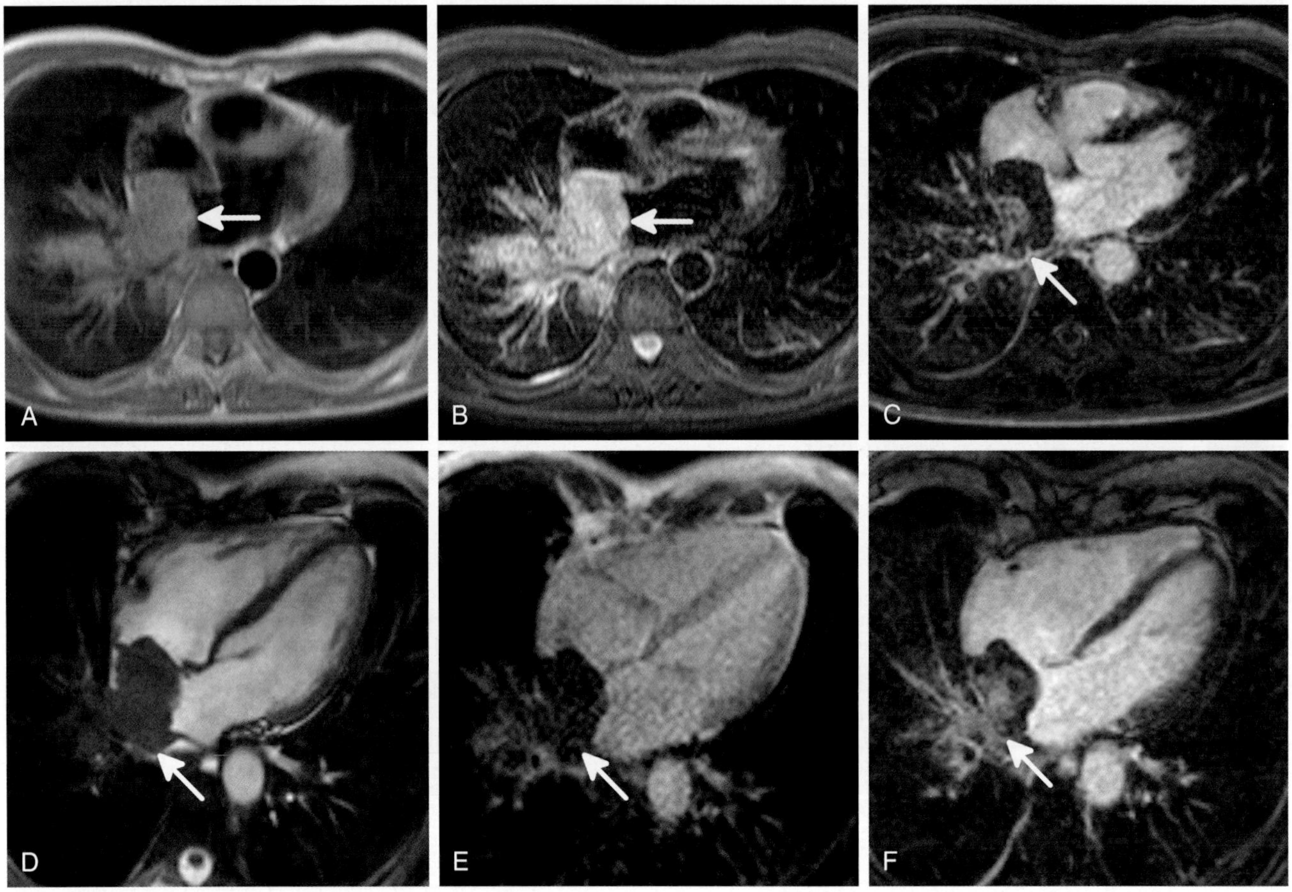

Figure 32.13 Lung cancer invading the heart. Arrows point at the tumor mass. (A) Axial blood-suppressed, T1-weighted turbo spin-echo (TSE) image. There is an intermediate signal intensity mass in the left atrium with ill-defined borders, extending across the interatrial septum into the right atrium. (B) Axial blood-suppressed, T2-weighted spectral inversion recovery TSE image. There is nonhomogeneous increased signal intensity. (C) Axial delayed enhancement inversion recovery image 10 to 20 minutes after contrast administration using inversion times to null the myocardium. The malignancy shows nonhomogeneous contrast enhancement. (D) Four-chamber (4CH) steady-state free precession end-diastolic frame. There is an intermediate T2-/T1-weighted signal in the mass. (E) 4CH first-pass perfusion frame showing nonhomogeneous contrast uptake during administration of extracellular IV contrast material (Gd-DO3A-butrol). (F) Delayed enhancement inversion recovery turbo field-echo image taken 10 to 20 minutes after contrast administration using inversion times to null the myocardium. Invading lung cancer shows nonhomogeneous contrast enhancement.

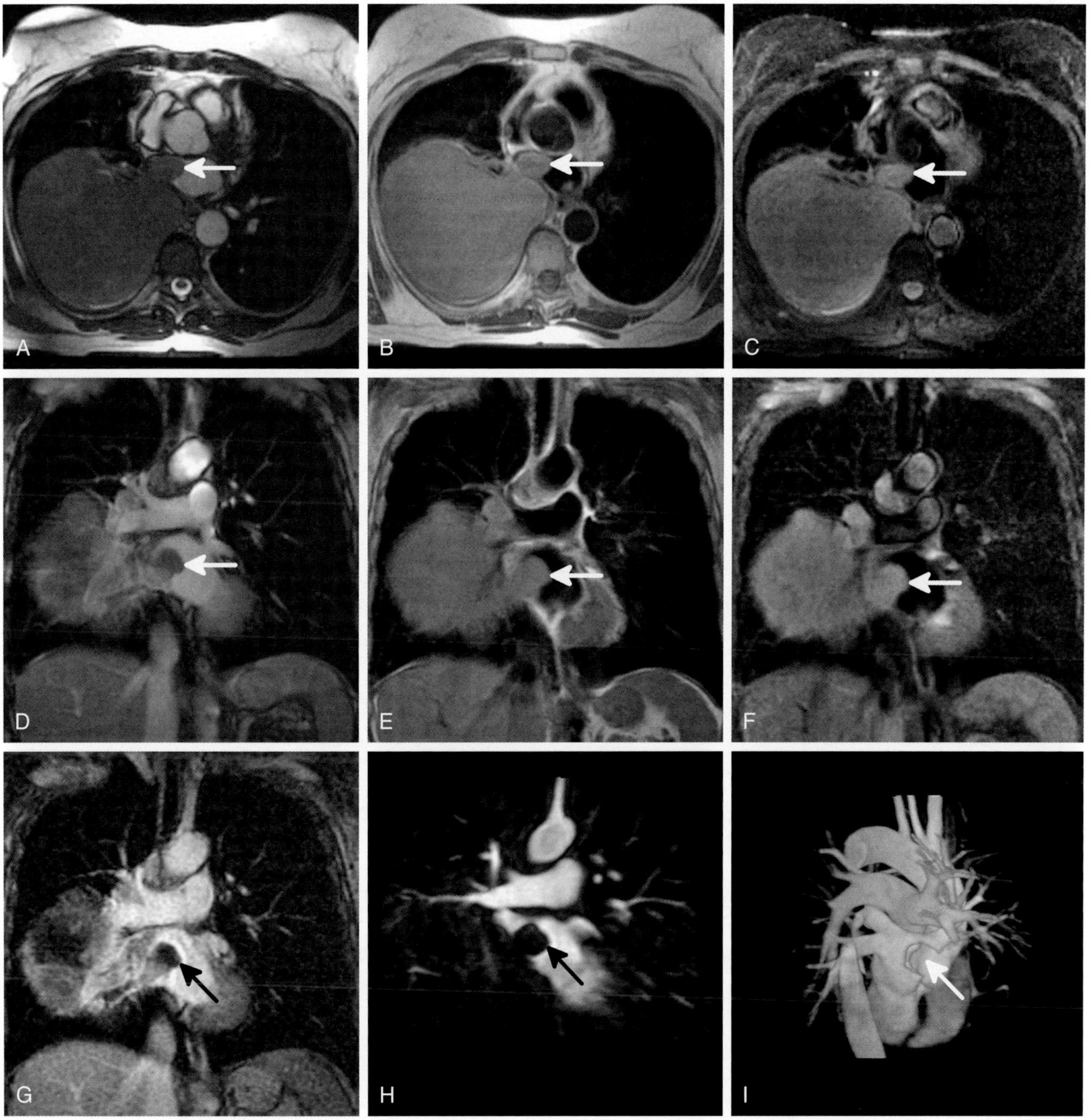

Figure 32.14 Lung cancer invading the left atrium. White arrows point to the intracardiac extension of the malignant lesion. (A) Axial cine steady-state free precession (SSFP) end-diastolic frame. There is an intermediate, slightly nonhomogeneous T2-/T1-weighted signal intensity in the tumor extending from the right lung into the left atrium. (B) Axial blood-suppressed, T1-weighted turbo spin-echo (TSE) image, intermediate heterogenous signal intensity. (C) Axial T2-weighted, black blood, fat-suppressed image, nonhomogeneous, slightly increased T2-weighted signal intensity. (D) Coronal cine SSFP end-diastolic frame, lobulated extension of the tumor into the left atrium via the right superior pulmonary vein. (E) Coronal blood-suppressed, T1-weighted TSE image, intermediate, heterogenous signal intensity. (F) Coronal T2-weighted, black blood, fat-suppressed TSE image, nonhomogeneous, slightly increased T2-weighted signal intensity. (G) Coronal early enhancement inversion recovery turbo field-echo image taken 3 to 8 minutes after contrast administration using intentionally long inversion times. Invading lung cancer shows nonhomogeneous contrast enhancement. Nonenhancing component at the tip of the invading tumor may represent thrombus *(black arrow)*. (H) Coronal thin slab maximum intensity projection of a three-dimensional contrast-enhanced magnetic resonance angiography (CE-MRA) scan taken in end-inspiration during the first pass of the extracellular gadolinium contrast agent. The black arrow points to the filling defect caused by the left atrial metastatic lesions. (I) Volume-rendered reconstruction of the CE-MRA dataset. The white arrow points to the filling defect created by the lesion.

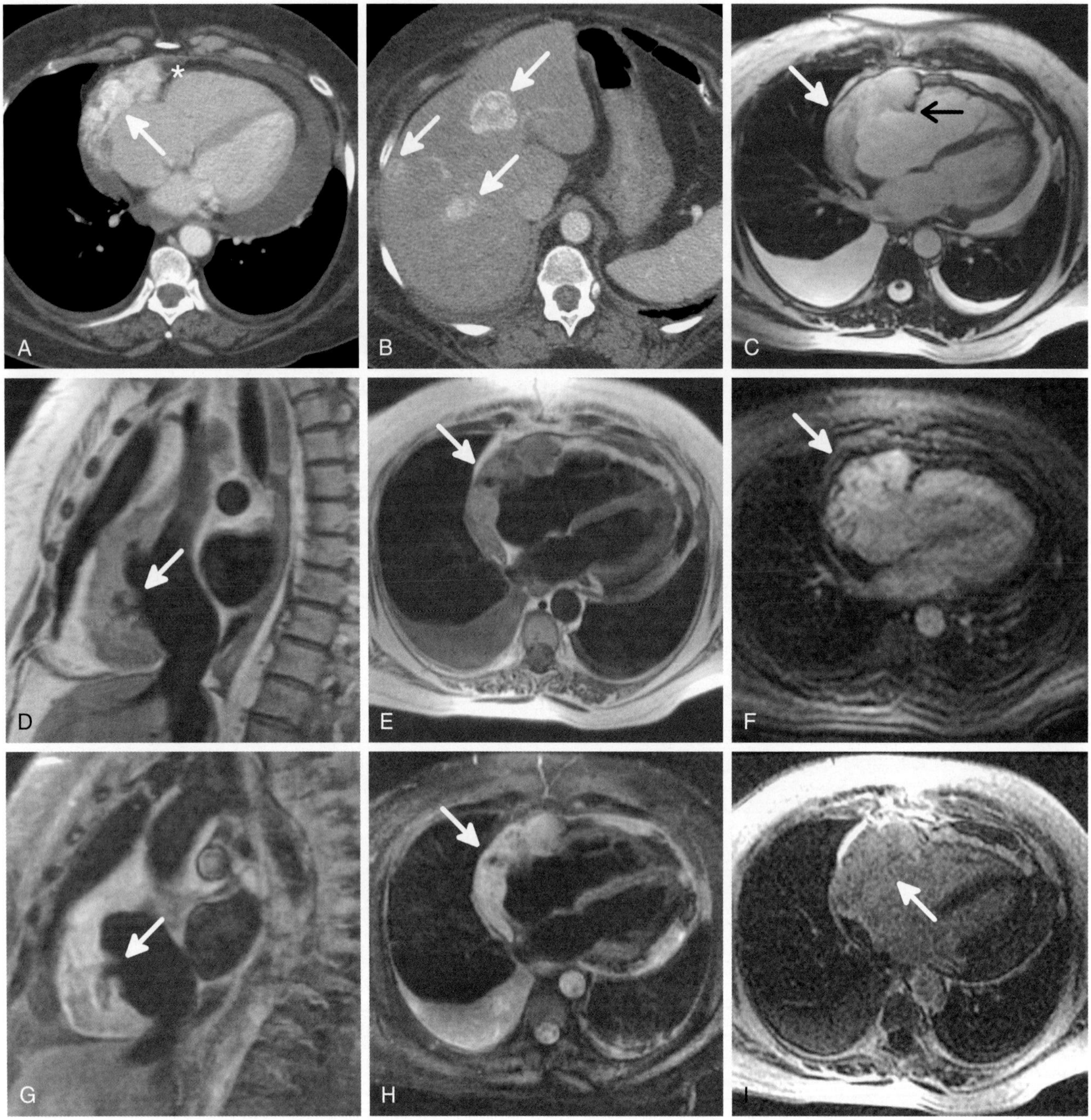

Figure 32.15 Angiosarcoma of the right atrium. (A) Axial contrast-enhanced CT image of the chest. The arrow points to the highly enhancing lesion arising from the lateral wall of the right atrium, extending through the epicardial fat, which is widened *(asterisk)* into the pericardium. Note pericardial effusion. (B) Axial contrast-enhanced CT image of the abdomen. The arrows point to hypervascular metastatic lesions of the liver. (C) Axial steady-state free precession end-diastolic frame. An angiosarcoma *(white arrow)* arising from the lateral and posterior wall of the right atrium extends to the right atrioventricular groove *(black arrow)*. (D) Sagittal T1-weighted black blood fast spin-echo (FSE) image showing the angiosarcoma arising from the right atrium *(arrow)*. (E) Axial T1-weighted, black blood FSE image. The signal void in the tumor *(arrow)* is due to the vascular spaces within. (F) First-pass perfusion image taken during extracellular contrast material administration (gadodiamide), with high-contrast uptake *(arrow)*. (G) Sagittal T2-weighted black blood FSE fat-suppressed (triple) image. Heterogeneously increased signal intensity within the tumor *(arrow)*, volcano-like extension into the right atrial chamber. (H) Axial T2-weighted, black blood FSE, fat-suppressed (triple) image. The tumor is hyperintense *(arrow)*, with pericardial and pleural effusion. (I) Axial late enhancement magnitude image, with inversion time set to null the myocardium. The tumor's contrast material accumulation is similar to the blood pool *(arrow)*.

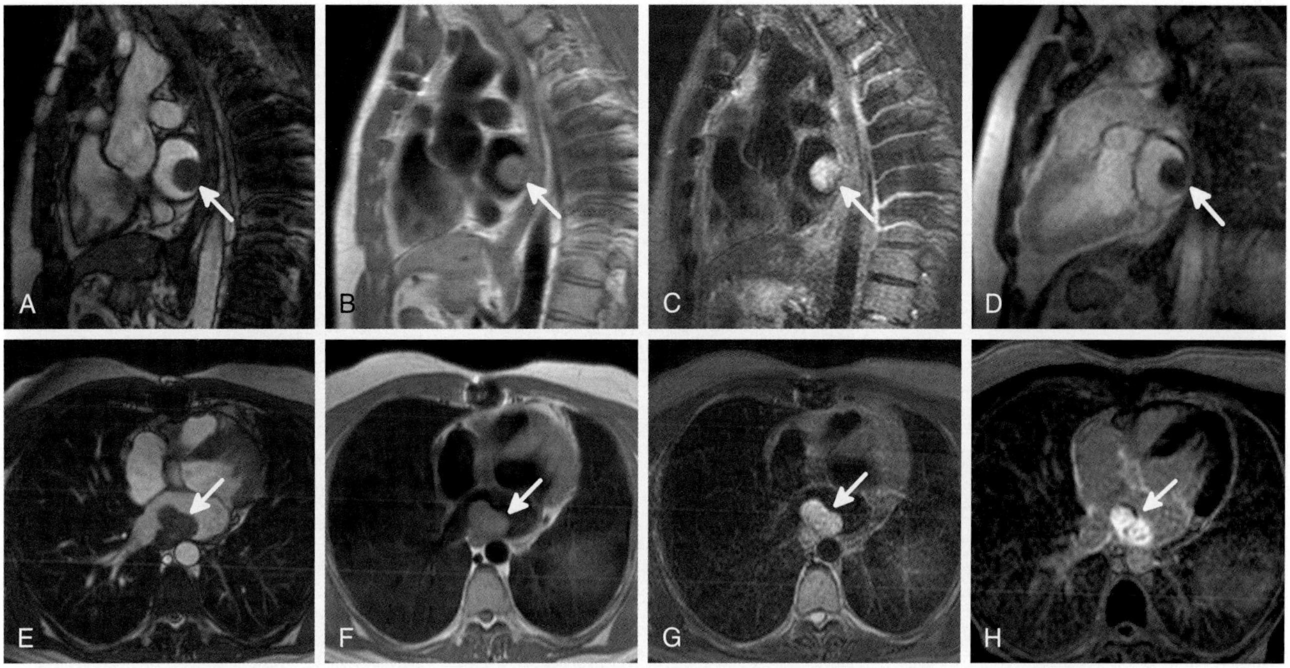

Figure 32.16 Recurrent high-grade myxofibrosarcoma of the left atrium. There was previous left atrial high-grade myxofibrosarcoma removal. Arrows point at the sarcoma. (A) Sagittal steady-state free precession. There is an intermediate T2-/T1-weighted signal intensity lesion arising from the posterior wall of the left atrium. (B) Sagittal blood-suppressed, T1-weighted turbo spin-echo (TSE) image, with intermediate signal intensity of the same lesion. (C) Sagittal black blood, T2-weighted TSE image, with inhomogeneously increased T2-weighted signal intensity. (D) First-pass perfusion frame in a two-chamber view showing nearly absent contrast uptake during IV administration of extracellular contrast material (Gd-DO3A-butrol). (E) Axial cine balanced steady-state free precession end-diastolic frame, intermediate signal intensity lobulated lesion. (F) Axial blood-suppressed, T1-weighted TSE image. The lesion is isointense to muscle. (G) Axial black blood, T2-weighted, spectral inversion recovery TSE image. There is nonhomogeneous increased T2-weighted signal intensity. (H) Axial delayed enhancement inversion recovery image taken 10 to 20 minutes after contrast administration using inversion times to null the myocardium. Recurrent myxofibrosarcoma shows marked late gadolinium accumulation.

Angiosarcomas usually present with right-sided heart failure, hemorrhagic pericardial effusions, and metastasis. Microscopically, angiosarcomas are comprised of rapidly proliferating anaplastic cells derived from blood vessels and line irregular, fluid-filled spaces. There are usually extensive areas of hemorrhage and necrosis in the tumor. Macroscopically, there are two morphologic variants, the focal type, which is a well-defined intracavitary mass protruding into the right atrium, and the diffuse type, which rapidly involves the right ventricle and pericardium and presents with right heart failure and cardiac tamponade.

Imaging

On imaging, angiosarcomas may appear as well-defined or diffusely infiltrating right-sided masses, depending on the subtype. Pericardial involvement appears as thickening, effusion, nodularity, or frank disruption of fat planes. On MRI, the tumors demonstrate heterogeneous T1 and T2 signals due to tumor necrosis or hemorrhage, avid enhancement on first-pass perfusion due to vascularity, and heterogeneous enhancement on delayed hyperenhancement images. Osteosarcomas demonstrate surface calcifications on CT. Other sarcomas usually appear as broad-based filling defects. Several of these arise from the left atrium, a rather common site of origin for sarcomas, and may involve the pulmonary veins (Figs. 32.16 and 32.17).

Lymphoma

Description

Lymphomatous involvement of the heart is usually a component of disseminated disease, and primary cardiac lymphoma is rare, accounting for about 1% of primary cardiac tumors, making it the second most common primary malignancy of the heart. Most of these tumors are of the B cell phenotype. There has been a slight increase in primary cardiac lymphoma in recent years due to association with Epstein-Barr virus–related-lymphoproliferative disorders, which occur in patients with HIV infection and transplant recipients. However, overall, more primary cardiac lymphomas occur in immunocompetent patients than in immunocompromised individuals.

Imaging

Lymphomas usually manifest as diffuse infiltrating microlobulated masses with patchy enhancement, often with associated pericardial effusion (Figs. 32.18 and 32.19). The most common sites of involvement are the atria, with

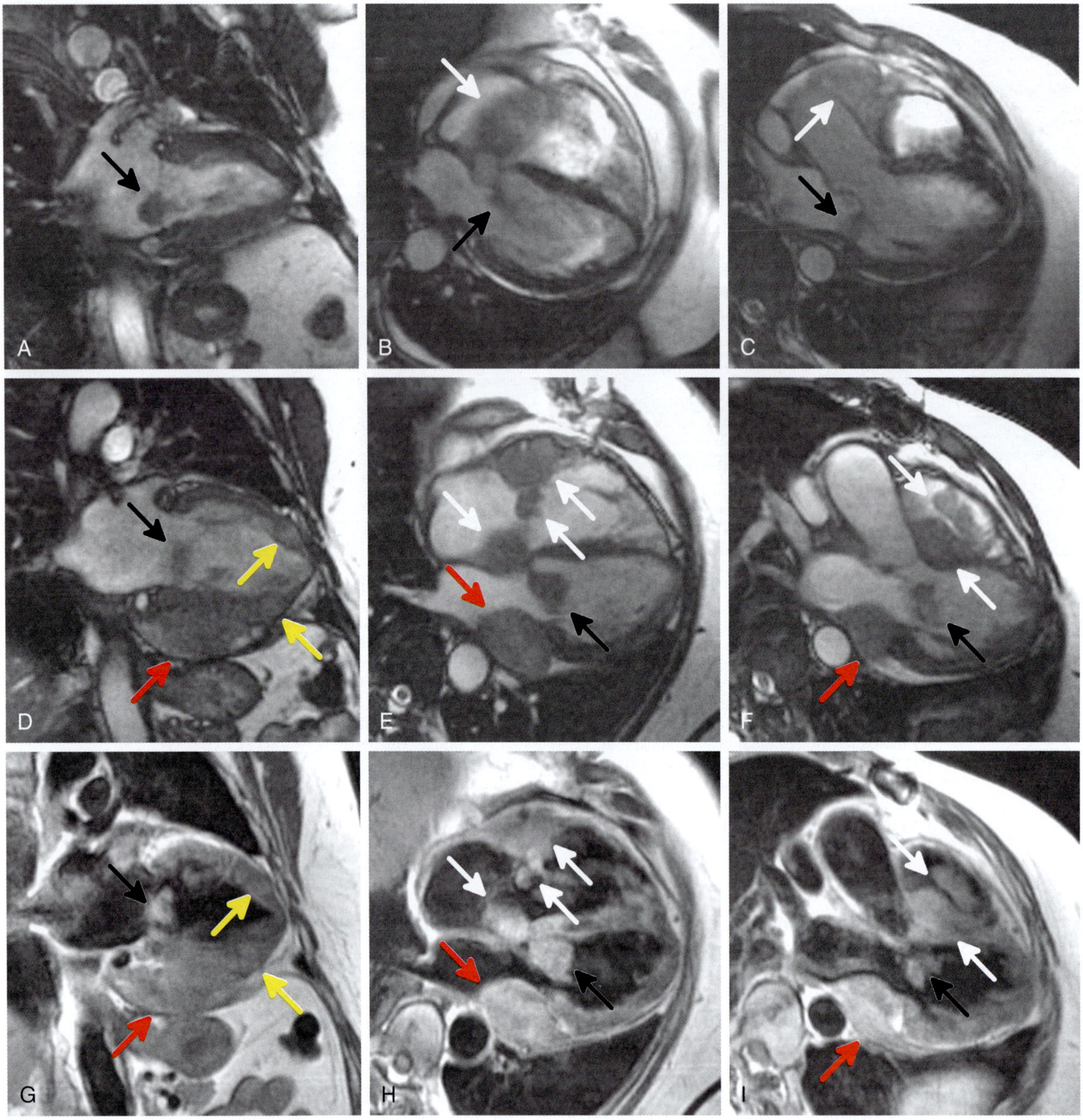

Figure 32.17 Synovial fibrosarcoma. (A–C) Initial examination. Two-chamber (2CH; A), four-chamber (4CH; B) and three-chamber (3CH; C) steady-state free precession (SSFP) images. This tumor on the mitral valve is projecting into the left atrium *(black arrow)*. A bulky tumor, also on the tricuspid valve, is extending into the right ventricular outflow tract (RVOT; *white arrow*). The patient refused all treatment options. (D-I) Follow-up examination 8 months later. The patient agreed to get treatment, but it was too late by that time. (D) Follow-up 2CH SSFP, end-systolic frame. A new lesion showed up in the anteroapical wall and apex *(yellow arrows)*. Another new bulky lesion can be spotted in the left and inferior pericardial space, extending into the left atrioventricular groove *(red arrow)*. (E) Follow-up 4CH SSFP, end-systolic frame. The tricuspid lesion *(white arrows)* has become larger and has spread to the right atrioventricular groove. The mitral lesion is much larger *(black arrow)*. Note a new lesion in the left atrioventricular groove, contiguous with the pericardial lesion *(red arrow)*. (F) 3CH SSFP image. Invasion of the RVOT has progressed *(white arrows)*, with enlargement of the mitral lesion *(black arrow)*. A new lesion in the left atrioventricular groove is contiguous with the pericardial lesion *(red arrow)*. (G) 2CH, T1-weighted black blood fast spin-echo (FSE) image. The left ventricular anteroapical lesions *(yellow arrows)* and the pericardial space lesions *(red arrow)* show slightly inhomogeneous, intermediate signal intensity. Note the heterogenous mitral lesion *(black arrow)*. (H) 4CH T2-weighted, black blood FSE fat-suppressed image. Heterogeneously increased signal intensity within the tricuspid lesion is now extending into the right atrioventricular groove *(white arrows)*. The mitral lesion is much larger *(black arrow)*. Note a new lesion in the left atrioventricular groove contiguous with the pericardial lesion *(red arrow)*. (I) 3CH T2-weighted, black blood FSE fat-suppressed image. There is inhomogeneous signal intensity of the lesions, mostly higher compared to the myocardium. Invasion of the RVOT has progressed *(white arrows)*. There is enlargement of the mitral lesion *(black arrow)*. A new lesion in the left atrioventricular groove is contiguous with the pericardial lesion *(red arrow)*.

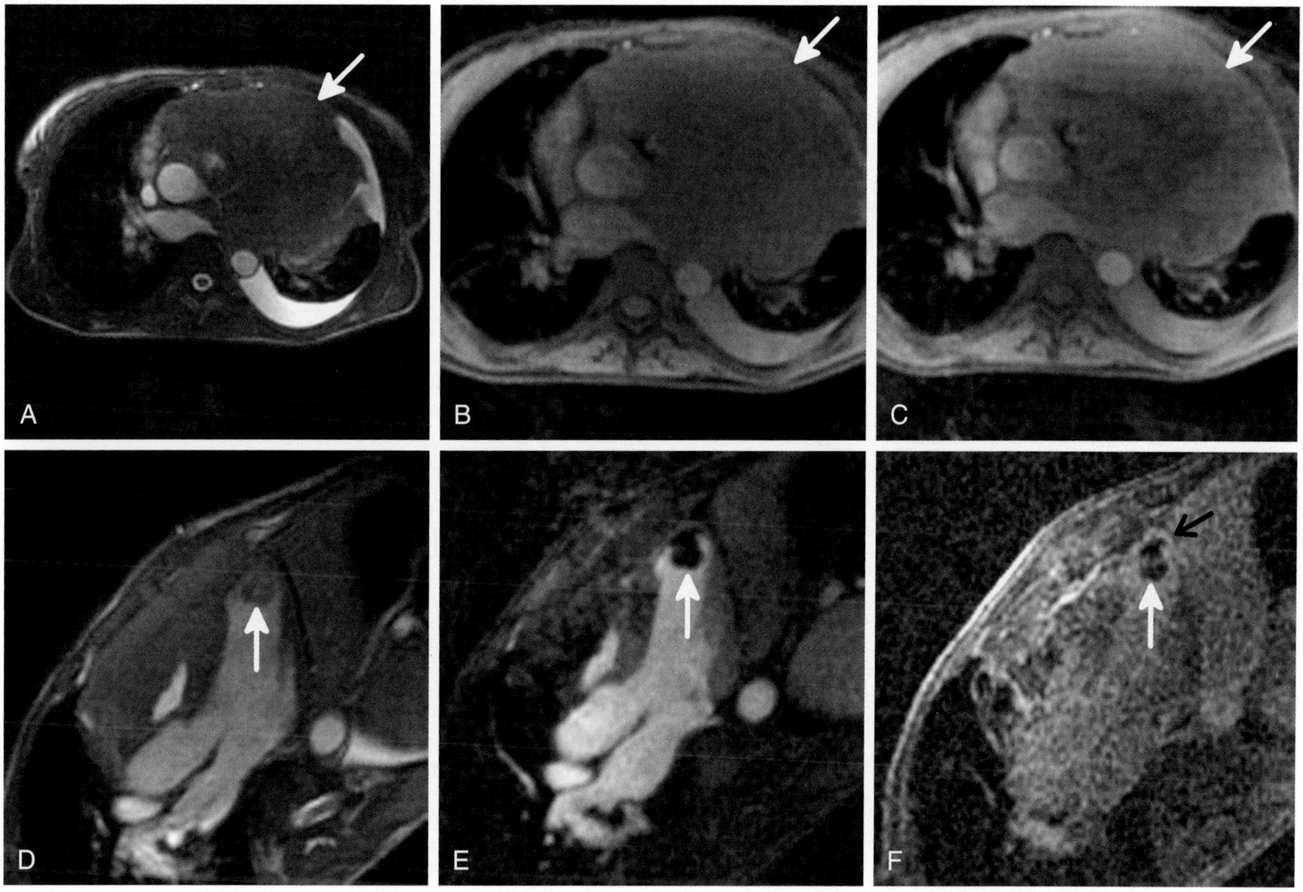

Figure 32.18 Diffuse large cell non-Hodgkin lymphoma. The patient also has an apical infarct, with a thrombus. (A) Axial fast imaging employing steady-state acquisition (FIESTA) end-diastolic frame. A large mediastinal tumor *(white arrow)* is encasing the aortic root, the left main coronary artery, and its bifurcation. Pleural effusion on the left side. (B) Axial fat suppressed gradient echo (GRE) image before contrast administration. There is a heterogeneous intermediate signal in the tumor *(white arrow)*. (C) Axial fat-suppressed GRE image after contrast administration (extracellular gadolinium), with nonhomogeneous enhancement in the tumor mass *(white arrow)*. (D) Three-chamber (3CH) FIESTA, end-diastolic frame. There is an apical filling defect *(white arrow)*. The apical myocardium is thin and was akinetic. (E) 3CH early enhancement image, with no contrast uptake in the apical abnormality, represents a thrombus *(white arrow)*. (F) 3CH late enhancement image Hyperenhancement of the apex *(black arrow)* represents an infarct; the thrombus *(white arrow)* is adjacent to the infarct.

the right atrium more common than the left. Within the right atrium, the free wall is the most common site of involvement. A right atrial lymphoma may extend into the right ventricle across the atrioventricular groove, with encasement of the right coronary artery. Angiosarcoma of the heart may have a similar pattern of involvement; a clue to distinction on imaging is that involvement of the intervening valve favors angiosarcoma. Valves lack lymphatics and are therefore spared in lymphoma.

Metastatic lesions and Erdheim-Chester disease are other entities that cross the right atrioventricular groove. In the heart, involvement of the right-sided chambers is usually a sign of malignancy (Fig. 32.20). On CT, lymphoma appears as hypoattenuating or isoattenuating masses relative to the myocardium, which demonstrate heterogeneous enhancement. On MRI, these lesions are isointense to hypointense on T1-weighted images and isointense to hyperintense on T2-weighted images. Although cardiac lymphoma is usually associated with pericardial effusion, a variant known as *primary effusion lymphoma* presents as pericardial effusion only. The effusion in these cases is usually large, may progress to cardiac tamponade, and is associated with a concomitant diagnosis of Kaposi sarcoma.

■ Anatomic Variants and Mimics

Anatomic Variants

Crista terminalis is a well-defined fibromuscular ridge along the posterior wall of the right atrium that extends from the superior vena cava to the IVC; it marks the fusion plane of the smooth posterior wall and trabeculated anterior wall of the right atrium (Fig. 32.21). In the adult, the crista terminalis acts as the anatomic boundary between the right atrium and right atrial appendage and

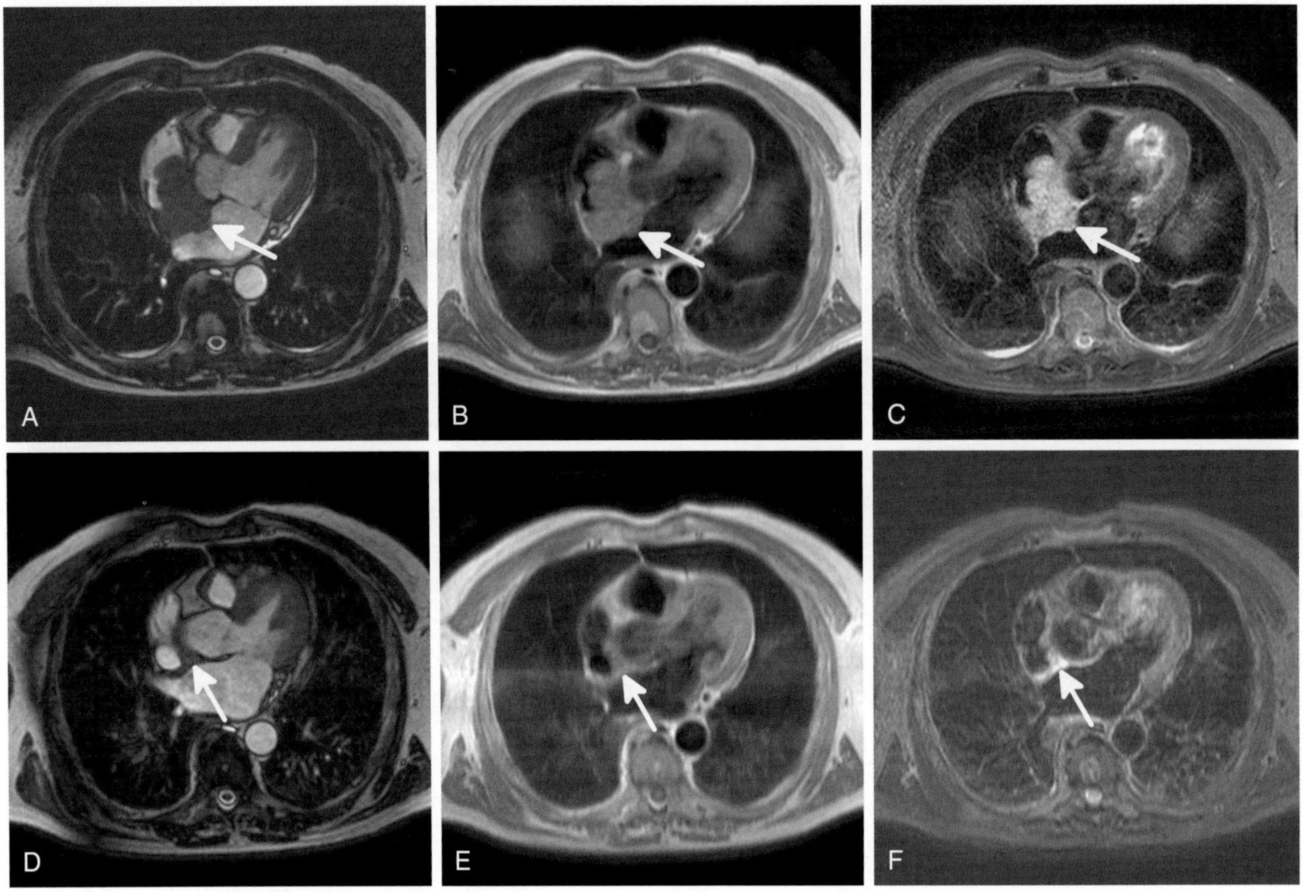

Figure 32.19 Large B cell lymphoma *(arrows)* before (A–C) and after (D–F) chemotherapy. Cardiac MRI demonstrates a good response, with a small residual mass. (A) Axial balanced steady-state free precession (b-SSFP) end-systolic frame. Tumor involves the right atrium, extends into the interatrial septum and left atrium, and surrounds the aortic root. The T2-/T1-weighted signal is roughly similar to the myocardium. (B) Axial T1-weighted, black blood, turbo spin-echo (TSE) image. Nonhomogeneous intermediate signal intensity can be visualized. (C) Axial T2-weighted, black blood TSE, spectral inversion recovery (SPIR) image. The tumor demonstrates high signal intensity. (D) Axial b-SSFP end-systolic frame. There is a significant reduction in size due to chemotherapy. (E) Axial T1-weighted, black blood, TSE image. There is a very small residual tumor in the interatrial septum. (F) Axial T2-weighted, black blood TSE, SPIR image. There is a very small residual tumor tumor in the interatrial septum

serves as the point of attachment of the anterior pectinate muscles. The taenia sagittalis are the most prominent of these pectinate muscles and appear as chords arising from the crista terminalis, coursing anteriorly. The CT scan can have a wide range of appearances, from stubby to long and thin. Crista terminalis may be mistaken for thrombus or tumor, particularly on echocardiography, but is easily characterized on CT and MRI by its typical location and appearance.

A remnant of the fetal eustachian valve may be seen at the junction of the IVC with the right atrium. The thebesian valve is seen at the junction of the coronary sinus with the right atrium in about 40% of cases. Awareness of these valves and their anatomic location allows distinction from masses.

A coumadin ridge is the junction of the left superior pulmonary vein and left atrial appendage; it may be mistaken for a mass when it is bulbous.

Thrombus

A thrombus is the most common intracardiac space-occupying lesion. The most common site is in the left atrial appendage, but it can occur anywhere. Thrombi may be seen in low-flow states associated with intracardiac aneurysms and pseudoaneurysms in the ventricles or in cardiomyopathies, or they may be attached to indwelling catheters and lines that terminate in the heart (Fig. 32.22). Thrombi may also form on the surface of intracardiac neoplasms. Thrombi are typically homogenous and nonenhancing on CT. Left atrial appendage thrombi are distinguished from slow flow by delayed-phase imaging, where a thrombus persists as a filling defect. Blooming of blood products in conjunction with nonenhancement on the postgadolinium sequences helps make a confident diagnosis (Fig. 32.23). Chronic thrombi may demonstrate calcification or some degree of neovascularity.

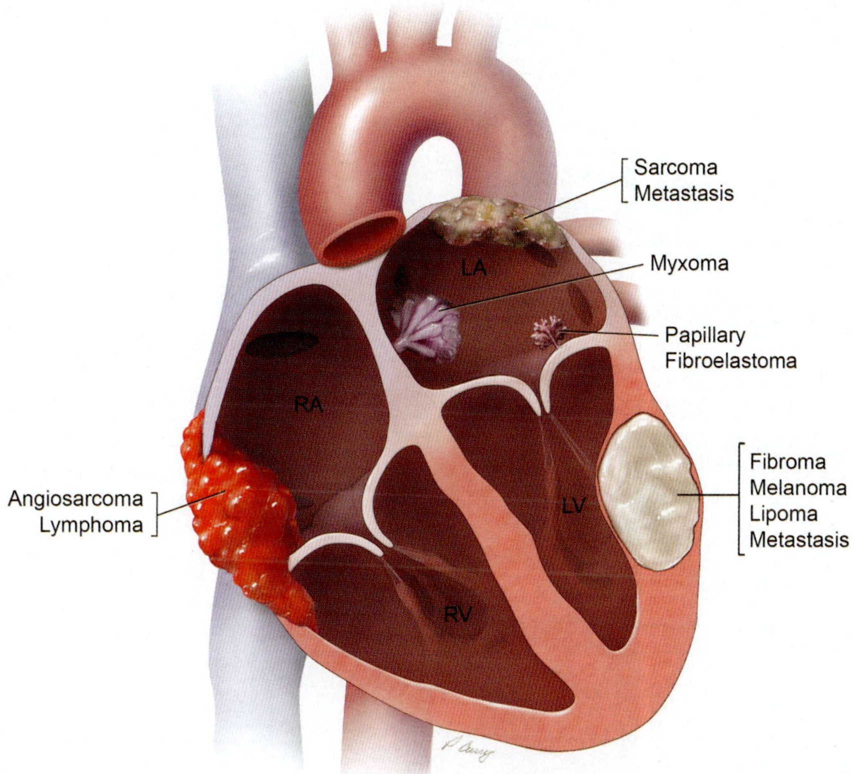

Figure 32.20 Common tumors of the heart and their typical locations. Angiosarcoma and lymphoma can occur in the free wall of the right atrium *(RA)*, extending into the right ventricle *(RV)*. Other tumors and their locations: other sarcomas, posterior wall of left ventricle *(LV)*; melanomas and metastasis, can occur anywhere; myxoma, left atrium *(LA)* attached to the fossa ovalis; papillary fibroelastoma on valves; fibroma, lipoma, intramural, often in the LV. (Courtesy Pam Curry, UT Southwestern Medical Center, Dallas.)

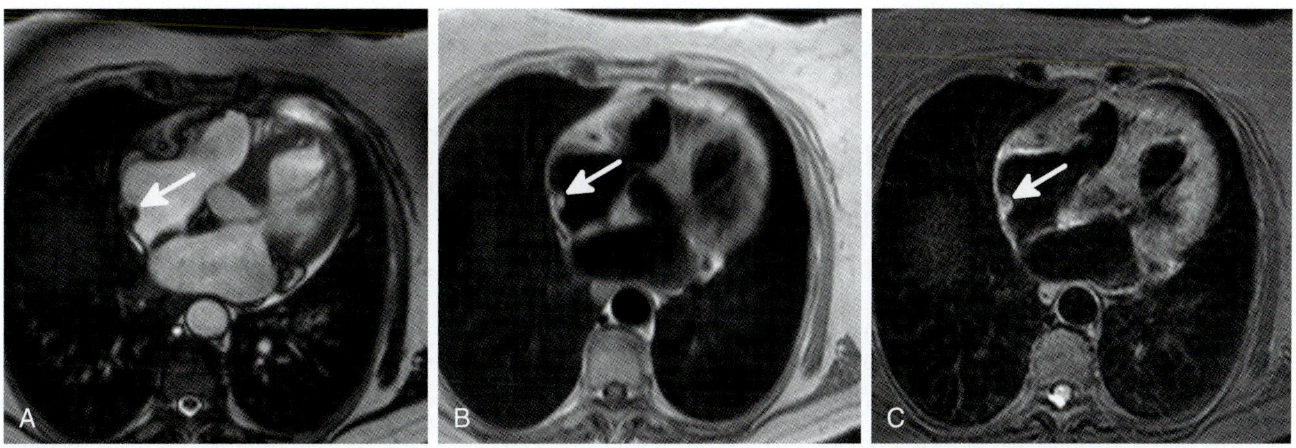

Figure 32.21 Crista terminalis. This echocardiogram raised the suspicion of a right atrial tumor. Cardiac MRI scans demonstrate a normal anatomic structure crista terminalis *(arrows)* along the posterior wall of the right atrium. Sometimes it can appear as a craniocaudal stringlike structure separated from the right atrial wall, called *taenia sagittalis*. (A) Axial balanced steady-state free precession end-systolic frame. (B) Axial T1-weighted black blood turbo spin-echo (TSE) image. (C) Axial T2-weighted black blood TSE spectral inversion recovery for fat suppression image.

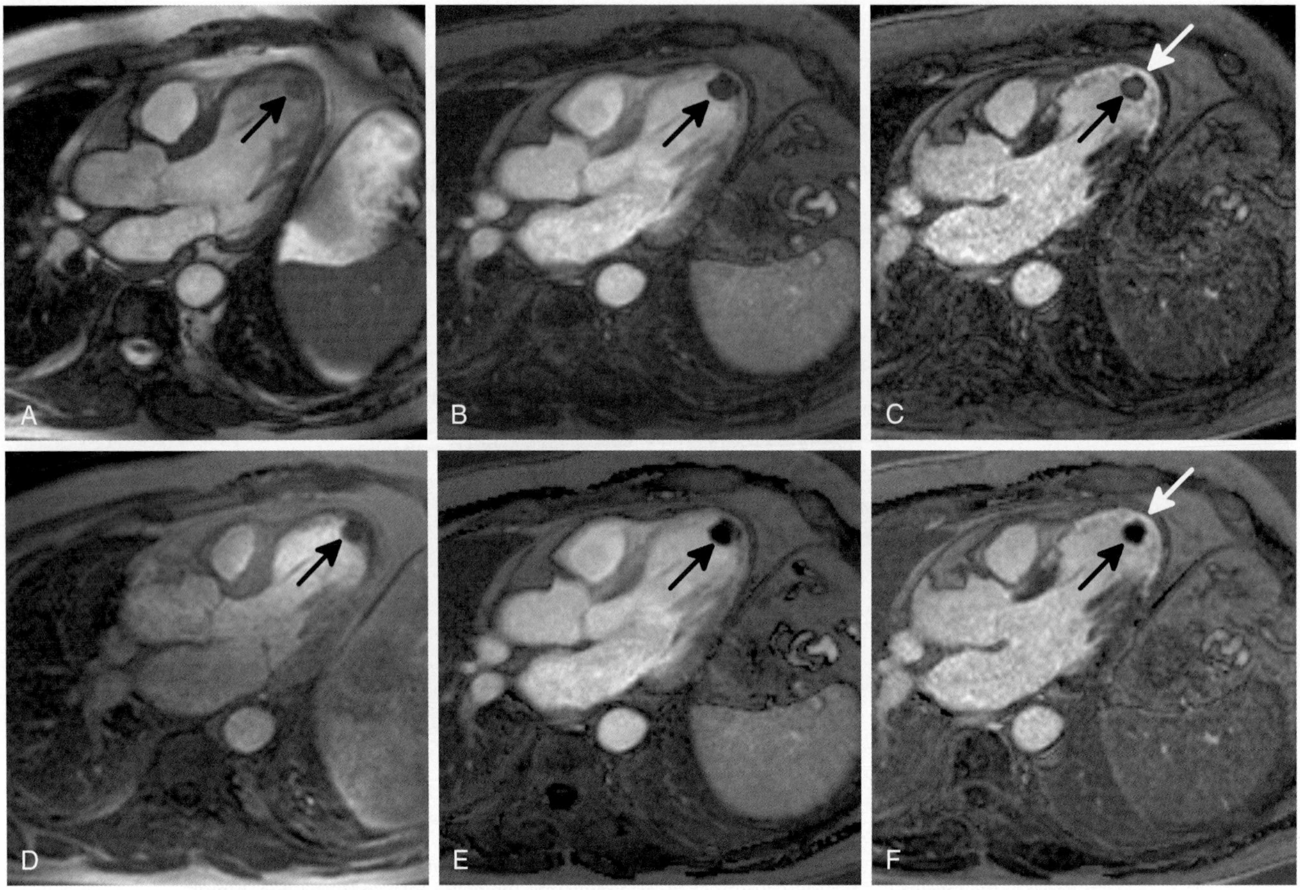

Figure 32.22 Apical thrombus (dark signal; *black arrows*) after an apical myocardial infarction in left anterior descending artery territory in a patient with left ventricular noncompaction and an apical infarction scar (bright enhancement; *white arrows*). (A) Left ventricular outflow tract (LVOT) balanced steady-state free precession end-diastolic frame. (B) LVOT early enhancement magnitude image. (C) LVOT late enhancement magnitude image. (D) First-pass perfusion, k-t BLAST, balanced turbo field-echo image showing lack of first-pass uptake in the thrombus *(black arrow)* and the apical infarction scar. (E) LVOT early enhancement phase-sensitive inversion recovery (PSIR) image. (F) LVOT delayed enhancement PSIR image. It is important to examine PSIR images because a thrombus may show increased signal on magnitude images due to the relatively short inversion time used. Do not be fooled by the bright signal in the middle of a thrombus on the magnitude image (C); a negative signal can cause this. Rely on the PSIR images instead.

Caseous Mitral Annular Calcification

A caseous mitral annular calcification usually involves the posterior mitral annulus and may be mistaken for a mass. CT is the definitive modality for diagnosis and shows a peripheral rim of calcification and central lower density homogenous (caseous) material that represents liquefied calcium and tissue. Caseous mitral annular calcification is also referred to as a *toothpaste tumor* by surgeons because of the intraoperative appearance of the caseous material (Figs. 32.24 and 32.25).

Hypertrophic Cardiomyopathy

A focal, masslike, and apical type of cardiomyopathy may present with localized thickening of the myocardium on imaging. In hypertrophic cardiomyopathy, this so-called lesion will follow the myocardium on all imaging sequences and may demonstrate some contractility on cine MRI evaluation.

Erdheim-Chester Disease

Erdheim-Chester disease, or syndrome (also known as *polyostotic sclerosing histiocytosis*), is a non–Langerhans cell histiocytosis characterized by a mononuclear infiltrate consisting of lipid-laden foamy histiocytes. It is a multisystem disease that may involve the heart, usually the pericardium, right atrium, and atrioventricular groove. Another pattern of involvement is the periarterial type, which, in the heart, manifests as soft tissue infiltration around the coronary arteries or around the aorta. There is almost always associated characteristic bony involvement, with bilaterally symmetric, lower extremity, long bone diaphyseal and metaphyseal sclerosis and relative sparing of the epiphysis. Other sites of involvement are the central

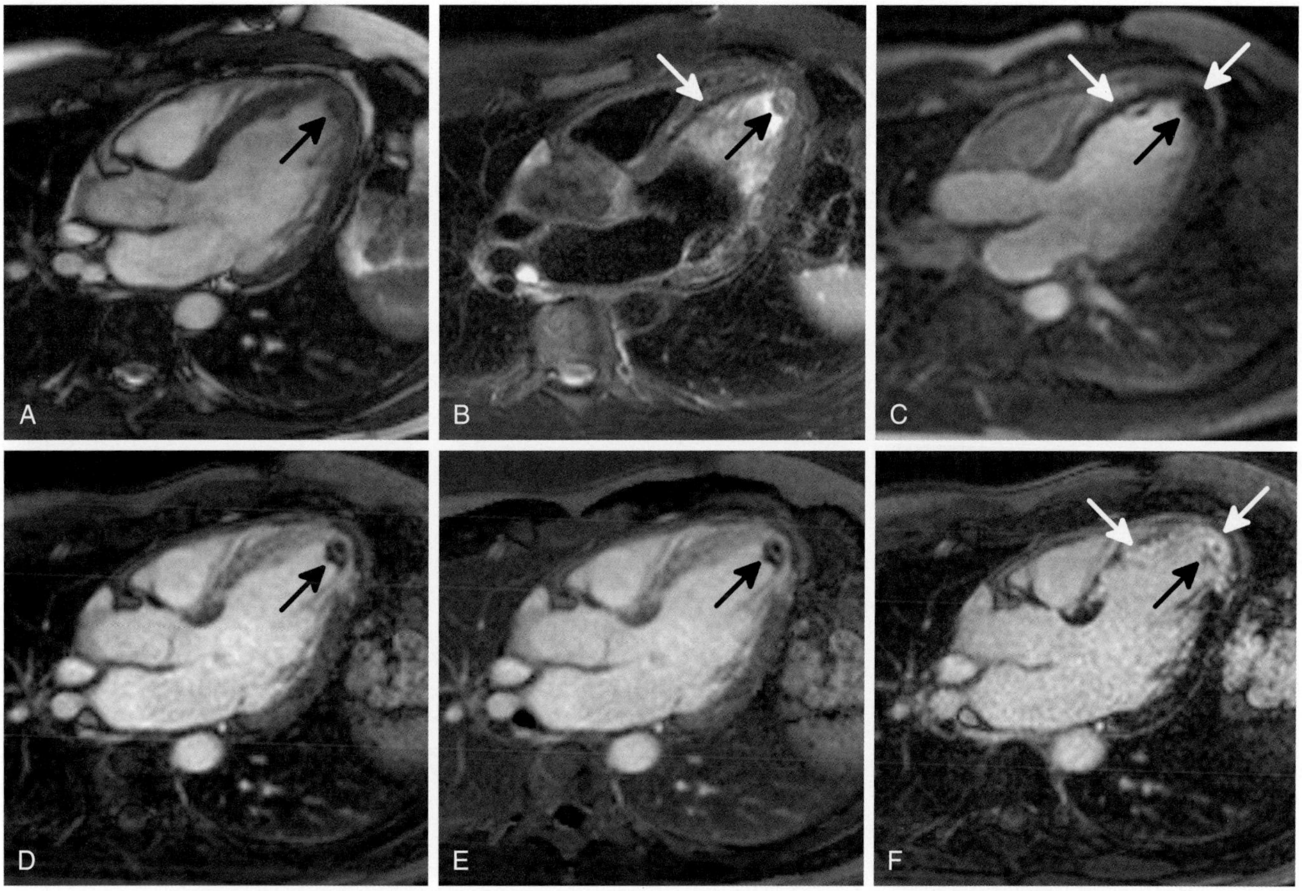

Figure 32.23 Organized apical thrombus in left anterior descending artery territory infarction; apical thrombus (dark signal, *black arrow*), infarcted myocardium *(white arrow)*. (A) Left ventricular outflow tract (LVOT) balanced steady-state free precession end-diastolic frame. (B) LVOT T2-weighted black blood spectral inversion recovery for fat suppression image. An apical bright signal is caused by slow-flowing blood in the apex due to the wall motion abnormality caused by the infarction. The white arrow points to the infarction scar; chronic infarcts contain dense connective tissue. (C) First-pass perfusion k-t BLAST balanced turbo field-echo LVOT image showing lack of first-pass uptake in the thrombus *(black arrow)* and apical infarction scar *(white arrows)* as well. (D) LVOT early enhancement magnitude image, with inner bright signal in the middle of the thrombus. (E) LVOT early enhancement phase-sensitive inversion recovery image, with an inner signal in the thrombus. (F) LVOT delayed enhancement magnitude image. The thrombus almost completely accumulated contrast material in the late phase. This is the sign of an organized thrombus. Compare this enhancement to the apical thrombus shown before.

nervous system, orbits, lungs, adrenal glands, and kidneys. Diagnosis is confirmed by biopsy (Fig. 32.26).

Pericardial Neoplasms

Pericardial Cysts

Description

Pericardial cysts, also termed *mesothelial cysts,* are congenital lesions, formed due to aberrant formation of the somatic cavities. They are generally unilocular and are lined by a single layer of mesothelial cells, supported by an outer layer of thick connective tissue. The most common location of pericardial cysts is the right cardiophrenic angle, followed by the left cardiophrenic angle and then by locations elsewhere in the mediastinum.

Imaging

Pericardial cysts are usually found incidentally on imaging. On CT, they appear as well-defined, nonhomogeneous, fluid-attenuating lesions that contain no internal septa. On MRI, cysts demonstrate low signal on T1-weighted sequences and high signal on T2-weighted sequences and are typically nonenhancing (Fig. 32.27). Pericardial cysts with proteinaceous material or hemorrhagic material demonstrate an intermediate signal on CT and high to intermediate signal on T1-weighted images.

Pericardial Mesothelioma

Description

Primary pericardial mesothelioma is extremely rare, but is the most common primary malignancy of the

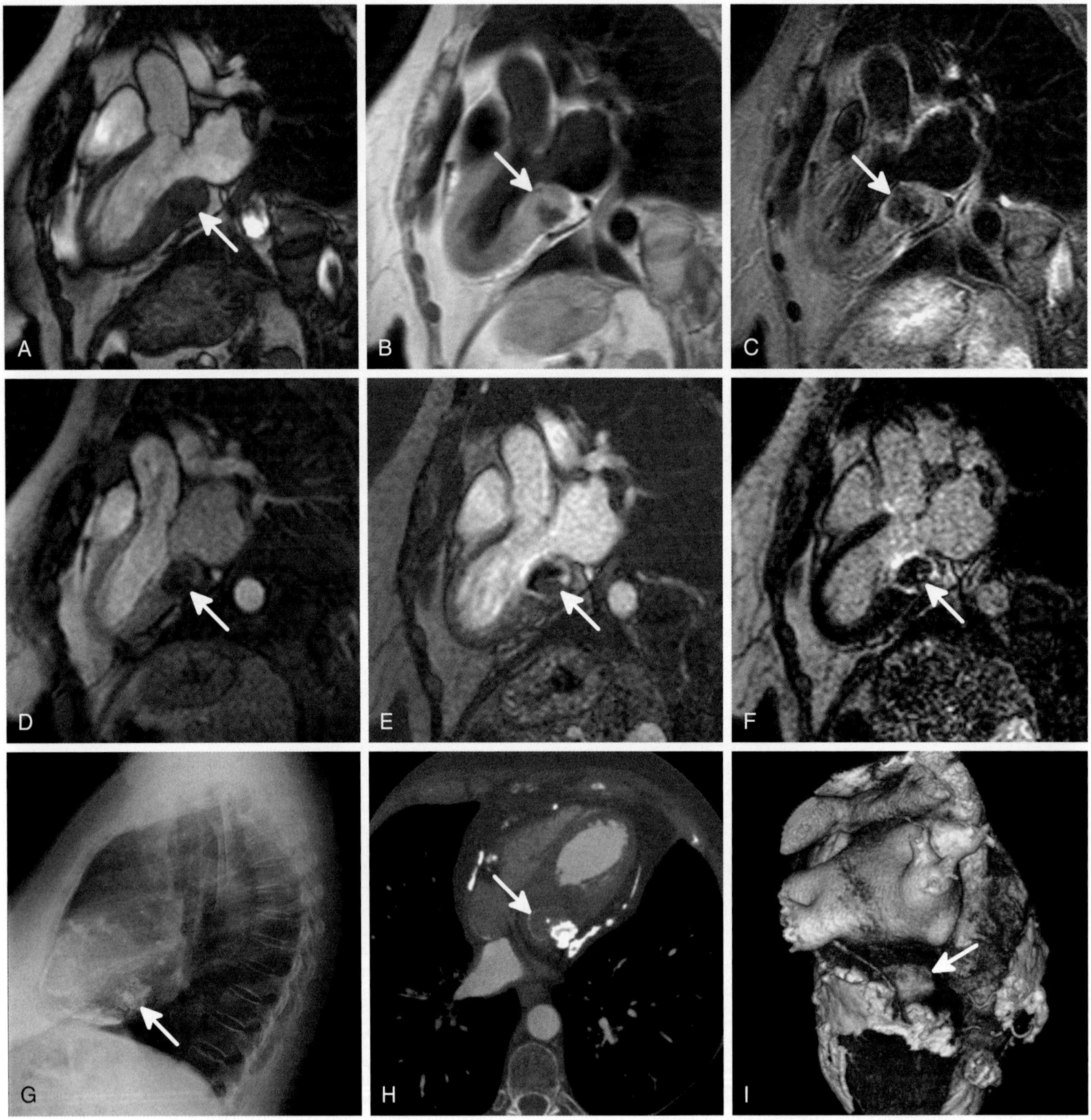

Figure 32.24 Caseous mitral annular calcification. The arrows point to the caseous mitral annular calcification. (A) Left ventricular outflow tract (LVOT) balanced steady-state free precession end-diastolic frame; slightly low T2-/T1-weighted signal. (B) LVOT T1-weighted black blood turbo spin-echo (TSE) image. The outer border has increased signal in contrast to the central dark signal. (C) LVOT T2-weighted black blood TSE spectral inversion recovery for fat suppression image. The abnormality has an increased signal compared to the myocardium. The outer rim shows a slightly increased signal. (D) First-pass perfusion k-t BLAST balanced turbo field-echo LVOT image, with lack of first-pass uptake. (E) LVOT early enhancement magnitude image. The outer rim shows enhancement and nearly completely absent inner uptake. (F) LVOT delayed enhancement magnitude image, enhancement of the outer border with no central uptake. (G) Lateral chest x-ray. The basal inferolateral calcification is delineated. Coarse pericardial calcification is also present. (H) Axial image of the cardiac CT examination. Inferolateral mitral calcification and pericardial calcium both can be seen. (I) Volume-rendered reconstruction of a cardiac CT scan; pericardial and mitral annular calcifications.

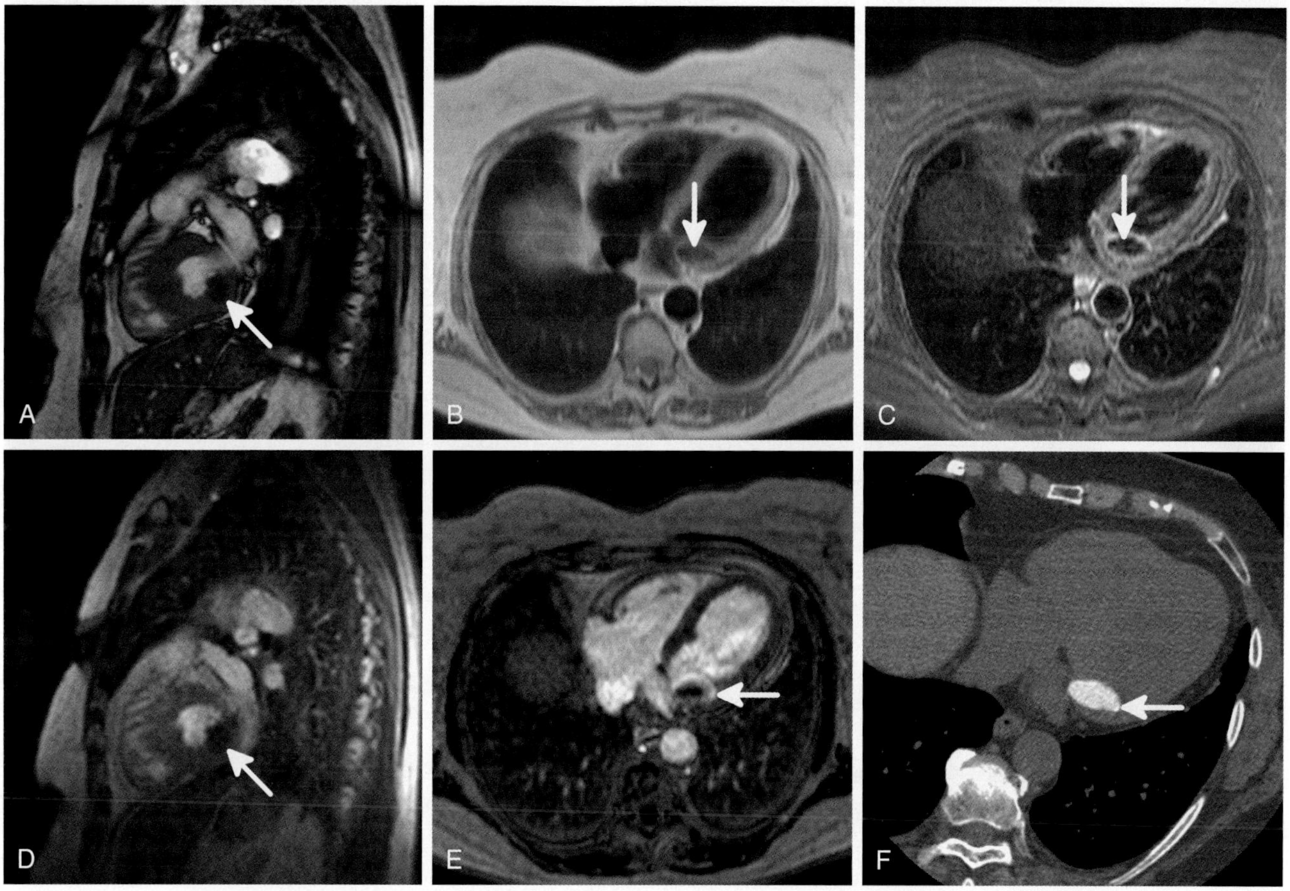

Figure 32.25 Caseous mitral annular calcification *(arrows)*. (A) Sagittal (left ventricular outflow tract) balanced steady-state free precession end-diastolic frame. There is a lower T2-/T1-weighted signal compared to the myocardium. (B) Axial T1-weighted black blood turbo spin-echo (TSE) image, with reduced signal centrally. (C) Axial T2-weighted black blood TSE spectral inversion recovery for fat suppression image. The abnormality has increased signal compared to the myocardium; the outer rim shows slightly increased signal. (D) First-pass perfusion k-t BLAST balanced turbo field-echo sagittal image with lack of first-pass uptake. (E) Axial late enhancement magnitude image, with delayed enhancement of the outer border with lack of central uptake. (F) Axial image of the cardiac CT examination. Inferolateral calcification can be clearly differentiated.

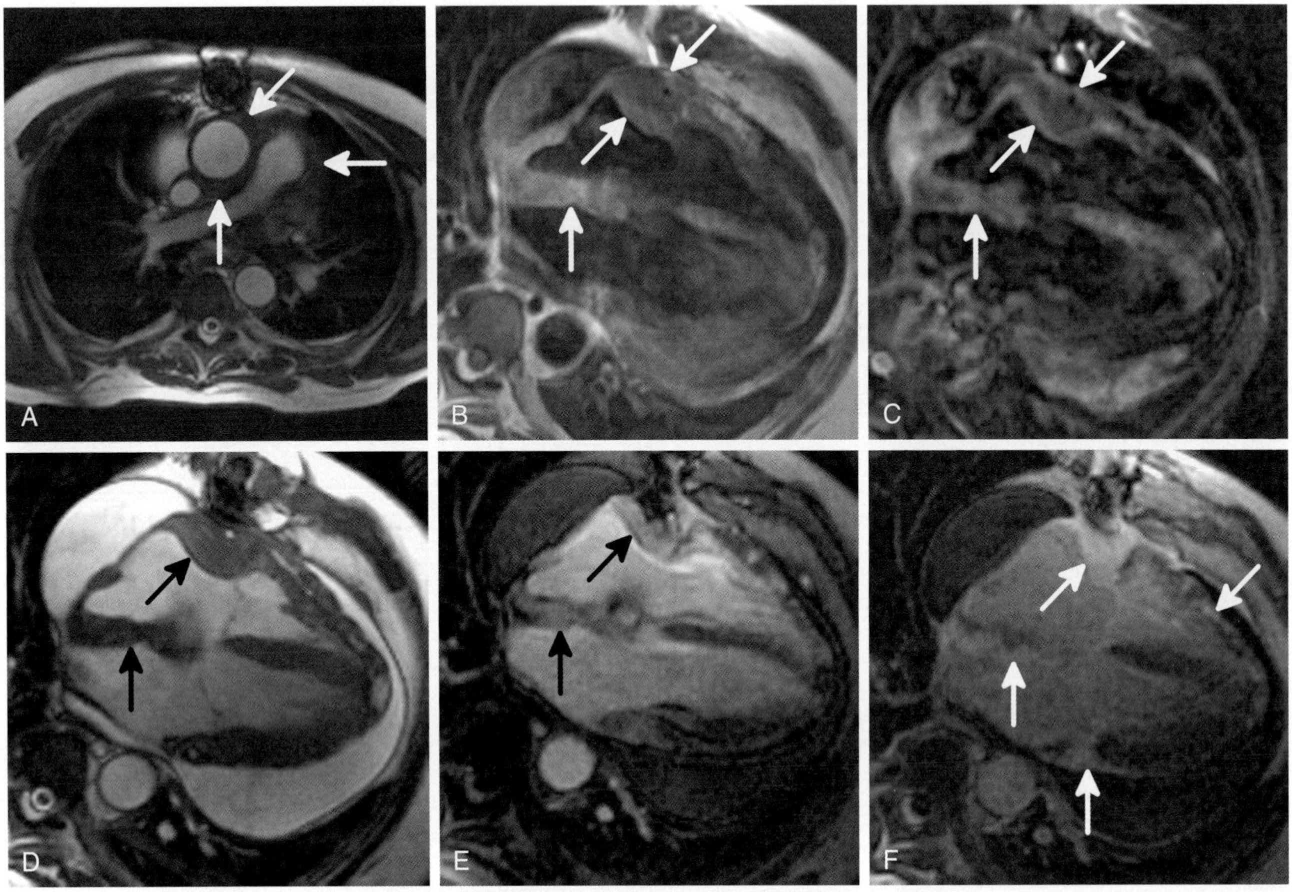

Figure 32.26 Erdheim-Chester disease. The patient had bilateral exophthalmus for years and pericardial effusion refractory to treatment. Pericardial window surgery raised the suspicion of a disseminated tumor. Cardiac MRI scan showed multilocular involvement of the cardiovascular structures caused by non-Langerhans cell histiocytosis. Black and white arrows point to the diffusely infiltrative disease. (A) Axial fast imaging employing steady-state acquisition (FIESTA) end-diastolic frame, thickening of the ascending aorta and pulmonary trunk. This is called the *coated aorta sign*. (B) Four-chamber (4CH) T1-weighted black blood fast spin-echo (FSE) image. There is thickening of the interatrial septum and involvement of the atrioventricular groove. Note thickening along the right atrioventricular groove, usually a sign of malignancy, but also seen in Erdheim-Chester disease. (C) 4CH T2-weighted black blood FSE fat-suppressed (triple) image. There is heterogeneously increased signal because of the infiltration. (D) 4CH FIESTA end-diastolic frame. The T2-/T1-weighted signal is similar to that of the myocardium. (E) 4CH early enhancement image, increased early uptake in the thickened structures. (F) 4CH late enhancement image, marked delayed enhancement of the thickened atrial wall and atrioventricular groove. There are also spots of enhancement along the right ventricular surface.

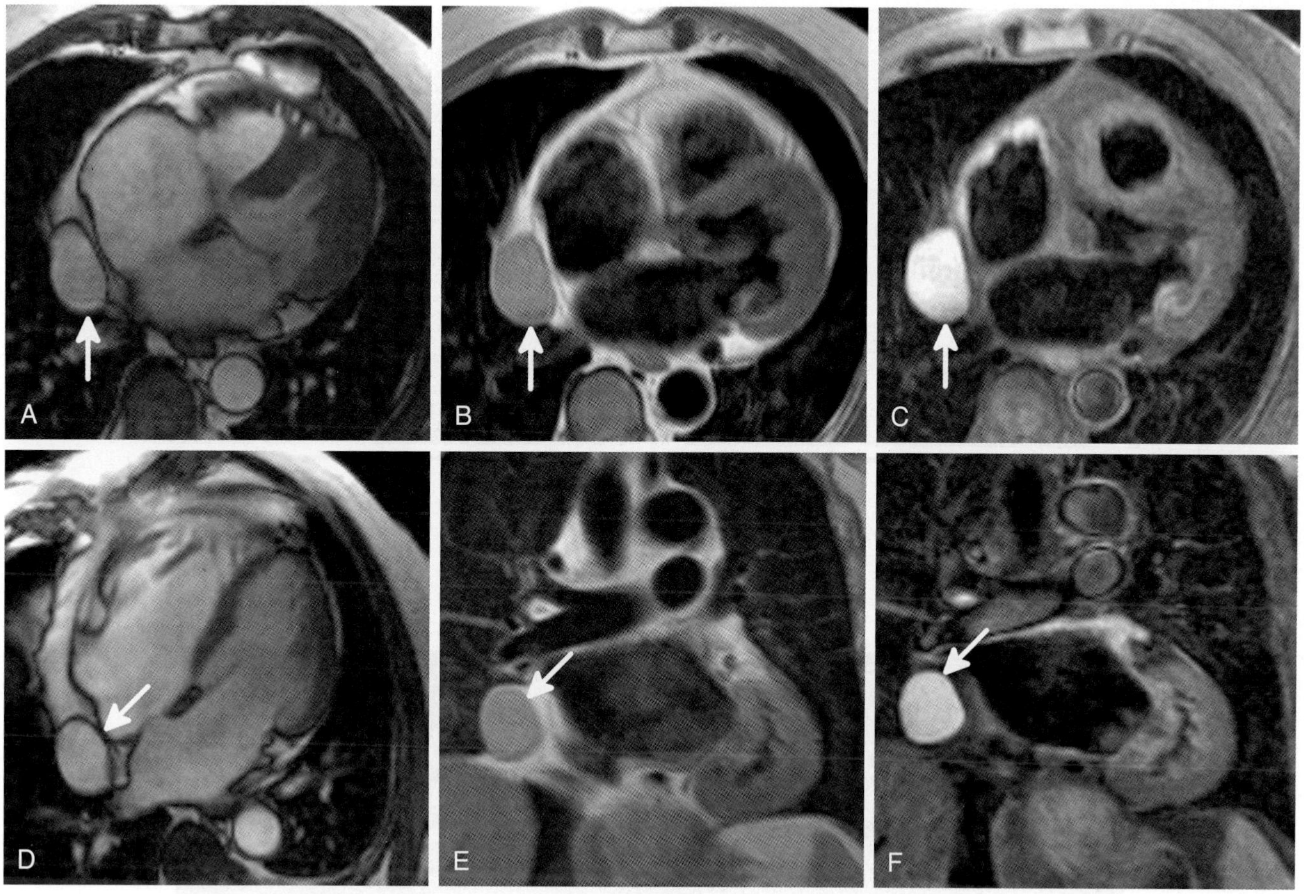

Figure 32.27 Pericardial cyst, with sharp borders and homogeneous signal intensity *(arrows)*. (A) Axial fast imaging employing steady-state acquisition (FIESTA) end-diastolic frame. The high T2-/T1-weighted signal is equivalent to fluid signal. (B) Axial T1-weighted black blood fast spin-echo (FSE) image, intermediate signal intensity due to the protein content. (C) Axial T2-weighted black blood FSE fat-suppressed (triple) image. The high T2-/T1-weighted signal is equivalent to fluid signal. (D) Four-chamber FIESTA end-diastolic frame. The high T2-/T1-weighted signal is equivalent to fluid signal. (E) Coronal T1-weighted black blood FSE image, with intermediate signal intensity due to the protein content. (F) Coronal T2-weighted black blood FSE fat-suppressed (triple) image. The high T2-/T1-weighted signal is equivalent to fluid signal.

pericardium. Unlike pleural mesothelioma, the relationship with asbestosis is uncertain.

Imaging

On both CT and MRI, pericardial mesothelioma appears as a heterogeneously or nodular enhancing mass along the pericardium, which involves the visceral and parietal layers, with possible invasion of adjacent structures. Metastatic disease is found in approximately 50% of patients. Distinction from the more common pericardial metastasis is challenging on imaging (Fig. 32.28).

Pericardial Metastasis

Pericardial metastasis is much more common than primary pericardial malignancy. Carcinoma of the lung and breast, lymphoma, and leukemia is most likely to metastasize to the pericardium. Pericardial metastasis appears as nodular or smooth thickening and enhancement of both the parietal and visceral layers of the pericardium.

■ Vascular Neoplasms

Vascular malformations and neoplasms are a heterogeneous group of lesions that affect the arterial, capillary, venous, or lymphatic system. They encompass a wide range of lesions, syndromes, and masses. Due to the heterogeneity of the lesions, several classifications systems have been proposed; the system originally proposed by Mulliken and Glowacki has now been modified, expanded, and adopted by the International Society for the Study of Vascular Anomalies (Table 32.1). Benign vascular tumors include a variety of hemangiomata and pyogenic granulomas. Locally aggressive or borderline vascular tumors include kaposiform, retiform, or composite hemangioendothelioma, papillary intralymphatic angioendothelioma, and Kaposi sarcoma. Malignant vascular tumors include angiosarcoma and epithelioid hemangioendothelioma.

Intracardiac vascular malformations are histologically classified into capillary, cavernous, arteriovenous, or more commonly, mixed types (Fig. 32.29).

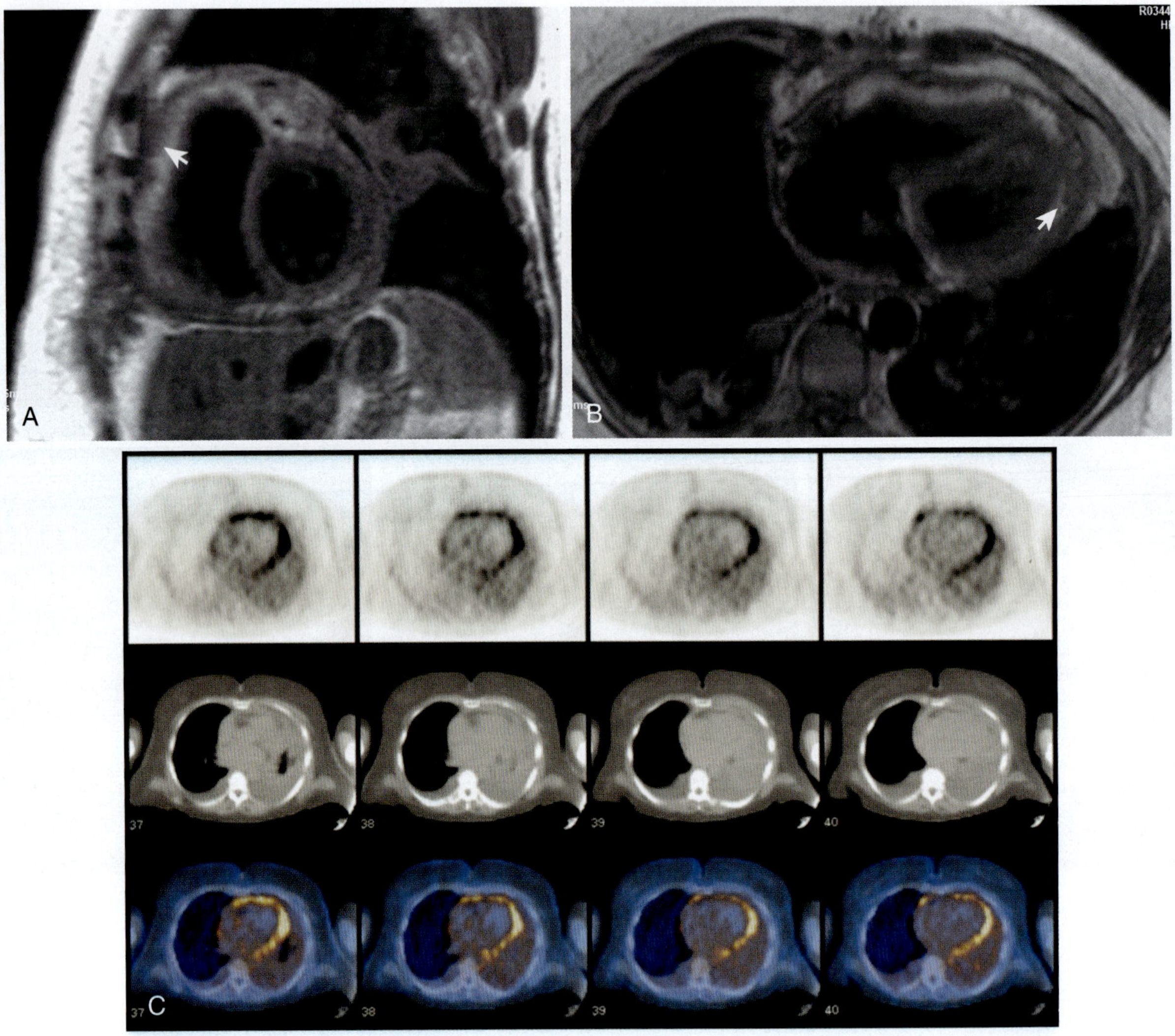

Figure 32.28 Primary pericardial mesothelioma on short-axis (A) and axial (B) black blood, T1-weighted MRI scans through the heart. There is diffuse nodularity of the pericardium *(arrows)* infiltrating the epicardial fat. On imaging alone, this would be difficult to distinguish from pericardial metastasis. Confirmed by biopsy. (C) Axial images from positron emission tomography–computed tomography (PET-CT). There is diffuse uptake in the pericardium along the tumor. *Top row,* Axial PET images; *middle row,* axial CT; *bottom row,* fused PET-CT images. There are bilateral pleural effusions.

TABLE 32.1 Classification of Vascular Anomalies

	VASCULAR MALFORMATIONS			
VASCULAR TUMORS	**SIMPLE**	**COMBINED**	**OF MAJOR NAMED VESSELS**	**ASSOCIATED WITH OTHER ANOMALIES**
Benign	Capillary malformations	Combined (two or more vascular malformations in one lesion)	Affect lymphatics, veins, arteries, anomalies of origin	Klippel-Trenaunay syndrome
Locally aggressive or borderline	Lymphatic malformations	Capillary-venous, capillary-lymphatic, capillary-AV, lymphatic-venous, capillary-lymphatic-venous, capillary-venous-AV, or capillary-lymphatic-venous-AV malformation	Course	
Malignant	Venous malformations		Number	
	AV malformations		Length	
	AV malformations and fistulae (high flow)		Diameter • Aplasia • Hypoplasia • Stenosis • Ectasia • Aneurysm	
			Valves	
			Communication	
			Persistence of embryonic vessel	

AV, Arteriovenous.
Modified from International Society for the Study of Vascular Anomalies. Classification of vascular anomalies. http://www.issva.org/classification.

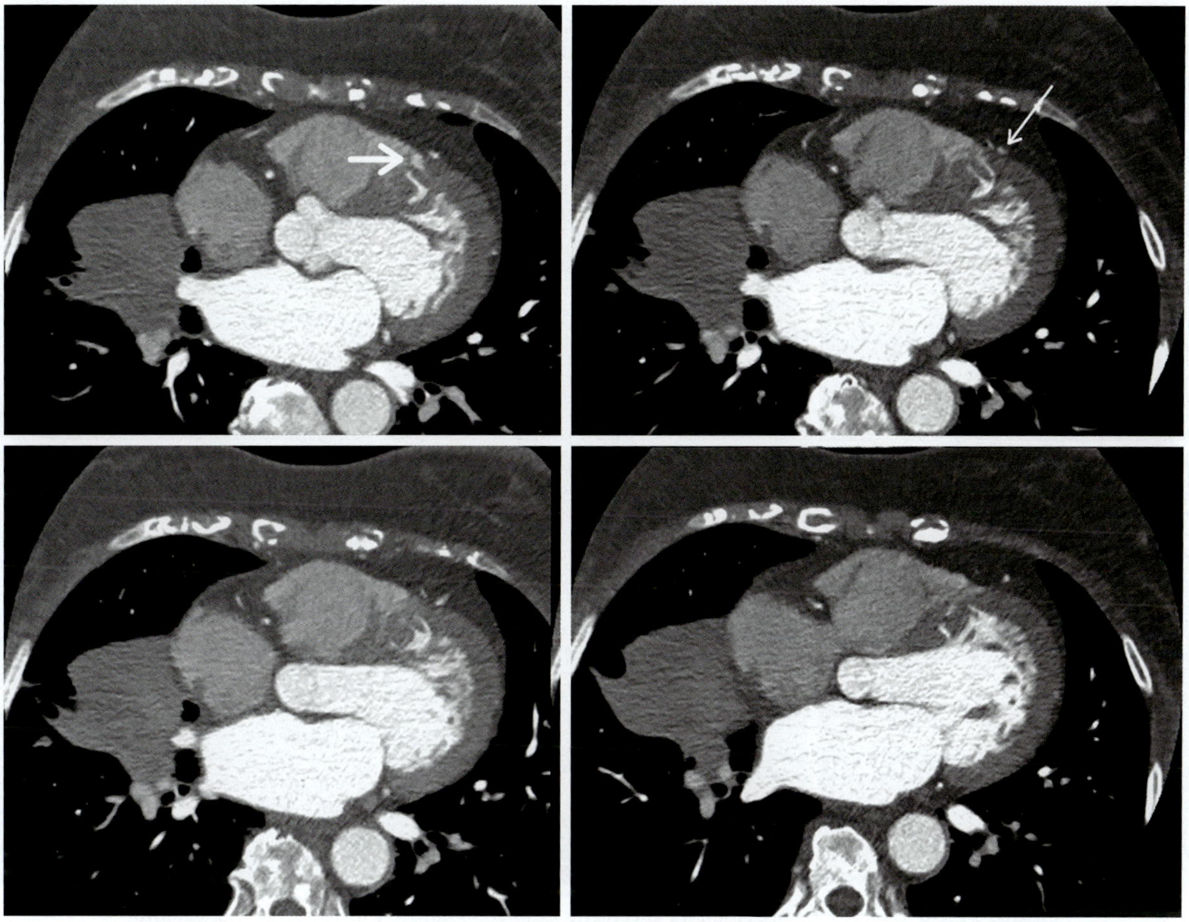

Figure 32.29 Axial cardiac CT images demonstrate an intracardiac, high-flow arteriovenous malformation centered in the interventricular septum supplied by the left anterior descending artery *(long thin arrow)*, demonstrating a nidus *(thick horizontal arrow)* and draining via vascular channels into the left ventricle.

Lymphangioma (Lymphatic Malformations)

Description

Lymphangioma occurs as lobulated, fluid-filled, nonenhancing cystic spaces, with septations. The current preferred terminology is lymphatic malformations (LMs). They are classified as macrocystic LMs (maximum cyst diameter >1 cm) and microcystic LMs (maximum cyst diameter <1 cm). These lesions manifest as localized masses, which may infiltrate between tissue planes. They may also present with fluid leakage, such as chylous fluid in body cavities or weeping from skin vesicles. Skin and subcutaneous tissues are usually affected, LMs may also involve muscle, bones, or viscera. Lymphangiomas have been described nearly everywhere in the body, related to the ubiquitousness of the lymphatic system.

Imaging

LMs are best visualized on ultrasonography and MRI. The cystic components of macrocystic LMs are easily visualized, whereas the microcystic types are predominantly solid lesions. Fluid-fluid levels in cysts result from the layering of protein or blood. MRI better demonstrates the deeper, more infiltrative LMs.

Intravenous Leiomyomatosis

An intravenous leiomyomatosis is a rare tumor that originates from a uterine leiomyoma. There is intravascular proliferation of smooth muscles cells beyond the boundary of the leiomyoma. Extension into the iliac veins and IVC is common, but it usually remains intravascular and tends not to invade tissue. Extension into the IVC occurs in about 30% of cases and intracardiac extension (usually the right atrium) occurs in 10% of cases (Fig. 32.30).

Intravenous Leiomyosarcoma

An intravenous leiomyosarcoma is a rare tumor that arises from the smooth muscle cells in a vessel wall. Leiomyosarcoma of the venous system involves the IVC in 50% of cases. Most of the tumors have a predominantly extravascular growth pattern, although an intravascular variant does exist. The extravascular variant can completely efface the lumen, the so-called imperceptible lumen sign.

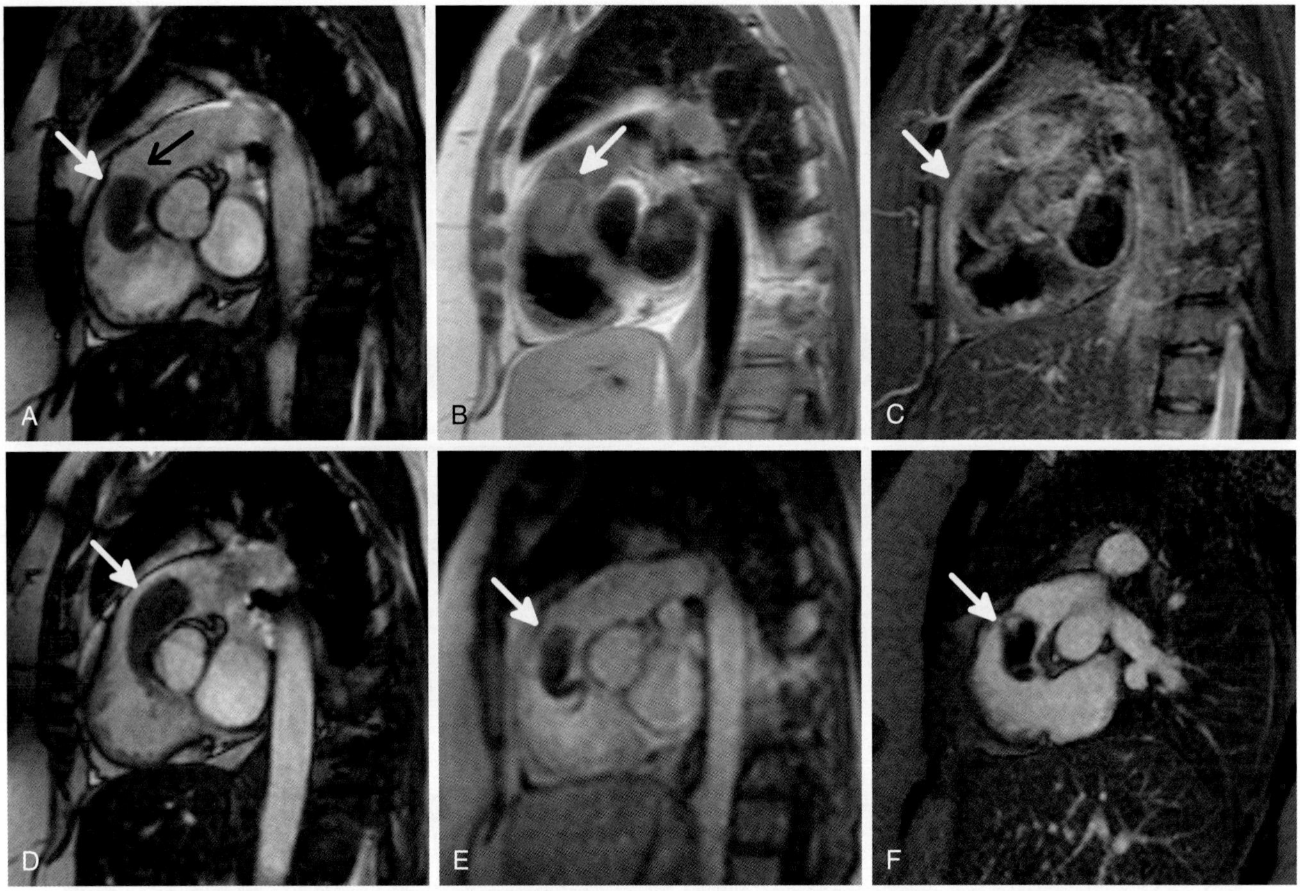

Figure 32.30 Leiomyomatosis. Histology after uterus extirpation showed a malignant type of leiomyomatosis. Echocardiographic follow-up raised the suspicion of a metastasis in the right ventricular outflow tract (RVOT) or a thrombus. White arrows indicate the tumor. (A) RVOT balanced steady-state free precession (b-SSFP) end-diastolic frame. Attached near the aortic root, the lesion was located below the pulmonary valve *(black arrow)* in diastole. (B) RVOT T1-weighted, black blood turbo spin-echo (TSE) image. The intermediate signal is very close to that of the myocardium. (C) RVOT T2-weighted black blood TSE spectral inversion recovery for fat suppression image. There is relatively low signal intensity compared to the myocardium. (D) RVOT b-SSFP end-systolic frame. The bulky portion of the tumor has marked displacement over the cardiac cycle; it protrudes 1 inch above the pulmonary valve in systole. (E) RVOT first-pass perfusion k-t BLAST saturation recovery balanced turbo field-echo image. The bulky portion shows some partial first-pass uptake. (F) RVOT delayed enhancement image. There are spots of extracellular gadolinium contrast material accumulation.

Bibliography

Antunes C, Graça B, Donato P. Thoracic, abdominal and musculoskeletal involvement in Erdheim-Chester disease: CT, MR and PET imaging findings. *Insights Imaging*. 2014;5(4):473–482.

Beroukhim RS, Prakash A, Buechel ER, et al. Characterization of cardiac tumors in children by cardiovascular magnetic resonance imaging: a multicenter experience. *J Am Coll Cardiol*. 2011;58(10):1044–1054.

Broderick LS, Brooks GN, Kuhlman JE. Anatomic pitfalls of the heart and pericardium. *Radiographics*. 2005;25(2):441–453.

Burke A, Virmani R. Pediatric heart tumors. *Cardiovasc Pathol*. 2008;17(4):193–198.

Chiles C, Woodard PK, Gutierrez FR, Link KM. Metastatic involvement of the heart and pericardium: CT and MR imaging. *Radiographics*. 2001;21(2): 439–449.

Cho JM, Danielson GK, Puga FJ, et al. Surgical resection of ventricular cardiac fibromas: early and late results. *Ann Thorac Surg*. 2003;76(6):1929–1934.

Di Vito A, Mignogna C, Donato G. The mysterious pathways of cardiac myxomas: a review of histogenesis, pathogenesis and pathology. *Histopathology*. 2015;66(3):321–332.

Haroche J, Cluzel P, Toledano D, et al. Images in cardiovascular medicine. Cardiac involvement in Erdheim-Chester disease: magnetic resonance and computed tomographic scan imaging in a monocentric series of 37 patients. *Circulation*. 2009;119(25):e597–e598.

International Society for the Study of Vascular Anomalies. Classification of vascular anomalies. http://www.issva.org/classification.

Jeudy J, Kirsch J, Tavora F, et al. From the radiologic pathology archives: cardiac lymphoma: radiologic-pathologic correlation. *Radiographics*. 2012;32(5):1369–1380.

John PR. Vascular anomalies. In: Abbara S, Kalva SP, eds. *Problem Solving in Cardiovascular Imaging*. Philadelphia: Elsevier; 2013:813–834.

Khosa F, Magoon P, Bedi H, Khan AN, Otero H, Yucel K. Primary and metastatic vascular neoplasms: imaging findings. *AJR Am J Roentgenol*. 2012;198(3):700–704.

Maleszewski JJ, Larsen BT, Kip NS, et al. PRKAR1A in the development of cardiac myxoma: a study of 110 cases including isolated and syndromic tumors. *Am J Surg Pathol*. 2014;38(8):1079–1087.

Motwani M, Kidambi A, Herzog BA, Uddin A, Greenwood JP, Plein S. MR imaging of cardiac tumors and masses: a review of methods and clinical applications. *Radiology*. 2013;268:26–43.

Mulliken JB, Glowacki J. Classification of pediatric vascular lesions. *Plast Reconstr Surg*. 1982;70(1):120–121.

Nascimento AF, Winters GL, Pinkus GS. Primary cardiac lymphoma: clinical, histologic, immunophenotypic, and genotypic features of 5 cases of a rare disorder. *Am J Surg Pathol*. 2007;31(9):1344–1350.

O'Donnell DH, Abbara S, Chaithiraphan V, et al. Cardiac tumors: optimal cardiac MR sequences and spectrum of imaging appearances. *AJR Am J Roentgenol*. 2009;193(2):377–387.

Patel R, Lim RP, Saric M, et al. Diagnostic performance of cardiac magnetic resonance imaging and echocardiography in evaluation of cardiac and paracardiac masses. *Am J Cardiol*. 2016;117(1):135–140.

Randhawa JS, Budd GT, Randhawa M, et al. Primary cardiac sarcoma: 25-year Cleveland Clinic experience. *Am J Clin Oncol*. 2016;39(6):593–599.

Singhal P, Luk A, Rao V, Butany J. Molecular basis of cardiac myxomas. *Int J Mol Sci*. 2014;15(1):1315–1337.

Tao TY, Yahyavi-Firouz-Abadi N, Singh GK, Bhalla S. Pediatric cardiac tumors: clinical and imaging features. *Radiographics*. 2014;34(4):1031–1046.

Wang JG, Han J, Jiang T, Li YJ. Cardiac paragangliomas. *J Card Surg*. 2015;30(1):55–60.

Webb EM, Wang ZJ, Westphalen AC, Nakakura EK, Coakley FV, Yeh BM. Can CT features differentiate between inferior vena cava leiomyosarcomas and primary retroperitoneal masses? *AJR Am J Roentgenol*. 2013;200(1):205–209.

SECTION 5

Entities by Anatomic Region

CHAPTER 33
Diaphragm and Chest Wall

Cameron Hassani and Christopher Lee

CHAPTER OUTLINE

■ Diaphragm

Relevant Anatomy

The diaphragm is a dome-shaped muscle with a central noncontractile tendon. Anteriorly and laterally, the diaphragm attaches to the body wall (ribs, costal cartilages, inferior sternum, and xiphoid process) via muscular diaphragmatic slips (Fig. 33.1A). Posteriorly, musculotendinous crura attach the diaphragm to the posterior body wall (lower thoracic and lumbar vertebrae). The right crus is typically larger and longer than the left. The right and left crura are joined by the median arcuate ligament, just anterior to the aorta (see Fig. 33.1B).

The phrenic nerve is the motor and sensory nerve of the diaphragm. The phrenic nerves originate from C3, C4, and C5, traveling in the lateral compartment of the neck to the thoracic inlet. The right phrenic nerve descends laterally along the superior vena cava, right atrium, and inferior vena cava (IVC), branching to innervate the cranial surface of the diaphragm. The left phrenic nerve descends laterally along the aortic arch and left heart border before branching at the superior surface of the diaphragm. After branching, both phrenic nerves pass through the IVC hiatus and further innervate the inferior surface of the diaphragm.

There are three important openings related to the diaphragm—the vena caval hiatus, esophageal hiatus, and aortic hiatus. The vena caval hiatus is located within the midportion of the diaphragm, at the T8 vertebral level, allowing the IVC to pass from the abdomen to the thorax. Branches of the right phrenic nerve and lymphatics also pass through this hiatus. The esophageal hiatus is located within the muscle fibers of the right crus, at the T10 level, allowing for the passage of the esophagus, vagus nerve, and lymphatics. The aortic hiatus, despite its name, is not a true opening in the diaphragm. It is actually located posterior to the diaphragm, between the left and right crura, typically at the T12 level. This hiatus allows the aorta to pass posteriorly without being affected by muscular diaphragmatic contraction. The thoracic duct, and sometimes the azygous vein, also passes through the aortic hiatus.

The sternocostal triangles, or foramina of Morgagni, are small gaps on both sides of the medial anterior diaphragm, between the sternal and costal attachment points of the diaphragm, and are not openings within the diaphragm itself. The epigastric vessels and lymphatic channels pass through these foramina. Diaphragmatic hernias (i.e., Morgagni hernia) can occur at these sites.

Function

The diaphragm is the primary muscle of respiration, innervated by the phrenic nerve. Central contraction increases craniocaudal thoracic volume and decreases thoracic pressure, resulting in the inspiration of air. Relaxation of the diaphragm allows for passive expiration secondary to elastic recoil of the lungs and pleura. Variable levels of muscle contraction induce forced air expiration and also aid in nonrespiratory functions, such as vomiting, defecation, and childbirth.

During inspiration, the three diaphragmatic hiatus change shape in different ways. The caval hiatus dilates, allowing increased blood flood through the IVC; the esophageal hiatus constricts, acting as a sphincter for the

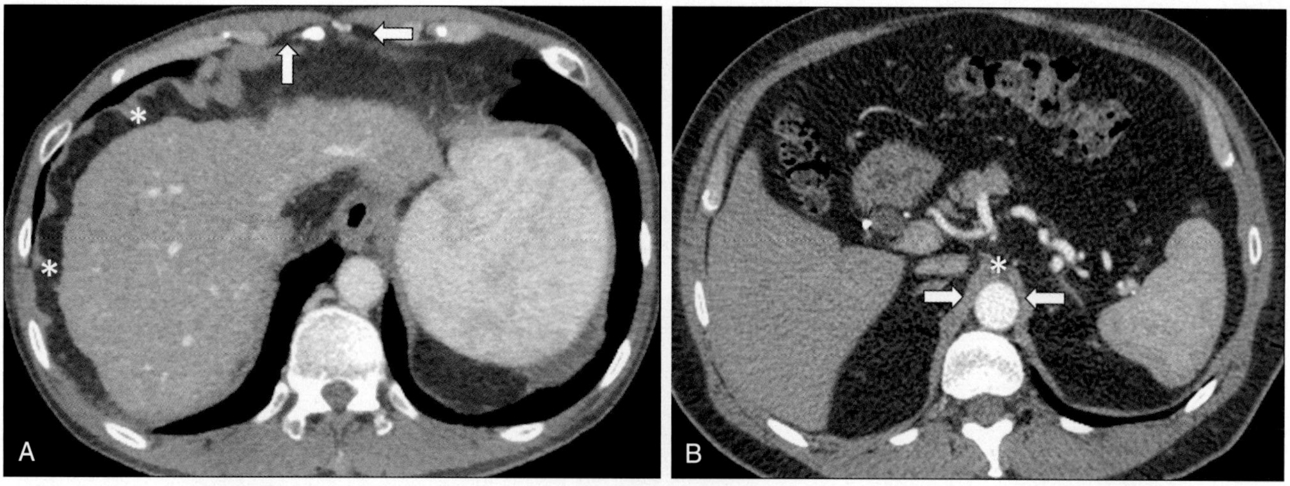

Figure 33.1 Normal appearance of the diaphragm on CT. (A) Diaphragmatic slips *(asterisks)* attach to the ribs and sternum. Note the fat- and vessel-containing sternocostal triangles *(arrows)*, anterior to the diaphragm, between the sternum and ribs. (B) Left and right crura of the diaphragm *(arrows)* arch anterior to the aorta to join at the median arcuate ligament *(asterisk)*.

esophagus. Diaphragm contraction has no effect on the size and shape of the aortic hiatus.

Flattening of the diaphragm from increased lung volumes or emphysema will restrict the normal function of the diaphragm, limiting the degree of available excursion.

Imaging

Techniques That Best Image the Diaphragm

The diaphragm is well seen on plain radiography, fluoroscopy, ultrasonography (US), computed tomography (CT), and magnetic resonance imaging (MRI). Chest radiography is often the initial modality for the evaluation of diaphragmatic disease. Not only is it the initial modality of choice, but it is also the most common modality for detecting disease, with up to 90% sensitivity. The frontal chest radiograph provides excellent assessment of diaphragmatic position and contour. The lateral view confirms the contour of the diaphragm and provides additional information for the diagnosis of eventration—relative elevation of one diaphragmatic segment. Radiographs, however, are not specific enough to differentiate between most causes of nontraumatic and traumatic elevation.

Fluoroscopy (the so-called sniff test) provides real-time imaging of diaphragmatic motion. Typically, continuous fluoroscopic imaging is performed while the patient takes several normal tidal breaths, followed by several deep breaths. The patient is finally instructed to take short rapid sniffs through the nostrils, with real-time images obtained in both the frontal and lateral projections. Differing behaviors of the diaphragm during these maneuvers offer clues to the underlying disease, as discussed later.

US is a useful modality that also provides real-time imaging of the diaphragm, with the added benefits of portability (beneficial in the intensive care unit setting) and lack of ionizing radiation. Limitations of US include technologist's experience, small field of view, and artifacts due to overlying air within the lung or bowel. US can be used to evaluate diaphragmatic excursion and thickness, with breathing maneuvers similar to those for fluoroscopic evaluation. Low-frequency (1–3 MHz) probes, which offer greater depth, are used to evaluate motion and excursion, whereas high-frequency (7–18 MHz) probes offer improved spatial resolution, thus allowing accurate measurements of muscle thickness.

CT has a limited role in demonstrating diaphragmatic functional abnormalities. However, it is useful in identifying potential causes of dysfunction, such as malignancy. CT also readily identifies nondiaphragmatic causes of perceived elevation, such as pleural effusion, lung processes, and abdominal processes. CT with multiplanar reformats is critical for the assessment of the diaphragm in the trauma setting due to its high specificity for detecting rupture.

MRI is not commonly used for diaphragmatic assessment, mainly due to equipment availability, imaging time, low resolution, and radiologist inexperience. Dynamic MRI may have an increased role in the future due to its ability to perform real-time imaging without the need for ionizing radiation.

Normal Appearance of the Diaphragm on Imaging

On frontal and lateral radiographs, the diaphragm should be smooth and dome-shaped, with the peak of the dome at least 1.5 cm above a line connecting the costophrenic angle and ipsilateral cardiophrenic angle. The right hemidiaphragm is usually higher than the left, typically between the sixth and seventh anterior ribs on an end-inspiratory frontal radiograph. The contours of the diaphragm should be sharp and visible through the heart as they contact the lower lobes of both lungs (Fig. 33.2). Obscuration of this contour, known as the *silhouette sign*, suggests pathology in either lower lobe.

CT demonstrates similar findings as chest radiographs, with a sharp, smoothly marginated interface between

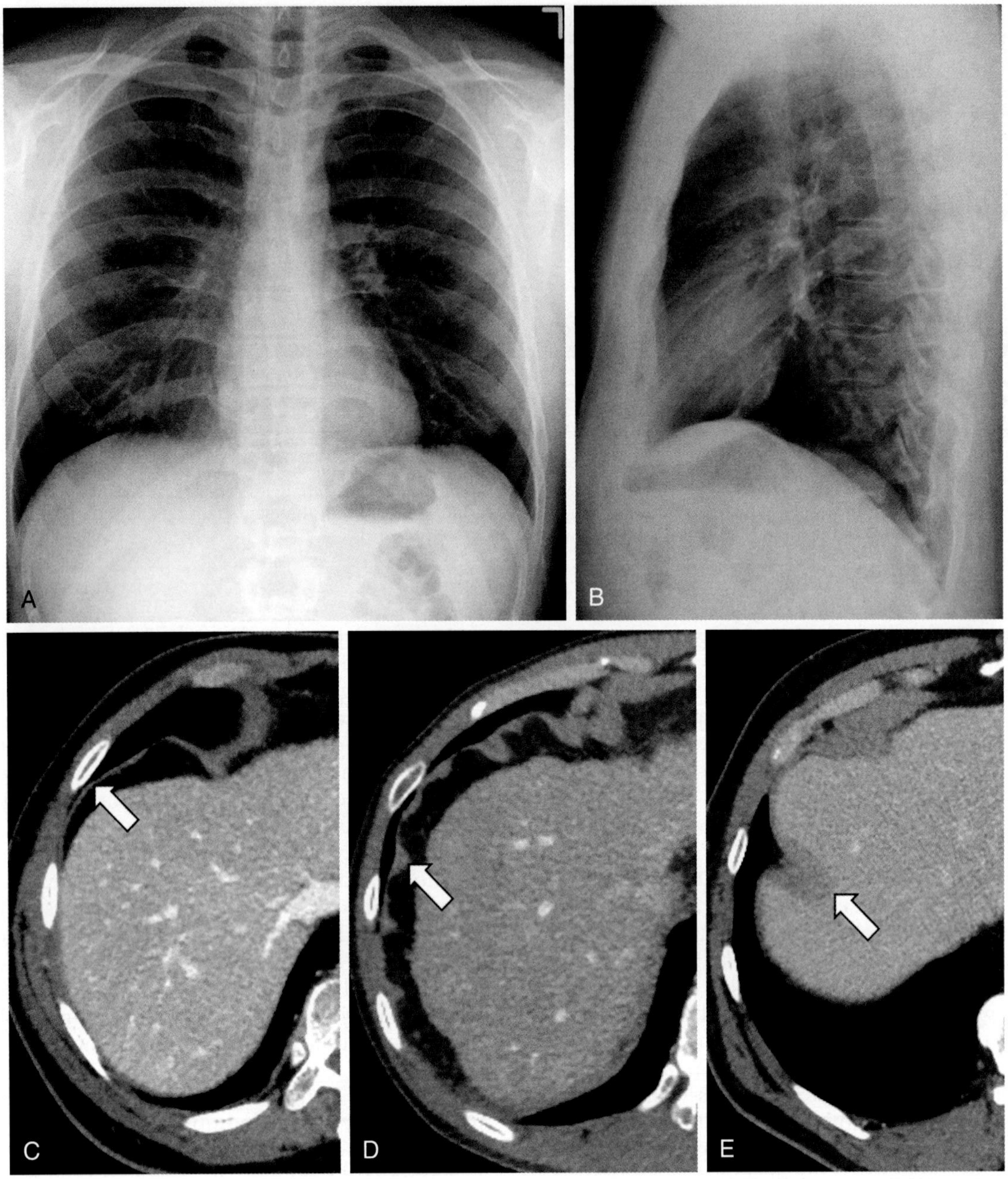

Figure 33.2 Normal appearances of diaphragm. Frontal (A) and lateral (B) radiographs. The diaphragm appears as a smooth, dome-shaped structure with symmetric height on both sides. On CT, diaphragm can be smooth (C) or nodular in contour (D), depending on the phase of respiration *(arrows)*. (E) Prominent diaphragmatic folds may simulate masses in the adjacent liver or spleen.

the diaphragm and adjacent fat, lung, and abdominal organs. Scalloping is a commonly encountered normal variant, in which individual slips of muscle invaginate and indent the liver surface; this should not be confused with a hepatic mass (see Fig. 33.2). Scalloping is often accentuated on deep inspiration. The median arcuate ligament appears as a thin band of ligamentous tissue arching over the aorta. In certain cases, this ligament impinges on the celiac artery as it arises from the aorta, which may result in median arcuate ligament syndrome (Fig. 33.3).

On real-time fluoroscopy or US, the diaphragm moves caudally during inspiration and cranially with expiration. Excursion of the diaphragm is most pronounced at the posterior periphery.

On US, the diaphragm appears as an echogenic band that normally thickens during inspiration. The thickening ratio can be calculated as follows:

(Thickness at inspiration – thickness at expiration)/(thickness at expiration)

Thickening <20% and/or end-expiration thickness <0.2 cm is suggestive of paralysis. Excursion can also be objectively measured between inspiration and expiration, with an excursion >2.5 cm considered normal. Excursion

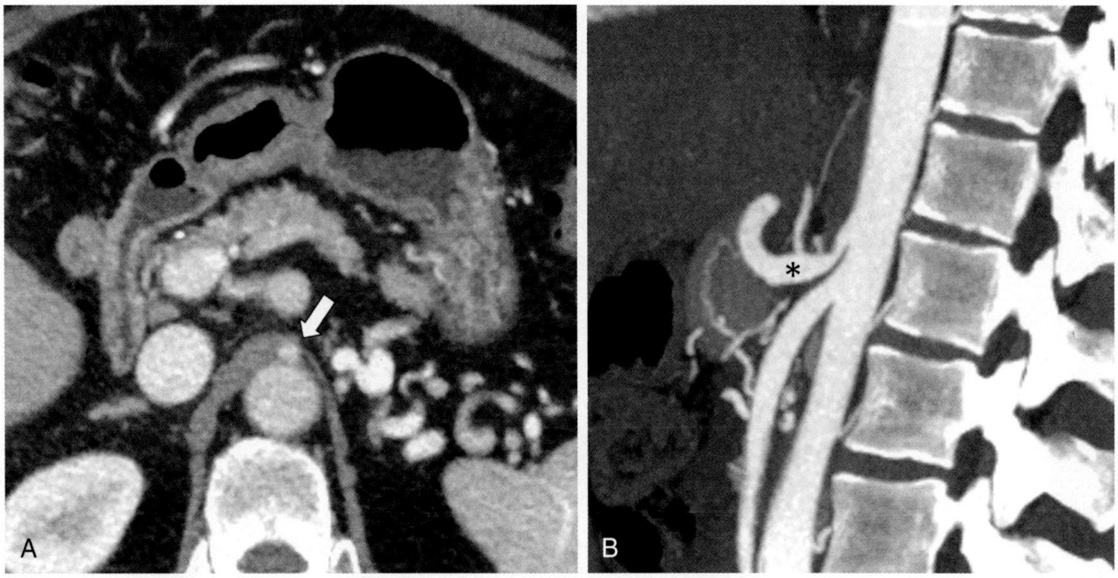

Figure 33.3 Median arcuate ligament syndrome. Axial (A) and sagittal (B) CT scans demonstrate a narrowed celiac artery at the commissure of the left and right crura of the diaphragm, the median arcuate ligament *(arrow)*, with poststenotic dilation of a J-shaped celiac artery *(asterisk)*.

<2.5 cm and paradoxic motion of any degree are considered abnormal.

Diagnostic Approach to an Elevated Diaphragm

Evaluation of an elevated diaphragm should always be performed within the clinical context. In the asymptomatic patient, unilateral elevation is usually due to eventration. In a patient who has evidence of sternotomy, paralysis should be considered.

Eventration

This is a focal weakness of an otherwise intact diaphragm resulting in a focal elevation. Eventration is caused by the replacement of normal muscular diaphragmatic tissue with fibrous tissue. The underlying cause may be congenital or acquired, with congenital muscular insufficiency being more common. In the adult, eventration is virtually always asymptomatic (discovered incidentally) and is generally unilateral. It usually affects the anteromedial portion of the diaphragm. Diagnosis can be confidently made on the lateral chest radiograph, which demonstrates relative elevation of the anterior portion (Fig. 33.4A–C). Real-time fluoroscopic or US imaging shows reduced excursion of the elevated segment, with normal movement of the remainder of the diaphragm. No follow-up imaging or treatment is needed in most cases.

In patients without imaging findings characteristic of eventration, possibilities include diaphragm paralysis or paresis, elevation due to mass effect or perceived elevation with normal position of the diaphragm. Radiograph can exclude lung volume loss. CT can be performed to rule out displacement due to mass effect from abdominal process. After exclusion of other causes, dynamic fluoroscopy or US can diagnose diaphragmatic paresis or paralysis.

Diaphragmatic Paralysis

This is commonly encountered after surgical interruption of the phrenic nerve. Less commonly, it is due to phrenic nerve invasion by neck and/or mediastinal malignancy, extrinsic nerve compression, neuropathy, or idiopathic causes. Paralysis is usually unilateral and asymptomatic but can be bilateral, in which case the clinical presentation may range from dyspnea to respiratory failure. Imaging demonstrates elevation of the entire diaphragm, as opposed to eventration, in which only a part of the diaphragm is elevated (see Fig. 33.4D and E). On real-time fluoroscopy or US, the paralyzed diaphragm will exhibit reduced or absent caudal excursion during tidal and deep breathing. During a rapid sniff, characteristic paradoxic cranial motion of the affected diaphragm is observed, while the contralateral normal diaphragm descends. If both hemidiaphragms are affected, paradoxic motion may not be immediately recognized due to their symmetric movement. Any cranial movement of the diaphragm during a sniff should alert the radiologist to the presence of paralysis. On ultrasound, the paralyzed diaphragm is typically thinned, measuring <0.2 cm at end-expiration. Furthermore, real-time US can show a lack of normal thickening during breathing (<20% thickening between end-inspiration and end-expiration).

Diaphragmatic Paresis

This indicates weakness of the diaphragm (not to be confused with paralysis). Similar to paralysis, the entire hemidiaphragm is elevated, with reduced or delayed excursion during tidal breathing, with paradoxic motion on rapid sniff. However, if some degree of caudal motion of the diaphragm is seen during deep inspiration, then a diagnosis of paresis is made rather than paralysis.

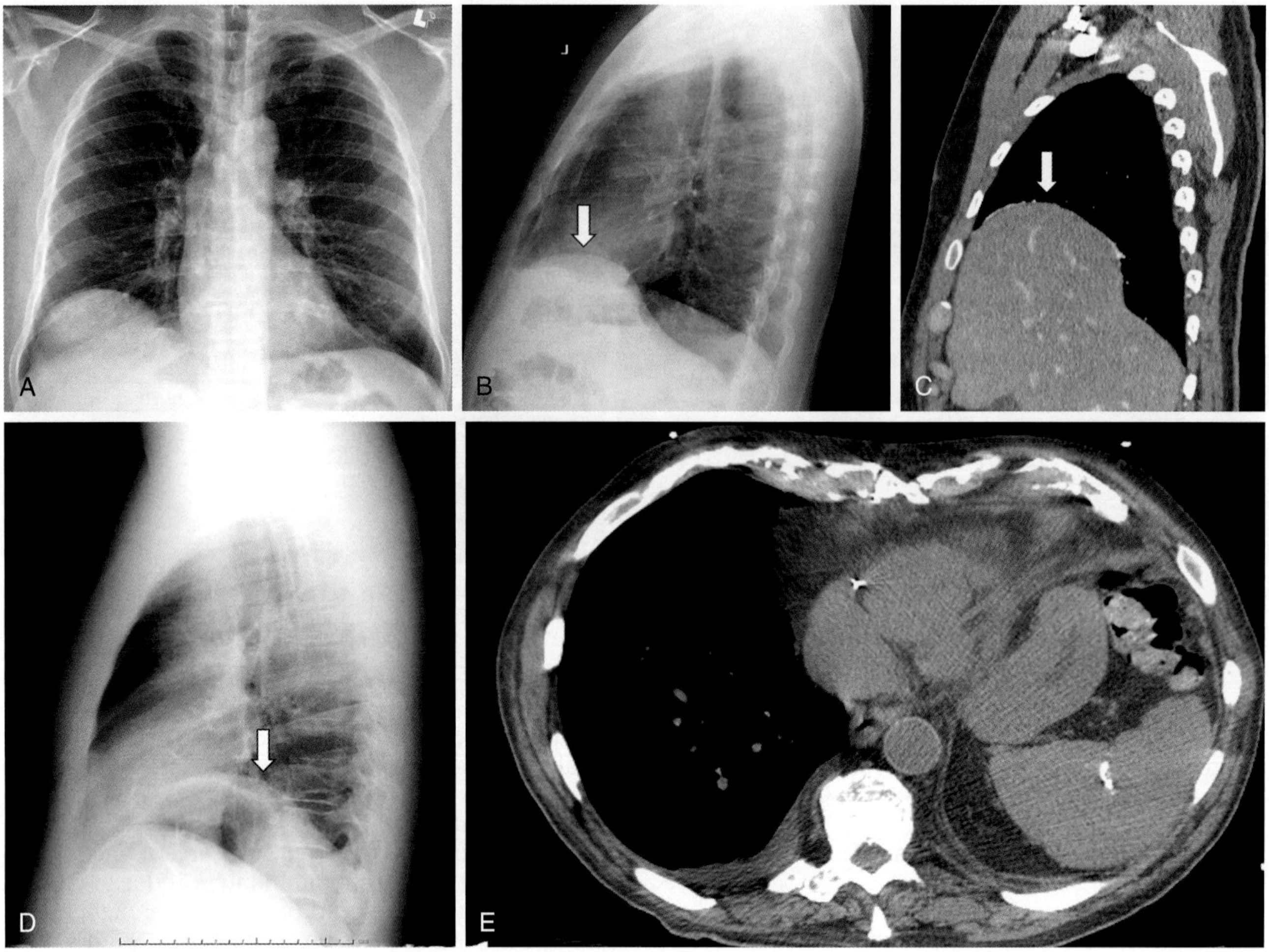

Figure 33.4 Elevated diaphragm. (A) Frontal radiograph demonstrates elevation of the right hemidiaphragm relative to the left, but it is nonspecific for cause. Lateral radiograph (B) and sagittal CT scan (C) demonstrate a humplike elevation of the anterior portion of the right hemidiaphragm *(arrows)*, consistent with eventration. (D) Lateral radiograph in a different patient demonstrates elevation of the entire left hemidiaphragm *(arrow)*, in this case secondary to paralysis. (E) Axial CT scan through the lower chest demonstrates asymmetric presence of abdominal viscera on the left, which should alert the radiologist to diaphragmatic elevation, in this case due to paralysis.

Causes of Elevation of the Diaphragm That Mimic Primary Diaphragmatic Disease

The diaphragm can be elevated without the presence of a structural or functional abnormality, such as with normal exhalation, increased abdominal pressure (e.g., with obesity, hepatosplenomegaly, ascites, Valsalva maneuver), or decreased lung volume (atelectasis or lung resection). Muscle weakness related to lupus myositis is also a well-known cause of diaphragmatic elevation.

Causes of Perceived Elevation of the Diaphragm

A well-described cause of perceived elevation of the diaphragm is a subpulmonic pleural effusion, which is a pleural fluid that resides between the lung base and diaphragmatic surface. In this case, the diaphragm is not actually elevated but merely appears elevated on chest radiographs due to silhouetting of the diaphragm by the pleural fluid and a new air interface created more superiorly by the effusion. On frontal radiographs, a helpful hint is lateral displacement of the central peak of the perceived diaphragm (Fig. 33.5). When the subpulmonic effusion is located on the left, increased distance between the stomach bubble and lung is often observed. A subpulmonic pleural effusion should also silhouette the pulmonary vasculature projecting through the perceived diaphragmatic contour. On the lateral radiograph, the *Rock of Gibraltar sign* may be seen—broad flattening of the posterior diaphragm with a sharp clifflike downstroke of the most anterior portions of the diaphragm.

Causes of Flattening of the Diaphragm

Flattening of the diaphragm is usually the result of lung hyperinflation, such as with emphysema, obstructive airway disease, or cystic lung disease. It is also seen in cases of increased thoracic pressure caused by a large pneumothorax or pleural effusion.

Nontraumatic Defects

Nontraumatic defects of the diaphragm include congenital diaphragmatic hernia (CDH), hiatal hernia (HH), and

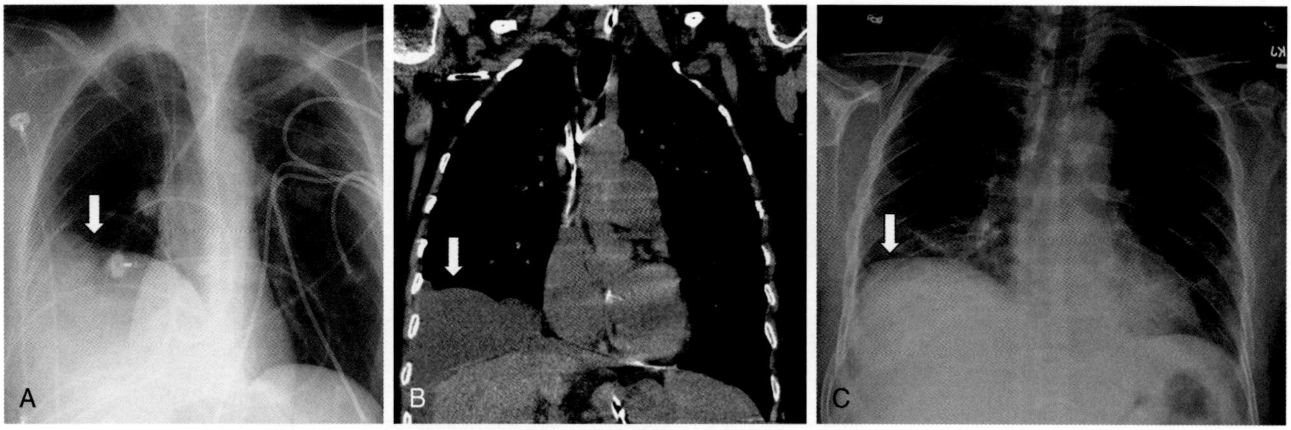

Figure 33.5 Subpulmonic pleural effusion. Frontal radiograph (A) and coronal CT scan (B) demonstrate apparent elevation of the right hemidiaphragm, with lateralization and meniscal appearance of the diaphragmatic peak *(arrows)*. (C) Small, subtle, subpulmonic pleural effusion on a frontal radiograph in a different patient, with apparent elevation of the right hemidiaphragm and lateralization of the peak *(arrow)*.

surgical defects. CDH includes Bochdalek hernia (BH) and Morgagni hernia (MH), with BH being more common. In adults, these are usually detected incidentally. Large hernias can result in pulmonary, gastrointestinal, or genitourinary symptoms secondary to mass effect. It has been found that up to 50% of CDHs are detected prenatally.

BH results from failure of fusion of the posterolateral pleuroperitoneal membranes. It is usually left-sided and seen posteriorly on the lateral radiograph. On the frontal view, there is a focal apparent elevation of the diaphragm due to herniated fat and, occasionally, other abdominal contents (Fig. 33.6).

In contrast, MH is typically right-sided and anteromedial in location, located at the cardiophrenic angle in 90% of cases. It usually contains omentum and colon but has been reported to contain solid viscera. Similar to BH, the frontal radiograph demonstrates focal apparent elevation of the diaphragm. The lateral view usually shows a well-defined mass overlying the heart. MH can be distinguished from eventration by obscuration of a portion of the diaphragmatic contour by herniated abdominal contents.

HH is the result of widening of the esophageal hiatus, allowing a portion or the entirety of the stomach to pass into the thorax. The two major types of HH are sliding (gastroesophageal junction herniates into the chest) and paraesophageal (gastroesophageal junction remains in its normal location) hernias. HH of either the sliding or paraesophageal type typically appears on the frontal radiograph as a mass to the left of the spine, with obscuration or displacement of the azygoesophageal interface. On the lateral projection, the mass is visible posterior to the heart, often with a characteristic air-fluid level.

Features of Trauma

Diaphragmatic rupture is rare, occurring in 0.8% to 8% of cases of blunt or penetrating injury to the lower thorax or upper abdomen, usually after a motor vehicle accident. Most injuries occur posterolaterally and are 10 cm or longer. The left side is more common than the right, likely due to the presence of the liver on the right. The posterolateral portion is most often affected due to relative weakness of the musculotendinous junction; central tendon injury is rare. The presence of a preexisting CDH increases the likelihood of diaphragmatic rupture. Rupture is difficult to diagnose clinically, and many are initially undetected, making imaging the primary diagnostic tool. Delayed rupture of the diaphragm has also been reported, with imaging findings occurring after initial presentation.

The chest radiograph is usually abnormal but not specific for the detection of injury. The most reliable signs of injury are enteric air—stomach, small bowel, colon—above the expected location of the diaphragm, especially in conjunction with adjacent rib fractures or pleural effusion. The presence of a nasogastric tube is especially helpful in confirming the abnormal position of the stomach above the diaphragm. Additional nonspecific signs include elevation of the hemidiaphragm and contour obscuration.

CT is the primary modality for assessing diaphragmatic trauma; however, much of the diaphragm is in-plane on axial CT, making multiplanar (sagittal and coronal) evaluation necessary. The most specific CT signs of diaphragmatic rupture are diaphragmatic discontinuity, what is called the *dangling diaphragm sign*, *dependent viscera sign*, and *collar sign*, and the presence of abdominal contents in the thorax. The dangling diaphragm sign represents a free edge of the torn diaphragm that moves or curls medially, away from its normal course along the chest wall (Fig. 33.7A and B). The dependent viscera sign refers to herniated abdominal organs directly apposed to the posterior chest wall (see Fig. 33.7C). Finally, the collar sign (also known as the *hourglass sign*) represents a waistlike configuration of herniated organs as they pass through a diaphragmatic defect, best seen on coronal and sagittal reformations (see Fig. 33.7D). Less specific signs include relative thickening of the affected diaphragm compared to the contralateral side, diaphragmatic elevation, or associated injuries,

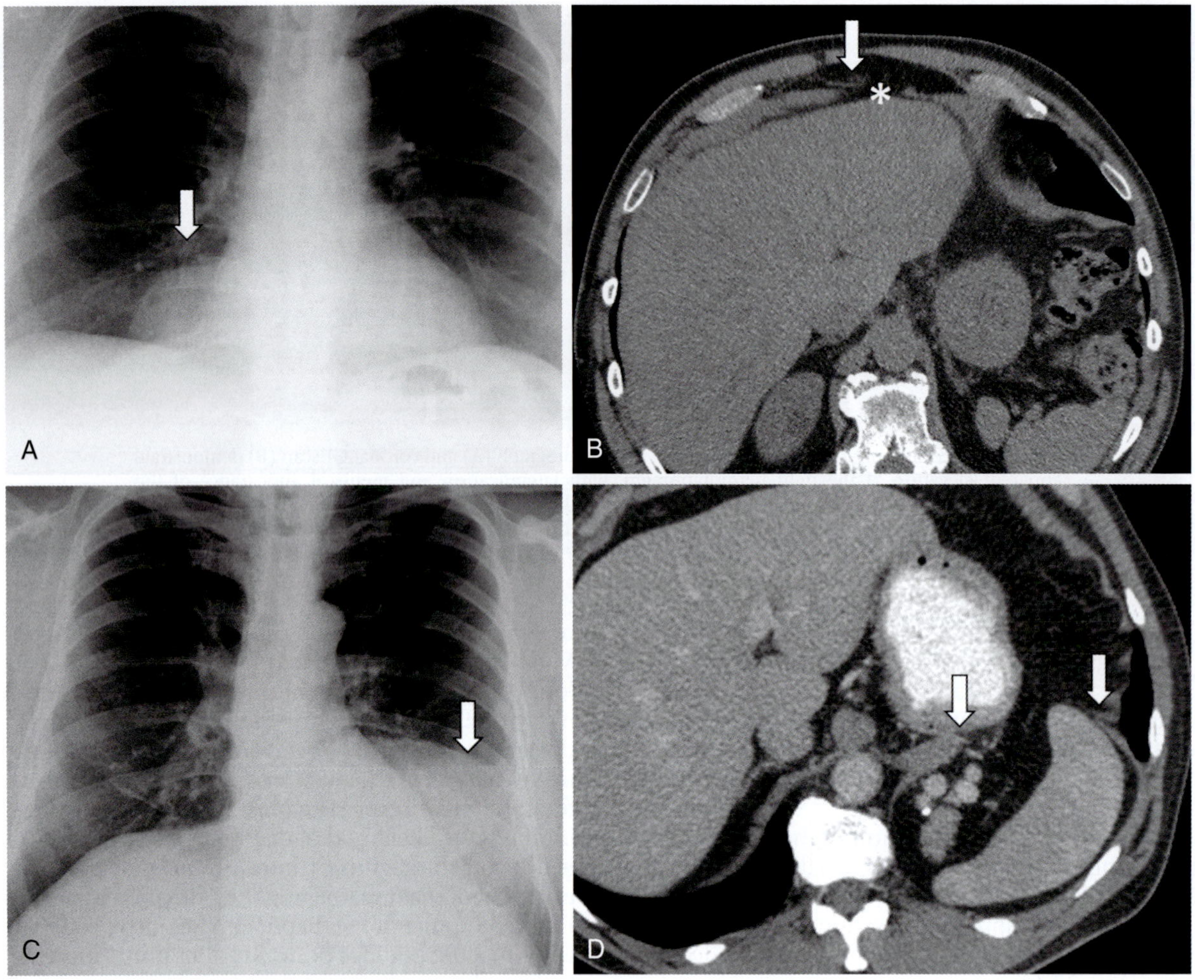

Figure 33.6 Congenital diaphragmatic hernia. (A) Frontal radiograph demonstrates a well-defined right cardiophrenic angle mass *(arrow)*. (B) Axial CT scan in the same patient demonstrates an open defect in the anterior diaphragm *(asterisk)*, with herniation of omental fat and vessels *(arrow)* into the mediastinum, consistent with Morgagni hernia. (C) Bochdalek hernia in a different patient is seen on a frontal radiograph as a left lower thoracic opacity, which silhouettes the diaphragm *(arrow)*. (D) Axial CT scan in the same patient shows a large defect in the posterior diaphragm *(arrows)*, with herniation of the spleen, mesenteric vessels, and pancreatic tail into the thorax.

such as osseous fracture, pneumothorax, hemothorax, pneumoperitoneum, or hemoperitoneum.

US has been used to evaluate the diaphragm in the trauma setting but has significant limitations due to bowel gas artifacts, which tend to be pronounced in cases of diaphragmatic rupture. MRI can reliably depict signs of trauma, similar to CT, but is usually not practical in the acute trauma setting.

Fluoroscopy with enteric contrast is not commonly used but can demonstrate narrowing of bowel as it passes through the site of injury into the thorax (collar sign).

Masses That Can Occur in the Diaphragm

Although overall very rare, both benign and malignant masses can involve the diaphragm. Benign lesions are more common.

The most common benign lesions are cysts. Bronchogenic, mesothelial, teratoid, and hydatid cysts all can involve the diaphragm. On CT, cysts appear as uniform, well-defined, water attenuation lesions without enhancement. Wall calcifications may or may not be present. MRI demonstrates a homogeneous T2 signal, indicating fluid. Cysts on US typically appear as thin-walled, hypoechoic or anechoic lesions that demonstrate posterior acoustic enhancement, with or without wall calcification. In the unique case of a hydatid cyst, multiple vesicles can be seen within the cyst on US or MRI. CT can also demonstrate a cyst with internal vesicles, larger loculations, or a heterogeneous mass with both solid and cystic components. In adults, cysts can become symptomatic, presenting as chest pain, upper abdominal discomfort, or dyspnea. Surgical removal of a diaphragmatic cyst is recommended when symptomatic, when concerning for hydatid infection, or when the diagnosis is unclear.

Lipoma is the second most common benign primary lesion of the diaphragm. Lipomas are encapsulated, homogeneous, fat-containing lesions that usually arise from the posterior left hemidiaphragm (Fig. 33.8A). They

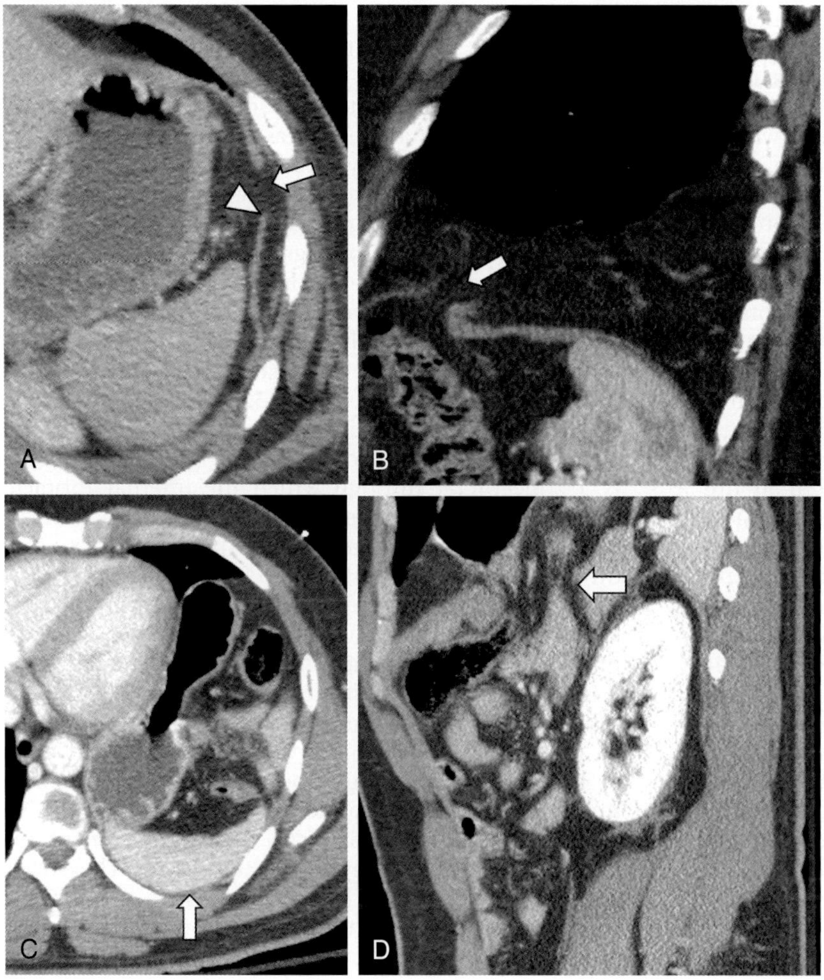

Figure 33.7 Diaphragmatic rupture. Axial (A) and sagittal (B) CT images demonstrate discontinuity of the diaphragm *(arrows)* and a dangling diaphragm sign *(arrowhead)*, consistent with rupture. (C) In a different patient with diaphragmatic rupture, the spleen and abdominal organs are laying dependently *(arrow)* on the posterior chest wall without support of the diaphragm, consistent with the dependent viscera sign. (D) Sagittal CT scan in another patient demonstrates diaphragmatic discontinuity and the collar sign *(arrow)*. The small bowel and stomach are narrowed as they pass through the defect, as if surrounded by a collar.

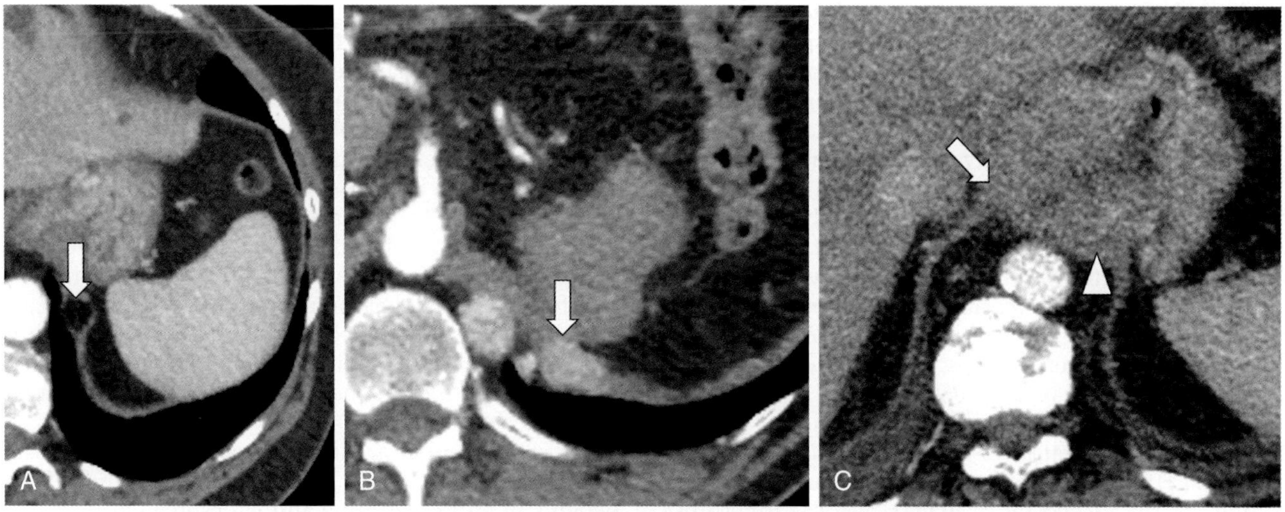

Figure 33.8 Diaphragmatic masses. (A) Axial CT scan demonstrates a small, fat-containing mass within the left posterior hemidiaphragm, one of the most common locations for a diaphragmatic lipoma *(arrow)*. (B) Axial CT scan in a different patient reveals an enhancing nodule within the body of the left hemidiaphragm in a patient with metastatic renal cell carcinoma *(arrow)*. (C) Axial CT scan in a patient with gastric cancer reveals a gastric mass that directly invades the left *(arrowhead)* and right *(arrow)* crura of the diaphragm, evidenced by the loss of fat planes between the diaphragm and mass.

are usually found in obese patients. Differentiation of a lipoma from malignant liposarcoma can be difficult, but large lesions with scattered thick septations, nodules, and ipsilateral pleural effusion should raise concern for liposarcoma. A lipoma should not be confused with a BH, which also occurs along the posterior hemidiaphragm. A lipoma should be surrounded by diaphragmatic muscle or tissue, whereas a BH is seen as fat protruding through a defect that is not completely surrounded by diaphragm.

Other exceedingly rare benign primary tumors of the diaphragm include fibroma, hemangioma, schwannoma, chondroma, hamartoma, and leiomyoma, among others. Benign endometrial implants on the diaphragm have also been reported, which may present as catamenial pneumothorax.

Most malignant masses of the diaphragm are due to secondary involvement, either via direct invasion or metastatic spread. Direct invasion can occur from lung cancer, mesothelioma, esophageal cancer, or an upper abdominal malignancy (see Fig. 33.8C). Common sources of metastatic disease include thymoma (in the form of drop metastases to the pleural space) and ovarian cancer (see Fig. 33.8B).

Primary malignant lesions are rare and usually sarcomas (typically rhabdomyosarcoma or fibrosarcoma and, less commonly, liposarcoma). Imaging characteristics are nonspecific, with heterogeneous appearance and variable enhancement as the most commonly reported features. When the mass is large, it can be difficult to diagnose diaphragmatic origin of the tumor.

■ Chest Wall

Important Anatomy

The chest wall is a cylinder of bone, muscle, cartilage, and fat that encases and protects the internal organs. Functionally, the chest wall facilitates upper extremity and torso movement and breathing. The spine, ribs, and costal cartilages form the core of the thoracic cylinder and provide the innermost defense for the central vital organs. There are normally 12 ribs, which converge anteriorly at the sternum and manubrium. Between the ribs are 11 intercostal spaces, each of which contains muscle, fat, and a neurovascular bundle of nerve, artery, and vein. The neurovascular bundle usually courses high (cranially) in the intercostal space, along the caudal surface of each rib, adjacent to the parietal pleura.

The region between the chest wall and pleura is known as the extrapleural space (EPS). The EPS is comprised of three components, from deep to superficial: (1) deep extrapleural fat (a fat layer in contact with the parietal pleura); (2) endothoracic fascia (a loose connective tissue lining the rib and costal cartilage); and (3) innermost intercostal muscle. On CT, the EPS is seen as a thin stripe, of either fat or soft tissue attenuation, directly lining the pleura. This stripe has been called the *extrapleural stripe* and represents a combination of the endothoracic fascia and innermost intercostal muscle. The deep extrapleural fat may be seen as a part of this stripe or, when prominent, a layer of fat between the stripe and the pleura (Fig. 33.9A and B). The EPS can become prominent due to inflammation or infiltration by adjacent disease, such as empyema, interstitial lung disease, or cancer. If the EPS is prominent but of mostly fat attenuation, considerations should include obesity or chronic steroid use (see Fig. 33.9C). This is often confused with pleural thickening, particularly on chest radiographs. The EPS can also become expanded by hematoma or air, usually secondary to trauma or iatrogenic dissection of the space. The EPS should not normally contain visible lymph nodes; prominent lymph nodes are usually due to inflammation or metastatic disease (see Fig. 33.9D).

Within the anterior intercostal spaces, between the sternum and the ribs and deep to the intercostal muscle, is a zone of fat through which the internal thoracic artery, also termed the *internal mammary artery,* courses. The internal thoracic arteries are paired arteries, one on each side of the chest, which supply the anterior chest wall and breasts, terminating at the seventh costal cartilage. Adjacent to the internal thoracic arteries are internal thoracic veins and lymph nodes. Internal thoracic artery lymph nodes are important markers of metastatic disease in cases of breast cancer or transthoracic spread of abdominal cancers.

The radiologist should be aware of the sternalis muscle, a normal anatomic variant seen in about 5% of the population, which can appear prominent on mammography and may be mistaken for a chest wall mass. The sternalis muscle may be unilateral or bilateral. It appears as a relatively narrow band of muscle running anterior to the pectoralis major muscle, from the jugular notch to the inferior sternum. If a convex mass is evident along the chest wall in the craniocaudal mammogram, the radiologist should recognize this as a normal variant.

Imaging

Techniques That Best Image the Chest Wall

MRI is the most reliable imaging tool to depict and characterize the chest wall and its abnormalities. MRI depicts tumor size, morphology, vascularity, and extent of involvement better than CT. Cardiac and/or respiratory gating has been used to reduce or eliminate motion-related artifacts. In the case of breast masses, the time course of lesion enhancement can be used to differentiate benign from malignant masses. MRI is especially important for the detection of small and occult masses. Breast MRI is not recommended for routine surveillance but does have a role in screening women who are considered high risk (e.g., *BRCA* gene mutations or a strong family history).

CT can also offer accurate assessment of tumor size, morphology, vascularity, and extent, with the added benefits of rapid scan time and widespread availability. However, CT is limited in tissue plane distinction compared to MRI.

Plain radiography can be useful in the detection of osseous and soft tissue abnormalities but has a limited role in characterizing or delineating the extent of disease.

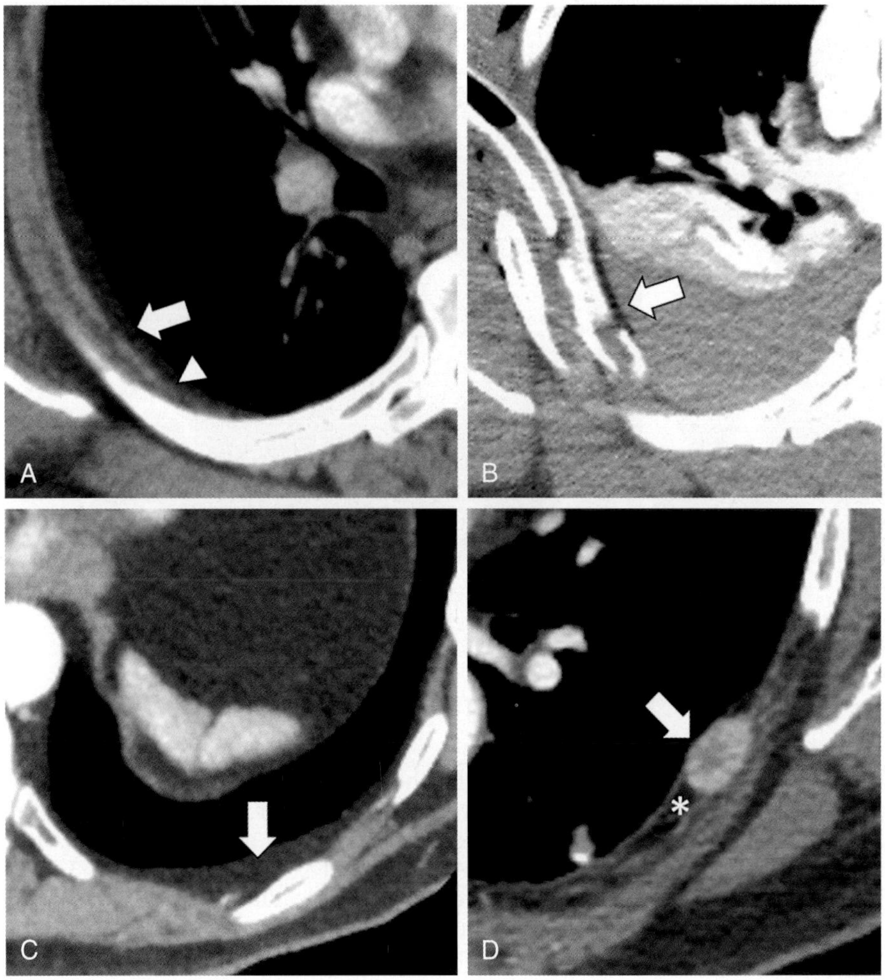

Figure 33.9 Extrapleural space (EPS). (A) Axial CT scan demonstrates the normal EPS: (1) thin layer of deep extrapleural fat *(arrow)* and (2) extrapleural stripe *(arrowhead)*, which is a combination of the endothoracic fascia and innermost intercostal muscle. (B) Axial CT scan in another patient shows a thoracostomy tube localized to the EPS by the thin layer of extrapleural fat *(arrow)* deep to the tube. (C) Axial CT scan in a different patient reveals prominent extrapleural fat *(arrow)* in a patient on chronic steroids. (D) Extrapleural metastatic lymphadenopathy, external to the thickened parietal pleura *(arrow)* and centered in the extrapleural fat *(asterisk)*.

The role of positron emission tomography (PET)-CT is primarily in the detection of primary or metastatic chest wall malignancy and assessment of treatment response.

US is routinely used to evaluate breast masses and is especially important in differentiating solid and cystic masses, as well as guiding percutaneous needle biopsies. Contrast-enhanced US has been emerging as a promising technique for the evaluation of sarcomatous lesions and other solid masses.

Determining Chest Wall Invasion by Lung or Pleural Disease

Determination of chest wall invasion by intrathoracic malignancy is a primary part of tumor staging. Establishing chest wall invasion is also important when evaluating pulmonary or pleural infections as invasion is indicative of aggressive infection. The best indicator of invasion is rib destruction and/or involvement of the chest wall musculature (Fig. 33.10A). In challenging cases where rib or muscle involvement is not evident, the EPS can be a very useful landmark. Any obliteration or obscuration of the EPS should raise concern for chest wall invasion. A mass contiguous with the extrapleural fat or innermost intercostal muscle is also suggestive of chest wall invasion (see Fig. 33.10B). In the case of a lesion arising from the chest wall, such as hematoma or tumor, if a stripe of fat is seen between the lesion and lung, the lesion remains within the chest wall (the stripe of fat represents the EPS).

Common Congenital and Developmental Anomalies

The most common congenital anomalies include cervical ribs, pectus excavatum, pectus carinatum, cleidocranial dysostosis, and Poland syndrome.

Cervical ribs, also called *accessory ribs,* are supernumerary ribs arising from the C7 vertebral body. They are of variable size (short riblet or full-sized jointed rib) and number, often seen bilaterally. Most cases are asymptomatic. The most common associated complication is thoracic outlet syndrome secondary to compression of adjacent vessels (subclavian artery or vein) and/or nerves (brachial plexus). Cervical ribs can be identified on frontal radiographs as ribs arising from the cervical spine, with characteristic horizontal or caudally angled medial portions as they extend off the vertebral body.

Pectus excavatum, the most common congenital deformity of the sternum, refers to inward concave depression of the sternum, colloquially termed *funnel chest.* Frontal chest radiographs demonstrate indistinctness

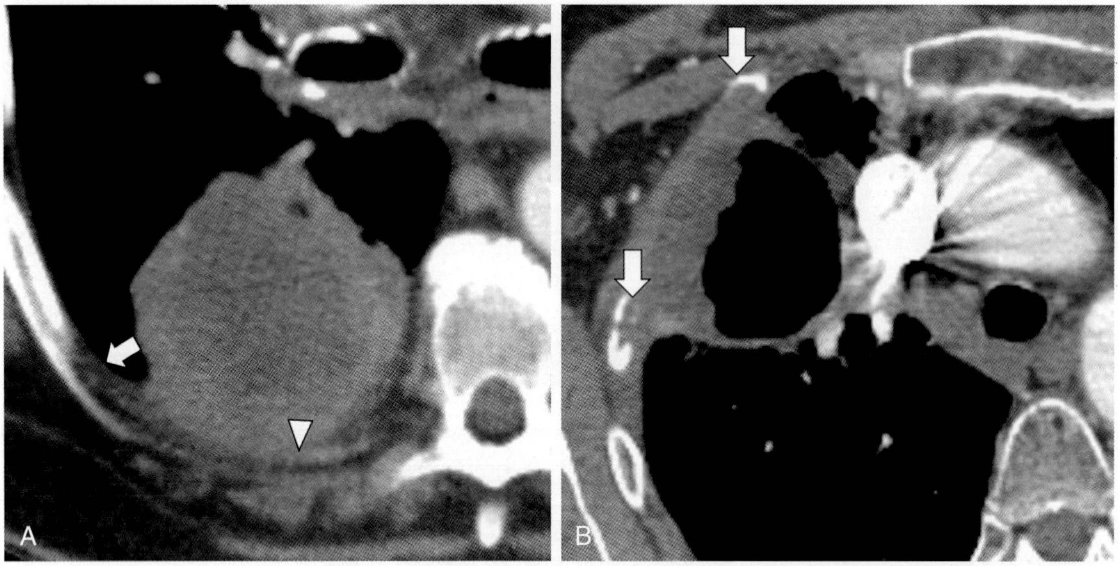

Figure 33.10 Chest wall invasion. (A) Axial CT scan demonstrates right lower lobe lung cancer with invasion of the chest wall. The mass is closely apposed with the extrapleural stripe *(arrowhead)*, with obliteration of the extrapleural fat plane *(arrow)*. (B) Axial CT scan in a different patient reveals a right upper lobe pulmonary abscess, also with invasion of the chest wall, most clearly evidenced by rib destruction *(arrows)*.

of the right heart border with displacement of the heart to the left and downward-sloping anterior ribs. Lateral radiographs reveal the characteristic inward and concave depression of the sternum relative to the anterior ribs (Fig. 33.11A and B). CT can be used to obtain accurate measurements for Haller index (HI) calculation (see next section) and to assess for complications related to the chest wall deformity (see Fig. 33.11C).

Pectus carinatum, the opposite of pectus excavatum, and colloquially termed *pigeon chest,* represents anterior sternal protrusion with associated convex deformity of adjacent costal cartilages. Pectus carinatum is usually of the chondrogladiolar type (involvement of the sternal body) and, more rarely, the chondromanubrial type (involvement of the manubrium). Pectus carinatum cannot be reliably identified on frontal radiographs but is well visualized on lateral radiographs or CT scans. Similar to pectus excavatum, the degree of deformity can be calculated using the HI (see next section).

Cleidocranial dysostosis is a hereditary disease of delayed ossification of midline structures. In the thorax, it is marked by partial or total absence of the clavicles, supernumerary ribs, and spondylosis. Chest radiographs demonstrate the absence of clavicles, with radiolucent lung apices due to the absence of overlying bone.

Poland syndrome represents unilateral absence of the pectoralis muscles and ipsilateral syndactyly. There may be associated ipsilateral hypoplasia of the ribs as well. Chest radiographs commonly show a unilateral hyperlucent hemithorax; CT demonstrates unilateral absence of the pectoralis musculature.

Important Measurements in Pectus Excavatum

In assessing pectus excavatum, surgical planning is, in part, predicated on the precise measurement of the HI. The HI is the ratio of the lateral distance between the inner rib margins and the shortest distance between the anterior vertebral body and sternum. For pectus excavatum, the HI should be determined at the most depressed part of the sternum. A normal HI is 2.5, whereas HI >3.25 is considered severe pectus excavatum. The HI is considered in conjunction with clinical and cosmetic considerations in the decision-making process for operative repair. It can be calculated as follows:

(Transverse distance between the inner rib margins)/
(Anteroposterior distance from the inner margin of the sternum to the anterior margin of the vertebral body)

Important Findings in the Setting of Trauma

The thorax is the third most common site of traumatic injury after the head and extremities. CT is superior to chest radiography for the detection of thoracic injury. Thoracic trauma can be classified as blunt or penetrating, with penetrating injuries typified by a tract between the inner thorax and skin (e.g., stabbing, gunshot wound). Blunt trauma causes 90% of thoracic injuries.

Rib fractures are the most common injuries resulting from blunt thoracic trauma. Fractures of the relatively unprotected fourth through eighth ribs are most common. Higher impact forces are usually required to injure the upper ribs. Rib fractures are often associated with intrathoracic injury. For example, 52% of cardiac contusion cases are associated with rib fractures. Furthermore, the fractured ribs themselves can cause adjacent injury, such as pneumothorax, hemothorax, or pulmonary contusion. Up to 15% of cases of upper rib fracture have associated injuries to the subclavian vessels and/or brachial plexus. One important traumatic injury is flail chest. Flail chest

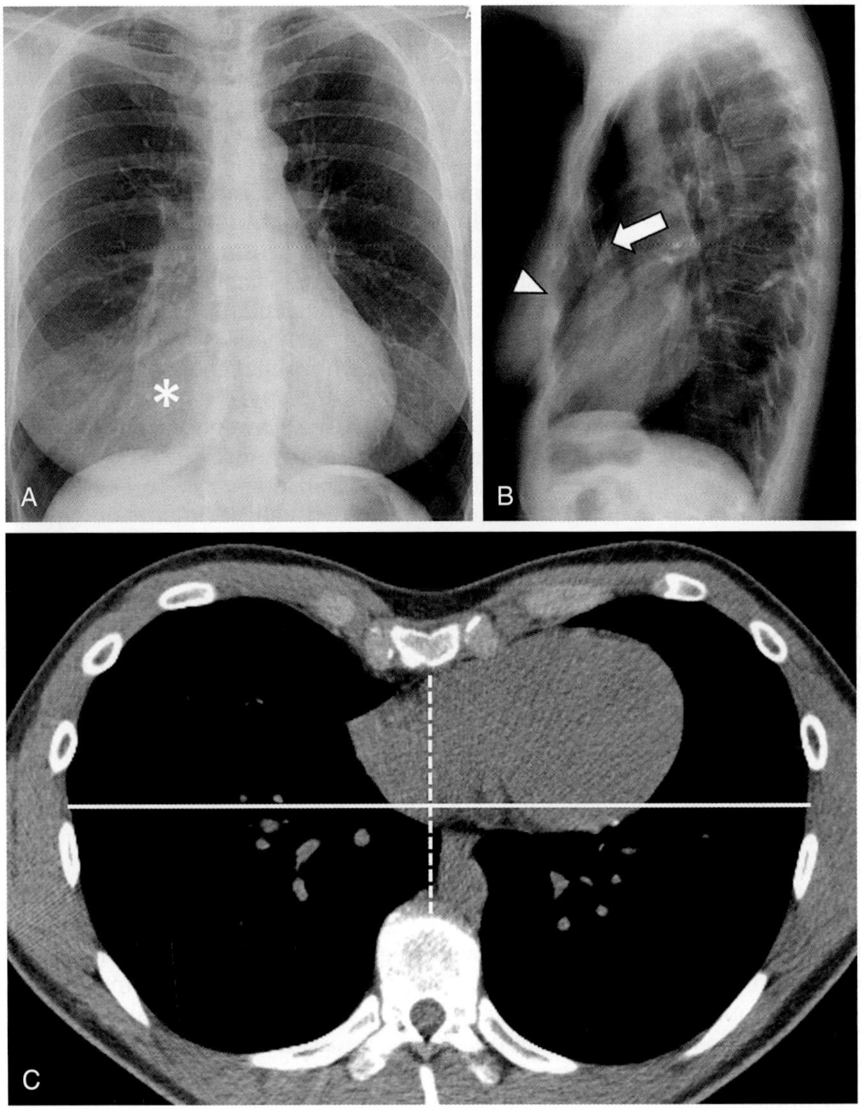

Figure 33.11 Pectus excavatum. Frontal (A) and lateral (B) chest radiographs show a hazy opacity that silhouettes the right cardiac border *(A, asterisk)*. (B) Lateral view demonstrates inward displacement of the sternum *(arrow)* relative to the anterior ribs *(arrowhead)*, confirming pectus excavatum. (C) Axial CT scan demonstrates proper measurement of the Haller index. Measurements are taken at the narrowest anteroposterior (AP) distance between the sternum and spine. *Solid line,* Transverse distance between ribs; *dashed line,* AP distance between the sternum and spine.

occurs when three contiguous ribs are fractured in two or more places. The result of this fracture pattern is a segment of the chest wall that is completely independent of the remainder of the chest wall, allowing for free paradoxic movement during breathing. Most flail chests require surgical treatment and prolonged mechanical ventilation.

Sternal fractures are due to direct blunt anterior trauma (e.g., seatbelt or air bag injury during a motor vehicle accident). Associated injuries can include retrosternal mediastinal hematoma, pulmonary contusion, myocardial contusion, and spinal injury. Sternoclavicular joint dislocation can also be present, with the anterior dislocation more common and usually better tolerated. Posterior sternoclavicular dislocation can be associated with injuries to the adjacent mediastinal vessels, trachea, and esophagus.

Scapular fractures are rare and are usually the result of more severe injury. As such, they are typically associated with other injuries, such as rib fracture, pneumothorax, or pulmonary contusion. Spinal fractures are also rare and are usually of the hyperflexion or axial loading type. There may be associated spinal cord injury, and evaluation with MRI is recommended when there is concern for cord injury.

Soft tissue hematoma is seen as a high-density (i.e. 30–80 Hounsfield units [HU]) fluid collection within the chest wall fat or musculature. Hematoma can result from arterial or venous bleeding. High-attenuation contrast material within or near a hematoma is suggestive of an arterial source of hematoma, for which evaluation with arteriography and possible embolization is warranted. Extrapleural hematomas occur in the EPS and are almost always accompanied by adjacent rib fractures. A helpful sign of extrapleural hematoma is the extrapleural fat sign. This sign refers to accumulation of blood within the EPS, which displaces the extrapleural fat away from the ribs and toward the pleura and lung.

Subcutaneous emphysema (SE) is air between and within the fascial planes of the chest wall. In the trauma setting, the air can arise from the mediastinum (pneumomediastinum), pleural space (pneumothorax), or an open wound secondary to penetrating injury.

Masses in the Chest Wall

Soft Tissue Masses

Chest wall masses are generally uncommon and usually of soft tissue or osseous origin. Soft tissue masses can be further divided into benign and malignant lesions. Imaging characteristics are protean, with overlap between specific pathologic entities; however, the hallmark of benign lesions is slow or no growth. Rapid growth of a lesion should raise suspicion for malignancy. Bone scalloping or mild osseous erosion can be seen in benign slow-growing lesions, whereas frank bone invasion suggests malignancy.

The most common soft tissue masses include lipoma, hematoma, peripheral nerve sheath tumor, metastasis, liposarcoma, elastofibroma dorsi, lymphoma, hemangioma, desmoid tumor, and malignant fibrous histiocytoma (MFH).

LIPOMAS AND LIPOSARCOMAS

These are benign, encapsulated, fat-containing masses that occur more frequently in older and obese patients (Fig. 33.12A). The true prevalence of lipomas is impossible to gauge because they are often incidentally detected on imaging without further workup, but they likely represent the most common chest wall mass. On CT and MRI, these appear as homogeneous, fat attenuation/intensity lesions, without large or nodular areas of enhancement. Small thin septations can be present that demonstrate faint enhancement on CT or MRI, with corresponding low signal on nonenhanced T1-weighted images. Uniform signal loss on fat-suppressed T1-weighted MRI is a hallmark of lipoma. Any area of increased attenuation on CT (relative to adjacent subcutaneous fat) and calcification or ossification, thick septations, or nonuniform fat suppression on MRI suggests a soft tissue component, thus raising suspicion for a malignant liposarcoma (see Fig. 33.12B). Lesions larger than 10 cm in size are also suggestive of liposarcoma, although this finding is of low specificity. Liposarcomas display a spectrum of homogeneous to heterogeneous signal intensities on T1- and T2-weighted MRI, depending on pathologic subtype. Well-differentiated lesions contain more fat (high T1 and T2 signal), whereas dedifferentiated or undifferentiated liposarcomas have greater soft tissue components and a resulting heterogeneous signal. Any contrast enhancement should be considered abnormal and a sign of malignancy. The accurate diagnosis of liposarcoma is important because it usually presents as a painless chest wall mass.

HEMATOMAS

These are collections of blood in the chest wall and present as a mass of high attenuation (30–70 HU) on noncontrast CT (see Fig. 33.12C). Some hematomas will demonstrate a fluid-hematocrit level. Hematomas are usually seen after surgery (with damage of chest wall vasculature) or in patients who are on anticoagulation therapy. Hematomas that do not resolve may form a chronic expanding hematoma. Hematomas with associated contrast enhancement should raise suspicion for a bleeding soft tissue neoplasm, or ruptered vessel in the setting of trauma.

PERIPHERAL NERVE SHEATH TUMOR

Another common soft tissue tumor of the chest wall is a peripheral nerve sheath tumor (PNST), a neurogenic tumor arising from a peripheral nerve. Up to 27% of PNSTs have been reported to originate within the chest wall. Schwannoma is the most common PNST (85%), followed by neurofibroma. Chest wall PNSTs arise from nerve roots, either in the intercostal spaces from intercostal nerves or spinal nerve roots or in the axilla from the brachial plexus. These lesions can be benign or malignant, without specific imaging characteristics to differentiate between them reliably. However, any rapid change in size of a suspected PNST should raise concern for malignancy.

On CT or MRI, PNSTs are typically smoothly demarcated, round, or ovoid masses. Schwannomas are typically isointense or hyperintense to muscle on T1-weighted images and heterogeneously hyperintense on T2-weighted images. Neurofibromas are usually isointense or hypointense to muscle on T1 and hyperintense on T2-weighted images, with a characteristic target pattern of peripheral T2 hyperintensity relative to the center sometimes evident. Generally, schwannomas and neurofibromas demonstrate avid enhancement on postcontrast CT and MRI, with neurofibromas occasionally exhibiting a target-like appearance of peripheral enhancement. Smaller lesions exhibit more uniform enhancement, whereas larger lesions show more heterogeneous enhancement. Malignant PNSTs frequently demonstrate areas of necrosis and hemorrhage, marked by areas of nonenhancement. Up to 75% of schwannomas can appear low attenuation on CT due to the presence of lipid-rich Schwann cells, thus potentially being mistaken for a lipoma. Enhancement remains a key distinguishing factor, along with high T2 signal on MRI scans. Tissue biopsy is usually required for diagnosis but may not be needed in the presence of multiple skin lesions, which would support the diagnosis of neurofibromatosis.

OTHER TUMORS AND LESIONS

Vascular tumors of the chest wall include benign hemangioma, glomus tumor, and malignant angiosarcoma. Hemangiomas are uncommon benign masses that can arise in the intramuscular, intercostal, or subcutaneous spaces. They present in younger patients as painful masses. Hemangiomas are composed of blood vessels that create specific imaging characteristics. On CT, they are usually heterogeneous in attenuation, with up to 30% of lesions containing calcifications; CT detects intratumoral calcifications better than MRI. Due to their vascular nature, hemangiomas enhance significantly following contrast administration. On MRI, these lesions follow fat signal intensity on T1- and T2-weighted sequences (due to fibrofatty components). Signal voids corresponding to dilated tortuous vessels may be seen, and marked contrast enhancement is observed. Malignant angiosarcomas present as large painful masses with a rapid growth rate. They can develop within the chest wall following radiation therapy (e.g., for breast cancer), in cases of chronic lymphedema, or after chemical exposure.

Elastofibroma dorsi is a benign lesion in the posterolateral chest wall, with a characteristic infrascapular location between the serratus anterior muscle and ribs. They are more common in females and bilateral in up

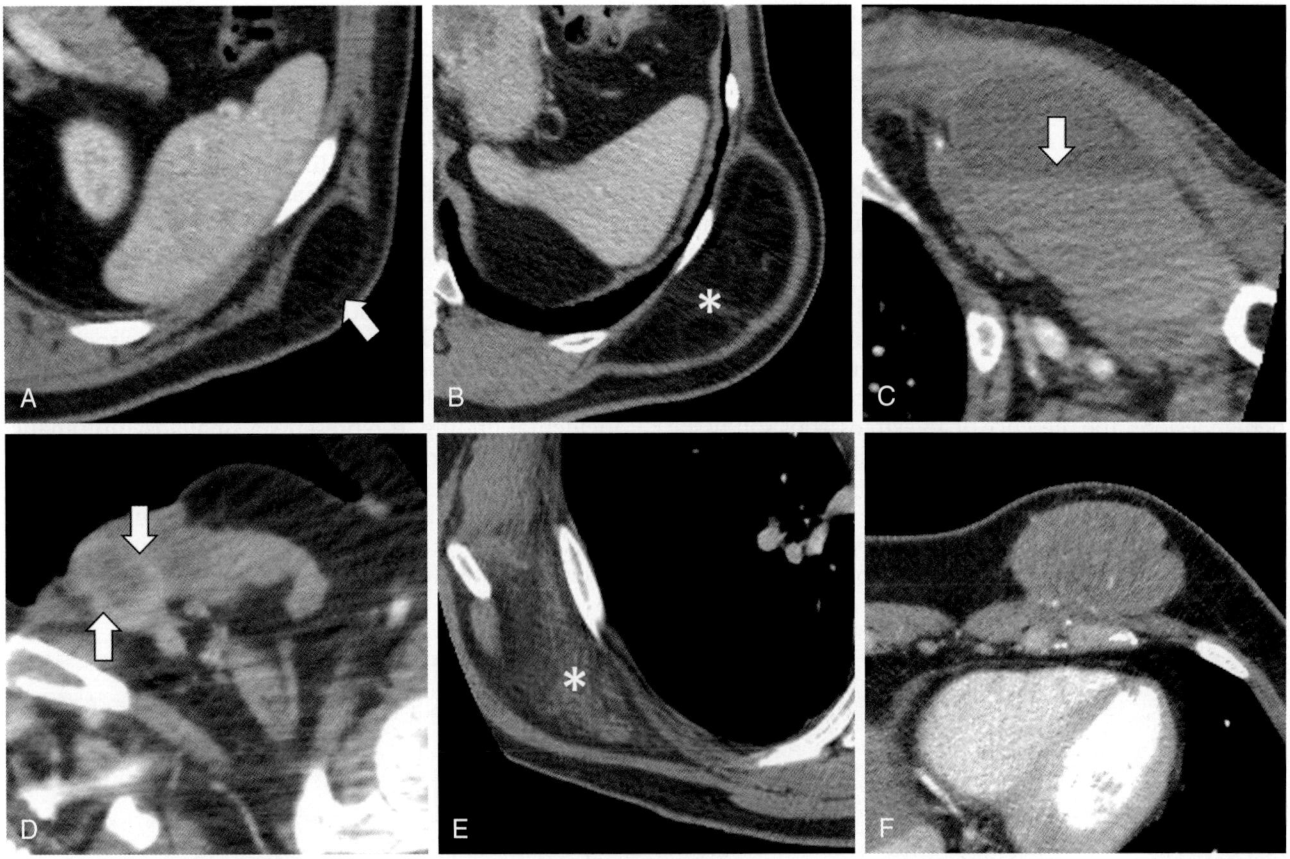

Figure 33.12 Soft tissue masses. (A) Axial CT scan demonstrates an encapsulated, homogeneously fat attenuation mass *(arrow)* consistent with a lipoma. (B) Axial CT scan in another patient reveals an encapsulated fat attenuation mass with thick internal septations *(asterisk)* compatible with liposarcoma. (C) Axial CT scan in a patient on anticoagulation demonstrates a well-defined mass in the left anterior chest wall with a fluid-hematocrit level *(arrow)*, consistent with hematoma. (D) Axial CT scan demonstrates a mass in the anterior left chest wall with central low attenuation and peripheral nodular enhancement *(arrow)*, consistent with malignant fibrous histiocytoma. (E) Axial CT scan demonstrates a mass *(asterisk)* in the posterolateral chest wall in the infrascapular region. This mass has a striated appearance, with a mixture of fat and soft tissue characteristic of elastofibroma dorsi. (F) Axial CT scan in a different patient shows a heterogeneously enhancing mass within the anterior chest wall compatible with metastasis in a patient with extensive metastatic melanoma.

to 60% of cases. On CT, these appear as poorly defined masses of muscle attenuation, with linear or heterogeneous internal low attenuation (representing fibrous or fatty components; see Fig. 33.12E). On MRI, a low signal mass of similar signal intensity to muscle is seen with intralesional areas of high T1 and T2 signal. These lesions may demonstrate mild to moderate hypermetabolic activity on PET-CT.

Chest wall metastases are uncommon and often reflect advanced extensive malignancy. Lung cancer, breast cancer, and mesothelioma metastases usually result from direct extension or lymphangitic spread, whereas melanoma and renal cell carcinoma are spread hematogenously (see Fig. 33.12F).

Soft tissue sarcomas are rare malignancies. Fibrosarcoma and MFH develop in adults; rhabdomyosarcoma occurs in children. Other than liposarcomas, there are no specific imaging characteristics to distinguish the various types of sarcomas. MFH has been reported to demonstrate central low attenuation on CT, corresponding to its myxoid matrix, with more peripheral nodular enhancement (see Fig. 33.12D). On MRI, these lesions possess variable signal characteristics and exhibit heterogeneous enhancement.

Similarly, lymphoma and other hematologic malignancies (e.g., myeloma, plasmacytoma) are rare entities in the chest wall. Secondary chest wall involvement by direct extension is more common than primary chest wall malignancy. Large B cell lymphoma is the most common primary chest wall lymphoma, whereas Hodgkin lymphoma is the most common secondary malignancy (usually from the mediastinum or axilla). Chest wall lymphoma presents as a well-defined mass of soft tissue attenuation that spreads to and encases adjacent structures, such as bone or cartilage. CT demonstrates a soft tissue mass with mild contrast enhancement. MRI characteristics include a variable T1 signal relative to muscle and T2 hyperintensity. Lymphomas can exhibit central necrosis, which appears as heterogeneous decreased enhancement on CT or MRI.

Plasmacytoma when seen as a soft tissue mass, is termed the extramedullary form of plasmacytoma.

However, osseous plasmacytoma can also have a prominent soft tissue component. The soft tissue lesions are usually well-defined lobulated masses of relatively uniform enhancement on CT and MRI.

Osseous Masses

Similar to the soft tissue masses, chest wall lesions arising from the bones can be benign or malignant. Benign osseous tumors include osteochondroma, aneurysmal bone cyst, fibrous dysplasia, ossifying fibromyxoid tumor, giant cell tumor, and chondromyxoid fibroma. Malignant lesions include chondrosarcoma, myeloma or plasmacytoma, osteosarcoma, and Ewing sarcoma. Although malignant lesions may be challenging to distinguish from benign lesions, the presence of an extraosseous soft tissue component is highly suggestive of malignancy.

BENIGN OSSEOUS LESIONS

Osteochondroma is the most common benign bone tumor and the most common benign tumor of the ribs. In the chest, they most often arise from the rib or scapula, typically at the costochondral junction. On imaging, they appear as pedunculated lesions with characteristic continuity between the medullary cavity of the lesion and the originating bone (Fig. 33.13A). Osteochondroma sometimes exhibits a hyaline cap, which is seen as a well-defined, radiodense margin on radiographs and CT; the hyaline cap demonstrates high T2 signal on MRI. Thickening of the cap >2 mm, bone erosion, and/or increasing pain at the lesion site are suggestive of malignant transformation. Most osteochondromas are solitary but can be multiple in osteochondromatosis, also called *multiple hereditary exostoses.*

Enostosis, also known as a *bone island,* is a very common incidental finding. It represents a small, asymptomatic, non-neoplastic focus of compacted bone. It is typically 1 cm (ranging from 2 mm to 2 cm), hyperdense, ovoid, and located within the medullary space (see Fig. 33.13B and C). On chest radiographs, enostoses within the ribs can be confused for pulmonary nodules; they sometimes

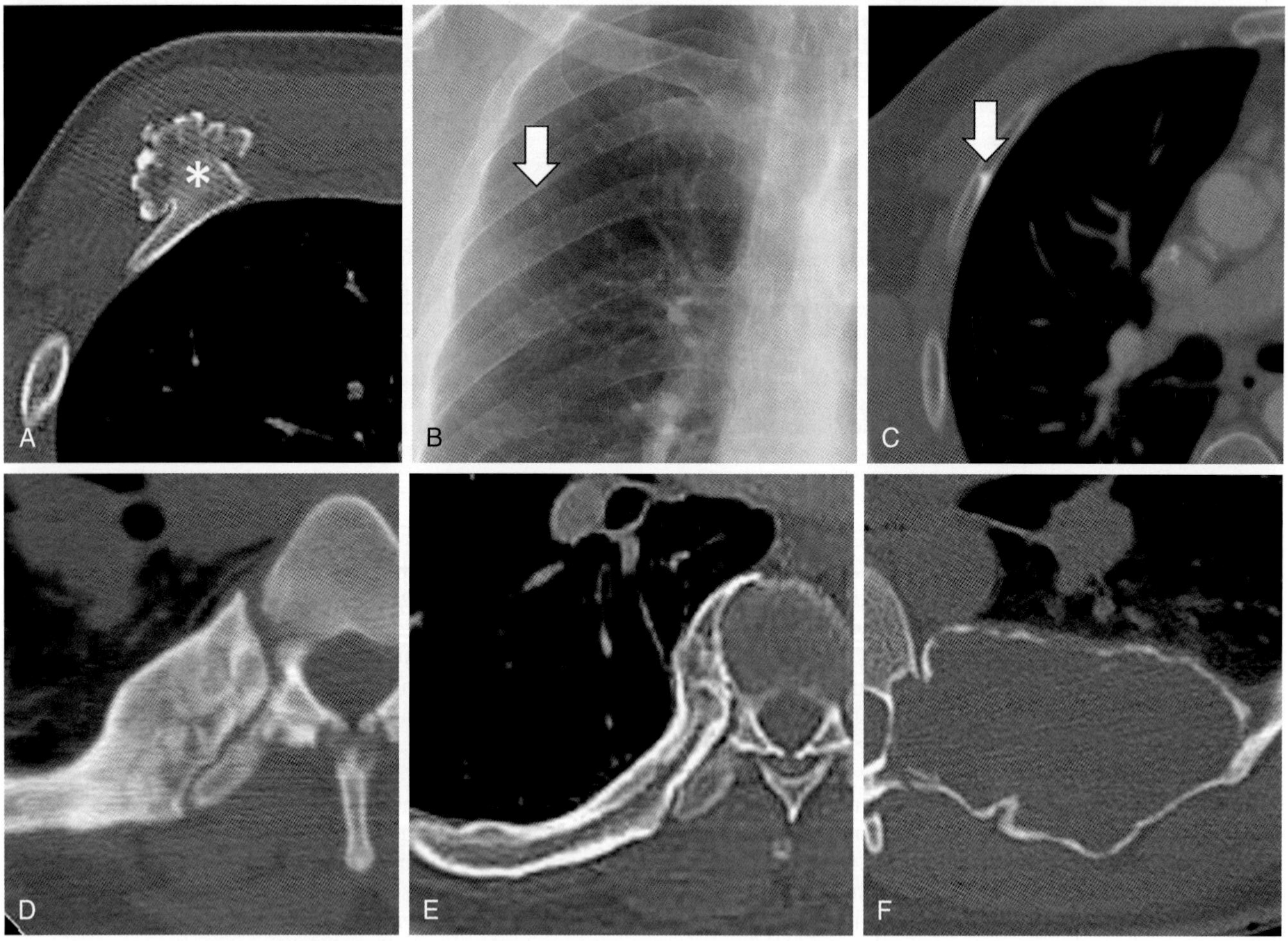

Figure 33.13 Benign osseous lesions. (A) Axial CT scan demonstrates a pedunculated lesion arising from an anterior rib with characteristic continuity between the medullary cavity of the lesion and rib, compatible with an osteochondroma *(asterisk)*. Frontal radiograph (B) reveals a nodular density *(arrow)* projecting over the right upper lobe, which on axial CT scan (C) corresponds to a focal sclerotic lesion within the right third anterior rib *(arrow)*, compatible with enostosis or bone island. Enostosis can be confused for a pulmonary nodule on chest radiographs. Fibrous dysplasia has a variety of appearances on CT scan, usually as an expansile ground-glass lesion (D), but also as cortical thickening (E). (F) Axial CT scan shows an expansile lytic lesion located eccentrically in the posterior elements of a midthoracic vertebral body and adjoining rib, compatible with an aneurysmal bone cyst.

demonstrate spiculated margins. MRI demonstrates decreased signal on T1- and T2-weighted sequences. On CT, a mean attenuation value >885 is highly suggestive of a bone island in ovoid medullary lesions measuring between 2 mm and 2 cm, and is a useful tool to differentiate bone island from metastatic disease.

Fibrous dysplasia (FD) is another commonly encountered benign osseous lesion. The vast majority are monostotic, but polyostotic disease can occur. FD usually arises from the rib but has also been reported to originate from the clavicle. FD can be asymptomatic or present with pain and fracture. Characteristically, the lesion appears as a slow-growing, expansile, fusiform mass with a central soap bubble or ground-glass appearance on radiographs and CT scans (see Fig. 33.13D). However, there is a range of appearances, including cortical thickening and increased trabeculation mimicking Paget disease (see Fig. 33.13E). Irregular calcifications can be seen within the lesion. These lesions demonstrate variable T2 signal and predominantly low T1 signal on MRI. FD can show increased radiotracer uptake on bone scintigraphy.

Aneurysmal bone cyst (ABC) is a benign but rapidly growing lesion. Imaging characteristically demonstrates an expansile and lytic lesion, typically eccentric in location (see Fig. 33.13F). ABCs have a predilection for the posterior elements of the spine. They occasionally demonstrate soft tissue extension beyond the bone, making it difficult to distinguish them from malignancy. Identification of a fluid level within the lesion, corresponding to hemorrhage, may be helpful but is not specific for ABC.

Enchondroma is a rare, usually painless lesion. It is located within the medullary cavity of tubular bones, commonly within the ribs. These are typically small, 1- to 2-cm lesions, which are lucent but contain central chondroid calcifications that appear as rings and arcs. Enchondroma can be complicated by malignant transformation into low-grade chondrosarcoma. Any pain that is associated with these lesions should raise suspicion for malignancy.

Paget disease is a chronic disorder of bone resorption and remodeling that results in thickened, yet fragile bones. Although rare in the thorax, there is a predilection for spinal involvement. Imaging demonstrates cortical and trabecular thickening, which may be hypermetabolic on PET-CT. Sarcomatous degeneration has been reported.

MALIGNANT OSSEOUS LESIONS

Metastases are the most common malignant lesions of the ribs. Common primary malignancies include the lung, breast, thyroid, kidney, and prostate gland. Metastases have a variety of appearances and may be focal, diffuse, osteolytic, or osteoblastic, with or without associated soft tissue components.

Chondrosarcoma is the most common primary malignant tumor of the chest wall. It most commonly arises from the anterior ribs, costochondral junctions, or sternum. They are twice as common in men, usually in patients younger than 20 or older than 40 years. On radiographs or CT scans, they appear as slow-growing, expansile, intramedullary lesions with bone destruction. Intralesional calcifications may be present, which may be linear, ring, or arc-shaped, with stippled or dense configuration (Fig. 33.14A). On MRI, these lesions demonstrate a variable T1 signal but increased T2 signal. Areas of intralesional calcifications remain low signal on all sequences. There is usually variable contrast enhancement on CT or MRI; peripheral rim enhancement can be present, which can be confused for an abscess (see Fig. 33.14B and C).

Plasmacytoma and myeloma are plasma cell neoplasms originating from bone marrow. These lesions typically present at 50 to 70 years of age, more often in men. Plasmacytoma is the solitary form of disease, whereas multiple lesions are present in multiple myeloma. Plasmacytoma presents as a painful, expansile, lytic mass, often located in a vertebral body. Extraosseous plasmacytoma has a similar presentation but can be seen as a purely soft tissue lesion, without direct osseous involvement. Multiple myeloma is a systemic disease that manifests as multifocal osteolysis and lucencies, usually quite discrete, sometimes mistaken for generalized osteopenia (see Fig. 33.14D). MRI demonstrates low T1 signal and high T2 signal, with diffuse enhancement.

Osteosarcoma is a rare thoracic mesenchymal tumor with a predilection for the ribs, scapulae, and clavicles. The osseous form of disease is more common in younger patients, whereas the extraosseous form is seen in patients around 50 years of age. Chest wall osteosarcoma commonly presents as a painful mass with local extension and metastatic spread to the lungs and lymph nodes. Radiographs and CT scans demonstrate a soft tissue mass containing osteoid matrix; the mineralization is, importantly, central in location (see Fig. 33.14F). MRI features are variable but predominantly high T1 and T2 signal intensity, with heterogeneous enhancement.

Chest Wall Infections

Chest wall infections represent a broad spectrum of disease, including soft tissue infections such as cellulitis, phlegmon, abscess, pyomyositis, and necrotizing fasciitis and bone and joint infections such as osteomyelitis and septic arthritis. Infections are usually secondary to invasive procedures (e.g., thoracostomy tube placement for empyema), with resulting phlegmon or abscess. Chest wall infections usually occur in immunocompromised individuals, diabetics, and postoperative patients. The most common causative organisms of pyogenic infection are *Staphylococcus aureus* and *Pseudomonas aeruginosa*. In the immunocompromised patient, additional common organisms include *Actinomyces*, *Aspergillus*, and mycobacterial species. A chest wall phlegmon or abscess appears as a fluid or soft tissue attenuation mass. In the case of abscess a peripheral rim of enhancement is seen (Fig. 33.15A and B). Chronic or aggressive infections can erode or invade the ribs. Sinus tracts or fistulas can also been seen in the chronic setting. Adjacent empyema or pneumonia may also be present. Necrotizing fasciitis is an infection involving the intermuscular fascial layers. CT features are nonspecific but generally consist of fluid and, sometimes, air within the intermuscular fascia. MRI better demonstrates fluid as increased T2 signal within the fascial layers and surrounding muscles; postcontrast,

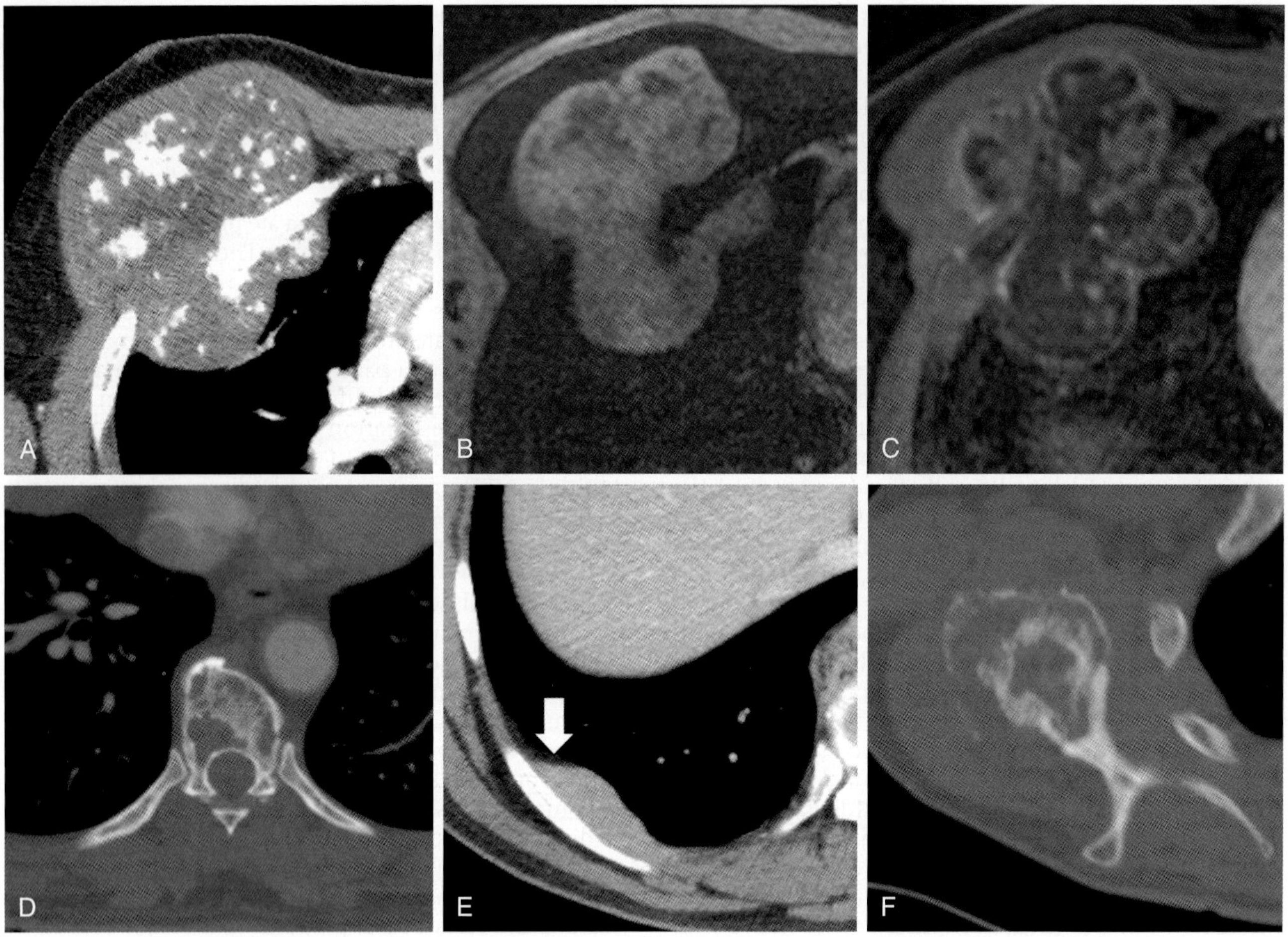

Figure 33.14 Malignant bone masses. (A) Chondrosarcoma on a CT scan appears as an expansile destructive mass arising from the anterior rib with irregular, intralesional chondroid matrix. On MRI, this lesion demonstrates increased signal on T2-weighted images (B) and peripheral enhancement on postcontrast T1-weighted images (C). In a different patient (D), multiple lytic lesions in the thoracic spine are consistent with multiple myeloma. (E) In contradistinction, extramedullary plasmacytoma on CT scan appears as a well-defined enhancing mass along the rib-intercostal space, displacing the extrapleural fat *(arrow)* without adjacent bone destruction. (F) Osteosarcoma of the right scapula presenting as an expansile lytic mass with cortical destruction mixed areas of lucency and sclerosis.

T1-weighted images demonstrate associated abscess formation as rim-enhancing fluid collections.

Empyema necessitans is a subtype of empyema, defined as direct extension of infection out of the pleural space and into the chest wall (see Fig. 33.15C). The most commonly causative organisms are *Mycobacterium tuberculosis, Actinomyces,* and *Aspergillus* species.

Osteomyelitis in the chest wall usually involves the sternum, ribs, or sternoclavicular joints. Sternal osteomyelitis can occur as a complication of cardiothoracic surgery or, less commonly, as a complication of intravenous drug abuse. Imaging findings of osteomyelitis on radiography and CT include osteopenia, cortical erosion, periosteal reaction, and mixed lucency-sclerosis of the bone. MRI findings include high T2 signal and low to intermediate T1 signal from marrow edema.

Pyogenic arthritis is rare but can occur in the thorax, especially at the sternoclavicular joint. The most common organisms are *P. aeruginosa* and *S. aureus*; 95% of cases of sternoclavicular pyogenic arthritis are unilateral. CT or MRI typically reveals osteolysis of the affected bones, which progresses to sclerosis and cortical thickening. There may be an associated soft tissue mass surrounding the bone or joint; adjacent inflammatory infiltration of fat and muscle assists in differentiating this entity from malignancy.

Costochondritis is a localized infection of the costochondral junction, which may be secondary to adjacent pulmonary infection, postoperative infection, or hematogenous infection. On CT, costochondritis manifests as focal soft tissue swelling at the costochondral junction, with or without destruction. This is in contradistinction to Tietze syndrome, which is a benign costochondritis not due to infection, that also manifests as soft tissue thickening at the costochondral junction.

Inflammatory Disorders That Can Result in Muscle Atrophy

Polymyositis and dermatomyositis are autoimmune diseases that affect the skeletal muscles. When polymyositis

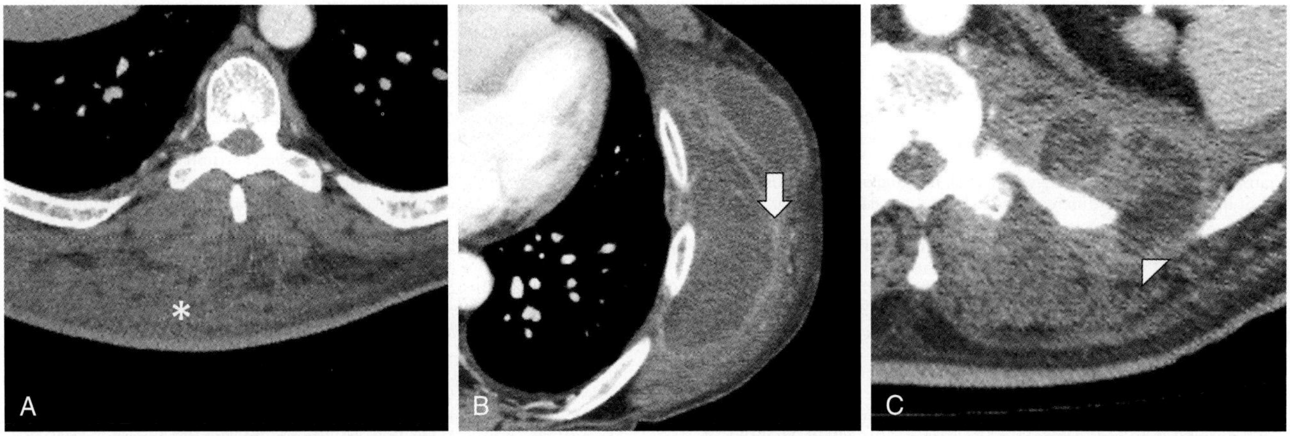

Figure 33.15 Various types of infection in the chest wall. (A) Axial CT scan demonstrates skin thickening and subcutaneous masslike infiltration *(asterisk)* compatible with cellulitis and phlegmon. (B) Axial CT scan in a different patient shows a lateral chest wall mass with rim enhancement *(arrow)* compatible with abscess. (C) Axial CT scan in another patient reveals a left-sided empyema with extension of the fluid beyond the ribs, indicating chest wall extension *(arrowhead)*, called *empyema necessitans.*

is associated with a skin rash, it is called *dermatomyositis.* These disorders are typified by muscle atrophy, fibrosis, and soft tissue calcifications. Early in the disease course, there is increased muscular bulk and increased density, with thickening of surrounding subcutaneous fat secondary to inflammatory infiltration. Amorphous and irregular soft tissue calcifications are seen in up to 70% of children but in only 10% of adults and correlates with disease severity. CT is the preferred modality for depicting calcifications, but MRI is superior in demonstrating soft tissue edema, muscular thickening, muscular atrophy, and fibrosis.

Subcutaneous Emphysema

Subcutaneous emphysema (SE) is air beneath the skin. SE is usually traumatic or iatrogenic. Following penetrating injury, air tracks from outside the patient into the subcutaneous tissues. Iatrogenic SE may be postsurgical or postprocedural, such as from central vascular access, chest tube placement, or thoracic surgery. Increasing SE in the setting of recent thoracic surgery should raise suspicion for an air leak from the lung through the surgical opening, occasionally requiring pneumolysis. SE is frequently associated with pneumothorax or pneumomediastinum. In the case of pneumomediastinum, air tracks through the thoracic inlet and into the neck and subcutaneous tissues of the chest wall.

SE in the chest wall is best visualized on radiographs as abnormal lucencies not confined to the lungs, with a fine wispy, linear, or globular appearance. These lucencies often outline the contours of muscles and muscle fibers with a branching appearance likened to a Ginkgo leaf (called the *Ginkgo leaf sign*).

In situ SE can be observed, rarely, in cases of necrotizing fasciitis of the chest wall, the result of so-called flesh-eating bacteria, usually beta-hemolytic *Streptococcus*. This is a life-threatening disease and usually occurs in immunocompromised patients. Although more commonly occurring in the lower extremities or abdomen, necrotizing fasciitis can occur in the thorax after chest drainage or thoracic surgery.

SE has also been reported in rare cases of necrotizing lung and/or pleural infections that invade the chest wall and create a fistulous communication of air between these compartments and the chest wall.

Bibliography

Abbey-Mensah GN, Waite S, Reede D, Hassani C, Legasto A. Diaphragm appearance: a clue to the diagnosis of pulmonary and extrapulmonary pathology. *Curr Probl Diagn Radiol.* 2017;46(1):47–62.

Bergin D, Ennis R, Keogh C, et al. The "dependent viscera" sign in CT diagnosis of blunt traumatic diaphragmatic rupture. *AJR Am J Roentgenol.* 2001;177(5): 1137–1140.

Birnbaum DJ, D'Journo XB, Casanova D, Thomas PA. Necrotizing fasciitis of the chest wall. *Interact Cardiovasc Thorac Surg.* 2010;10(3):483–484.

Boon AJ, Harper CJ, Ghahfarokhi LS, et al. Two-dimensional ultrasound imaging of the diaphragm: quantitative values in normal subjects. *Muscle Nerve.* 2013;47(6):884–889.

Bradley FM, Hoover HC Jr, Hulka CA, et al. The sternalis muscle: an unusual normal finding seen on mammography. *AJR Am J Roentgenol.* 1996;166(1):33–36.

Brink JA, Heiken JP, Semenkovich J, et al. Abnormalities of the diaphragm and adjacent structures: findings on multiplanar spiral CT scans. *AJR Am J Roentgenol.* 1994;163(2):307–310.

Carter BW, Benveniste MF, Betancourt SL, et al. Imaging evaluation of malignant chest wall neoplasms. *Radiographics.* 2016;36(5):1285–1306.

Chelli Bouaziz M, Jelassi H, Chaabane S, et al. Imaging of chest wall infections. *Skeletal Radiol.* 2009;38(12):1127–1135.

Ch'en Y, Armstrong JD. Value of fluoroscopy in patients with suspected bilateral hemidiaphragmatic paralysis. *Am J Roentgenol.* 1993;160(1):29–31.

Chetta A. Chest radiography cannot predict diaphragm function. *Respir Med.* 2005;99:39–44.

Chung JH, Carr RB, Stern EJ. Extrapleural hematomas: imaging appearance, classification, and clinical significance. *J Thorac Imaging.* 2011;26:218–223.

Cohn D, Benditt JO, Eveloff S, McCool FD. Diaphragm thickening during inspiration. *J Appl Physiol (1985).* 1997;83(1):291–296.

David EA, Marshall MB. Review of chest wall tumors: a diagnostic, therapeutic, and reconstructive challenge. *Semin Plast Surg.* 2011;25(1):16–24.

Desser TS, Edwards B, Hunt S, et al. The dangling diaphragm sign: sensitivity and comparison with existing CT signs of blunt traumatic diaphragmatic rupture. *Emerg Radiol.* 2010;17(1):37–44.

Goretsky MJ, Kelly RE Jr, Croitoru D, Nuss D. Chest wall anomalies: pectus excavatum and pectus carinatum. *Adolesc Med Clin.* 2004;15(3):455–471.

Hammerman AM, Susman N, Strzembosz A, Kaiser LR. The extrapleural fat sign: CT characteristics. *J Comput Assist Tomogr.* 1990;14(3):345–347.

Iochum S, Ludig T, Walter F, et al. Imaging of diaphragmatic injury: a diagnostic challenge? *Radiographics.* 2002;22(Spec No):S103–S116, discussion S116–S118.

Jeung MY, Gangi A, Gasser B, et al. Imaging of chest wall disorders. *Radiographics.* 1999;19(3):617–637.

Kaya SO, Karabulut N, Yuncu G, et al. Sinus cut-off sign: a helpful sign in the CT diagnosis of diaphragmatic rupture associated with pleural effusion. *Eur J Radiol.* 2006;59(2):253–256.

Keats T, Anderson M. *Atlas of Normal Roentgen Variants That May Simulate Disease.* 9th ed. Philadelphia: Elsevier/Saunders; 2013.

Kerns SR, Gay SB. CT of blunt chest trauma. *AJR Am J Roentgenol.* 1990;154(1):55–60.

Kim MP, Hofstetter WL. Tumors of the diaphragm. *Thorac Surg Clin.* 2009;19(4): 521–529.

Kransdorf MJ, Bancroft LW, Peterson JJ, et al. Imaging of fatty tumors: distinction of lipoma and well-differentiated liposarcoma. *Radiology.* 2002;224(1):99–104.

Kuhlman JE, Bouchardy L, Fishman EK, Zerhouni EA. CT and MR imaging evaluation of chest wall disorders. *Radiographics.* 1994;14(3):571–595.

Lennon EA, Simon G. The height of the diaphragm in the chest radiograph of normal adults. *Br J Radiol.* 1965;38(456):937–943.

Levine BD, Motamedi K, Chow K, et al. CT of rib lesions. *AJR Am J Roentgenol.* 2009;193(1):5–13.

Lichtenberger JP 3rd, Carter BW, Abbott GF. Pitfalls in imaging of the chest wall. *Semin Roentgenol.* 2015;50(3):251–257.

Mak SM, Bhaludin BN, Naaseri S, Di Chiara F, Jordan S, Padley S. Imaging of congenital chest wall deformities. *Br J Radiol.* 2016;89(1061):20150595.

Moore K, Agur A. *Essential Clinical Anatomy.* 4th ed. Baltimore: Lippincott Williams & Wilkins; 2011.

Mullan CP, Madan R, Trotman-Dickenson B, et al. Radiology of chest wall masses. *AJR Am J Roentgenol.* 2011;197(3):W460–W470.

Muller N. *High-Yield Imaging: Chest.* Philadelphia: Saunders/Elsevier; 2010.

Nason LK, Walker CM, McNeeley MF, et al. Imaging of the diaphragm: anatomy and function. *Radiographics.* 2012;32(2):E51–E70.

Ontell FK, Moore EH, Shepard JA, Shelton DK. The costal cartilages in health and disease. *Radiographics.* 1997;17(3):571–577.

O'Sullivan P, O'Dwyer H, Flint J, et al. Soft tissue tumours and mass-like lesions of the chest wall: a pictorial review of CT and MR findings. *Br J Radiol.* 2007;80(955):574–580.

Pierce JC 3rd, Henderson R. Hypermetabolism of elastofibroma dorsi on PET-CT. *AJR Am J Roentgenol.* 2004;183(1):35–37.

Poole DC, Sexton WL, Farkas GA, et al. Diaphragm structure and function in health and disease. *Med Sci Sports Exerc.* 1997;29(6):738–754.

Ulano A, Bredella MA, Burke P, et al. Distinguishing untreated osteoblastic metastases from enostoses using CT attenuation measurements. *AJR Am J Roentgenol.* 2016;207(2):362–368.

Urschel JD, Takita H, Antkowiak JG. Necrotizing soft tissue infections of the chest wall. *Ann Thorac Surg.* 1997;64(1):276–279.

Wanek S, Mayberry JC. Blunt thoracic trauma: flail chest, pulmonary contusion, and blast injury. *Crit Care Clin.* 2004;20(1):71–81.

Weksler B, Ginsberg RJ. Tumors of the diaphragm. *Chest Surg Clin North Am.* 1998;8(2):441–447, Review.

Wiener MF, Chou WH. Primary tumors of the diaphragm. *Arch Surg.* 1965;90:143–152.

Worthy SA, Kang EY, Hartman TE, et al. Diaphragmatic rupture: CT findings in 11 patients. *Radiology.* 1995;194(3):885–888.

Yamaguchi M, Yoshino I, Fukuyama S, et al. Surgical treatment of neurogenic tumors of the chest. *Ann Thorac Cardiovasc Surg.* 2004;10(3):148–151.

CHAPTER 34

Problem Solving in the Mediastinum

Jeanne B. Ackman

CHAPTER OUTLINE

Mediastinal Lesions

Although it may not be difficult to identify a mediastinal mass on cross-sectional imaging, it can be challenging to determine its nature. Diagnostic specificity is critical to prevent unnecessary intervention and its associated morbidity and expenditure. The aim of this chapter is to serve as a guide toward maximizing the benefit of current diagnostic imaging tools for mediastinal lesions to improve diagnostic accuracy and clinical management in the interests of patient care. Emphases will be placed on anterior mediastinal lesions, which have historically been a source of confusion, and on thoracic MRI, which has heretofore been underutilized.

Current primary diagnostic imaging tools for the mediastinum include chest radiography (CXR), contrast esophagography, chest computed tomography (CT), 18-fluorodeoxyglucose positron emission tomography (^{18}FDG-PET), and thoracic magnetic resonance imaging (MRI). These diagnostic imaging tools can occasionally supplant endoscopic evaluation, surgical exploration, and biopsy when used to their full potential.

Mediastinal lesions are often detected incidentally on chest imaging performed for an unrelated reason. Alternatively, patient symptoms or signs can lead to a clinical suspicion of a mediastinal mass, whether due to gradual enlargement or rapid lesion enlargement because of hemorrhage or lesion rupture, the occurrence of which may lead to airway, vascular, esophageal, or nerve root compression. Presenting symptoms and signs may include shortness of breath, dysphagia, chest pain, hoarseness (from recurrent laryngeal nerve involvement), hemidiaphragmatic paralysis (from phrenic nerve involvement), and, rarely, a radiculopathy.

Designating the mediastinal compartment from which a mass arises is the first step toward narrowing the differential diagnosis because it leads to consideration of the structures that dwell in that particular space and their cellular composition. Both the center method and structure displacement method can be helpful for this analysis. The center method presumes that the center of the largest part of the lesion on an axial image designates the compartment of origin. The structure displacement method is based on the premise that a large lesion typically displaces anatomic structures from other compartments adjacent to its own.

The second step toward narrowing the differential diagnosis is tissue characterization. Overall, CXR does this least well, CT is better, and MRI is best to characterize tissue.

The third and last step is consideration of statistical probability and clinical context. Therefore the questions to ask when presented with a mediastinal lesion are as follows:

1. Which compartment?
2. What tissue type?
3. What is the most likely lesion, both statistically and contextually?

The recently proposed tricompartmental definition of mediastinal compartments by Carter et al. and the International Thymic Malignancy Interest Group published in the *Journal of Thoracic Oncology* will be used for the purposes of lesion compartmentalization in this chapter. This updated definition of mediastinal compartments is

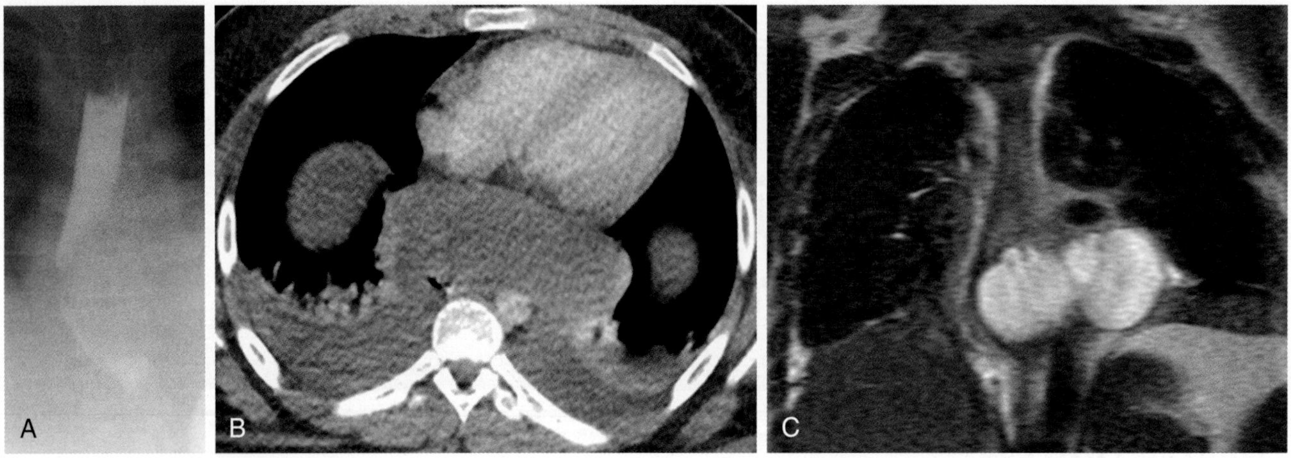

Figure 34.1 A 16-year-old young man with epigastric pain. (A) Iopamidol esophagram revealing marked rightward displacement and compression of the esophagus by a large middle mediastinal mass. (B) Axial chest CT scan with IV contrast reveals a heterogeneous attenuation mass displacing the esophagus posteriorly and to the right. (C) Coronal single-shot, fast spin-echo T2-weighted MRI scan reveals the mass to represent a complex multilocular cyst, with the esophagus draped around its right lateral margin. The mass proved to be an infected esophageal duplication cyst on surgical resection.

based on their delineation by cross-sectional imaging, rather than by CXR. All three mediastinal compartments are described to extend from the thoracic outlet to the diaphragm. The anterior mediastinal, or prevascular, compartment is defined as all structures posterior to the sternum and anterior to the pericardium. The middle mediastinum, or visceral compartment, extends from the anterior margin of pericardium posteriorly to a vertical line traversing the junction between the anterior and middle thirds of the thoracic vertebrae. The posterior mediastinum, or paravertebral compartment, contains all mediastinal structures posterior to the above-mentioned vertical line and is contained by the inner margin of the chest wall, extending posterolaterally to the lateral margin of thoracic spinal transverse processes.

■ Problem Solving With Imaging

Chest Radiography

On CXR, the first indication of a mediastinal mass may be the shift, deformation, or silhouetting of mediastinal anatomy, contours, or lines or, alternatively, the obliteration of spaces typically filled with air, such as the retrosternal clear space. These mediastinal lines have been discussed earlier in Chapter 2. For example, widening or thickening of the anterior junction line may be an early indication of an anterior mediastinal or prevascular mass on a frontal CXR. Anterior mediastinal masses may also be detected when soft tissue attenuation replaces the normally air-filled retrosternal clear space. Middle mediastinal or visceral compartmental masses may be detected by silhouetting of the paratracheal stripes, fill-in of the aortopulmonary window, or distortion of the azygoesophageal recess. Posterior or paravertebral compartmental mediastinal masses may be deduced if the mass silhouettes the paraspinal lines or vertebrae.

Although the CXR may suggest a mediastinal mass, it seldom can achieve diagnostic specificity because of the lack of soft tissue contrast between mediastinal structures on CXR. Therefore, once a mediastinal mass is suggested by CXR, cross-sectional imaging is usually the next step, whether by chest CT or MRI.

Contrast Esophagography

Contrast esophagography may depict a mediastinal mass directly or incidentally infer the presence of a mediastinal mass by outlining an intraluminal mass, by highlighting an aberrant course of the esophagus, or by demonstrating mass effect on the esophagus by an adjacent mass (Fig. 34.1).

Contrast esophagography can be quite helpful when there is concern for esophageal fistulae and perforation. It is performed most safely with a low-osmolar, iodinated contrast agent such as iopamidol, with administration of barium sulfate reserved for cases in which the initial low-osmolar contrast agent esophagram is negative. CT and MRI may also depict these findings (Figs. 34.2 and 34.3).

Chest CT

Chest CT not only more readily depicts the mediastinal compartment in which the lesion resides, but also provides some insight into the nature of the tissue, including better delineation of lesion morphology than CXR, some indication of the lesion's cystic or solid nature and enhancement, heterogeneity versus homogeneity of attenuation, the presence or absence of gross fat and calcification, and lesion invasiveness.

Dual-energy CT with IV contrast may offer some advantage over standard, single-energy CT in differentiating cystic from solid lesions because of the material decomposition

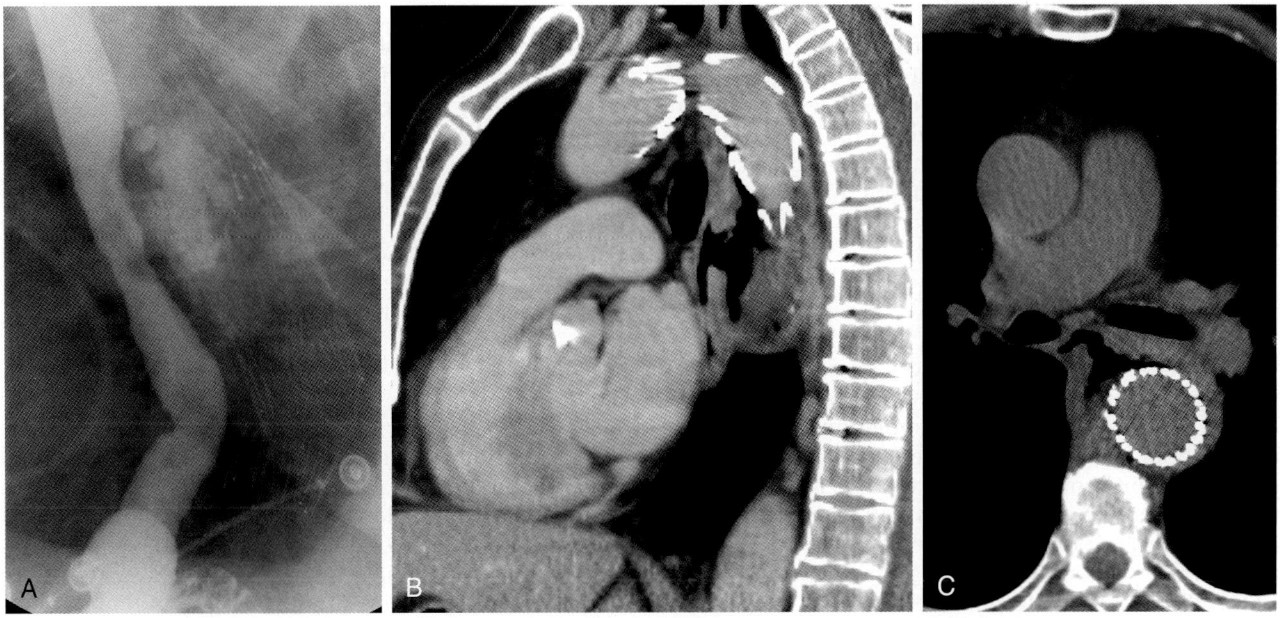

Figure 34.2 A 64-year-old man status post thoracic endovascular aortic repair of a nonruptured thoracic aortic aneurysm complicated by a polymicrobial abscess and persistent aortoesophageal fistula. (A) Contrast esophagram. (B) Sagittal chest CT scan with IV contrast. (C) Axial noncontrast chest CT scan revealing an aortoesophageal fistula.

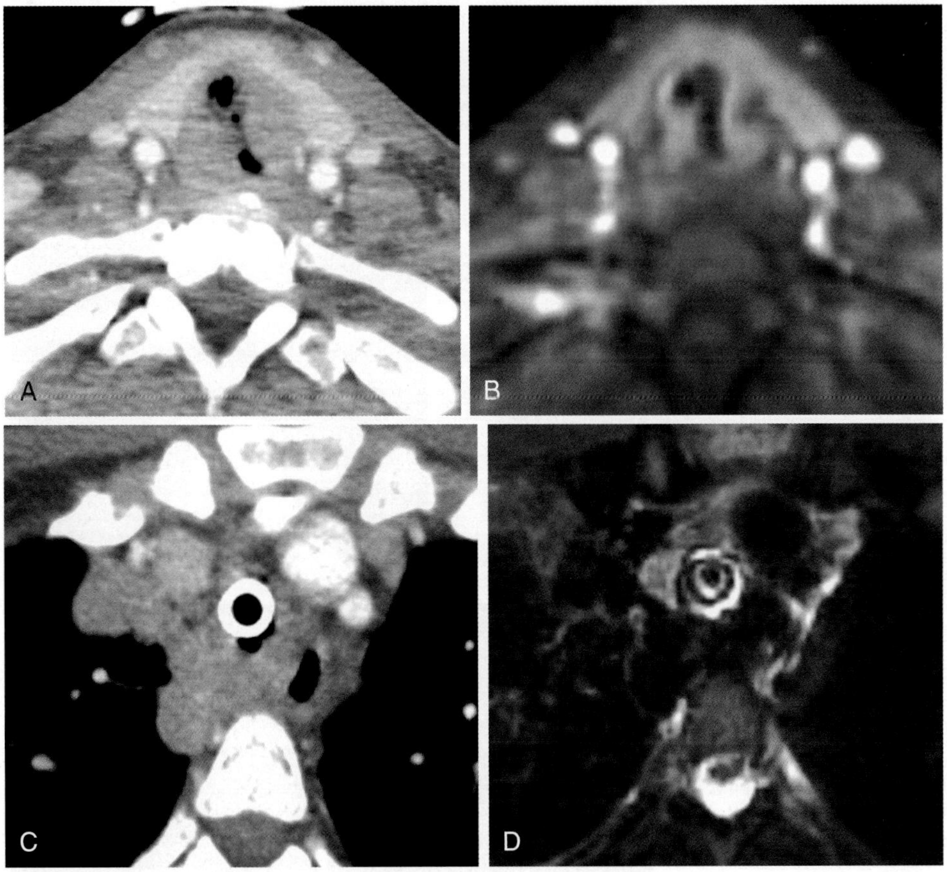

Figure 34.3 A 32-year-old woman with chronic fibrosing mediastinitis whose endoscopic biopsy caused a tracheoesophageal fistula (TEF). (A) Axial CT scan with IV contrast and matched axial three-dimensional, ultrafast gradient echo, fat-saturated, T1-weighted MR image, (B) demonstrate the TEF. (C) Axial CT scan with IV contrast and matched axial, radially acquired, respiratory-triggered, fat-saturated, T2-weighted MR image, (D) demonstrating the contiguous, more bulky component of the mass in the upper chest. This infiltrative mass insinuates between the left posterolateral trachea and esophagus and partially fills the medial right apical extrapleural space. The marked T2 hypointensity of this mass on MRI reflects its fibrous nature, a tissue characteristic not appreciable by CT. If MRI had been performed prior to biopsy, the interventionist would have had a better sense of the nature of tissue (hard, resistant) to undergo sampling and might have approached it differently, avoiding the iatrogenic TEF.

images it provides. Region of interest (ROI) assessment of attenuation is not absolute with this form of CT, however. These images are generated by the subtraction of two basis materials (e.g., water, calcium, iodine). The water images, also known as *virtual noncontrast images*, are generated by digitally subtracting iodine (IV contrast) from the image, aiding discrimination of enhancing from nonenhancing lesions and allowing quantification of water content in mg/mL. The water images also facilitate the differentiation of calcium from iodine on postcontrast chest CT. The iodine images can also help differentiate high-attenuation hemorrhage and other nonenhancing tissues from enhancing tissue. Dual-energy CT enables lower IV contrast doses because its images can be reconstructed at several different virtual monoenergetic levels, ranging from 40 to 190 keV, with the lower keV images yielding better iodine contrast and the higher keV images exhibiting diminished noise and artifacts.

FDG-PET

Beyond its seminal role in cancer staging, ^{18}FDG-PET imaging has a limited role in the evaluation of mediastinal lesions. Its strength is its ability to demonstrate the level of metabolic activity within a lesion and to ferret out clinically significant lesions that are difficult to detect by CT, either because they are very small but metabolically active or because of their isoattenuation with adjacent tissue. Many lesions may be too small to detect with ^{18}FDG-PET imaging, despite their malignant nature, if they are insufficiently metabolically active. In addition, many benign mediastinal lesions, including thymic hyperplasia and inflammatory mediastinal cysts, demonstrate ^{18}FDG-PET avidity (Fig. 34.4) and can therefore be misinterpreted as malignant or, at least, meriting resection to exclude malignancy. Even a normal thymus may be ^{18}FDG-PET–avid. In cases of indeterminate mediastinal lesions on CT, it is often valuable to perform MRI prior to consideration of PET to ascertain if there are lesion features favoring a benign diagnosis, instead of referring the patient directly for ^{18}FDG-PET imaging. MRI in select cases has the potential to spare the patient morbidity and radiation exposure and our health care system the cost of unnecessary surgery. PET is substantially more expensive and time-consuming than MRI and exposes the patient to a significant dose of radiation (effective dose range of 8–26 mSv), unlike MRI.

Thoracic MRI

The superior tissue contrast of MRI and resultant superior tissue characterization, when compared with CT, enables the following: (1) definitive discernment between cystic and solid lesions (Fig. 34.5); (2) demonstration of the simplicity or complexity of a cystic lesion, (3) detection of blood products (Figs. 34.6 and 34.7); (4) discernment of the presence of smooth muscle and collagenous and fibrous material based on relative or actual T2 hypointensity (Figs. 34.8 and 34.9; see Fig. 34.3); (5) delineation of the enhancement pattern of a lesion by dynamic contrast enhancement (DCE; Fig. 34.10); and (6) demonstration of the degree of restricted diffusion with

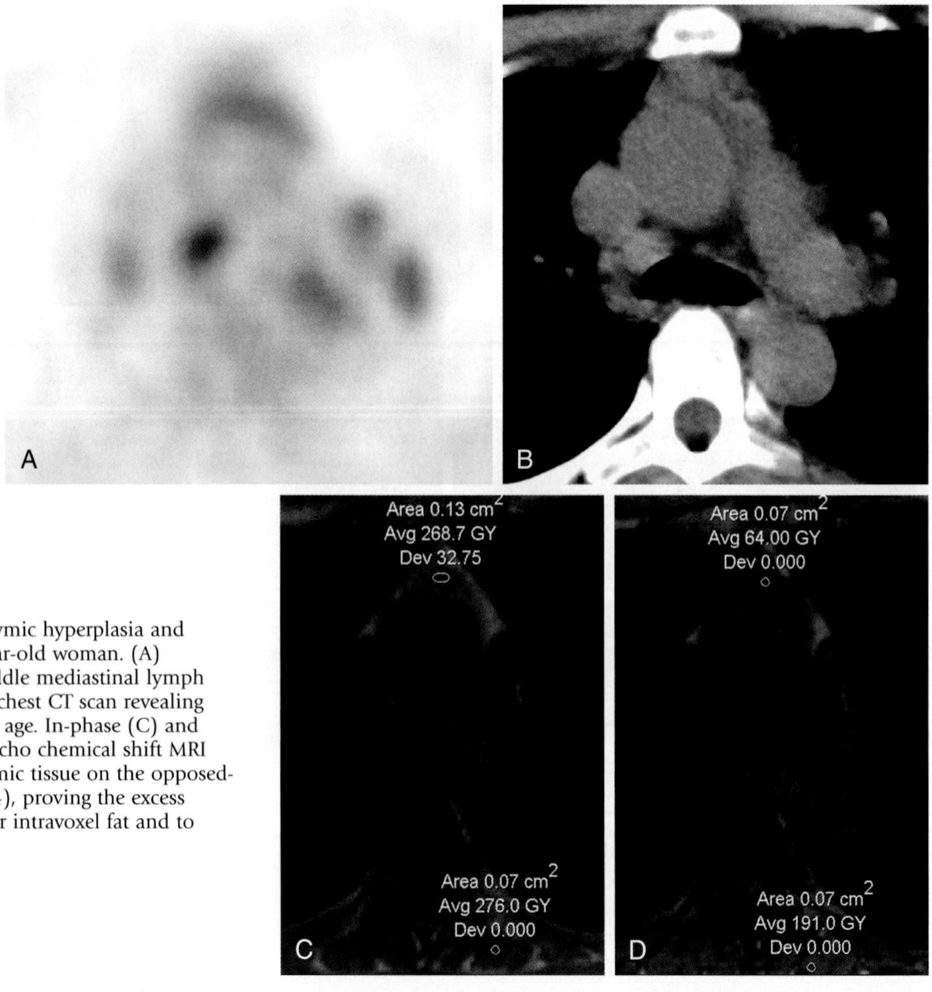

Figure 34.4 ^{18}FDG-PET–positive thymic hyperplasia and lymph nodes of sarcoidosis in a 42-year-old woman. (A) ^{18}FDG-PET–avid thymic tissue and middle mediastinal lymph nodes of sarcoidosis. (B) Noncontrast chest CT scan revealing excess soft tissue in the thymic bed for age. In-phase (C) and opposed-phase (D) ultrafast gradient echo chemical shift MRI reveals marked suppression of the thymic tissue on the opposed-phase image (chemical shift ratio = 0.4), proving the excess thymic tissue to contain microscopic or intravoxel fat and to therefore represent thymic hyperplasia.

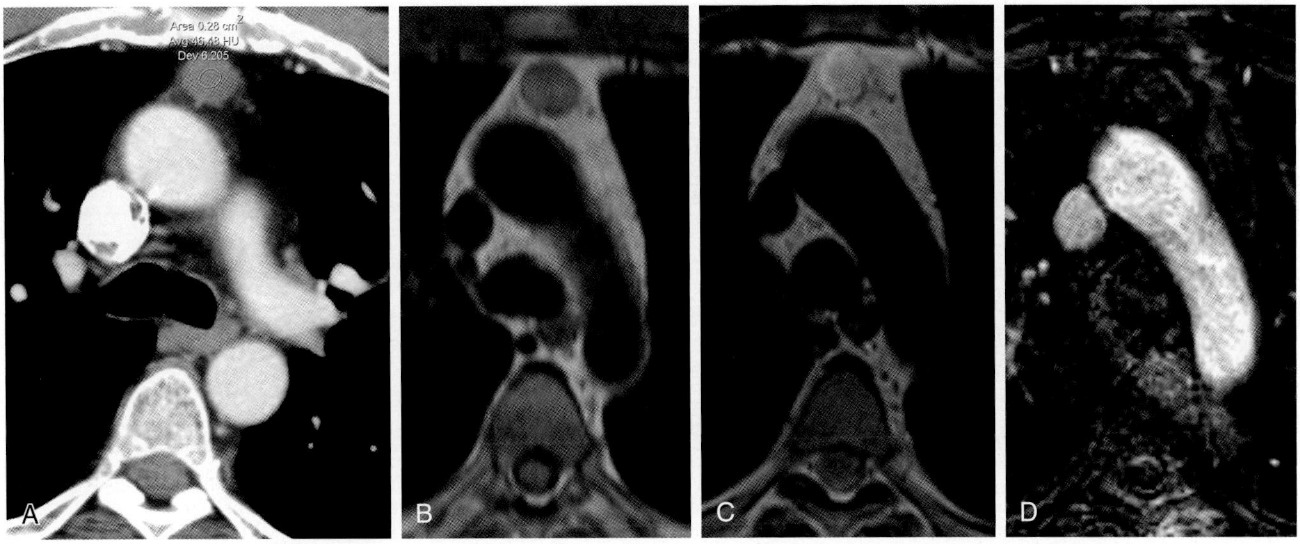

Figure 34.5 Thymic cyst in a 52-year-old man. (A) Axial chest CT scan with IV contrast revealing a solitary, 46-HU nodule in the thymic bed. It is unclear by CT whether this lesion is a cyst or a solid thymic neoplasm. (B–D) Axial breath-hold, cardiac-gated, double inversion recovery T1-weighted, T2-weighted, and postprocessed, postcontrast, subtracted three-dimensional ultrafast gradient echo fat-saturated T1-weighted MR images demonstrating a T1- and T2-hyperintense, nonenhancing thymic nodule, with a thin smooth wall, compatible with a thymic cyst. (From Ackman JB. A practical guide to nonvascular thoracic magnetic resonance imaging. *J Thorac Imaging.* 2014;29(1):17–29.)

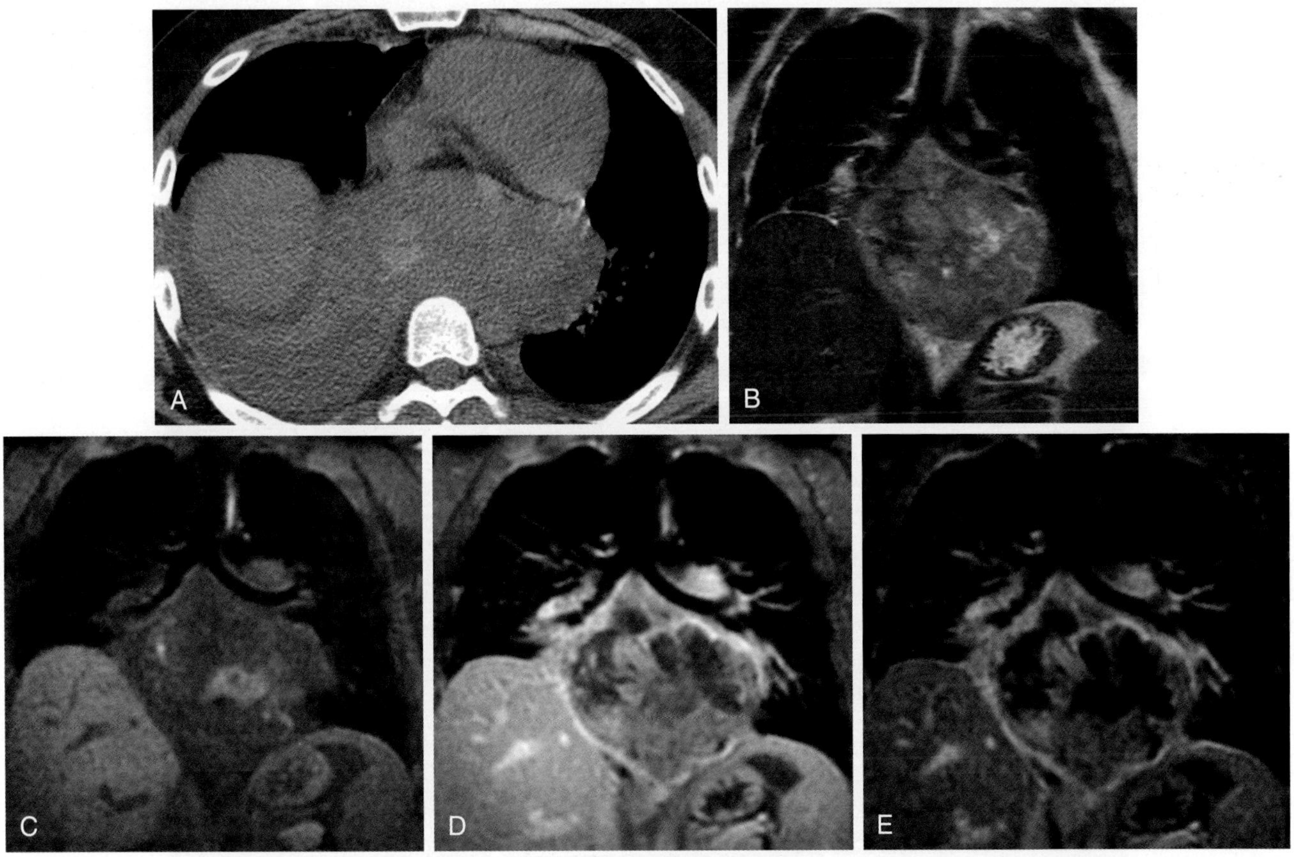

Figure 34.6 Large hemorrhagic, undifferentiated small round cell sarcoma arising from the middle mediastinum in a 24-year-old man with a 3-week history of dyspnea and palpitations. (A) Axial and coronal images from chest CT with IV contrast revealing a large, heterogeneous middle mediastinal mass and associated right pleural effusion. It is unclear whether this tissue is primarily hemorrhagic or solid and impossible to be certain where the solid components lie. (B–E) Coronal breath-hold single-shot, fast spin-echo, T2-weighted, precontrast ultrafast gradient echo (GRE), fat-saturated T1-weighted, postcontrast ultrafast GRE, fat-saturated, and postcontrast, postprocessed subtracted MRI scans, respectively, revealing the heterogeneous T1/T2 signal mass to be mixed hemorrhagic, necrotic, and solid. The postprocessed subtracted image clearly demonstrates the enhancing solid components and provides the endoscopist with important information—that subcarinal bronchoscopic biopsy should yield diagnostic tissue.

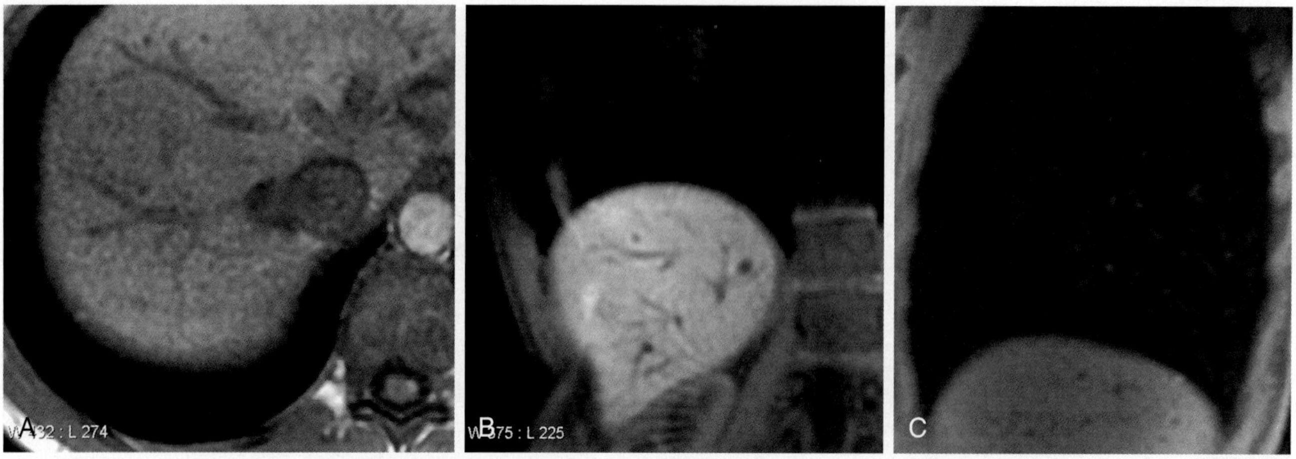

Figure 34.7 A 4-mm endometrioma along the right posterolateral hemidiaphragmatic pleura of a 24-year-old woman with pleuritic chest pain during menses over the past 2 years. Axial (A), coronal (B), and sagittal (C) ultrafast three-dimensional gradient echo, fat-saturated T1-weighted MRI scans revealing a tiny, T1-hyperintense, round, well-circumscribed lesion that appeared during menses when the patient was symptomatic. This lesion was not identifiable on an earlier MRI scan when this patient was between menstrual cycles.

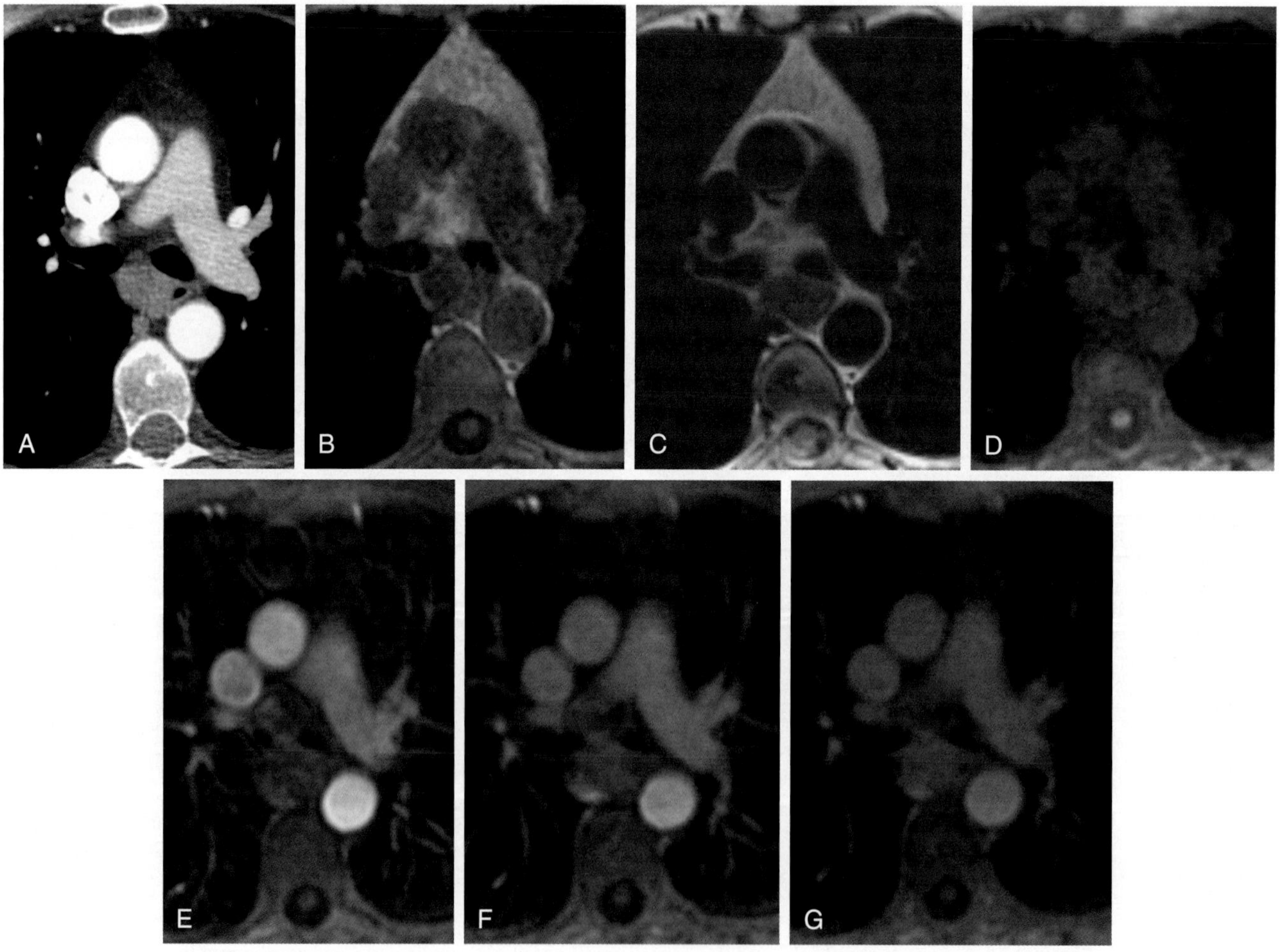

Figure 34.8 Esophageal leiomyoma in a 63-year-old woman. (A) Axial chest CT scan demonstrating a right midparaesophageal mass of soft tissue attenuation. Its tissue composition is indeterminate by CT and may be cystic or solid. (B and C) Axial breath-hold in-phase T1-weighted and cardiac-gated double inversion recovery, T2-weighted MRI scans, respectively, reveal the lesion to be of low-intermediate T1 and T2 signal, favoring the presence of smooth muscle, collagenous, and/or fibrous material. Axial breath-hold precontrast (D) and postcontrast (E–G) three-dimensional ultrafast gradient echo fat-saturated, T1-weighted 20-second, 1-minute, and 5-minute MRI scans reveal very mild, gradual enhancement of this solid lesion. The MRI features and location are most consistent with an esophageal leiomyoma, as proven by a subsequent endoscopic fine needle biopsy.

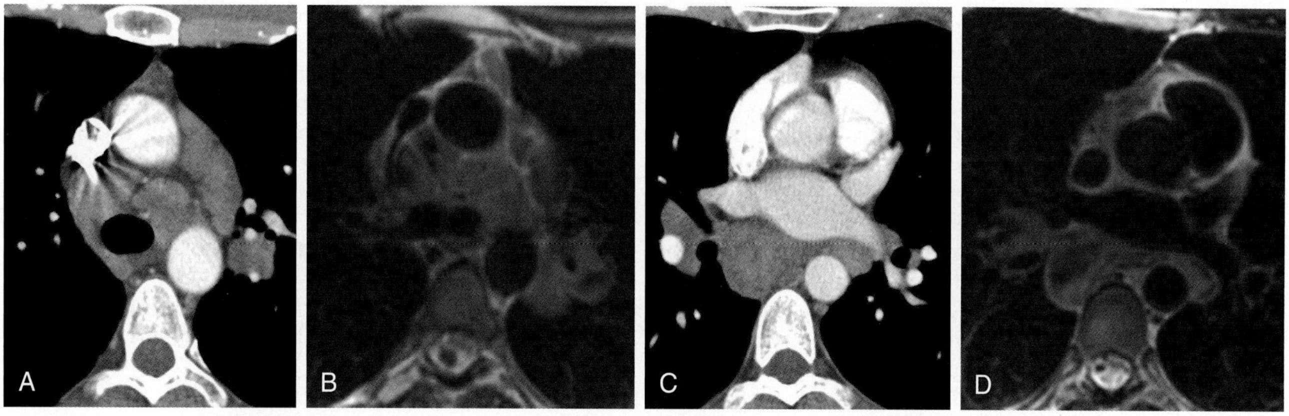

Figure 34.9 The dark lymph node sign of sarcoidosis. Matched axial contrast-enhanced chest CT (A, C) and cardiac-gated double inversion recovery T2-weighted MRI images (B, D) reveal the noncalcified lymphadenopathy on CT at two distinct axial levels to exhibit areas of low T2 signal on MRI, compatible with fibrotic changes observed in old granulomas—in this case, sarcoidosis.

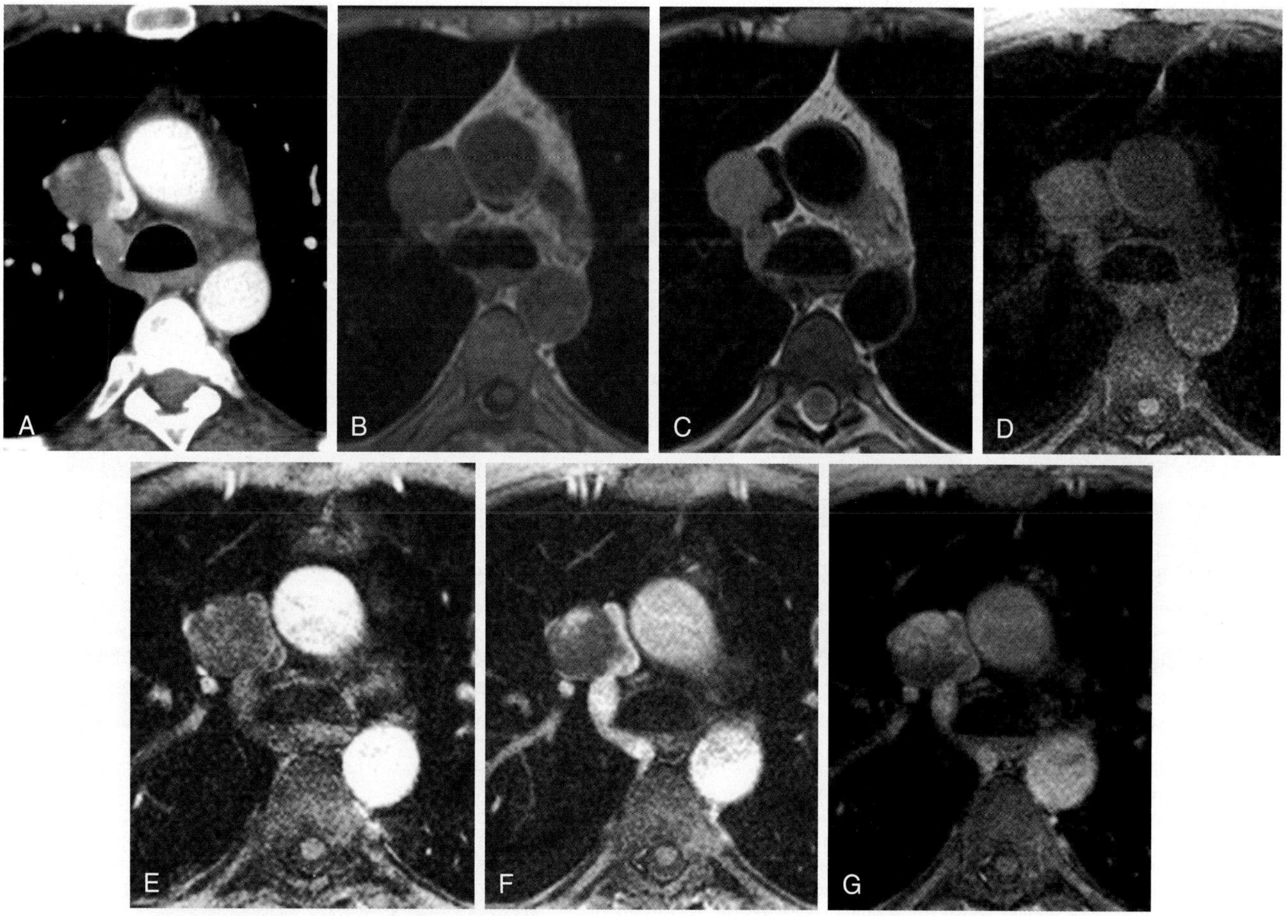

Figure 34.10 Hemangioma in the middle mediastinum of a 57-year-old man. (A) Axial chest CT scan revealing a 30-HU, round, well-circumscribed lesion compressing and indenting the superior vena cava, with a peripheral hyperattenuating focus, whether calcification or focal enhancement. (B) Axial in-phase ultrafast gradient echo (GRE) T1-weighted and cardiac-gated T2-weighted MRI (C) scans reveal the lesion to be mildly and homogeneously T1-hyperintense and T2-hyperintense. (D–G) Axial pre- and postcontrast ultrafast three-dimensional GRE fat-saturated T1-weighted images at 20 seconds, 1 minute, and 5 minutes reveal the lesion to demonstrate peripheral nodular enhancement, with partial fill-in over time. The signal characteristics and dynamic contrast enhancement pattern of this lesion are compatible with a hemangioma, with the diagnosis proven at surgery; the surgery was performed secondary to concern for eventual superior vena cava syndrome.

apparent diffusion coefficient (ADC) mapping (see Fig. 34.8), all without any radiation exposure. The high soft issue contrast of MRI may demonstrate chest wall and neurovascular invasion better. Free breathing steady-state free precession (SSFP) MRI and cardiac tagging by MRI can further assist in the assessment of mediastinal mass invasion of adjacent structures. MRI may also demonstrate the compartment in which a lesion resides better, changing the differential diagnosis. For example, it can be difficult to discern whether a lesion is mediastinal or paramediastinal, not only by CXR, but also by CT. In such cases, the higher soft tissue contrast and superior definition of soft tissue planes by MRI can be helpful (Fig. 34.11). MRI does not readily demonstrate calcifications, however. When present, calcifications on MR are usually T2-hypointense. These capabilities of MRI often lead to greater diagnostic specificity in the evaluation of mediastinal lesions and may provide additional valuable information for clinical management, whether medical or surgical.

Because of its lack of ionizing radiation, MRI may be used to screen for or follow up lymphadenopathy in young, pregnant, and/or radiation-averse patients with lymphoma and chronic lymphocytic leukemia, melanoma metastases in pregnant patients (without IV gadolinium administration), endometriomas, paragangliomas and teratomas in patients with predisposing genetic mutations (e.g., a mutation in the succinate dehydrogenase complex, subunit D integral membrane protein *[SDHD]* gene), and teratomas in patients with anti-*N*-methyl-D-aspartate receptor antibodies, respectively. For sample mediastinal and thymic MRI protocols, see Table 34.1 and Box 34.1.

Mediastinal Lesions by Compartment

Table 34.2 provides a list of mediastinal lesions categorized by compartment, whether prevascular, visceral, or paravertebral.

Prevascular or Anterior Mediastinal Compartment

Normal anatomic structures in the prevascular compartment of the mediastinum include the thymus, lymphatics, lymph nodes, vessels, and fat. Therefore lymphadenopathy, whether from an inflammatory, metastatic, or lymphoproliferative cause, and thymic lesions comprise the bulk of lesions in this compartment. Thymic lesions include benign nonneoplastic lesions such as thymic hyperplasia

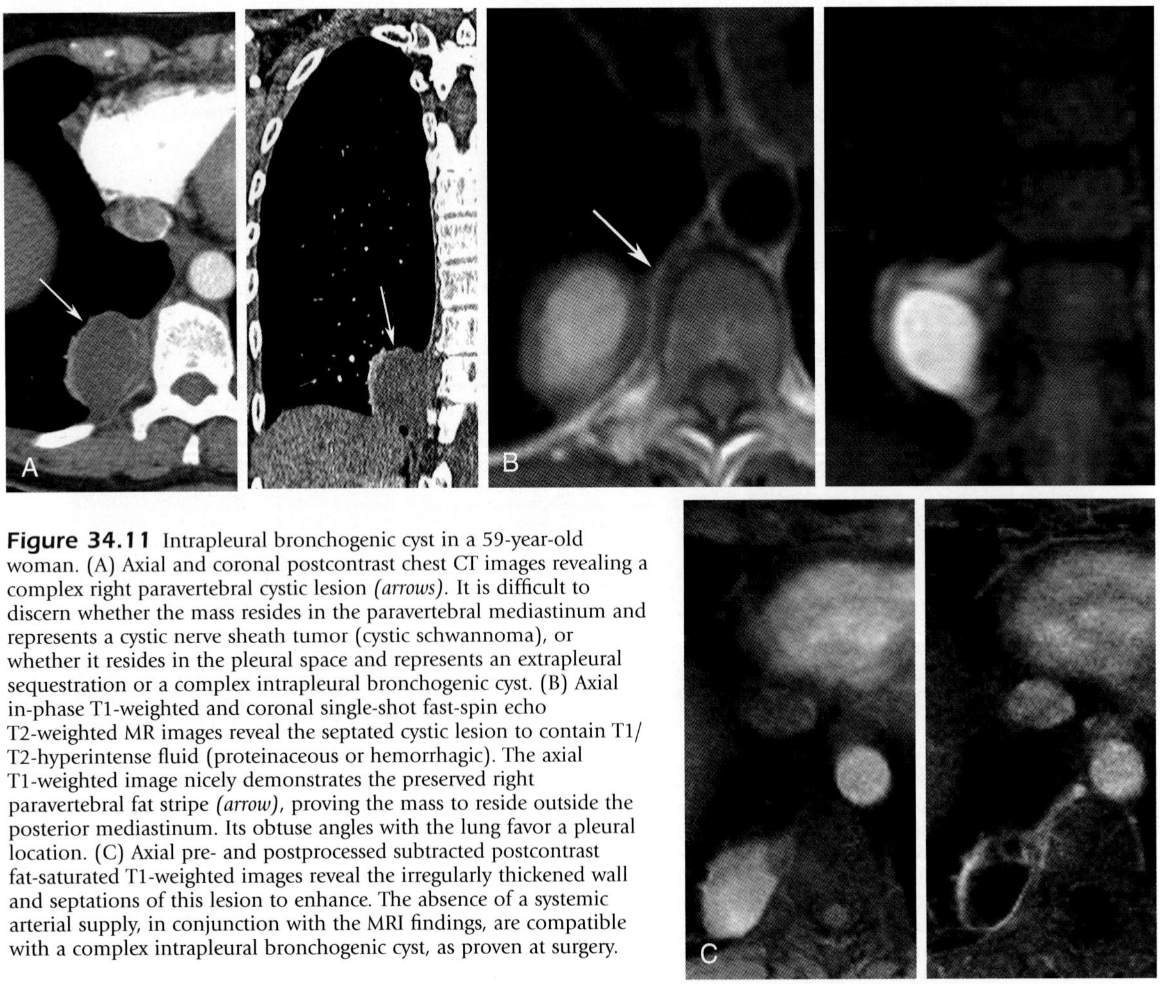

Figure 34.11 Intrapleural bronchogenic cyst in a 59-year-old woman. (A) Axial and coronal postcontrast chest CT images revealing a complex right paravertebral cystic lesion *(arrows)*. It is difficult to discern whether the mass resides in the paravertebral mediastinum and represents a cystic nerve sheath tumor (cystic schwannoma), or whether it resides in the pleural space and represents an extrapleural sequestration or a complex intrapleural bronchogenic cyst. (B) Axial in-phase T1-weighted and coronal single-shot fast-spin echo T2-weighted MR images reveal the septated cystic lesion to contain T1/T2-hyperintense fluid (proteinaceous or hemorrhagic). The axial T1-weighted image nicely demonstrates the preserved right paravertebral fat stripe *(arrow)*, proving the mass to reside outside the posterior mediastinum. Its obtuse angles with the lung favor a pleural location. (C) Axial pre- and postprocessed subtracted postcontrast fat-saturated T1-weighted images reveal the irregularly thickened wall and septations of this lesion to enhance. The absence of a systemic arterial supply, in conjunction with the MRI findings, are compatible with a complex intrapleural bronchogenic cyst, as proven at surgery.

TABLE 34.1 Mediastinal MRI Protocol

	MANUFACTURER		
PULSE SEQUENCE[a]	**GE**	**SIEMENS**	**PHILIPS**
BH axial and sagittal SSFP balanced GRE	FIESTA	True FISP	BFFE
BH coronal ultrafast spin-echo T2	SSFSE	HASTE	UFSE
BH sagittal ultrafast spin-echo fat-saturated T2	SSFSE	HASTE	UFSE
BH axial in- and out-of-phase T1 (chemical shift) ultrafast GRE	FSPGR	Turbo FLASH	TFE
BH cardiac-gated double IR T2	Double IR FSE T2	Double IR TSE T2	Double IR UFSE T2
BH pre- and post–three-dimensional ultrafast GRE (with postgadolinium imaging) acquired at 20 s (axial), 1 min (axial), 3 min (sagittal), and 5 min (axial)[b]	LAVA	VIBE	THRIVE
Optional coronal/sagittal BH STIR	Fast STIR	Turbo STIR	STIR TSE
Optional diffusion-weighted echoplanar imaging with b values of 50, 400, 800	eDWI	DWI	DWI
Optional BH cardiac-gated double IR	Double IR prep FSE T1	Double IR prep TSE T1	Double IR prep UFSE T1
Optional BH cardiac-gated sagittal double IR fat-saturated T2	Double IR FSE fat-saturated T2	Double IR TSE fat-saturated T2	Double IR UFSE fat-saturated T2
Optional respiratory-triggered radially acquired FSE T2 (periodically rotated overlapping parallel lines with enhanced reconstruction)	PROPELLER	BLADE	MultiVane
Optional respiratory-triggered radially acquired FSE fat-saturated T2 (periodically rotated overlapping parallel lines with enhanced reconstruction)	PROPELLER	BLADE	MultiVane
Optional respiratory-triggered axial-driven equilibrium T2	FRFSE	RESTORE	DRIVE
Optional respiratory-triggered axial-driven equilibrium fat-saturated T2	FRFSE	RESTORE	DRIVE

[a]Default slice thickness is 4 mm for all pulse sequences.
[b]Option to add, for example, postgadolinium axial imaging 2 and 4 minutes after injection. Imaging planes can be changed to optimize lesion characterization.
BH, Breath-hold; *FSE*, fast spin-echo; *GRE*, gradient echo; *IR*, inversion recovery; *SSFP*, steady-state free precession.
Modified from Ackman JB. A practical guide to non-vascular thoracic magnetic resonance imaging. *J Thorac Imaging*. 2014;29(1):17–29.

BOX 34.1 Noninvasive Thymic Lesion Protocol[a]

Breath-hold (BH) axial steady-state free precession imaging
BH axial in- and out-of-phase ultrafast gradient echo (GRE) T1
BH, electrocardiographic-gated axial double inversion recovery T2
If needed,[b] BH pre- and post–three-dimensional ultrafast GRE with automated subtraction (postgadolinium imaging) acquired at 20 seconds (axial), 1 minute (axial), 3 minutes (sagittal), and 5 minutes (axial)

[a]Default slice thickness is 4 mm for all pulse sequences.
[b]If the thymic lesion uniformly suppresses on opposed-phase imaging, with a chemical shift ratio ≤0.7 or signal intensity index >10%, no IV contrast administration is needed.

and thymic cysts, benign neoplastic lesions such as a mature teratoma and thymolipoma, and malignant neoplastic lesions, the most common of which is a thymoma. More rare thymic neoplasms include thymic carcinoma and thymic neuroendocrine tumor (formerly referred to as thymic carcinoid). Germ cell tumors are less common than most of the above-mentioned thymic lesions, with mature teratoma representing the most common germ cell tumor. Lymphangiomas and hemangiomas may also reside in the prevascular compartment in adults, although they are rare lesions.

Normal Anterior Mediastinal Structures

Normal anterior mediastinal structures are sometimes misinterpreted as abnormal, and vice versa.

PERICARDIAL FAT PAD VERSUS PERICARDIAL CYST

On CXR, when it is difficult to ascertain whether an apparent cardiophrenic angle mass represents a pericardial fat pad or pericardial cyst, it is reasonable to perform mediastinal MRI to avert radiation exposure and answer the clinical question definitively (Fig. 34.12). Chest CT may alternatively be performed. Pericardial cysts may change location and morphology between examinations and are typically of water attenuation on CT and T1-hypointense and T2-hyperintense on MRI. Their CT attenuation and MR T1-weighted signal may be increased in rare cases of intralesional hemorrhage. Typically there is no appreciable wall enhancement of pericardial (mesothelial) cysts on CT or MRI.

TABLE 34.2 Mediastinal Mass Location by Mediastinal Compartment

ANTERIOR MEDIASTINUM, PREVASCULAR COMPARTMENT[a]	MIDDLE MEDIASTINUM, VISCERAL COMPARTMENT	POSTERIOR MEDIASTINUM, PARAVERTEBRAL COMPARTMENT
Lymphadenopathy	Lymphadenopathy	Lymphadenopathy
Thymic lesions (cyst, hyperplasia, neoplasms)		
Thyroid and parathyroid lesions	Thyroid lesions Ascending aortic aneurysm Aortic arch aneurysm Dilated main pulmonary artery Aberrant right or left subclavian artery Tracheal lesions Esophageal lesions Paraganglioma and other neurogenic tumors Descending aortic aneurysm	Neurogenic tumors including neurofibroma, schwannoma, paraganglioma Lateral meningocele
Germ cell tumors	Pancreatic pseudocyst	Pancreatic pseudocyst
Pericardial or mesothelial[b] cysts	Mesothelial cysts	Mesothelial cysts Extramedullary hematopoiesis
Morgagni hernia	Hiatal hernia	Bochdalek hernia
Bronchogenic cysts (rarely)	Foregut duplication cysts	Foregut duplication cysts
Abscess	Abscess	Abscess
Hematoma	Hematoma	Hematoma
Fibrosing mediastinitis	Fibrosing mediastinitis	Fibrosing mediastinitis
Hemangioma	Hemangioma	Hemangioma
Lymphangioma	Lymphangioma	Lymphangioma
Sarcoma	Sarcoma	Sarcoma

[a]Based on the new International Thymic Malignancy Interest Group classification scheme of mediastinal compartments referenced at the end of this chapter as Carter et al. A modern definition of mediastinal compartments. *J Thorac Oncol.* 2014;9(9):S97–S101.
[b]Mesothelial cysts can theoretically be found anywhere in the body where mesothelium exists.
From Ackman JB. A practical guide to nonvascular thoracic magnetic resonance imaging. *J Thorac Imaging.* 2014;29(1):17–29.

NORMAL THYMUS

The normal adult thymus is not visible on CXR. On chest CT or MRI, it may be triangular or arrowhead in shape or quadrilateral in configuration, with or without intercalated gross fat. Occasionally, the upper aspect of the thymus, particularly in young adults, may be rounded or lobulated. The upper limit of normal maximal thymic lobe thickness was reported by Baron et al. in 1982 to be 1.8 cm from age 6 to19 years and 1.3 cm from age 20 years onward. In 2013 Ackman et al. demonstrated a sex difference in normal thymic appearance in 20- to 30-year-old adults, with the thymus of young women often exhibiting a fuller, more quadrilateral shape and higher attenuation than that of men. Awareness of this sex difference should reduce misinterpretation of a normal thymus as thymic hyperplasia or neoplasm in these young women. This study also found that the upper limit of normal maximal thymic lobar thickness for a triangular thymus in this young adult age group was 1.6 cm, rather than 1.3 cm. If the thymus were quadrilateral in configuration, the upper limit of normal was 2.2 cm in 20- to 30-year-olds. Until further research proves otherwise for adults older than 30 years, 1.3 cm should continue to be used as the upper limit for normal maximal thymic lobe thickness in older adults. On CT, normal thymic soft tissue is isoattenuating to muscle, without appreciable enhancement. On MRI, normal thymic tissue is T1-isointense and T2-hyperintense to muscle, and its enhancement is appreciable.

Age matters when distinguishing a normal from a hyperplastic thymus. The thymus reaches maximal weight at puberty and then involutes over time, becoming mostly fatty by age 40 years and almost completely fatty by age 60, although reticulonodular strands of tissue and nodules up to 7 mm can remain. Excess tissue for age, with normal thymic morphology, thickness, and CT attenuation or MR signal, indicates thymic hyperplasia.[18]FDG-PET imaging can yield confusing results in the thymus. Both normal and hyperplastic thymus may be FDG-PET–avid. In such cases, thymic morphology, thickness, CT attenuation, and, when relevant, MR signal must all be taken into account to determine whether FDG-PET–avid thymic tissue is normal or abnormal.

Nonneoplastic Anterior Mediastinal Masses

THYMIC HYPERPLASIA VS. THYMIC TUMOR (PITFALL: NONSUPPRESSING NORMAL THYMUS)

Thymic hyperplasia can be difficult to discern from thymic tumors, whether lymphoma or thymoma. In 2007 Inaoka et al. reported that the demonstration of microscopic fat

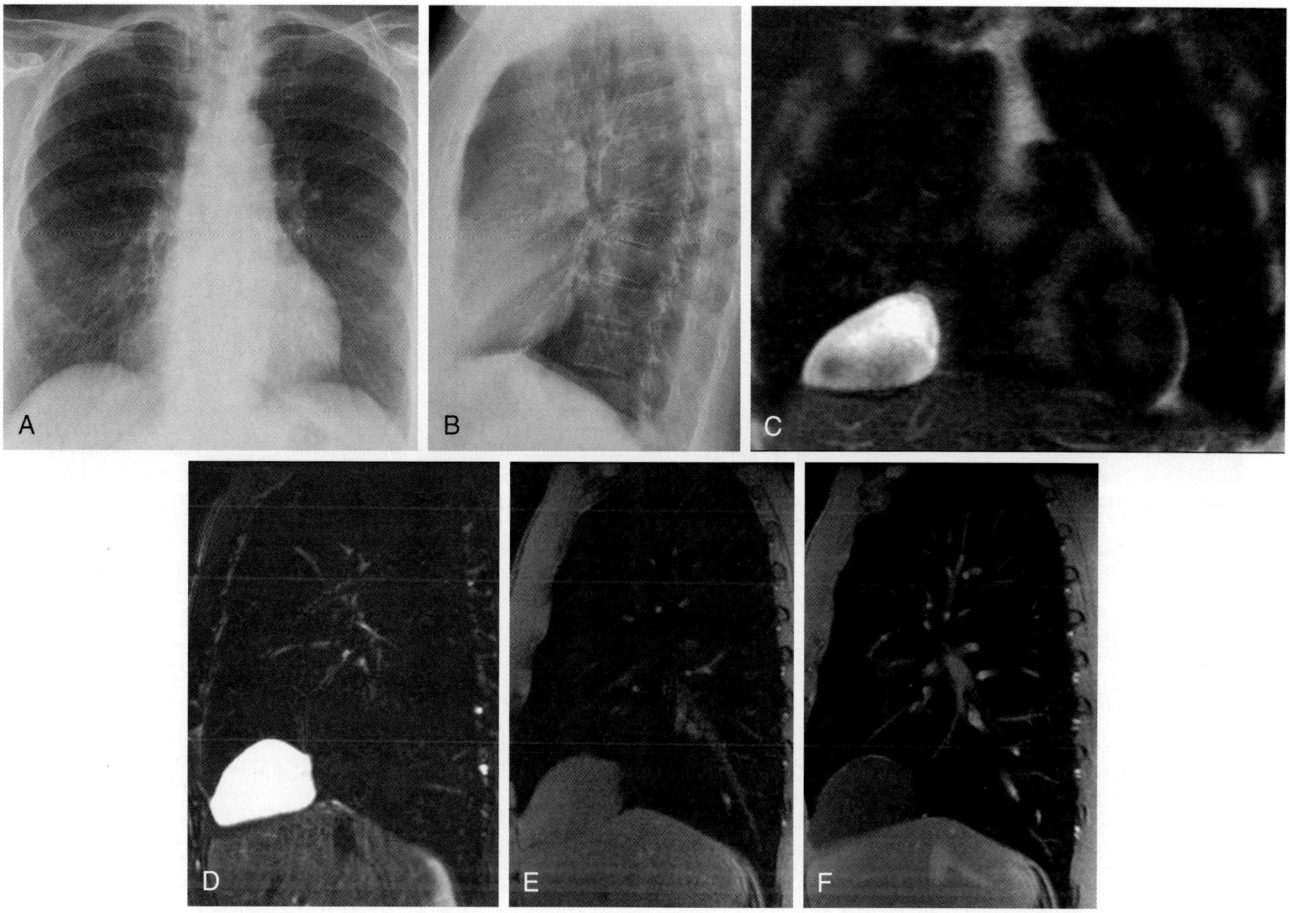

Figure 34.12 Pericardial cyst in a 66-year-old woman. Posteroanterior (A) and lateral (B) chest x-rays reveal a fairly lucent, dextroconvex right cardiophrenic angle mass. The tissue composition of this mediastinal mass is unclear by chest radiography and may be fluid, fatty, or other soft tissue composition. (C) Coronal single-shot fast spin-echo T2-weighted, sagittal single-shot fast-spin echo fat-saturated T2-weighted (D), and precontrast (E) and postcontrast (F) ultrafast three-dimensional gradient echo, fat-saturated T1-weighted images, revealing a homogeneously T1-hypointense, markedly T2-hyperintense, nonenhancing right cardiophrenic angle mass with a barely perceptible wall. Bandlike enhancing tissue along the anterosuperior aspect of the mass represents compressive atelectasis. The patchy low T2 signal in the mass on the coronal image represents proton spin dephasing within the jiggling, or secondarily pulsating, fluid because of the adjacent beating heart.

in solid thymic tissue with a chemical shift MRI confirms the diagnosis of thymic hyperplasia (or normal thymus, depending on thymic morphology, thickness, and CT attenuation or MR signal for age). Often, detection of microscopic fat on the opposed-phase chemical shift MR image can be made qualitatively based on an overt drop in signal when compared with the in-phase image (Fig. 34.13). Occasionally, however, the reduction in signal is not appreciable to the naked eye. When not appreciable, simple quantitative assessment of signal dropout by the calculation of a chemical shift ratio (CSR) or signal intensity index (SII) can be made. The CSR calculation is as follows:

$$\text{CSR} = \frac{\text{OP SI thymus/OP SI paraspinal muscle}}{\text{IP SI thymus/IP SI paraspinal muscle}}$$

where IP = in-phase, OP = opposed-phase, and SI = signal intensity as measured by the ROI.

A CSR ≤ 0.7 is consistent with a normal or hyperplastic thymus (see Fig. 34.13). A CSR ≥ 1.0 is indicative of thymic neoplasm in most cases, with 0.8 and 0.9 representing indeterminate values.

Provided the in-phase and opposed-phase images are obtained by a dual-echo chemical shift MRI acquisition, an SII can be calculated to assess the degree of fat suppression (see below) and solely requires ROI placement over the thymic tissue in question, not the paraspinal musculature. The SII can be calculated as follows:

$$\text{SII} = [(\text{IP SI thymus} - \text{OP SI thymus})/\text{IP SI thymus}] \times 100$$

A SII >9% is compatible with a normal thymus or thymic hyperplasia, rather than tumor.

No test is perfect, however. There occasionally may be insufficient microscopic fat in the thymic tissue of a young adult to yield suppression on opposed-phase chemical shift MRI, as there was in the 21-year-old woman whose MRI scans are depicted in Fig. 34.14.

For this reason, one must always be circumspect and try to determine if other imaging findings and the clinical

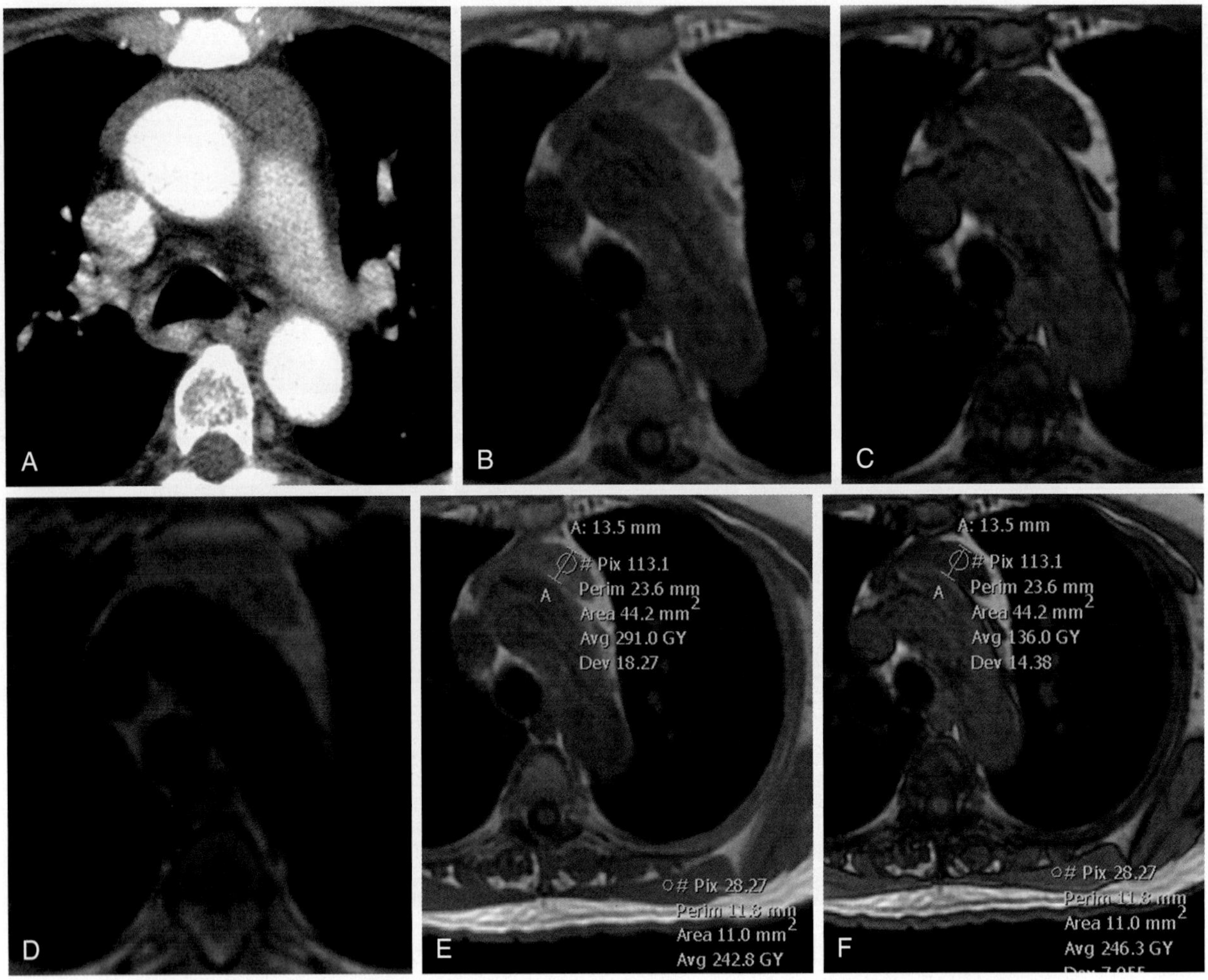

Figure 34.13 Thymic hyperplasia in a 64-year-old woman with severe hyperthyroidism. (A) Axial chest CT scan with IV contrast revealing excess thymic soft tissue for age, with a maximal thymic lobe thickness of 1.6 cm. (B) Axial in-phase ultrafast gradient echo (GRE) T1-weighted, opposed-phase ultrafast GRE T1-weighted (C), and cardiac-gated double inversion recovery T2-weighted (D) images reveal the thymic tissue to suppress homogeneously on opposed-phase images, indicating the diffuse presence of microscopic fat. The thymic tissue is mildly T2-hyperintense. (E and F) Chemical shift ratio (CSR) calculation. Axial in-phase ultrafast GRE T1-weighted (E) and opposed-phase ultrafast GRE T1-weighted (F) images with region of interest placement for CSR calculation on the thymic tissue and a chest wall muscle on the same image. CSR = ([opposed-phase thymic tissue/opposed-phase chest wall muscle] ÷ [in-phase thymic tissue/in-phase chest wall muscle]) = 136/246 ÷ 291/243 = 0.5.

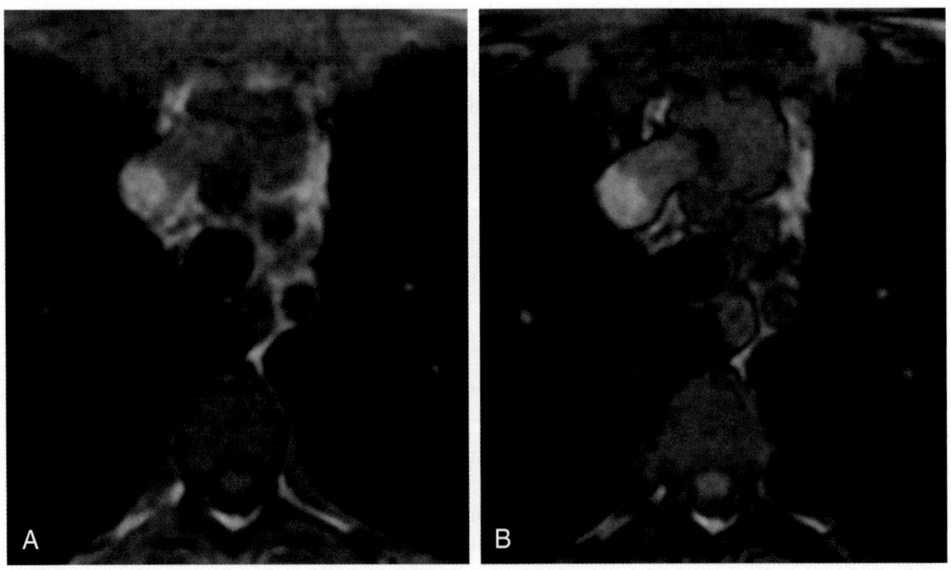

Figure 34.14 Nonsuppressing normal thymus in a 21-year-old woman presenting with syncope and an arrhythmia, proven histopathologically. (A) In-phase ultrafast gradient echo (GRE) T1-weighted image and opposed-phase ultrafast GRE T1-weighted image (B) reveal no suppression of signal on the opposed-phase image. Although microscopic fat was present in the histopathologic specimen, it was an insufficient amount to elicit signal suppression on opposed-phase chemical shift MRI. (Modified from Ackman JB, Mino-Kenudson M, Morse CR. Nonsuppressing normal thymus on chemical shift magnetic resonance imaging in a young woman. *J Thorac Imaging.* 2012;27:W196–W199.)

context still favor normal or hyperplastic thymus over tumor. If CSR or SII results in conflict with an otherwise normal or hyperplastic thymic appearance, serial non-contrast MRI follow-up can be helpful, beginning at 3 to 6 months and with a doubling of subsequent follow-up intervals, provided that there is no concerning change in the appearance of the thymic tissue over time. If the thymic tissue involutes (Fig. 34.15) and/or suppresses over time, it can be deduced that it represents a normal or hyperplastic thymus, and surgical resection will have been averted.

THYMIC CYST: DISCERNMENT FROM SOLID THYMIC LESION

If a lesion in the thymic bed is round, oval, or saccular, well-circumscribed, noninvasive, homogeneous in attenuation, and measures up to 100 Hounsfield units (HU) on CT, the lesion may represent a benign thymic cyst or, less likely, a unilocular lymphangioma, rather than a solid lesion. In such a case, thymic MRI can make this distinction. The hyperattenuation on CT is usually due to hemorrhagic content and on MRI may yield T1 hyperintensity of the lesion (see Fig. 34.5). MRI may also detect subtle lesion complexity within a cyst, such as enhancing mural nodularity and/or septations, in which case the lesion is presumed to be a cystic thymoma, until proven otherwise; such lesions can be inflammatory, however. Thymic cysts may be unilocular or multilocular and can coexist with thymic hyperplasia and thymic neoplasms. These benign cysts may fluctuate both in size and attenuation over time on account of spontaneous hemorrhage and resorption.

LYMPHANGIOMAS AND HEMANGIOMAS

Lymphangiomas and hemangiomas may occur in the anterior mediastinum and in other mediastinal compartments, although they are rare. Lymphangiomas usually present as unilocular or multilocular cysts and may be of water or higher attenuation. They may appear solid on CT on account of myriad small cysts and can contain enhancing septations. Despite their benign nature, they can be large (Fig. 34.16) and infiltrative.

It is difficult to make a definitive diagnosis of a mediastinal hemangioma on CT because standard chest CT is not routinely performed with DCE because of radiation exposure and lack of necessity in most cases. MRI can diagnose hemangiomas in the mediastinum when a T2-hyperintense lesion with peripheral nodular enhancement and fill-in or partial fill-in over time on DCE imaging is found. An example of a mediastinal hemangioma was provided earlier (see Fig. 34.10). As in the liver, however, not all hemangiomas exhibit this pattern of enhancement. Mediastinal hemangiomas can exhibit a crumbly, fatty-intercalated morphology and texture, or they can be well-circumscribed, without fatty intercalation.

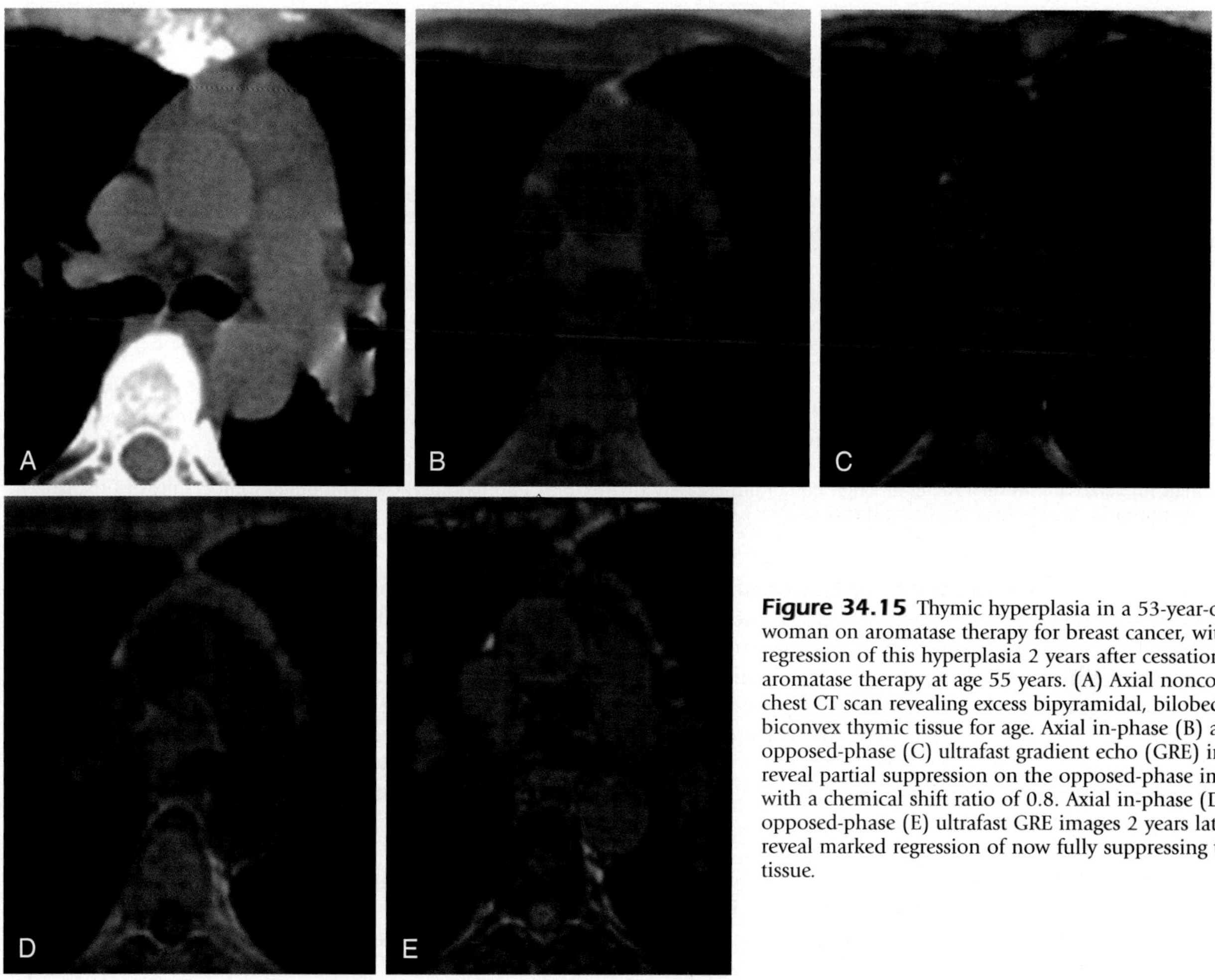

Figure 34.15 Thymic hyperplasia in a 53-year-old woman on aromatase therapy for breast cancer, with regression of this hyperplasia 2 years after cessation of aromatase therapy at age 55 years. (A) Axial noncontrast chest CT scan revealing excess bipyramidal, bilobed, biconvex thymic tissue for age. Axial in-phase (B) and opposed-phase (C) ultrafast gradient echo (GRE) images reveal partial suppression on the opposed-phase image, with a chemical shift ratio of 0.8. Axial in-phase (D) and opposed-phase (E) ultrafast GRE images 2 years later reveal marked regression of now fully suppressing thymic tissue.

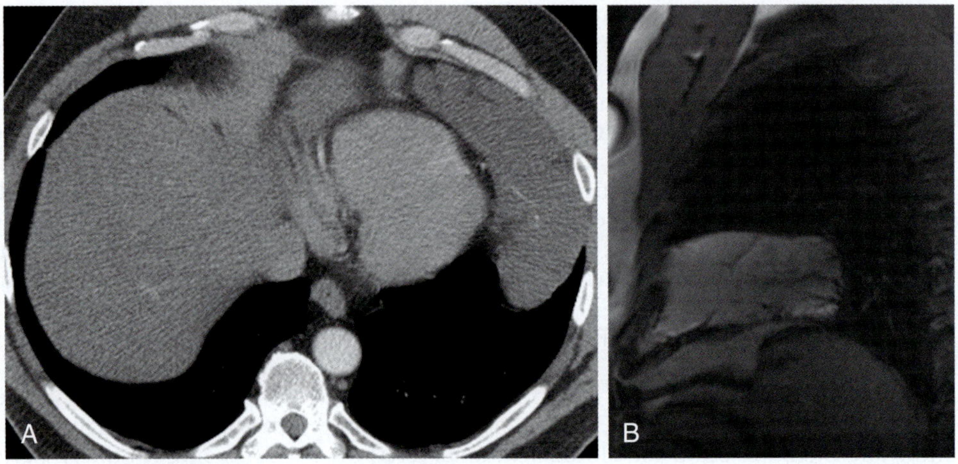

Figure 34.16 Multilocular lymphangioma with calcified septation in a 46-year-old man. (A) Axial contrast-enhanced chest CT scan demonstrating a multilocular cystic mass with a finely calcified septation in the left cardiophrenic angle. (B) Sagittal steady-state free precession image revealing marked hyperintensity of this cystic lesion on this water-weighted sequence. This noncontrast MRI scan demonstrates the multiple septations within this lesion that are virtually invisible by CT.

TABLE 34.3 Differentiating Features of Thymoma, Lymphoma, Thymic Hyperplasia, and Thymic Bed Cysts[a,b]

LESIONAL AND PERILESIONAL CT FEATURES	THYMOMA	LYMPHOMA	THYMIC HYPERPLASIA	THYMIC BED CYST	*P* VALUE
Off-midline	32/39[a] (82%)	5/19[a] (26%)	1/10 (10%)	4/9[a] (44%)	< .0001
Bipyramidal	0/42 (0%)	0/31 (0%)	6/10 (60%)	0/10 (0%)	< .0001
Quadrilateral, triangular, bilobed	0/42 (0%)	0/31 (0%)	10/10 (100%)	0/10 (0%)	< .0001
Round, oval, or saccular	20/42 (48%)	5/31 (16%)	0/10 (0%)	10/10 (100%)	< .0001
Lobulated	19/42 (45%)	23/31 (74%)	0/10 (0%)	1/10 (10%)[c]	< .0001
Lobulated and multinodular	4/42 (10%)	8/31 (26%)	0/10 (0%)	0/10 (0%)	< .0001
Amorphous	0/42 (0%)	3/31 (10%)	0/10 (0%)	0/10 (0%)	< .0001
Well-defined	39/42 (93%)	17/31 (55%)	10/10 (100%)	10/10 (100%)	< .001
Homogeneous attenuation	14/42 (33%)	4/31 (13%)	3/10 (30%)	10/10 (100%)	< .0001
Intercalated fat or marbling	0/42 (0%)	0/31 (0%)	5/10 (50%)	0/10 (0%)	< .0001
Associated lymphadenopathy	5/42 (12%)	10/31 (32%)	0/10 (0%)	0/10 (0%)	< .001
Overt pericardial involvement	0/42 (0%)	7/31 (22%)	0/10 (0%)	0/10 (0%)	< .001
Mass effect	12/42 (28%)	23/31 (74%)	0/10 (0%)	1/10 (10%)	< .0001

[a]That achieved statistical significance.
[b]The fraction denominators for midline analysis vary from the total number of thymoma, lymphoma, thymic hyperplasia, and thymic bed cyst cases with available imaging (n = 39, 19, 10, and 9 rather than n = 42, 31, 10, and 10, respectively) because in several cases (particularly the lymphoma cases), the lesion could not be definitively characterized as midline or off-midline.
[c]One of 10 thymic bed cysts was both oval and lobulated.
From Ackman JB, Verzosa S, Kovach AE, et al. High rate of unnecessary thymectomy and its cause. Can computed tomography distinguish thymoma, lymphoma, thymic hyperplasia, and thymic cysts? *Eur J Radiol.* 2015;84(3):524–533.

Prevascular or Anterior Mediastinal Neoplasms

Although the finding of a large, irregular, heterogeneously enhancing, at least partially solid mass in the anterior mediastinum, with or without lymphadenopathy or invasion of adjacent structures, provides an opportunity for an academic discussion regarding the differential diagnosis, it usually requires resection, regardless of its nature, unless lymphoma is a consideration.

DISTINGUISHING THYMIC HYPERPLASIA, THYMIC CYSTS, AND LYMPHOMA FROM THYMOMA

One of the most difficult problems regarding image interpretation in the anterior mediastinum arises from efforts to distinguish thymic hyperplasia, thymic cysts, and lymphoma, which usually do not require resection, from thymic tumors that do require resection. Many unnecessary thymectomies have been performed because of this interpretative difficulty. In fact, unnecessary or nontherapeutic thymectomy rates of 22% to 68% have been reported in the literature. Therefore the focus of our problem-solving effort in the prevascular or anterior mediastinum will be to distinguish these entities from one another.

In research involving a recent 6-year study cohort (Table 34.3), Ackman et al. found these lesions to differ significantly on CT and, by inference, on MRI regarding the following:

1. Location with respect to midline
2. Morphology

3. Circumscription or definition
4. Homogeneity versus heterogeneity of attenuation
5. Presence or absence of:
   a. Intercalated gross fat or marbling
   b. Associated lymphadenopathy
   c. Overt pericardial involvement
   d. Mass effect

THYMIC HYPERPLASIA. Thymic hyperplasia is most typically midline, often bipyramidal, and usually quadrilateral, triangular, and/or bilobed in configuration. Well-defined borders are usual, allowing for a crumbly consistency that can manifest when there is gross fatty intercalation encircling islands or small reticulonodular strands of hyperplastic (or normal) thymic tissue. Gross fatty intercalation or fatty marbling (Fig. 34.17) is specific for thymic hyperplasia, although not present in every case (see Figs. 34.13 and 34.14). Pure thymic hyperplasia does not cause mass effect. Thymic lesions with coexistent thymic hyperplasia may do so.

THYMIC CYSTS. Thymic cysts are more apt to be midline than off-midline in location. They are well-defined and round, oval, or saccular in configuration. Not infrequently, they exhibit the expected morphology of a sac of fluid in response to gravity and may mimic the configuration of a hot water bottle placed on a horizontal surface (Fig. 34.18).

Like other cysts, thymic cysts can deform or change in morphology between examinations on account of their fluid nature and differences in respiratory phase during imaging. Their attenuation is almost always homogeneous, with CT attenuation values ranging from those of water up to 100 HU. It is critical to recognize that CT attenuation values of 20 through 100 HU do not automatically confer a diagnosis of a solid mass on CT (Fig. 34.19).

Thymic cysts have been repeatedly misinterpreted as thymomas on CT because of a lack of awareness that lesions measuring greater than water attenuation may be cystic, rather than solid. True thymic cysts have not been reported to yield mass effect on adjacent structures. Larger cysts in the thymic bed, such as large mesothelial cysts, can cause mass effect, however (Fig. 34.20).

Recognition of the possibility of a thymic bed cyst in the differential diagnosis of anterior mediastinal lesions is critical to averting unnecessary thymectomy. In the

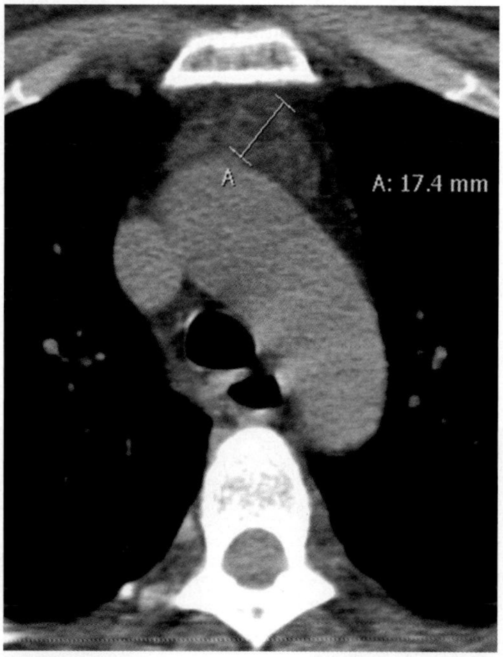

Figure 34.17 Thymic hyperplasia with gross fatty intercalation in a 51-year-old woman with lymphoid follicular hyperplasia on axial CT without IV contrast.

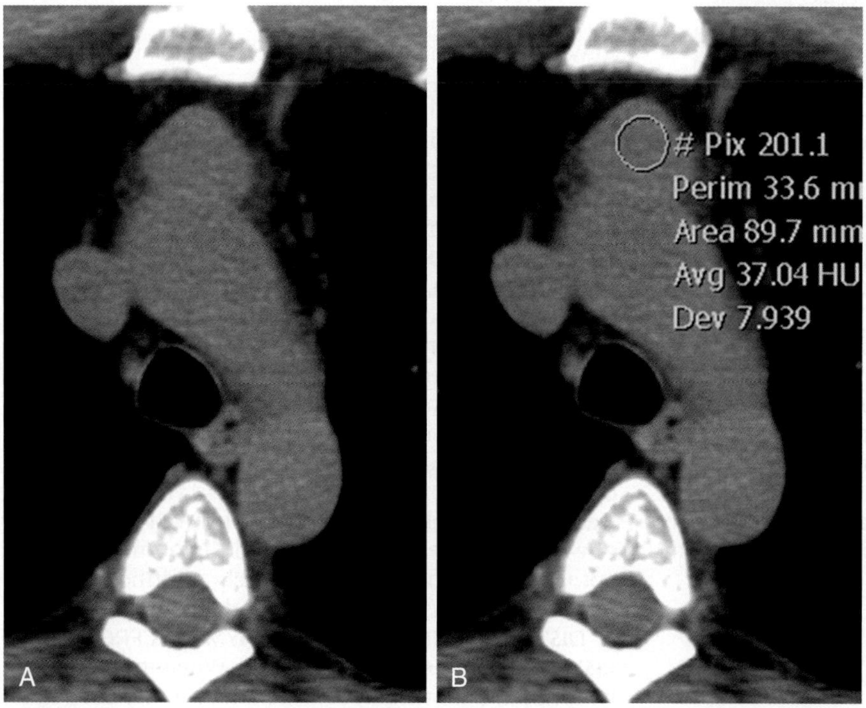

Figure 34.18 Thymic cyst in a 61-year-old woman exhibiting a saccular or hot water bottle configuration. (A and B) Axial noncontrast chest CT measured 37 HU, with and without region of interest placement. This woman underwent median sternotomy and thymectomy for this benign thymic cyst. Had she undergone a preoperative MRI, the surgery might have been averted.

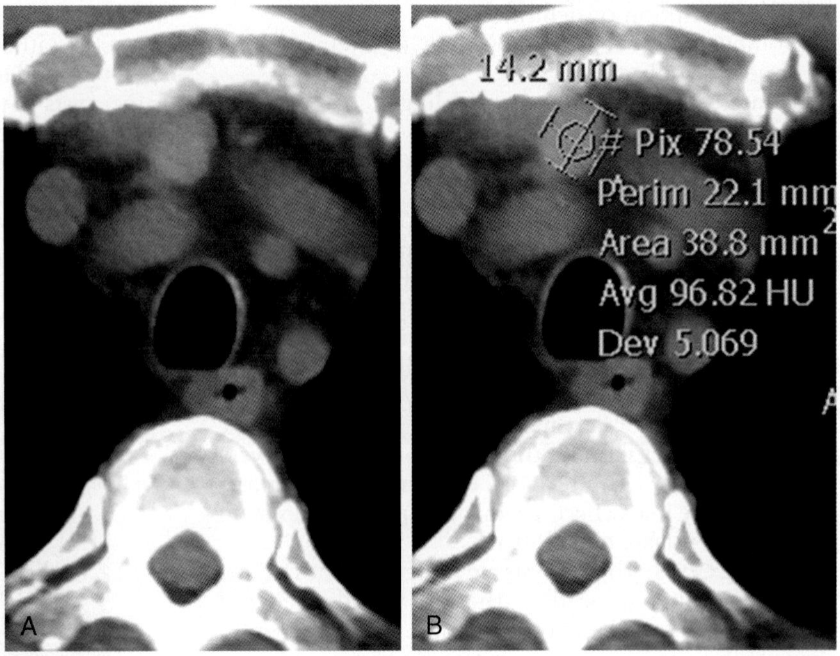

Figure 34.19 Thymic cyst measuring 97 HU in a man in his seventh decade on axial noncontrast CT without (A) and with (B) region of interest placement.

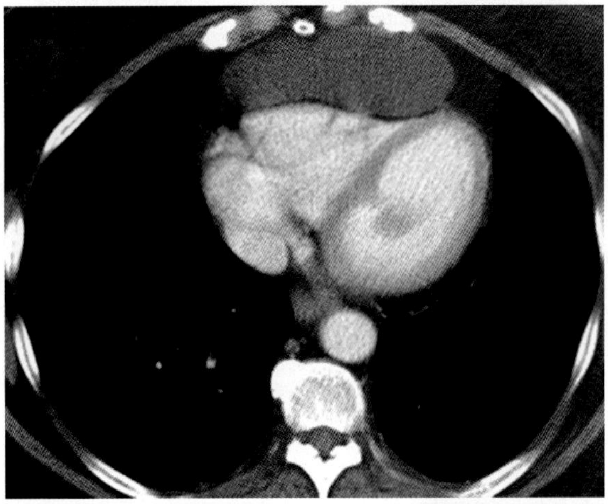

Figure 34.20 Large prevascular mesothelial cyst exerting mass effect on the right ventricle on an axial chest CT scan with IV contrast.

study cohort of Ackman et al., benign thymic bed cysts comprised 53% of the inadvertent benign thymectomy specimens over a 6-year period at their quaternary referral hospital because they were misinterpreted as thymomas on chest CT. In the same cohort, thymic hyperplasia comprised 38% and reactive and atrophic tissue comprised the rest of the unnecessary thymectomies. When the possibility of a cyst is recognized, thymic MRI can make the distinction among a simple cyst,[a] which can be followed to ensure benignity over time; a complex cyst, which can be followed or resected; and a solid lesion in need of resection.

[a]The term "simple cyst" as used here includes protein- or hemorrhage-containing and otherwise simple thymic cysts with thin, smooth walls, no enhancing internal septations.

LYMPHOMA. Primary anterior mediastinal lymphoma can be difficult to characterize as midline or off-midline but, when it can be characterized, is more apt to span both sides of the midline than a thymoma. Lobulated and combined lobulated-multinodular morphology is common in anterior mediastinal lymphoma. A multinodular component to the lobulation, secondary to multiple coalescing lymph nodes, is nearly specific for lymphoma when compared with thymoma (Fig. 34.21). Associated lymphadenopathy is also much more common in lymphoma than thymoma. Mass effect and overt pericardial involvement were also much more common in a series for lymphoma than for thymoma; however, this may have been because of the higher proportion of low-risk thymoma than high-risk thymoma in the cohort studied.

THYMOMA. Thymomas are most typically off-midline in location, round in configuration, well defined, and heterogeneous in attenuation (Fig. 34.22). If a round, well-circumscribed mass in the thymic bed of homogeneous attenuation is found, consideration of the possibility that the lesion may represent a thymic cyst, rather than a thymoma, must be made and, when possible, an MRI performed to differentiate between a cystic and solid lesion and avert unnecessary diagnostic intervention, including thymectomy. In the series by Ackman et al., which included more low-risk than high-risk thymomas, lobulated morphology was observed in just under 50% of cases, and combined lobulated-multinodular morphology was very uncommon for thymomas. Lymphadenopathy was unusual, and mass effect was observed in just under one-third of cases. More advanced thymomas are more apt to be lobulated, although rarely multinodular, and usually exhibit associated lymphadenopathy.

DISTINGUISHING LOW-RISK THYMOMA FROM HIGH-RISK THYMOMA AND LYMPHOMA. When thymoma and lymphoma both remain considerations in the differential

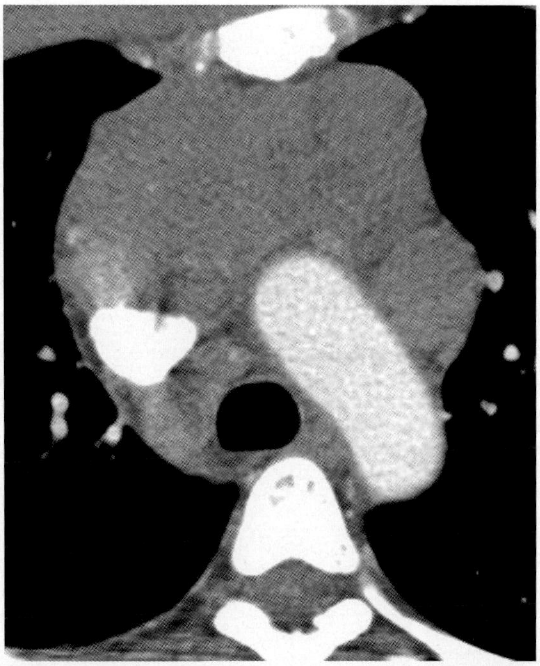

Figure 34.21 Primary mediastinal large B cell lymphoma in a 43-year-old woman on a chest CT scan with IV contrast. The anterior mediastinal mass is lobulated and multinodular, with associated, in some cases contiguous, middle mediastinal lymphadenopathy

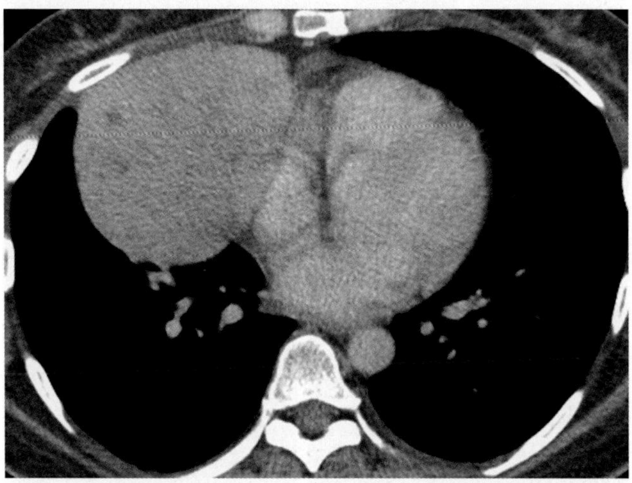

Figure 34.22 Low-grade thymoma, World Health Organization classification type A, in a 46-year-old woman. A chest CT scan with IV contrast reveals the large mass to be round, well circumscribed, heterogeneous in attenuation, and off-midline, with mild mass effect on the right cardiac chambers.

diagnosis for an anterior mediastinal lesion, dynamic, contrast-enhanced MRI can be performed to help differentiate these entities. In 2002, Sakai et al. found that thymomas exhibited more rapid time to peak enhancement than nonthymomas, including lymphoma, thymic carcinoma, and germ cell tumors. They also demonstrated that low-risk thymomas enhanced more rapidly than high-risk thymomas. The mean time to peak enhancement for low-risk thymomas was 1.3 minutes (Fig. 34.23), that for high-risk thymomas was 2.5 minutes, and that for nonthymomas was 3.2 minutes.

When discernment of a low-risk from a high-risk thymoma is desired to help with treatment planning, diffusion-weighted imaging with ADC mapping may also be helpful, although biopsy is preferred if definitive assessment is needed. In 2009, Abdel Razek et al. showed in their institutional cohort that an ADC value of 1.25 $\times 10^{-3}$ mm^2/s could be used as a threshold value to distinguish these entities, with ADC values less than 1.25 $\times 10^{-3}$ mm^2/s typical of high-risk thymomas and thymic carcinoma and higher ADC values typical of low-risk thymomas. This ADC cutoff value may only be used as a rough guide, however.

FATTY ANTERIOR MEDIASTINAL MASSES

The finding of an anterior mediastinal mass containing confluent gross fat or a microscopically fatty, liquid component (latter detectable by MRI), excluding fatty intercalated thymic hyperplasia, usually indicates the presence of a dermoid cyst or mature teratoma. Both thymolipomas and liposarcomas may contain fat and soft tissue components, but neither should contain the fat-fluid levels or microscopically fatty fluid virtually pathognomonic for teratomas (Fig. 34.24); both of these tumors are rare.

The soft tissue component of a thymolipoma represents thymic tissue. Within liposarcomas, increasing amounts of soft tissue typically indicate a higher grade of liposarcoma. Differentiating features between thymolipoma and liposarcoma include the usual conformity of thymolipomas to adjacent anatomic structures and their relatively nonaggressive, noninfiltrative appearance. Thymolipomas do not typically insinuate between and splay visceral and vascular structures, however liposarcomas will do this (Fig. 34.25).

ALGORITHM FOR PREVASCULAR MEDIASTINAL MASS MANAGEMENT

Fig. 34.26 presents an algorithm regarding prevascular mediastinal mass management.

Visceral or Middle Mediastinal Compartment

Because the central airways, esophagus, heart and great vessels (including all of the ascending and descending thoracic aorta), pericardium, nerves (e.g., vagus, recurrent laryngeal, phrenic), paraganglia, and lymphatics reside in the visceral compartment, masses arising from this compartment include lymphadenopathy, whether from an inflammatory, metastatic, or lymphoproliferative cause, tracheal and esophageal masses, foregut duplication cysts, mesothelial or pericardial cysts, benign and malignant cardiac masses (whether primary or metastatic malignancy), vascular aneurysms, and neurogenic tumors (e.g., neurofibromas, schwannomas, paragangliomas), lymphangiomas, and hemangiomas.

Normal Middle Mediastinal Structures Sometimes Misinterpreted as Abnormal

Occasionally, normal middle mediastinal findings on CXR may be misinterpreted as abnormal. An example includes the normal main pulmonary artery in young women,

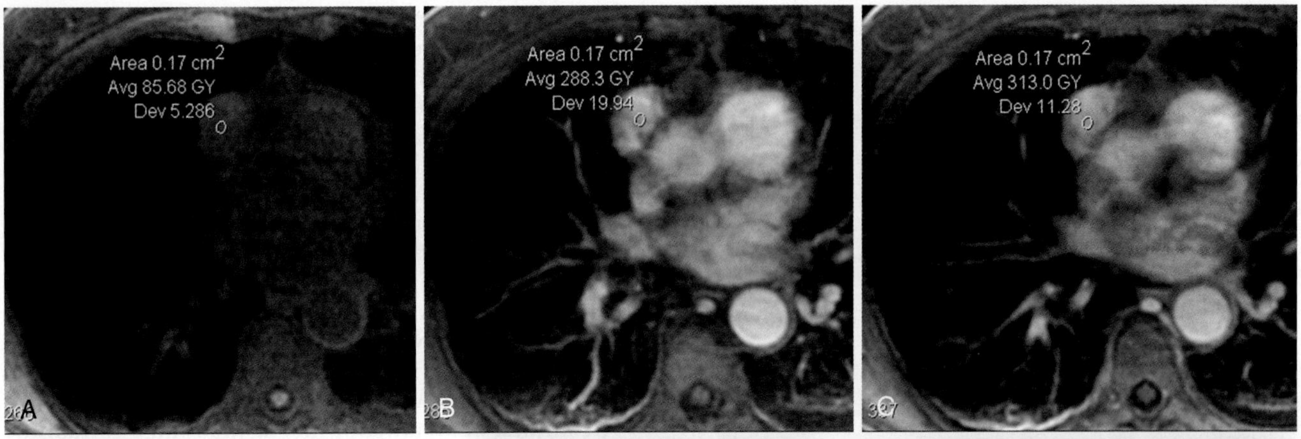

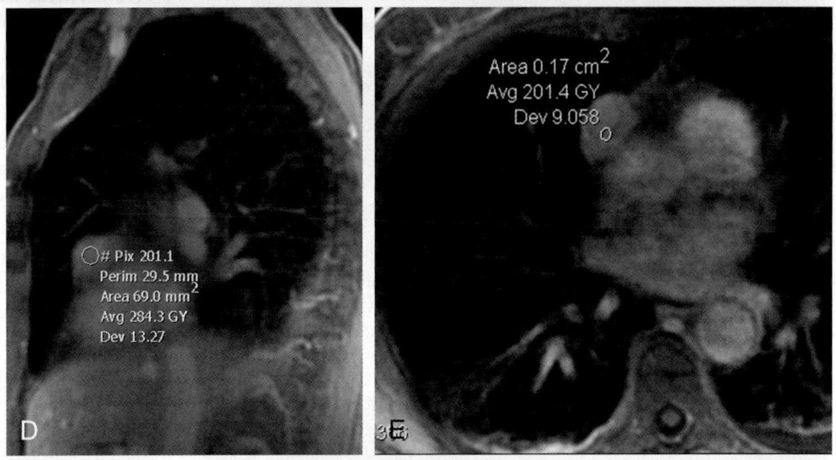

Figure 34.23 The rapid time-to-peak enhancement of a low-grade thymoma (World Health Organization type AB) in a 67-year-old woman on pre- and postcontrast three-dimensional ultrafast gradient echo fat-saturated T1-weighted dynamic contrast enhancement MRI, with region of interest (ROI) values of 86, 288, 313, 284, and 201 at precontrast (A), 20 seconds (B), 1 minute (C), 3 minutes (D), and 5 minutes (E), respectively, with the 3-minute evaluation slightly limited by the fact that the sagittal ROI may not be located at precisely the same place as those on the axial images. The rapid time-to-peak enhancement, location, and morphology (mildly lobulated, ovoid, well circumscribed) of this lower right thymic bed mass favor thymoma over lymphoma.

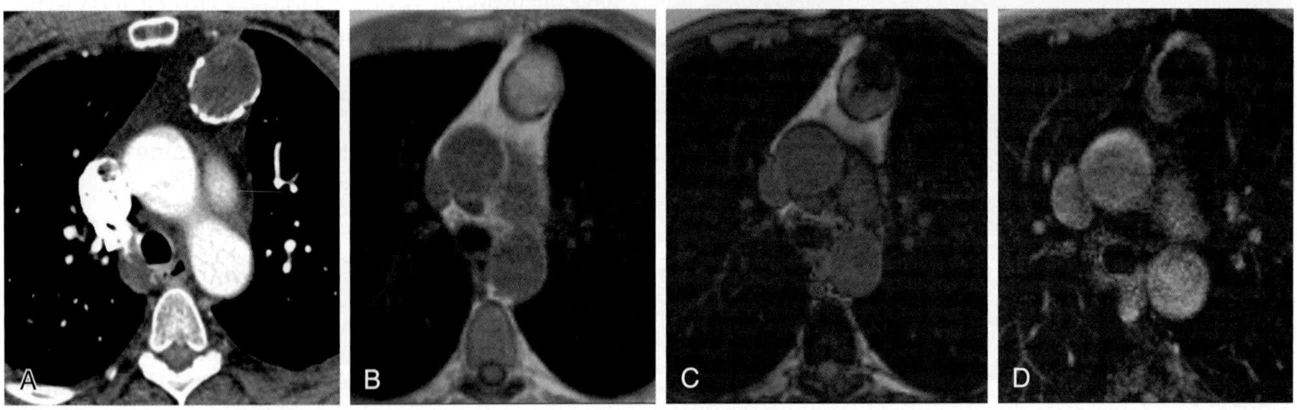

Figure 34.24 Dermoid cyst or teratoma in a 59-year-old woman. (A) Chest CT scan with IV contrast reveals a partially rim-calcified, well-circumscribed, ovoid mass of heterogeneous attenuation in the left thymic bed. In-phase (B) and opposed-phase (C) ultrafast gradient echo (GRE) T1-weighted MRI, and postcontrast, postprocessed, subtracted ultrafast three-dimensional GRE fat-saturated T1-weighted MRI (D) reveal suppression of the nondependent component of this lesion on the opposed-phase images, with no internal enhancement and with irregular wall enhancement of this lesion. The suppression on the opposed-phase image indicates the presence of microscopic fat mixed with fluid in a component of this complex cyst. The wall calcification of this lesion, although visible on CT, is undetectable on the MR images. These findings are pathognomonic for a teratoma.

which can be prominent on CXR and mimic pathology, whether due to true main pulmonary enlargement or lymphadenopathy. Although chest CT can readily make this distinction, MRI can do so without radiation and just as quickly, with a single 8- to 10-second breath-hold axial steady-state free precession pulse sequence and should be considered an alternative option (Fig. 34.27).

Congenital Developmental Lesions of the Visceral Mediastinum

Foregut duplication cysts in the visceral mediastinum (typically bronchogenic cysts and esophageal duplication cysts) may be of water attenuation or may reach attenuation values up to 100 HU on CT. When of higher attenuation, they can mimic a solid lesion. Performance of MRI is instrumental

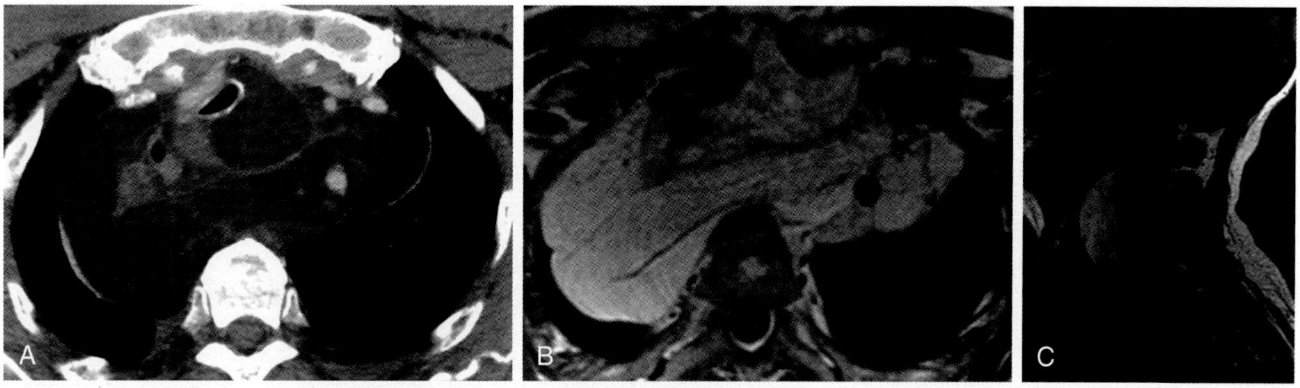

Figure 34.25 Large liposarcoma extending from the chest into the prevertebral neck, insinuating between, displacing, and splaying the trachea, esophagus, and great vessels. (A) Axial chest CT scan with IV contrast. (B) Axial T1-weighted MR image of the chest and sagittal T1-weighted MR image of the neck (C).

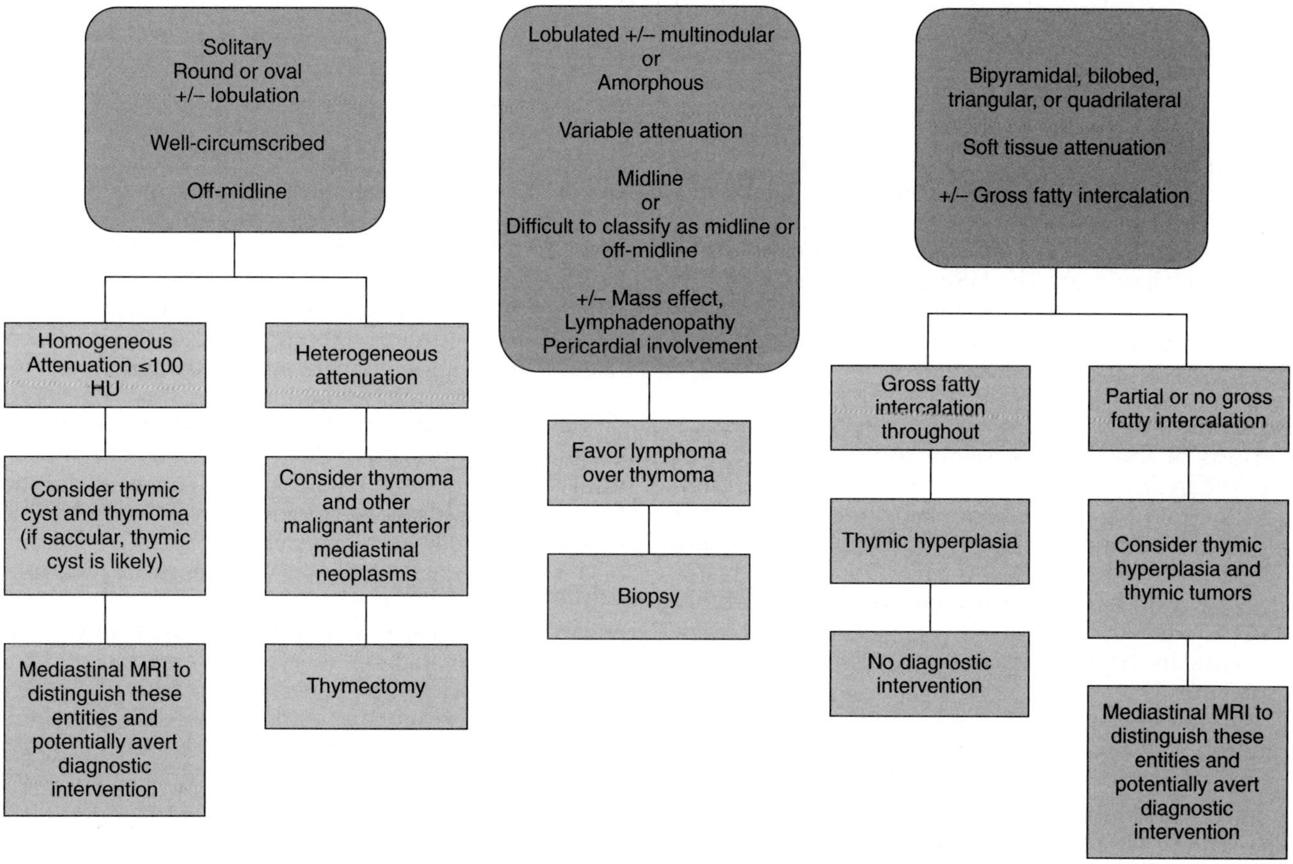

Figure 34.26 Algorithm for prevascular or anterior mediastinal mass management.

to distinguish cystic from solid lesions (Fig. 34.28) in this context and in many others throughout the body.

When uncomplicated, foregut duplication cysts are typically round or ovoid, well circumscribed, and homogenous in attenuation and MRI signal. On MRI they may be of low, intermediate, or high T1 signal and are markedly T2-hyperintense (isointense to cerebrospinal fluid). They may exhibit no enhancement or thin, smooth wall enhancement. Esophageal duplication cysts should be in close contact with the esophagus, may have a slightly thicker wall than bronchogenic cysts, and may be more oblong or tubular in shape, with a vertical orientation. Both can occur in the subcarinal space and azygoesophageal recess, however. Hemorrhage, infection (see Fig. 34.1), and perforation of these cysts may occur, in part due to the occasional presence of ectopic gastric mucosa within these cysts. The differential diagnosis for these foregut duplication cysts includes lymphangiomas and pleuropericardial or mesothelial cysts. If the cyst exhibits a direct relationship with the spinal canal, and/or a coexistent vertebral anomaly is present at the same level, a neuroenteric cyst can be specifically diagnosed.

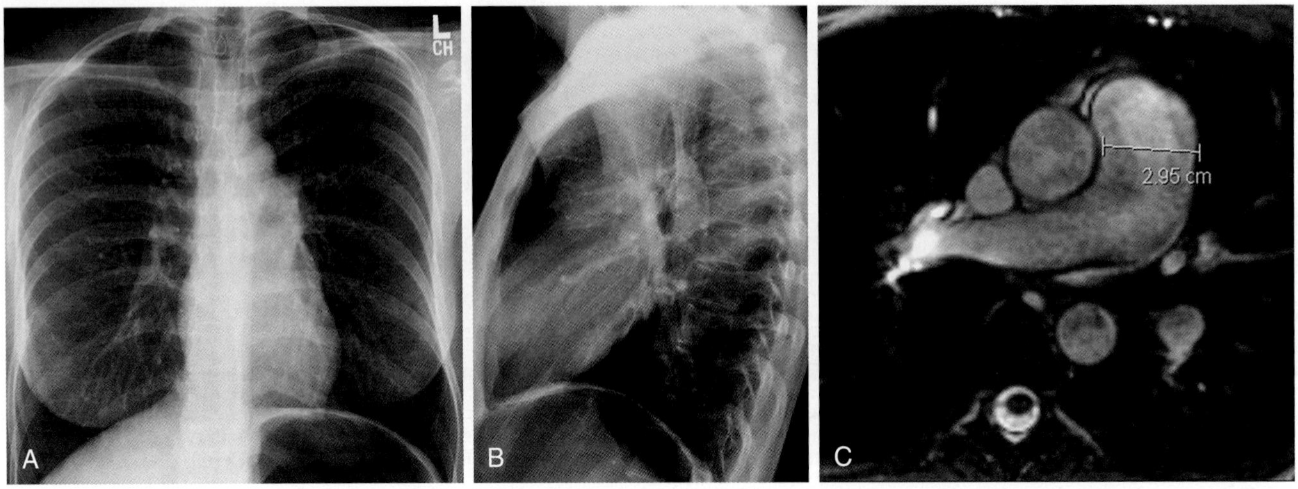

Figure 34.27 Prominent left hilum in a 26-year-old woman on posteroanterior (A) and lateral (B) chest x-rays proven by an 8- to 10-second breath-hold axial steady-state free precession (white blood gradient echo without IV contrast). (C) MRI through the hila represents a main pulmonary artery at the upper limit of normal in diameter, with no lymphadenopathy.

Hemangiomas and lymphangiomas have been discussed earlier in the context of anterior mediastinal lesions. Fig. 34.10 demonstrates the CT and MRI characteristics of a pathology-proven hemangioma found in the middle or visceral mediastinum. The MRI characteristics of low to intermediate T1 signal, T2 hyperintensity, and peripheral nodular enhancement over time may be pathognomonic, as they are for hepatic hemangiomas.

Posttraumatic, Postsurgical, and Inflammatory Lesions of the Visceral Mediastinum

The differential diagnosis of a widened mediastinum on CXR not only includes lymphadenopathy and other solid and cystic masses but also mediastinal hematomas, which are often readily deduced by clinical context—for example, shortly after cardiac bypass surgery or other trauma. When the diagnosis is not evident by CXR, chest CT is usually the next step, with MRI reserved for further problem solving.

The finding of pneumomediastinum, pneumopericardium, and other unusual air tracts on CXR elicits a broad differential diagnosis, which can be reduced by consideration of the clinical context. Pneumomediastinum due to asthma or coughing is a diagnosis of exclusion. Consideration must be made of tracheal and esophageal perforation, tracking of peritoneal or retroperitoneal air into the mediastinum, tracheoesophageal fistulae (see Fig. 34.3), esophagobronchial or pleural fistulae, and esophagopericardial fistulae (Fig. 34.29), depending on the clinical scenario, location and morphology of the air, and presence or absence of pleural effusions or other fluid.

Other inflammatory lesions of the visceral mediastinum include fibrosing mediastinitis and large-vessel vasculitides. Fibrosing mediastinitis is not recognizable as a specific entity by CXR, although it may present on CXR with mediastinal widening and lymphadenopathy, with or without calcification. It may resemble a focal mass or infiltrative lesion on CT or MRI, vary in calcification and enhancement, and encase and narrow bronchovascular structures, mimicking a neoplasm. MRI may add diagnostic specificity when there is sufficient fibrotic or collagenous material to yield T2 hypointensity within the lesion, as is often the case in chronic fibrosing mediastinitis (see Fig. 34.3). Acute mediastinitis is T2-hyperintense, however.

Large vessel vasculitides may thicken vessel walls and mimic chronic thromboembolic pulmonary hypertension (Fig. 34.30), pulmonary angiosarcoma, an infiltrative lymphoma, and fibrosing mediastinitis on CT (see Fig. 34.3).

Mediastinal MRI with DCE may be helpful to distinguish these entities, not only by discernment of intraluminal from intramural lesions, but by T2 signal (chronic fibrosing mediastinitis is typically T2-hypointense, unlike neoplasms) and by the enhancement pattern. The degree of vessel wall enhancement on MRI reportedly correlates with disease activity. Intraluminal thrombus should not enhance, unless organized and infiltrated with cellular material. In 2004, Yi et al. demonstrated the primary differentiating features between a pulmonary artery sarcoma and pulmonary embolism on CT to be the presence of a low-attenuation filling defect that filled the entire luminal diameter of a proximal pulmonary artery, expansion of the artery, and extraluminal extension. In their study, pulmonary artery sarcoma manifested as a low-attenuation lesion, despite IV contrast administration. The higher soft tissue contrast of an MRI scan than a CT scan may distinguish pulmonary embolism from pulmonary sarcoma by demonstrating the enhancement of these pulmonary arterial neoplasms better, in contrast to a bland thromboembolism.

Neoplasms in the Visceral or Middle Mediastinum

Visceral mediastinal neoplasms include lymphoma, neoplasms arising from the tracheobronchial tree and esophagus, nerve sheath tumors arising along middle mediastinal nerves, including the phrenic, vagus, and recurrent laryngeal nerves, paragangliomas usually arising in the middle mediastinum from aortopulmonary paraganglia (and in the posterior or paravertebral mediastinum

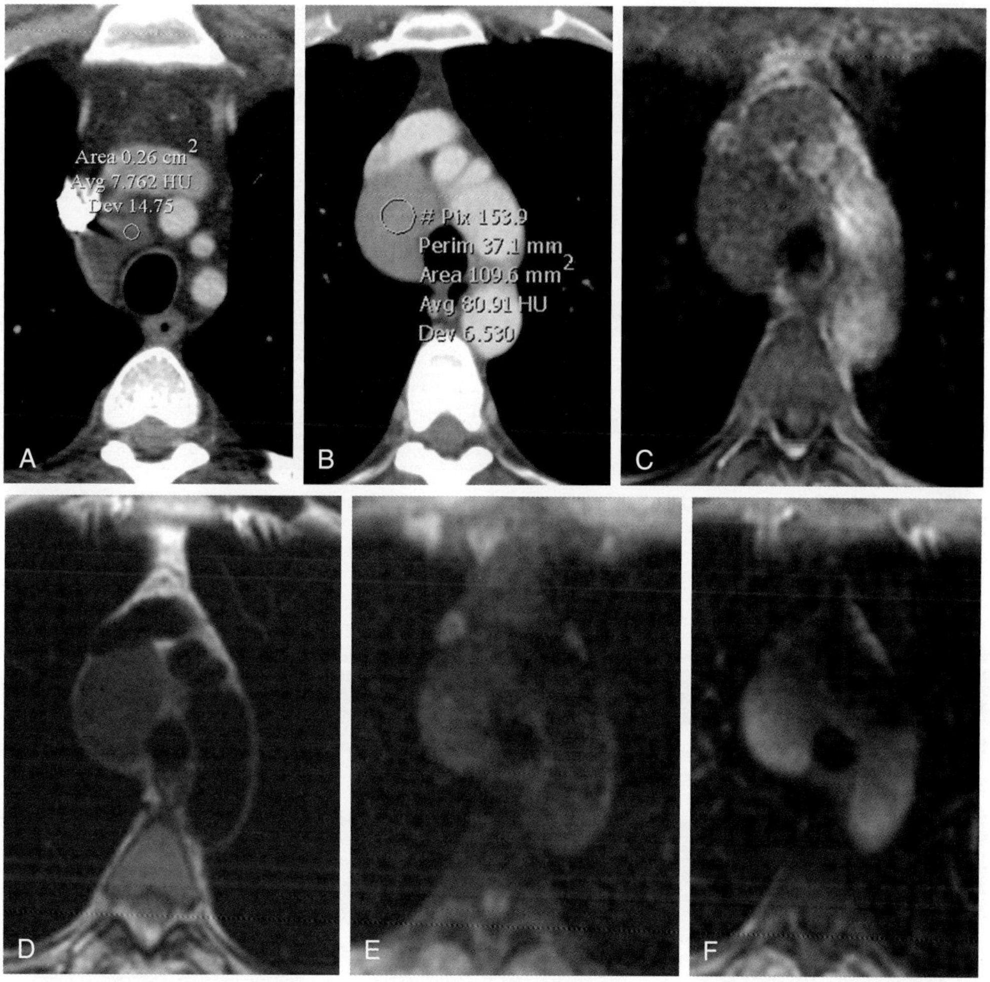

Figure 34.28 Cystic versus solid lesions in the middle mediastinum. (A and B) Axial chest CT scans with IV contrast of two separate adults with homogeneous attenuation and well-circumscribed lesions filling the right paratracheal space in a manner mimicking that of fluid, with the lesion in (A) measuring water attenuation (8 HU) and the lesion in (B) measuring 81 HU. The lesion in (A) was thought to represent a bronchogenic or mesothelial cyst. Given that the lesion in (B) could be cystic or solid (bronchogenic cysts measuring up to 100 HU have been found), MRI was performed. (C and D) Axial in-phase T1-weighted and cardiac-gated double inversion recovery T2-weighted images of the mass in (B) reveal it to be of intermediate T1 signal and low-to-intermediate T2 signal, with the lack of T2 hyperintensity making a cyst very unlikely, unless there is T2 shading from blood products, as seen with endometriomas. (E) Precontrast and 5-minute postcontrast (F) three-dimensional gradient echo, fat-saturated, T1-weighted MRI scans reveal the right paratracheal mass in (B) to enhance moderately, confirming its solid nature. The constellation of findings, aside from location, favor a mesenchymal tumor containing fibrous material (solitary fibrous tumor of the mediastinum) or densely packed smooth muscle. A rare right paratracheal leiomyoma was found at histopathology on surgical resection. (From Levesque MH, Aisagbonhi O, Digumarthy S, et al. Primary paratracheal leiomyoma: Increased preoperative diagnostic specificity with magnetic resonance imaging. *Ann Thorac Surg.* 2016;102:e151–e154.)

from sympathetic paraganglia), and rare lesions, including sarcomas. Upper endoscopy is the mainstay of esophageal lesion diagnosis, although contrast esophagography continues to have a role, particularly as an initial screening or overview examination after a finding of equivocal esophageal wall thickening on CT. Chest CT remains the modality of choice for the initial evaluation and staging of most clinically or radiographically suspected middle mediastinal neoplasms. MRI can add diagnostic specificity regarding the differentiation of paragangliomas and nerve sheath tumors from lymph nodes and other masses. Paragangliomas or extraadrenal pheochromocytomas are markedly T2-hyperintense on MRI and enhance vigorously, as opposed to most lymph nodes. They may or may not exhibit the classically described salt-and-pepper appearance on spin-echo T1-weighted MRI, with areas of low signal due to vessel flow voids within this hypervascular tumor; this latter finding has been more commonly observed in large paragangliomas. (The imaging appearance of nerve sheath tumors will be discussed in the next section, "Paravertebral or Posterior Mediastinal Compartment.") When mediastinal lesions are indeterminate on CT, MRI can be used to determine the consistency of these lesions, whether comprised of fluid, solid tissue, or both. MRI can also better designate the location of solid components and determine whether they are within reach of less invasive means of diagnostic intervention, such as endoscopic biopsy (see Fig. 34.6).

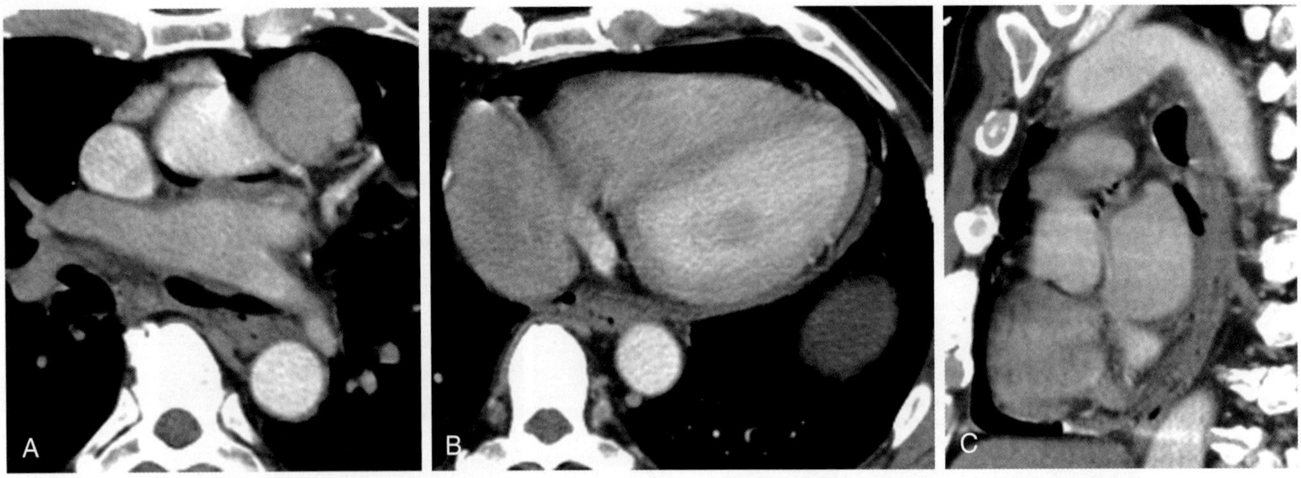

Figure 34.29 Esophagopericardial fistula in a 65-year-old man status post pulmonary vein ablation and prior esophageal stricture dilations. (A and B) Axial chest CT images at upper and lower levels, revealing two possible sites for the fistula, in addition to pneumopericardium. (C) Corresponding sagittal CT scan with IV contrast.

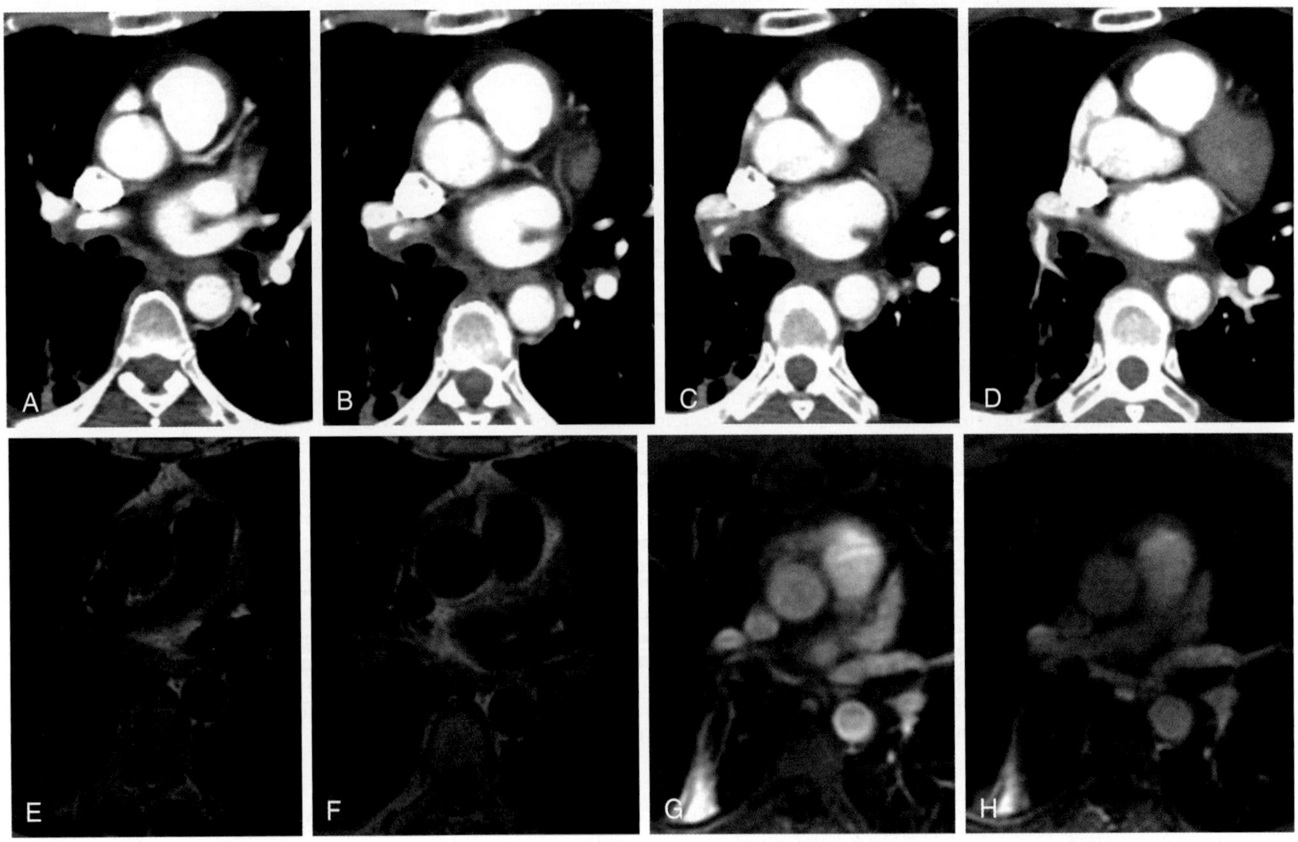

Figure 34.30 Takayasu arteritis involving the distal right main and right interlobar arteries and proximal right interlobar branches in a 49-year-old woman with worsening pleuritic chest pain over a few months. (A–D) Consecutive axial contrast-enhanced chest CT images (2.5-mm slices) through the distal right main and interlobar pulmonary artery revealing excess abnormal soft tissue eccentrically located along the vessel wall, focal pulmonary arterial narrowing, and dependent right lower lobe opacity. It is unclear whether these findings represent chronic pulmonary embolism, a vasculitis, or an infiltrative tumor. (E and F) Two consecutive cardiac-gated double inversion recovery, T1-weighted images (4-mm slices) revealing apparent abnormal thickening of the vessel wall, as confirmed by axial postcontrast ultrafast three-dimensional gradient echo, fat-saturated, T1-weighted 20-second (G) and 5- minute (H) MR images. The 20-second image reveals the markedly stenotic pulmonary arterial segment (3–4 mm lumen) through which high-signal IV contrast passes. The 5-minute image reveals enhancement of the stenotic vessel wall, with now more dilute gadolinium passing through the stenotic segment. The lower signal of the intraluminal contrast at 5 minutes may also be attributable to spin dephasing from turbulence. On all images, a wedge-shaped, dependent right lower lobe opacity is present. Given its marked, homogenous enhancement on postcontrast MRI scans, it is more likely to represent atelectasis than a pulmonary infarct.

Paravertebral or Posterior Mediastinal Compartment

Because vessels, lymphatics, sympathetic paraganglia, intercostal nerves, and spinal nerve roots reside in the paravertebral compartment, vascular masses (Fig. 34.31), lymphadenopathy, and neurogenic tumors most typically arise here. Extramedullary hematopoiesis, lymphangiomas, and hemangiomas may also arise in this compartment.

Previously Described Lesions Also Occurring in the Paravertebral Mediastinum

Most of the lesions that can arise in the paravertebral mediastinal compartment, including foregut duplication cysts, lymphangiomas, and hemangiomas, inflammatory lesions, vascular lesions, and neoplasms, have been mentioned, discussed, and/or depicted in earlier sections of this chapter. Thus the focus of this section will be how imaging, and in particular MRI, can be used to distinguish neurogenic tumors, the most common type of posterior mediastinal mass, from one another. The extent of neurogenic tumors and their relationship to nerve roots are also better depicted by MRI than CT.

Neurogenic Tumors

Neurofibromas and schwannomas appear similarly on CT. Both are well circumscribed, low- to intermediate-attenuation lesions. On MRI, whereas both neurofibromas and schwannomas are of low to intermediate T1 signal, their T2 signal characteristics usually differ. Neurofibromas are nonencapsulated or pseudoencapsulated, are typically centrally T2-hypointense and peripherally T2-hyperintense (so-called target appearance), and exhibit limited enhancement (Fig. 34.32). Neurofibromas rarely contain cystic elements. When cystic change, increased heterogeneous T2 signal, and increased enhancement develop in a previously observed neurofibroma, degeneration into a malignant peripheral nerve sheath tumor

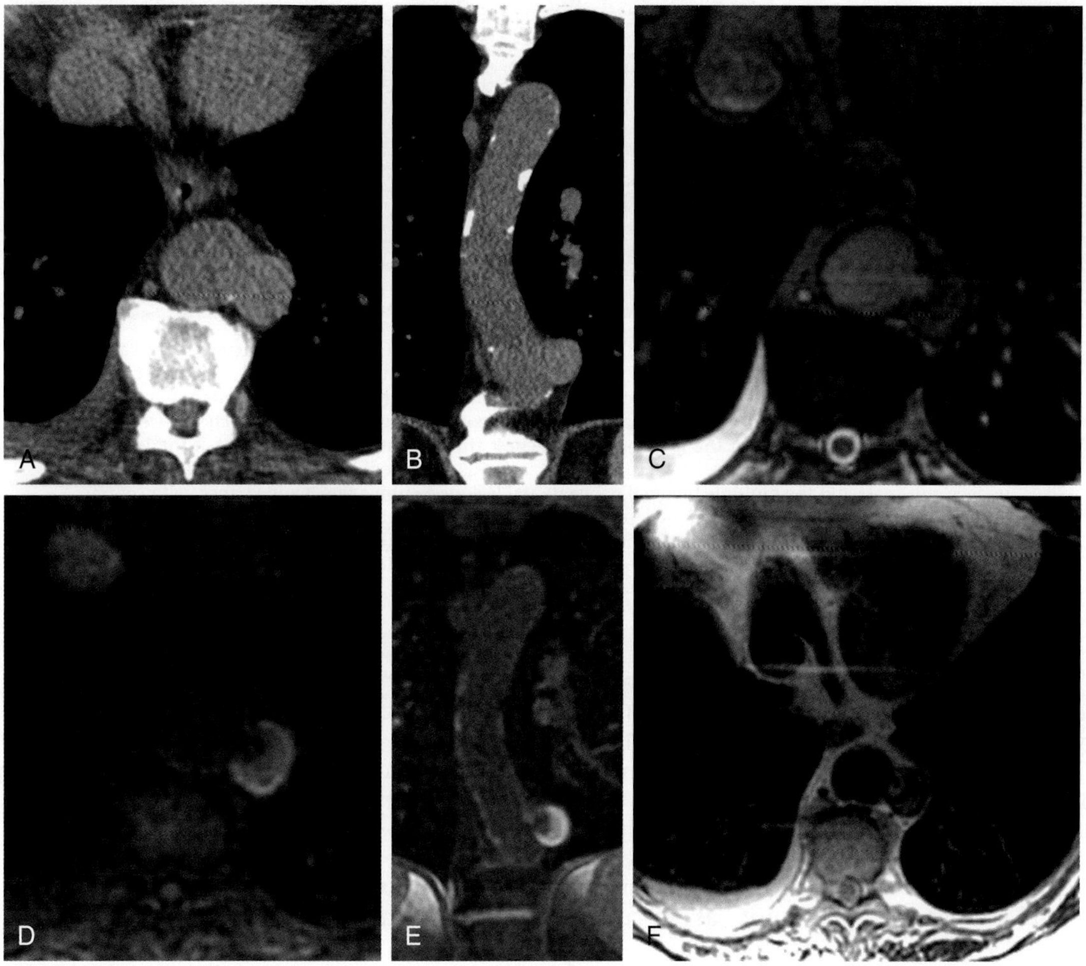

Figure 34.31 Saccular aortic pseudoaneurysm with mural thrombus in a 70-year-old man with hypertension, coronary artery disease, and renal insufficiency whose follow-up chest CT without IV contrast (A and B) revealed a gradually enlarging, now 2-cm left paraaortic mass along the lower descending aorta on CT. It is unclear whether this mass is truly left paraaortic and represents a pathologically enlarged lymph node or neoplasm, or whether it represents a vascular lesion arising from the aorta. (C–F) Axial steady-state free precession (C, bright blood gradient echo [GRE]), axial and coronal ultrafast three-dimensional GRE fat-saturated T1-weighted (D, E), and axial cardiac-gated double inversion recovery T2-weighted MR images without IV contrast (F) reveal the indeterminate lesion on CT to represent a saccular pseudoaneurysm containing T1/T2-hyperintense mural thrombus.

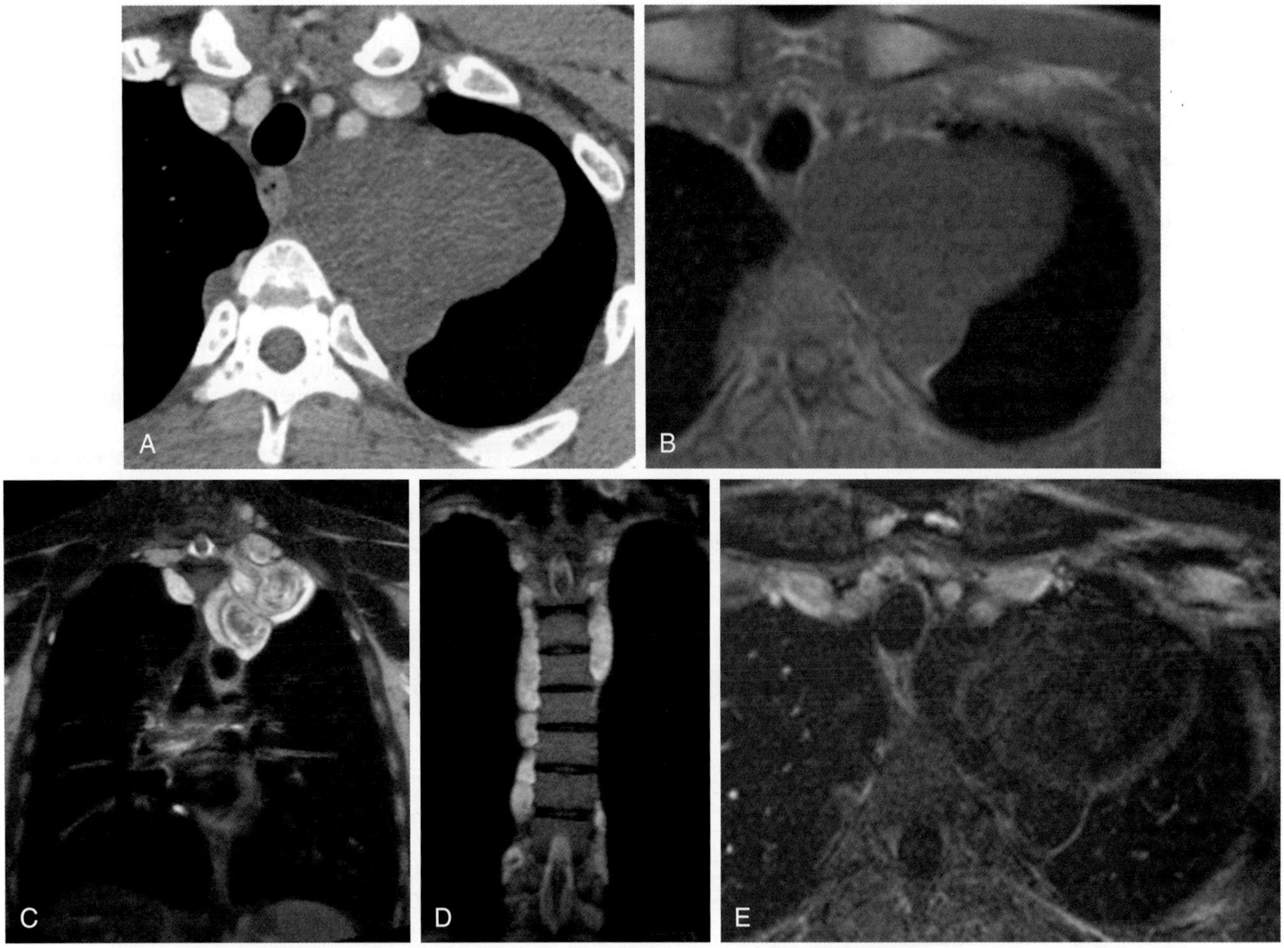

Figure 34.32 Neurofibromatosis in a 21-year-old man. (A) Axial CT scan with IV contrast revealing a large, lobulated soft tissue mass in the left mid-to-posterior mediastinum, mildly displacing the adjacent trachea, esophagus, and great vessels. A much smaller right paravertebral soft tissue mass is present. (B–D) Single axial in-phase T1-weighted image (B) and two coronal single shot fast spin-echo T2-weighted MRI images (C, D) with (C) at the level of the mid-chest (from front to back) and (D) at the level of the thoracic spine. The left upper mediastinal mass exhibits intermediate T1 signal. On T2-weighted images, this mass and the multiple bilateral paravertebral lesions exhibit a target appearance, with central T2 hypointensity and peripheral T2 hyperintensity, findings characteristic of neurofibromas. (E) Axial postprocessed, postcontrast ultrafast three-dimensional gradient echo fat-saturated T1-weighted image reveals very limited enhancement and the absence of cystic or necrotic change, as is typical of a benign neurofibroma.

should be considered. Schwannomas are encapsulated and are typically centrally T2-hyperintense, whether or not they are cystic. Schwannomas moderately enhance (Fig. 34.33).

Paragangliomas differ from other neurogenic tumors in appearance because of their marked T2 hyperintensity and vivid enhancement, with or without the classically described salt-and-pepper appearance, as discussed earlier.

Ganglioneuromas are indolent benign tumors of intermediate T1 and T2 signal on MRI. They may exhibit a whorled appearance on T1- and T2-weighted images because of low-signal curvilinear bands in the tumor (Fig. 34.34). By contrast, ganglioneuroblastomas and neuroblastomas may exhibit a homogeneous or heterogeneous signal and enhancement, may contain hemorrhage, may metastasize, and typically present in younger adults and the pediatric population.

Pitfalls and Remedies

Some common pitfalls of mediastinal lesion interpretation and their remedies are listed in Table 34.4.

Appropriate Diagnostic Imaging Examination Selection

Selection of the appropriate diagnostic imaging test should be tailored to the nature of the mass and the individual patient. When a mediastinal mass is found on CXR, cross-sectional imaging is usually the next step unless there is a suggestion of achalasia or concern of esophageal perforation, in which case contrast esophagography may be preferred. The decision whether to proceed to chest CT or directly to mediastinal MRI on the suggestion of a mediastinal mass on CXR, should be based on patient age,

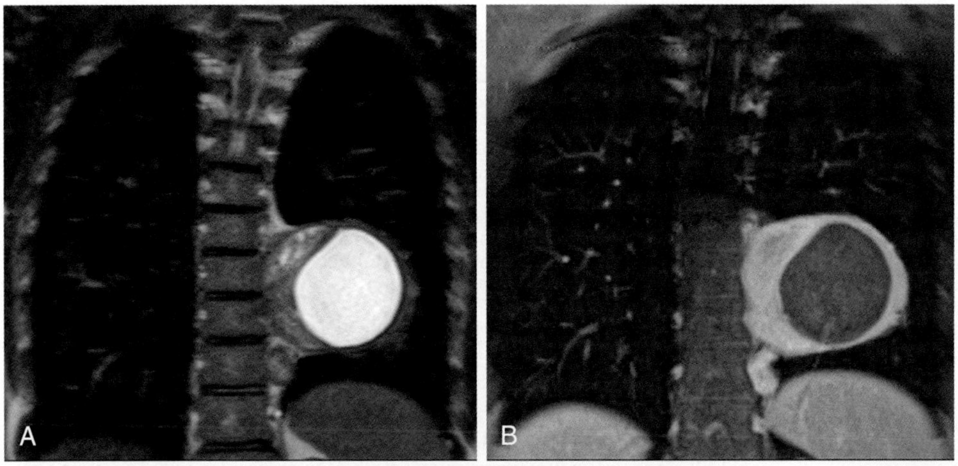

Figure 34.33 Tandem left paraspinal schwannomas, one cystic, the other solid, in a 36-year-old man with a paternal history of neurofibromatosis type 1. (A) Coronal single-shot fast spin-echo T2-weighted image and coronal postcontrast ultrafast three-dimensional gradient echo fat-saturated T1-weighted image (B) revealing both lesions to exhibit peripheral T2 hypointensity, central T2 hyperintensity, and substantial enhancement, in contradistinction to neurofibromas.

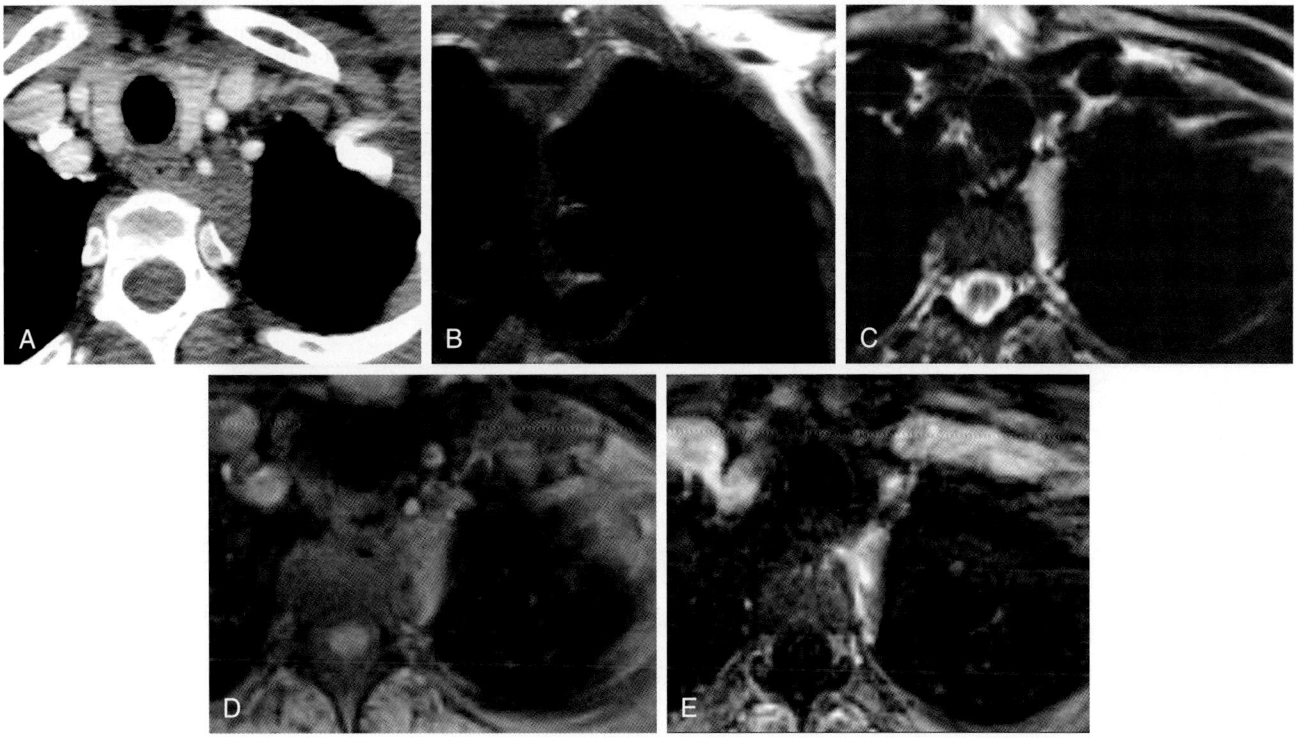

Figure 34.34 Left posterior mediastinal ganglioneuroma in a 55-year-old woman, presenting as an incidental finding on chest CT performed for cough and recent pneumonia. (A) Axial chest CT scan revealing a homogeneous attenuation, 38 HU, plaquelike, somewhat infiltrative-appearing soft tissue mass along the medial left lung apex and left paravertebral space, with a differential diagnosis of infiltrative lymphoma and plaquelike, possibly invasive lung cancer, in addition to a neurogenic tumor. (B) Coronal T2-weighted image reveals an increased T2 signal lesion clearly embedded in the left apical extrapleural or posterior mediastinal fat and much more well circumscribed than implicated on CT. (C) Axial, more heavily T2-weighted image. (D and E) Pre- and postprocessed, subtracted ultrafast three-dimensional gradient echo fat-saturated T1-weighted images revealing intermediate T1 signal precontrast and whorled, heterogeneous enhancement postcontrast. The oft-described whorled appearance of ganglioneuromas on T1- and T2-weighted precontrast images is not present in this case.

concerns about radiation exposure, and whether the mass is deemed solitary and unrelated to any primary malignancy.

Although it is not currently routine practice to proceed directly to MRI, most suspected solitary, incidentally discovered, mediastinal masses can be evaluated more thoroughly and definitively by MRI. Particularly in younger, otherwise healthy adults, for whom the suspicion for metastatic disease, fine and micronodular lung parenchymal abnormalities, and primary lung cancer is low, it is reasonable to proceed directly from CXR to MRI, bypassing CT.

A summary of each modality's strengths and weaknesses is provided next.

Summary of Strengths and Weaknesses of Each Imaging Modality

Table 34.5 summarizes the strengths and weaknesses of each imaging modality discussed with regard to problem solving in the mediastinum. These strengths

TABLE 34.4 Common Pitfalls and Remedies in Imaging Interpretation of Mediastinal Lesions

PITFALL	REMEDY
Misinterpretation of cystic mediastinal lesions as solid on CT	Mediastinal MRI is helpful when an indeterminate, well-defined, homogenous attenuation, round, ovoid, or saccular mediastinal lesion measuring up to 100 HU is found on CT and, additionally, when discernment of fluid from solid components of a mass is needed to optimize the diagnostic yield of a minimally invasive biopsy.
Misinterpretation of ^{18}FDG-PET–avid normal thymus or thymic hyperplasia as lymphoma, recurrent lymphoma after treatment, or a thymic neoplasm	Refer to appearance of thymic tissue on concurrent CT, if available; if indeterminate or unavailable, MRI should be used to distinguish between these entities.
Misinterpretation of normal thymus in young women as thymic hyperplasia or tumor	Recognize that a normal thymus in young women may exhibit a fuller, more quadrilateral shape, higher soft tissue attenuation on CT, and occasionally lack of signal suppression on opposed-phase chemical shift MRI.
Misuse of chemical shift ratio assessment on cystic lesions, leading to misinterpretation of these lesions as thymic tumors	Avoid the use of a chemical shift ratio when evaluating the cystic component of mediastinal lesions. Fluid in cysts should not suppress on opposed-phase MRI scans unless it contains microscopic or intravoxel fat, with the latter pathognomonic for a dermoid cyst or teratoma.
Failure to understand the difference between macroscopic and microscopic fat suppression on MRI	Gross fat is T1/T2-hyperintense on T1- and T2-weighted fast spin-echo MRI scans and saturates or drops in signal on fat-saturated images. Microscopic or intravoxel fat (admixed with soft tissue or fluid) suppresses or drops in signal on opposed-phase gradient echo chemical shift MRI.
Misinterpretation of chronic thromboembolic pulmonary disease as pulmonary artery sarcoma or large-vessel vasculitis (or the converse) on CT	Focused thin section (3–4 mm) cardiac-gated MRI with dynamic contrast enhancement and postprocessed subtraction can help distinguish between these entities.
Misinterpretation of a small paraganglioma as a lymph node on CT	MRI signal characteristics and dynamic contrast enhancement pattern can help distinguish these entities.

TABLE 34.5 Strengths and Weaknesses of Imaging Modalities[a]

IMAGING MODALITY	STRENGTHS	WEAKNESSES
Chest x-ray	Reasonable initial evaluation in a patient with symptoms or signs referable to a mediastinal mass Preliminary placement of a lesion within one of the three mediastinal compartments, slightly narrowing the differential diagnosis	Poor soft tissue contrast, near-complete lack of diagnostic specificity Radiation exposure
Contrast esophagography	Confirmation of esophageal mucosal or luminal involvement, fistula, tract, or perforation Secondary inference of mediastinal mass location	No tissue characterization May not demonstrate submucosal or intramural lesions Radiation exposure
Chest CT	Better mediastinal mass compartmentalization and tissue characterization than chest radiography	Inferior tissue characterization to MRI, with exception of calcification detection Radiation exposure
^{18}FDG-PET	The only listed imaging modality depicting metabolic activity of a lesion Can be positive in normal and benign disease (e.g., normal and hyperplastic thymus) Can be negative in malignant disease (e.g., indolent tumors)	Limited tissue characterization beyond metabolic activity, unless accompanied by diagnostic CT Labor- and time-intensive Most radiation exposure of all listed imaging modalities Most expensive of all listed imaging modalities
MRI	Superior soft tissue contrast resulting in superior mediastinal mass compartmentalization and tissue characterization than CT, with the exception of calcification detection May offer better surgical guidance than CT with respect to lesion compartment placement, lesion characteristics, and bronchovascular, neurovascular, and chest wall invasion or involvement Lower rate of contrast allergy to gadolinium than iodinated contrast Offers a means of serial follow-up of indeterminate and probably benign lesions without radiation exposure, often without IV contrast, in young and pregnant patients and others No radiation	Generally much longer scan time than CT, although shorter than PET-CT Slightly more expensive than CT

[a]With regard to problem solving in the mediastinum.
From Ackman JB. High rate of unnecessary thymectomy and its cause. Can computed tomography distinguish thymoma, lymphoma, thymic hyperplasia, and thymic cysts? *Eur J Radiol.* 2015;84:524–533.

and weaknesses must be weighed against the effect of radiation exposure and cost over a given patient's care cycle, rather than the cost of the individual test. For example, if MR performance has averted unnecessary surgery, it has yielded great cost savings.

■ Conclusion

Specific characterization of a mediastinal lesion requires placement of the lesion within one of the three mediastinal compartments, tissue characterization, and subsequent gauging of what lesion is most apt to be, both statistically and contextually. Virtual biopsy with diagnostic imaging is the goal. When a lesion is indeterminate on CT, performance of MRI may add diagnostic specificity. Awareness of the capabilities, strengths, and weaknesses of currently used radiologic imaging modalities is critical to improve the diagnostic specificity when characterizing mediastinal lesions and may secondarily reduce unnecessary surgery and health care costs.

Bibliography

Abdel Razek AA, Khairy M, Nada N. Diffusion-weighted MR imaging in thymic epithelial tumors: correlation with World Health Organization classification and clinical staging. *Radiology*. 2014;268–275.

Ackman JB. A practical guide to nonvascular thoracic magnetic resonance imaging. *J Thorac Imaging*. 2014;29(1):17–29.

Ackman JB. MR imaging of mediastinal masses. *Magn Reson Imaging Clin North Am*. 2015;23(2):141–164.

Ackman JB, Calkins JC, Risacher S, Shepard JA. A 4-year retrospective review of our experience developing a successful non-vascular thoracic MR practice. *J Thorac Imaging*. 2013.

Ackman JB, Mino-Kenudson M, Morse CR. Nonsuppressing normal thymus on chemical shift magnetic resonance imaging in a young woman. *J Thorac Imaging*. 2012;27(6):W196–W198.

Ackman JB, Verzosa S, Kovach AE, et al. High rate of unnecessary thymectomy and its cause. Can computed tomography distinguish thymoma, lymphoma, thymic hyperplasia, and thymic cysts? *Eur J Radiol*. 2015;84(3):524–533.

Ackman JB, Wu CC, Halpern EF, et al. Nonvascular thoracic magnetic resonance imaging: the current state of training, utilization, and perceived value: survey of the Society of Thoracic Radiology membership. *J Thorac Imaging*. 2014;29(4):252–257.

Agarwal PP, Seely JM, Matzinger FR. Wandering pleuropericardial cyst. *J Comput Assist Tomogr*. 2006;30(2):276–278.

Balcombe J, Torigian DA, Kim W, Miller WT Jr. Cross-sectional imaging of paragangliomas of the aortic body and other thoracic branchiomeric paraganglia. *AJR Am J Roentgenol*. 2007;188(4):1054–1058.

Baron RL, Lee JK, Sagel SS, Peterson RR. Computed tomography of the normal thymus. *Radiology*. 1982;142(1):121–125.

Brix G, Lechel U, Glatting G, et al. Radiation exposure of patients undergoing whole-body dual-modality 18f-FDG PET/CT examinations. *J Nucl Med*. 2005;46(4):608–613.

Carter BW, Tomiyama N, Bhora FY, et al. A modern definition of mediastinal compartments. *J Thorac Oncol*. 2014;9(9):S97–S101.

Charruau L, Parrens M, Jougon J, et al. Mediastinal lymphangioma in adults: CT and MR imaging features. *Eur Radiol*. 2000;10(8):1310–1314.

Choe YH, Han BK, Koh EM, et al. Takayasu's arteritis: assessment of disease activity with contrast-enhanced MR imaging. *AJR Am J Roentgenol*. 2000;175(2):505–511.

Chung JH, Cox CW, Forssen AV, et al. The dark lymph node sign on magnetic resonance imaging: a novel finding in patients with sarcoidosis. *J Thorac Imaging*. 2014;29(2):125–129.

Chung MH, Lee HG, Kwon SS, Park SH. MR imaging of solitary pulmonary lesion: emphasis on tuberculomas and comparison with tumors. *J Magn Reson Imaging*. 2000;11(6):629–637.

Coursey CA, Nelson RC, Boll DT, et al. Dual-energy multidetector CT: how does it work, what can it tell us, and when can we use it in abdominopelvic imaging? *Radiographics*. 2010;30(4):1037–1055.

Diaz A, Black E, Dunning J. Is thymectomy in non-thymomatous myasthenia gravis of any benefit? *Interact Cardiovasc Thorac Surg*. 2014;18(3):381–389.

Gawande RS, Khurana A, Messing S, et al. Differentiation of normal thymus from anterior mediastinal lymphoma and lymphoma recurrence at pediatric PET/CT. *Radiology*. 2012;262(2):613–622.

Hahn HP, Fletcher CD. Primary mediastinal liposarcoma: clinicopathologic analysis of 24 cases. *Am J Surg Pathol*. 2007;31(12):1868–1874.

Jerushalmi J, Frenkel A, Bar-Shalom R, et al. Physiologic thymic uptake of 18F-FDG in children and young adults: a PET/CT evaluation of incidence, patterns, and relationship to treatment. *J Nucl Med*. 2009;50(6):849–853.

Jeung MY, Gasser B, Gangi A, et al. Imaging of cystic masses of the mediastinum. *Radiographics*. 2002;22 Spec No:S79–S93.

Johnson TR. Dual-energy CT: general principles. *AJR Am J Roentgenol*. 2012;199(5 suppl):S3–S8.

Kent MS, Wang T, Gangadharan SP, Whyte RI. What is the prevalence of a "nontherapeutic" thymectomy? *Ann Thorac Surg*. 2014;97(1):276–282.

McNeeley MF, Chung JH, Bhalla S, Godwin JD. Imaging of granulomatous fibrosing mediastinitis. *AJR Am J Roentgenol*. 2012;199(2):319–327.

Munden RF, Nesbitt JC, Kemp BL, et al. Primary liposarcoma of the mediastinum. *AJR Am J Roentgenol*. 2000;175(5):1340.

Nakazono T, White CS, Yamasaki F, et al. MRI findings of mediastinal neurogenic tumors. *AJR Am J Roentgenol*. 2011;197(4):W643–W652.

Olsen WL, Dillon WP, Kelly WM, et al. MR imaging of paragangliomas. *AJR Am J Roentgenol*. 1987;148(1):201–204.

Priola A, Priola S, Ciccone G, et al. Differentiation of rebound and lymphoid thymic hyperplasia from anterior mediastinal tumors with dual-echo chemical-shift MR imaging in adulthood reliability of the chemical-shift ratio and signal intensity index. *Radiology*. 2015;274(1):238–249.

Rosado-de-Christenson ML, Pugatch RD, Moran CA, Galobardes J. Thymolipoma: analysis of 27 cases. *Radiology*. 1994;193(1):121–126.

Sakai S, Murayama S, Murakami J, et al. Bronchogenic carcinoma invasion of the chest wall: evaluation with dynamic cine MRI during breathing. *J Comput Assist Tomogr*. 1997;21(4):595–600.

Sakai S, Murayama S, Soeda H, et al. Differential diagnosis between thymoma and non-thymoma by dynamic MR imaging. *Acta Radiol*. 2002;43(3):262–268.

Seo JS, Kim YJ, Choi BW, Choe KO. Usefulness of magnetic resonance imaging for evaluation of cardiovascular invasion: evaluation of sliding motion between thoracic mass and adjacent structures on cine MR images. *J Magn Reson Imaging*. 2005;22(2):234–241.

Singla S, Litzky LA, Kaiser LR, Shrager JB. Should asymptomatic enlarged thymus glands be resected? *J Thorac Cardiovasc Surg*. 2010;140(5):977–983.

Sugita R, Morimoto K, Yuda F. Intrapleural bronchogenic cyst. *Eur J Radiol*. 1999;32(3):204–207.

Tanaka O, Kiryu T, Hirose Y, et al. Neurogenic tumors of the mediastinum and chest wall: MR imaging appearance. *J Thorac Imaging*. 2005;20:316–320.

Vinee P, Stover B, Sigmund G, et al. MR imaging of the pericardial cyst. *J Magn Reson Imaging*. 1992;2(5):593–596.

Yi CA, Lee KS, Choe YH, et al. Computed tomography in pulmonary artery sarcoma: distinguishing features from pulmonary embolic disease. *J Comput Assist Tomogr*. 2004;28(1):34–39.

CHAPTER 35

The Pleura

Matthew P. Moy, Gerald F. Abbott, and Subba R. Digumarthy

CHAPTER OUTLINE

Pleural Anatomy

The pleura is a stroma supported by the mesothelial lining of the thoracic cavity. It is composed of two layers: an inner visceral pleura and an outer parietal pleura. The visceral pleura lines the lungs and their fissures. The visceral pleura is supplied by pulmonary arterioles, with drainage via the pulmonary veins. The parietal pleura lines the chest wall, diaphragm, and mediastinum. The parietal pleura is supplied by the systemic circulation and drains via the azygos, hemiazygos, and internal mammary veins.

Pleural Space and Its Normal Contents

The pleural space is the potential space between the visceral and parietal pleura. The right and left pleural spaces do not communicate. Although the pleura is permeable to gas and liquid, there is no gas within the pleural space under normal conditions. In contrast, the pleural space contains approximately 5 mL of physiologic pleural fluid, which acts as a lubricant. Pleural fluid is produced at a rate of up to 100 mL of fluid/h, and the pleural space can absorb fluid at a rate of approximately 300 mL/h. Lymphatic drainage of the pleural space, which allows for clearance of cells, protein, and other particulate matter, occurs through the stoma in the parietal pleura, which leads to lymphatic vessels in the chest wall and ultimately the thoracic duct. The lymphatic drainage of the visceral pleura occurs via the lymphatics in the pulmonary interstitium and drains into hilar nodes.

Imaging the Pleura: Indications and Advantages of Different Modalities

Evaluation of Pleura

The pleura and pleural space can be directly visualized and, if required, sampled by video-assisted thoracic surgery or open surgery. These procedures are invasive and can lead to complications. Imaging allows noninvasive evaluation of the pleura and is useful for diagnosis, procedural planning, and, if required, image-guided intervention.

Indications for Plain Radiography

Plain radiography is useful as a low-cost screening evaluation of the pleura and pleural space and can detect some different pathologies, including pneumothorax, effusion, and pleural masses, although characterization of abnormality is limited due to poor contrast resolution. The margins of the pleura are delineated by the interface of air in the lungs and soft tissue density along the chest wall, mediastinum, and diaphragm. Pleural abnormalities can be suspected when this interface is obscured or when abnormal soft tissue contours are seen along the chest wall or mediastinum. For example, dependent pleural fluid collects in characteristic locations on upright (costophrenic angles) and decubitus radiography, although loculated fluid may have a fixed masslike shape (Fig. 35.1). Plain radiography is also useful in following known pleural pathology, such as monitoring pleural effusion or pneumothorax size.

Indications for Ultrasound

Ultrasound differentiates between fluid and solid tissue and can be used as a troubleshooting tool in the further evaluation of radiographic abnormalities. Sonography is particularly suited for the evaluation of pleural effusion and image-guided thoracentesis. Effusions appear as anechoic collections, which are easily distinguished from the echogenic ribs and dirty shadowing from the air-containing lungs. Echogenic septations may be seen on ultrasound, which are not evident on other imaging modalities (Fig. 35.2). In patients who have failed blind thoracentesis, sonography is useful for localizing loculated collections of fluid. Ultrasound guidance reduces the risk of complication from thoracentesis. Also, ultrasound can be performed at the bedside, allowing assessment of critically ill patients who may not be stable enough to travel to the radiology department.

Indications for Computed Tomography

CT provides superior spatial resolution and excellent contrast resolution in the evaluation of thoracic structures, including the pleura, particularly when IV contrast is administered. The major strengths of CT include not only the detection of an abnormality, but also compositional analysis and precise localization (pleural, extrapleural, or parenchymal). CT is the most sensitive modality for the detection of pleural effusion and pneumothorax and is also sensitive for the detection of pleural masses, pleural thickening, and calcification. In contrast to plain radiography, CT allows cross-sectional evaluation of the entire pleural space, as well as adjacent thoracic structures. Multiplanar reconstruction can be achieved with a single sequence of image acquisition. IV contrast can help differentiate solid from cystic lesions and an empyema from a lung abscess. CT is the modality of choice in the routine evaluation of pleural masses, pleural malignancy, degree and extent of pleural thickening, and asbestos-related pleural disease.

Indications for Magnetic Resonance Imaging

The role of routine MRI of the pleura is limited. Although MRI has superior soft tissue contrast in comparison with CT, the spatial resolution, acquisition time, and cost of MRI prohibits its routine use in the evaluation of pleural disease. MRI is a useful adjunct to CT in the evaluation

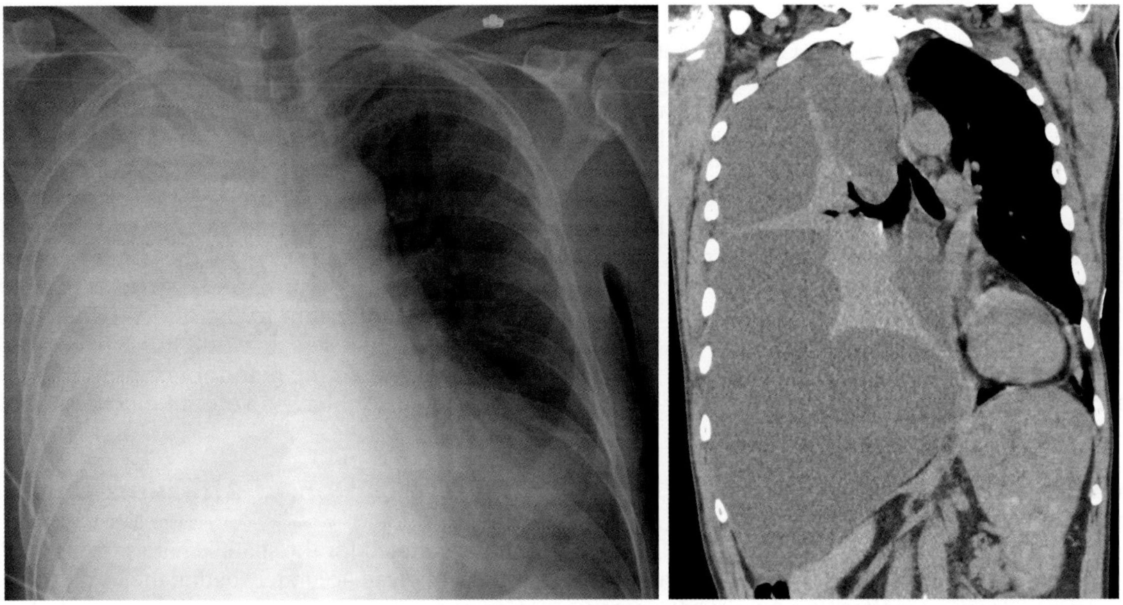

Figure 35.1 Loculated pleural effusion. This composite image of a posteroanterior chest radiograph *(left)* and coronal chest CT scan *(right)* shows a large, loculated right pleural effusion that opacifies the entire hemothorax on the radiograph. CT reveals the large effusion, with multiple areas of loculation, and compressive (relaxation) atelectasis of the entire right lung. The large effusion has displaced the right hemidiaphragm inferiorly and flattened its contour.

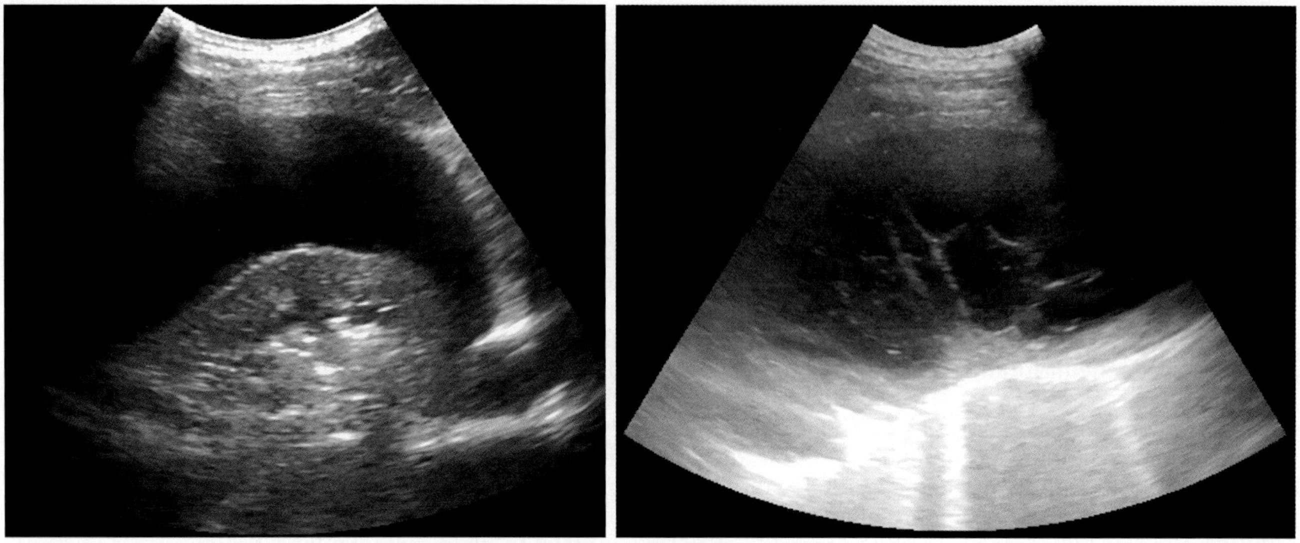

Figure 35.2 Ultrasound of pleural effusion. This composite image of ultrasound findings in two patients, one with a purely anechoic fluid collection *(left)*, and the other with multiple septations *(right)*, indicates loculations within the pleural effusion. Septations may be detected in noninfected parapneumonic pleural effusions or within infected fluid collections (e.g., empyema). If a bronchopleural fistula develops, air may form multiple air-fluid levels separated by septations within the infected pleural fluid collection.

of pleural masses and malignancy because it is more accurate and sensitive than other modalities in the detection of the chest wall, mediastinal, and diaphragmatic invasion. Lung and pleural pathology in the apices are often better visualized on MRI than on CT. Some studies have suggested that MRI can also be helpful in elucidating the cause of pleural effusion. However, the MRI signal characteristics are usually nonspecific.

Indications for Positron Emission Tomography

Positron emission tomography (PET) with fluorodeoxyglucose (FDG) can be a useful problem-solving tool in the evaluation of certain pleural diseases, especially in combination with diagnostic quality CT. PET-CT is more accurate than CT, MRI, or PET alone for the staging of malignancy (including malignant mesothelioma), is superior in the detection of intrathoracic and extrathoracic lymphadenopathy, and can be used to assess response to treatment. It can also be used to differentiate malignant mesothelioma and pleural metastasis from most benign pleural diseases. Malignancy usually demonstrates higher FDG avidity, although infection or talc pleurodesis can also be intensely hypermetabolic.

■ Pleural Effusion

Importance of the Size of Pleural Effusion

Although size does not necessarily correlate with the patient's symptoms, it does affect the perceived severity of disease, and larger pleural effusions are more likely to be symptomatic. Effusion size is also a predictor of ease of thoracentesis and can help assess the need for image guidance. Small pleural effusion size (measuring <1 cm on a lateral decubitus radiograph, which corresponds to an approximate volume <300 mL) is a relative contraindication to thoracentesis. However, the percutaneous sampling of small effusions can provide essential diagnostic information. If a small effusion is identified, performing thoracentesis with image guidance can increase the success of sampling and minimize complications.

Pleural effusion volume can be estimated by plain radiography and CT. The minimum fluid volume that can be detected on a lateral decubitus radiograph is approximately 10 mL, and therefore any visible pleural effusion must measure at least 10 mL in volume. On the lateral projection, blunting of the posterior costophrenic angle occurs with an effusion volume of at least 50 mL. On the posteroanterior (PA) view, at least 200 mL of fluid is needed to obscure the lateral costophrenic angle, and at least 500 mL is required to obscure the normal diaphragmatic contour. On CT, effusion volume can be estimated on the axial image superior to the hemidiaphragm in which the effusion appears largest. Effusions occupying less than 25% of the anteroposterior (AP) dimension of the hemithorax, or measuring less than 3 cm in AP dimension in the midclavicular line, correspond to a volume less than 300 mL. Effusions occupying more than 50% of the hemithorax, or more than 10 cm in AP dimension, have a volume more than 1000 mL.

Characterization of Effusions on CT

CT is well suited for the spatial characterization of pleural effusion and can accurately define the location and extent of pleural effusions. Free-flowing pleural fluid layers dependently and often has a crescentic shape in the axial plane. Loculated effusions, in contrast, have a lenticular shape and can displace adjacent lung parenchyma. In challenging cases, additional imaging in the prone or

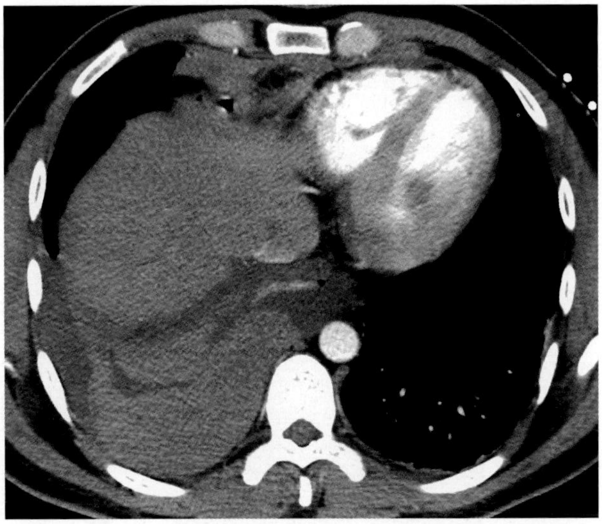

Figure 35.3 Acute hemothorax. This axial contrast-enhanced CT shows a large area of high attenuation within a right pleural effusion, diagnostic of hemothorax in this patient, who has been receiving warfarin (Coumadin) therapy. The attenuation matches that of the adjacent right hepatic dome and measures within the range of CT attenuation for blood (+35 to +45 HU), as compared to the pleural effusion demonstrated along the medial and lateral aspects of the hemothorax.

decubitus position can help differentiate simple effusions from loculated effusions.

Although some specific types of pleural effusion can be readily diagnosed by CT, in general, the modality is limited in characterizing the cause of pleural fluid. Acute hemothorax is most easily identified by CT and demonstrates high attenuation, usually from 35 to 70 Hounsfield units (HU) (Fig. 35.3). Occasionally, a hematocrit effect (a fluid-fluid layer with higher density in the dependent layer) is seen. As hemothorax evolves, fluid attenuation more closely approximates water and is more difficult to discriminate from other causes of effusion. Chylothorax rarely can present as a low-attenuation effusion (<0 HU) or with a fat-fluid layer. However, its attenuation usually approximates water due to an averaging of fat and protein. CT cannot reliably differentiate exudative and transudative effusions. Although certain features, such as loculation, pleural thickening, and pleural nodularity, are more common in exudative effusions, the findings are nonspecific and cannot replace pleural fluid laboratory analysis.

■ Empyema

Imaging Features of Empyema

Empyema usually presents as a pleural effusion in a febrile patient. The most common imaging appearance of empyema is an uncomplicated pleural effusion. Loculated pleural effusions are less common but are an important sign of increased complexity that should elevate the level of suspicion for infection, particularly in a patient with persistent fever and leukocytosis of unknown origin. On CT, the visceral and parietal pleura surrounding each side of the empyema are visible and uniformly thickened, a finding known as the *split pleura sign*. Both pleural layers typically enhance with the administration of IV contrast.

Effect of Multiloculation on Management

Treatment of empyema includes an extended course of antibiotics and percutaneous drainage of pus. It is important to identify and describe every loculated collection seen because each one will likely require separate drainage. If the patient is reimaged after draining thoracostomy tubes are inserted, careful attention should be paid to any undrained or inadequately drained collections. Occasionally, a single locule can require multiple tubes due to high-viscosity pus or septations that cannot be visualized by CT.

Significance of Air in an Empyema

Spontaneous air in an empyema (or any pleural effusion) indicates the presence of a bronchopleural fistula (Fig. 35.4). A bronchopleural fistula may occur as a complication of infection (particularly tuberculosis), recurrent spontaneous pneumothorax, or chemoradiation for lung cancer. If a bronchopleural fistula is present, adequate drainage of the empyema is essential to ensure adequate healing and prevent back-spillage into the bronchial tree, which can result in diffuse pneumonitis. Occasionally, tube thoracostomy is insufficient, and surgical drainage or repair is required. Bronchopleural fistula may also occur as a postoperative complication following pneumonectomy when an air leak at the bronchial stump communicates with the pleural space.

■ Pneumothorax

Signs of Tension Pneumothorax

Tension pneumothorax refers to an increasing accumulation of air within the pleural space (usually increasing with inspiration, without egress of air from the pleural space on expiration) causing contralateral mediastinal displacement and, ultimately, leading to respiratory failure from compression of the ipsilateral and contralateral lungs and diminished return of blood to the right heart. It is primarily a clinical diagnosis, but there are several radiographic findings associated with tension pneumothorax that should prompt urgent communication with the referring provider. Any mass effect on the mediastinum, such as a contralateral mediastinal shift or tracheal deviation, should raise suspicion for tension pneumothorax (Fig. 35.5). However, in patients maintained on positive-pressure ventilation, mediastinal shift may not be evident, even if tension pneumothorax is present. Inversion of the ipsilateral hemidiaphragm or a widened ipsilateral intercostal space are also concerning signs of increasing intrathoracic pressure and tension. The degree

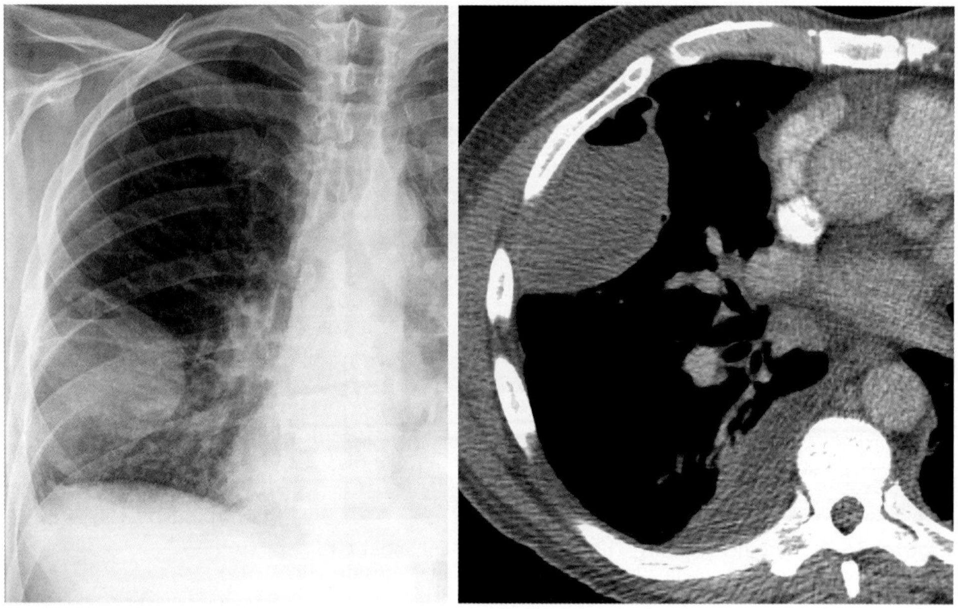

Figure 35.4 Empyema with bronchopleural fistula. This composite image of a posteroanterior (PA) chest radiograph *(left)* and contrast-enhanced axial chest CT scan *(right)* shows a loculated pleural fluid collection with an air-fluid level in the lateral aspect of the right hemithorax and a second collection along the paraspinal region. Air within a loculated pleural effusion is usually due to a bronchopleural fistula. On the PA radiograph, the loculated fluid collection manifests with incomplete borders, a radiographic sign of an extrapulmonary lesion, typically of pleural or chest wall origin.

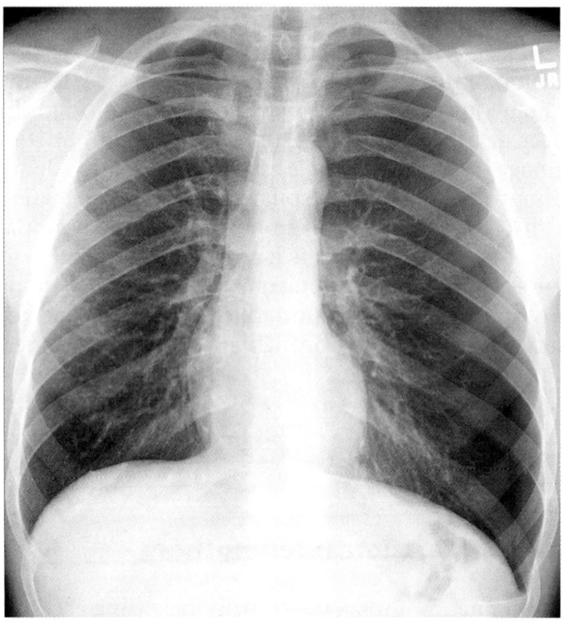

Figure 35.5 Tension pneumothorax. This posteroanterior chest radiograph shows abnormal lucency on the outer aspect of the left hemithorax and a sharp pleural line along the edge of the collapsing left lung. There is a shift of the heart to the contralateral side, inferior displacement of the left hemidiaphragm, and abnormal lucency within the left lateral costophrenic sulcus (called the *deep sulcus sign*).

of ipsilateral lung collapse is not a reliable sign of tension because underlying lung disease or pleural scarring can prevent collapse of some areas of the lung.

Importance of Apical Emphysema or Apical Bullae

Prominent apical emphysema or apical bullae predispose a patient to spontaneous pneumothorax, which can be recurrent. These patients often benefit from bullectomy (in combination with pleurodesis), so identification of these dilated air spaces can help guide management and prevent future pneumothoraces. Also, the identification of concurrent contralateral bullae will affect surgical planning because both sides may be targeted for surgical treatment. Apical bullae are usually well visualized in the coronal plane on CT. Placement of a thoracostomy tube into an apical bulla can cause a bronchopleural fistula and should be avoided.

■ Lipoma and Liposarcoma

Imaging Features Concerning for Liposarcoma

Lipomas are the most common benign tumor of the chest wall and diaphragm and typically present as incidental findings in asymptomatic patients. Most lipomas are composed almost entirely of fat, have a thin capsule, and may have thin internal fibrous bands. Any thickened bands of soft tissue attenuation, nodular soft tissue, or large soft tissue components within a fatty mass are suspicious for liposarcoma, a relatively rare malignant tumor of fat. These findings are best assessed by CT, and the soft tissue components often enhance with IV contrast. Large fat-containing lesions must also raise suspicion of malignancy, although lipomas can also grow to a large size over time.

Usefulness of MRI

MRI can characterize soft tissue accurately and will demonstrate similar findings to those seen on CT. Fat components are easily differentiated from soft tissue components. Fat demonstrates T1 and T2 hyperintensity, with loss of signal on fat saturation sequences. Soft tissue has variable T1 and T2 signals but will enhance with gadolinium contrast. MRI can also be used to define the extent of involvement for surgical planning. If CT findings are indeterminate, MRI is useful for identifying other masses, such as intramuscular neurofibromas, and for evaluating the extent of neurogenic tumors.

Asbestos-Related Pleural Disease

Types of Benign Asbestos-Related Pleural Disease

Although prior asbestos exposure is concerning due to significantly increased risks of interstitial lung disease, lung cancer, and malignant mesothelioma, benign asbestos-related pleural disease is far more common. The four types of benign disease are noncalcified pleural plaques, calcified pleural plaques, benign asbestos pleural effusion, and diffuse pleural fibrosis.

Pleural plaques are the most common of the benign entities and develop approximately 20 to 30 years after the initial asbestos exposure. The plaques are composed of fibrohyaline tissue and form within the parietal pleura, manifesting with characteristic radiographic and CT findings (Fig. 35.6). On radiography, pleural plaques manifest as discontinuous areas of pleural thickening that may be calcified or noncalcified, with incomplete borders, and characteristically distributed along the costal, diaphragmatic, and paravertebral pleural surfaces. They typically spare the pleural surfaces in the lung apices and costophrenic sulci.

Noncalcified pleural plaques are often visible on plain radiography and may display incomplete borders. Radiographic visibility is increased when the plaques calcify, a finding that occurs in approximately 50% of cases. The calcification pattern can be nodular, sheetlike, amorphous, and ill-defined. The lateral radiograph is especially useful for identifying plaques along the diaphragmatic pleura. CT is much more sensitive than plain radiography in the detection of noncalcified and calcified plaques.

Benign asbestos pleural effusion is a dose-related reaction to asbestos exposure and occurs earlier than other asbestos-related manifestations, often within 10 years, but occasionally as early as 1 year after exposure. Effusions are typically unilateral and exudative on fluid analysis, and they can be hemorrhagic. The detection of an effusion, in combination with a history of asbestos exposure and exclusion of other causes of effusion (particularly malignancy), confirms the diagnosis.

Diffuse pleural fibrosis is believed to occur after a previous asbestos-related pleural effusion or pleurisy. Diffuse smooth pleural thickening is seen without nodularity, and the costophrenic angles are typically obliterated on plain radiography (Fig. 35.7). Pleural plaques, in contrast, usually do not obliterate the costophrenic angles. Fibrosis also involves the visceral pleura and underlying lung parenchyma, and subpleural fibrous bands are often visible on CT.

Holly Leaf Pattern of Pleural Calcification

Calcified asbestos-related pleural plaques, when visualized en face on the PA radiograph, appear denser along their lateral borders and demonstrate a serpentine calcified edge, which has been likened to the shape of a holly leaf (see Fig. 35.6). This occurs when the plaques are located on the anterior or posterior pleura, and the pattern of calcification is characteristic of asbestos-related plaques.

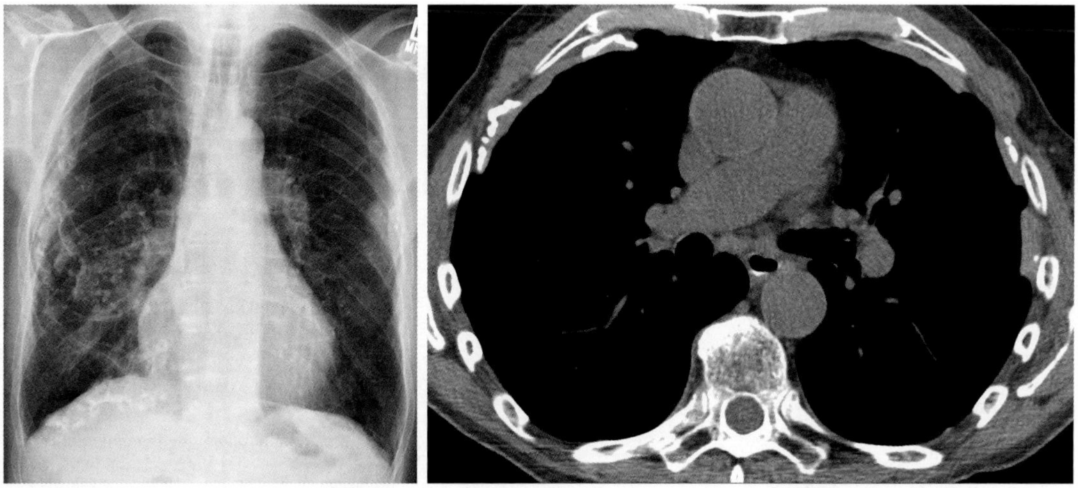

Figure 35.6 Pleural plaques. This composite image of a posteroanterior chest radiograph *(left)* and CT scan *(right)* shows the characteristic appearances of asbestos-related pleural plaques. On radiography, pleural plaques manifest as discontinuous areas of pleural thickening that may be calcified or noncalcified, with incomplete borders and characteristically distributed along the costal, diaphragmatic, and paravertebral pleural surfaces. CT better delineates the calcified and noncalcified pleural plaques and their typical distribution adjacent to ribs; lower sections showed similar plaques along the diaphragmatic and lower right paravertebral pleural surfaces.

Mesothelioma

Imaging Features Concerning for Malignant Mesothelioma

Mesothelioma is the most common primary malignant neoplasm of the pleura, with approximately 2500 new cases annually in the United States, and is the second most common malignancy of the pleura, after metastasis. It arises from mesothelial cells of the pleura, usually of the parietal rather than the visceral layer. Prior asbestos exposure is the strongest predisposing risk factor and is dose-related. There are several findings on plain radiography and CT that should raise suspicion of pleural malignancy, whether primary (e.g., mesothelioma) or metastatic:

- Pleural thickening >1 cm in thickness, pleural nodularity, circumferential growth pattern within the involved hemithorax, and involvement of the mediastinal pleura (which is typically spared in fibrothorax) may be seen.
- Pleural plaques are demonstrated in approximately 25% of patients with mesothelioma and are considered a marker of their previous asbestos exposure.
- Diffuse pleural thickening can be seen in 60% of patients with malignant mesothelioma.
- Discrete pleural masses are present in about 50% of all cases (Fig. 35.8).
- Ipsilateral hemithoracic volume loss, often in combination with circumferential pleural thickening, may occur secondary to lung encasement by tumor.
- Ipsilateral pleural effusion is a common manifestation of mesothelioma.
- Concurrent mediastinal or thoracic lymphadenopathy occurs, an uncommon finding in benign pleural disease.

MRI and PET-CT are more sensitive than CT alone in the assessment of local invasion (malignant mesothelioma is intensely FDG-avid). PET-CT is also superior to all other modalities in the detection of lymphadenopathy and accuracy of staging.

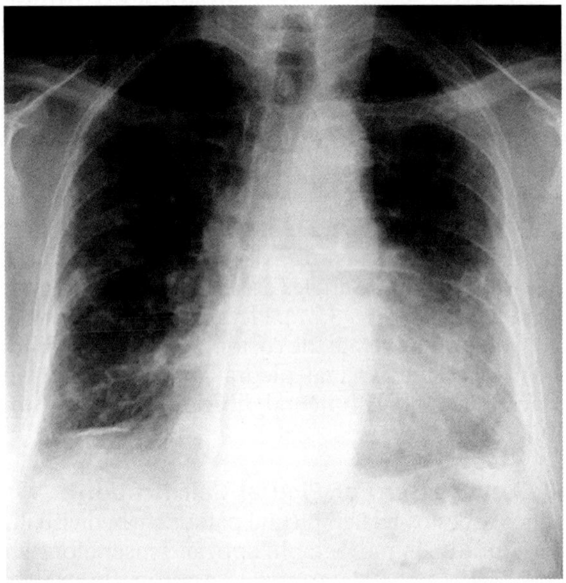

Figure 35.7 Diffuse pleural thickening. This posteroanterior chest radiograph shows bilateral pleural thickening within the lateral costophrenic sulci and coexistent bilateral calcified pleural plaques along the costal, diaphragmatic, and right paravertebral pleural surfaces. Pleural plaques typically spare the pleural surface in the lung apices and costophrenic sulci, whereas diffuse pleural thickening characteristically manifests as unilateral or bilateral involvement of the costophrenic sulci, often a result of asbestos-related pleural effusion.

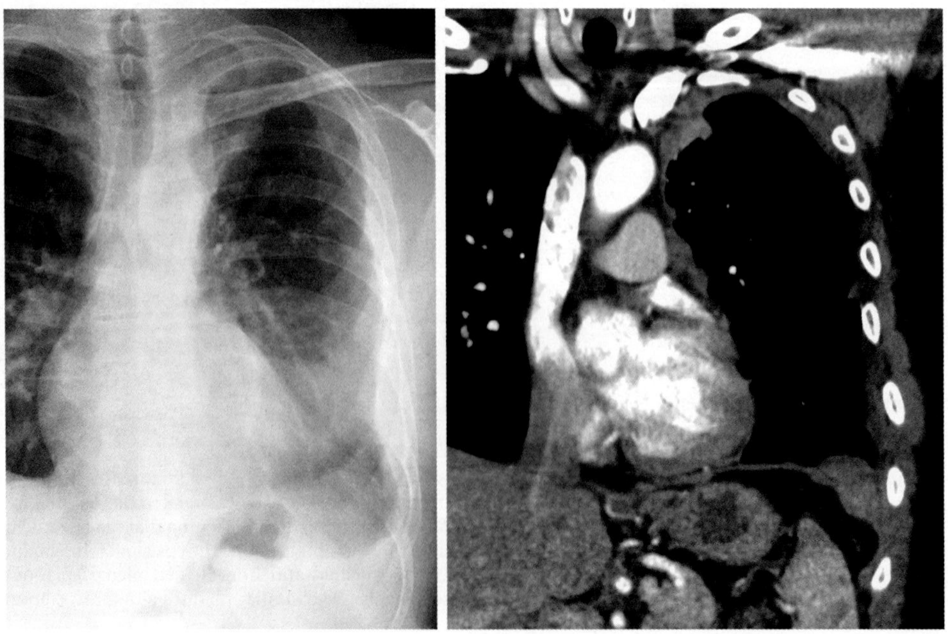

Figure 35.8 Malignant mesothelioma. This composite image of a posteroanterior chest radiograph *(left)* and coronal CT reformation *(right)* shows pleural thickening in the left hemithorax, with CT features suggesting pleural malignancy: (1) pleural thickening >1 cm; (2) nodularity; (3) circumferential growth pattern; and (4) involvement of the mediastinal pleura. These findings occur in primary and secondary pleural malignancies. Pleural plaques are demonstrated in approximately 25% of patients with mesothelioma and are considered to be a marker of their previous asbestos exposure.

Problem-Solving Issues

Imaging Features That Help Distinguish a Subpulmonic Pleural Effusion From Low Lung Volumes

A subpulmonic pleural effusion is an effusion located between the lung base and diaphragm. Radiographically, the interface between the fluid and lung parenchyma can mimic an elevated hemidiaphragm, a finding that has been called a *pseudohemidiaphragm*. Several radiographic features can suggest the presence of a subpulmonic effusion (Fig. 35.9). On a PA chest radiograph, the apex of a right subpulmonic effusion forms a pseudohemidiaphragm that is more laterally positioned than the expected position of a true right hemidiaphragm. On the lateral view, a right subpulmonic effusion may manifest with a flat horizontal interface beneath the lower lobe and an oblique interface anteriorly that conforms to the major fissure at that level, with an abrupt descent to the anterior costophrenic sulcus (called the *Rock of Gibraltar sign*). In the case of a left pleural effusion, the pseudohemidiaphragm is abnormally separated from the gastric bubble. A gastric bubble to diaphragm distance more than 2 cm is suggestive of a subpulmonic effusion.

Imaging Features That Suggest the Presence of a Malignant Pleural Effusion

Although there are no reliable imaging findings that can differentiate exudative and transudative effusions (malignant effusions are usually exudative), there are some features that are more commonly seen in malignant effusions. A very large pleural effusion size, particularly if unilateral, is concerning for malignancy. Pleural nodules and nodular pleural thickening are the most sensitive and specific CT findings of malignant effusion, although smooth pleural thickening may also occur (Fig. 35.10). Contrast-enhanced CT improves visualization of pleural thickening and nodules. Coronal or sagittal reformations are best for evaluation of the diaphragmatic pleura, an area where small nodules are commonly missed. Associated findings of a pulmonary mass, chest wall mass, or mediastinal or extrapleural lymphadenopathy can help support concerns for malignant effusion. MRI is comparable to CT in detecting pleural changes associated with malignancy, but the relatively high cost and long acquisition time of MRI favors CT as the modality of choice for the routine evaluation of malignant pleural involvement. Malignant effusions are associated with increased pleural FDG avidity, and PET can be useful to assess pleural involvement in patients with known malignancy or to exclude malignant effusion. False-positives may occur in the setting of infection or prior talc pleurodesis, which are also hypermetabolic. A suspicion of a malignant effusion will prompt cytologic analysis of the pleural fluid and should be communicated to the referring provider.

Imaging Features That Help Differentiate Empyema From a Lung Abscess

Empyema is centered in the pleural space (peripheral to lung parenchyma) and usually has an elongated or lenticular shape, forms tapered obtuse margins with the

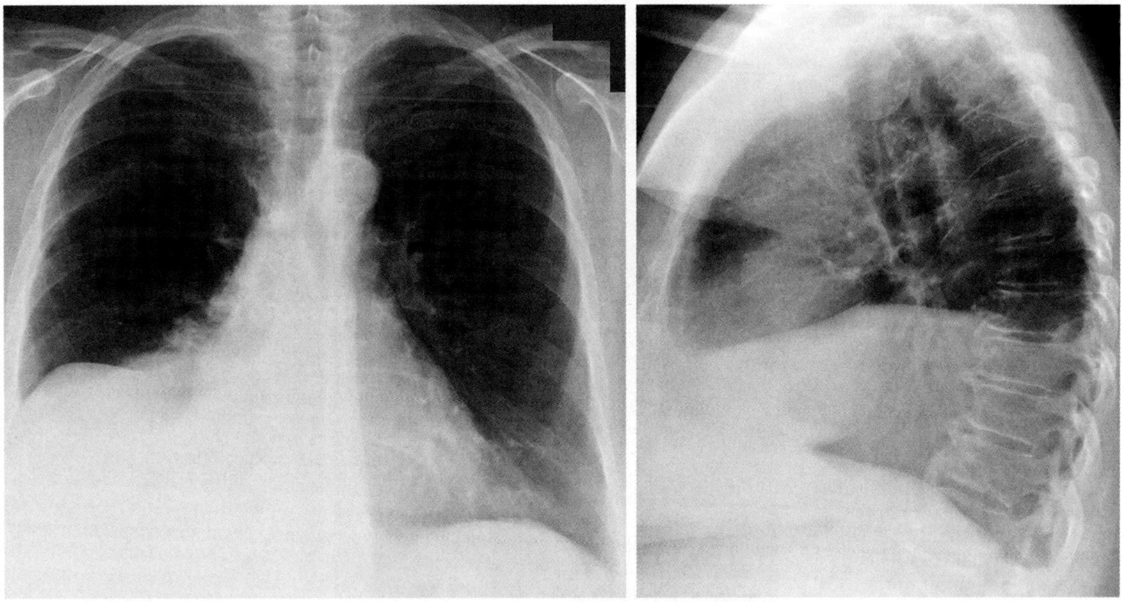

Figure 35.9 Subpulmonic effusion (composite posteroanterior [PA] and lateral radiographs). This PA chest radiograph *(left)* shows the sharp border of a pseudohemidiaphragm with its apex more laterally positioned than the expected position of the apex of a true right hemidiaphragm. The lateral view *(right)* shows a well-defined horizontal interface between the subpulmonic effusion and right lower lobe and an oblique interface anteriorly that conforms to the major fissure at that level. The findings on the lateral radiograph have been likened to the profile of the Rock of Gibraltar.

noninvolved pleura, and displaces the adjacent lung away from the chest wall. If an air-fluid level is present in an empyema, orthogonal radiographic views may show a discrepancy in the length of the air-fluid level as compared between PA and lateral radiographs. By contrast, a lung abscess typically has a round or spherical morphology and, if an air-fluid level is present, its length on orthogonal radiographs should be approximately equal (Fig. 35.11). An abscess will also form more acute margins with the pleura and will not displace the lung parenchyma away from the pleura.

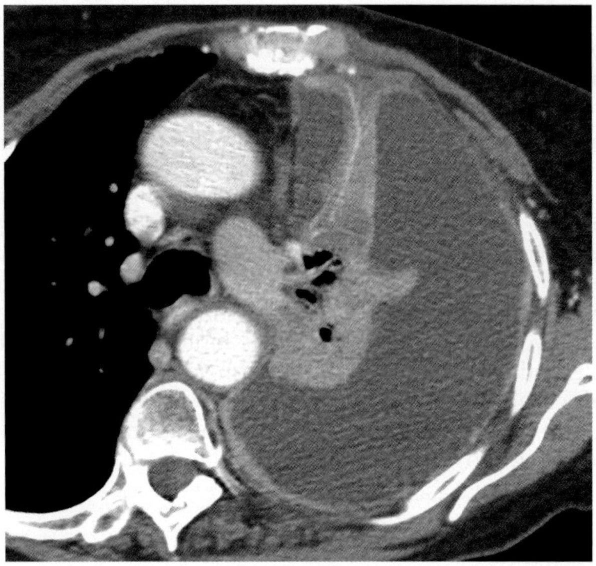

Figure 35.10 Malignant pleural effusion. This contrast-enhanced axial CT scan of a patient with lung cancer shows a very large left pleural effusion, with areas of smooth pleural thickening laterally and along the left paraspinal and mediastinal pleura. A large unilateral pleural effusion should raise the possibility of malignant pleural effusion, a suspicion that is further supported by the detection of associated pleural thickening, which may be smooth and nodular. In this case, a central low-attenuation mass in the hilar aspect of the atelectatic left upper lobe represents a primary lung cancer.

Distinguishing Talc Pleurodesis From Pleural Calcification

Talc is often used as a chemical agent for pleurodesis to treat recurrent pneumothorax and malignant pleural effusion. It can be administered as a slurry through a thoracostomy tube or in a powder form during thoracoscopy. On CT, talc appears radiodense secondary to its magnesium content and can mimic pleural calcification (Fig. 35.12). The CT attenuation of talc is approximately 300 to 350 HU. Talc has a clustered or fine linear appearance and is not visible on plain radiography. In contrast, calcification from asbestos-related pleural disease, prior hemothorax, or prior empyema is usually more extensive and platelike and may be visible on plain radiography.

Imaging Features That Help Differentiate a Skin Fold From Pneumothorax

An overlying skin fold or article of clothing may manifest as a band-line interface on chest radiography that may mimic a pneumothorax, especially if aligned parallel to a pleural surface (Fig. 35.13). Skin folds usually have a black or lucent edge, whereas a pneumothorax has a white or radiodense edge due to the visceral pleural reflection. If the edge continues beyond the ribs, one can confidently call the finding a skin fold. Similarly, if pulmonary vascular markings are seen between the edge and chest wall, the edge is caused by a skin fold rather than a pneumothorax.

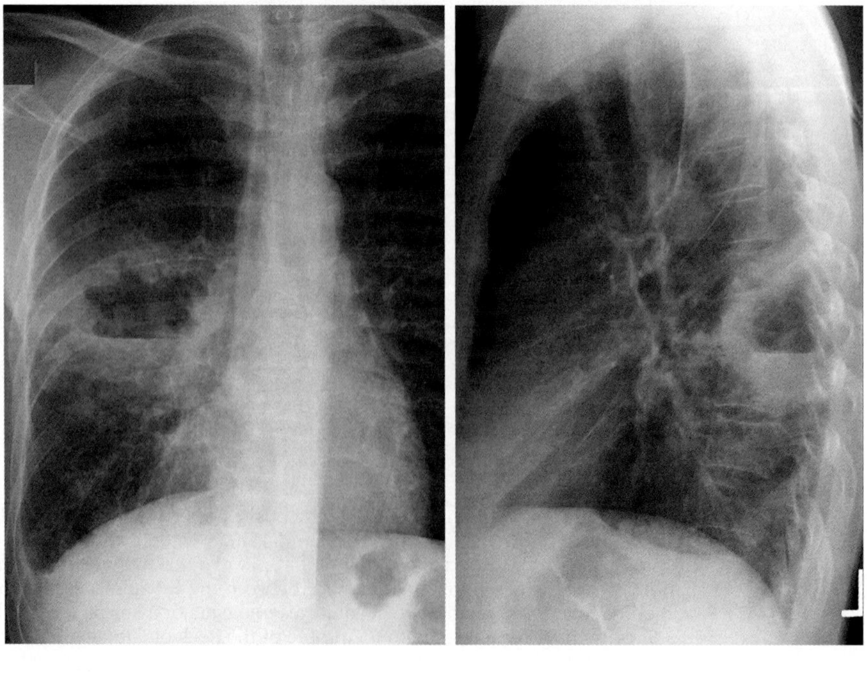

Figure 35.11 Lung abscess—empyema versus abscess. These composite posteroanterior (PA) *(left)* and lateral *(right)* chest radiographs demonstrate a cavitary mass in the superior segment of the right lower lobe, with an internal air-fluid level that exhibits approximately equal lengths on both orthogonal views, a finding that suggests the spherical morphology of a lung abscess. By contrast, an empyema with a bronchopleural fistula typically demonstrates a disparity in the length of an associated air-fluid level when measured on PA and lateral chest radiographs, a manifestation of the lenticular shape that is more characteristic of pleural fluid collections.

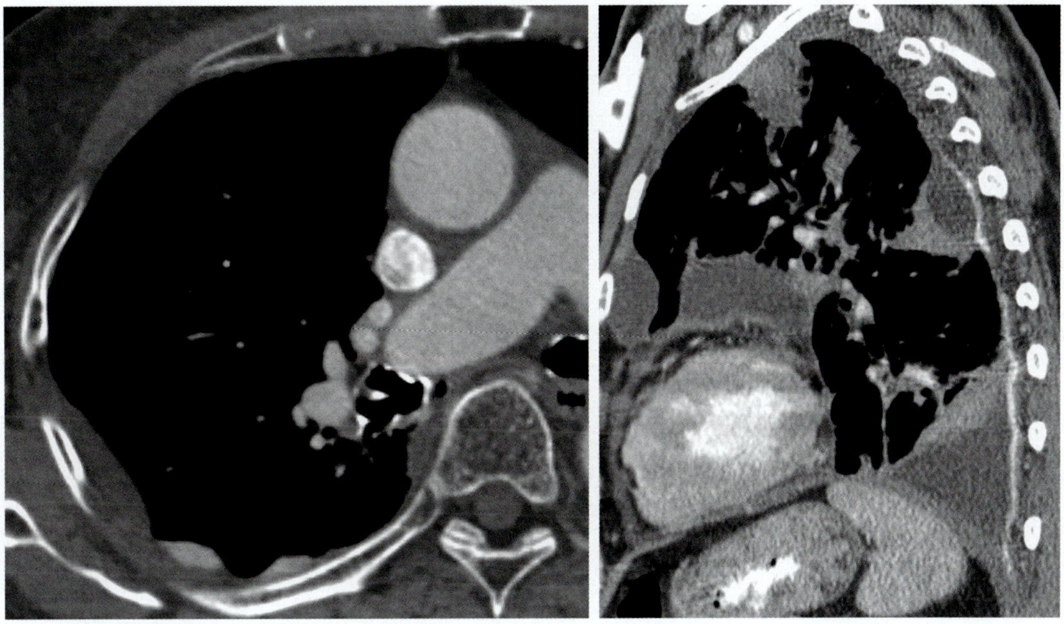

Figure 35.12 Talc pleurodesis for malignant pleural effusion. This composite image of an axial CT scan of a 77-year-old woman *(left)* and sagittal reformatted CT of a 73-year-old man *(right)*, both of whom were treated by pleurodesis for intractable malignant pleural effusions, shows characteristic CT findings. Focal and sheetlike areas of high-attenuation pleural thickening represent magnesium deposits from talc pleurodesis. The sagittal image *(right)* also shows multiple areas of loculated pleural effusion. The CT attenuation of talc is approximately 300 to 350 HU. Talc is typically not visible by plain radiography, in contrast to calcified pleural plaques (see Fig. 35.6).

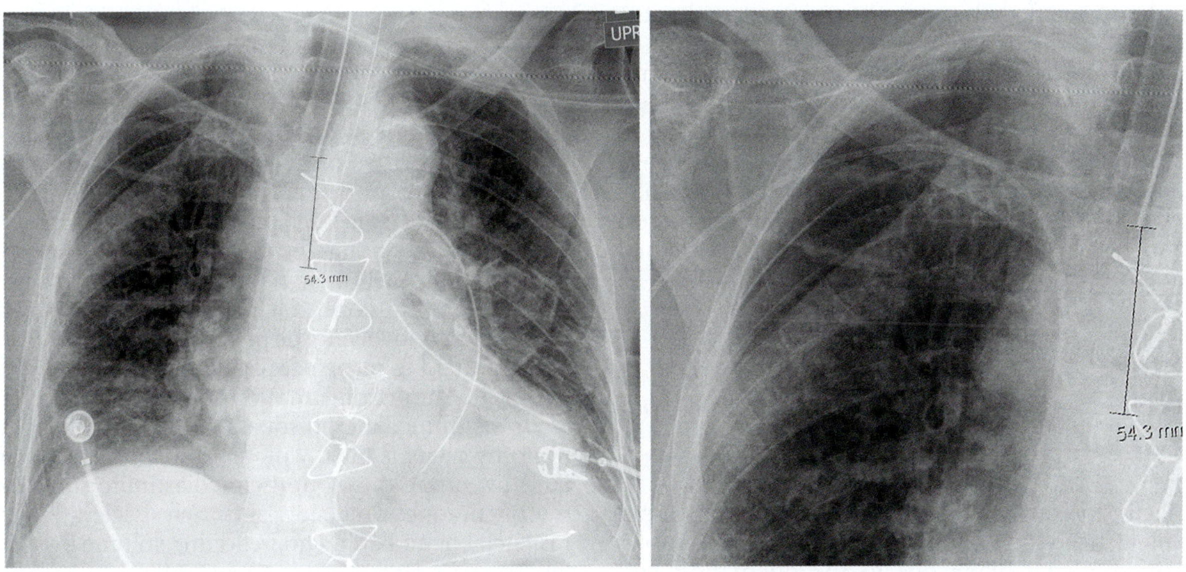

Figure 35.13 Skin fold mimics pneumothorax. This posteroanterior chest radiograph *(left)* and detail of the same view *(right)* shows an oblique bandlike opacity with a sharp outer border that mimics a pneumothorax. On the detailed view *(right)*, lung markings are clearly visible in the peripheral lung, extending beyond the sharp border, which represents the edge of a skin fold.

Imaging Features That Help Characterize and Differentiate Lesions as Parenchymal, Pleural, or Extrapleural

Lesions in the pleural space, extrapleural space, and subpleural lung parenchyma can sometimes be difficult to localize. The distinction has important implications in the differential diagnosis of the imaging findings. Several radiographic features are helpful in the precise localization of abnormality, although there can be some overlap between extrapleural and pleural lesions or between pleural and parenchymal lesions. In many cases, biopsy is necessary for a definitive diagnosis.

Extrapleural lesions displace the visceral and parietal pleura and thus form an obtuse angle with lung parenchyma. Radiographic findings of rib destruction or muscle

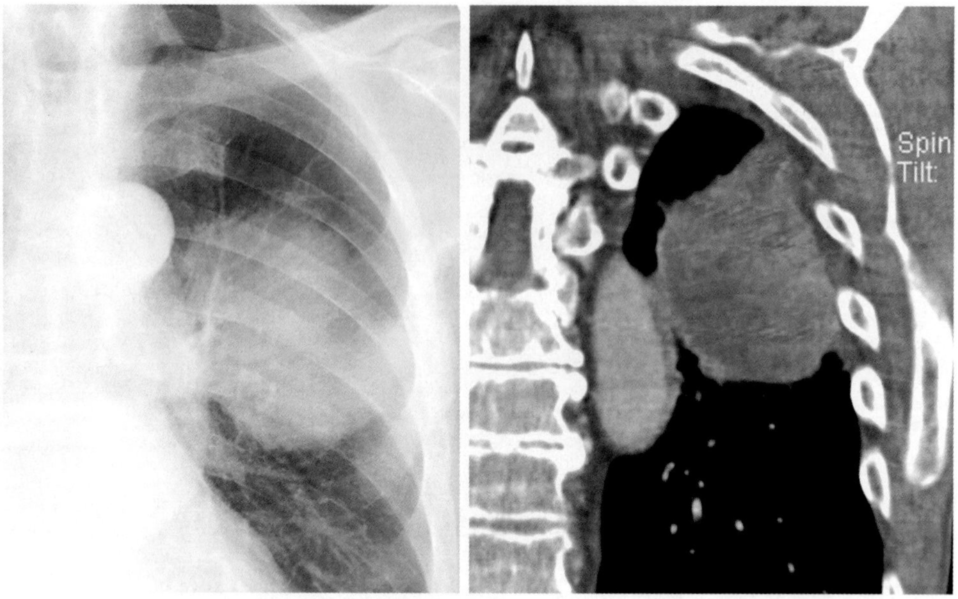

Figure 35.14 Lung cancer with incomplete borders. This composite image of a posteroanterior (PA) chest radiograph *(left)* and coronal reformatted CT scan *(right)* shows a left upper lobe mass. On PA radiography, the mass has visible borders inferiorly and superomedially, but indistinct and incomplete borders along its peripheral aspect. Parenchymal lesions that involve the pleura may exhibit the incomplete border sign, which is more characteristic of pleural lesions (e.g., pleural tumor, loculated fluid). The incomplete border sign suggests the presence of an extrapulmonary lesion in the thorax, usually involving the pleura or chest wall.

infiltration are not always present but confirm an extrapleural location.

Most pleural lesions also form an obtuse angle with lung parenchyma and demonstrate an incomplete border sign on plain radiography. However, if a pleural lesion is large or pedunculated, it may form an acute angle with the lung. The presence of pleural fibrosis or prior pleurodesis can affect the appearance of a pleural mass, causing it to form an acute angle with the lung.

Parenchymal lesions are centered in the lung and form an acute angle with the adjacent normal lung parenchyma. However, obtuse angles can be formed in the setting of pleural or chest wall invasion, and those lesions may manifest with incomplete borders on chest radiography (Fig. 35.14). An associated finding of pulmonary vessel engulfment helps confirm the location as parenchymal and does not occur with an extrapulmonary mass.

■ Pitfalls

Pleural Effusion Versus Ascites

Pleural effusion can be difficult to distinguish from upper abdominal ascites on CT. This can be particularly troublesome in the axial plane due to the orientation and thinness of the diaphragm. However, several clues can help differentiate the two:

- Pleural effusion displaces the diaphragmatic crus anteriorly.
- The interface of pleural fluid and liver or spleen is indistinct due to volume averaging with the diaphragm, whereas the interface between ascites and the liver or spleen is sharp and well defined.
- Pleural effusion preferentially accumulates within the costophrenic sulci and thus is seen peripherally in the hemithorax. The hemidiaphragm is a domed convex superiorly, so ascites will accumulate centrally in the axial plane (Fig. 35.15).
- Pleural fluid appears progressively smaller on axial images when moving caudally, whereas the opposite is true for ascites.
- If the hemidiaphragm is inverted, though, the last two findings are reversed and can be a cause of confusion. In this case, coronal and sagittal reconstructions can be helpful to differentiate pleural effusion from ascites.

Pneumonectomy

Patients who have undergone pneumonectomy, either for treatment of benign or malignant disease, have a characteristic postoperative appearance that can mimic pleural pathology on plain radiography if the patient's history is not known. With surgical removal of the lung, the hemithorax becomes completely opacified, which can be confused with a large pleural effusion. Additionally, there are postoperative complications involving the pneumonectomy cavity, which are important to recognize. Of note, the parietal pleura is left in situ during pneumonectomy.

In the immediate postoperative period, the pneumonectomy cavity is filled with air and appears similar to a large pneumothorax, but the mediastinum shifts toward the pneumonectomy side, and there is elevation of the ipsilateral hemidiaphragm, reflecting volume loss. Gradually, the air is reabsorbed and replaced by serosanguineous fluid, giving the appearance of a progressively rising air-fluid level until the pneumonectomy cavity is completely opacified, which usually occurs within weeks to months. Findings of volume loss remain with ipsilateral mediastinal shift, posterior rotation of the heart, and anterior herniation of the remaining lung across the midline. At this point, the postpneumonectomy appearance can easily be distinguished from a large pleural effusion or hydrothorax based on the volume loss. An abnormal fluid accumulation would cause a contralateral mediastinal shift.

There are also some important complications involving the pneumonectomy cavity that are important to be aware of and recognize.

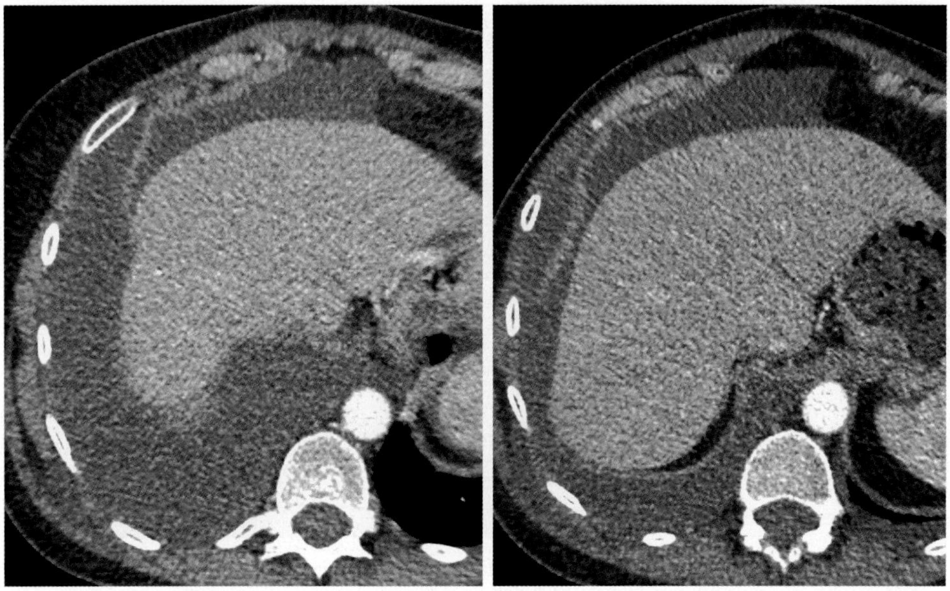

Figure 35.15 Pleural effusion and ascites. This composite image of two adjacent axial CT images in the lower thorax *(left)* and upper abdomen *(right)* shows adjacent fluid collections representing ascites and pleural effusion, distinguished by their location with respect to the thin hemidiaphragm. Pleural effusion accumulates in the costophrenic sulci and is therefore located peripherally to the hemidiaphragm, whereas abdominal ascites accumulate medially. The interface between pleural fluid and liver is indistinct (seen posterolaterally in the left image), whereas the interface between ascites and the liver is well defined (seen anteriorly in the left image and anterolaterally and posterolaterally in the right image).

Bronchopleural Fistula

This is a potentially fatal complication that occurs from bronchial stump leak, with an incidence rate of 2% to 13% and mortality rate of 16% to 70%. This is usually an early postoperative complication (within the first week) but can occur as a later complication secondary to infection or recurrent malignancy. A bronchopleural fistula will cause an inferior drop in the air-fluid level in the pneumonectomy cavity on upright radiography and contralateral mediastinal shift. Reemergence of an air-fluid level after normal opacification of the pneumonectomy cavity has occurred is a sign of late bronchopleural fistula formation.

Esophagopleural Fistula

This is a less common complication (approximate incidence <1%), with similar radiographic findings as a bronchopleural fistula in the early and late postoperative settings. It occurs from direct esophageal injury or perioperative ischemia. CT is especially useful for distinguishing between the two entities.

Empyema

This occurs with similar frequency to bronchopleural fistula. Similarly, it manifests as a drop in the air-fluid level, contralateral mediastinal shift, or reemergence of an air-fluid level after complete opacification. The source of infection may be from direct contamination or hematogenous seeding, and empyema may coexist with bronchopleural and esophagopleural fistula. Risk factors include a right pneumonectomy, completion pneumonectomy after prior lobectomy, neoadjuvant radiation therapy, gross contamination of the pleura, sepsis, mediastinal lymph node dissection, and postoperative mechanical ventilation. CT can be useful for further evaluation and will demonstrate pleural thickening or nodularity, as well as identification of concurrent bronchopleural or esophagopleural fistula.

Chylothorax

This is a rare complication (incidence ≅1%) that occurs from injury to the thoracic duct. Chylothorax will cause fluid accumulation, with a contralateral mediastinal shift. It is radiographically indistinguishable from hydrothorax or hemothorax, and direct sampling is needed to confirm the diagnosis.

Another potential pitfall in postoperative imaging can occur in the setting of pneumothorax of the nonoperative side. Mediastinal shift away from the remaining lung is normal after pneumonectomy, so even small pneumothoraces can mimic a tension pneumothorax if the patient's surgical history is unknown to the interpreting radiologist. In rare cases, there can be an illusion of a bilateral pneumothorax secondary to anterior herniation of the nonoperative pleural space across the midline. Communication with the referring provider and clinical assessment of the patient are essential. CT can resolve any remaining doubts in case of an incomplete surgical history by clearly defining the postoperative anatomy.

Pseudotumor (Interlobar Pleural Effusion)

A pleural fluid collection within the major or minor fissure is sometimes referred to as a *pseudotumor* because it can mimic a lung mass on plain radiography. It is usually seen in the setting of heart failure, although renal failure and hepatic hydrothorax can also cause preferential accumulation of fluid in the fissures. Typically interlobar fluid collections manifest as ovoid or lenticular-shaped homogeneous opacities without air bronchograms (Fig. 35.16). A pseudotumor is always located along the distribution of the minor fissure or, less commonly, the major fissure. The lateral projection is useful for localization, and interlobar fluid will change shape and orientation between orthogonal views, whereas a true mass will not. Decubitus views will cause the fluid to

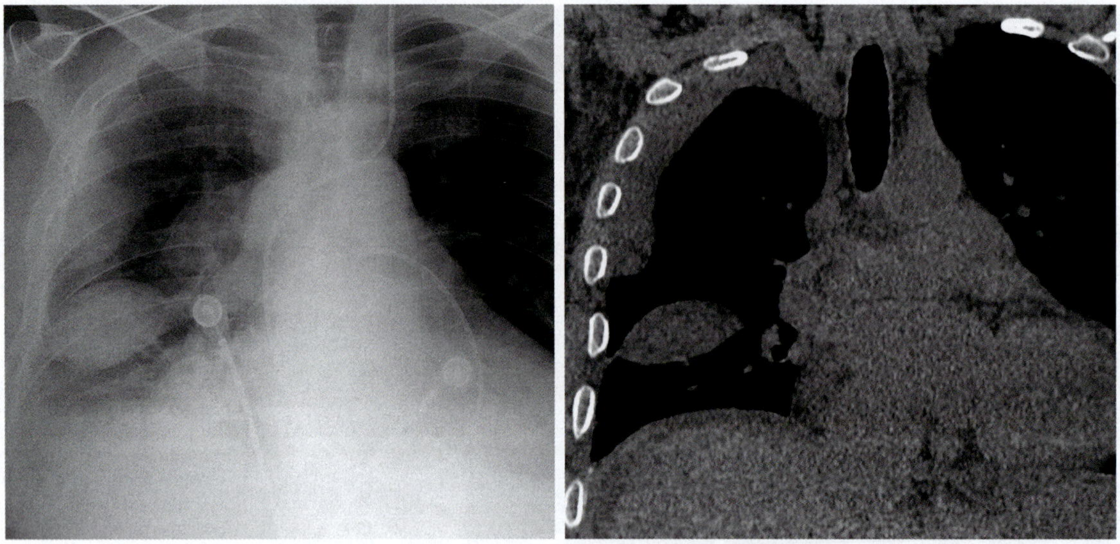

Figure 35.16 Pseudotumor. This composite image of posteroanterior chest radiograph *(left)* and coronal CT reformation *(right)* shows a lenticular-shaped mass extending along the minor fissure representing a fluid collection that resolved following treatment of the patient's heart failure. Similar accumulations may occur along the major interlobar fissures. In both cases, localization is often more clearly defined on lateral chest radiography.

flow out of the fissures. Concomitant findings of heart failure, such as cardiomegaly and cardiogenic pulmonary edema, help support the diagnosis.

Solitary (Localized) Fibrous Tumor of the Pleura

A solitary fibrous tumor of the pleura is a rare primary pleural neoplasm arising from submesothelial connective tissue. Most are benign, although a small percentage can be malignant. Although smaller pleural masses form obtusely angled interfaces with the adjacent lung parenchyma and often exhibit incomplete borders on radiography, larger pleural tumors usually form acutely angled interfaces with the lung parenchyma and, less frequently, demonstrate the incomplete border sign. Solitary fibrous tumors are variable in size, and larger tumors manifest as a single lobulated mass, without associated lymphadenopathy (Fig. 35.17). Some may arise within an interlobar fissure, and approximately 80% of all solitary fibrous tumors of the pleura involve the lower thorax. Larger tumors may exhibit positional changes if the mass is pedunculated. On CT, small masses have homogeneous soft tissue attenuation, whereas large masses are heterogeneous, with a whorled appearance, and may demonstrate cystic areas or, less commonly, calcification. Heterogeneous enhancement is seen with the administration of IV contrast material on both CT and MRI.

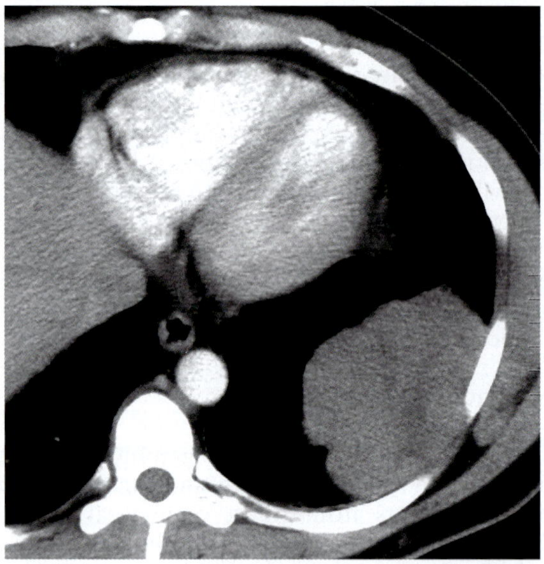

Figure 35.17 Solitary fibrous tumor. This contrast-enhanced axial chest CT scan shows a lobulated heterogeneous mass extending along the pleural surface in the left lower hemithorax, characteristic imaging features of a solitary fibrous tumor of the pleura.

Fibrothorax

Fibrothorax is a fibrotic reaction of the pleura as a result of prior infection, hemothorax, autoimmune disorder, uremia, or drug reaction. It manifests as unilateral, diffuse, pleural thickening and calcification, with ipsilateral hemithoracic volume loss on plain radiography, and can resemble malignant mesothelioma (Fig. 35.18). However, fibrothorax is not a malignant entity and is only treated with decortication in symptomatic patients with normal underlying lung parenchyma. Fibrothorax tends to form extensive, dense, circumferential pleural calcification (>25% of the pleural surface). Malignant mesothelioma can have calcifications in approximately 20% of cases from the engulfment of asbestos-related pleural plaques. CT is particularly useful in identifying fibrothorax because the calcification typically involves both the parietal and visceral pleural surfaces—often separated by fluid and

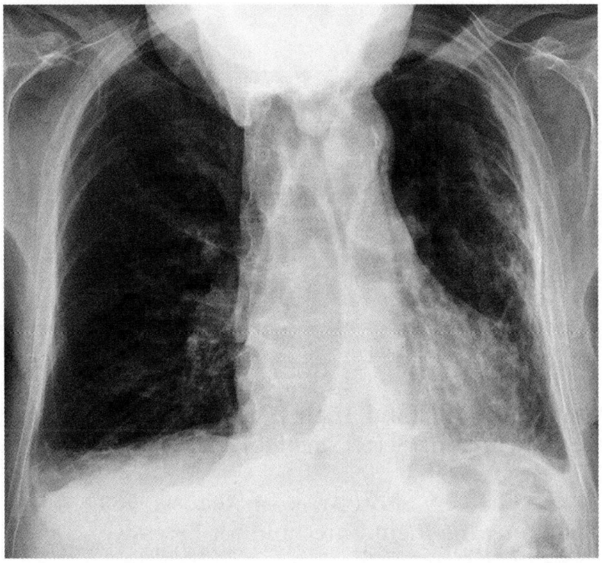

Figure 35.18 Fibrothorax. This posteroanterior chest radiograph shows calcified pleural thickening extending along the left lateral hemithorax and loss of volume in the left lung. The patient had a history of prior hemothorax related to trauma.

soft tissue attenuation—and characteristic sparing of mediastinal pleura (88% of cases) is often demonstrated. Contrast-enhanced CT can be helpful to identify enhancing pleural nodules, which would suggest malignancy rather than fibrothorax.

Bibliography

Chae EJ, Seo JB, Kim SY, et al. Radiographic and CT findings of thoracic complications after pneumonectomy. *Radiographics*. 2006;26:1449–1467.

Cugell DW, Kamp DW. Asbestos and the pleura: a review. *Chest*. 2004;125:1103–1117.

McLoud TC. The pleura. In: McLoud TC, Boiselle PM, eds. *Thoracic Radiology: the Requisites*. 2nd ed. Philadelphia: Mosby Elsevier; 2010:379–399.

Moy MP, Levsky JM, Berko NS, Godelman A, Jain VR, Haramati LB. A new, simple method for estimating pleural effusion size on CT scans. *Chest*. 2013;143(4):1054–1059.

Murray JG, Patz EF, Erasmus JJ, Gilkeson RC. CT appearance of the pleural space after talc pleurodesis. *AJR Am J Roentgenol*. 1997;169:89–91.

Nadich DP, Webb WR, Muller NL, et al. Pleura, chest wall, and diaphragm. In: Nadich DP, Webb WR, Muller NL, et al, eds. *Computed Tomography and Magnetic Resonance of the Thorax*. 4th ed. Philadelphia: Lippincott Williams & Wilkins; 2007:769–883.

Nickell LT, Lichtenberger LP, Khorashadi L, Abbott GF, Carter BW. Multimodality imaging for characterization, classification, and staging of malignant pleural mesothelioma. *Radiographics*. 2014;34:1692–1706.

Rosado-de-Christenson ML, Abbott GF, Strollo DC. Neoplasms of the lung, pleura, and chest wall. In: Gourtsoyiannis NC, Ros PR, eds. *Radiologic-Pathologic Correlations: From Head to Toe*. Berlin: Springer; 2005:165–184.

Stark DD, Federle MP, Goodman PC, Podrasky AE, Webb WR. Differentiating lung abscess and empyema: radiography and computed tomography. *AJR Am J Roentgenol*. 1983;141:163–167.

Walker CM, Takasugi JE, Chung JH, et al. Tumorlike conditions of the pleura. *Radiographics*. 2012;32(4):971–985.

CHAPTER 36

Trachea and Bronchi

Pierluigi Ciet, Benedikt H. Heidinger, Nihara Chakrala, and Diana Litmanovich

CHAPTER OUTLINE

■ Central Airway Anatomy and Physiology: Essentials for the Radiologist

Anatomy

The trachea is a cartilaginous and fibromuscular conduct extending from the lower border of the larynx (2 cm below the vocal cords, at the level of spinal C6) to the carina (at the level of spinal T5), where it bifurcates into the main stem bronchi. The trachea ranges from 10 to 12 cm in length, with an extrathoracic portion above the sternal manubrium that ranges from 2 to 4 cm. Sagittal and coronal tracheal diameters vary according to patient height, weight, age, and sex. The sagittal diameter ranges from 13 to 27 mm in males and 10 to 23 mm in females, and the coronal diameter ranges from 13 to 25 mm and 10 to 21 mm, respectively.

C-shaped cartilaginous rings, from 16 to 22 rings, define the anterior and lateral contours of the trachea. Cartilaginous rings reinforce the tracheal wall and maintain lumen patency during expiration. These cartilaginous rings tend to calcify with advanced age, particularly in women, and in patients on long-standing warfarin therapy. The posterior portion of the tracheal wall, also known as *pars membranacea,* is a thin fibromuscular membrane closely connected to the anterior esophageal wall. Constantly in motion, the pars membranacea assumes a convex and concave shape at end-inspiration and end-expiration, respectively, and contains a small amount of smooth muscle, often referred to as *tracheal muscle*. The tracheal muscle has an inner circular muscle layer and an external longitudinal, layer. These layers are similar to those of the esophagus, having a common embryologic origin, although constrictor capacity is limited. Main stem and lobar bronchi also have cartilaginous and fibromuscular elements, but the cartilaginous support varies while moving distally toward the lung periphery, with more irregularly shaped cartilage plates at more peripheral levels.

Branches of the inferior thyroid arteries and extreme right intercostal artery provide blood to the trachea superiorly, whereas blood is provided inferiorly by branches of the bronchial arteries and third intercostal artery. Branches of the vagus and recurrent laryngeal nerves and sympathetic trunks innervate the trachea, and the parasympathetic nervous system is the main pathway in control of airway smooth muscle and vessels. These nerves cause bronchoconstriction, mucus secretion, and bronchial vasodilation.

The trachea is lined with pseudostratified, columnar, ciliated epithelium containing goblet cells, which produce mucins, the main component of mucus, to moisten and protect the airways. Mucus and cilia execute the mucociliary function—that is, the excretion of inhaled foreign particles that are pushed toward the larynx and then the pharynx, where they can be swallowed or expelled as phlegm.

Physiology

Tracheal anatomy is related to its functions. First, because the trachea is an airway conductor, its structure must be elastic so it can sustain the conformational changes occurring during the breathing cycle. The trachea elongates at end-inspiration with a three-dimensional (3D) change in size and location, and elastic recoil of the trachea restores its original length and position with the C-shaped cartilages, preventing collapse during expiration. In the general population, there is a large variability in the range of central airways collapse, with studies showing up to 78% collapse in healthy subjects. More detailed description of central airways collapse assessment is given in the following sections. Second, the ciliated mucous membrane of the trachea plays a crucial role in tracheobronchial clearance, the mechanism for clearing the airways. This mechanism is assisted by the coughing reflex, which pushes out the mucus eventually expelled as phlegm through the mouth or swallowed down the esophagus. Mucus film also represents the first barrier of the immune system because it contains glycoproteins, immunoglobulins, albumin, lipids, enzymes, antienzymes, antibacterials, cell products, and mediators. Finally, the central airways contribute to the air-conditioning capacity of the upper respiratory tract, mainly carried out in the nasal cavity. The capacity to heat and humidify the air mainly occurs during normal mouth breathing during exercise and during pathologic mouth breathing resulting from nasal obstructions, such as the flu.

■ Appropriateness of Imaging Modalities: Determining Which Technique Should Be Used

Chest X-Ray

A chest x-ray (CXR) represents a fast, low-cost, and low-radiation modality that offers a preliminary assessment of central airway pathology; however, the purpose is mainly to exclude parenchymal or other sources of clinical symptoms.

In a CXR, the trachea appears as a flipped Y structure that is darker compared to the surrounding mediastinal tissue due to the air content. Well-defined tracheal lines, called *paratracheal stripes*, delimit the tracheal contours and are crucial for the assessment of central airways. The right paratracheal stripe is normally seen in the frontal CXR as a line that extends from the level of the clavicles to the right tracheobronchial angle at the level of the azygos arch. This stripe is easily identified by the presence of air on both sides (lung and trachea lumen) and consists of the right tracheal wall, adjacent pleural surfaces, and mediastinal fat. The paratracheal stripe has a thickness of 3 to 4 mm; thickening can be an expression of a different pathology, such as lipomatosis, paratracheal lymphadenopathy, thyroid, parathyroid, or tracheal malignancy, and pleural effusion. Similarly, the left paratracheal stripe represents the left trachea wall, the pleural surface between the left upper lobe and the adjacent mediastinal fat, and is seen less frequently in the frontal CXR than the right paratracheal stripe.

Computed Tomography

CT is the most accurate noninvasive modality for assessing not only the airways, but also the entire thorax. CT provides better characterization of CXR abnormalities, such as abnormal tracheal contours, atelectasis, or diffuse parenchymal disease, that can involve the airways. Nowadays, CT is also frequently performed in patients before interventional bronchoscopic procedures to obtain precise preprocedural anatomic correlation and biopsy guidance of peripheral lung lesions. Finally, CT is routinely used in the follow-up of patients undergoing medical and surgical treatment of airway disease. The only major limitation of CT is radiation exposure, which can be problematic, especially in pediatric patients, who are more sensitive to radiation than adults. This problem has been partially overcome by the new generation of CT scanners, which use automatic exposure control devices that can reduce the dose to less than 3 mSv.

POTENTIAL PROBLEM: HOW TO DESIGN AND REVIEW APPROPRIATE CT AIRWAY IMAGING PROTOCOLS

SOLUTION. Routine CT protocol for central airways assessment includes high-resolution axial images, which provide precise information about the size and shape of the airway lumen, presence and location of abnormalities, and mediastinal, hilar, and pulmonary associated abnormalities. Typical scan parameters and postprocessing reconstruction settings are described in Tables 36.1 and 36.2. Axial images are also indicated to assess direct and indirect signs of airway diseases, such as bronchial wall thickening and bronchiectasis or trapped air. In cases of suspected airway malignancy or infection, IV contrast

TABLE 36.1 Standard Scan Parameters for Multidetector CT

Scanner	Multidetector CT
kVp, mAs	110–140, 50–80
Pitch	≥1
Field of view	Lung apices to bases or to the first or second branching of the main bronchi
Acquisition	End-inspiration; end-expiration[a] with lower kV and mA settings; forced expiration[a] with lower kV and mA settings

[a]When tracheomalacia is suspected.

TABLE 36.2 Standard Multiplanar Two-Dimensional (2D) and Three-Dimensional (3D) Reconstructions

POSTPROCESSING RECONSTRUCTION SETTINGS	FEATURES
2D reconstructions	1 mm thickness—axial, coronal, and sagittal
2D thick MPRs	1–10 mm thickness, coronal, ± MinIP algorithm
3D surface rendering	Surface rendering of trachea and main bronchi
3D virtual bronchoscopy	Internal surface rendering of the trachea and main bronchi

MinIP, Minimum intensity projection; *MPRs,* multiplanar reconstructions.

administration is preferred; otherwise, an unenhanced study would be sufficient.

However, axial images are usually combined with two-dimensional (2D) and 3D multiplanar reconstructions (MPRs) of the airways. 2D and 3D reconstructed images enhance the identification of subtle and short-segment airway stenosis. Curved MPRs are useful to measure cross-sectional diameters or the area of nonlinear structures (e.g., stenosis located in a bent or kinked trachea). The minimum intensity projection technique is useful for displaying the distribution of air trapping and emphysema in the lung parenchyma. These MPRs are complementary and do not substitute axial images by providing additional information needed for a complete overview of the complex central airway anatomy.

CT assessment of the central airways begins with visualization of the native axial images. Interpretation should begin with assessment of the tracheal and bronchial lumen and walls, followed by the surrounding mediastinal and hilar structures. It is very important to use consistent lung window settings for airway assessment because bronchial wall thickening can vary significantly using different settings. Recommended window settings for lung and mediastinum assessment are as follows: (1) lung setting, and window level (WL), −450 to −700 HU; window width (WW), 1200 to 1500 HU, (2) mediastinal setting, WL, 40 to 50 HU, WW, 350 to 400 HU.

Magnetic Resonance Imaging

In the last two decades, MRI technology has largely improved, allowing for the introduction of MRI into airway imaging. The main advantage of using MRI over CT is the lack of ionizing radiation, which makes MRI valuable for the pediatric population and repeated follow-up imaging. Moreover, MRI offers the possibility to study airway dynamics by cine mode acquisitions.

A second important advantage of MRI over CT is its intrinsic high tissue characterization. By using different tissue weighting (T1, T2, proton density), MRI can distinguish between different tissue compositions, such as fat and water. Finally, MRI allows the assessment of thoracic vessels without the use of contrast material with either bright contrast using a steady-state free precession readout or dark contrast using a single-shot, turbo spin-echo readout with a black blood preparation.

Spatial resolution with MRI is lower than with CT, usually with collections of isotropic voxels ranging from 2 to 5 mm^3. The most frequently used sequence is 3D gradient echo (GRE) in breath-hold conditions. It can be acquired using a phase array torso or head-neck-spine coil. The latter setting allows for the improvement of spatial resolution with isotropic voxels around 1 mm^3. The preferred tissue weighting for central airway imaging is proton density, which enhances the signal of the central airways wall, minimizing the brightness of the mediastinal fat. T2 weighting can be obtained with 2D single-shot fast spin-echo or 3D turbo spin-echo techniques. 3D acquisition enables 3D postprocessing techniques similar to those obtained with CT.

POTENTIAL PROBLEM: HOW TO DESIGN AND REVIEW APPROPRIATE MR AIRWAY IMAGING PROTOCOLS

SOLUTION. For central airway assessment, single-voxel thick (1–10 mm) 2D MPRs are usually displayed simultaneously in the coronal, sagittal, and oblique planes. Thick-slab 2D MPRs can be used with a minimum intensity projection algorithm, a technique that improves the visibility of the airways from the surrounding lung parenchyma by highlighting the lowest attenuation voxels (i.e., air). 2D MPRs improve the detection and assessment of airway stenoses, longitudinal extent of airway stenoses, and complex congenital airway abnormalities. These reconstructions are sometimes combined with curved planar reformats performed along the lumen of an airway, allowing for the depiction of multiple contiguous airway segments on a single plane (Fig. 36.1).

3D reconstruction can be external or internal renderings of the airways. External or surface rendering displays the outer surface of the airways and its relationship with the adjacent mediastinal and lung structures. This technique allows selectively segmenting the central airways, giving a rapid anatomic overview of potential pathologies. 3D surface rendering improves the detection of mild and focal airway stenosis and improves confidence of the findings seen on axial images. Internal 3D rendering, or virtual bronchoscopy, supplies an endoluminal view similar to conventional bronchoscopy. This technique allows visualization of the lumen of central airways until the sixth to seventh order of subdivisions. Virtual bronchoscopy is useful for assessing airway stenosis, guidance of transbronchial biopsy, and foreign body (FB) aspiration. It can be used in situations where conventional bronchoscopy is not desirable (e.g., young children) or feasible (e.g., high-grade obstructing stenosis, beyond which a conventional bronchoscope cannot pass).

The MRI protocol for central airways frequently includes a multiphase dynamic acquisition, performed during specific breathing maneuvers, such as forced expiration, cough, or hyperpnea. These dynamic acquisitions are usually performed to assess tracheobronchomalacia (TBM). Typical sequences used to assess dynamic tracheal collapsibility are 2D axial and sagittal steady-state free precession techniques, 3D GRE multiphase with parallel imaging, or the time-resolved imaging of contrast kinetics (TRICKS) platform. Basic MRI scan parameters for 1.5-T MRI are described in Table 36.3.

Central airway assessment using MRI is similar to CT, except that with MRI different tissue weighting provides different information. For example,T1 weighting is normally used for vessel visualization, T2 weighting for bronchi, and PD weighting for lung parenchyma and central airways. Therefore, once the abnormality is detected, it is important to assess signal characteristics with different tissue weighting. Moreover, in MRI, different window settings will influence lumen appearance and size, so it is important to keep a constant window setting (average, maximum intensity projection, minimum intensity projection), especially for the assessment of tracheal collapsibility. However, unlike CT, there are no well-defined window settings for MRI. We recommend using an average algorithm and similar WW and WL between end-inspiration and end-expiration (or dynamic) acquisitions.

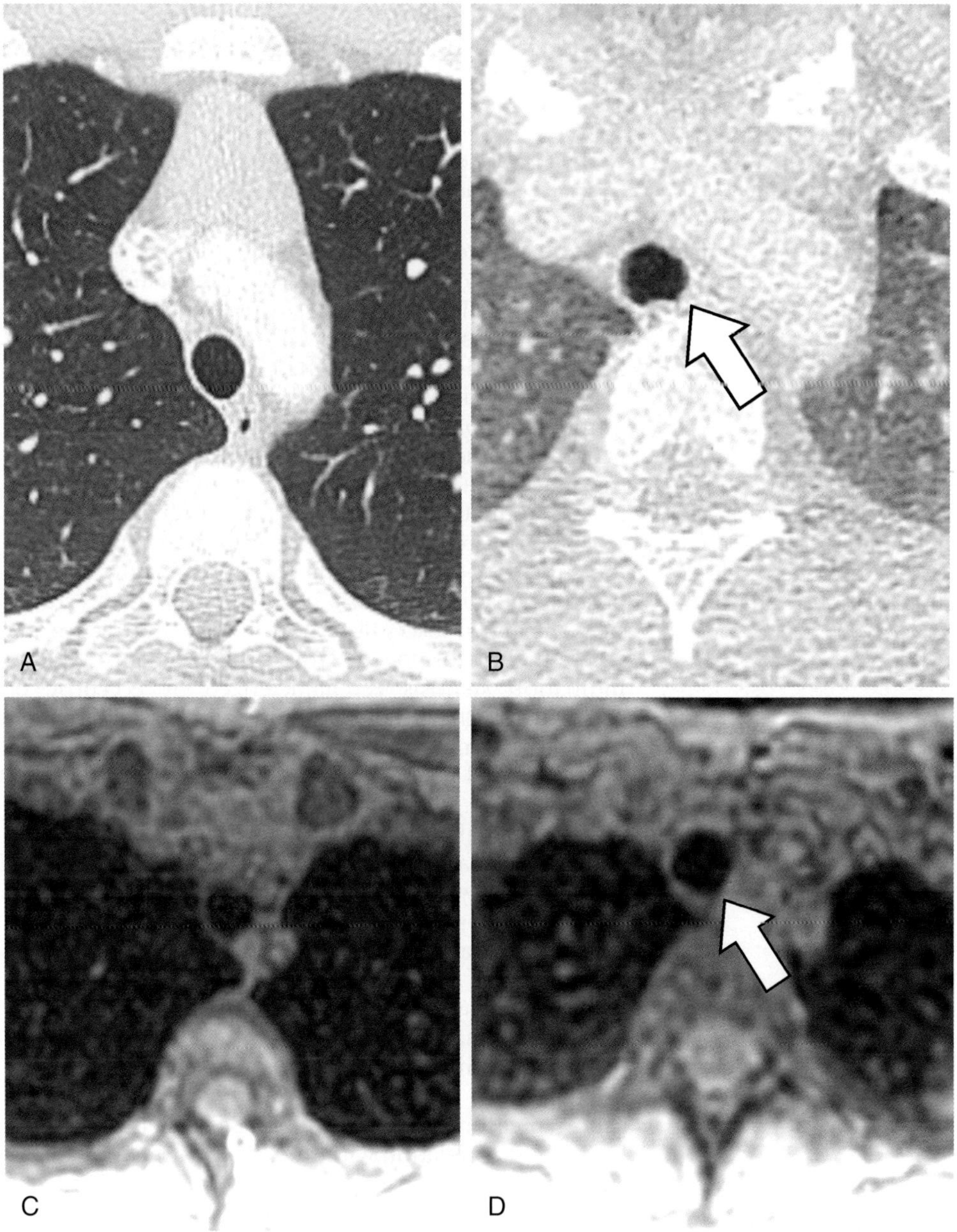

Figure 36.1 A 43-year-old healthy man. Axial end-inspiratory (A) and end-expiratory (B) CT images. Axial end-inspiratory (C) and end-expiratory (D) reformats, three-dimensional radiofrequency spoiled gradient echo sequence. Note the variable shape of the trachea in expiration *(arrows)* and increased density of lung parenchyma in expiration (B and D).

Despite these advantages, MRI still has lower spatial and temporal resolution than CT, and MRI is more difficult and time-consuming than CT. Finally, the lack of standard MRI protocols between centers limits the experience with this modality in thoracic imaging, so that MRI is still not routinely used in clinical practice for airway imaging.

POTENTIAL PROBLEM: HOW TO PREPARE THE PATIENT FOR AIRWAY CT OR MRI

SOLUTION. Any patient that undergoes airways imaging must be adequately prepared for the breathing maneuvers performed during the scans. Assessment of pathology, such as for TBM, requires dedicated expiratory imaging with both CT and MRI. For CT, there are two main types of acquisitions: (1) paired end-inspiratory and end-expiratory CT; and (2) paired end-inspiratory and dynamic expiratory CT. The first type consists of an acquisition at total lung capacity (TLC) and one at residual volume (RV). In this case, the subjects are coached prior to the scan to reach TLC, RV, and breath-holding for a few seconds. The breath-hold time is longer for MR imaging, up to 8 to 12 seconds. The second type consists of an acquisition at TLC and one during forced expiration, which replicates the peak flow maneuver (forced expiratory volume in 1 second [FEV_1]). For this dynamic acquisition, patients are trained to reach TLC and blow all air out as fast as they can. Possible variance of this dynamic acquisition is the coughing maneuver, in which the patient is asked to cough out air from the TLC. The aim of these dynamic maneuvers is to elicit the collapse point of the trachea during expiration. One should stress that the patient should exhale without pursing the lips because doing so artificially increases the intraluminal tracheal pressure, which may prevent the manifestation of subtle TBM.

Prior to the scan, the CT or MRI technologist can help the patient rehearse these breathing maneuvers and, if possible, may be assisted by a dedicated technician. This training is crucial for pediatric patients because it reduces the anxiety related to the MRI investigation, improves the efficiency of the MRI time, and increases the number of children who successfully complete the MRI investigation. More recently, some centers have introduced the use of CT and MRI compatible spirometers which improves the reproducibility of these breathing maneuvers and allows acquisition of the images when the patient is at end-inspiration and end-expiration.

Pathology

Classification of central airway diseases is relatively complex. Three main classification systems exist: (1) pathology-based, benign and malignant; (2) cause-based, congenital and acquired; and (3) anatomy-based, local and diffuse. For practical clinical purposes, the anatomic classification will be discussed in this chapter (Table 36.4). In each group, the description follows a frequency order, from the most common to the least common.

TABLE 36.3 Standard Scan Parameters for 1.5-T MRI Scanners

PARAMETER	BREATH-HOLD ACQUISITION[a]	DYNAMIC EXPIRATORY
Sequence	Radiofrequency-spoiled gradient echo sequence (SPGR)[b]	Time-resolved imaging of contrast kinetics scan (TRICKS)[b]
Repetition time	1.4 ms	2.1 ms
Echo time	0.6 ms	0.8 ms
Flip angle	2–3 degrees	2–3 degrees
Voxel size	2–3 mm isotropic	3 mm isotropic
Acquisition time	8–12 s (± parallel imaging)	48 phases in 19 s

[a]End-inspiratory and end-expiratory.
[b]General Electric brand names; comparable MRI sequences have different names with other vendors.

Common Localized Central Airway Diseases

Iatrogenic Stenosis

Iatrogenic stenosis includes postintubation and posttransplant stenosis. Postintubation stenosis represents the most common cause of acquired focal airways stenosis and can occur after endotracheal intubation or tracheostomy tube placement. This type of stenosis was frequent before the introduction of the low-pressure cuff endotracheal tube, which has reduced its prevalence to less than 1%. However, the prevalence of tracheal stenosis in a long-standing tracheostomy tube placement is still around 30%.

The most frequent site of stenosis after intubation is the subglottic region, at the level of the cuff, whereas posttracheostomy stenosis usually occurs at the stoma site. The most susceptible portions of the trachea are where the mucosa overlies the cartilaginous ring. Postintubation stenosis is characterized by eccentric or concentric tracheal wall thickening and luminal narrowing, with a craniocaudal length ranging between 1.5 and 2.5 cm. Typical symptoms are dyspnea on exertion, stridor, and wheezing. On CT, the axial image shows focal and circumferential luminal narrowing that can produce the typical hourglass appearance (Fig. 36.2).

Additionally, posttransplantation bronchial anastomotic stenosis is relatively frequent. In patients for whom lung transplantation is complicated by infection and rejection, the prevalence is even higher. Patients present with symptoms in the first month after transplantation, characterized by a failure to improve and decline of pulmonary function tests (PFTs), especially FEV_1. On CT, focal narrowing at the anastomotic site can be measured to assess the grade of stenosis, which has a good correlation with the PFT. Treatment of airway stenosis includes bronchoscopic interventions, such as dilation and stenting, and surgical procedures.

TABLE 36.4 Focal and Diffuse Central Airway Diseases

LOCALIZED	DIFFUSE
Iatrogenic (postintubation stenosis, posttransplantation stenosis)	Tracheobronchomalacia (classification, congenital or primary form, acquired or secondary form)
Traumatic	Saber-sheath trachea
Neoplasm (mimickers, benign, primary malignant, secondary malignant)	Excessive dynamic airway collapse
Congenital (tracheal bronchus, bronchial atresia)	Sarcoidosis
Idiopathic laryngotracheal stenosis	Granulomatosis with polyangiitis (Wegener)
Extrinsic compression	Tracheobronchomegaly
Broncholithiasis	Relapsing polychondritis
Anthracofibrosis	Tracheobronchopathia osteochondroplastica
Foreign body	Amyloidosis
Infection (fungal, rhinoscleroma, tuberculosis)	Inflammatory bowel disease

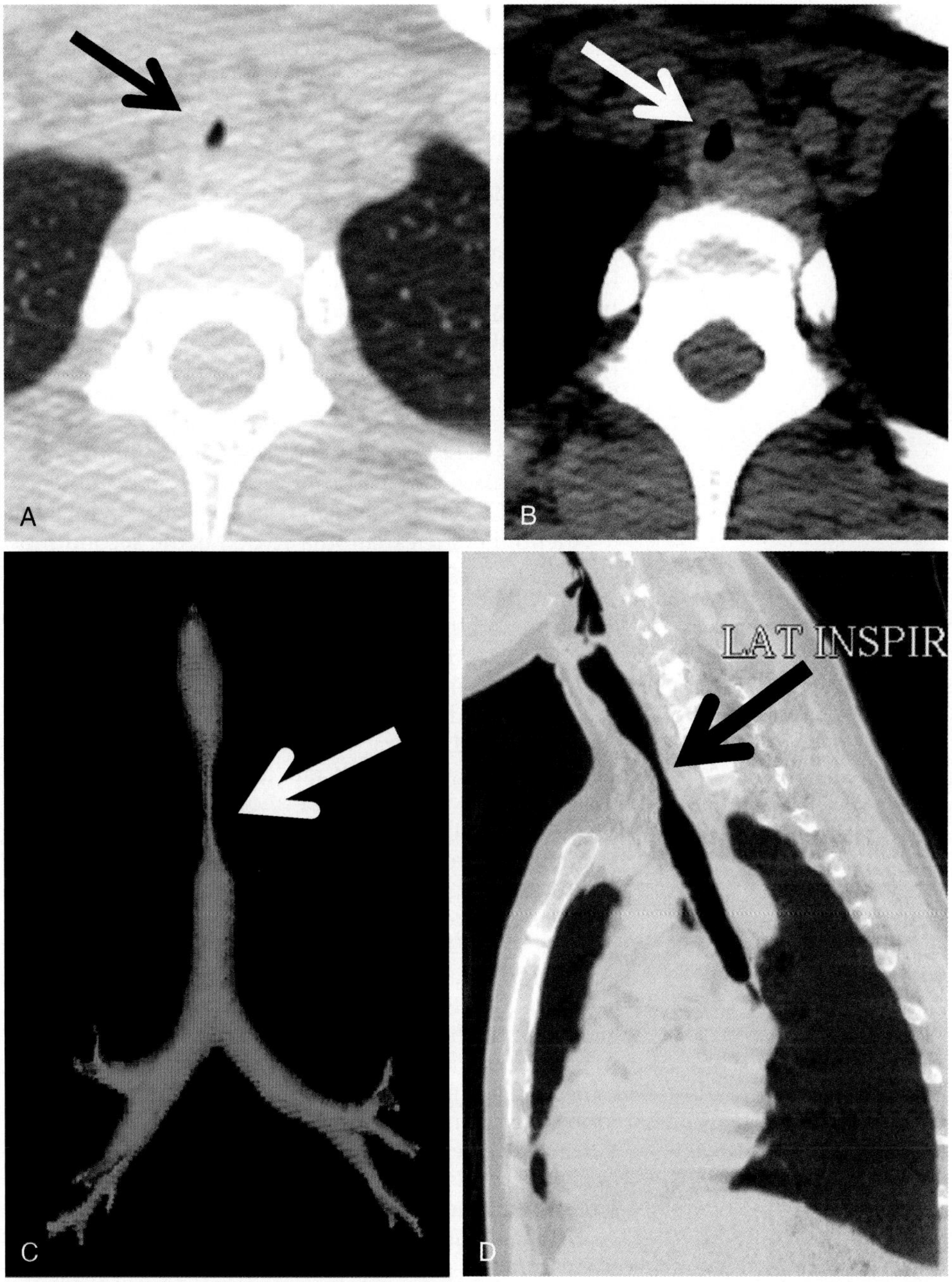

Figure 36.2 A 21-year-old female patient with postintubation stenosis at a typical location in the upper portion of the intrathoracic trachea. Axial CT images in lung (A) and mediastinal (B) window settings show severe circumferential narrowing *(arrows)* of the trachea with wall thickening. Sagittal minimum intensity projection reformation CT (C), and three-dimensional reconstruction (D) images show typical hourglass-like narrowing *(arrows)* of the trachea.

Trauma

Airways trauma can be caused by tracheal wall perforation during intubation, direct blunt trauma, or tearing injury of the main stem bronchi at the level of the hilar attachment to the pleura. Regardless of the cause of the trauma, all these lesions tend to heal with stenosis, which can assume the typical hourglass appearance. CT is the method of choice to assess location, morphology, extension, and coexisting complications.

Neoplasm

Central airway neoplasms can be malignant or benign (Box 36.1). Malignant neoplasms are far more common than benign neoplasms and predominate in adults. They are primarily due to local invasion or hematogenous metastatic spread. Benign neoplasms are more common in children and young adults. Central airways tumors are characterized by symptoms of obstruction, such as chronic cough, dyspnea, recurrent infection, and hemoptysis. Dyspnea occurs only in advanced neoplasms, when the airway lumen is substantially narrowed.

SECONDARY MALIGNANT NEOPLASMS

Secondary malignant neoplasms can be the result of local invasion or hematogenous metastatic spread. Local invasion can be from cancers of the thyroid, esophagus, lung, or larynx. Signs of direct tracheal invasion on CT are an endoluminal mass near the primary tumor, cartilage destruction, and fistulization (Figs. 36.3 and 36.4). Tumors that frequently metastasize to the central airways

BOX 36.1 Classification of Central Airway Neoplasms

Epithelial Neoplasms

Malignant

Squamous cell carcinoma[a]
Adenocarcinoma
Large cell carcinoma
Neuroendocrine tumors
Carcinoids (typical and atypical)
Large cell neuroendocrine tumor
Small cell carcinoma

Benign

Papilloma
Papillomatosis

Salivary Glands

Malignant

Adenoid cystic carcinoma
Mucoepidermoid carcinoma
Carcinoma

Benign

Adenoma pleomorphic
Adenoma, mucous gland
Myoepithelioma
Oncocytoma

Mesenchymal Neoplasms

Malignant

Soft tissue sarcomas
Chondrosarcoma
Lymphomas

Benign

Lipoma
Fibroma
Fibromatosis
Histiocytoma
Hemangioma
Hemangiopericytoma
Chemodectoma
Leiomyoma
Granular cell tumor
Schwann cell tumor
Chondroma
Chondroblastoma

Secondary Neoplasm

Direct Invasion

Esophagus, thyroid, larynx, lung

Hematogenous Metastasis

Breast, colorectal, renal, ovarian, uterine, testicular, melanomas, and sarcomas

[a]Squamous cell carcinoma and adenoid cystic carcinoma represent 86% of malignant neoplasms of central airways.

are breast, colorectal, renal, lung, ovary, thyroid, uterine, testicular, melanoma, and sarcoma. On CT, hematogenous metastases appear as endoluminal nodules or eccentric thickening of the airway wall, with soft tissue density and contrast enhancement (Fig. 36.5).

PRIMARY MALIGNANT NEOPLASMS

Squamous cell carcinoma (SCC) is the most frequent primary neoplasm of the trachea, with a predominance in males (M:F, 2–4 : 1) in the age range of 50 to 60 years. It is highly associated with smoking. Up to 40% of patients with SCC of the trachea develop other smoking-related cancers, such as head and neck or lung cancer. SCC tends to extend locally. When it extends to the esophagus, a tracheoesophageal fistula (TEF) is frequent. CT findings of SCC include a polypoid intraluminal mass, with soft tissue density and irregular and lobulated borders. SCC shows high FDG avidity on PET imaging.

Adenoid cystic carcinoma (ACC) is the second most common malignant neoplasm and originates from the salivary glands. There is no association with smoking habit or sex predominance. The age of occurrence is earlier than that for SCC, usually in the fourth decade of life. ACC appears as an intraluminal focal mass, mostly located in the trachea and main bronchi, with circumferential wall thickening and infiltrative growth along the submucosa. ACC has a slower growth rate and a lesser tendency to invade locally than SCC. CT shows a well-defined soft tissue mass infiltrating the airway wall and, in the late stages, the surrounding mediastinal fat. Circumferential wall thickening can produce localized stenosis, which is better appreciated in the coronal and sagittal MPR images. PET-CT shows high FDG-avidity in ACC.

A third malignant neoplasm is mucoepidermoid carcinoma (MEC). MEC arises from the minor salivary glands lining the tracheobronchial tree. It typically occurs in patients younger than 40 years. MEC is usually located in more distal airways compared to SCC and ACC, commonly involving the lobar and segmental bronchi. The CT appearance of MEC is an oval or lobulated endobronchial mass, with mild contrast enhancement (differential diagnosis with carcinoid).

Carcinoid tumors are rare neuroendocrine neoplasms that range from low-grade (typical) to intermediate-grade (atypical) to high-grade small cell carcinomas. Like MEC, carcinoid neoplasms affect patients in their 40s. Carcinoid is the most frequent bronchial tumor in childhood and may produce hormones and neuroamines (e.g., adrenocorticotropic hormone, serotonin, somatostatin). Symptoms related to airway obstruction, such as chronic cough, recurrent infection, and hemoptysis, are more frequent than symptoms produced by hormone secretion. On CT, carcinoid appears as a smooth rounded intraluminal or lobulated mass that may contain calcifications (Fig. 36.6). Carcinoid tumors may have low FDG avidity on a PET-CT scan. Other imaging modalities include somatostatin receptor scintigraphy and Octreoscan, a nuclear medicine technique that uses a somatostatin-radiolabeled analogue (octreotide).

BENIGN NEOPLASMS

Benign neoplasms are less frequent than malignant ones, accounting for less than 2% of all lung neoplasms. On

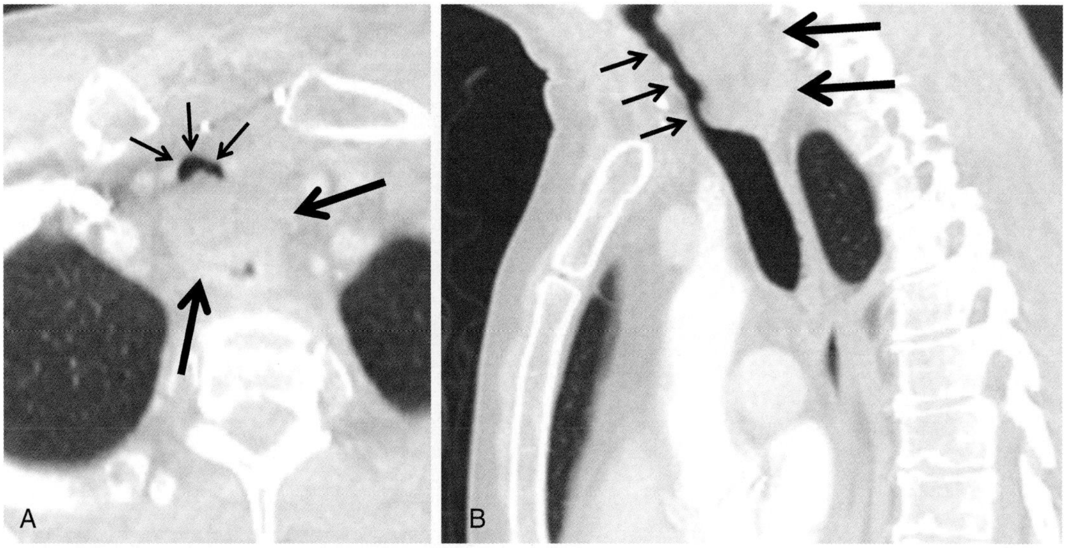

Figure 36.3 A 50-year-old man with anaplastic thyroid cancer invading the trachea. Axial (A) and coronal reformation (B) CT images show a soft tissue mass *(large arrows)* next to the trachea. The mass invades the trachea, causing luminal narrowing *(small arrows)*.

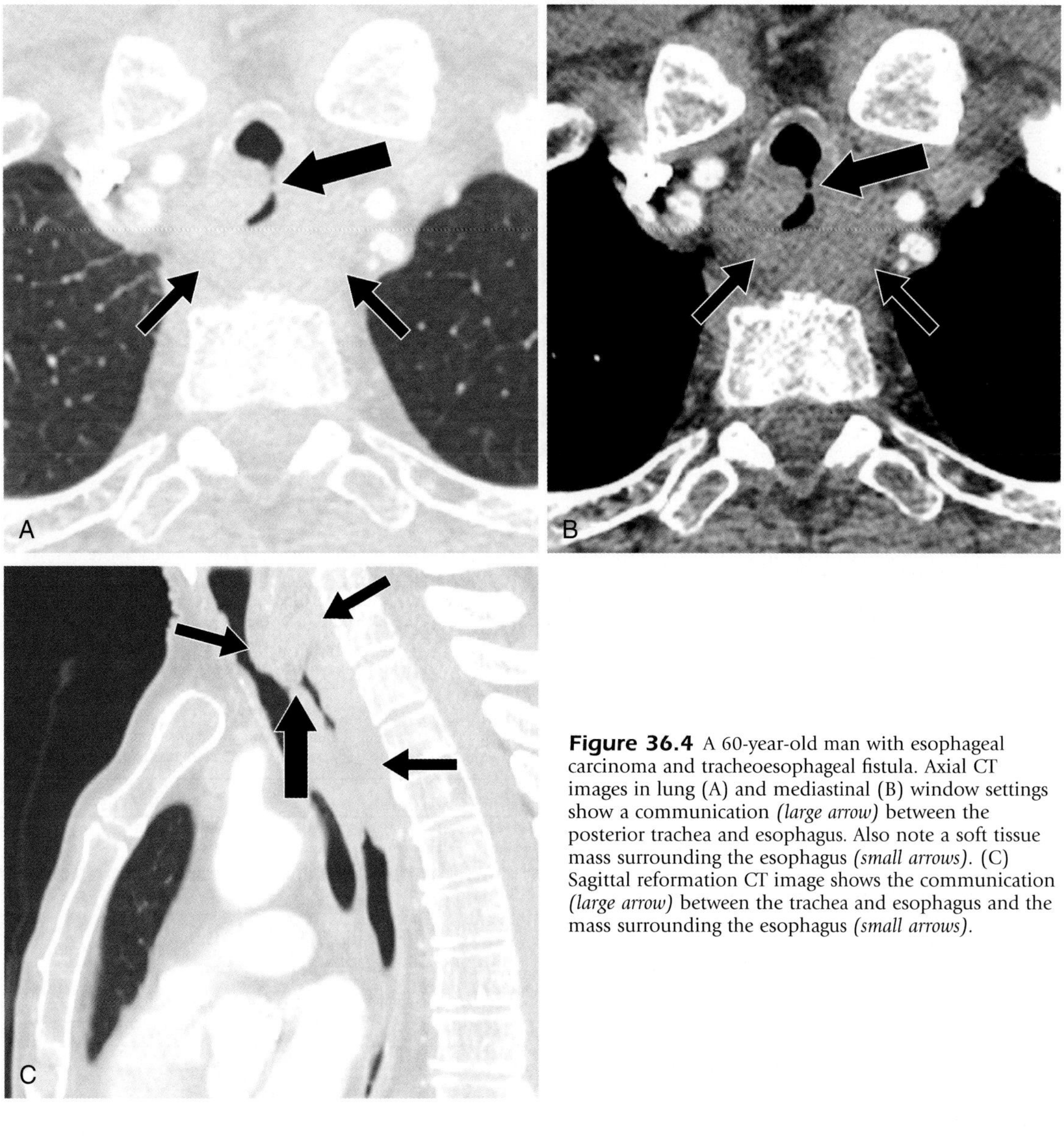

Figure 36.4 A 60-year-old man with esophageal carcinoma and tracheoesophageal fistula. Axial CT images in lung (A) and mediastinal (B) window settings show a communication *(large arrow)* between the posterior trachea and esophagus. Also note a soft tissue mass surrounding the esophagus *(small arrows)*. (C) Sagittal reformation CT image shows the communication *(large arrow)* between the trachea and esophagus and the mass surrounding the esophagus *(small arrows)*.

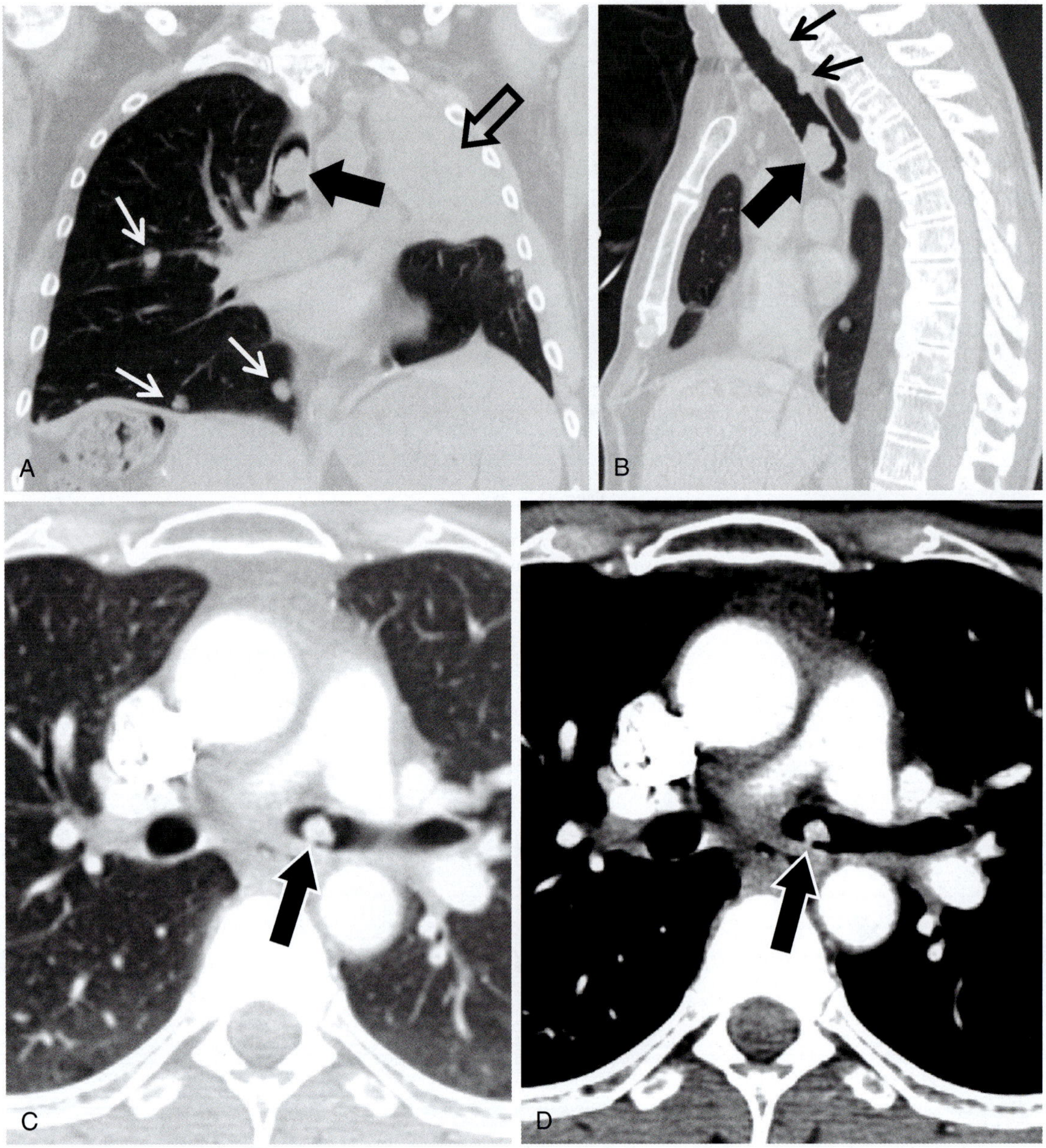

Figure 36.5 Central airway metastases. (A and B) A 60-year-old man with rectal cancer metastases. The coronal reformation CT image (A) shows a soft tissue mass *(black solid arrow)* in the trachea. Note postobstructive atelectasis *(open black arrow)* of the left upper lobe and multiple nodules *(white arrows)* in the lung parenchyma. (B) Sagittal CT reformation image shows the soft tissue mass in the nondependent *(large arrow)* trachea and a second soft tissue mass *(small arrows)* in the dependent trachea. (C and D) A 48-year-old woman with breast cancer metastasis. Axial CT images in lung (C) and mediastinal (D) window settings show a round soft tissue mass *(arrows)* in the left main stem bronchus.

CT, benign tumors appear as masses that are within the tracheobronchial lumen and do not show local invasion or distant metastases. Some of these tumors have typical features that help their characterization on CT (Table 36.5).

Squamous cell papillomas and hamartomas are the most common benign neoplasms of the central airways. Squamous cell papillomas can be single or multiple. The single form frequently involves the larynx and bronchi, less commonly the trachea, in male adults and is associated with smoking. Multiple papillomas, also known as *laryngotracheal papillomatosis*, are associated with human

TABLE 36.5 Typical Features of Airway Tumors

FEATURE	TUMOR TYPE
Fat-contacting lesions	Lipoma, hamartochondroma
Intralesional calcifications	Hamarthoma, chondroma, carcinoid
Fat and calcifications contacting lesions	Hamartoma
High contrast enhancing tumors	Carcinoid, hemangioma, fibroma and glomus tumor

papilloma virus infection (types 6 and 11). It is usually acquired at birth, leading to a high incidence in young children. On CT, papillomas appear as pedunculated lobulated nodules within the airways, without calcification or fatty content (Fig. 36.7). When involving the lung, papillomatosis produces multiple lung nodules, with a predominantly posterior lung distribution that can cavitate. Lung lesions can degenerate to carcinoma, so continuous follow-up is warranted.

Hamartomas are neoplasms containing a mixture of fat, cartilage, fibrous tissue, and epithelial components. These tumors are usually located in the lung parenchyma; the most common airway location is in the segmental bronchi. On CT, they appear as well-circumscribed lesions ranging from a few millimeters to 2 to 3 cm (Fig. 36.8). Hypodense and hyperdense foci within the lesion can represent fat and calcifications.

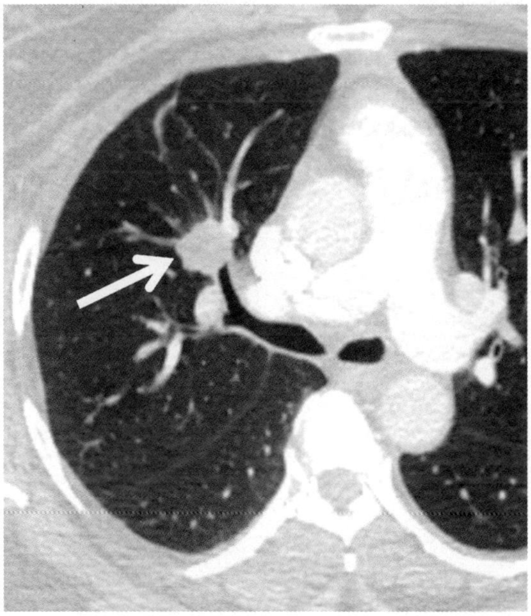

Figure 36.6 A 48-year-old woman with carcinoid. This axial CT image shows a soft tissue spiculated mass *(arrow)* obstructing the right upper lobe bronchus proximally (positive bronchus sign).

Lipomas account for less than 0.1% of the benign lung tumors. On CT, these tumors appear as well-defined, intraluminal, low-density masses, frequently associated with signs of bronchial obstructions such as atelectasis and postobstructive pneumonitis.

Myoblastomas are uncommon benign neoplasms that usually affect the head and neck region and, rarely, the central airway. These neoplasms occur most frequently in women in their 40s. On CT, they have the common appearance of polypoid intraluminal masses, with soft tissue density associated with signs of bronchial obstructions.

Schwannomas are rare neurogenic tumors originating from the schwann cells of the nerve sheath. On CT, they appear as well-circumscribed, low tissue density masses, with strong contrast enhancement.

Leiomyomas are more frequently found in the bronchi than in the trachea. On CT, leiomyomas usually appear as oval lesions, with associated postobstructive changes and mild contrast enhancement.

Neoplasm mimickers are soft tissue masses resembling a neoplasm. Mucus is the most common neoplasm mimicker found in the airways (Fig. 36.9). In most cases, it can be differentiated from a neoplasm because of its low-attenuation air bubble content, location in dependent airway portions, and mobility after coughing. However, when thick and strongly adhering to the airway wall, it may be difficult to distinguish from a neoplasm. If it persists after follow-up imaging, bronchoscopy is recommended for the differential diagnosis. Other neoplasm mimickers are broncholithiasis, tracheobronchopathia osteoplastica, amyloidosis, and focal infection, which will be discussed in the following sections.

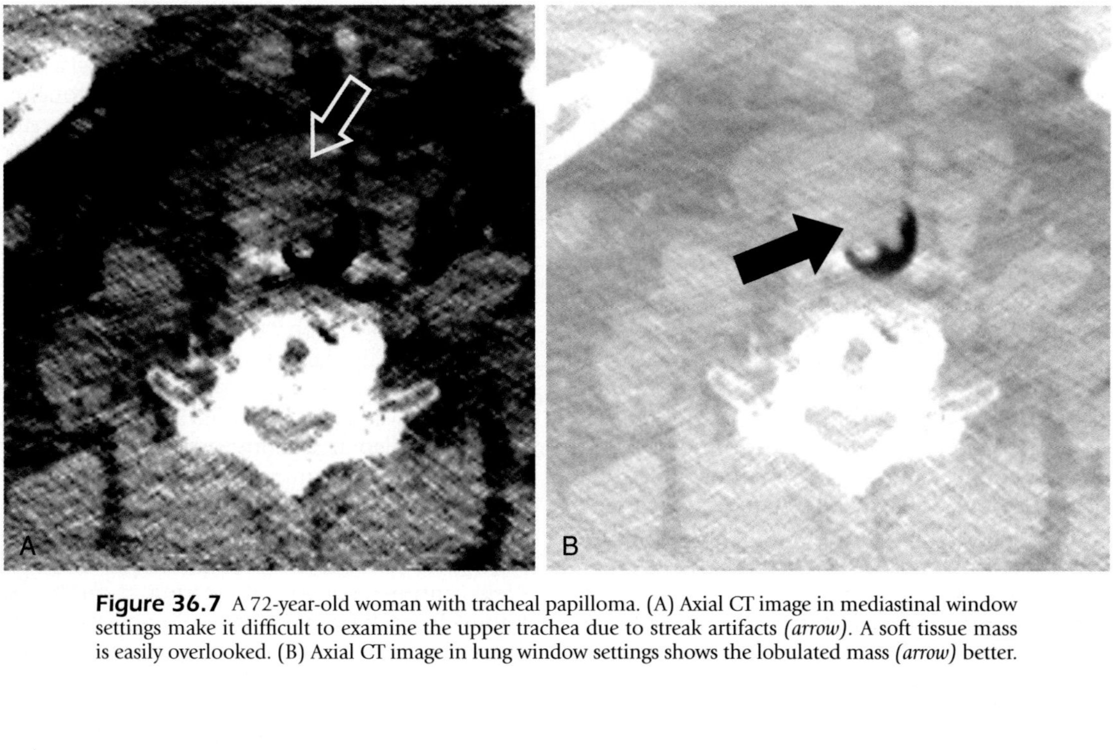

Figure 36.7 A 72-year-old woman with tracheal papilloma. (A) Axial CT image in mediastinal window settings make it difficult to examine the upper trachea due to streak artifacts *(arrow)*. A soft tissue mass is easily overlooked. (B) Axial CT image in lung window settings shows the lobulated mass *(arrow)* better.

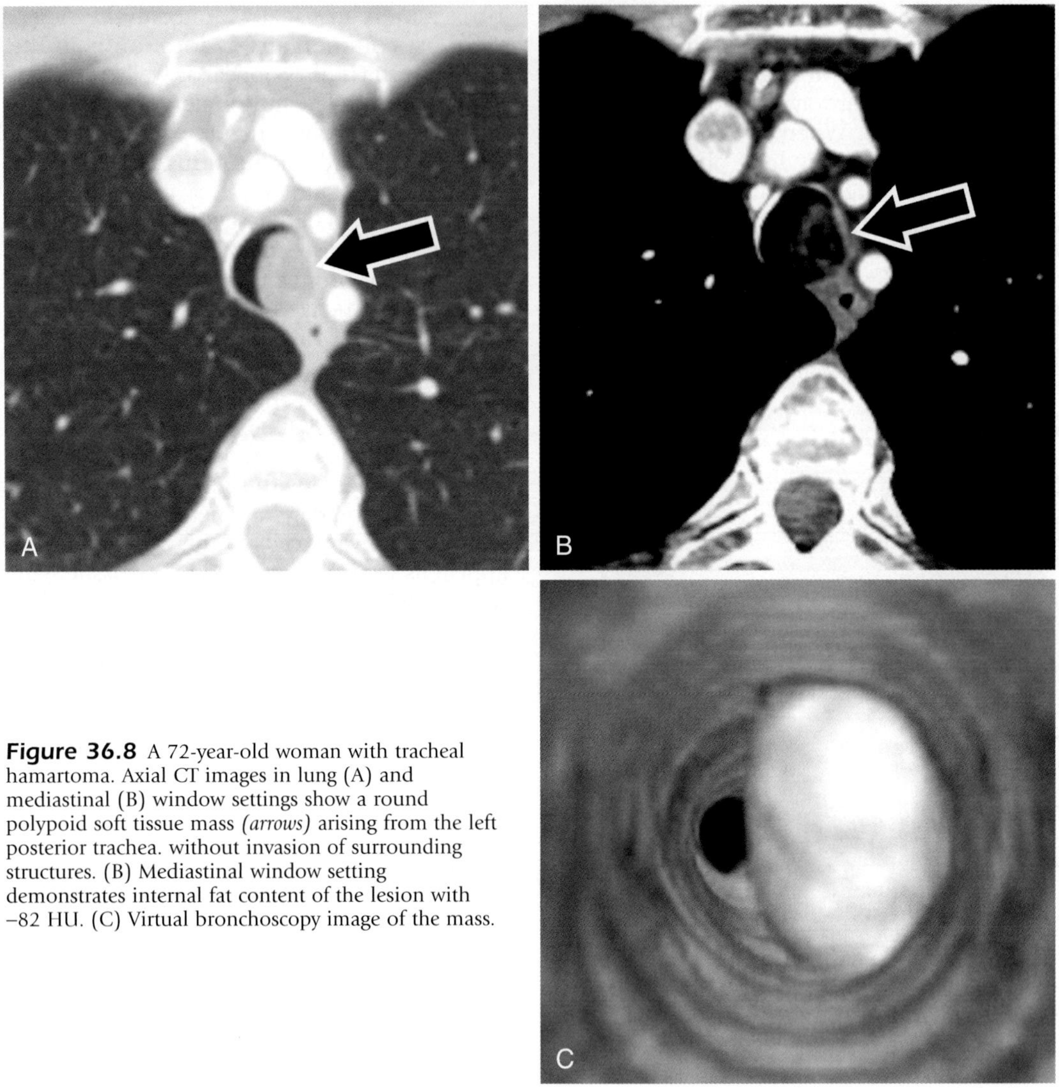

Figure 36.8 A 72-year-old woman with tracheal hamartoma. Axial CT images in lung (A) and mediastinal (B) window settings show a round polypoid soft tissue mass *(arrows)* arising from the left posterior trachea. without invasion of surrounding structures. (B) Mediastinal window setting demonstrates internal fat content of the lesion with –82 HU. (C) Virtual bronchoscopy image of the mass.

Focal Congenital Anomalies

Congenital tracheobronchial variants are frequently found in clinical practice, with a prevalence ranging from 1% to 12%. They are frequently asymptomatic and may be associated with cardiovascular (e.g., pulmonary artery slings, right-sided aortic arch anatomy) or other anomalies. However, severe congenital anomalies of the central airways, including tracheal agenesis and TEF, are rare and present early in life.

Bronchial atresia is the focal and mostly juxtahilar lack of a segmental bronchus, associated with normal distal airways. The most common site of bronchial atresia is the left upper lobe, especially the apicoposterior segmental bronchus. The bronchi distal to a site of atresia may be filled with mucus and dilate, forming a bronchocele. The alveoli distal to the site of bronchial atresia are ventilated through collateral ventilation, which may produce focal hyperinflation or trapped air. CXR findings include perihilar tubular opacity, with or without an air-fluid level, and surrounding hyperlucency due to trapped air (Fig. 36.10). On CT, it appears as tubular or ramified mucus-filled bronchus with distal trapped air, which is better depicted on the expiratory scan. If collateral ventilation is missing, bronchial atresia may cause atelectasis or cystic dilation of the lobe. Bronchial atresia is usually asymptomatic and incidentally diagnosed, although recurrent infection or pneumothorax can occur.

Congenital tracheobronchial stenosis is characterized by lumen reduction greater than 50%. It is usually due to tracheobronchial wall anomalies (e.g., disproportionate cartilage) or an intraluminal diaphragm. Most frequently, stenosis is focal (type 3), but can also be diffuse (type 1) or funnel-like (type 2). Tracheobronchial stenosis can also be caused by extrinsic compression from surrounding structures such as vascular rings, displaced innominate arteries, and vascular slings (Fig. 36.11). Tracheobronchial stenosis is also frequently associated with congenital lobar emphysema and venolobar syndrome.

Primary tracheobronchial diverticulum is an interrupted division of the primary lung bud. It is usually encountered at the level of the trachea, originating from the right side a few centimeters above the carina. It can be associated with TEF, tracheal stenosis, and congenital pulmonary airway malformation. The differential diagnosis must

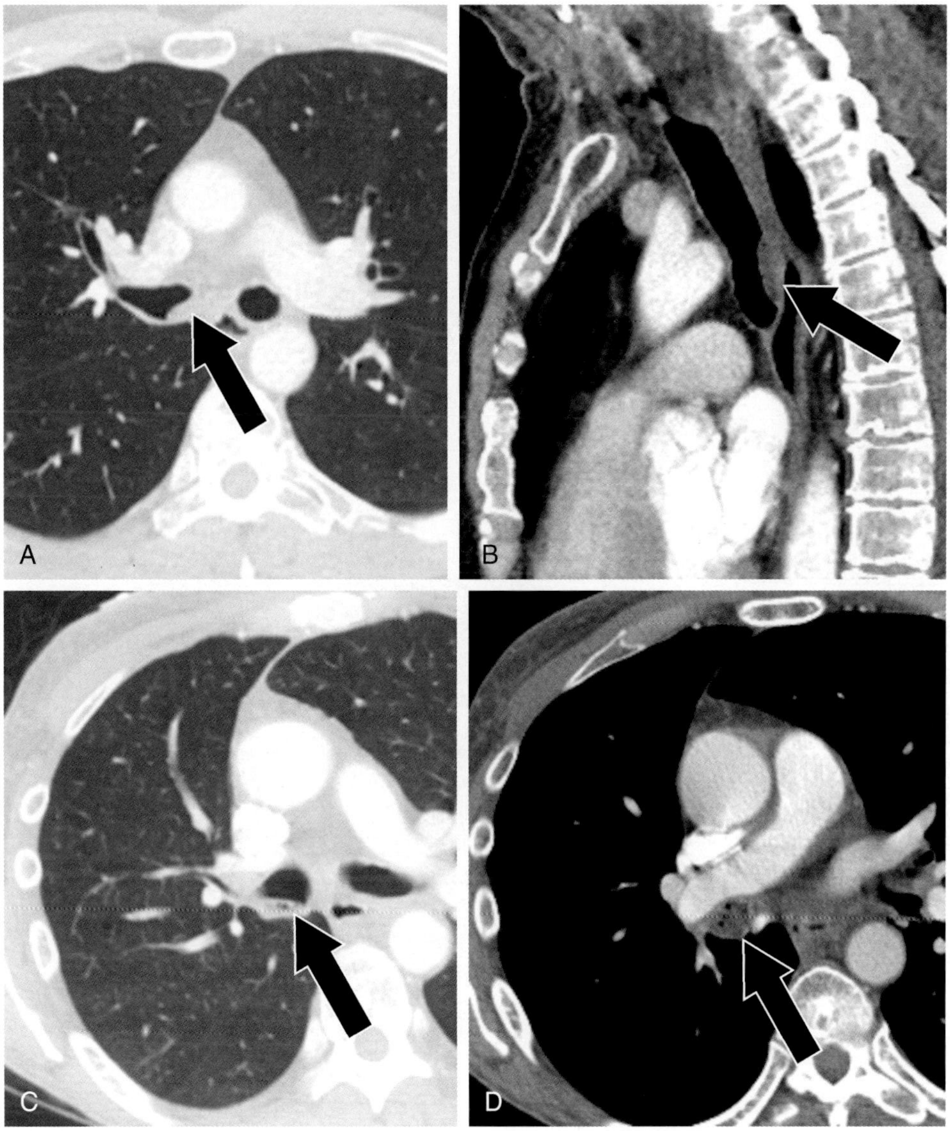

Figure 36.9 (A and B) Mucous secretions in a 50-year-old woman. (A) Axial and sagittal reformation (B) CT images show a soft tissue mass *(arrows)* in the dependent portion of the trachea (B) extending down to the right main stem bronchus (A). (C and D) Axial CT images in a 44-year-old man show a soft tissue mass with air bubbles *(arrows)* in the dependent portion (C) of the right main stem bronchus, causing bronchial obstruction (D).

be made with acquired diverticula such as tracheocele, laryngocele, Zenker diverticulum, and bronchogenic cyst.

Tracheal bronchus (TB) describes an abnormal bronchus usually originating from the distal trachea and directed toward the right upper lobe (Fig. 36.12). TB can be rudimentary, forming a blind pouch. Displaced bronchi occur more frequently than a supernumerary TB. When the entire right upper lobe bronchus is displaced, it is referred to as a *pig bronchus*. This may cause a correctly positioned endotracheal tube to undergo segmental or lobar collapse. TB is normally asymptomatic but may produce recurrent infection, cough, stridor, and hemoptysis. Clinical symptoms are more frequent in supernumerary TB and those occurring to the left. Bronchiectasis, atelectasis, focal emphysema, and cystic lung malformation can be present. TB is also associated with other congenital anomalies, including supernumerary lobes, tracheal stenosis, partial anomalous pulmonary venous return, and other congenital heart diseases.

An accessory cardiac bronchus (ACB) usually originates from the inner wall of the bronchus intermedius or, less frequently, from the right main bronchus. If ACBs have a blind extremity, the presence of airway cartilage can help differentiate ACBs from diverticulum. ACBs are usually incidentally discovered but may cause recurrent infections, cough, or hemoptysis. ACBs are associated with tracheal bronchi and bronchiectasis.

A bridging bronchus (BB) is an extremely rare airway abnormality characterized by an anomalous bronchus crossing the midline of the mediastinum from one side to the other. There are two types of BB. In the first classic type, the right lower lobe is ventilated by a bronchus originating from the medial aspect of the left main bronchus. In this type, the right main bronchus may be missing or may be represented by a short diverticulum. This is frequently associated with tracheal stenosis or lung hypoplasia. However, the right main bronchus may also be present at the level of the carina, ventilating the right upper lobe.

In the second type of BB, the right lower lobe is ventilated by a bronchus originating from the distal anterior aspect of the carina. This is called an *anterior*

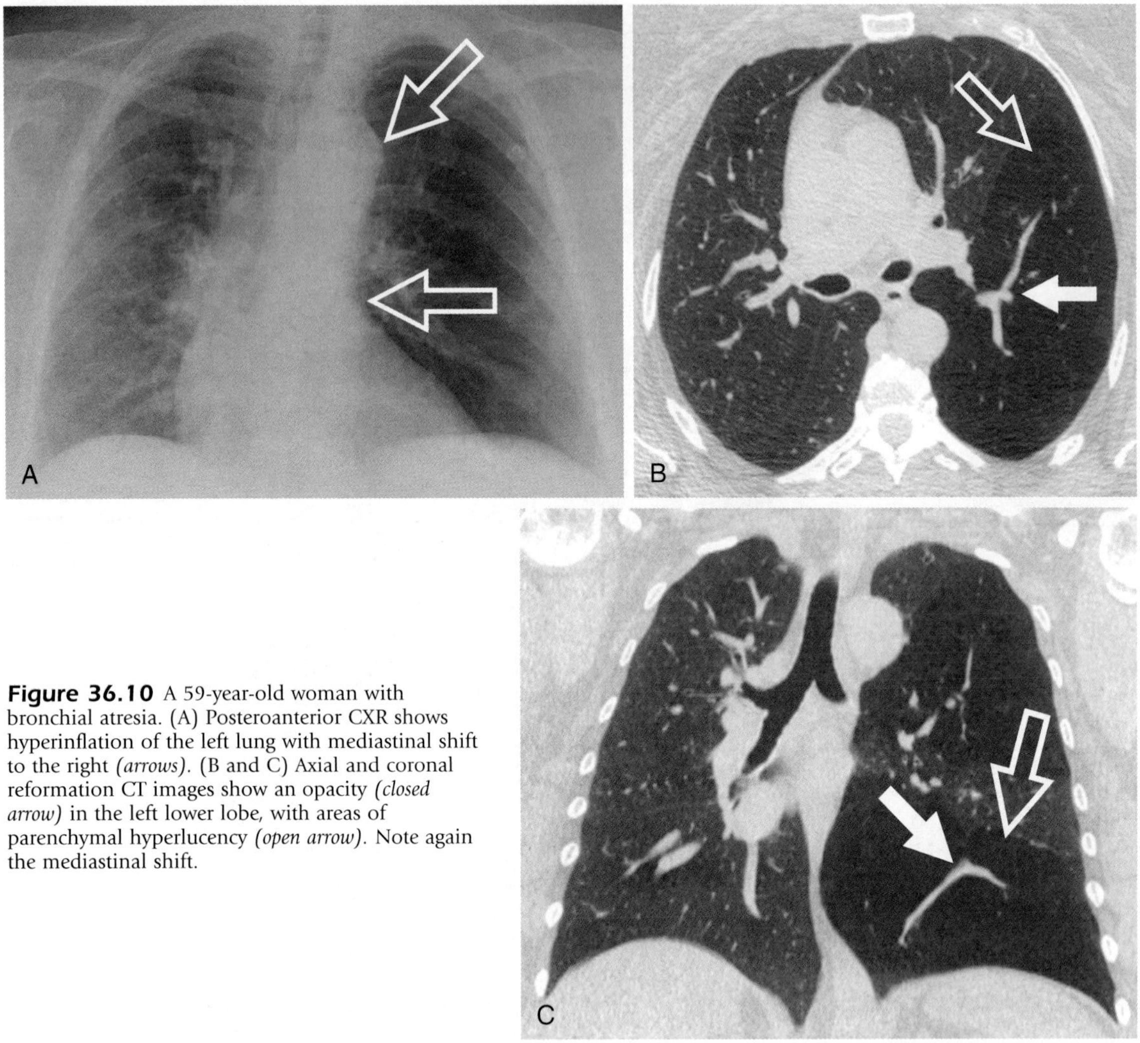

Figure 36.10 A 59-year-old woman with bronchial atresia. (A) Posteroanterior CXR shows hyperinflation of the left lung with mediastinal shift to the right *(arrows)*. (B and C) Axial and coronal reformation CT images show an opacity *(closed arrow)* in the left lower lobe, with areas of parenchymal hyperlucency *(open arrow)*. Note again the mediastinal shift.

bridging bronchus. It is important to differentiate BB from TB because BB is frequently associated with tracheal and bronchial stenosis, along with other congenital abnormalities.

BB creates a so-called pseudocarina located to the left of the midline of the trachea at T5–T7 as compared to the normal level of the carina at T4–T5. The course of the BB is more horizontal than the right main bronchus. The BB is usually accompanied by other malformations, such as vascular anomalies, pulmonary anomalous venous return (PAVR), and cardiac malformations. BB is usually symptomatic, presenting with recurrent lung infection, respiratory distress due to airway stenosis, and signs of obstruction, such as atelectasis and bronchiectasis.

Acquired Airway Diverticula

Acquired diverticula are protrusions of the mucosa through a weak point of the posterolateral wall (e.g., between the cartilaginous rings). They are usually located on the right side, at the level of the thoracic inlet. Acquired diverticula are frequently encountered in patients with chronic obstructive pulmonary disease (COPD), asthma, or congenital airway dilation (e.g., tracheobronchomegaly of Mounier-Kuhn disease). Less frequently, they can be due to the traction mechanism of adenopathy or fibrosis. Acquired diverticula are frequently asymptomatic and an incidental finding, but sometimes can present with nonspecific symptoms, such as cough, recurrent infection, hemoptysis, and stridor. The typical CT appearance is of a focal outpouching of the air adjacent to the main airway (Fig. 36.13). It is difficult to differentiate between primary and secondary diverticula, although position and the presence of cartilage may favor the diagnosis of congenital diverticula.

Broncholithiasis

Broncholithiasis is the presence of calcified or ossified material in the airway lumen. Most frequently, this is caused by erosion and extrusion of a calcified adjacent lymph node into the airway lumen, usually associated with chronic necrotizing granulomatous diseases. Other less common causes are as follows: (1) aspiration of bone tissue or endobronchial calcification of a chronic FB; (2) erosion and extrusion of calcified bronchial cartilage plates; and (3) migration of calcified material into the bronchus from a remote site, such as pleural plaque or kidneys through a nephrobronchial fistula. The most

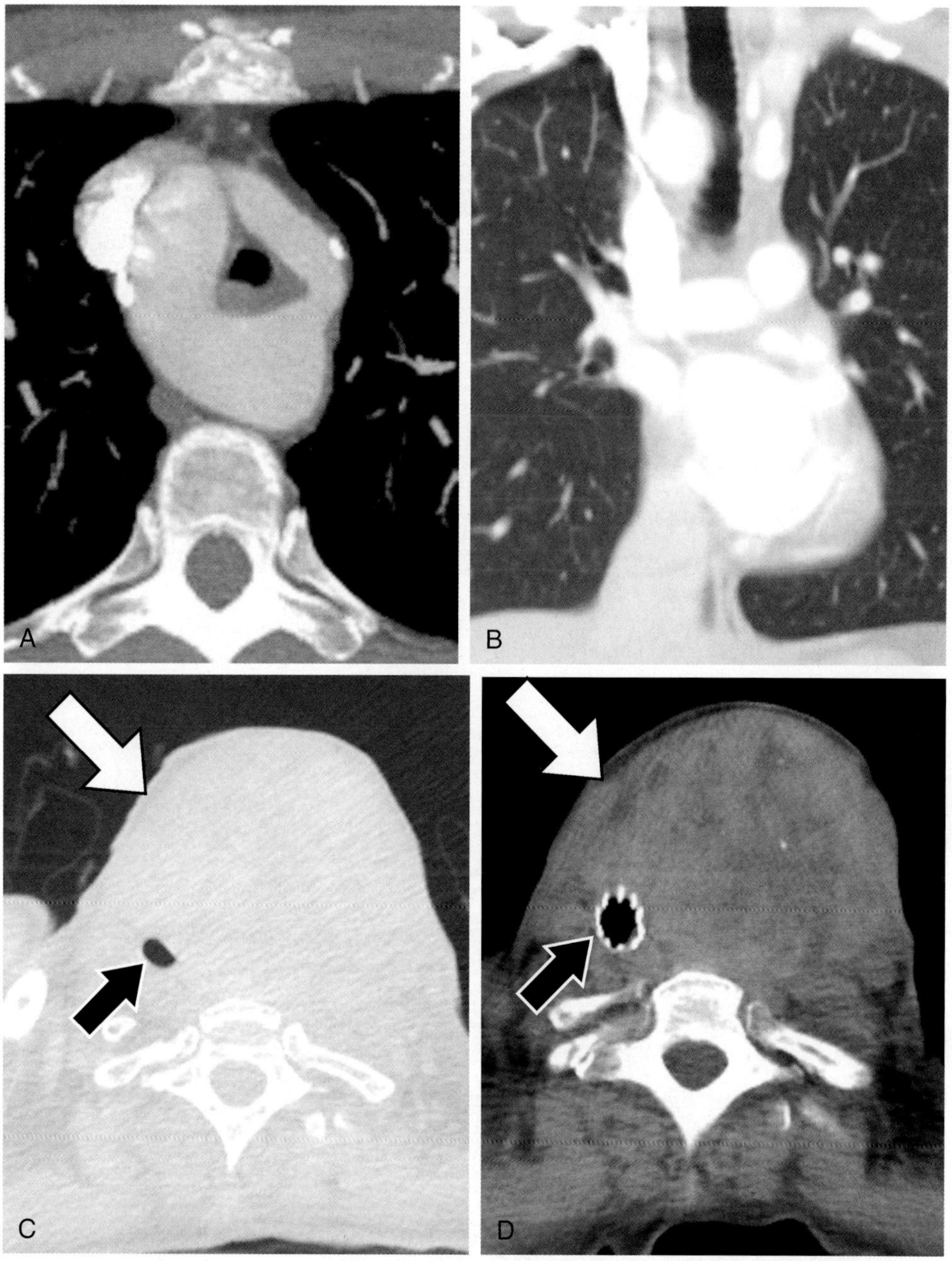

Figure 36.11 (A and B) Extrinsic airway compression in a 64-year-old man with a double aortic arch. (A) Axial minimum intensity projection and coronal (B) reformation CT images show a vascular ring encompassing the trachea, causing luminal narrowing. (C and D) An 82-year-old woman with goiter. Axial CT images show a large cervical soft tissue mass *(white arrows)* compressing the trachea *(black arrows)*. (D) This was treated by endoluminal stenting.

common symptoms of broncholithiasis are nonproductive cough, hemoptysis, and recurrent infection. Some patients may expectorate calcified material (lithoptysis), therefore facilitating the diagnosis. Rare complications are bronchoesophageal or bronchoaortic fistulas. On CXR, signs of obstruction, such as atelectasis, mucus impaction, and bronchiectasis, more frequently depict calcified material, in particular when small. A possible indirect sign of broncholithiasis at CXR is the disappearance or dislocation of a previously identified calcified focus on serial radiographs. On CT, the endobronchial or peribronchial calcified nodule can be identified along with signs of obstructions such as atelectasis, bronchiectasis, mucus impaction, and obstructive pneumonitis. To differentiate endobronchial from peribronchial calcified nodules, MPR with a bone or wide window setting (e.g., WL, 300 HU; WW, 1800–2000 HU) is used.

Anthracofibrosis

Bronchial anthracofibrosis (BAF) is a rare disorder of the central airways, with an unknown cause. BAF is characterized by bronchial inflammatory narrowing produced by submucosal anthracotic (from the Greek *ánthrakos*, meaning "coal") material. BAF is more common in Asian countries and tends to affect mostly nonsmoking females. BAF is associated with *Mycobacterium tuberculosis* infection and the inhalation of biomass fuel smoke. Symptoms are not specific and include cough, dyspnea, and chest pain. On CT, the bronchial narrowing produced by BAF is usually multifocal (one to five segments) and often bilateral (segmental or lobar). The trachea and main bronchi are usually not involved. Associated findings are atelectasis, consolidation, interstitial changes, and calcified or noncalcified lymphadenopathy. The right middle lobe is the most commonly affected site, followed by the right

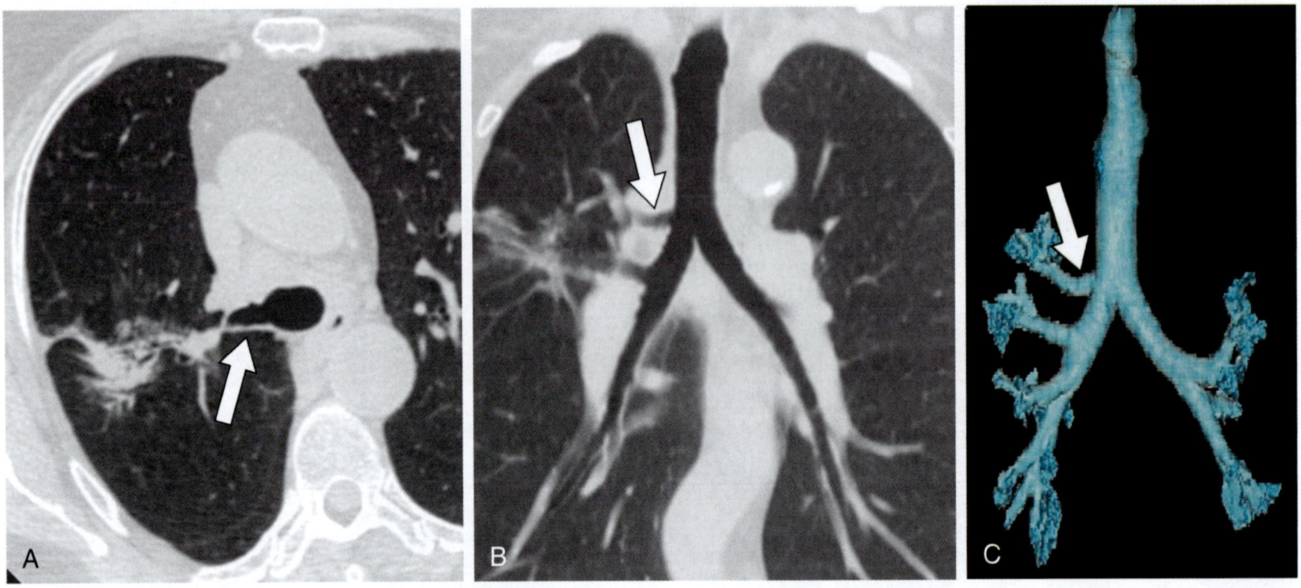

Figure 36.12 A 77-year-old woman with tracheal bronchus. Axial (A), coronal reformation CT (B), and three-dimensional reconstruction images (C) show a bronchus *(arrows)* arising from the trachea at the level of the carina, supplying the apical segment of the right upper lobe.

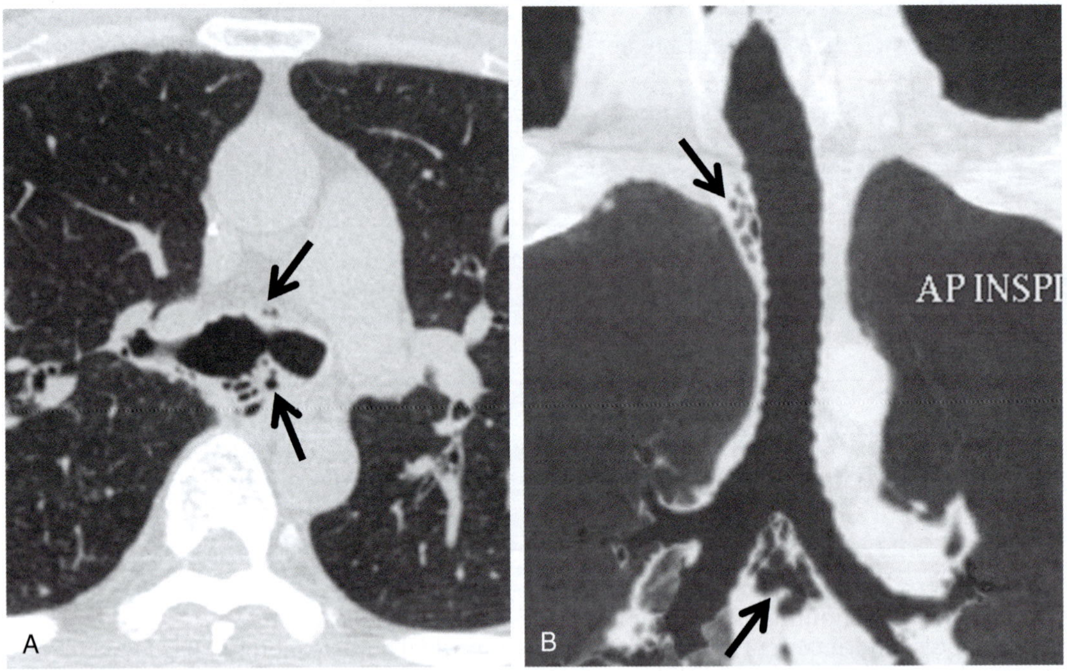

Figure 36.13 A 46-year-old man with airway diverticulosis. Axial (A) and coronal minimum intensity projection reformation (B) CT images show multiple diverticula *(arrows)* arising from the trachea and bronchi.

upper and left upper lobes. However, imaging findings are nonspecific and difficult to differentiate from bronchogenic carcinoma and tuberculosis. Thus, diagnosis is typically made via bronchoscopy and biopsy.

Foreign Bodies

Aspiration of an FB is more common in children than adults. In adults, FB aspiration tends to occur in subjects with neurologic abnormalities or drug or alcohol addictions that impair the swallowing reflex. Patients present with a sudden attack of coughing, choking, and dyspnea, with or without vomit. This clinical presentation is also called *penetration syndrome* and represents the most predictive factor in the clinical suspicion of FB aspiration. Other associated symptoms are recurrent and unresolved pulmonary infection, severe respiratory distress, cyanosis, and respiratory muscle retraction. Symptoms depend on FB location; when located more distally in the lobar or subsegmental bronchi, they can be minimal or absent. In adults, the FB is usually located in the right bronchial tree due to the acute angle of the right main bronchus; in children, both sides are affected equally.

On CXR, FB can be directly seen only if radiopaque (Fig. 36.14). However, FBs are frequently not radiopaque, and therefore only indirect signs, such as atelectasis, hyperinflation, mediastinal shift, and obstructive emphysema, may be present. In almost half of patients (40%), the CXR is normal. In those cases, a high clinical suspicion should prompt a bronchoscopic evaluation. Bronchoscopy is considered the reference standard for the diagnosis of tracheobronchial FB and is used for the removal of the FB. Therefore it is usually preferred over cross-sectional imaging modalities. CT is used to assess missed or retained FBs after initial bronchoscopy.

Infection

Several types of infection can affect the central airways. Here the most frequent types that result in short focal segment stenosis—endobronchial tuberculosis (EBTB), scleroma, and fungal infections—will be discussed.

EBTB is an infection of the tracheobronchial tree by *M. tuberculosis*. Bronchial stenosis is present in up to 68% of patients with EBTB in the acute stage and in up to 90% of patients in the chronic stage. The most common site of involvement is the right upper lobe and right main bronchus. EBTB accompanies lung parenchymal TB in 10% to 40% of patients suffering with tuberculosis. It has different clinical presentations depending on the site, extent of involvement, and stage. Respiratory symptoms are usually not specific, such as a chronic cough that does not respond to antitussive medication and progresses over months. Occasionally, patients may have bronchorrhea, hemoptysis, and chest pain. Examination of sputum samples results in variable diagnostic yields, whereas PFTs are commonly restrictive. The CXR is abnormal in less than 10% of patients, so CT is the primary modality used because it allows for the detection and assessment of focal lobar or segmental bronchial stenosis with secondary collapse, hyperinflation, or obstructive pneumonia (Fig. 36.15). A lobar tree-in-bud appearance is a sign of bronchogenic dissemination. CT can also be valuable for planning a bronchoscopy, which is allows for an accurate diagnosis via tissue biopsy.

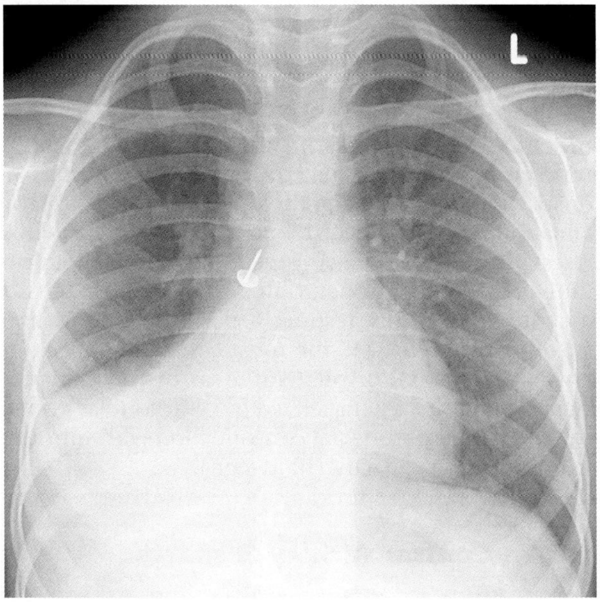

Figure 36.14 A 5-year-old boy with foreign body (FB) aspiration. This posteroanterior chest x-ray shows an opaque FB consistent with a pushpin in the bronchus intermedius. Note collapse of the right middle and right lower lobes.

Scleroma is a chronic granulomatous disease of the upper airways caused by *Klebsiella rhinoscleromatis*, a gram-negative bacterium. Scleroma infection is transmitted by air droplets and usually begins at the nose. It can, however, extend to the larynx, pharynx, and trachea. Scleroma infection progresses slowly over many years, with periods of remission and relapse. This disease is common in tropical and temperate zones such as Africa, Asia, South America, and Central America. Nasal and pharyngeal scleromas are more common in males, whereas laryngotracheal scleroma is more common in females; the age range of patients with scleroma is 20 to 40 years. Laryngotracheal scleroma is usually seen in the subglottic region at the fibrotic stage. Clinically, the most common symptoms are nasal obstruction, deformity, and epistaxis. The most frequent intrathoracic imaging finding is a symmetric or asymmetric circumferential subglottic stenosis, with extension into the trachea and the bronchi. Imaging is essential to narrow the differential diagnosis, but biopsy is usually needed to rule out other causes.

Endobronchial fungal infection is an underrecognized entity. Airway fungal colonization depends on environmental factors and host status. Risk factors are prolonged mechanical ventilation, steroid therapy, and lung transplantation. The most common agents, in decreasing order, are *Aspergillus* spp., *Coccidioides immitis*, fungi of the zygomycosis group, *Candida* spp., *Cryptococcus neoformans*, and *Histoplasma capsulatum*.

Aspergillus is a ubiquitous mold, without geographic predilections (Fig. 36.16). It represents the most common fungal airway colonizer in immunocompromised hosts. There are four different types of *Aspergillus* airway infection. Intracavitary aspergilloma is the most common type in immunocompetent hosts. The most important predisposing factor is the presence of a lung cavity, usually related to tuberculosis or sarcoidosis. Patients are often asymptomatic, with the most frequent sign being intermittent hemoptysis. CXR and CT show a cavity containing a soft tissue mass (fungus ball) producing the characteristic air crescent sign. When the aspergilloma fills the cavity, the lesion can be easily mistaken for a carcinoma. Allergic bronchopulmonary aspergillosis is a hypersensitivity reaction to *Aspergillus* characterized by excessive mucus production, abnormal mucociliary clearance, and mucoid impaction. The main predisposing factor is bronchial asthma. Patients present with symptoms of recurrent wheezing, low-grade fever, cough, increased sputum production, and chest pain. On CT, tubular mucoid filling involves the segmental and subsegmental bronchi, with a typical central distribution, and is seen more commonly in the upper lobes. Obstructed airways can induce atelectasis and areas of consolidation. When

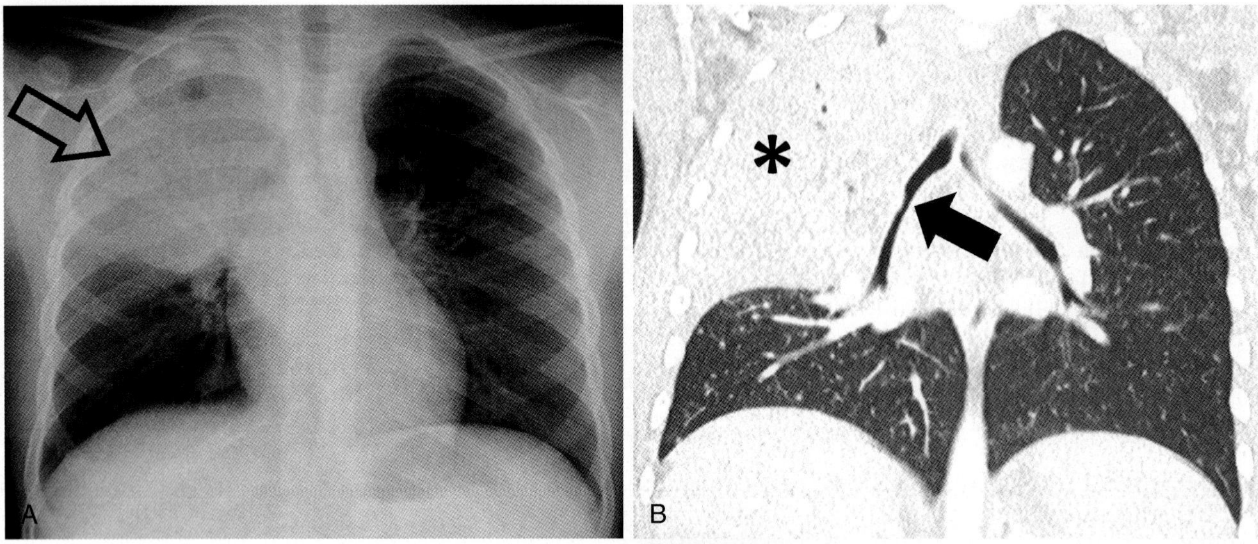

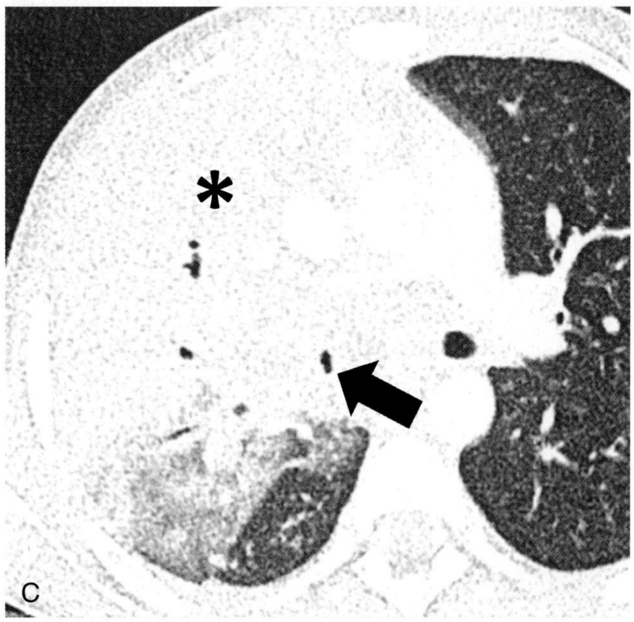

Figure 36.15 An 8-year-old boy with primary tuberculosis. (A) Posteroanterior CXR shows opacity *(arrow)* of the right upper lobe. Coronal reformation (B) and axial (C) CT images show narrowing *(arrows)* of the right main stem bronchus and opacity of the right upper lobe *(asterisks)*.

long-standing, the impacted bronchi can contain calcium deposits in 30% of patients.

Tracheobronchial aspergillosis usually occurs in lung transplant recipients, but also in other types of immunocompromised hosts, such as recipients of other solid organ transplants, patients with hematologic malignancies, and patients with HIV infection. Affected patients present with progressive dyspnea, cough, and hemoptysis. Occasionally, infected patients expectorate intraluminal mucus plugs. There are different patterns of *Aspergillus* tracheobronchitis. In obstructive bronchial aspergillosis, thick mucus plugs fill the airways, with little mucosal inflammation or invasion. In the ulcerative forms, there is focal invasion of the tracheobronchial mucosa. Finally, pseudomembranous tracheobronchitis is characterized by extensive inflammation and invasion of the tracheobronchial tree, with a pseudomembrane formation by necrotic debris and *Aspergillus* hyphae overlying the mucosa. On CT, it is difficult to detect *Aspergillus* tracheobronchitis, which can manifest as peribronchial thickening, small endobronchial nodules, and smooth or irregular bronchial narrowing. These findings are nonspecific; thus, to reach the diagnosis, bronchoscopy evaluation is usually needed. Invasive airways aspergillosis represents up to 10% of *Aspergillus* infections. It is commonly found in neutropenic and AIDS patients. Invasive aspergillosis typically results in peribronchial areas of consolidation. On CXR, the most common appearance is patchy unilateral or bilateral areas of consolidation, whereas on CT it is characterized by centrilobular nodular opacities and peribronchial consolidation with surrounding ground-glass opacity (halo sign).

Diffuse Central Airway Diseases

Long-segment airway involvement is seen in TBM, saber-sheath trachea, tracheobronchomegaly, sarcoidosis, granulomatosis with polyangiitis (GPA; Wegener granulomatosis), relapsing polychondritis (RP),

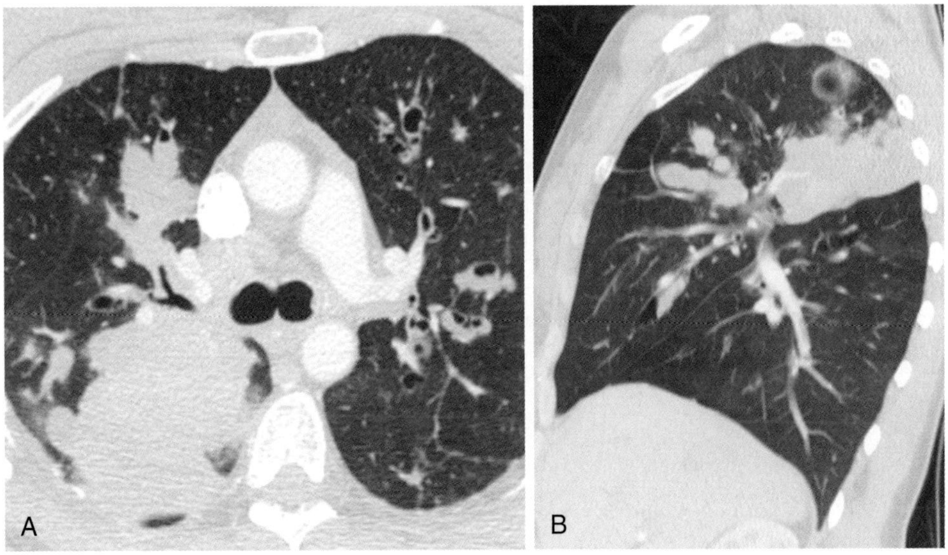

Figure 36.16 A 40-year-old woman with aspergillosis. Axial (A) and sagittal reformation (B) CT images show combination of cylindric bronchiectasis, endobronchial secretions, and large consolidation in the posterior segment of the right upper lobe. This combination of findings is consistent with allergic bronchopulmonary aspergillosis.

tracheobronchopathia osteoplastica, amyloidosis, and inflammatory bowel disease (IBD). The radiologic appearances of these diffuse airways diseases are summarized in Table 36.6.

Tracheobronchomalacia

TBM is a condition characterized by excessive tracheobronchial collapsibility. It is usually caused by weakness of the anterior and/or lateral airway walls caused by softening of the cartilage. These airway walls then bulge into the tracheal lumen with forced expiration or coughing (Fig. 36.17). Less frequently, in addition to the anterior and lateral parts, the posterior trachea is also involved, causing a concentric pattern of collapse. The cause of primary TBM is still unclear, although tracheal development abnormalities such as abnormal cartilaginous rings (e.g., decreased cartilage-to-muscle ratio or increased cartilaginous ring length) have been described. Primary TBM can also be associated with congenital anomalies such as TEF. Secondary (or acquired) TBM is associated with chronic endotracheal intubation, chronic airway inflammation, COPD, RP, and extrinsic compression. TBM is classified according to the severity of the collapse, location, and morphology (Table 36.7). A pathognomonic symptom is the so-called barking seal cough, which occurs in less than 5% of patients. More commonly, patients seek medical attention for recurrent respiratory tract infections, dyspnea on exertion, and wheezing. Consequently, TBM is frequently mistaken for asthma and should be considered in patients refractory to asthma therapy. Similarly, PFTs are specific but frequently normal.

The optimal threshold to define TBM is still a matter of debate. The most common criteria are based on a collapse exceeding 50% on bronchoscopy. Different studies, however, have shown airway collapsibility exceeding this threshold in healthy volunteers. Airway collapsibility depends on the breathing maneuver that the patient is performing during images acquisition. During dynamic expiration, the degree of tracheal collapse is greater than at end-expiration. Therefore, tracheal collapse should be measured in dynamic expiratory acquisitions, with a threshold of 70% to avoid an overdiagnosis of TBM.

POTENTIAL PROBLEM: HOW AND WHERE TO MEASURE CENTRAL AIRWAY COLLAPSIBILITY

SOLUTION. Multidetector CT (MDCT) is the imaging modality of TBM screening. Two CT protocols can be used for TBM: (1) end-inspiratory and end-expiratory acquisitions; and (2) end-inspiratory and dynamic expiratory acquisitions. End-expiratory and dynamic expiratory imaging can be acquired with low-dose settings to reduce the cumulative dose. The first protocol includes two breath-hold acquisitions at TLC and RV, whereas the second protocol includes acquisition during specific breathing maneuvers. These maneuvers can include peak flow (FEV_1) or coughing maneuvers. In these maneuvers, image acquisition is triggered when the patient is forcefully exhaling or coughing. Currently, dynamic acquisitions are preferred over breath-hold acquisition because they elicit TBM better. However, in noncompliant patients, such as young children or intubated adults, breath-hold acquisitions are still used. On CT, TBM assessment starts by identifying and measuring the cross-sectional area (CSA) of the narrowest tracheal lumen during expiratory imaging (end-expiration or dynamic expiration). The same tracheal section is then identified in the end-inspiratory acquisition using anatomic references and measured to compute airway collapse, according to this formula:

$$\Delta\text{Tracheal lumen } (\%) = ([CSA_{insp} - CSA_{exp}])/(CSA_{insp}) \times 100$$

Associated findings of bronchial wall thickening, mucus plugs, atelectasis, and/or consolidation are better assessed in the end-inspiratory acquisitions, whereas trapped air is more easily detected in the expiratory images.

TABLE 36.6 Radiologic Appearance of Diffuse Airway Diseases

DRAWING	DISEASE	MOST AFFECTED SITE	WALL THICKENING	CALCIFICATIONS	MALACIA	LUMINAL STENOSIS
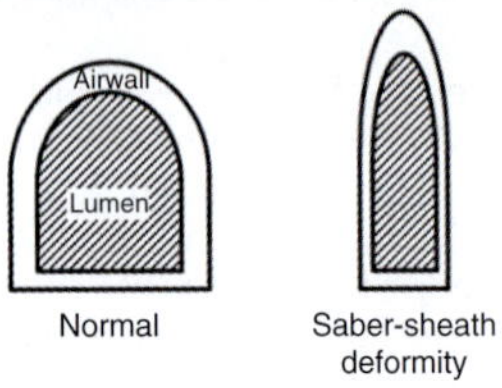 A	Saber-sheath deformity	Intrathoracic trachea	No	Possible	Yes	Yes
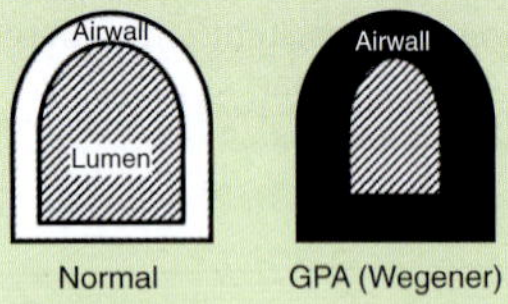 B	Granulomatosis with polyangiitis (GPA)	Subglottic	Nodular	Rare	Rare	Circumferential focal stenosis
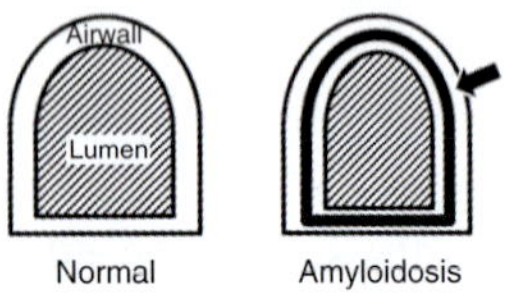 C	Amyloidosis	Tracheobronchial	Focal nodular or circumferential	Possible	Rare	Yes
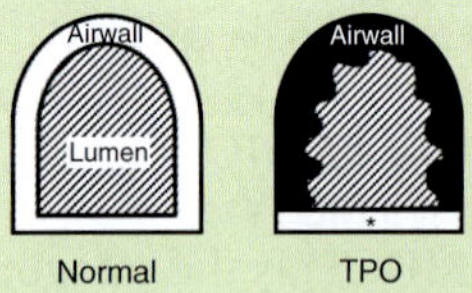 D	Tracheobroncho-pathia osteo-chondroplastica (TPO)	Lower two-thirds of the trachea and main bronchi	Diffusely nodular	Frequent	No	Yes
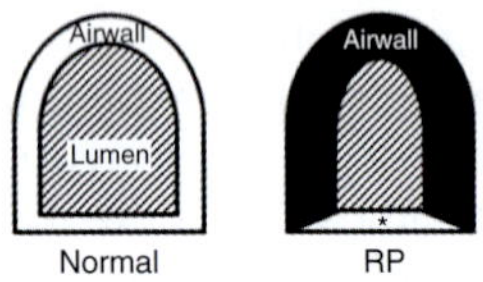 E	Relapsing polychondritis (RP)	Trachea	Both diffuse and smooth	Possible	Yes, frequent	Yes, especially in the acute phase
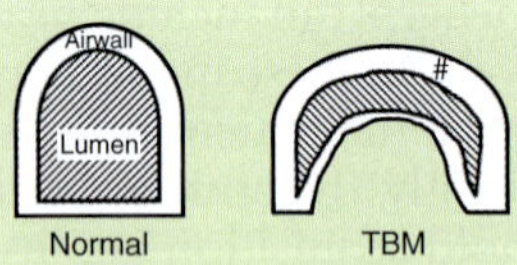 F	Tracheobroncho-malacia (TBM)	Trachea, main and lobar bronchi	Only present in case of recurrent infections	Possible, according to cause	Collapse >50% end-expiratory and >70% dynamic-expiratory imaging	Variable airway stenosis, worsened during physical exercise
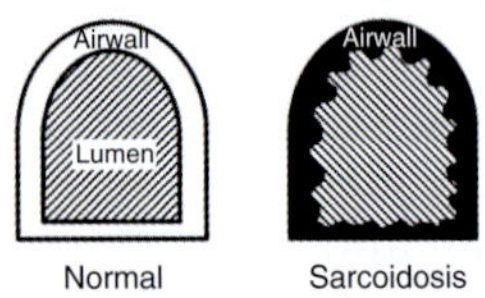 G	Sarcoidosis	Subglottic portion and proximal part of the trachea	Nodular thickening	Possible	Rare	Intrinsic or extrinsic

A, Coronal elongation in saber-sheath deformity; *B*, circumferential wall thickening in granulomatosis with polyangiitis; *C*, submucosa deposit of amyloid *(arrow)*; *D*, nodular thickening of the anterolateral wall *(black)* and sparing of posterior membrane *(asterisk)* in tracheobronchopathia osteochondroplastica; *E*, smooth anterolateral wall thickening, with sparing of the posterior membrane *(asterisk)* in relapsing polychondritis; *F*, frown appearance of tracheobronchomalacia (hashtag *[#]* represents possible thickening of the anterior wall in case of recurrent infection); *G*, irregular wall thickening in sarcoidosis.

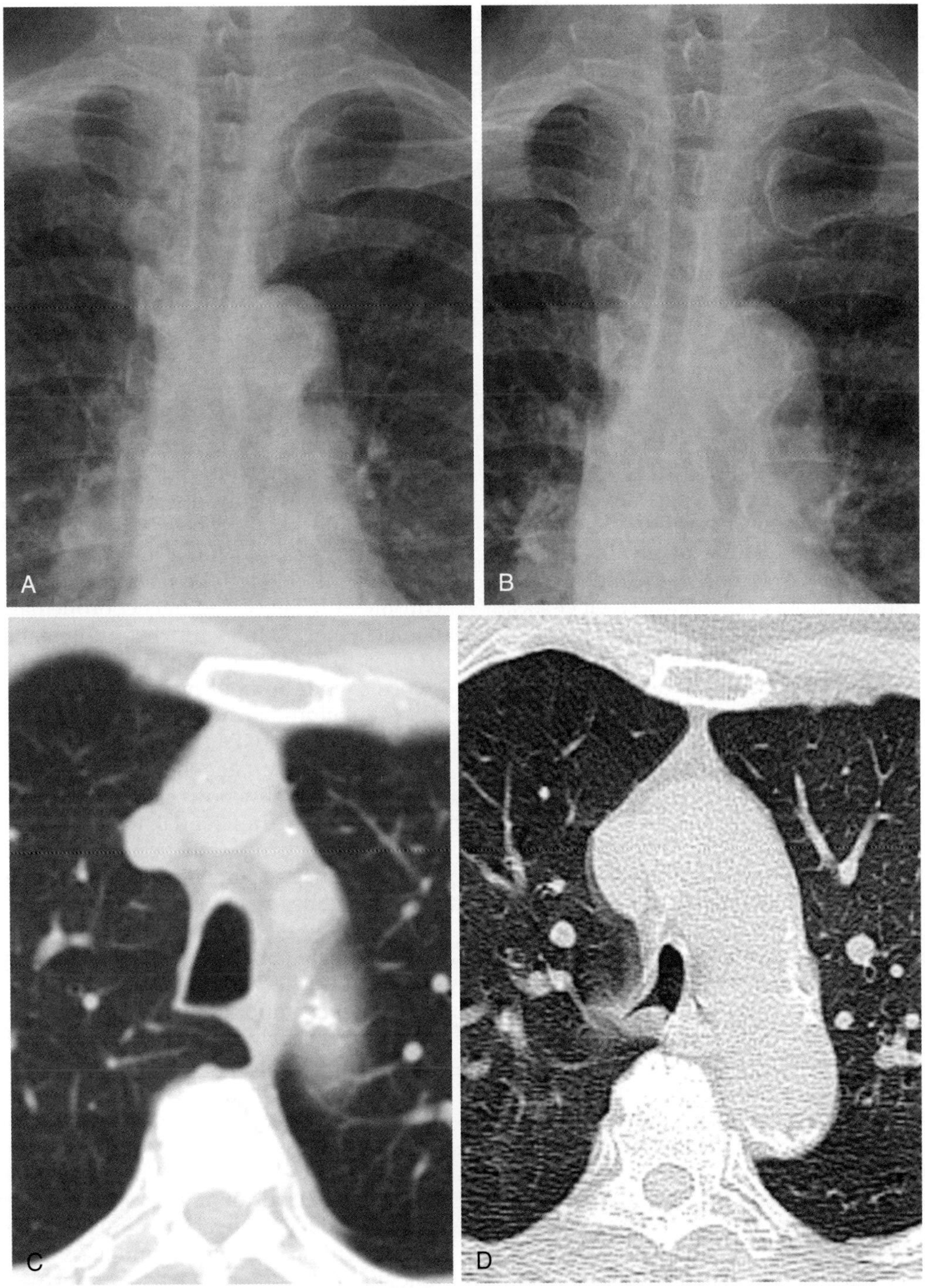

Figure 36.17 A 71-year-old patient with tracheobronchomalacia. Posteroanterior CXR shows normal configuration of the trachea in inspiration (A) and narrowing of the trachea in expiration (B). Axial CT images show saber-sheath configuration of the trachea in inspiration (C) and significant decrease of lateral tracheal diameter on expiration (D).

POTENTIAL PROBLEM: HOW TO DIFFERENTIATE TRACHEOBRONCHOMALACIA FROM EXCESSIVE DYNAMIC AIRWAY COLLAPSE

SOLUTION. Excessive dynamic airway collapse (EDAC) is a pathologic collapse of the airway lumen of more than 50%, which is entirely due to the laxity of the posterior wall membrane with structurally intact airway cartilage. EDAC is frequently misnamed as TBM, but it is pathophysiologically and morphologically different from TBM. Lung diseases most frequently associated with EDAC are COPD and asthma. The decreased transmural pressure and weakened posterior tracheal membrane facilitate collapse of the airways during coughing and/or forced expiration. A recent classification, based on bronchoscopic or radiographic studies, has graded EDAC according to functional status, extent, morphology, origin, and collapse severity. This classification not only allows

TABLE 36.7 Tracheobronchomalacia (TBM) Classifications

CRITERIA	CLASSIFICATION
Location	Type I, bronchus intermedius and left main bronchi Type II, trachea and proximal main bronchi Type III, intrapulmonary segmental and distal bronchi
Severity	Mild, 50%–70% collapse Moderate, 70%–90% collapse Severe, >90% collapse
Morphology	Inspiratory lunate configuration (coronal-sagittal diameter >1): highly specific for TBM Inspiratory biconvex ("fish mouth") configuration: frequently associated with TBM Saber-sheath deformity (coronal-sagittal diameter <0.6): TBM common in chronic obstructive pulmonary disease patients Expiratory crescentic configuration ("frown sign"): high specificity for TBM Circumferential

TBM to be distinguished from EDAC, but also to monitor the progression or improvement of the disease process after treatment.

Saber-sheath deformity is characterized by coronal narrowing and sagittal widening of the intrathoracic tracheal diameter, with a coronal-to-sagittal diameter ratio of <0.6. Different from tracheomalacia, saber-sheath deformity produces a fixed obstruction and affects only the intrathoracic portion of the trachea. This is partially explained by the strong association with COPD, where chronically overinflated lungs compress the trachea and produce coronal narrowing.

Sarcoidosis

Sarcoidosis is a multiorgan granulomatous disorder characterized by the presence of noncaseating granulomas in involved organs. It typically affects individuals between 20 and 60 years, although it is more common in young adults. It can present with one or more of the following abnormalities: bilateral hilar adenopathy, pulmonary opacities, and skin, joint, and eye lesions. The respiratory system is usually involved, where the most common findings are the hilar and mediastinal adenopathy, followed by the parenchymal changes.

Airway involvement is frequently underestimated and tends to increase, according to the severity of the parenchymal involvement. Airway involvement is a negative prognostic factor and is associated with morbidity and mortality. Sarcoidosis can cause compression of the airways by enlarged lymph nodes, bronchial wall thickening (due to edema, granuloma formation, and mucosal friability), airway stenosis, and traction bronchiectasis by parenchymal fibrosis. The trachea and main bronchi are less frequently involved than distal airways and seldom produce symptoms. The main symptoms of airway sarcoidosis are a chronic cough due to reduced mucociliary clearance, mucosal edema, and erythema. CT is most commonly used to assess parenchymal changes and lymphadenopathy and can be helpful to assess airway involvement (Fig. 36.18). However, it can overestimate airway involvement and may cause false-positive results in up to 15% of cases. Bronchoscopy with biopsy is the method of choice to diagnose airway sarcoidosis. Treatment for sarcoidosis includes corticosteroids and immunomodulators. Interventional bronchoscopy is sometimes used to relieve severe symptomatic airway stenosis.

Granulomatosis With Polyangiitis (Wegener Granulomatosis)

GPA is a multisystemic disease involving the lungs, small arteries, and kidneys. It is a chronic relapsing disease of unknown cause, with a median survival of 22 years. Three forms characterize respiratory tract involvement: chronic rhinosinusitis, tracheobronchial disease, and parenchymal nodules. Tracheobronchial disease occurs in 15% to 55% of GPA patients. It is characterized by stenosis, endoluminal mass lesions, and, occasionally, TBM. Subglottic stenosis is the most common airway manifestation in GPA. This can be the initial presentation or may occur later, during the course of the disease. Tracheobronchial stenosis can be solitary or multiple and is frequently circumferential, with progressive concentric luminal narrowing. Calcification of the tracheal rings and bronchiectasis are also possible. Associated parenchymal findings are nodules, consolidation, ground-glass opacities, and mediastinal lymphadenopathy. Common symptoms are cough, hoarseness, hemoptysis, dyspnea, stridor, and wheezing.

Imaging is important to narrow the differential diagnosis and is usually combined with bronchoscopy. CXR usually shows multiple lung opacity but is not useful to assess tracheobronchial GPA, which is assessed by CT. CT findings include endotracheal nodules or an asymmetric soft tissue mass, with alterations of the tracheal rings (Fig. 36.19). Diffuse bronchial wall thickening can lead to segmental and lobar atelectasis. Other radiographic findings include bilateral and diffuse lung nodules, which may cavitate, along with ground-glass opacities and consolidations. Treatment of tracheobronchial GPA includes immunosuppressive drugs, interventional bronchoscopy procedures, and surgery for airway obstructions. Despite proper immunosuppressive treatment, a large number of patients with GPA experience progressive airway diseases.

Tracheobronchomegaly

Tracheobronchomegaly is a diffuse dilation of the trachea, also known as Mounier-Kuhn syndrome. This disease is usually seen in males in the fourth to fifth decades of life and results from a connective tissue weakness that leads to central airways enlargement. The diagnosis is made when the tracheal diameter is larger than 3 cm, the right main stem bronchial diameter is more than 2.5 cm, and the left main stem bronchial diameter is more than 2 cm.

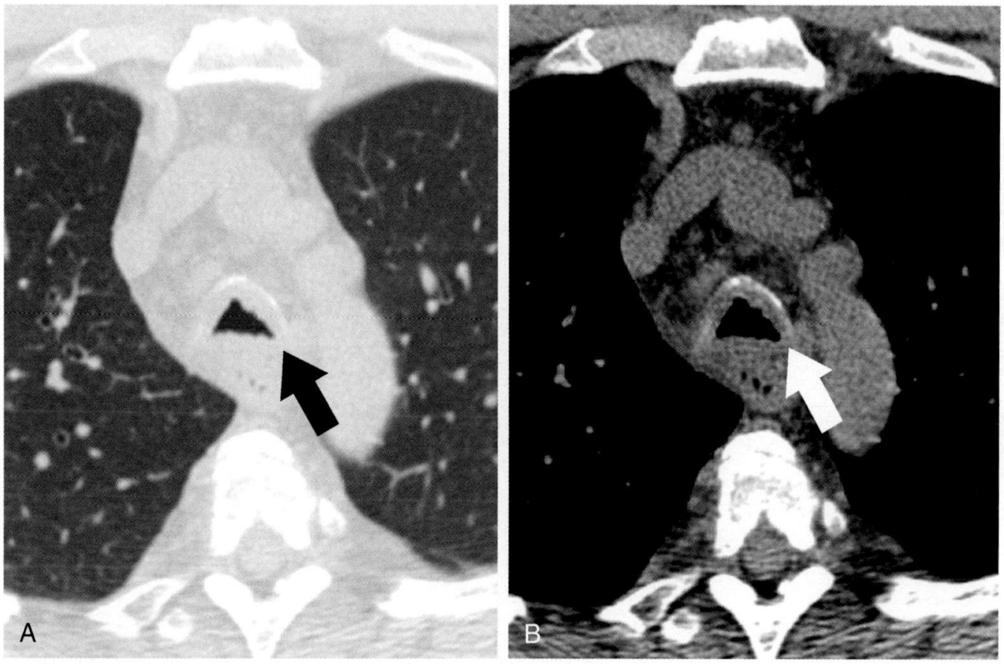

Figure 36.18 A 55-year-old man with sarcoidosis. Axial CT images in lung (A) and mediastinal (B) window settings show severe circumferential, irregular, wall thickening and luminal narrowing of the trachea *(arrows)*.

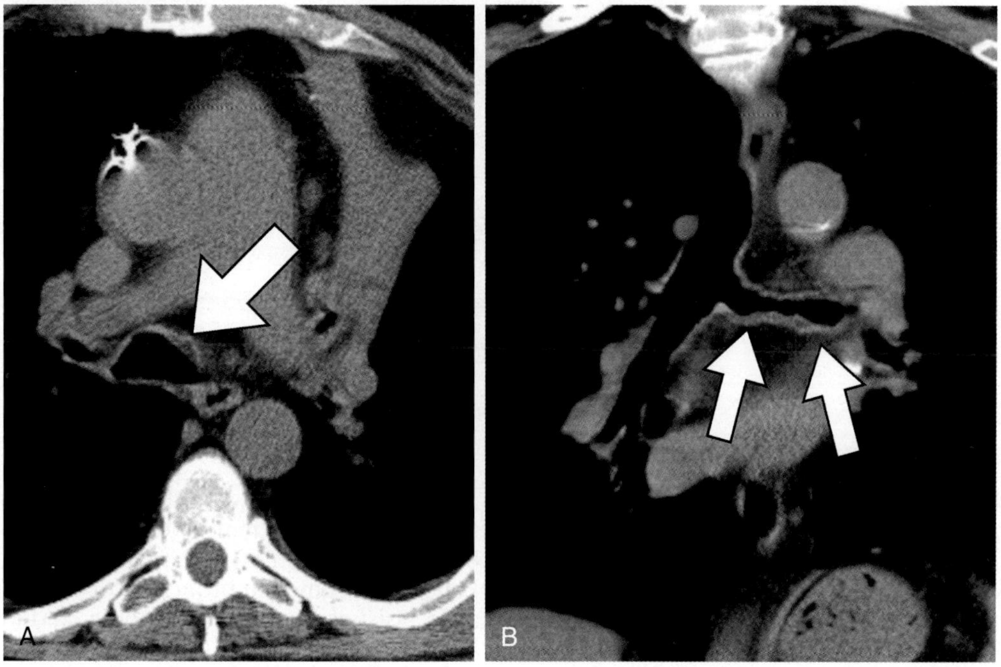

Figure 36.19 A 73-year-old man with granulomatosis with polyangiitis. Axial (A) and coronal reformation (B) CT images show wall thickening *(arrows)* of the left side of the trachea (A) and left main stem bronchi (B).

Increased flaccidity of the tracheal wall may result in expiratory collapse. Moreover, bronchiectasis and bronchial diverticula are common. Tracheobronchomegaly can also be seen in patients with cutis laxa or Ehlers-Danlos syndrome. Patients with tracheobronchomegaly are prone to recurrent respiratory infection due to reduced mucociliary clearance. Paired end-inspiratory and expiratory or dynamic expiratory CT is the modality of choice to diagnose tracheobronchomegaly and associated TBM (Fig. 36.20). Less frequently, diffuse tracheal dilation may also be the result of traction from fibrosis in severe idiopathic pulmonary fibrosis, end-stage sarcoidosis, postprimary tuberculosis, radiation therapy, fungal diseases, and pneumonectomy.

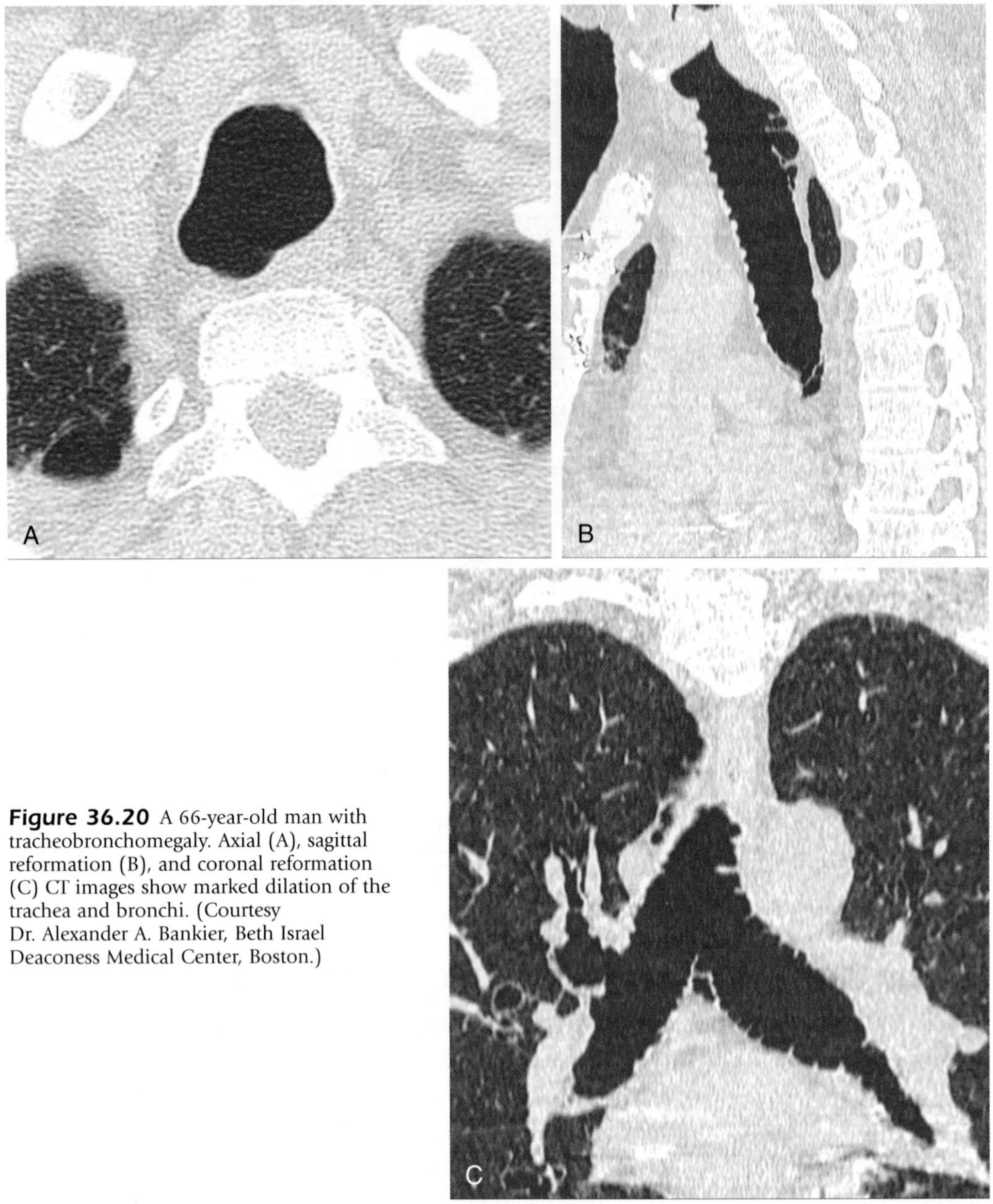

Figure 36.20 A 66-year-old man with tracheobronchomegaly. Axial (A), sagittal reformation (B), and coronal reformation (C) CT images show marked dilation of the trachea and bronchi. (Courtesy Dr. Alexander A. Bankier, Beth Israel Deaconess Medical Center, Boston.)

Relapsing Polychondritis

RP is a chronic multiorgan disease characterized by recurrent cartilage inflammation involving the ears, nose, joints, airways, and vessels. This disease has a female predominance and can affect patients of any age. Central airway involvement is present in 20% to 50% of patients. Patients with RP present with symptoms of airway obstruction, such as dyspnea, cough, stridor, and hoarseness. Airway obstruction is related to different mechanisms according to the disease stage—airway edema in the active stage and dynamic collapse due to cartilage destruction and stenosis in the fibrous stage.

On chest radiographs, RP can show long-segment tracheal stenosis and secondary signs of obstructions (e.g., pneumonia, atelectasis). CT is the preferred modality to assess RP, and dynamic expiratory imaging is recommended to assess the common findings of TBM better. Other important CT findings are multifocal or diffuse airway stenosis, airway wall thickening, calcification of the airway cartilage typically sparing the posterior membranous wall, and secondary air trapping (Fig. 36.21). Lobar and segmental bronchi obstruction may produce atelectasis, obstructive pneumonia, and bronchiectasis. Bronchoscopy in RP is used to assess the disease stage and severity of airway involvement.

Tracheobronchopathia Osteochondroplastica

Tracheobronchopathia osteochondroplastica (TPO) is a rare benign disease of unknown cause, with an overall prevalence of 0.12%. It has been described in association with chronic inflammation and infection, atrophic rhinitis, silicosis, amyloidosis, and mycobacterioses. The tracheobronchial abnormality in TPO consists of submucosal cartilaginous nodules connected to tracheal cartilage (ecchondromas), which subsequently undergo calcification and ossification. These cartilaginous or bony

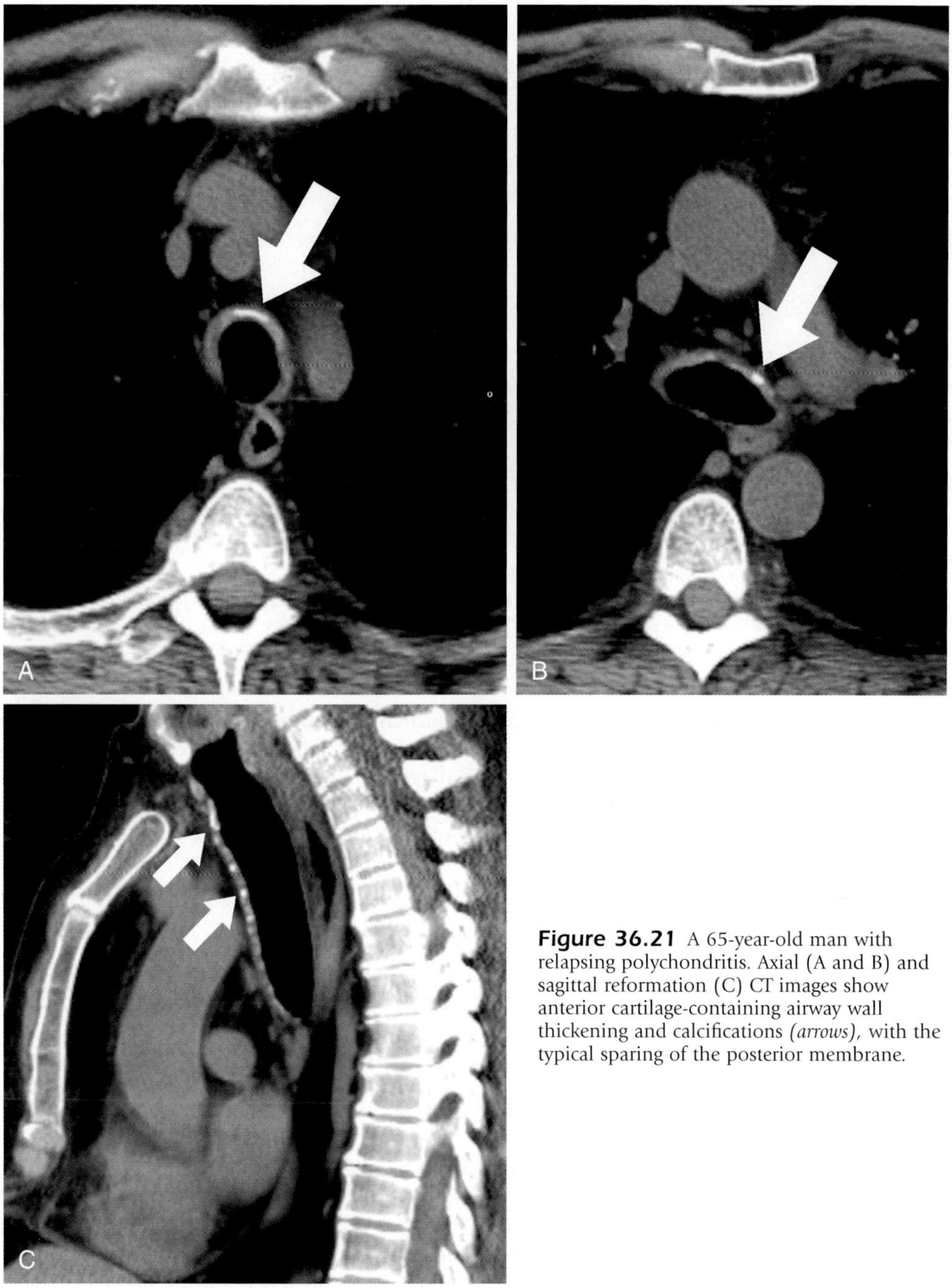

Figure 36.21 A 65-year-old man with relapsing polychondritis. Axial (A and B) and sagittal reformation (C) CT images show anterior cartilage-containing airway wall thickening and calcifications *(arrows)*, with the typical sparing of the posterior membrane.

submucosal nodules tend to increase in size and number over a period of years, obstructing the airway lumen. Interestingly, these nodules spare the posterior membrane of the trachea. Patients with TPO are usually in their sixth or seventh decade of life, although TPO has also been described in pediatric patients. TPO patients present with nonspecific symptoms, such as chronic cough, hoarseness, dyspnea, hemoptysis, and recurrent respiratory infection. Therefore, many patients are initially misdiagnosed as asthma or chronic bronchitis patients. Impairment of PFTs depends on the location and severity of the lesions. Moderately symptomatic patients can demonstrate an obstructive pattern, with abnormal flow-volume loops.

Imaging is important to narrow the differential diagnosis but can seldom lead to the diagnosis of TPO. CXR is usually negative although, rarely, airway calcification or findings related to airway obstruction (e.g., pneumonia, atelectasis, bronchiectasis) may be seen. CT typically shows numerous calcified or noncalcified cartilaginous nodules protruding in the airway lumen, with sparing of the membranous posterior wall (Fig. 36.22). When the posterior membrane is involved, other disease should be considered (e.g., amyloidosis). Other associated CT findings are bronchial wall thickening and a deformed tracheal cartilage, without external compression. Although bronchoscopy is the method of choice to confirm

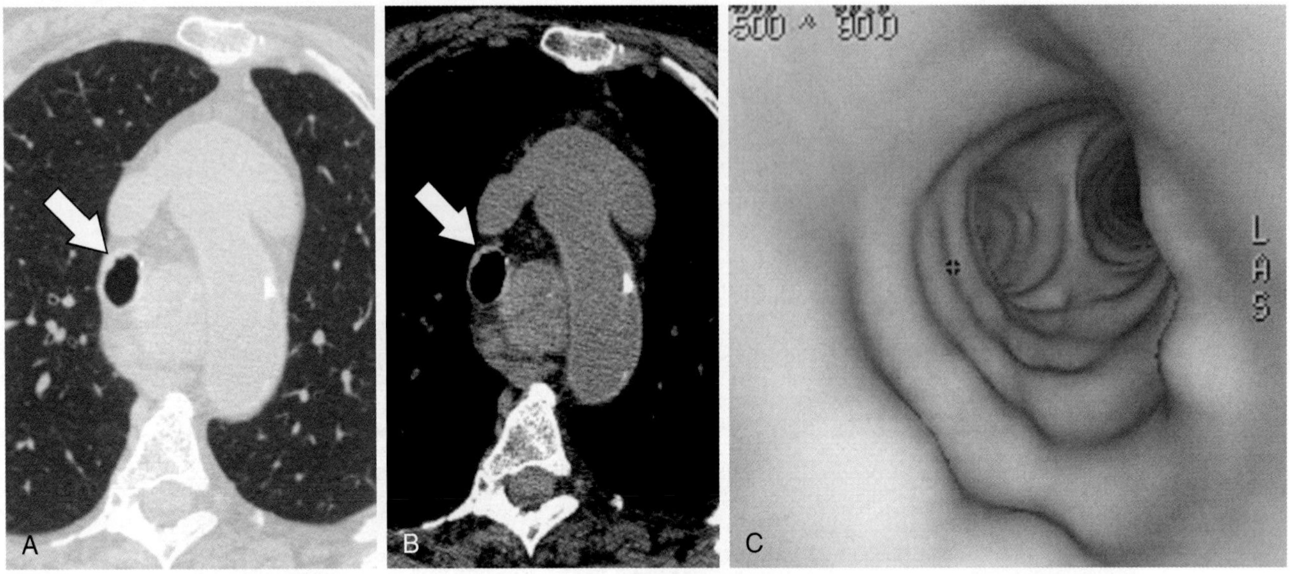

Figure 36.22 A 77-year-old woman with tracheobronchopathia osteochondroplastica. Axial CT images in lung (A) and mediastinal (B) window settings show nodular wall thickening *(arrows)* in the anterolateral trachea. (C) Virtual bronchoscopy shows nodular tracheal wall irregularities.

diagnosis, there is no curative treatment for TPO, so bronchoscopy is focused on improving the symptoms.

Tracheobronchial Amyloidosis

Tracheobronchial amyloidosis (TBA) is the most common of the three possible manifestations of pulmonary amyloidosis, which also include persistent diffuse interstitial deposit and parenchymal nodules (amyloidomas). Amyloidosis can be idiopathic or associated with various inflammatory, hereditary, or neoplastic diseases. TBA is more common in men after their fifth decade and can cause cough, hoarseness, stridor, airway obstruction, and occasionally hemoptysis. Airway obstruction can lead to atelectasis or recurrent pneumonia. Symptomatic TBA is usually characterized by focal airway abnormalities, which may warrant bronchoscopic or surgical resection. Diagnosis is usually obtained with biopsy and demonstration of a green birefringence on Congo red preparations.

On CT, TBA can be diffuse, infiltrative, with multifocal submucosal plaques, or nodular (Fig. 36.23). Diffuse irregular wall thickening with calcifications can involve any portion of the trachea to the segmental bronchi without sparing the posterior membrane (as seen in TPO). Associated findings are atelectasis, postobstructive pneumonia, and air trapping. In the differential diagnosis, MRI can be useful because amyloid deposits have an intermediate T1 signal intensity and low T2 signal intensity.

Inflammatory Bowel Diseases and Other Inflammatory Diseases

IBDs and other inflammatory diseases, such as Crohn disease, ulcerative colitis, and Behçet disease, can occasionally involve the airways. Among these diseases, ulcerative colitis is the most common. IBD airway involvement usually assumes an obliterative bronchiolitis pattern, but others, such as ulcerative tracheitis, tracheobronchitis, and bronchiectasis, have also been described. The diagnosis of airway IBD is frequently secondary to the gastrointestinal diagnosis. Imaging findings are not specific, and therefore the clinical history and bronchoscopy are important to reach the diagnosis. On CT, tracheobronchitis findings include concentric bronchial wall thickening, tracheal ring calcification, and bronchiectasis.

Potential Pitfalls and Their Solutions

Differentiating Secretions From True Endobronchial Lesions

Mucus plugs in the central airways can resemble endobronchial lesions. Some characteristics, such as low density (low HU), air bubble content, and dependent position, lean more toward mucus secretion diagnosis than to true lesions. However, in patients with chronic airway inflammation (e.g., COPD, cystic fibrosis), the secretions can demonstrate high CT density, without containing air, or may be located in nondependent areas in the airways. These can raise concern for malignant endobronchial lesions. In these cases, it is sufficient to reacquire end-inspiratory images after vigorous coughing and expectoration, which will move true secretions to a different location and upward. When there is no displacement, an endobronchial lesion should be considered, and further assessment by bronchoscopy is warranted.

Assessing Very Short Areas of Stenosis

As described, the craniocaudal extent of short-segment stenosis can be underestimated on axial images. In this case, MPR in the coronal and sagittal planes, along with

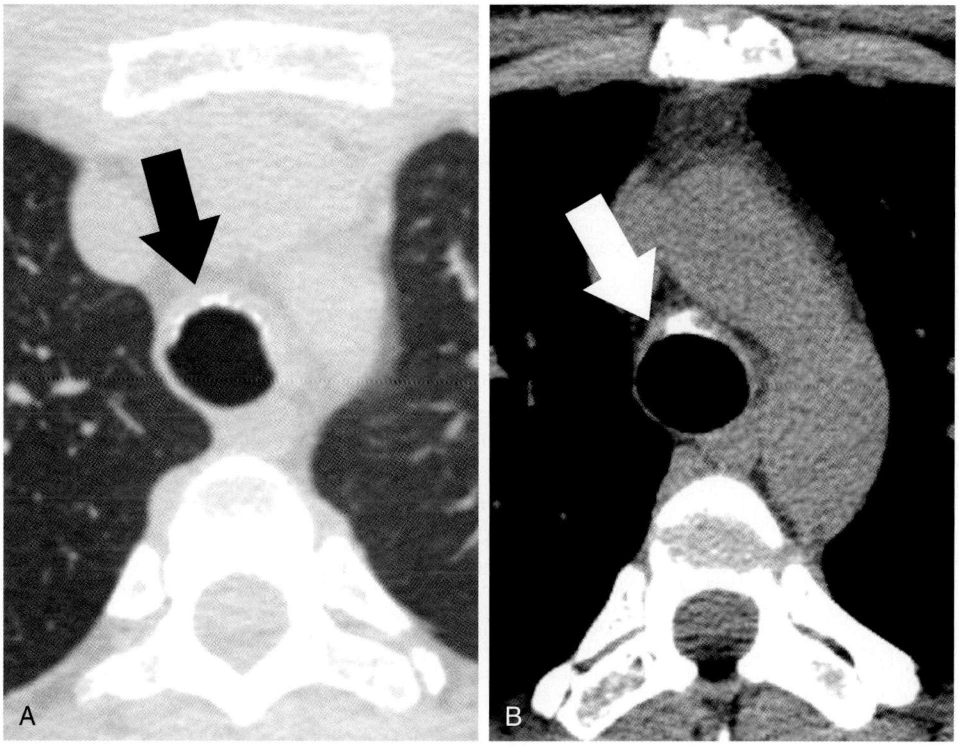

Figure 36.23 A 24-year-old woman with amyloidosis of the central airways. Axial CT images in lung (A) and mediastinal (B) window settings show severe smooth thickening *(arrows)* of the anterolateral trachea with calcifications.

curved planar reformats, will allow precise assessment of shape, extension, and relationship to surrounding structures of the stenosis.

Defining the Right Threshold for Excessive Collapsibility of the Airways in Healthy Individuals

The correct threshold to define TBM is still debated. The most used threshold of 50%, which derives from bronchoscopy evaluation, has not been proven to be useful. In fact, during dynamic expiratory imaging in adult healthy volunteers, a mean expiratory collapse of 54%, 67%, and 61% in the trachea, right, and left main stem bronchi, respectively, has been reported. This collapse can be even higher when forceful maneuvers such as coughing are used for expiratory imaging. In these cases, it is conceivable to use a higher threshold of up to 70% expiratory collapse to avoid TBM overdiagnosis. Finally, future studies are necessary to define the optimal threshold for TBM. The use of newer modalities in airway imaging, such as MRI, might help define this threshold, especially in the pediatric population, for whom CT radiation exposure remains a matter of concern.

Distinguishing Excessive Thickening of Cartilaginous Rings From Pathologic Narrowing

Excessive thickening of cartilaginous rings can be detected by comparison with adjacent tracheal rings. In pathologic conditions, an enlarged tracheal ring will appear larger and frequently distorted compared to the adjacent cartilaginous rings. This will also determine lumen narrowing, with the typical hourglass shape appearance of the stenosis in the coronal reformats.

■ Summary

Tracheobronchial imaging has been revolutionized by MDCT. 3D reconstruction and volume rendering techniques have overcome the limitations of axial image assessment. More recently, MRI has been introduced in airway imaging; its high tissue characterization and temporal resolution might improve diagnostic capability in airway imaging. Moreover, its free radiation technique may play a larger role in the pediatric population.

The trachea should be carefully visualized and scrutinized on CXR to detect possible abnormalities, which can be further investigated with CT and/or MRI. A higher detection rate of central airway diseases can be obtained when their classification in focal and diffuse pathology is better understood. This classification can help develop a practical diagnostic algorithm for evaluating central airway diseases.

Bibliography

Abdel Razek AA. Imaging of scleroma in the head and neck. *Br J Radiol.* 2012;85(1020):1551–1555.

Abu-Hijleh M, Lee D, Braman SS. Tracheobronchopathia osteochondroplastica: a rare large airway disorder. *Lung.* 2008;186(6):353–359.

Baughman RP, Culver DA, Judson MA. A concise review of pulmonary sarcoidosis. *Am J Respir Crit Care Med.* 2011;183(5):573–581.

Boiselle PM. Imaging of the large airways. *Clin Chest Med.* 2008;29(1):181–193.

Boiselle PM. Imaging of the large airways. *Clin Chest Med.* 2008;29(1):181–193, vii.

Boiselle PM, Lee KS, Ernst A. Multidetector CT of the central airways. *J Thorac Imaging*. 2005;20(3):186–195.

Brink JA, Amis ES Jr. Image wisely: a campaign to increase awareness about adult radiation protection. *Radiology*. 2010;257(3):601–602.

Carden KA, Boiselle PM, Waltz DA, et al. Tracheomalacia and tracheobronchomalacia in children and adults: an in-depth review. *Chest*. 2005;127(3):984–1005.

Cataneo AJ, Reibscheid SM, Ruiz Júnior RL, et al. Foreign body in the tracheobronchial tree. *Clin Pediatr (Phila)*. 1997;36(12):701–706.

Chung MP, Lee KS, Han J, et al. Bronchial stenosis due to anthracofibrosis. *Chest*. 1998;113(2):344–350.

Ciet P, Wielopolski P, Manniesing R, et al. Spirometer-controlled cine magnetic resonance imaging used to diagnose tracheobronchomalacia in paediatric patients. *Eur Respir J*. 2014;43(1):115–124.

Desir A, Ghaye B. Congenital abnormalities of intrathoracic airways. *Radiol Clin North Am*. 2009;47(2):203–225.

Ernst A, Feller-Kopman D, et al. Central airway obstruction. *Am J Respir Crit Care Med*. 2004;169(12):1278–1297.

Ernst A, Rafeq S, Boiselle P, et al. Relapsing polychondritis and airway involvement. *Chest*. 2009;135(4):1024–1030.

Eslamy HK, Newman B. Imaging of the pediatric airway. *Paediatr Anaesth*. 2009;19(suppl 1):9–23.

Franquet T, Müller NL, Oikonomou A, et al. *Aspergillus* infection of the airways: computed tomography and pathologic findings. *J Comput Assist Tomogr*. 2004;28(1):10–16.

Franquet T, Serrano F, Giménez A, et al. Necrotizing aspergillosis of large airways: CT findings in eight patients. *J Comput Assist Tomogr*. 2002;26(3):342–345.

Gibbs JM, Chandrasekhar CA, Ferguson EC, et al. Lines and stripes: where did they go? From conventional radiography to CT. *Radiographics*. 2007;27(1):33–48.

Gillmore JD, Hawkins PN. Amyloidosis and the respiratory tract. *Thorax*. 1999;54(5):444–451.

Gómez-Seco J, Pérez-Boal I, Guerrero-González J, et al. Anthracofibrosis or anthracostenosis. *Arch Bronconeumol*. 2012;48(4):133–136.

Goske MJ, Applegate KE, Bulas D, et al. Alliance for radiation safety in pediatric imaging. Image gently: progress and challenges in CT education and advocacy. *Pediatr Radiol*. 2011;41(suppl 2):461–466.

Grenier PA, Beigelman-Aubry C, Brillet PY. Nonneoplastic tracheal and bronchial stenoses. *Radiol Clin North Am*. 2009;47(2):243–260.

Gross RE. Arterial malformations which cause compression of the trachea or esophagus. *Circulation*. 1955;11(1):124–134.

Han FF, Yang TY, Song L, et al. Clinical and pathological features and imaging manifestations of bronchial anthracofibrosis: the findings in 15 patients. *Chin Med J*. 2013;126(14):2641–2646.

Ingegnoli A, Corsi A, Verardo E, et al. Uncommon causes of tracheobronchial stenosis and wall thickening: MDCT imaging. *Radiol Med*. 2007;112(8):1132–1141.

Kang EY. Large airway diseases. *J Thorac Imaging*. 2011;26(4):249–262.

Karnak D, Avery RK, Gildea TR, et al. Endobronchial fungal disease: an under-recognized entity. *Respiration*. 2007;74(1):88–104.

Kim YJ, Jung CY, Shin HW, et al. Biomass smoke induced bronchial anthracofibrosis: presenting features and clinical course. *Respir Med*. 2009;103(5):757–765.

Ko JM, Jung JI, Park SH, et al. Benign tumors of the tracheobronchial tree: CT-pathologic correlation. *AJR Am J Roentgenol*. 2006;186(5):1304–1313.

Kwong JS, Müller NL, Miller RR. Diseases of the trachea and main-stem bronchi: correlation of CT with pathologic findings. *Radiographics*. 1992;12(4):645–657.

Lee KS, Boiselle PM. Update on multidetector computed tomography imaging of the airways. *J Thorac Imaging*. 2010;25(2):112–124.

Lee KS, Kim TS, Fujimoto K, et al. Thoracic manifestation of Wegener's granulomatosis: CT findings in 30 patients. *Eur Radiol*. 2003;13(1):43–51.

Murgu S, Colt H. Tracheobronchomalacia and excessive dynamic airway collapse. *Clin Chest Med*. 2013;34(3):527–555.

Ngo AV, Walker CM, Chung JH, et al. Tumors and tumorlike conditions of the large airways. *AJR Am J Roentgenol*. 2013;201(2):301–313.

Park CM, Goo JM, Lee HJ, et al. Tumors in the tracheobronchial tree: CT and FDG PET features. *Radiographics*. 2009;29(1):55–71.

Polychronopoulos VS, Prakash UB. Airway involvement in sarcoidosis. *Chest*. 2009;136(5):1371–1380.

Polychronopoulos VS, Prakash UB, Golbin JM, et al. Airway involvement in Wegener's granulomatosis. *Rheum Dis Clin North Am*. 2007;33(4):755–775, vi.

Prakash UB. Tracheobronchopathia osteochondroplastica. *Semin Respir Crit Care Med*. 2002;23(2):167–175.

Prince JS, Duhamel DR, Levin DL, et al. Nonneoplastic lesions of the tracheobronchial wall: radiologic findings with bronchoscopic correlation. *Radiographics*. 2002;22(Spec No):S215–S230.

Rafeq S, Trentham D, Ernst A. Pulmonary manifestations of relapsing polychondritis. *Clin Chest Med*. 2010;31(3):513–518.

Ridge CA, O'donnell CR, Lee EY, et al. Tracheobronchomalacia: current concepts and controversies. *J Thorac Imaging*. 2011;26(4):278–289.

Rikimaru T. Endobronchial tuberculosis. *Expert Rev Anti Infect Ther*. 2004;2(2):245–251.

Sebening C, Jakob H, Tochtermann U, et al. Vascular tracheobronchial compression syndromes—experience in surgical treatment and literature. *Thorac Cardiovasc Surg*. 2000;48(3):164–174.

Seo JB, Song KS, Lee JS, et al. Broncholithiasis: review of the causes with radiologic-pathologic correlation. *Radiographics*. 2002;22(Spec No):S199–S213.

Swanson KL. Airway foreign bodies: what's new? *Semin Respir Crit Care Med*. 2004;25(4):405–411.

Urban BA, Fishman EK, Goldman SM, et al. CT evaluation of amyloidosis: spectrum of disease. *Radiographics*. 1993;13(6):1295–1308.

Webb EM, Elicker BM, Webb WR. Using CT to diagnose nonneoplastic tracheal abnormalities: appearance of the tracheal wall. *AJR Am J Roentgenol*. 2000;174(5):1315–1321.

CHAPTER 37

Cardiac Valves

Ahmed H. El-Sherief, Rahul Renapurkar, and Michael Bolen

CHAPTER OUTLINE

■ Introduction

Echocardiography is the primary imaging modality used in the evaluation of cardiac valve morphology, function, and disease. This modality is broadly available and portable, and there is widespread clinical familiarity with the performance and interpretation of this modality. However, it is operator-dependent and is sometimes limited by suboptimal acoustic windows (e.g., patients affected by obesity). In certain patients, MRI may be used in the evaluation of cardiac valve morphology, function, and disease. MRI offers good morphologic assessment of valves and can provide quantitation of valve insufficiency (whereas echocardiography is semiquantitative), as well as a gold standard assessment of ventricular volume, mass, and ejection fraction. However, it is relatively expensive and time-consuming, and the skill set for performance and interpretation of these examinations is not widespread. In certain patients (e.g., evaluation of cardiac valves as part of preprocedural planning and assessment of postprocedural complications) CT is used to evaluate cardiac valve morphology, disease, and, in some cases, function.

■ Cardiac Valve Anatomy

There are four cardiac valves: two atrioventricular valves (tricuspid valve, mitral valve) and two semilunar valves (pulmonic valve, aortic valve). The atrioventricular valves regulate blood flow from the atrial chambers to the ventricular chambers, and the semilunar valves regulate blood flow from the ventricular chambers to the great vessels (pulmonary artery, thoracic aorta).

The inflow and outflow valves of the left ventricle (mitral valve, aortic valve) are in fibrous continuity, whereas the inflow and outflow valves of the right ventricle (tricuspid valve, pulmonic valve) are separated by the muscular infundibulum of the right ventricle, a point of interest in evaluating complex congenital cases.

Aortic Valve

The aortic root is located between the left ventricular chamber and the ascending aorta and supports and surrounds the aortic valve. The aortic root complex consists of the ventriculoarterial junction (also known as the *annulus*), aortic valve leaflets, aortic valve leaflet attachments, sinuses of Valsalva, aortic valve interleaflet trigones, and sinotubular junction (Fig. 37.1). The normal aortic valve consists of three leaflets (also described as cusps)—the right coronary, left coronary, and noncoronary leaflets. The leaflets extend from their basal attachments (within the left ventricle) to the sinotubular junction, attaching in a semilunar fashion. The semilunar attachment of the aortic valve leaflets creates triangular interleaflet spaces, with the apex of these triangles known as *commissures*.

During ventricular systole, the aortic valve leaflets open to allow blood flow from the left ventricular chamber into the aorta (Fig. 37.2). During ventricular diastole, the aortic valve leaflets close (or coapt) to prevent regurgitation of blood back into the left ventricular chamber (see Fig. 37.2).

Congenital variations of the aortic valve include a one-leaflet valve, a two-leaflet valve, and a four-leaflet valve.

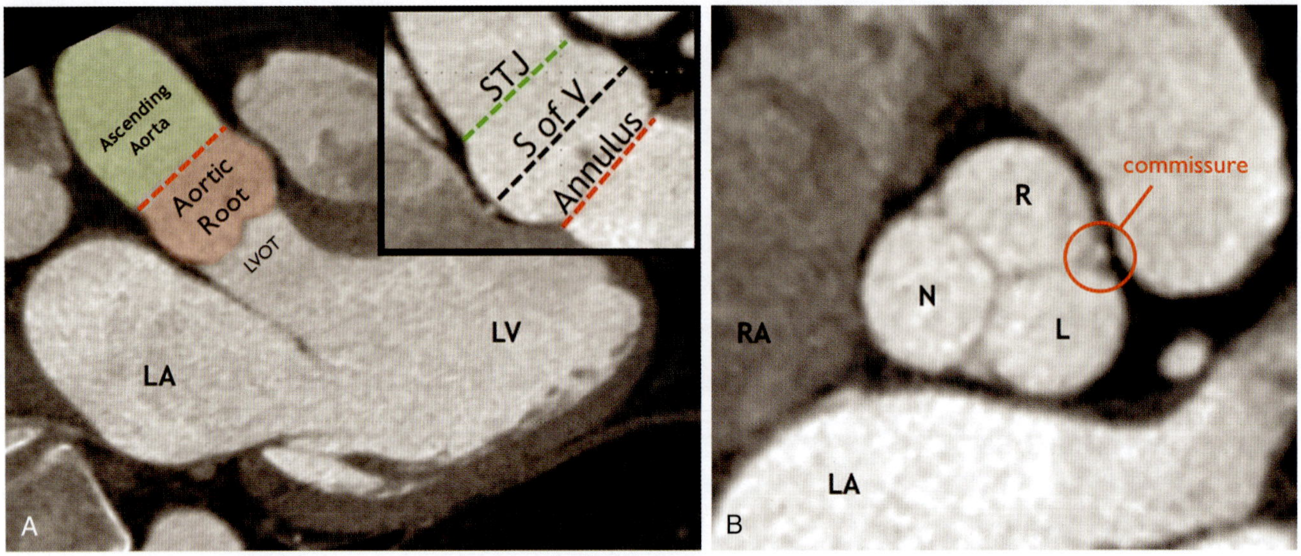

Figure 37.1 Aortic root complex. (A) Three-chamber view of the left ventricle *(LV)* on CT shows the aortic root complex, consisting of the annulus, aortic valve leaflets, aortic valve leaflet attachments, sinuses of Valsalva *(S of V)*, aortic valve interleaflet trigones, and sinotubular junction *(STJ)*. (B) Short-axis view of the aortic root at the level of the sinuses of Valsalva on CT shows the leaflets and commissures of the aortic valve. *L,* Left coronary leaflet or cusp; *LA,* left atrium; *LVOT,* left ventricular outflow tract; *N,* noncoronary leaflet or cusp; *R,* right coronary leaflet or cusp; *RA,* right atrium; *RV,* right ventricle.

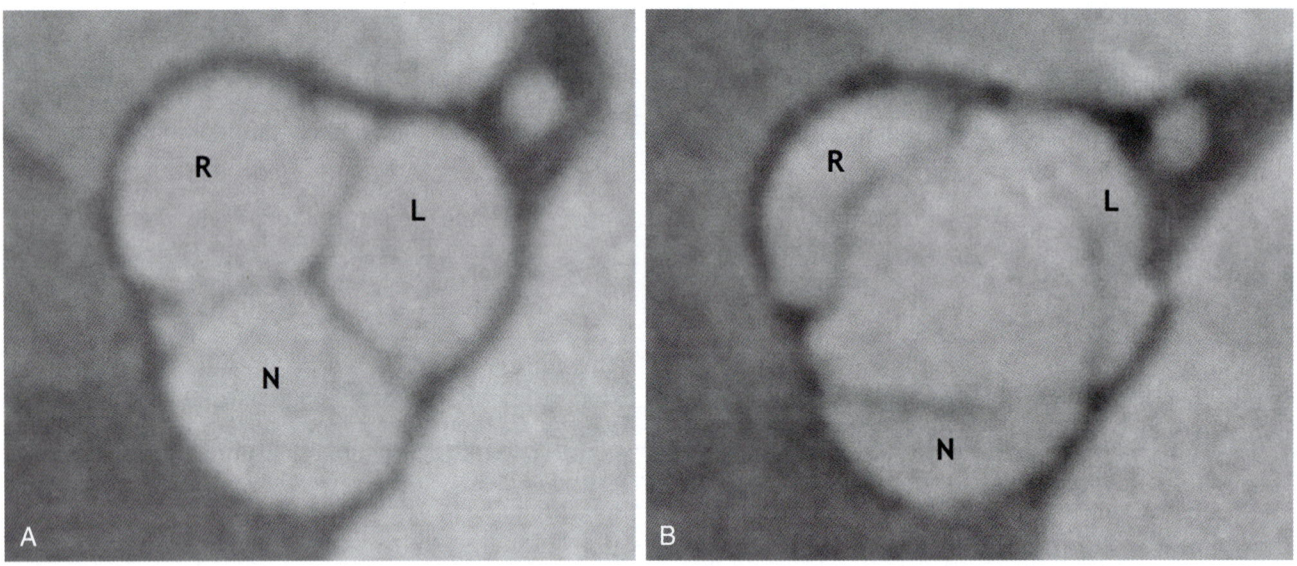

Figure 37.2 Aortic valve during ventricular end-diastole and ventricular end-systole. (A) Short-axis view of the aortic root at the level of the sinuses of Valsalva on CT shows closure or coaptation of the aortic valve leaflets or cusps during ventricular end-diastole. (B) Short-axis view of the aortic root at the level of the sinuses of Valsalva on CT shows opening of the aortic valve leaflets or cusps during ventricular end-systole. *L,* Left coronary leaflet or cusp; *N,* noncoronary leaflet or cusp; *R,* right coronary leaflet or cusp.

Mitral Valve

The mitral valve is located posteriorly and to the left of the aortic valve. The mitral valve complex consists of the mitral annulus, mitral valve leaflets, chordae tendineae, and papillary muscles (Fig. 37.3). The mitral annulus is a complex saddle-shaped fibrous ring that connects to the mitral leaflets. There are two mitral valve leaflets: the anterior and posterior mitral leaflets. The anterior leaflet of the mitral valve can be divided into three segments, and the posterior leaflet of the mitral valve can be divided into three scallops (anterior mitral leaflet, A1, A2, and A3; posterior mitral leaflet, P1, P2, and P3). The mitral valve leaflets attach to papillary muscles, the anterolateral and posterolateral papillary muscles, and to the left ventricular wall via the chordae tendineae.

During ventricular diastole, the mitral valve leaflets open to allow blood flow from the left atrial chamber

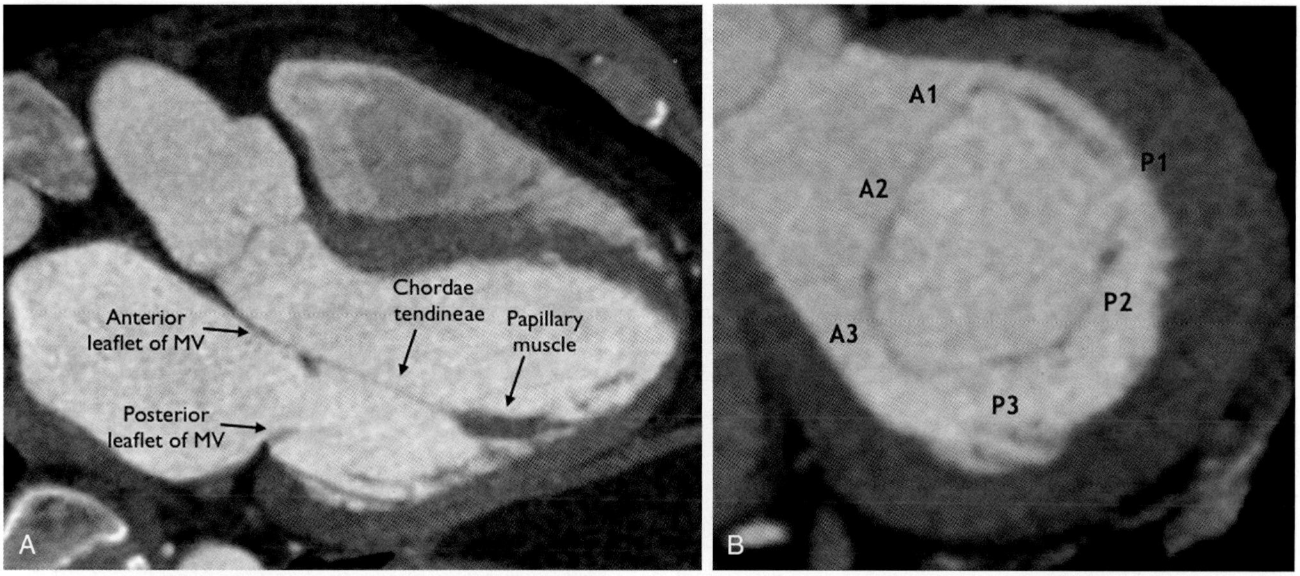

Figure 37.3 Mitral valve *(MV)* complex. (A) Three-chamber view of the left ventricle on CT shows the mitral valve complex consisting of the mitral annulus, mitral valve leaflets, chordae tendineae, and papillary muscles. (B) Short-axis view of the mitral valve complex at the level of the mitral annulus on CT shows segmental anatomy of the mitral valve leaflets. *A1*, Anterior segment of the anterior leaflet of mitral valve; *A2*, middle segment of see the anterior leaflet of the mitral valve; *A3*, posterior segment of the anterior leaflet of the mitral valve; *P1*, anterior scallop of the posterior leaflet of the mitral valve; *P2*, middle scallop of the posterior leaflet of the mitral valve; *P3*, posterior scallop of the posterior leaflet of the mitral valve.

into the left ventricular chamber. During ventricular diastole, the mitral valve leaflets close to prevent regurgitation of blood back into the left atrial chamber.

Congenital variations of the mitral valve complex include fusion of the papillary muscles, annulus with two orifices (also described as a *double-orifice mitral valve*), cleft leaflet, and supravalvar ring.

Pulmonic Valve

The pulmonic valve is located anteriorly, superiorly, and to the left of the aortic valve. The pulmonary root complex consists of the ventriculoarterial junction (also known as an *annulus*), pulmonic valve leaflets, pulmonic valve leaflet attachments, sinuses of Valsalva, pulmonic valve interleaflet trigones, and sinotubular junction. The normal pulmonic valve consists of three leaflets (also known as *cusps*).

During ventricular systole, the pulmonic valve leaflets open to allow blood flow from the right ventricular chamber into the pulmonary artery. During ventricular diastole, the pulmonic valve leaflets close to prevent regurgitation of blood back into the right ventricular chamber.

Congenital variations of the pulmonic valve include a two-leaflet valve, four-leaflet valve, and deficiency or absence of a valve leaflet (known as *atresia*).

Tricuspid Valve

The tricuspid valve is located posteriorly and to the right of the aortic valve. The tricuspid valve complex consists of the tricuspid annulus, tricuspid valve leaflets, chordae tendineae, and papillary muscles. There are three tricuspid valve leaflets: the anterior, posterior, and septal leaflets. The tricuspid valve leaflets attach to papillary muscles (usually three papillary muscles—anterior, posterior, and septal papillary muscles) via the chordae tendineae.

During ventricular diastole, the tricuspid valve leaflets open to allow blood flow from the right atrial chamber into the right ventricular chamber. During ventricular diastole, the tricuspid valve leaflets close to prevent regurgitant blood flow into the right atrial chamber.

Congenital variations of the tricuspid valve include deficiency or absence of a valve leaflet (atresia) or apical displacement and partial fusion of the septal and posterior tricuspid valve leaflets (Ebstein anomaly).

■ Valvular Regurgitation

Mitral Valve Regurgitation

Mitral valve regurgitation (MR) is the most common form of valvular heart disease. MR may be primary, due to inherent dysfunction of the valve leaflets, or subvalvular apparatus, the most common type of which is myomatous valve degeneration. This causes elongation of leaflets and chordae and may lead to prolapse (bowing of leaflets >2 mm into the left atrium) and MR. Flail mitral leaflet occurs when there is systolic eversion of the leaflet into the left atrial chamber secondary to a ruptured chordae or papillary muscle and is typically accompanied by significant MR (Fig. 37.4). MR may be characterized as

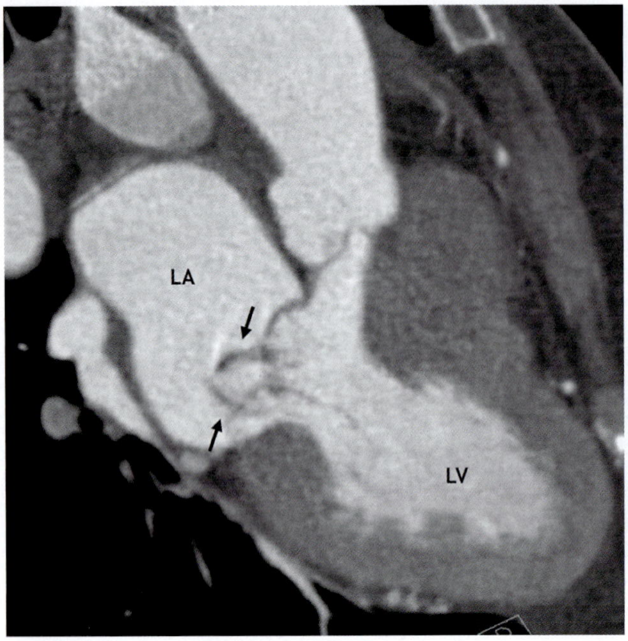

Figure 37.4 Flail mitral valve leaflet. Three-chamber view of the left ventricle *(LV)* on CT shows eversion of the posterior leaflet of the mitral valve into the left atrial chamber during systole (in between the *arrows*). *LA,* Left atrium.

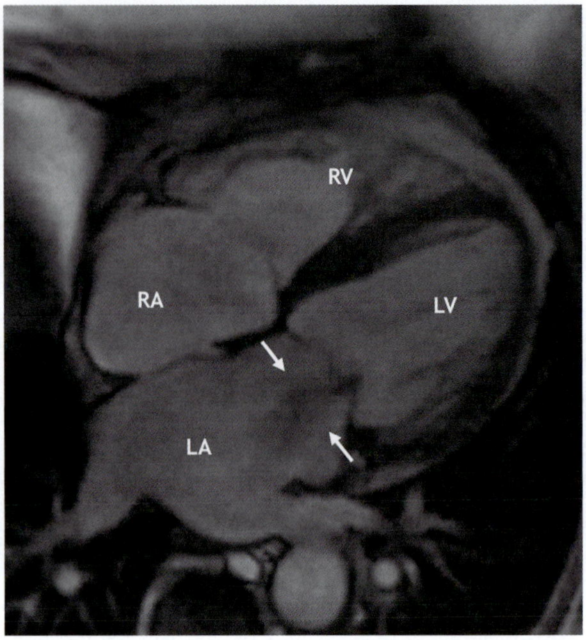

Figure 37.5 Mitral valve regurgitation. Four-chamber view on steady-state free precession MRI shows signal void (in between the *arrows*) that originates from the mitral valve and extends into the left atrial chamber during ventricular systole. *LA,* Left atrium; *LV,* left ventricle; *RA,* right atrium; *RV,* right ventricle.

functional (or secondary), where the leaflets and valve apparatus are normal, and changes in the left ventricle, usually due to ischemia or dilation, lead to annular enlargement or papillary muscle displacement, which results in tethering and tenting of the leaflets.

On CT and MRI, MR is identified as incomplete coaptation of the mitral valve leaflets during ventricular systole. On cine steady-state free precession (SSFP) MRI, MR is identified as a signal void that originates from the mitral valve and extends into the left atrial chamber during ventricular systole (Fig. 37.5).

Aortic Valve Regurgitation

Aortic valve regurgitation (AR) is caused by abnormalities in the aortic root complex: (1) abnormality of the annulus (e.g., annular dilation secondary to cystic medial degeneration); and (2) abnormality of a leaflet (e.g., leaflet thickening in rheumatic heart disease).

On CT and MRI, AR is identified as incomplete coaptation of the aortic valve leaflets during ventricular diastole (Fig. 37.6). On cine SSFP MRI, AR is identified as a signal void that originates from the aortic valve and extends into the left ventricular outflow tract–left ventricular chamber during ventricular diastole (see Fig. 37.6).

Pulmonic Valve Regurgitation

Pulmonic valve regurgitation (PR) is caused by abnormalities in the pulmonic root complex: (1) abnormality of the annulus (e.g., annular dilation secondary to severe pulmonary hypertension); or (2) abnormality of a leaflet (e.g., two-leaflet pulmonic valve). In clinical practice, significant PR is often seen in patients' status posttreatment for pulmonary stenosis and in patients' status posttreatment for tetralogy of Fallot.

On CT and MRI, PR is identified as incomplete coaptation of the pulmonic valve leaflets during ventricular diastole. On cine SSFP MRI, PR is identified as a signal void that originates from the pulmonic valve and extends into the right ventricular chamber during ventricular diastole.

Tricuspid Valve Regurgitation

Similar to the mitral valve, tricuspid valve regurgitation (TR) may be functional (secondary) or may be due to derangement of the leaflets themselves (primary); functional TR is more common in clinical practice. Functional TR is often due to right ventricular dilation, which disrupts the usual geometry and mechanics of the tricuspid valve and subvalvular apparatus. Right ventricular dilation, in turn, is usually due to left ventricular failure, but may also be noted in the setting of right ventricular infarction and cor pulmonale. Primary TR is less common and can be seen in the setting of rheumatic heart disease, endocarditis, and congenital scenarios such as Ebstein anomaly, where there is partial fusion of the septal and posterior leaflets of the tricuspid valve to myocardium, leading to partial atrialization of the inlet region of the right ventricle (Fig. 37.7).

On CT and MRI, TR is identified as incomplete coaptation of the tricuspid valve leaflets during ventricular systole. On cine SSFP MRI, TR is identified as a signal void that originates from the tricuspid valve and extends into the right atrial chamber during ventricular systole.

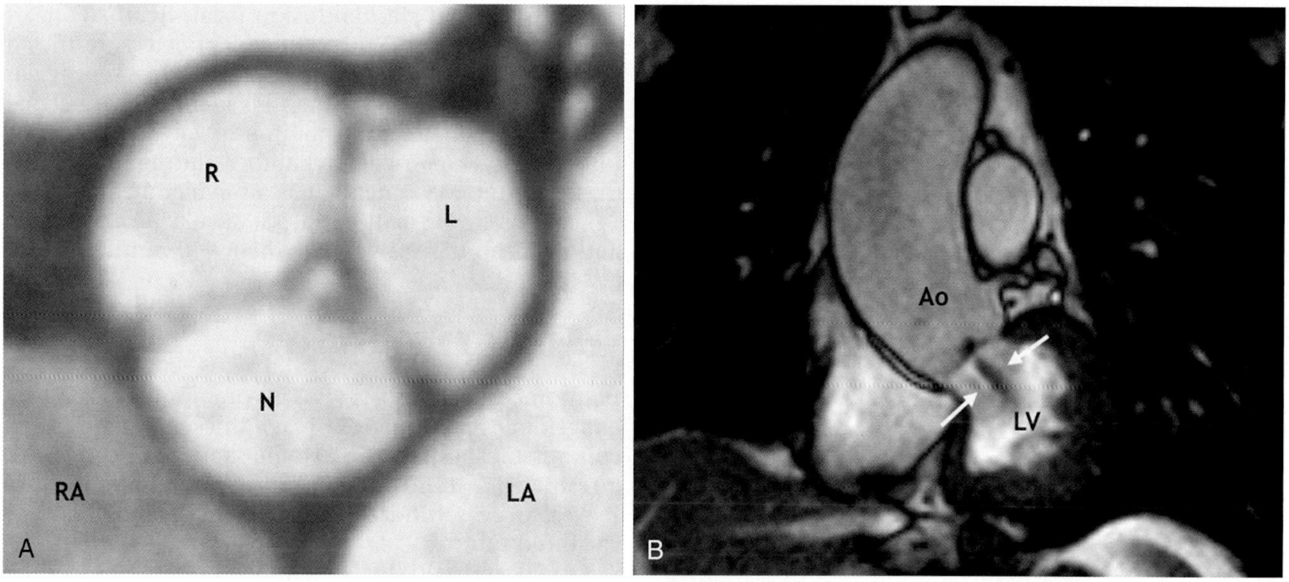

Figure 37.6 Aortic valve regurgitation. (A) Short-axis view of the aortic root at the level of the sinuses of Valsalva on CT shows incomplete coaptation of the aortic valve leaflets during ventricular diastole. (B) Coronal oblique view of the aortic root on steady-state free precession MRI shows a signal void (in between the *arrows*) that originates from the aortic valve and extends into the left ventricular outflow tract–left ventricular chamber during ventricular diastole. *Ao*, Aorta; *L*, left coronary leaflet or cusp; *LA*, left atrium; *LV*, left ventricle; *N*, noncoronary leaflet or cusp; *R*, right coronary leaflet or cusp; *RA*, right atrium.

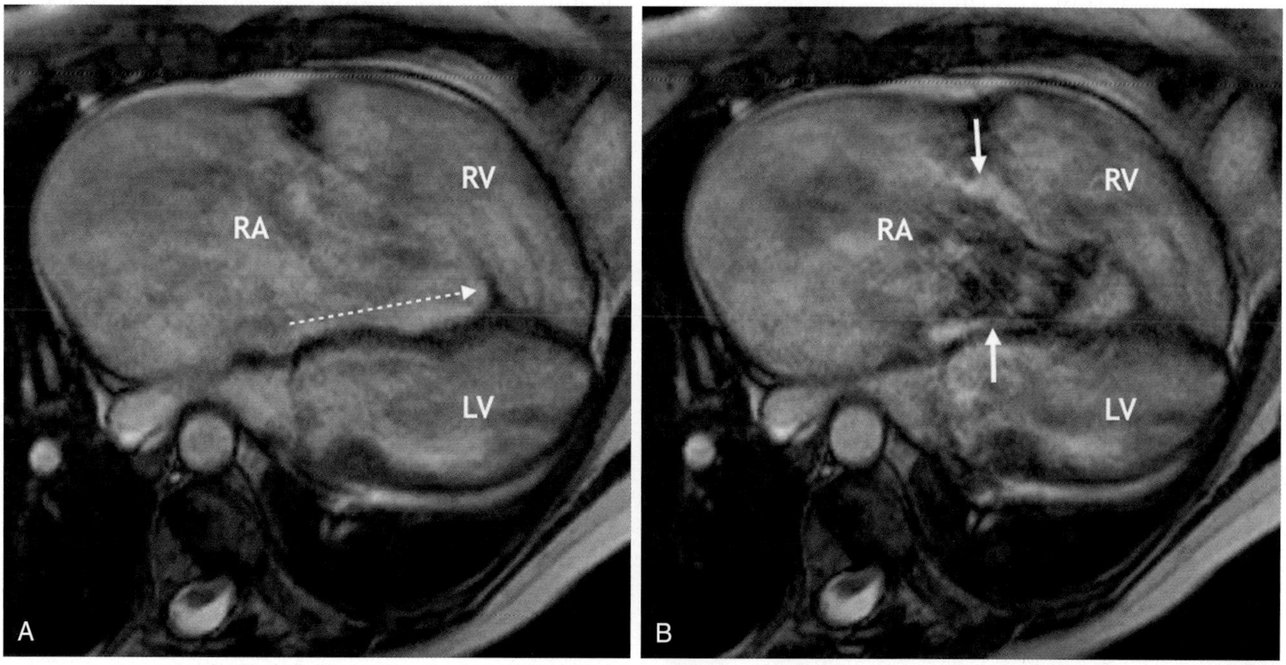

Figure 37.7 Ebstein anomaly. (A) Four-chamber view on steady-state free precession MRI shows partial atrialization of the right ventricle secondary to partial fusion of the septal and posterior leaflets of the tricuspid valve to myocardium (*dotted arrow*, apical displacement of the attachment of the septal leaflet of the tricuspid valve). (B) Four-chamber view steady-state free precession MRI shows tricuspid regurgitation manifesting as a signal void (in between the *arrows*) that originates from the tricuspid valve and extends into the right atrial chamber during ventricular systole. *LA*, Left atrium; *LV*, left ventricle; *RA*, right atrium; *RV*, right ventricle.

Quantification of Valve Regurgitation

Valve regurgitation can be quantified by MRI using velocity-encoded cine phase contrast imaging. This can be directly quantified in the case of AR and PR and indirectly quantified when assessing TR and MR (e.g., by subtracting the forward flow in the aorta from the left ventricular stroke volume to assess MR). This offers a potential benefit for the use of MRI in comparison to echocardiography, which by contrast provides a multiparametric semiquantitative assessment of valve insufficiency and may be hampered in the setting of eccentric insufficiency.

■ Valvular Stenosis

Aortic Valve Stenosis

Aortic valve stenosis (AS) is commonly caused by degeneration of the aortic valve or congenital malformation (e.g., bicuspid aortic valve) of the aortic valve (Fig. 37.8). On CT and MRI, AS is identified as narrowing of the aortic valve orifice area during ventricular systole. On cine SSFP MRI, AS is identified as a signal void that originates from the aortic valve and extends into the aortic root during ventricular systole. Mild AS is defined as a valvular area of >1.5 cm^2 but <2.5 cm^2; severe AS demonstrates a valvular area of <1.0 cm^2, aortic jet peak velocity >4.0 m/s, and/or a mean transvalvular gradient >40 mm Hg; critical stenosis demonstrates a valvular area <0.7 cm^2.

Mitral Valve Stenosis

Mitral valve stenosis (MS) is commonly caused by thickening and calcification of the mitral valve leaflets and commissural and chordal fusion from rheumatic heart disease. On CT and MRI, MS is identified as restricted opening of the mitral valve orifice during ventricular diastole. On cine SSFP MRI, MS is identified as a signal void that originates from the mitral valve and extends into the left ventricular chamber during ventricular diastole. Mild MS is defined as a valvular area of 1.5 to 2.5 cm^2; severe MS demonstrates a valvular area of <1 cm^2 and/or mean transvalvular gradient >10 mm Hg.

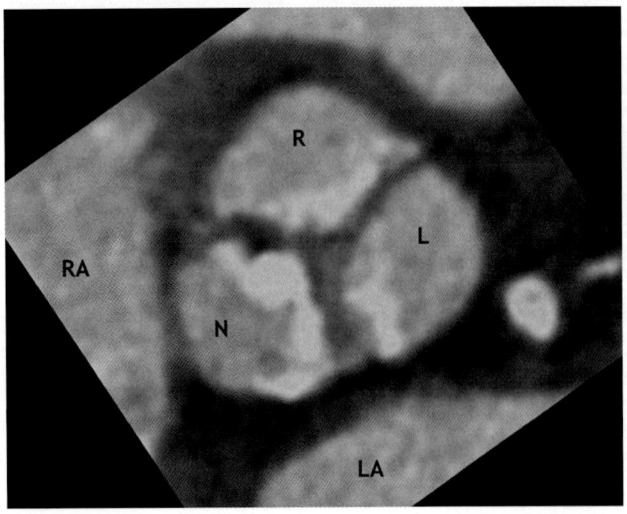

Figure 37.8 Calcific degeneration of the aortic valve. This short-axis view of the aortic root at the level of the sinuses of Valsalva on CT shows extensive calcification of the aortic valve leaflets. *L*, Left coronary leaflet or cusp; *LA*, left atrium; *N*, noncoronary leaflet or cusp; *R*, right coronary leaflet or cusp; *RA*, right atrium.

Pulmonic Valve Stenosis

Pulmonic valve stenosis (PS) is commonly caused by a congenital malformation (e.g., thickened and fused commissures resulting in a dome-shaped structure, with a restricted systolic opening) of the pulmonic valve. It may also be secondary to rheumatic heart disease or carcinoid tumor.

On CT and MRI, PS is identified as narrowing of the pulmonic valve orifice area during ventricular systole. Mild PS is defined as peak gradient <36 mm Hg, moderate PS >36 mm Hg to <64 mm Hg, and severe PS >64 mm Hg.

Quantification of Valve Stenosis

Careful planimetry on CT and MRI may be used to quantify the valve opening area (Fig. 37.9). Velocity-encoded phase contrast MRI may be used to estimate valve stenosis, but peak velocities often differ from those obtained by Doppler echocardiography.

■ Valvular Vegetation

Normal cardiac valves are resistant to the development of infectious vegetation (e.g., infectious endocarditis) or noninfectious vegetation (e.g., systemic lupus erythematosus). An acquired or congenital cardiac condition or direct trauma (e.g., catheter placement, cardiac valve repair or replacement) can lead to cardiac valve injury, creating an increased risk for vegetation development. Valvular leaflet thickening, retraction or shortening, or perforation may accompany valvular vegetation, leading to valvular regurgitation. Large vegetations are usually seen on CT or MRI, but vegetations that are smaller or more mobile may not be well depicted.

Vegetations usually occur on the upstream side of the valve (e.g., the ventricular side of the aortic valve and the atrial side of the mitral valve). Features that increase the likelihood of endocarditis include irregular margination, attachment to the free margin of the valve leaflet, and mobility independent of cardiac motion. In infective endocarditis, perivalvular spread of infection may occur and result in valve dehiscence, perivalvular abscess formation, or pseudoaneurysm formation, which may be well depicted by CT or MRI, given the wide field of view and potential for multiplanar reformatting of images (see Fig. 37.8). Prosthetic valves or other implanted hardware may lead to artifact on echocardiography, which may be less prominent on CT.

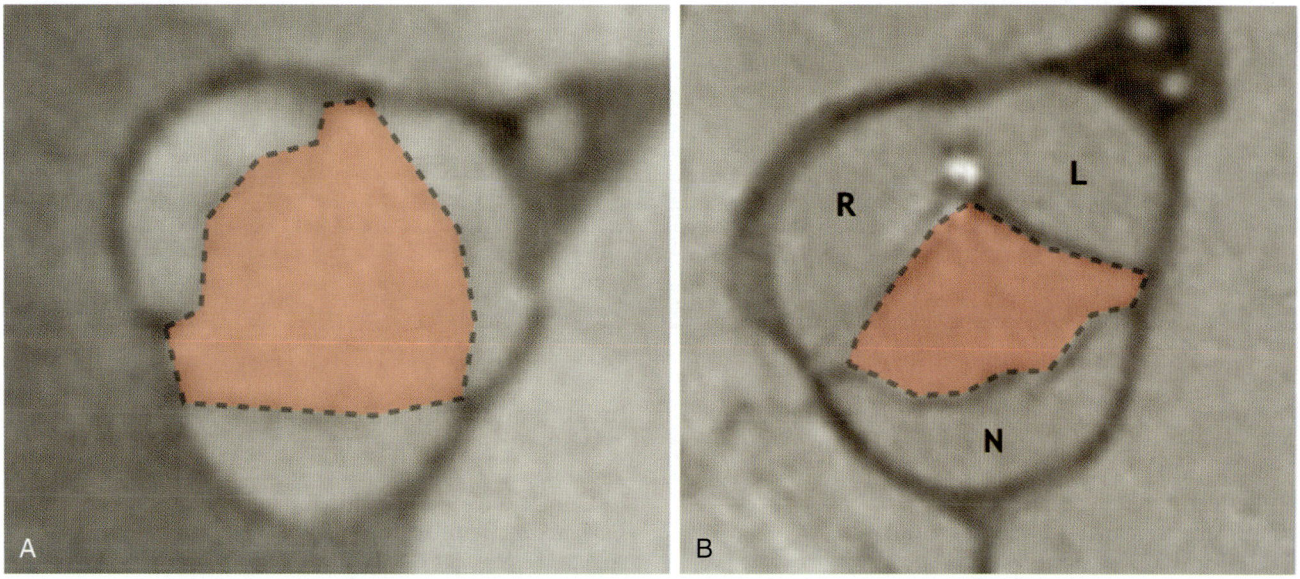

Figure 37.9 Valve planimetry. (A) Short-axis view of the aortic root at the sinuses of Valsalva on CT during ventricular end-systole shows valve area >2.5 cm^2 by planimetry. (B) Short-axis view of the aortic root at the sinuses of Valsalva on CT during ventricular end-systole shows valve area <2.5 cm^2 by planimetry (secondary to a functionally bicuspid aortic valve, where there is fusion of the right and left leaflets of the aortic valve). *L*, Left coronary leaflet or cusp; *N*, noncoronary leaflet or cusp; *R*, right coronary leaflet or cusp.

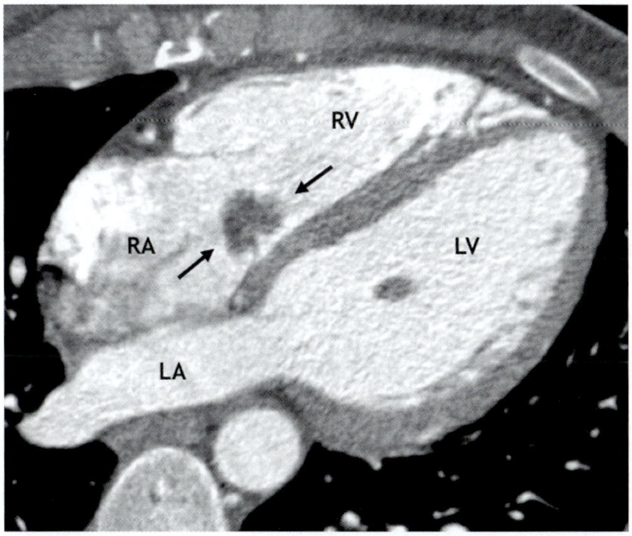

Figure 37.10 Papillary fibroelastoma. This multiplanar reconstructed CT image shows a frondlike and pedunculated mass on the tricuspid valve. The mass was surgically resected and pathologically confirmed to be a papillary fibroelastoma. *LA*, Left atrium; *LV*, left ventricle; *RA*, right atrium; *RV*, right ventricle.

■ Valvular Tumors

The most common primary valvular tumor is a papillary fibroelastoma. Papillary fibroelastomas usually occur on the aortic valve, followed by the mitral valve (anterior leaflet). They usually occur on the downstream side of the valve. These tumors are unusually small in diameter and usually appear frondlike, pedunculated, and mobile on imaging. Although papillary fibroelastomas are benign, they are associated with embolic events. Surgical resection is usually offered to symptomatic patients or asymptomatic patients with a tumor more than 10 mm in diameter. Large papillary fibroelastomas may be seen on CT or MRI (Fig. 37.10).

The second most common primary valvular tumor is a myxoma. Valvular myxomas usually occur on the mitral valve, followed by the tricuspid valve.

Bibliography

Anderson RH. The surgical anatomy of the aortic root. *Multimed Man Cardiothorac Surg*. 2007;2007(102):mmcts.2006.002527.

Bennett CJ1, Maleszewski JJ, Araoz PA. CT and MR imaging of the aortic valve: radiologic-pathologic correlation. *Radiographics*. 2012;32(5):1399–1420.

Bonow RO, Carabello BA, Chatterjee K, et al. 2008 focused update incorporated into the ACC/AHA 2006 guidelines for the management of patients with valvular heart disease: a report of the American College of Cardiology/American Heart Association task force on practice guidelines (writing committee to revise the 1998 guidelines for the management of patients with valvular heart disease): endorsed by the Society of Cardiovascular Anesthesiologists, Society for Cardiovascular Angiography and Interventions, and Society of Thoracic Surgeons. *Circulation*. 2008;118:e523–e661.

Charitos EI, Sievers HH. Anatomy of the aortic root: implications for valve-sparing surgery. *Ann Cardiothorac Surg*. 2013;2(1):53–56.

Chen JJ1, Manning MA, Frazier AA, et al. CT angiography of the cardiac valves: normal, diseased, and postoperative appearances. *Radiographics*. 2009;29(5):1393–1412.

Entrikin DW. Valves: computed tomography. In: Abbara S, Kalva S, eds. *Problem Solving in Cardiovascular Imaging*. Philadelphia: Saunders; 2012.

Gowda RM, Khan IA, Nair CK, et al. Cardiac papillary fibroelastoma: a comprehensive analysis of 725 cases. *Am Heart J*. 2003;146:404–410.

Halpern EJ, Zwas DR. Valve assessment. In: Halpern EJ, eds. *Clinical Cardiac CT Anatomy and Function*. New York: Thieme; 2008.

Morris MF1, Maleszewski JJ, Suri RM, et al. CT and MR imaging of the mitral valve: radiologic-pathologic correlation. *Radiographics*. 2010;30(6):1603–1620.

Piazza N, de Jaegere P, Schultz C, et al. Anatomy of the aortic valvar complex and its implications for transcatheter implantation of the aortic valve. *Circ Cardiovasc Interv*. 2008;1(1):74–81.

Ryan R, Abbara S, Colen RR, et al. Cardiac valve disease: spectrum of findings on cardiac 64-MDCT. *AJR Am J Roentgenol*. 2008;190(5):W294–W303.

Saremi F1, Gera A, Ho SY, et al. CT and MR imaging of the pulmonary valve. *Radiographics*. 2014;34(1):51–71.

Walker CM, Reddy GP. Valves: magnetic resonance imaging. In: Abbara S, Kalva S, eds. *Problem Solving in Cardiovascular Imaging*. Philadelphia: Saunders; 2012.

CHAPTER 38
Imaging of the Pericardium

Seth Kligerman

CHAPTER OUTLINE

Anatomy and Normal Appearance on Imaging

The pericardium is a fibrous sac that surrounds the heart and is composed of two distinct layers: the visceral pericardium and parietal pericardium. The visceral pericardium is the inner serous layer that consists of a very thin (<1 mm) layer of mesothelial cells. The visceral pericardium lines the epicardial surface of the heart and is separated from the cardiac surface by a layer of epicardial fat, which can vary dramatically in thickness. The parietal pericardium is itself composed of two layers: an outer fibrous layer and an inner serous layer. Similar to the visceral pericardium, the inner serous layer of the parietal pericardium is composed of a thin layer of mesothelial cells. The serosal pericardium is a closed sac composed of the serous layer of the parietal pericardium externally and the serous layer of the visceral pericardium internally and is itself within the fibrous pericardium. These two serous layers are continuous with each other at or near sites of attachments of the great vessels to the heart. The potential space where visceral and parietal serous layers are not attached is the pericardial cavity. The mesothelial cells of both serous layers secrete a small amount of fluid into the pericardial space to lubricate the cavity; therefore the space normally contains 15 to 35 mL of pericardial fluid. The fibrous layer of the parietal pericardium is attached to the mesothelial layer of the parietal pericardium and is composed of various layers of collagen and elastic fibers. Peripheral to those layers lies the pericardial connective tissue layer that contains large bundles of collagen, which form parts of the pericardial ligaments that anchor the pericardium to the manubrium, xiphoid process, and central tendon of the diaphragm loosely. Superiorly, the fibrous layer continues over the aortic arch, where it blends with the deep cervical fascia.

In normal individuals, the pericardium cannot be visualized by chest radiography. In certain disease processes, which will be discussed later, abnormalities of the pericardium can be visualized by radiography, although the evaluation is limited compared to cross-sectional imaging.

On CT, the pericardial sac is a thin curvilinear band of soft tissue that surrounds the heart and can be seen extending from the great vessels superiorly to the diaphragmatic surface inferiorly. It is best visualized anterior to the anterior wall of the right ventricle, where it is outlined by epicardial and mediastinal fat (Figs. 38.1 and 38.2). Although there may be certain areas where it is poorly visualized, such as overlying the lateral surface of the left ventricle, it is present, except in rare circumstances. It is often not possible to delineate the individual serous layers of the pericardium on cross-sectional imaging unless separated by fluid or thickened. The pericardium is often thin, measuring only 1 to 2 mm in thickness, although a thickness less than 4 mm is considered normal. Because fluid is often found in the pericardial sac, it is important not to confuse an effusion with pericardial thickening, although the delineation between the two may be difficult. Fluid in numerous pericardial sinuses and recesses, as discussed below, is common and should not be mistaken for pathology.

On MRI, the parietal pericardium will appear as a low-signal dark line surrounding the heart on T1- and T2-weighted dark blood imaging (Fig. 38.3). The pericardium is outlined by the high signal of surrounding epicardial and mediastinal fat. On steady-state free precession (SSFP) imaging, which is a mainstay in cine cardiac MRI, the pericardium still appears low in signal, although the intensity may not be as dark as that seen on T1- or T2-weighted imaging. However, it will still be outlined by adjacent fat on this sequence. The thickness of the pericardium may be overestimated on MRI due to a chemical shift artifact. Additional sequences can be used to visualize the pericardium, especially when certain diseases are suspected. Spatial modulation of

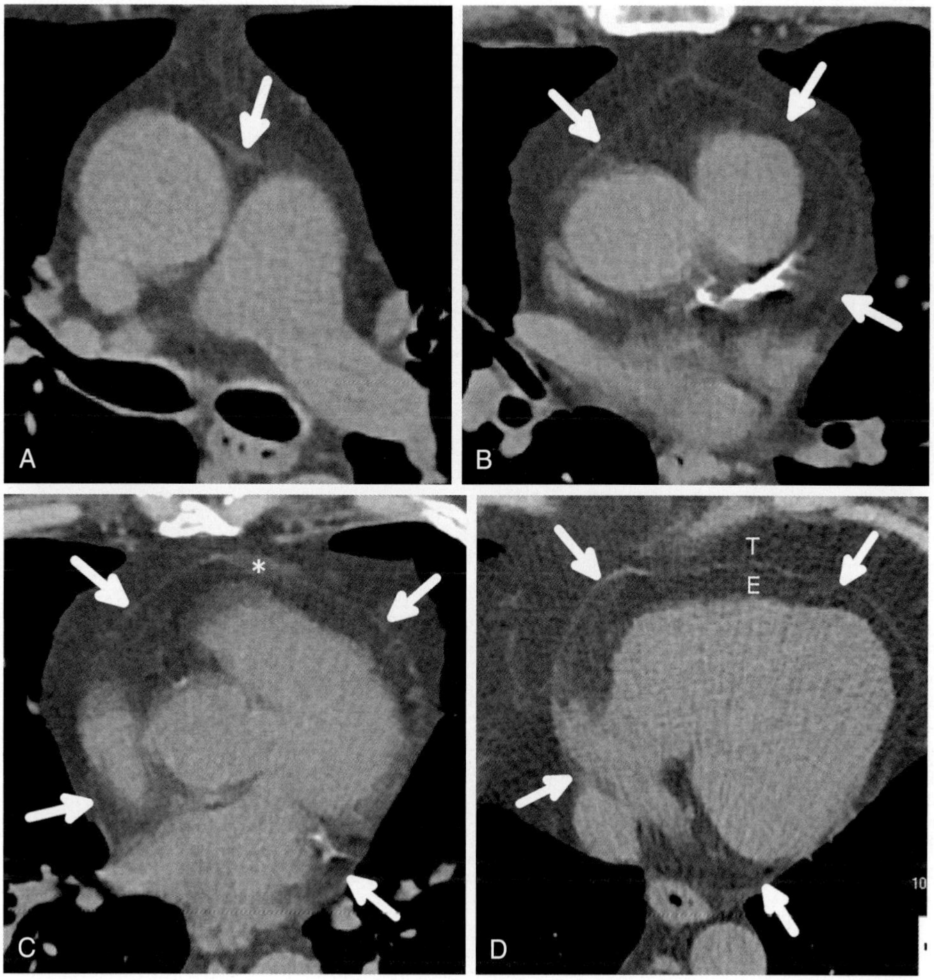

Figure 38.1 Normal pericardium on CT. Axial images at the level of the ascending aorta (A), main pulmonary artery (B), aortic root (C), and coronary sinus demonstrates a curvilinear band of soft tissue surrounding the heart from the level of the great vessels to the diaphgragm *(arrows)*. (D) The pericardium is best visualized when outlined by epicardial *(E)* and mediastinal *(T)* fat *(arrows)*. Although the entire pericardium is often difficult to visualize, it is almost always present. Up to 35 mL of fluid is normally found in the pericardial sac, and it is important not to confuse a small amount of physiologic fluid (*asterisk*, C) with pericardial thickening.

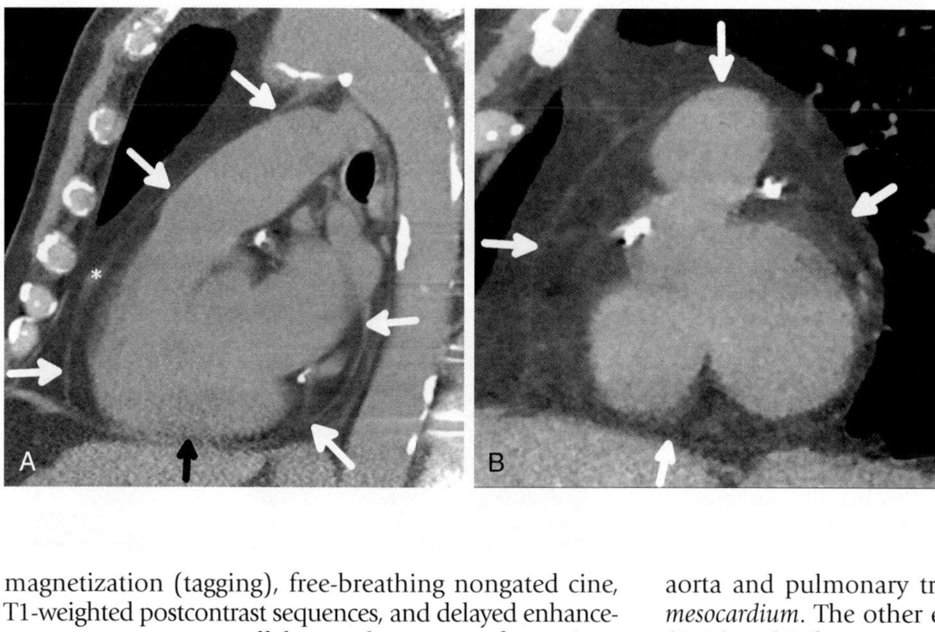

Figure 38.2 Normal pericardium on CT. A 5-mm thick ray-sum parasaggital image of the thorax (A) and 8-mm thick ray-sum short-axis image through the base of the left ventricle (B) show the extend of the pericardium, which encloses the heart *(white arrows)*. Although portions of the pericardium are not well seen, such as that along the diaphragmatic surface (*black arrow*, A), the pericardium is present. Fluid is normally present in the pericardium (*asterisk*, A) and should not be confused with pathologic thickening.

magnetization (tagging), free-breathing nongated cine, T1-weighted postcontrast sequences, and delayed enhancement sequences can all be used to assess for various pathologic processes and will be discussed below.

The portion of the visceral pericardium that covers the vessels is arranged in the form of two short tubes. One encloses the proximal portions of the ascending aorta and pulmonary trunk and is termed the *arterial mesocardium*. The other encloses the superior vena cava (SVC) and inferior vena cava (IVC) and the four pulmonary veins and is termed the *venous mesocardium*. The attachment of the venous mesocardium to the serous layer of the parietal pericardium occurs posterior to the left atrium and between the pulmonary veins in the shape

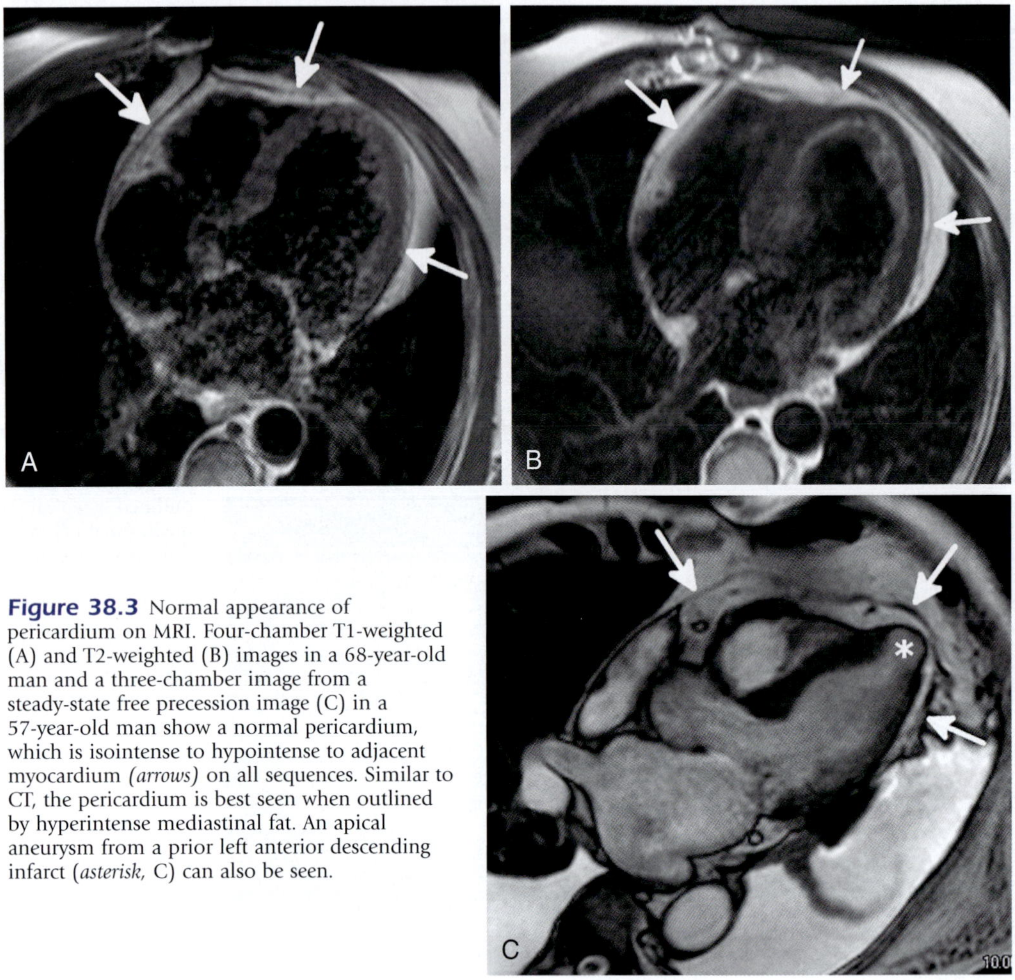

Figure 38.3 Normal appearance of pericardium on MRI. Four-chamber T1-weighted (A) and T2-weighted (B) images in a 68-year-old man and a three-chamber image from a steady-state free precession image (C) in a 57-year-old man show a normal pericardium, which is isointense to hypointense to adjacent myocardium *(arrows)* on all sequences. Similar to CT, the pericardium is best seen when outlined by hyperintense mediastinal fat. An apical aneurysm from a prior left anterior descending infarct (*asterisk*, C) can also be seen.

of an inverted U, forming the oblique sinus (Fig. 38.4). The oblique sinus is contiguous with the subcarinal region and forms a posterior pericardial recess.

Another serosal tunnel, the transverse sinus, is formed by a tunnel between the arterial mesocardium and venous mesocardia. Thus the transverse sinus lies superior to the left atrium and posterior to the aorta and main pulmonary artery (Fig. 38.5). As it does, it communicates with several recesses, including the superior aortic, inferior aortic, right pulmonic, and left pulmonic recesses. The left and right pulmonary recesses form the lateral extents of the transverse sinus. Each of these sinuses lies inferior to their respective pulmonary arteries (see Fig. 38.5). The superior aortic recess is a component of the transverse sinus that extends upward along the ascending aorta and is often visible on CT. The anterior portion of the superior aortic recess lies anterior to the ascending aorta and pulmonary artery and often has a triangular shape, but may be quite variable in appearance and extent (Fig. 38.6; see Fig. 38.5). The posterior portion of the superior aortic recess can be seen on CT as a crescent-shaped fluid collection posterior to the ascending aorta, usually at the level of the left pulmonary artery. This recess can be high riding and may extend superiorly into the right paratracheal region. Although this is a normal variant, the high-riding superior aortic recess

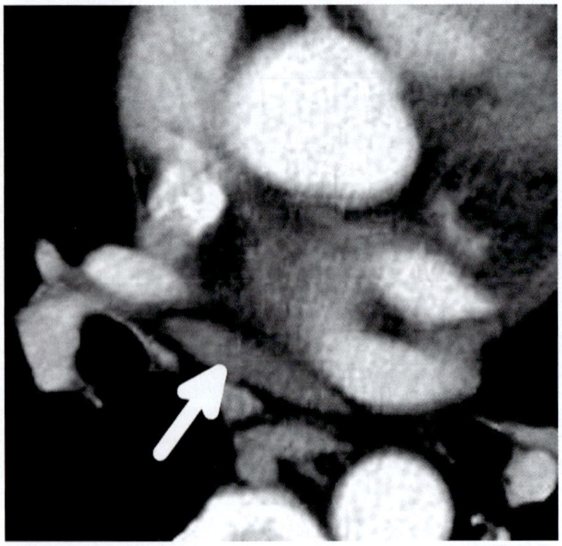

Figure 38.4 Axial CT image in a 44-year-old man demonstrates fluid in the oblique sinus *(arrow)*, which is located posterior to the left atrium.

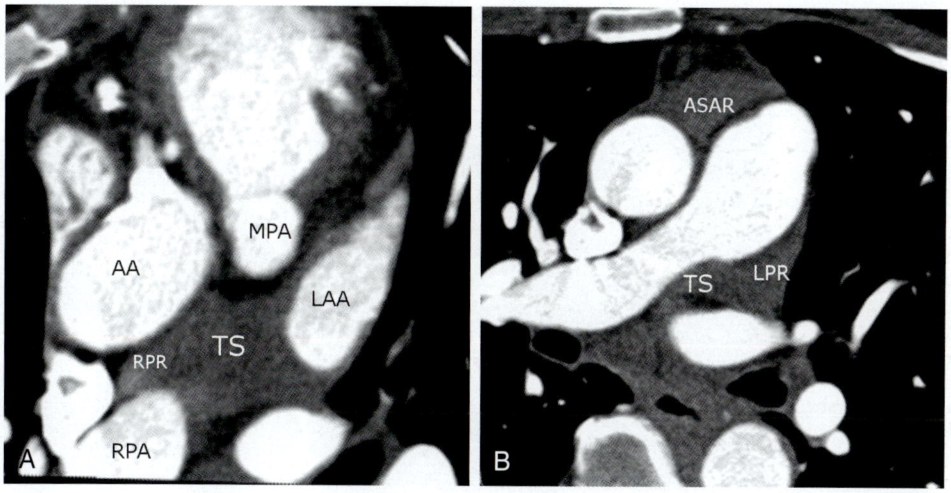

Figure 38.5 Fluid in the transverse sinus extending in the pulmonary recesses in a 59-year-old woman. (A) Axial oblique images show fluid in the transverse sinus *(TS)*, which is located between the ascending aorta *(AA)*, main pulmonary artery *(MPA)*, and left atrial appendage *(LAA)*. The TS is contiguous with fluid in the right pulmonary recess *(RPR)*, which is inferior to the right main pulmonary artery *(RPA)*. (B) More superior axial image shows fluid in the left pulmonary recess *(LPR)*, which is contiguous with the TS and is inferior to the left pulmonary artery. Fluid is also present in the anterior portion of the superior aortic recess *(ASAR)*.

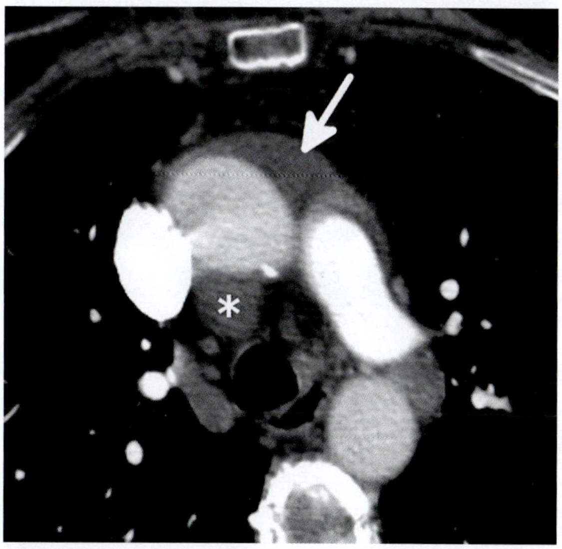

Figure 38.6 Fluid in the superior aortic recess in a 65-year-old man with lung cancer. This axial image at the level of the left pulmonary artery shows crescentic fluid in the anterior portion *(arrow)* and posterior portion *(asterisk)* of the superior aortic recess. Fluid in this location is common and should not be confused with adenopathy or other pathology.

can be confused for a mediastinal cyst mass, leading to unnecessary intervention (Fig. 38.7). The inferior aortic recess is located between the right lateral aspect of the ascending aorta and the right atrium, with its inferiormost extent at the level of the aortic annulus.

In addition to these, there are three additional recesses of the pericardial cavity proper. These include the postcaval recess, left pulmonary vein recess (Fig. 38.8), and right pulmonary vein recess (Fig. 38.9). The postcaval recess is posterior and right lateral to the SVC. The left and right pulmonary venous recesses are located between the superior and inferior pulmonary veins on each side. As the pulmonary veins extend through the fibrous pericardium to drain into the left atrium, serosal sleeves of pericardium invest the veins. On occasion, the sleeve around the right inferior pulmonary vein can be filled with fluid and can mimic adenopathy or a tumor (Fig. 38.10). Fluid in the sleeve will often be seen on both sides of the vein and does not narrow the vein. The characteristic location and fluid attenuation can help differentiate this from pathology.

Blood to the pericardium is supplied by branches from the thoracic aorta and pericardiophrenic arteries. Venous drainage is through the venae pericardial, which drain to the azygous vein, SVC, or brachycephalic veins. Innervation predominantly occurs through branches of the phrenic nerve, although vagal innervation from the esophageal plexus supplies some of the posterior pericardium. The lymphatic drainage of the pericardium is primarily directed toward the tracheobronchial nodes and, less frequently, toward the prepericardial lymphatic vessels and nodes (lymphatic drainage of the pericardium to the mediastinal lymph nodes).

■ Congenital Anomalies of the Pericardium

Pericardial Cyst

Pericardial cysts are benign congenital lesions lined by mesothelial cells. If a connection to the pericardium is present, they are termed *pericardial diverticula.* Pericardial cysts are uncommon lesions, occurring in 1 in 100,000 patients. Most occur at the cardiophrenic angles, on the right greater than the left. A minority occur in other parts

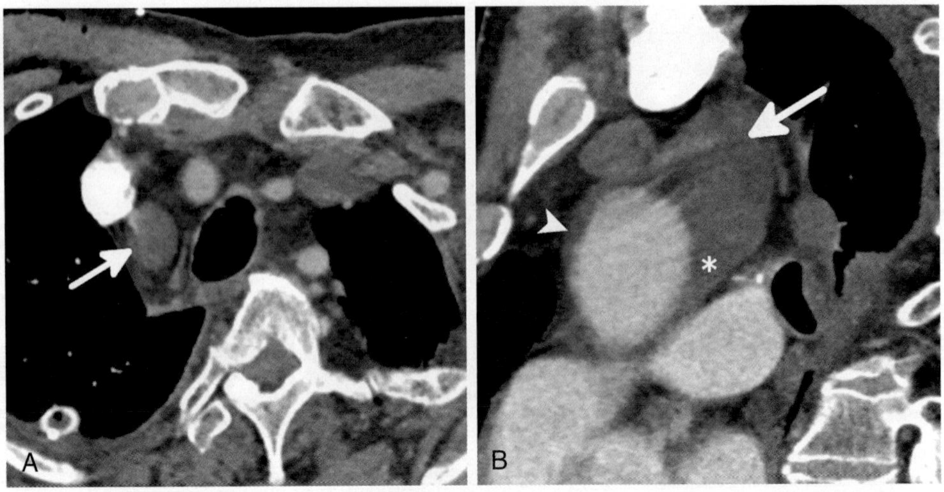

Figure 38.7 A 42-year-old man with high-riding superior pericardial recess mimicking a mediastinal cyst. (A) Axial image at the level of the aortic arch vessels shows a cystic mass in the right paratracheal region *(arrow)*. (B) Sagittal image shows that this fluid collection *(arrow)* communicates with the posterior *(asterisk)* and anterior *(arrowhead)* aspects of the superior aortic recess, consistent with a high-riding superior aortic recess. This anatomic variant can be easily confused with a mediastinal cystic mass, which could lead to unnecessary intervention.

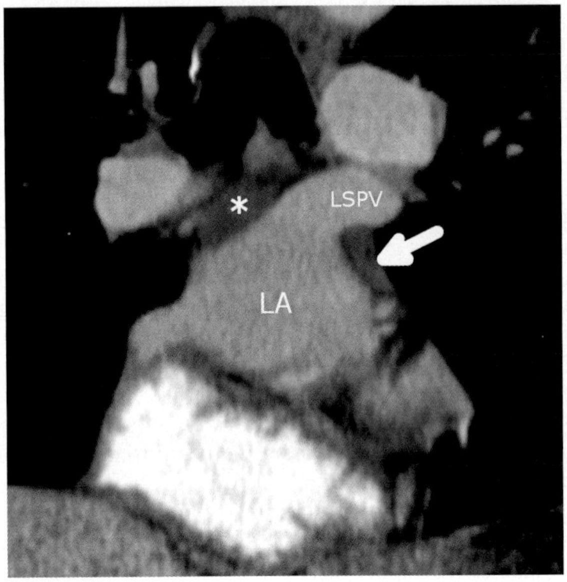

Figure 38.8 Coronal oblique multiplanar reformat demonstrates fluid in the left pulmonary venous recess *(arrow)*, which is located between the left superior pulmonary vein *(LSPV)* and left inferior pulmonary vein. A small amount of fluid is also seen in the superior aspect of the oblique sinus *(asterisk)*. *LA*, Left atrium.

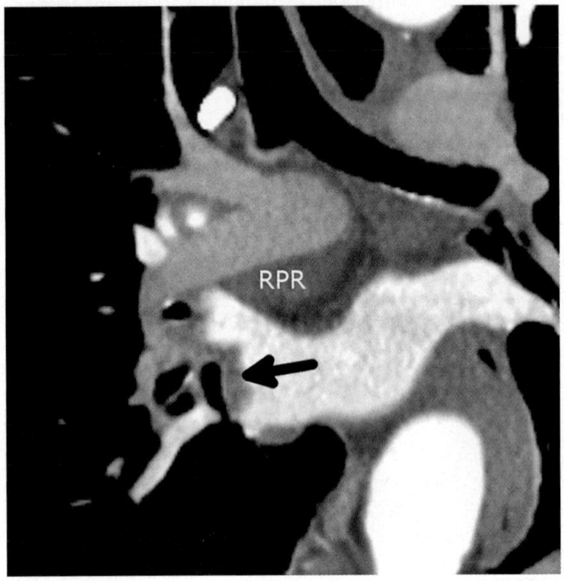

Figure 38.9 Coronal image in a 45-year-old woman with an aortic aneurysm shows fluid in the right pulmonary venous recess *(arrow)* between the right superior and inferior pulmonary veins. Fluid is also present in the right pulmonary recess *(RPR)*, inferior to the right pulmonary artery.

of the mediastinum, usually related to the pericardium. Most patients are asymptomatic, but up to one-third may present with chest pain, dyspnea, or cough, particularly if the cyst compresses adjacent structures.

Imaging features of pericardial cysts are often characteristic. On chest radiography, the cyst typically manifests as a rounded density that contacts the hemidiaphragm and anterior chest wall (Fig. 38.11). On CT, pericardial cysts typically appear as thin-walled round or ovoid lesions, with internal fluid attenuation. Proteinaceous material or hemorrhage can lead to increased attenuation on CT. If the diagnosis of a cyst cannot be definitively made on CT, MRI can help with the diagnosis. On T2-weighted images, pericardial cysts show homogeneous high signal intensity. On T1-weighted imaging, cysts will usually appear low signal, although an intermediate to high signal within the cyst can occur, depending on the degree of proteinaceous material. However, on both MRI and CT, internal septations should be absent. Additionally, although the wall of the cyst may enhance, no internal enhancement should be seen on CT or MRI. Internal enhancement, heterogeneous signal (MRI) or attenuation (CT), thickened wall, or numerous septations should raise the possibility of a cystic tumor.

Pericardial diverticula often cannot be distinguished from pericardial cysts but can be suspected if there is a direct connection of a cystlike structure to fluid in the pericardial space. Additionally, because of a retained connection with the pericardium, the fluid within a pericardial diverticulum can change over time. Most pericardial cysts and diverticula do not undergo treatment but symptomatic cysts may require aspiration or surgery.

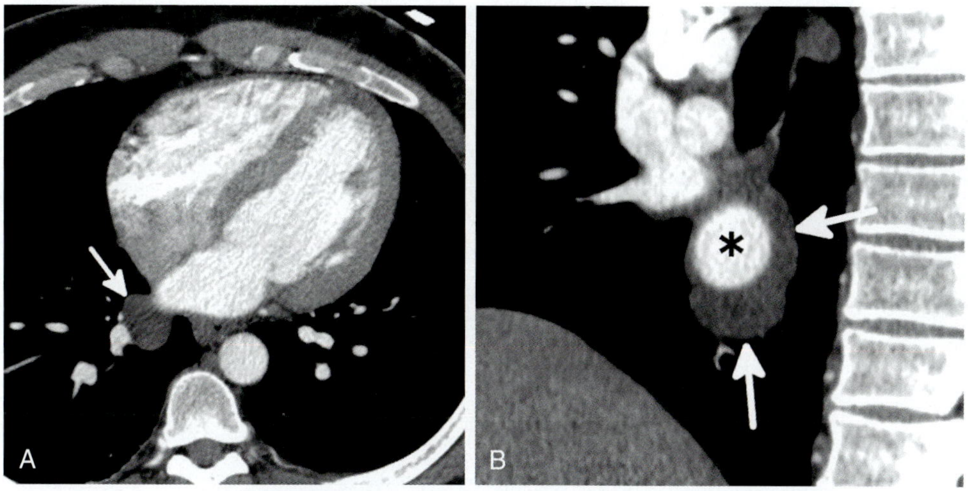

Figure 38.10 Axial oblique (A) and sagittal oblique (B) multiplanar reformats show fluid in a serosal sleeve *(arrows)* that surrounds the right inferior pulmonary vein (*asterisk,* B) in a 26-year-old man. This collection has a characteristic appearance and should not be confused with a mass or adenopathy.

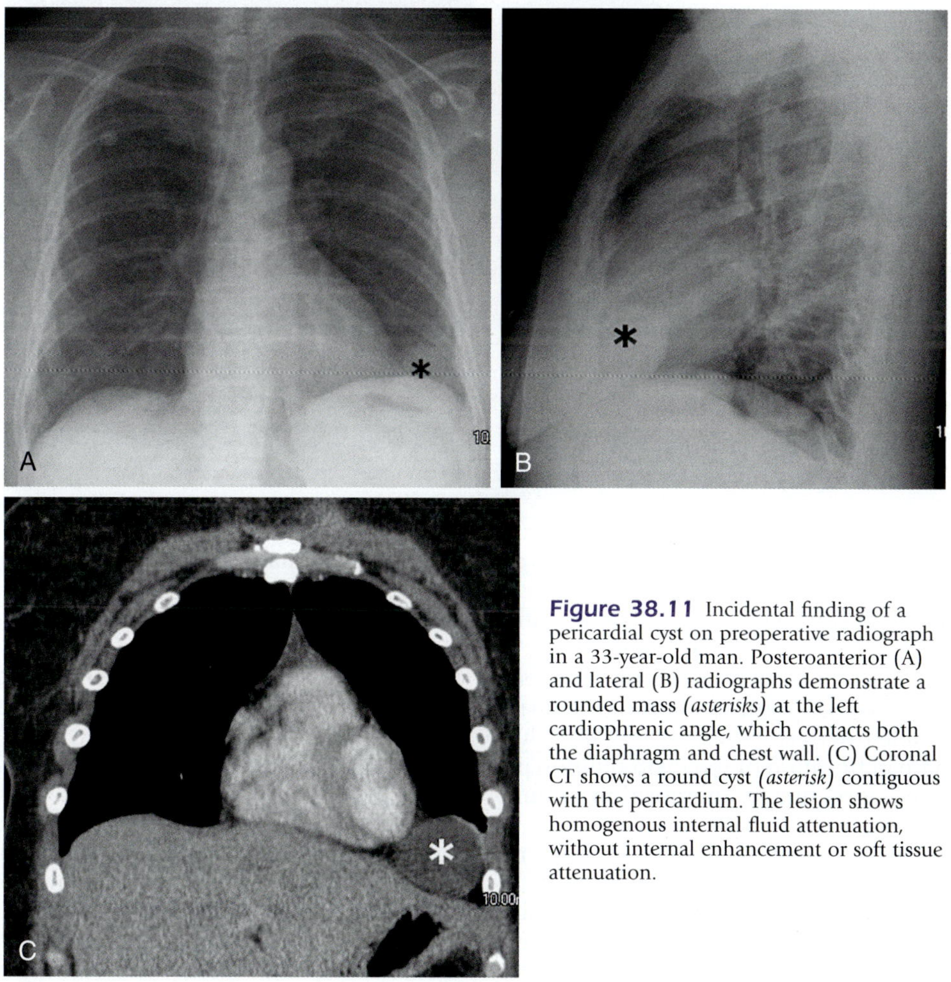

Figure 38.11 Incidental finding of a pericardial cyst on preoperative radiograph in a 33-year-old man. Posteroanterior (A) and lateral (B) radiographs demonstrate a rounded mass *(asterisks)* at the left cardiophrenic angle, which contacts both the diaphragm and chest wall. (C) Coronal CT shows a round cyst *(asterisk)* contiguous with the pericardium. The lesion shows homogenous internal fluid attenuation, without internal enhancement or soft tissue attenuation.

Pericardial Defect

Congenital absence of the pericardial is an uncommon abnormality that is estimated to occur in 1 in 7000 to 13,000 people. The defects can be partial or complete and are much more common on the left. One theory regarding cause postulates that the embryonic left common cardiac vein regresses earlier than normal, leading to a defect. Most pericardial defects are asymptomatic, and the finding is incidental. However, in very rare cases, portions of the left atrium can herniate through a partial defect and become incarcerated. This can lead to infarction of portions of the left atrium, most notably the left atrial appendage, with subsequent syncope and sudden death. Although these defects usually occur in isolation, 30% to 50% of patients will have an associated congenital

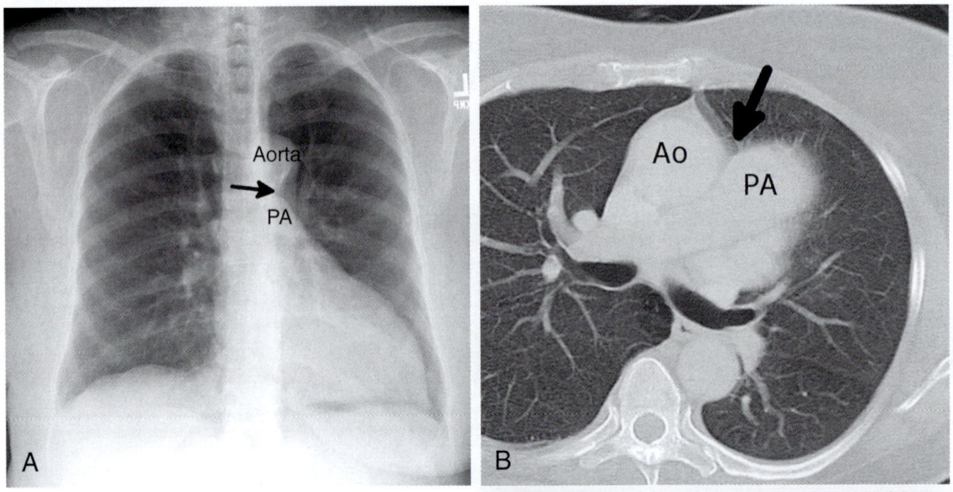

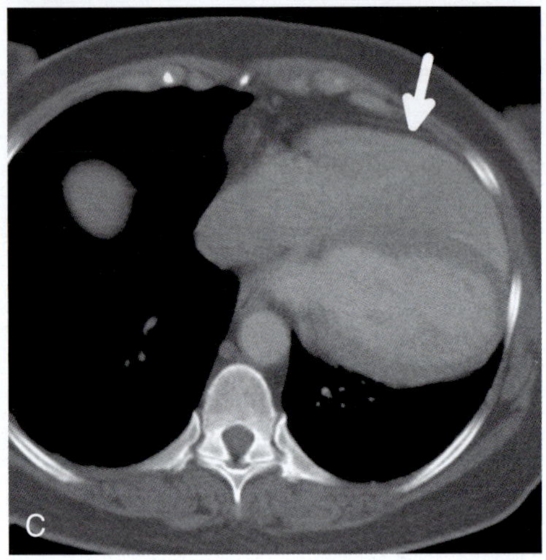

Figure 38.12 Incidental discovery of partial absence of the pericardium in a 55-year-old woman. (A) On posterior anterior radiograph, the main pulmonary artery *(PA)* is very well delineated because lung extends between the PA and aorta *(arrow)*. (B) Axial image through the PA shows lung herniating between the main PA and aorta *(Ao)*, a finding that is diagnostic of absence of the pericardium *(arrow)*. (C) Axial image through the ventricles shows leftward rotation of the heart due to partial absence. A portion of the pericardium can be seen overlying the right ventricle *(arrow)*.

anomaly. Cardiac anomalies include atrial septal defect, patent ductus arteriosus, and bicuspid aortic valve, or pulmonary abnormalities may be present. It can also be seen in patients with connective tissue disorders and characteristics suggestive of Marfan syndrome.

Absence of the pericardium can be a difficult diagnosis to make on radiography. Leftward rotation of the heart is present in left-sided defects. However, the best clue on x-ray is the sharp delineation of the main pulmonary artery and transverse aorta due to interposition of lung between these two structures (Fig. 38.12).

The appearance of a congenital absence of the pericardium on CT depends on whether the abnormality is partial or complete. In both partial and complete left-sided defects, there is leftward rotation of the heart into the left chest, with interposition of the lung between the aorta and pulmonary artery. If the defect is partial, the heart bulges leftward in the region of the left atrial appendage (see Fig. 38.12). The actual defect in partial absence of the pericardium may be difficult to visualize because the pericardium is usually absent over the lateral aspect of the left ventricle and, even under normal circumstances, the pericardium is often difficult to localize in this area. If the left-sided defect is complete, the entire heart is typically displaced to the left, and lung is interposed between the inferior margin of the heart and diaphragm.

On functional cine imaging, excessive motion of the cardiac apex has been observed in individuals with complete absence of the pericardium.

Acquired Pericardial Diseases

Pericardial Effusion

Pericardial effusions are commonly seen on imaging and represent an abnormal accumulation of fluid in the pericardial space. This collection may be characterized as transudative, exudative, hemorrhagic, or pyogenic (Fig. 38.13). Transudative effusion is a common finding in patients with congestive heart failure or other diseases or disorders that lead to increased right heart filling pressures. There are numerous causes of exudative effusions; these include acute infection, inflammation, malignancy, autoimmune disorders, and pericardial trauma. Exudative effusions are common in cases of pericarditis (see below). Blood products can also fill the pericardial space in cases of trauma or aortic dissection. In the pyopericardium, frank pus fills the pericardial space and carries a high mortality rate. Although most effusions are small in size and asymptomatic, symptomatology

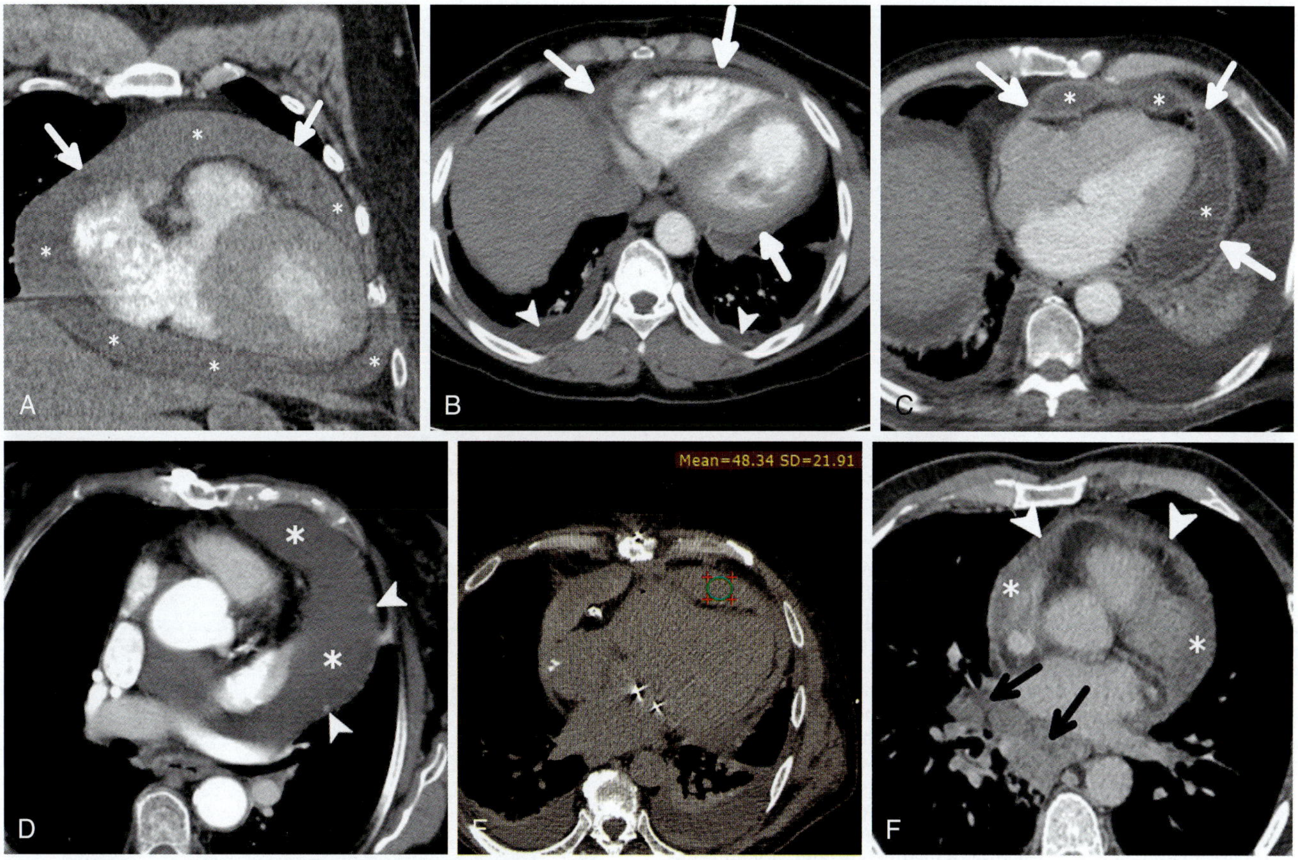

Figure 38.13 Types of material in pericardial effusions. (A) Coronal CT in a 36-year-old man with nephrotic syndrome demonstrates a large transudative effusion *(asterisks)*. The pericardium is not visibly thickened *(arrows)*. (B) Axial CT shows a sterile exudative effusion in a 32-year-old woman with lupus-related pleural *(arrowheads)* and pericardial *(arrows)* effusions. (C) Axial CT shows an exudative serosanguineous effusion *(asterisks)* with acid-fast bacilli, lymphocytes, and monocytes in a 27-year-old man with acute tuberculous pericarditis. There is associated pericardial thickening and enhancement *(arrows)*. (D) Axial oblique multiplanar reformat image from CT shows an effusion *(asterisks)* in a 65-year-old woman with renal cell carcinoma. Two small enhancing nodular foci of enhancement representing metastatic deposits are seen *(arrowheads)*. Pericardiocentesis demonstrated malignant cells. (E) Axial noncontrast CT in a 73-year-old patient with an acute type A dissection demonstrates high-attenuation pericardial fluid with an average CT density of 48.34 Hounsfield units (HU). Subsequent surgery confirmed the presence of hemopericardium. (F) Pyopericardium in a 44-year-old man with methicillin-resistant *Staphylococcus aureus* infection shows pericardial thickening *(arrowheads)* and bulky mediastinal adenopathy *(black arrows)*. Fluid in the pericardial space *(asterisks)* demonstrated an average CT attenuation of 34 HU, consistent with exudative material. Frank pus was removed during pericardiocentesis.

varies, depending on the cause of effusion and rapidity of accumulation.

The detection of a pericardial effusion on chest radiography can be difficult, especially if the effusion is small or moderate in size. Large effusions can often be suggested if the heart has an enlarged water bottle morphology on posteroanterior imaging or if there is a rapid increase in the size of the cardiac silhouette over a short period of time (Fig. 38.14). On the lateral radiograph, a fat pad sign (also referred to as the *Oreo cookie sign*), comprised of pericardial fluid outlined by lower attenuation mediastinal and epicardial fat, can help make the diagnosis (Fig. 38.15).

If a clinically significant pericardial effusion is suspected, echocardiography is often used as the initial technique but may be limited by poor acoustic windows or the location and characteristics of the pericardial collection. Both CT and MRI are valuable to quantify the pericardial effusion and may, in some cases, provide a degree of tissue characterization. On CT, an increase in density above that of simple fluid may indicate an exudative or hemorrhagic process, although there is overlap (see Fig. 38.13E and F). As discussed below in greater detail, patients with active pericardial inflammation will often demonstrate pericardial enhancement after the administration of IV contrast (see Fig. 38.13C and F). The presence of pericardial nodularity should raise concern for a malignant pericardial effusion (see Fig. 38.13D). In patients with a history of trauma, surgery, or aortic dissection, high-density fluid suggests hemopericardium (see Fig. 38.13).

MRI is also valuable to demonstrate the characteristics of pericardial effusion. Most effusions are high in signal on T2-weighted and SSFP sequences, even if the effusion is complex in nature. On T1-weighted sequences, simple transudative effusions typically display low signal

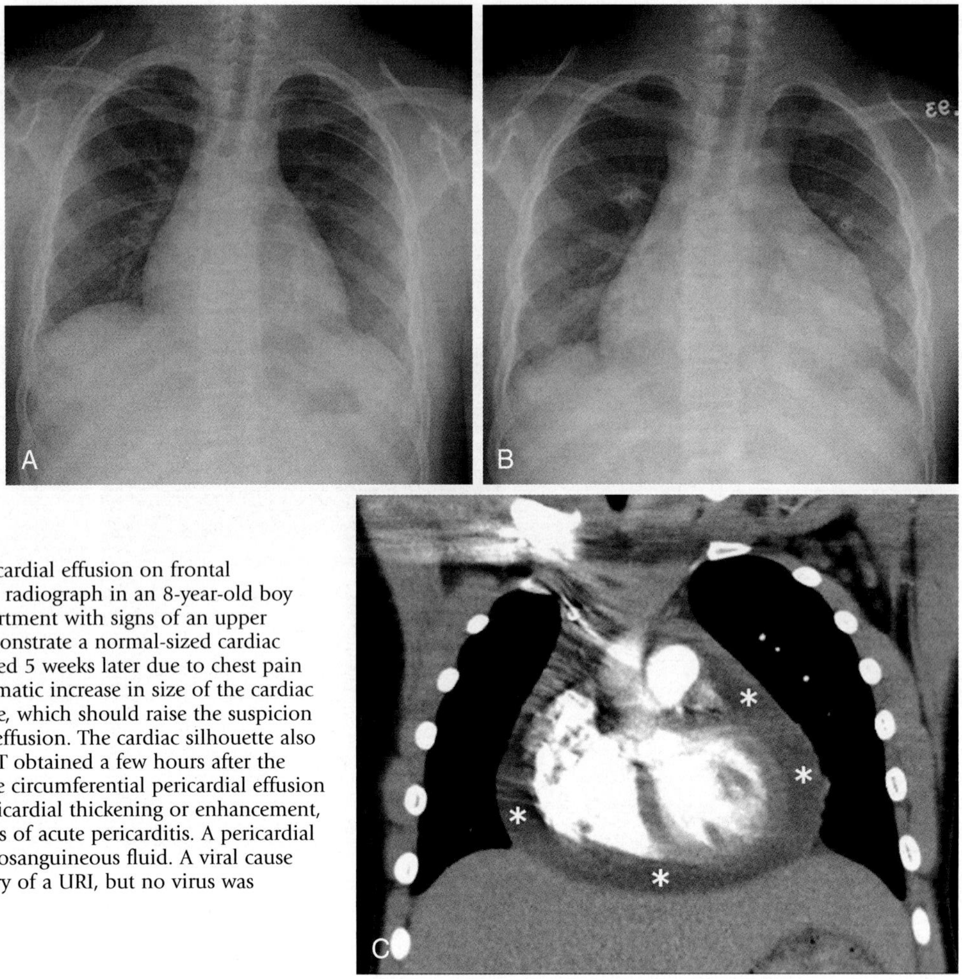

Figure 38.14 Diagnosis of a pericardial effusion on frontal radiograph. (A) Posteroanterior (PA) radiograph in an 8-year-old boy who presents to the emergency department with signs of an upper respiratory tract infection (URI) demonstrate a normal-sized cardiac silhouette. (B) PA radiograph obtained 5 weeks later due to chest pain and shortness of breath shows a dramatic increase in size of the cardiac silhouette over a short period of time, which should raise the suspicion of the development of a pericardial effusion. The cardiac silhouette also has a globular shape. (C) Coronal CT obtained a few hours after the chest radiograph in (B) shows a large circumferential pericardial effusion *(asterisks)*. There is no visualized pericardial thickening or enhancement, which does not exclude the diagnosis of acute pericarditis. A pericardial drain was placed, which revealed serosanguineous fluid. A viral cause was suspected given the recent history of a URI, but no virus was cultured from the fluid.

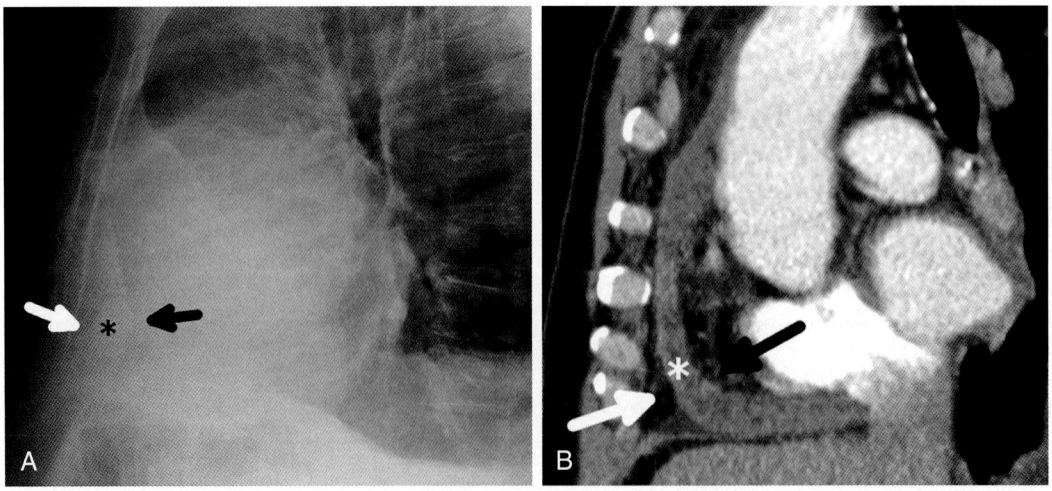

Figure 38.15 Fat pad sign on a lateral radiograph in a 59-year-old man with chronic renal failure. (A) Coned-down view of the heart on the lateral radiograph shows higher atteunation fluid *(asterisk)* outlined by epicardial fat centrally *(black arrow)* and mediastinal fat peripherally *(white arrow)*. (B) Corresponding CT shows the pericardial effusion *(asterisk)* outlined by epicardial *(black arrow)* and mediastinal *(white arrow)* fat, which correlates with the findings on the lateral radiograph.

intensity, whereas exudative or hemorrhagic effusions are more likely to demonstrate intermediate to high signal intensity. However, pericardial fluid characterization can be difficult, especially in cases of larger effusions, because the nonlinear motion of pericardial fluid during cardiac motion can lead to a falsely elevated high signal on T1-weighted images, even in the presence of a simple transudate (Fig. 38.16).

On delayed enhancement imaging, the appearance of a pericardial effusion will drastically differ, depending on whether the images are reconstructed using a magnitude or phase-sensitive inversion technique (PSIR). In essence, delayed imaging using a magnitude reconstruction represents an absolute value of longitudinal magnetization, whereas PSIR preserves its polarity. Therefore tissue whose longitudinal magnetization that lies off the null point will demonstrate increased signal, whether it lies above (z+) or below (z–), the set inversion time (TI). For example, if the TI is set to around 300 ms, which is a common time used to null myocardium, fat, whose T1 relaxation time is faster than normal myocardium, will have a magnetization above the null point (z+) and water, whose T1 relaxation is slower than that of myocardium, will have a magnetization below the null point (z–). However, because the magnitude reconstruction represents an absolute value, both fat and fluid will demonstrate high signal on magnitude imaging. Therefore it can be difficult to differentiate epicardial

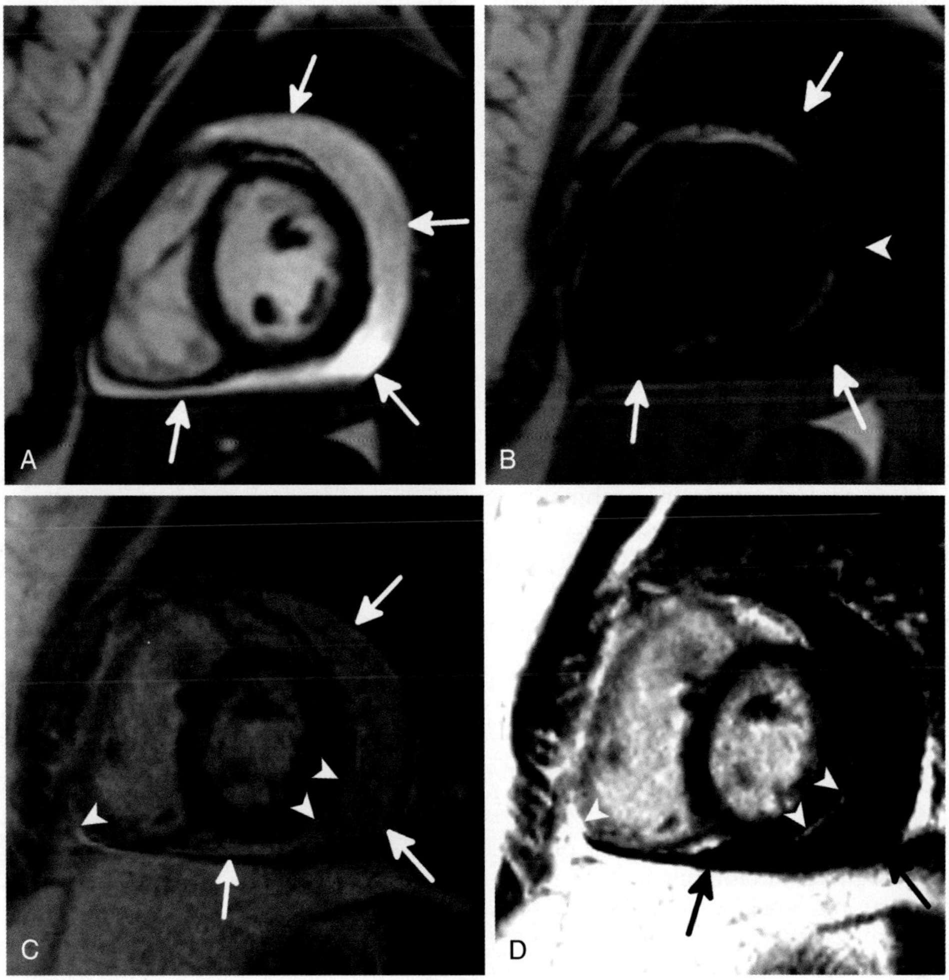

Figure 38.16 MRI of a transudative pericardial effusion in a 19-year-old woman with hypothyroidism, bipolar disorder, and chest pain. (A) Short-axis, steady-state free precession image through the midcavity level of the left ventricle shows a moderate-sized pericardial effusion that is homogenously high in signal *(arrows)*. (B) T1-weighted dark blood imaging at the same level shows a relatively homogenous, low-signal pericardial effusion *(arrows)*. An area of intermediate signal adjacent to the lateral segments *(arrowhead)* is a common finding in moderate to large effusions due to the nonlinear motion of the pericardial fluid but can lead to the misdiagnosis of an exudative effusion. Short-axis magnitude (C) and phase-sensitive inversion recovery (D) delayed gadolinium enhancement images set at an inversion time of 290 ms to null myocardium demonstrates the different appearance of the pericardial effusion between the two images. Because the magnitude reconstruction uses an absolute value of longitudinal magnetization (Mz), both fluid *(white arrows)* and epicardial fat *(white arrowheads)* appear similar in intensity. However, by preserving information about the polarity of Mz, pericardial fluid appears very dark *(black arrows)* because its T1 relaxation time is longer than the myocardium time; adjacent pericardial fat *(white arrowheads)* appears bright because its T1 relaxation time is shorter than the myocardium time.

fat from pericardial fluid using magnitude imaging (see Fig. 38.16C). However, PSIR preserves the information about the polarity of the longitudinal relaxation, so more negative values are ascribed darker pixels and more positive values are ascribed brighter pixels. Therefore, using the PSIR reconstruction, pericardial fluid will appear very dark, whereas epicardial fat will appear bright (see Fig. 38.16D). This is a useful tool that not only allows differentiation between tissues, but can also elucidate pathology, such as in the case of pericardial thickening or adjacent myocardial inflammation.

Pericardial Tamponade

Pericardial tamponade may complicate a pericardial effusion; it occurs when the pressure in the pericardial space exceeds that of the right ventricle. Due to decreased right ventricular filling, tamponade can lead to hemodynamic compromise and rapid death. The development of tamponade depends on the distensibility of the pericardium and rapidity in the accumulation of the pericardial fluid. The slow accumulation of fluid in a distensible pericardium can lead to accumulation of a large amount of pericardial fluid, without the development of tamponade. However, patients who rapidly develop an effusion are more susceptible to developing tamponade, especially if the pericardium is less compliant due to inflammation or scarring. In this case, as little as 100 to 200 mL of fluid can lead to tamponade. Tamponade is a clinical and physiologic diagnosis, and cross-sectional CT or MRI should not be the first imaging modality choice when assessing for tamponade. The diagnosis is usually made based on clinical criteria, in combination with characteristic cardiac findings on echocardiography, notably diastolic collapse of the right ventricular free wall, right atrial collapse, paradoxic motion of the interventricular septum, and a swinging motion of the heart in the pericardial sac. During inspiration, there will be an increase in flow across the tricuspid and pulmonic valves and decreased flow across the mitral and aortic valves, termed *flow velocity paradoxus.* Additional findings outside of the heart include dilation of the SVC and IVC and IVC plethora, all of which are due to increased right atrial pressure.

However, although CT and MRI should not play a primary role in the diagnosis of tamponade, associated findings on cross-sectional imaging may suggest the diagnosis. Typical findings include a moderate to large pericardial collection, with compression or flattening of the right atrium and/or right ventricular free wall (Fig. 38.17). Other nonspecific findings of increased right atrial pressure can be seen, including dilation of the SVC, IVC, and azygous vein, as well as reflux of contrast into the hepatic veins. Bowing of the interventricular septum toward the left can also occur but, again, is nonspecific, because it can be seen with any condition leading to severe pressure or volume overload of the right ventricle. Although effusions are the most common cause of tamponade, it is important to remember that large volumes of air within the pericardial sac can also lead to a tamponade physiology (Fig. 38.18).

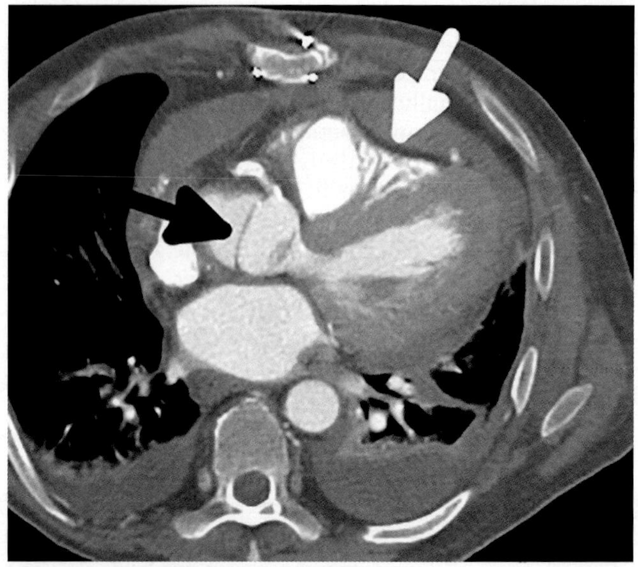

Figure 38.17 Cardiac tamponade in a 73-year-old patient with a type A dissection. This axial CT scan from a contrast-enhanced portion of a CT angiogram shows an intimal flap at the aortic root *(black arrow)*. The noncontrast portion from the same study (see Fig. 38.13E) demonstrated hemopericardium. Compression of the free wall of the right ventricle *(white arrow)* raises the concern for pericardial tamponade, which was confirmed on echocardiography.

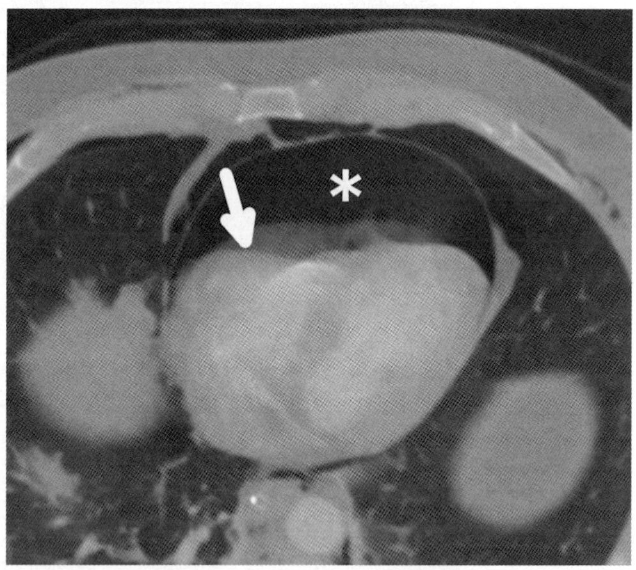

Figure 38.18 Cardiac tamponade due to pneumopericardium. This axial CT in a pedestrian who was struck by a motor vehicle shows a large volume of intrapericardial air *(asterisk)*, leading to compression of the right ventricle *(white arrow)*. The echocardiogram demonstrated tamponade physiology

Inflammation of the Pericardium

Acute Pericarditis

There are numerous causes of pericarditis. Although many cases are labeled as idiopathic, it is assumed that a large percentage of these are viral in cause (see Fig. 38.14).

However, pericarditis can be secondary to bacterial (see Fig. 38.13F), fungal, parasitic, or tuberculous (see Fig. 38.13C) infection. Other causes of acute pericarditis include postcardiac injury syndromes, such as those that occur after myocardial infarction (Fig. 38.19), connective tissue diseases (e.g., systemic lupus erythematosus [see Fig. 38.13B], rheumatoid arthritis, scleroderma), hypersensitivity reaction, radiation therapy, chronic renal failure, pericardial trauma, surgical manipulation, and malignancy (see Fig. 38.13D).

Although there are numerous causes of inflammation of the pericardium, its responses to injury are limited. In cases of acute inflammation, the pericardium reacts by releasing excess fluid, fibrin, or cells, in isolation or in combination, depending on the cause and severity of the insult. Similarly, the healing response can vary dramatically, depending on the underlying cause. For example, patients with acute pericarditis due to tuberculosis, radiation, chronic renal failure, or collagen vascular disease are more likely to develop chronic pericardial fibrosis and adhesions than patients who develop acute pericarditis secondary to viral infection, sarcoidosis, or hypersensitivity reactions. However, the severity of injury and patient-specific factors also play a role. Although some people with idiopathic or viral fibrinous pericarditis may develop permanent pericardial fibrous adhesions, pericardial thickening, or calcific pericarditis, others with a similar mechanism of injury may show resolution, without chronic impairment (Fig. 38.20).

In the acute setting, many patients with acute pericarditis experience sharp chest pain, which is usually worse on inspiration and when the patient is supine. A pericardial friction rub, due to fibrinous deposits, may be present on examination. Electrocardiographic changes are often present, and a small elevation of troponin levels is common.

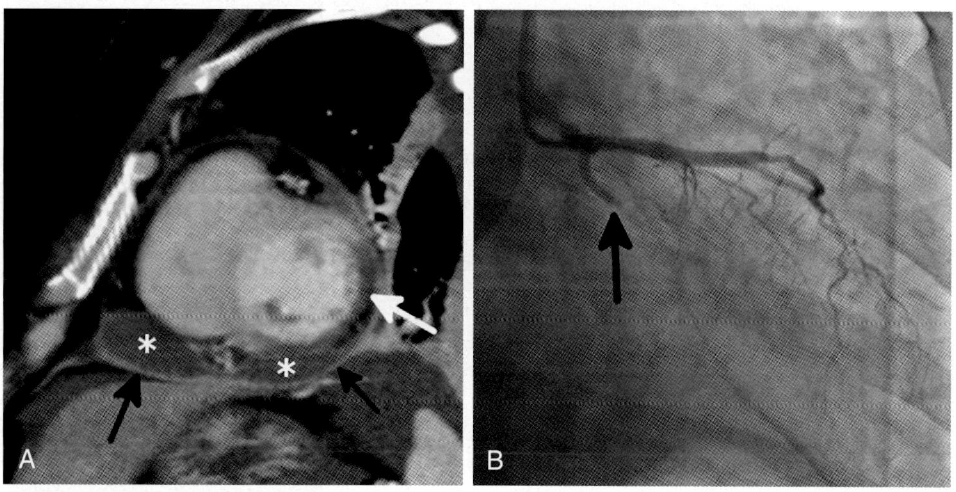

Figure 38.19 Dressler syndrome in a 55-year-old women who had a left circumflex (LCx) myocardial infarction 3 weeks prior. (A) Short-axis image of the heart through the midcavity level shows pericardial thickening and enhancement that is most pronounced along the interior walls of the left and right ventricles *(black arrows)*. There is an associated small to moderate pericardial effusion *(asterisks)* and a transmural lack of enhancement of the inferolateral segment of the left ventricle, consistent with prior infarction *(white arrow)*. (B) Coronary angiogram obtained during admission at the time of the acute myocardial infarction shows complete obstruction of the LCx *(arrow)*.

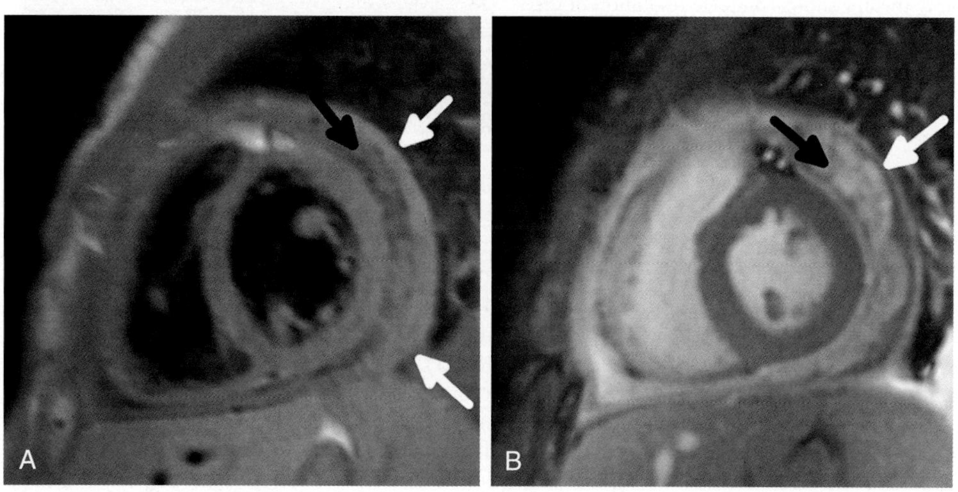

Figure 38.20 Idiopathic fibrinous pericarditis in a 21-year-old man with 5 weeks of chest pain. T1-weighted (A), steady-state free precession (SSFP; B), and spectral adiabatic inversion recovery (SPAIR) T2-weighted fat saturation

Continued

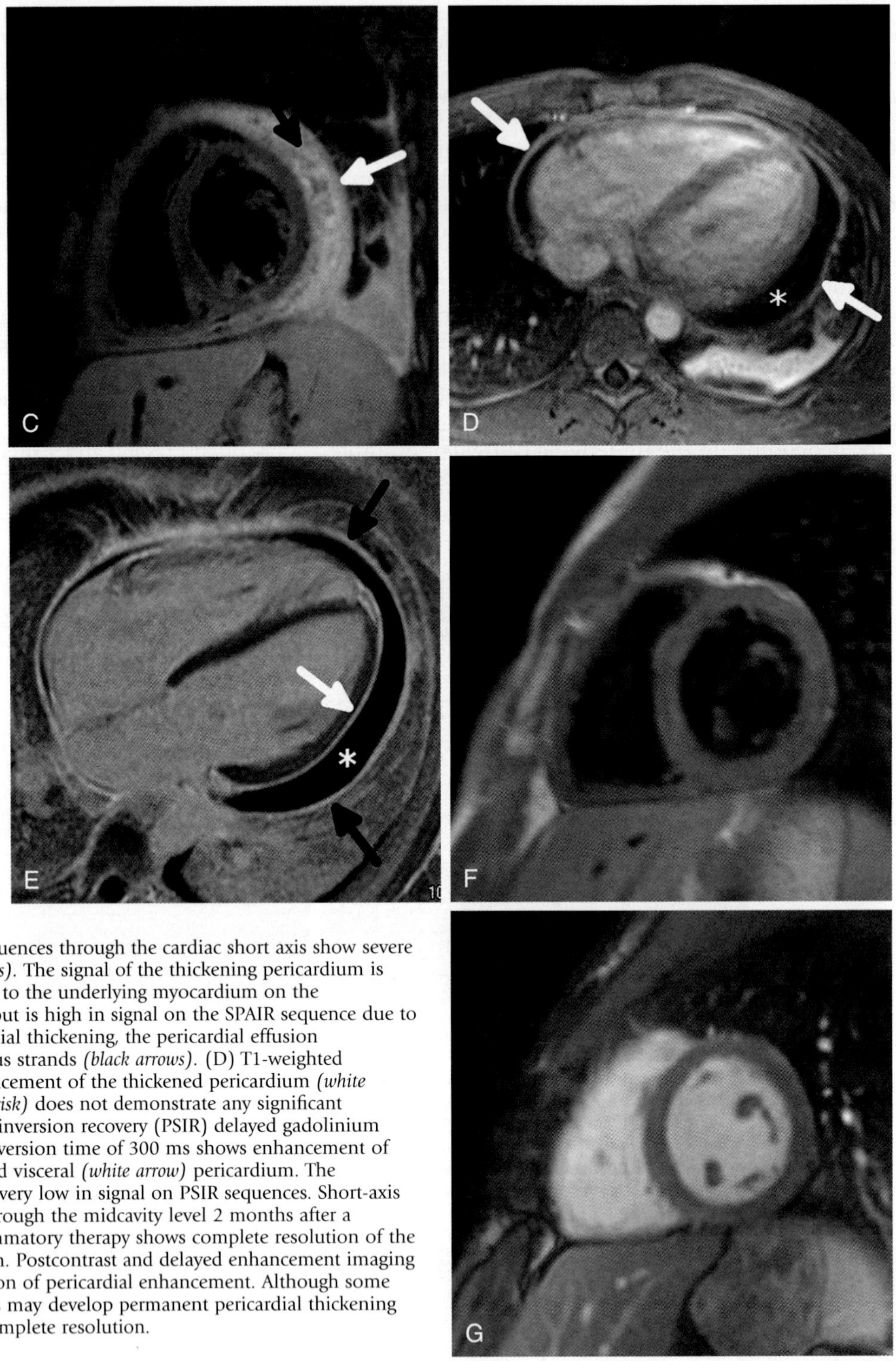

Figure 38.20, cont'd (C) sequences through the cardiac short axis show severe pericardial thickening *(white arrows)*. The signal of the thickening pericardium is isointense to slightly hyperintense to the underlying myocardium on the T1-weighted and SSFP sequences but is high in signal on the SPAIR sequence due to edema. In addition to the pericardial thickening, the pericardial effusion demonstrates pronounced fibrinous strands *(black arrows)*. (D) T1-weighted postcontrast imaging shows enhancement of the thickened pericardium *(white arrows)*. The pericardial fluid *(asterisk)* does not demonstrate any significant enhancement. (E) Phase-sensitive inversion recovery (PSIR) delayed gadolinium enhancement imaging set at an inversion time of 300 ms shows enhancement of both the parietal *(black arrows)* and visceral *(white arrow)* pericardium. The pericardial fluid *(asterisk)* appears very low in signal on PSIR sequences. Short-axis T1 (F) and SSFP (G) sequences through the midcavity level 2 months after a pericardial window and antiinflammatory therapy shows complete resolution of the pericardial thickening and effusion. Postcontrast and delayed enhancement imaging (not shown) also showed resolution of pericardial enhancement. Although some patients with fibrinous pericarditis may develop permanent pericardial thickening and fibrosis, others may have a complete resolution.

On CT, the pericardium is usually thickened to more than 4 mm in diameter and demonstrates smooth or nodular enhancement (see Figs. 38.13C, 38.13F, and 38.19). However, the lack of enhancement or thickening does not exclude the diagnosis of acute pericarditis (see Figs. 38.13B and 38.14). In many cases, there will be an associated pericardial effusion, which may help one visualize the pericardial inflammation. An effusion does not need to be present, especially if the pericardium is thickened, and the cavity has been obliterated by prior pericardial injury.

On MRI, the signal of the inflamed pericardium can vary, depending on the severity of disease and pulse sequence used (Fig. 38.20). On T1-weighted, T2-weighted, and SSFP sequences, the pericardium will appear intermediate (grayish) in signal and will be thickened. The signal of the pericardial effusion can vary, depending on the nature of the fluid. Edema-sensitive T2-weighted sequences, such

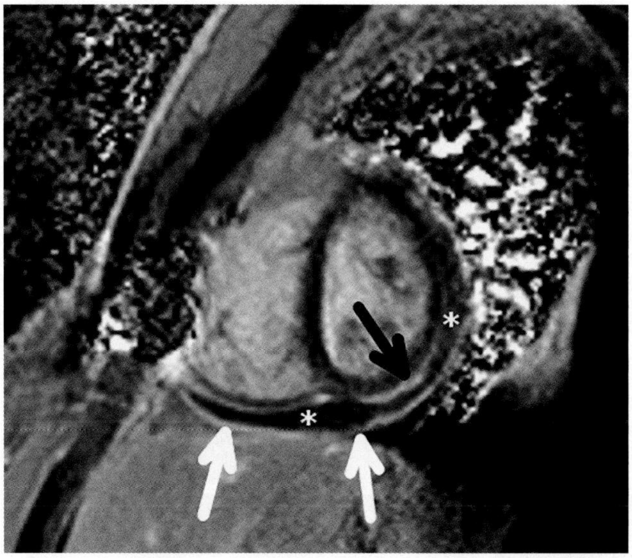

Figure 38.21 Myopericarditis in a 51-year-old man with an increase in troponin levels but normal coronary arteries on cardiac catheterization. Short-axis, phase-sensitive inversion recovery (PSIR), delayed gadolinium enhancement imaging set at an inversion time of 300 ms shows pericardial thickening and delayed enhancement, most notably the inferior and inferolateral aspects of the heart *(white arrows)*. The pericardial fluid appears very low in signal on PSIR sequences *(asterisks)*. There is delayed enhancement along the epicardium of the inferolateral wall of the left ventricle *(black arrow)*, consistent with associated myocarditis.

as a short tau inversion recovery sequence, may show pericardial edema and inflammation of the surrounding fat. In some cases, fibrinous bands can be seen in the pericardium. The pericardium will show enhancement on first-pass perfusion, postcontrast T1-weighted, and delayed contrast-enhanced sequences. Delayed enhancement can also be seen in the underlying myocardium, allowing for the diagnosis of myopericarditis (Fig. 38.21).

Fibrous Pericarditis

As discussed above, whereas in many cases the pericardium may return to normal after acute injury (see Fig. 38.20), in other cases the pericardium becomes permanently injured due to the deposition of fibrous tissue, with subsequent pericardial thickening. In addition, adhesions may develop between any layer of the pericardium, including between the epicardium of the heart and visceral layer of the pericardium, between the serosal layers of the visceral and parietal pericardium, and between the serosal and fibrous layers of the parietal pericardium. Although pericardial adhesions may be focal, in some cases the extent of adhesions is so extensive that the pericardial space becomes obliterated (Fig. 38.22). It should be noted that although pericardial thickening and adhesions often coexist, fibrous thickening can occur without the presence of adhesions, and adhesions can occur without fibrous thickening.

Although any cause of acute pericarditis can lead to fibrous pericarditis and/or adhesions, certain causes are more likely to lead to chronic fibrous thickening. These include conditions that lead to relapsing episodes of pericarditis, such as renal disease and certain collagen vascular diseases, such as rheumatoid arthritis, systemic lupus erythematosus, and scleroderma. Patients with idiopathic pericarditis have a relatively higher chance of developing thickening and adhesions. Other causes of fibrous pericardial disease include radiation, infections (most notably tuberculosis), and pericardial injury due to cardiac surgery or trauma.

Calcium deposition in the pericardium represents an end-stage reaction to pericardial injury. Although deposits may be focal (see Fig. 38.22E), extensive calcification can occur that can lead to encasement of the entire heart. The causes of calcific pericarditis are the same as those that lead to fibrous pericarditis.

On CT, fibrous pericarditis manifests as pericardial thickening, with a variably sized effusion. Conventionally, a threshold pericardial thickness value greater than 4 mm has been used to define pericardial thickening, but the limitations of such a sharp demarcation are evident. Pericardial enhancement may be absent. Calcifications are best visualized on CT, although extensive pericardial calcifications can be seen on chest radiography (Fig. 38.23).

On MRI, the pericardium will appear thickened and irregular, with variable early enhancement (Figs. 38.21 and 38.24). However, delayed hyperenhancement can be seen due to deposition of fibrous tissue. An MRI tagging sequence, which involves placing a grid of saturation lines over the heart and pericardium, can demonstrate adhesion between the visceral and parietal pericardium. In normal cases, the grid lines between the pericardial layers slip past each other during the cardiac cycle, and the grid lines break. When the visceral and parietal pericardium are adherent to one another, the grid lines in the area of adhesions will remain intact. Calcifications may be difficult to see, but the pericardium will appear low signal on all sequences, and enhancement within the areas of calcification will be absent. Although patients with pericardial fibrosis, adhesions, and calcification can remain asymptomatic, patients are at increased risk of developing physiologic constriction.

Constrictive Pericarditis

Constrictive pericarditis (CP) is a condition in which reduced compliance of the pericardium leads to elevated ventricular diastolic pressures. Although CP is occasionally secondary to acute or subacute pericarditis, it is typically the sequela of long-standing pericardial disease with pericardial fibrosis, adhesions, and/or calcification. There are numerous causes of CP, including infection (e.g., tuberculous), chronic renal disease, connective tissue disease, prior pericardial injury (e.g., trauma, cardiac surgery), or radiation. However, most cases of pericardial constriction are secondary to idiopathic pericarditis.

The pathophysiology of CP is secondary to the equalization of pressures in all cardiac chambers because the total cardiac volume is determined by the scarred and inelastic pericardium. Similar to tamponade, the heart

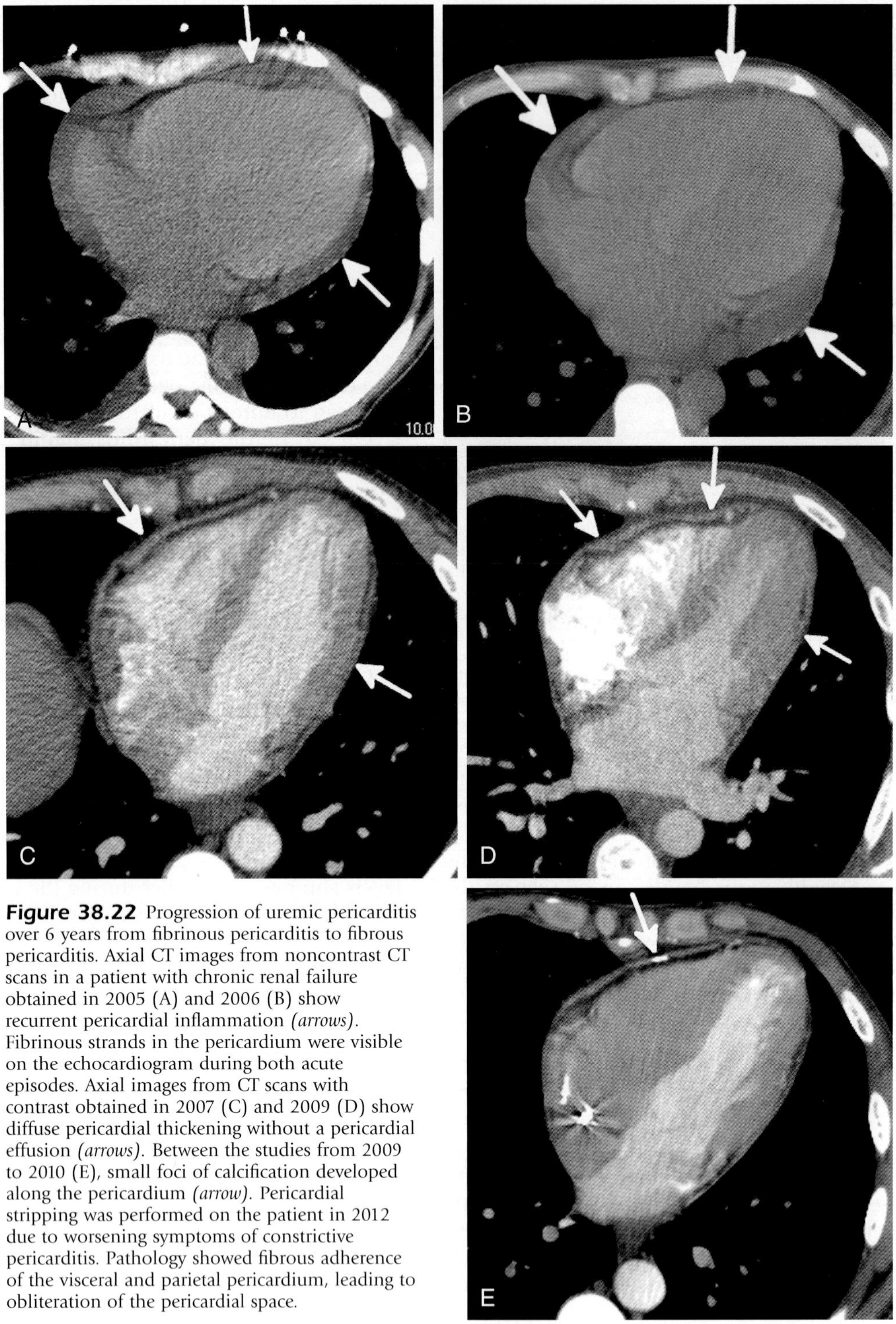

Figure 38.22 Progression of uremic pericarditis over 6 years from fibrinous pericarditis to fibrous pericarditis. Axial CT images from noncontrast CT scans in a patient with chronic renal failure obtained in 2005 (A) and 2006 (B) show recurrent pericardial inflammation *(arrows)*. Fibrinous strands in the pericardium were visible on the echocardiogram during both acute episodes. Axial images from CT scans with contrast obtained in 2007 (C) and 2009 (D) show diffuse pericardial thickening without a pericardial effusion *(arrows)*. Between the studies from 2009 to 2010 (E), small foci of calcification developed along the pericardium *(arrow)*. Pericardial stripping was performed on the patient in 2012 due to worsening symptoms of constrictive pericarditis. Pathology showed fibrous adherence of the visceral and parietal pericardium, leading to obliteration of the pericardial space.

is forced to operate in a noncompliant space, leading to elevated systemic and pulmonary venous pressures, which are required to maintain cardiac filling. The noncompliant space also leads to ventricular interdependence because the increased volume in one ventricle leads to decreased volume in the other ventricle.

CP typically manifests with symptoms of low cardiac output, which particularly affects the right side of the heart. Echocardiography is often performed initially and can demonstrate equalization of pressures during diastole. Additionally, the increased excursion velocity of the medial mitral annulus compared to the lateral mitral annulus (annulus paradoxus), and the decrease or reversal of blood flow in the hepatic veins during expiration, can be measured using Doppler and are highly suggestive of CP. However, in some cases, an echocardiogram is of limited diagnostic yield or the results are equivocal, and additional imaging may aid in the diagnosis.

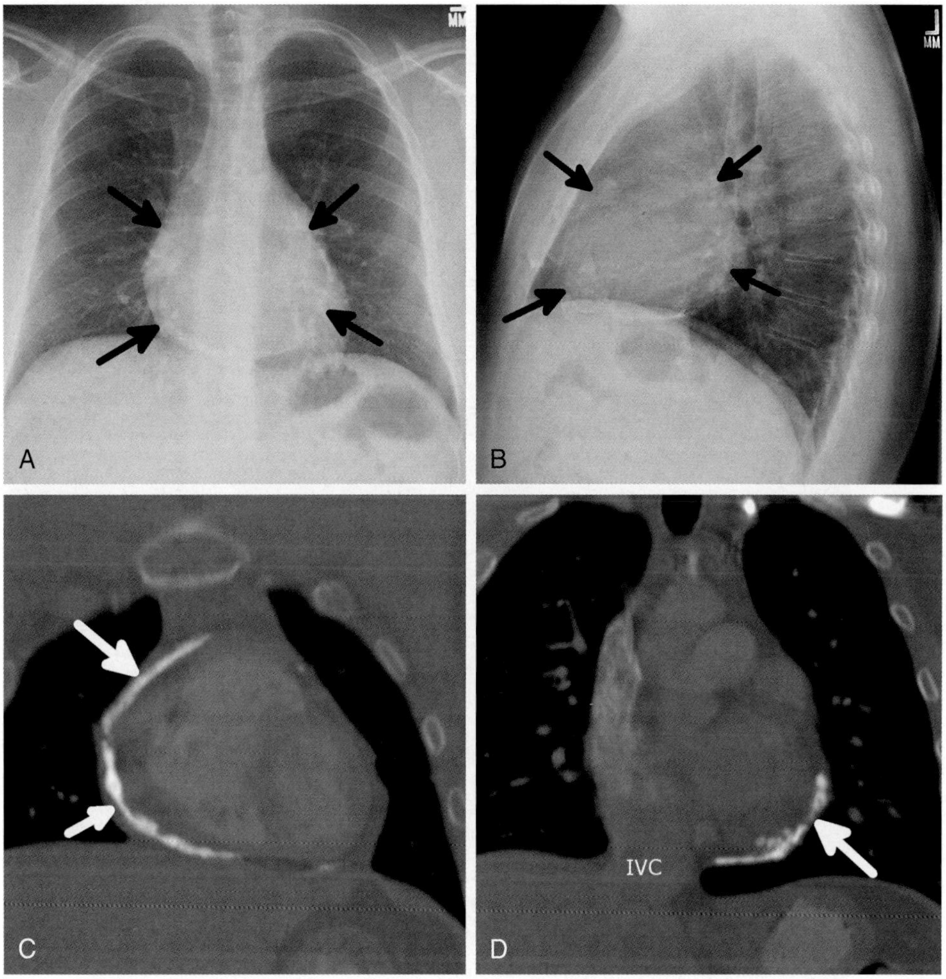

Figure 38.23 Diffuse pericardial calcification in a 66-year-old man with a history of tuberculous pericarditis and signs of constrictive pericarditis. Posteroanterior (A) and lateral (B) radiographs demonstrate extensive circumferential pericardial calcification *(black arrows)*. (C and D) Coronal images from contrast-enhanced CT show the diffuse calcification *(white arrows)*. The inferior vena cava (*IVC*) is severely dilated due to increased right atrial pressure from the diffuse calcific pericarditis.

CT and MRI are critical techniques in the diagnosis of CP. Thickening of the pericardium is well visualized with both techniques (Figs. 38.25 and 38.26; see Figs. 38.22 and 38.23). On CT, pericardial calcification is evident in up to 27% of patients with CP. Delayed gadolinium enhancement of the pericardium is present in approximately 50% of patients with CP and signifies greater fibroblastic proliferation and chronic inflammation of the pericardium.

However, although pericardial thickening is a common imaging feature, the absence of pericardial thickening does not exclude the diagnosis, because up to 28% of patients with CP demonstrate normal pericardial thickness on CT, and 18% have normal thickness on histology. Moreover, patients with end-stage CP are more likely than those with reversible CP to have a normal thickness of the pericardium.

Other morphologic features may be visible on CT or MRI. Poor compliance of the pericardium causes changes in the shape of the cardiac chambers. The ventricles may show a conical appearance, and there may be enlargement of one or both atria. Findings of elevated right-sided pressures are common, including dilation of the IVC and azygous vein, ascites, pleural effusions, and peripheral edema (see Figs. 38.25 and 38.26). However, these findings are nonspecific.

On retrospectively gated cine MRI or cardiac CT angiography, the noncompliant pericardium and ventricular interdependence lead to a classic septal bounce. In CP, rapid ventricular filling in early diastole is followed by abrupt termination of diastolic flow across the atrioventricular valves as the pericardial constraining volume is reached. Because right ventricular filling occurs slightly before left ventricular filling, this early increase in right ventricular pressures leads to a paradoxic leftward motion of the septum in early diastolic filing. The septum will then often rebound back toward the right during left ventricular filling and increased left ventricular pressures. This rightward and subsequent leftward motion of the septum creates a characteristic bounce. Although this early diastolic bounce can be seen in other conditions that lead to diastolic flattening of the interventricular septum, such as right ventricular volume overload, cor pulmonale, and in patients with bundle branch blocks, the septal bounce in CP tends to be more pronounced. Pericardial adhesions of tagging sequences provide an indirect clue to the diagnosis of CP, although patients with focal pericardial adhesions do not necessarily have constrictive physiology.

Due to pericardial adhesions, the excursion of the medial mitral annulus may be greater than the lateral mitral annulus (annulus paradoxus). Although this can

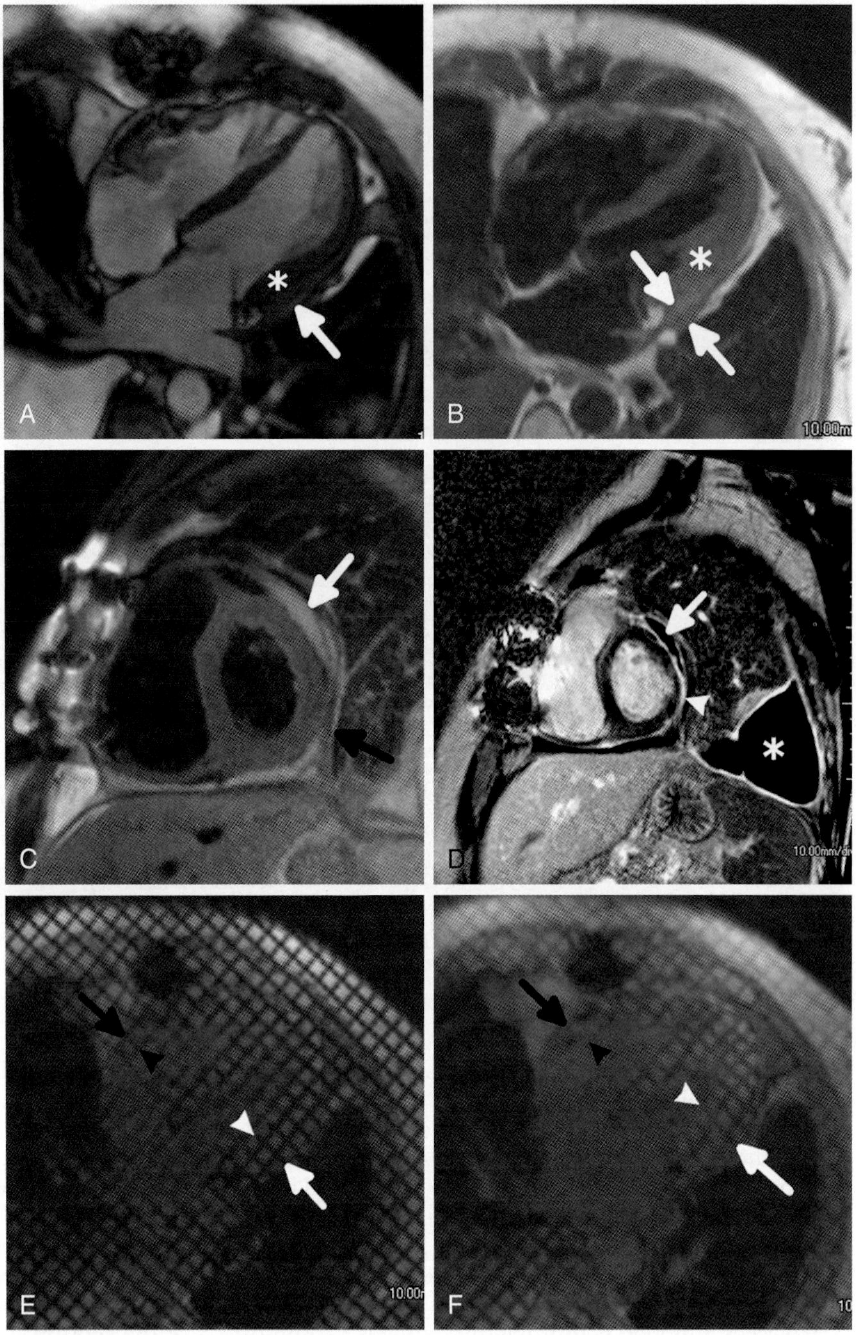

Figure 38.24 Focal fibrous pericarditis with pericardial adhesions in a 75-year-old man who developed hemopericardium after coronary artery bypass. Steady-state free precession (A) and T1-weighted (B) sequences in a four-chamber plane show focal pericardial thickening and fluid *(white arrows)* along the lateral aspect of the base of the left ventricle *(asterisk)*. (C) Short-axis, spectral adiabatic inversion recovery image through the base of the left ventricle shows pericardial thickening *(black arrow)* and some loculated pericardial fluid *(white arrow)*. (D) Short-axis, phase-sensitive inversion recovery (PSIR) delayed gadolinium enhancement imaging at the base set at an inversion time of 280 ms shows pericardial thickening and delayed enhancement along the anterolateral and inferolateral aspects of the left ventricle *(white arrowhead)*. The loculated pericardial fluid appears very low in signal on the PSIR sequence *(white arrow)*. Incidental note is made of a loculated pleural effusion *(asterisk)* with delayed pleural enhancement. (E) Image from a gradient echo tagging sequence in the four-chamber plane obtained during diastole shows multiple grid lines. The grid lines along the endocardial surface of the lateral wall of the left ventricle *(white arrowhead)* and epicardial surface of the left ventricle *(white arrow)* are intact. Similarly, the grid lines along the endocardial *(black arrowhead)* and epicardial *(black arrow)* surface of the right ventricle are intact. (F) During systole, the grid lines between the endocardial *(black arrowhead)* and epicardial *(black arrow)* surfaces of the right ventricle break as the pericardium slides freely along the surface of the heart. However, along the lateral wall of the left ventricle, the grid lines between the endocardial *(white arrowhead)* and epicardial *(white arrow)* surfaces remain intact, which signifies that the pericardium is scarred down and adherent to the underlying epicardium.

be measured using Doppler ultrasound, longitudinal motion of the mitral annulus can also be measured using SSFP imaging in the four-chamber axis; this has been shown to be have a high positive predictive value and specificity in the diagnosis of CP.

Phase contrast imaging can provide information on the flow of blood or tissue. Due to the high atrial pressures, CP leads to rapid early filling of the ventricles followed by rapid decrease in the rate of filling during later diastole. Phase contrast imaging performed across the mitral valve plane will show a narrow and high-velocity E wave during diastolic filling. The A wave, which corresponds to the filling of the ventricles during the atrial kick, will be diminished or absent. Unfortunately, this finding is also present in restrictive cardiomyopathy. To help in differentiation, a recent study demonstrated the utility of real-time, free-breathing, phase contrast imaging, which demonstrated a 25% increase in transmitral flow on expiration and a more than 45% increase in transtricuspid flow during inspiration in all patients with CP, but not in patients without CP or controls.

One of the best methods to diagnose CP on MRI is to demonstrate a respiratory variation of the diastolic bounce using nongated, free-breathing, cine MRI sequences (see Fig. 38.25). Due to the dissociation between intrathoracic and intracardiac pressures in CP, the negative intrathoracic pressures are not transmitted to the left heart chambers, which leads to decreased blood return from the lungs into

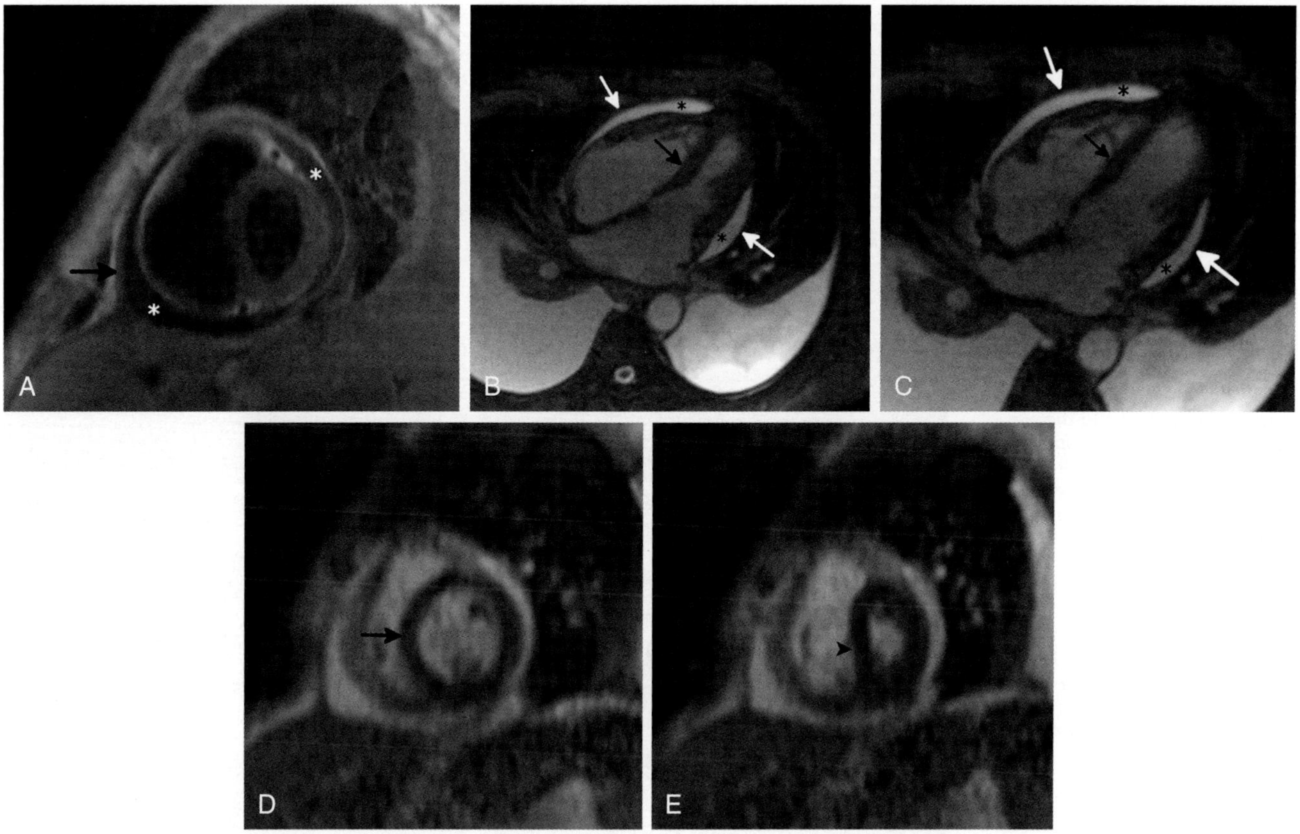

Figure 38.25 MRI findings in constrictive pericarditis (CP) in a 45-year-old man. (A) Short-axis T1-weighted image shows diffuse pericardial thickening best seen anteriorly *(arrow)*. A small to moderate pericardial effusion is present *(asterisks)*. (B) Four-chamber steady-state free precession images obtained during early diastole and middiastole (C) show a septal bounce, which is characteristic of CP. During early diastole, increased right ventricular (RV) pressures from early RV filling causes bowing of the septum to the left (*black arrow,* B). During middiastole, increased left ventricular (LV) pressures due to later LV filling cause the septum to bounce back to the right (*black arrow,* C). Pericardial thickening *(white arrows)* and an effusion *(asterisk)* are present. Free-breathing, nongated, short-axis cine images obtained during expiration (D) and inspiration (E) show the respiratory variation in septal morphology in CP. During expiration, LV pressures exceed RV pressures, and the septum has a normal appearance (*black arrow,* D). On early inspiration, rapid increase of RV pressures due to increased right-sided venous return leads to dramatic flattening of the septum (*arrowhead,* E).

the pulmonary veins. Therefore in patients with CP, the negative intrathoracic pressure on inspiration increases venous return to the right heart. However, because right ventricular motion is limited by the noncompliant pericardium, the increased right ventricular pressures lead to marked flattening of the interventricular septum. On expiration, the opposite occurs as positive intrathoracic pressure increases pulmonary return, resulting in a normal configuration of the septum of septal bowing to the right. This finding will be absent in restrictive cardiomyopathy and can help differentiate between the two.

Although pericardial thickening is a common finding in CP, pericardial effusions are usually not large. However, in rare cases, a patient may present with a large pericardial effusion, leading to a tamponade physiology, superimposed on a stiff noncompliant pericardium, leading to a constrictive physiology. Even after the pericardial fluid is removed, constrictive physiology persists. This syndrome is referred to as *effusive-constrictive pericarditis* and is a rare entity, occurring in less than 7% of patients presenting with pericardial tamponade. Similar to other forms of pericarditis, it is usually idiopathic, but can also occur due to radiation, malignancy, or infection.

■ Pericardial Tumors

Primary pericardial tumors are quite rare and, unlike their cardiac counterparts, are more likely to be malignant. Because the serous layers of the pericardium are layered by mesothelial cells, it is not surprising that primary pericardial mesothelioma accounts for 50% of primary pericardial neoplasms. However, it is still extremely rare and, in a necropsy series of 500,000 cases, the incidence was less than 0.0022%. Although highly associated with pleural mesothelioma, the association between asbestos exposure and pericardial mesothelioma is unclear. However, in approximately one-third of cases, patients have had a known exposure to asbestos. Similar to pleural mesothelioma, pericardial mesothelioma can be epithelioid, sarcomatoid, or biphasic on pathology. Early in the disease, CT and MRI demonstrate complex

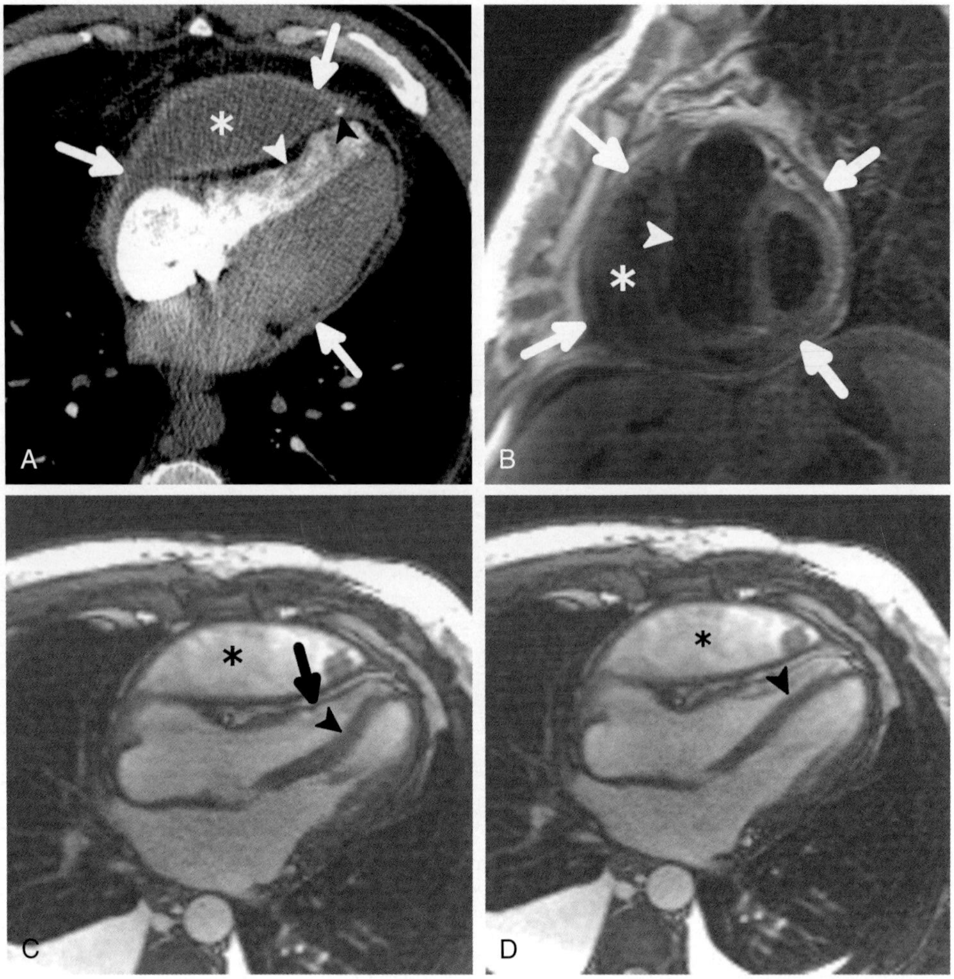

Figure 38.26 Constrictive pericarditis (CP) in a 40-year-old man with a history of a pericardial hematoma. (A) Axial CT image shows diffuse pleural thickening *(white arrows)* with a focus of pericardial calcification *(black arrowhead)*. In addition, there is a larger loculated pericardial fluid collection *(asterisk)* leading to compression of the anterior wall of the right ventricle *(white arrows)*, causing tamponade. (B) Short-axis T1-weighted image shows diffuse pericardial thickening *(arrows)* and the anteriorly located collection *(asterisk)* compression of the anterior wall of the right ventricle *(white arrowhead)*. Four-chamber steady-state free precession images obtained during early diastole (C) and middiastole (D) show a septal bounce, which is characteristic of CP. During early diastole, the septum is bowed to the left (*black arrowhead,* C) and, during middiastole, the septum bounces back to the right (*black arrowhead,* D). In addition, the heterogeneously located pericardial fluid collection *(asterisks)* causes compression of the anterior wall of the right ventricle *(black arrow)*, consistent with cardiac tamponade. (Courtesy Dr. Travis Henry.)

pericardial effusions and pericardial thickening that early in the disease may be mistaken for acute or chronic pericarditis. Unfortunately, cytologic evaluation of the pericardial fluid only demonstrates malignant cells in 20% of patients. As the disease progresses, masses fill the pericardium, often invading surrounding structures, including the heart and vasculature (Fig. 38.27). Prognosis is poor, and few patients survive longer than 12 months after diagnosis.

In addition to mesothelioma, primary pericardial malignancies include sarcomas, lymphoma, and germ cell tumors. Primary pericardial sarcomas can have numerous histologic subtypes, including angiosarcoma, synovial sarcoma, fibrosarcoma, liposarcoma, rhabdomyosarcoma, and undifferentiated sarcoma. Although most lymphomas that involve the pericardium represent part of a systemic disease, primary pericardial lymphoma can occur. Its appearance is widely variable; it can appear as a solitary mass, which can mimic other tumors (Fig. 38.28). Additionally, a primary effusion lymphoma can occur in patients with HIV infection and appear as a large pericardial effusion (Fig. 38.29). Most intrapericardial germ cell tumors occur in children and are benign teratomas. However, malignant germ cell tumors do occur and should be considered in any pediatric patient with a heterogeneous intrapericardial mass (Fig. 38.30).

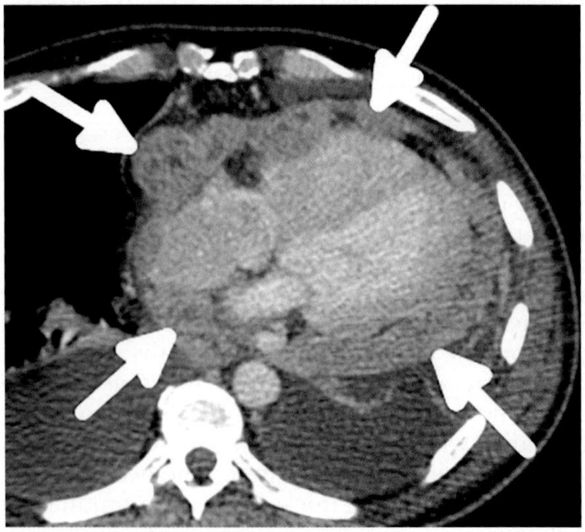

Figure 38.27 Pericardial mesothelioma in a 61-year-old man with shortness of breath. This axial CT image shows numerous pericardial masses and a complex pericardial effusion *(arrows)*. Pericardial mesothelioma, although rare, is the most common primary pericardial tumor. (Courtesy Dr. Travis Henry.)

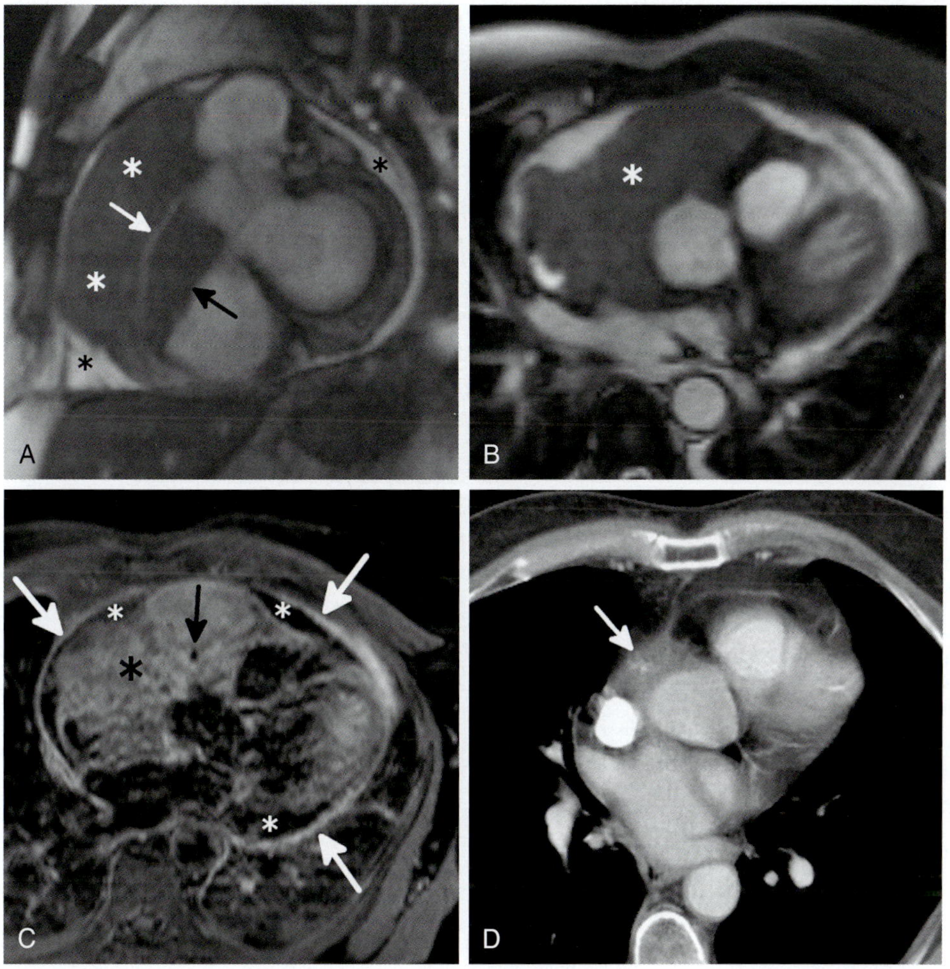

Figure 38.28 Pericardial lymphoma in a 62-year-old man. (A) Short-axis steady-state free precession (SSFP) image shows a large homogeneous mass centered in the right atrioventricular groove *(white asterisks)*, which is encasing the right coronary artery *(white arrow)*. There is also invasion of the right atrium *(black arrow)*. A small pericardial effusion is present *(black asterisk)*. (B) Four-chamber SSFP image shows that the bulk of the mass *(asterisk)* is in the pericardial cavity. (C) T1-weighted postcontrast image shows diffuse enhancement of the mass *(black asterisk)*, which enhances the right coronary artery *(black arrow)*. There is associated pericardial thickening *(white arrows)* and a small effusion *(white asterisks)*. Although the mass was thought to represent an angiosarcoma based on imaging, pathology showed a diffuse, large, B cell lymphoma. There was no disease elsewhere. (D) Axial image from a CT scan 6 years later shows a small amount of soft tissue in the pericardium with an associated central calcification *(arrow)*, consistent with posttreatment changes.

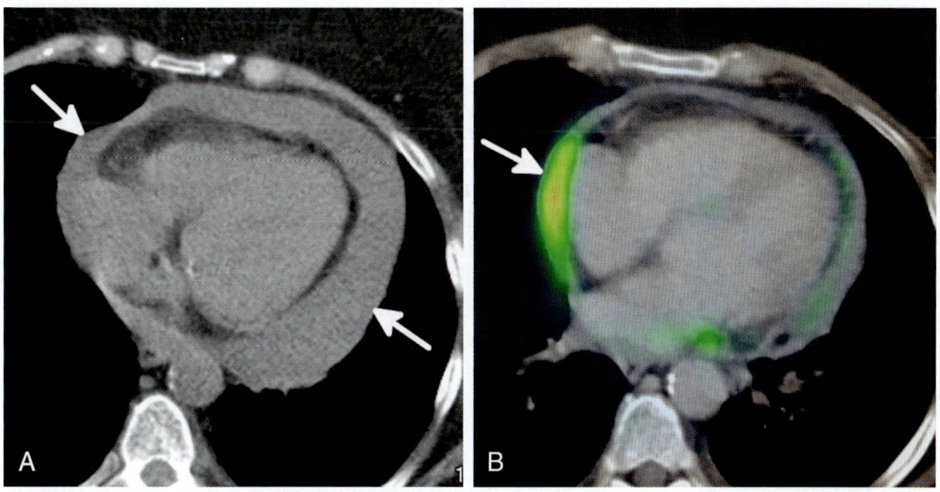

Figure 38.29 Primary pericardial effusion lymphoma in a 57-year-old woman with HIV infection. (A) Axial image from a noncontrast CT scan shows a moderate-sized pericardial effusion *(arrows)*. A pericardiocentesis was performed, which showed hemorrhagic fluid with numerous atypical lymphocytes, consistent with a B cell lymphoma. (B) Axial image from fused PET-CT performed after pericardiocentesis shows a residual pericardial effusion with multiple areas of increased fluorodeoxyglucose uptake *(arrow)* due to malignancy. No disease was present elsewhere.

There are a wide variety of benign intrapericardial tumors, which are all rare. If fat is present in an intrapericardial tumor, teratomas or lipoblastomas should be considered in the pediatric population. In nonpediatric patients, if the lesion is composed entirely of fat, the diagnosis of a lipoma can be made (Fig. 38.31). Paragangliomas in the thorax usually occur in the anterior mediastinum. However, intrapericardial paragangliomas do occur and, although these lesions are benign, they can invade into surrounding structures. These tumors demonstrate avid enhancement on CT and MRI and are intensely bright on T2-weighted sequences (Fig. 38.32).

The secondary spread of tumors to the pericardium is much more common than primary pericardial neoplasms. The most common malignancies to metastasize to the pericardium include lung cancer, breast cancer, and

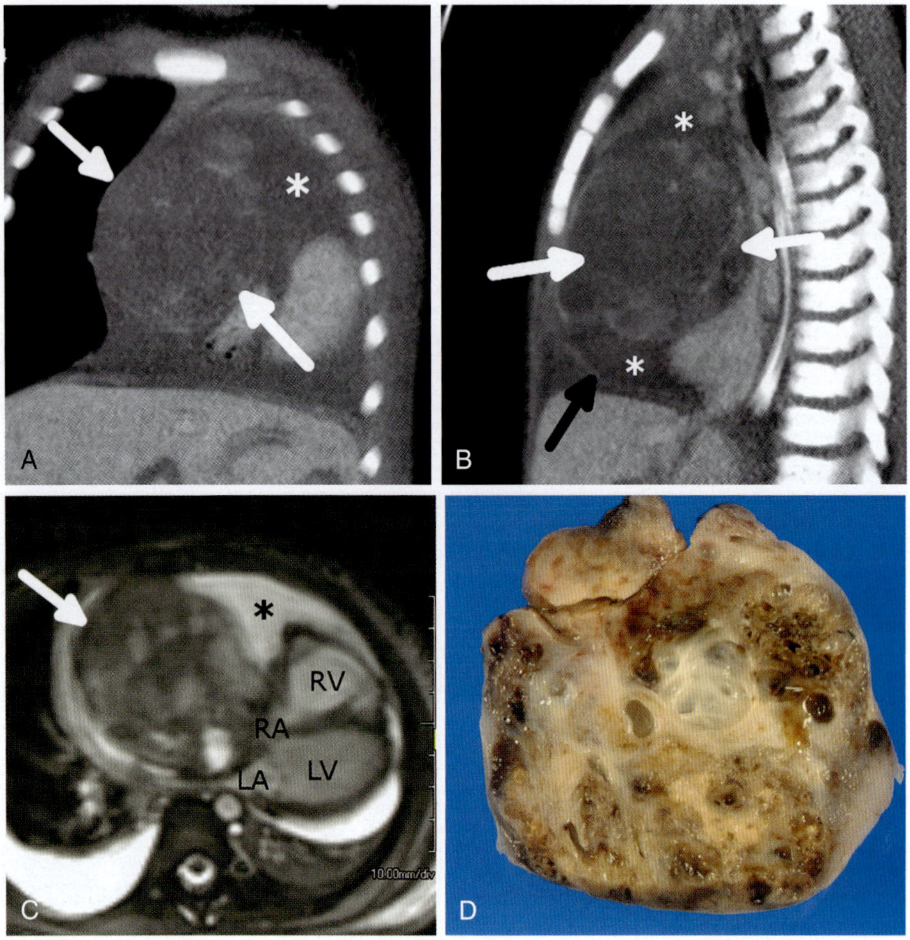

Figure 38.30 Malignant yolk sac tumor of the pericardium in a 21-month-old girl who presented with cardiac tamponade and an elevated AFP. Sagittal (A) and coronal (B) images from a contrast-enhanced CT scan of the chest show a soft tissue and cystic mass *(white arrows)* in the pericardium (B, *black arrow*). There was a large associated pericardial effusion (*asterisk*, A and B). (C) Four-chamber steady-state free precession image shows a part solid, part cystic heterogeneous mass in the pericardium *(white arrow)* and a large associated effusion *(asterisk)*. The mass leads to near-complete obliteration of the right atrium *(RA)* and severe compression of the right ventricle *(RV)* and left atrium *(LA)*. The left ventricle *(LV)* is displaced laterally. The patient was taken to surgery soon after the MRI was performed due to cardiac arrest. (D) Gross pathologic image shows a mixed cystic and solid lesion corresponding to findings on imaging.

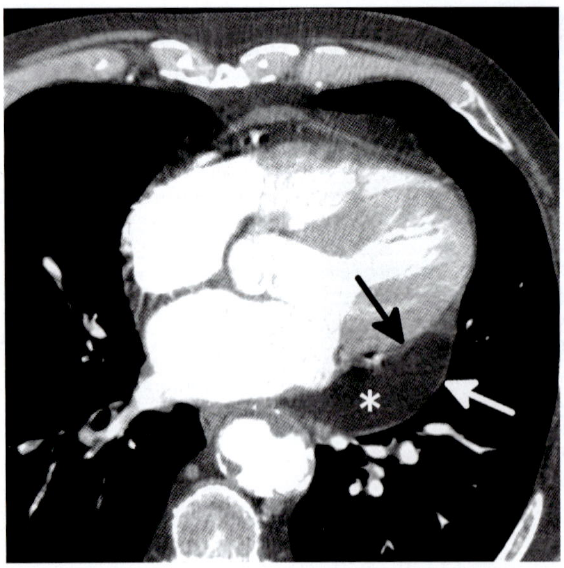

Figure 38.31 Incidental finding of an intrapericardial lipoma in a 78-year-old man. This axial CT shows a fatty mass *(asterisk)* located between the visceral *(black arrow)* and parietal *(white arrow)* layers of the pericardium. Lipomas are benign lesions and can be located in the pericardium, heart, or mediastinum.

lymphoma. Metastatic disease can occur by lymphatic extension, hematogenous spread, or direct contiguous extension. Lymphatic pathways represent a common route of spread of pericardial metastases because the visceral pericardium contains abundant lymphatic channels. Many tumors, such as breast cancer and lymphoma, seed the pericardium through lymphatic channels. Melanoma usually spreads hematogenously and is usually associated with diffuse disease elsewhere. Renal cell carcinoma is also associated with hematogenous metastases (Fig. 38.33). Direct extension usually occurs from lung cancer but can be seen with esophageal cancer, mediastinal lymphoma, or even breast cancer.

Symptoms of pericardial involvement by tumor are related to the extent of disease. Nonspecific symptoms of chest pain and shortness of breath are frequent. Effusions are often hemorrhagic and can be quite large, leading to tamponade in 16% of patients. Diffuse involvement can encase the heart, leading to pericardial constriction. CT and MRI may show the primary site of disease, as well as the extent of pericardial involvement. Typically, pericardial thickening is present, with a variable amount of pericardial nodularity. However, thickening may be absent, and the only finding is a pericardial effusion that may represent a mixture of fluid and hemorrhage (Fig. 38.34). Enhancement of portions of the pericardium may be present after contrast administration via CT or MRI.

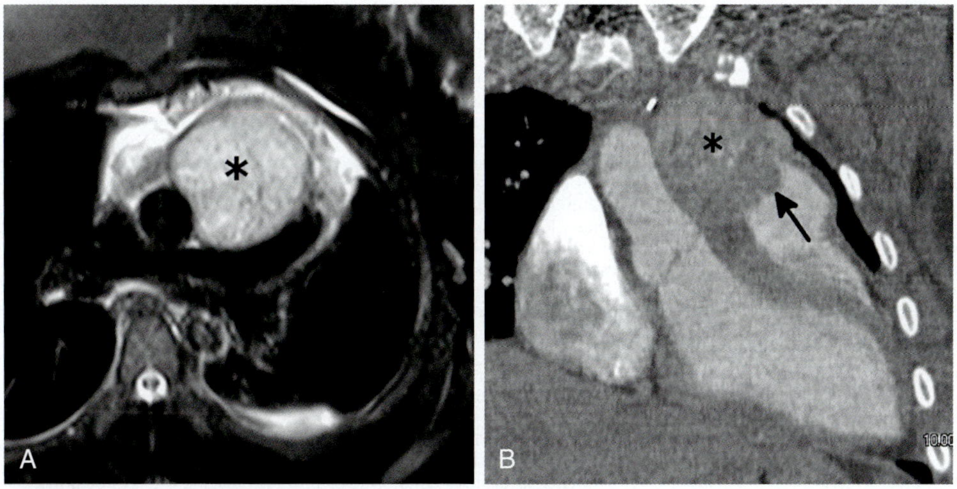

Figure 38.32 Intrapericardial paraganglioma in a 32-year-old woman with uncontrolled hypertension. (A) Axial image from a T2-weighted sequences shows a mass located between the aorta and pulmonary artery *(asterisk)*. This mass is intensely bright on T2-weighted sequences. (B) Coronal oblique multiplanar reformat obtained 10 months later, after an unsuccessful attempted resection, shows the enhancing mass *(asterisk)* invading into the pulmonary artery *(arrow)*. Although paragangliomas are benign, they can be locally aggressive and invade surrounding structures.

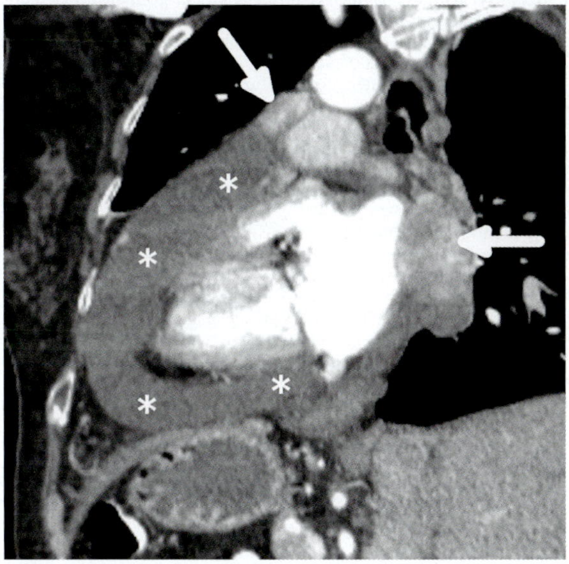

Figure 38.33 Pericardial metastases from renal cell carcinoma in a 71-year-old woman. This sagittal oblique multiplanar reformat shows a large pericardial effusion *(asterisks)*. Two dominant enhancing pericardial masses are present *(arrows)*. Therapeutic pericardiocentesis showed numerous malignant cells. Pericardial metastases are much more common than primary pericardial tumors.

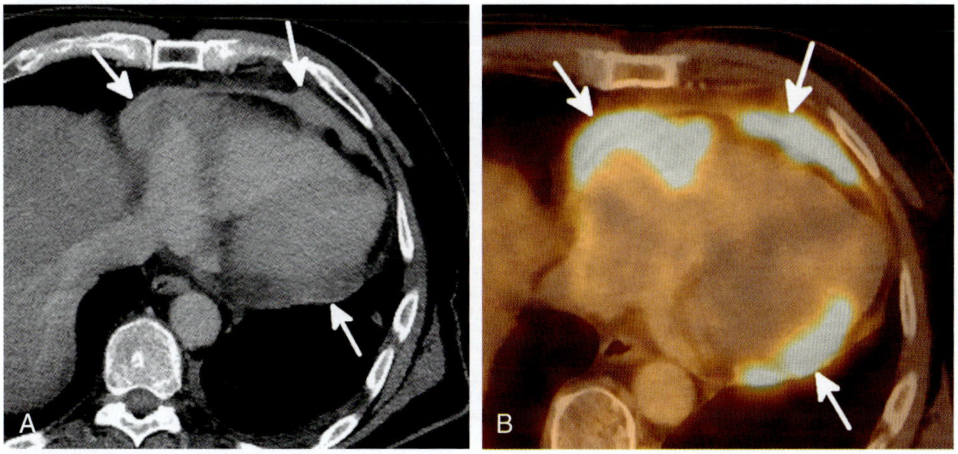

Figure 38.34 Lymphoma metastases to the pericardium in a 44-year-old man with a history of diffuse large B cell lyphoma. (A) Axial CT image shows nodular thickening of the pericardium *(arrows)*. (B) Fused image from PET-CT at the same level shows marked fluorodeoxyglucose uptake in the areas of pericardial nodularity *(arrows)*. A pericardial lymphoma was diagnosed on biopsy.

Bibliography

Abbas AE, Appleton CP, Liu PT, Sweeney JP. Congenital absence of the pericardium: case presentation and review of literature. *Int J Cardiol.* 2005;98:21–25.

Akiba T, Marushima H, Masubuchi M, et al. Small symptomatic pericardial diverticula treated by video-assisted thoracic surgical resection. *Ann Thorac Cardiovasc Surg.* 2009;15:123–125.

Alter P, Figiel JH, Rupp TP, et al. MR, CT, and PET imaging in pericardial disease. *Heart Fail Rev.* 2013;18:289–306.

Bertog SC, Thambidorai SK, Parakh K, et al. Constrictive pericarditis: cause and cause-specific survival after pericardiectomy. *J Am Coll Cardiol.* 2004;43:1445–1452.

Bogaert J, Francone M. Cardiovascular magnetic resonance in pericardial diseases. *J Cardiovasc Magn Reson.* 2009;11:14.

Bogaert J, Francone M. Pericardial disease: value of CT and MR imaging. *Radiology.* 2013;267:340–356.

Bull RK, Edwards PD, Dixon AK. CT dimensions of the normal pericardium. *Br J Radiol.* 1998;71:923–925.

Burazor I, Aviel-Ronen S, Imazio M, et al. Primary malignancies of the heart and pericardium. *Clin Cardiol.* 2014;37:582–588.
Carretta A, Negri G, Pansera M, et al. Thoracoscopic treatment of a pericardial diverticulum. *Surg Endosc.* 2003;17:158.
Carsky EW, Mauceri RA, Azimi F. The epicardial fat pad sign: analysis of frontal and lateral chest radiographs in patients with pericardial effusion. *Radiology.* 1980;137:303–308.
Caudron J, Fares J, Bauer F, Dacher JN. Evaluation of left ventricular diastolic function with cardiac MR imaging. *Radiographics.* 2011;31:239–259.
Chiles C, Woodard PK, Gutierrez FR, Link KM. Metastatic involvement of the heart and pericardium: CT and MR imaging. *Radiographics.* 2001;21:439–449.
Choe YH, Im JG, Park JH, et al. The anatomy of the pericardial space: a study in cadavers and patients. *AJR Am J Roentgenol.* 1987;149:693–697.
Choi YW, McAdams HP, Jeon SC, et al. The "high-riding" superior pericardial recess: CT findings. *AJR Am J Roentgenol.* 2000;175:1025–1028.
Chong HH, Plotnick GD. Pericardial effusion and tamponade: evaluation, imaging modalities, and management. *Compr Ther.* 1995;21:378–385.
Cohen R, Mirrer B, Loarte P, Navarro V. Intrapericardial mature cystic teratoma in an adult: case presentation. *Clin Cardiol.* 2013;36:6–9.
Cracknell BR, Ail D. The unmasking of a pyopericardium. *BMJ Case Rep.* 2015;2015.
Eisenberg MJ, Dunn MM, Kanth N, et al. Diagnostic value of chest radiography for pericardial effusion. *J Am Coll Cardiol.* 1993;22:588–593.
Faridah Y, Julsrud PR. Congenital absence of pericardium revisited. *Int J Cardiovasc Imaging.* 2002;18:67–73.
Feigin DS, Fenoglio JJ, McAllister HA, Madewell JE. Pericardial cysts. A radiologic-pathologic correlation and review. *Radiology.* 1977;125:15–20.
Feng D, Glockner J, Kim K, et al. Cardiac magnetic resonance imaging pericardial late gadolinium enhancement and elevated inflammatory markers can predict the reversibility of constrictive pericarditis after antiinflammatory medical therapy: a pilot study. *Circulation.* 2011;124:1830–1837.
Francone M, Dymarkowski S, Kalantzi M, Bogaert J. Real-time cine MRI of ventricular septal motion: a novel approach to assess ventricular coupling. *J Magn Reson Imaging.* 2005;21:305–309.
Francone M, Dymarkowski S, Kalantzi M, et al. Assessment of ventricular coupling with real-time cine MRI and its value to differentiate constrictive pericarditis from restrictive cardiomyopathy. *Eur Radiol.* 2006;16:944–951.
Frank H, Globits S. Magnetic resonance imaging evaluation of myocardial and pericardial disease. *J Magn Reson Imaging.* 1999;10:617–626.
Groell R, Schaffler GJ, Rienmueller R. Pericardial sinuses and recesses: findings at electrocardiographically triggered electron-beam CT. *Radiology.* 1999;212:69–73.
Hammer MM, Raptis CA, Javidan-Nejad C, Bhalla S. Accuracy of computed tomography findings in acute pericarditis. *Acta Radiol.* 2014;55:1197–1202.
Hynes JK, Tajik AJ, Osborn MJ, et al. Two-dimensional echocardiographic diagnosis of pericardial cyst. *Mayo Clin Proc.* 1983;58:60–63.
Ishihara T, Ferrans VJ, Jones M, et al. Histologic and ultrastructural features of normal human parietal pericardium. *Am J Cardiol.* 1980;46:744–753.
Jeudy J, Kirsch J, Tavora F, et al. From the radiologic pathology archives: cardiac lymphoma: radiologic-pathologic correlation. *Radiographics.* 2012;32:1369–1380.
Kalam K, Harmse W, Merchant N, Fu W. The role of cardiac MR in identifying annulus paradoxus, a specific marker for constrictive pericarditis. *J Cardiovasc Magn Reson.* 2015;17:P362.
Kellman P, Arai AE, McVeigh ER, Aletras AH. Phase-sensitive inversion recovery for detecting myocardial infarction using gadolinium-delayed hyperenhancement. *Magn Reson Med.* 2002;47:372–383.
Klein AL, Abbara S, Agler DA, et al. American Society of Echocardiography clinical recommendations for multimodality cardiovascular imaging of patients with pericardial disease: endorsed by the Society for Cardiovascular Magnetic Resonance and Society of Cardiovascular Computed Tomography. *J Am Soc Echocardiogr.* 2013;26:965–1012 e15.
Kodama F, Fultz PJ, Wandtke JC. Comparing thin-section and thick-section CT of pericardial sinuses and recesses. *AJR Am J Roentgenol.* 2003;181:1101–1108.
Kojima S, Yamada N, Goto Y. Diagnosis of constrictive pericarditis by tagged cine magnetic resonance imaging. *N Engl J Med.* 1999;341:373–374.
Lee KY, Oh YW, Noh HJ, et al. Extraadrenal paragangliomas of the body: imaging features. *AJR Am J Roentgenol.* 2006;187:492–504.
Leeman DE, Levine MJ, Come PC. Doppler echocardiography in cardiac tamponade: exaggerated respiratory variation in transvalvular blood flow velocity integrals. *J Am Coll Cardiol.* 1988;11:572–578.
LeWinter MM. Clinical practice. Acute pericarditis. *N Engl J Med.* 2014;371:2410–2416.
Little WC, Freeman GL. Pericardial disease. *Circulation.* 2006;113:1622–1632.
Maisch B, Seferovic PM, Ristic AD, et al. Guidelines on the diagnosis and management of pericardial diseases executive summary; the task force on the diagnosis and management of pericardial diseases of the European Society of Cardiology. *Eur Heart J.* 2004;25:587–610.
Myers RB, Spodick DH. Constrictive pericarditis: clinical and pathophysiologic characteristics. *Am Heart J.* 1999;138:219–232.
Nasser WK. Congenital diseases of the pericardium. *Cardiovasc Clin.* 1976;7:271–286.
Natanzon A, Kronzon I. Pericardial and pleural effusions in congestive heart failure—anatomical, pathophysiologic, and clinical considerations. *Am J Med Sci.* 2009;338:211–216.
Nishimura RA. Constrictive pericarditis in the modern era: a diagnostic dilemma. *Heart.* 2001;86:619–623.
Oh KY, Shimizu M, Edwards WD, et al. Surgical pathology of the parietal pericardium: a study of 344 cases (1993-1999). *Cardiovasc Pathol.* 2001;10:157–168.
O'Leary SM, Williams PL, Williams MP, et al. Imaging the pericardium: appearances on ECG-gated 64-detector row cardiac computed tomography. *Br J Radiol.* 2010;83:194–205.
Peebles CR, Shambrook JS, Harden SP. Pericardial disease—anatomy and function. *Br J Radiol.* 2011;84(Spec3):S324–S337.
Psychidis-Papakyritsis P, de Roos A, Kroft LJ. Functional MRI of congenital absence of the pericardium. *AJR Am J Roentgenol.* 2007;189:W312–W314.
Pugatch RD, Braver JH, Robbins AH, Faling LJ. CT diagnosis of pericardial cysts. *AJR Am J Roentgenol.* 1978;131:515–516.
Rajiah P. Cardiac MRI: part 2, pericardial diseases. *AJR Am J Roentgenol.* 2011;197:W621–W634.
Restrepo CS, Lemos DF, Lemos JA, et al. Imaging findings in cardiac tamponade with emphasis on CT. *Radiographics.* 2007;27:1595–1610.
Restrepo CS, Vargas D, Ocazionez D, et al. Primary pericardial tumors. *Radiographics.* 2013;33:1613–1630.
Rienmuller R, Groll R, Lipton MJ. CT and MR imaging of pericardial disease. *Radiol Clin North Am.* 2004;42:587–601, vi.
Riquet M, Le Pimpec-Barthes F, Hidden G. Lymphatic drainage of the pericardium to the mediastinal lymph nodes. *Surg Radiol Anat.* 2001;23:317–319.
Roberts WC. Pericardial heart disease: its morphologic features and its causes. *Proc (Bayl Univ Med Cent).* 2005;18:38–55.
Sagrista-Sauleda J, Angel J, Sanchez A, et al. Effusive-constrictive pericarditis. *N Engl J Med.* 2004;350:469–475.
Scheuermann-Freestone M, Orchard E, Francis J, et al. Images in cardiovascular medicine. Partial congenital absence of the pericardium. *Circulation.* 2007;116:e126–e129.
Shabetai R, Meaney E. Proceedings: haemodynamics of cardiac restriction and tamponade. *Br Heart J.* 1975;37:780.
Shah AB, Kronzon I. Congenital defects of the pericardium: a review. *Eur Heart J Cardiovasc Imaging.* 2015.
Sharma R, Harden S, Peebles C, Dawkins KD. Percutaneous aspiration of a pericardial cyst: an acceptable treatment for a rare disorder. *Heart.* 2007;93:22.
Spodick DH. Macrophysiology, microphysiology, and anatomy of the pericardium: a synopsis. *Am Heart J.* 1992;124:1046–1051.
Suman S, Schofield P, Large S. Primary pericardial mesothelioma presenting as pericardial constriction: a case report. *Heart.* 2004;90:e4.
Talreja DR, Edwards WD, Danielson GK, et al. Constrictive pericarditis in 26 patients with histologically normal pericardial thickness. *Circulation.* 2003;108:1852–1857.
Thavendiranathan P, Verhaert D, Walls MC, et al. Simultaneous right and left heart real-time, free-breathing CMR flow quantification identifies constrictive physiology. *JACC Cardiovasc Imaging.* 2012;5:15–24.
Thomason R, Schlegel W, Lucca M, et al. Primary malignant mesothelioma of the pericardium. Case report and literature review. *Tex Heart Inst J.* 1994;21:170–174.
Thurber DL, Edwards JE, Achor RW. Secondary malignant tumors of the pericardium. *Circulation.* 1962;26:228–241.
Truong MT, Erasmus JJ, Gladish GW, et al. Anatomy of pericardial recesses on multidetector CT: implications for oncologic imaging. *AJR Am J Roentgenol.* 2003;181:1109–1113.
Truong MT, Erasmus JJ, Sabloff BS, et al. Pericardial "sleeve" recess of right inferior pulmonary vein mimicking adenopathy: computed tomography findings. *J Comput Assist Tomogr.* 2004;28:361–365.
Verhaert D, Gabriel RS, Johnston D, et al. The role of multimodality imaging in the management of pericardial disease. *Circ Cardiovasc Imaging.* 2010;3:333–343.
Vesely TM, Cahill DR. Cross-sectional anatomy of the pericardial sinuses, recesses, and adjacent structures. *Surg Radiol Anat.* 1986;8:221–227.
Vogiatzidis K, Zarogiannis SG, Aidonidis I, et al. Physiology of pericardial fluid production and drainage. *Front Physiol.* 2015;6:62.
Waller BF, Taliercio CP, Howard J, et al. Morphologic aspects of pericardial heart disease: part I. *Clin Cardiol.* 1992;15:203–209.
Wang ZJ, Reddy GP, Gotway MB, et al. CT and MR imaging of pericardial disease. *Radiographics.* 2003;23(Spec No):S167–S180.
Welch TD, Ling LH, Espinosa RE, et al. Echocardiographic diagnosis of constrictive pericarditis: Mayo Clinic criteria. *Circ Cardiovasc Imaging.* 2014;7:526–534.
Yared K, Baggish AL, Picard MH, et al. Multimodality imaging of pericardial diseases. *JACC Cardiovasc Imaging.* 2010;3:650–660.
Zurick AO, Bolen MA, Kwon DH, et al. Pericardial delayed hyperenhancement with CMR imaging in patients with constrictive pericarditis undergoing surgical pericardiectomy: a case series with histopathological correlation. *JACC Cardiovasc Imaging.* 2011;4:1180–1191.

SECTION 6

Special Situations

CHAPTER 39

Intensive Care Imaging

Steven Zangan and Rishi Ramakrishna

CHAPTER OUTLINE

■ Value of a Routine Daily Chest Radiograph in the Intensive Care Unit

Determining Who Needs Imaging

Imaging of an intensive care unit (ICU) patient can be a difficult task that relies on cooperation and teamwork among many members of the clinical care team and technologist. The complexity of these critically ill patients, many of whom have numerous support devices, has led to the practice of daily routine chest radiography, especially of the mechanically ventilated, to assess for changes or complications. However, recent studies have shown that the elimination of daily routine chest radiography does not significantly affect mortality or length of stay in the hospital. According to the American College of Radiology appropriateness criteria, there is no specific need to obtain daily routine chest radiographs. Rather, imaging should be performed when there is a change in clinical status or after initial placement of an endotracheal tube, nasogastric tube, Swan-Ganz catheter, central venous catheter, chest tube, or other life support device due to the risk of complications associated with placement. Follow-up imaging of these support devices is then dependent on the clinical status or concern for new complication rather than on a routine basis.

■ Respiratory

Location of Endotracheal and Tracheostomy Tubes

A wide variety of endotracheal tubes exist; the size is chosen based on the patient body habitus. The width is optimally one-half to two-thirds the width of the trachea. Most have an inflatable cuff that seals the trachea, prevents air leaks, and reduces the risk of aspiration. Endotracheal tube position is commonly described as the distance of the tube tip to the carina. The carina normally lies at the level of T4–T5 (Fig. 39.1A) or the undersurface of the aortic arch; these are useful landmarks when the

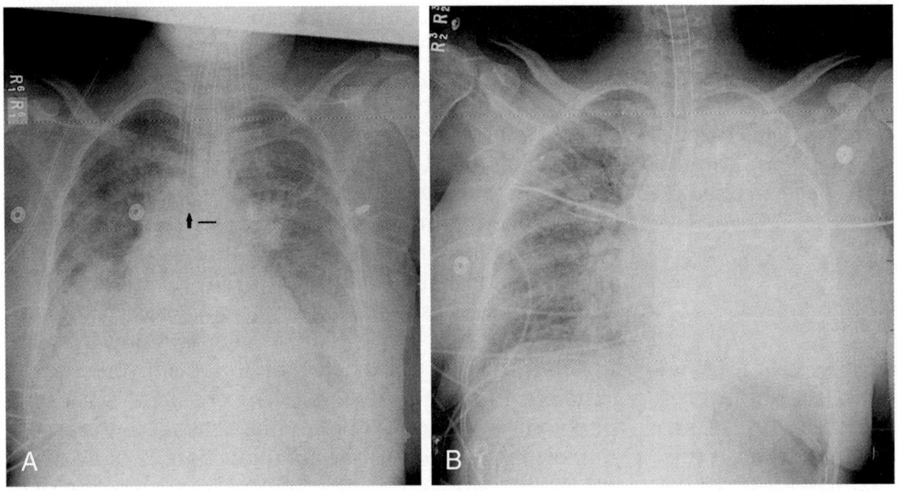

Figure 39.1 (A) Portable chest radiograph demonstrates the endotracheal tube tip approximately 2 cm above the carina *(arrow)*, which is at the level of T5 (*black line* denotes inferior endplate of T5). A nasogastric tube is also noted within the stomach. A left subclavian dual-lumen chest port has its tip at the superior cavoatrial junction. Cardiomegaly, pulmonary edema, pleural effusions, and nonspecific basilar consolidation suggest congestive heart failure. (B) Advancement of the endotracheal tube into the right main stem bronchus results in left lung atelectasis.

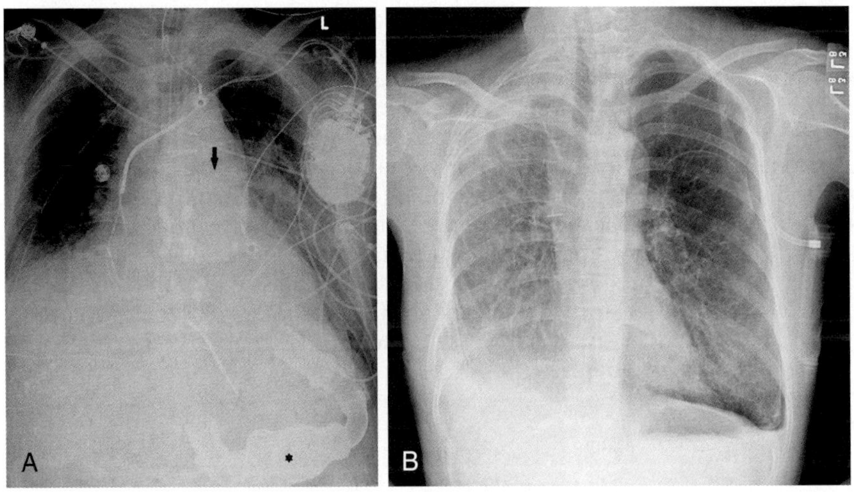

Figure 39.2 (A) Portable chest radiograph demonstrating a dual-chamber endotracheal tube with the left-sided tube in the left main stem bronchus *(arrow)* and the right-sided tube above the right main stem bronchus orifice. A left ventricular assist device is present *(asterisk)*. Automatic implantable cardioverter-defibrillator leads are in the right atrial appendage and right ventricular apex. A right chest tube is directed toward the right apex. (B) This portable chest radiograph demonstrates a left-sided chest tube outside the pleural space with a persistent left pneumothorax.

carina is not well seen. Ideally, the tube is positioned in the midtrachea, and the tip lies 3 to 6 cm above the carina. Because flexion and extension of the neck may result in a roughly 2-cm descent and ascent of the tube, respectively, some variability in position is not uncommon on serial radiographs. In select circumstances, dual-chamber endotracheal tubes are used and allow selective decompression or aeration of each lung (Fig. 39.2). In patients with tracheostomy tubes, the tip is ideally one-half to two-thirds of the width of the trachea and one-half to two-thirds of the distance from the stoma to the carina. The tip should not be resting against the tracheal wall.

When an endotracheal tube is advanced too inferiorly, the tip preferentially enters the right main stem bronchus because it is more vertically oriented. This may result in left lung atelectasis (see Fig. 39.1B). When advanced farther, the tip will enter the bronchus intermedius and obstruct the right upper lobe bronchus, resulting in right upper lobe atelectasis. When the tube is not deep enough, the tip may enter the esophagus. Close attention to the relationship of the tube and tracheal air column is mandatory. When in the esophagus, the tube may be left lateral to the tracheal margins, and the stomach may be distended with air. A right posterior oblique or lateral radiograph may provide better delineation of the pertinent anatomy. If the tube is outside the confines of the tracheal air column and not within the esophagus, tracheal rupture should be considered, especially in the setting of pneumothorax, pneumomediastinum, or subcutaneous emphysema. Overinflation of the tube cuff or balloon, which may manifest as bulging of the tracheal wall, may acutely lead to tracheal perforation or chronically result in stricture or scarring.

Positioning of Chest Tubes

The desired position of a chest tube is heavily dependent on the goals of tube placement and the physical properties of air and fluid. Because air accumulates anteriorly and superiorly, chest tubes placed primarily for a pneumothorax should be positioned accordingly. Conversely, free fluid settles in the dependent and posterior portions of the lung, and tubes placed for pleural effusions or hemothorax are directed toward the base. Finally, loculated fluid collections may require more directed placement.

Most large-bore chest tubes have a radiopaque line denoting the point just distal to the last fenestration in the tube (see Fig. 39.2A). This line should be in the thoracic cavity. If the side hole is outside the pleural space, tube function may be compromised, and subcutaneous emphysema may result (see Fig. 39.2B). Tubes within the fissures may also function poorly as the pleural surfaces appose and obstruct the tube.

Location of Enteric Tubes

Nasogastric and orogastric tubes can be used for feeding or decompression. The side port of the tube should be below the gastroesophageal (GE) junction to ensure proper function and reduce the risk of aspiration. If the sideport is not well visualized, approximately 10 cm of the tube should be below the GE junction. Tubes used for feeding often have a weighted tip. This tip should be postpyloric.

The course of any tube with the tip above the diaphragm should be closely evaluated to ensure that it is not within the trachea or esophagus (Fig. 39.3). A tube with a completely vertical orientation in the abdomen may suggest perforation. In cases such as esophagectomy with gastric interposition, an intrathoracic tube location may be desired. A hiatal hernia or intrathoracic stomach may also lead to an altered tube location.

Cardiovascular

Ideal Location for a Central Venous Catheter

The ideal location for the tip of a central venous catheter depends on its intended use and varies according to professional societal guidelines. Although there is no consensus, the cavoatrial junction is a commonly accepted landmark signifying appropriate positioning. A catheter with a high tip may have poorer flow rates and be more prone to malfunction and thrombosis. There is also a risk of superior vena cava (SVC) erosion, especially with a short left-sided catheter, when the tip and catheter course are relatively perpendicular to the caval wall. With a low tip, there is a risk of arrhythmia, and reports of cardiac tamponade due to gradual vascular erosion have been presented, although many of these reports were older studies with more rigid catheters that are no longer commonly in use. The SVC empties into the right atrium through a thickened ring of tissue formed by the crista terminalis and dividens. The cristae represent the embryonic transition from the sinus venosus to the atrium and form the anatomic cavoatrial junction. Because this is not visible radiographically, landmarks such as the right tracheobronchial angle and carina serve as surrogates. The cavoatrial junction typically resides 3 to 4 cm below these structures. There can be great variability in apparent tip position, with severe under- or overinflation or projectional differences in radiographs.

Catheters that take a vertical course but are to the left of the spine may reside in a left or double SVC, mediastinal or internal mammary vein, or the aorta, or they may be extravascular (Fig. 39.4). When the tip is directed posterolaterally, the catheter may have entered the azygos vein (Fig. 39.5). Mediastinal widening, loss of the aortic silhouette, an apical cap, or mass effect on surrounding structures may be seen in cases of mediastinal hematoma. An apical cap can also be secondary to an extrapleural hematoma.

Common Complications of Central Venous Catheter Insertion

Catheters should be traced to their source to evaluate for kinking or fragmentation. Catheter pinch-off occurs

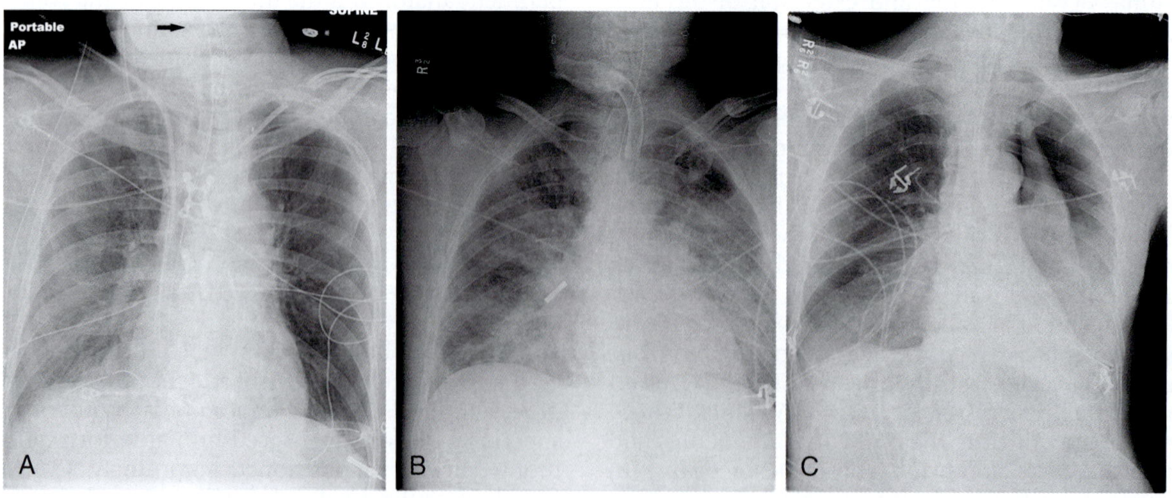

Figure 39.3 (A) Portable chest radiograph demonstrating a nasogastric tube coiled in the hypopharynx (*arrow*). The endotracheal tube tip is above the carina. A Swan-Ganz catheter is within the main pulmonary artery. Bilateral chest tubes are present. (B) Portable chest radiograph demonstrating a Dobhoff feeding tube entering the right main stem bronchus. (C) Portable chest radiograph demonstrates a nasogastric tube entering the left lung. This resulted in injury to the airway and a left pneumothorax.

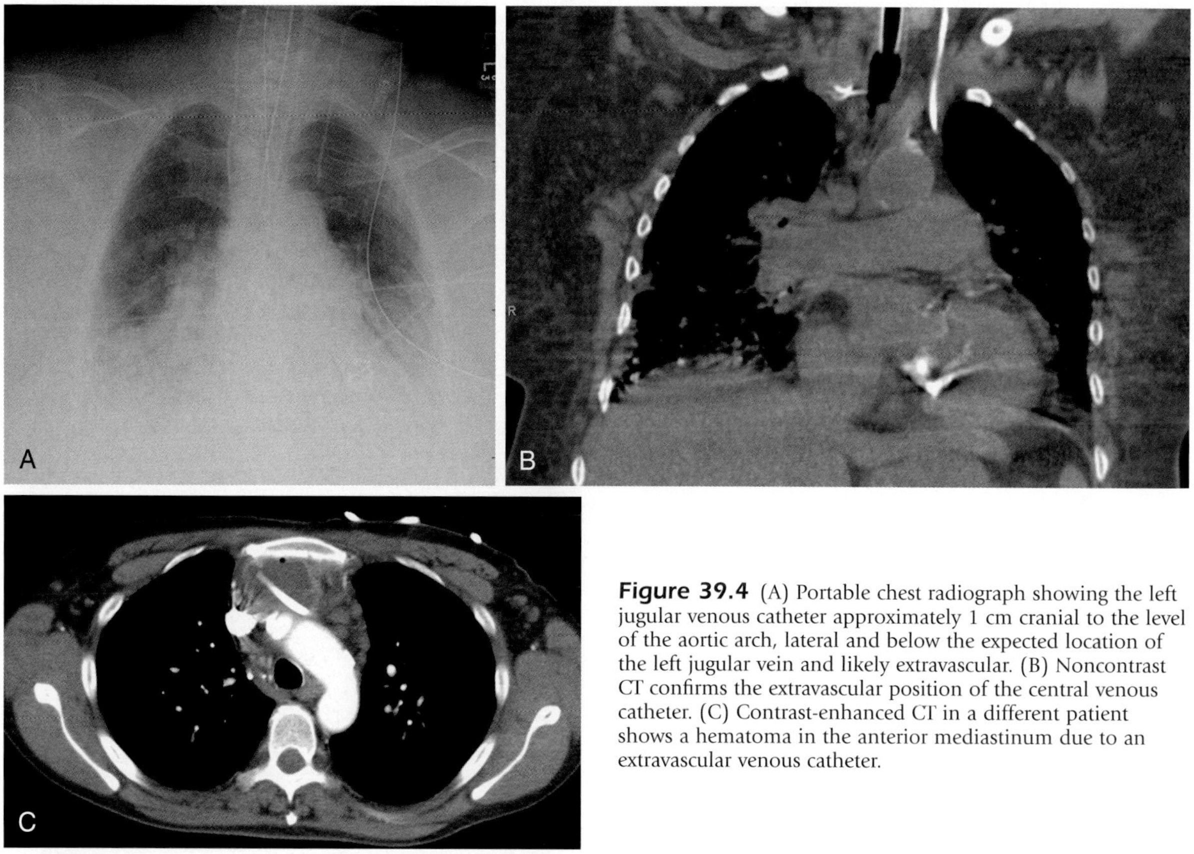

Figure 39.4 (A) Portable chest radiograph showing the left jugular venous catheter approximately 1 cm cranial to the level of the aortic arch, lateral and below the expected location of the left jugular vein and likely extravascular. (B) Noncontrast CT confirms the extravascular position of the central venous catheter. (C) Contrast-enhanced CT in a different patient shows a hematoma in the anterior mediastinum due to an extravascular venous catheter.

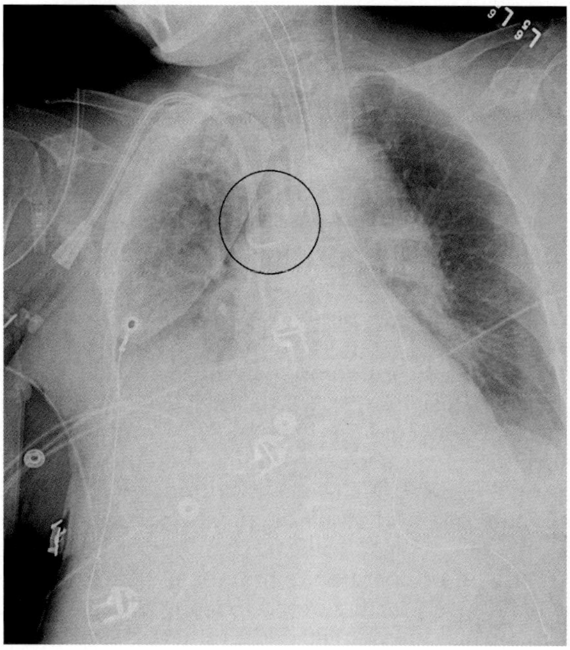

Figure 39.5 Anteroposterior chest radiograph demonstrates a left-sided central venous catheter with the tip in the azygos arch *(circle)*. Note the straight course of the appropriately positioned right jugular split tip dialysis catheter.

with subclavian lines near the junction of the first rib and clavicle. Repetitive compression by the costoclavicular ligament and subclavius muscle results in catheter fatigue. Initially, distortion is present without luminal narrowing, although this can progress to luminal narrowing or catheter transection or fracture. The distal tip may embolize to the heart or pulmonary artery (Fig. 39.6).

Following new central venous catheter insertion, the radiograph must be carefully evaluated for a pneumothorax on both sides. Although a new catheter may be present on one side, failed attempts at contralateral placement with errant needlesticks are a distinct possibility. A new pleural effusion suggests a hemothorax.

Pacemakers and Implantable Cardioverter-Defibrillators

Situating Pacemaker Leads

The specific model and configuration of the pacemaker will depend on the indication. The leads are typically introduced via the left subclavian vein. The initial post-placement radiograph should be closely examined for the presence of pneumothorax or hemothorax and appropriate lead course (Fig. 39.7A). One electrode will be directed toward the right ventricular apex. It courses along the base of the right ventricle, left of the midline on the frontal view and anteriorly and inferiorly directed on the lateral

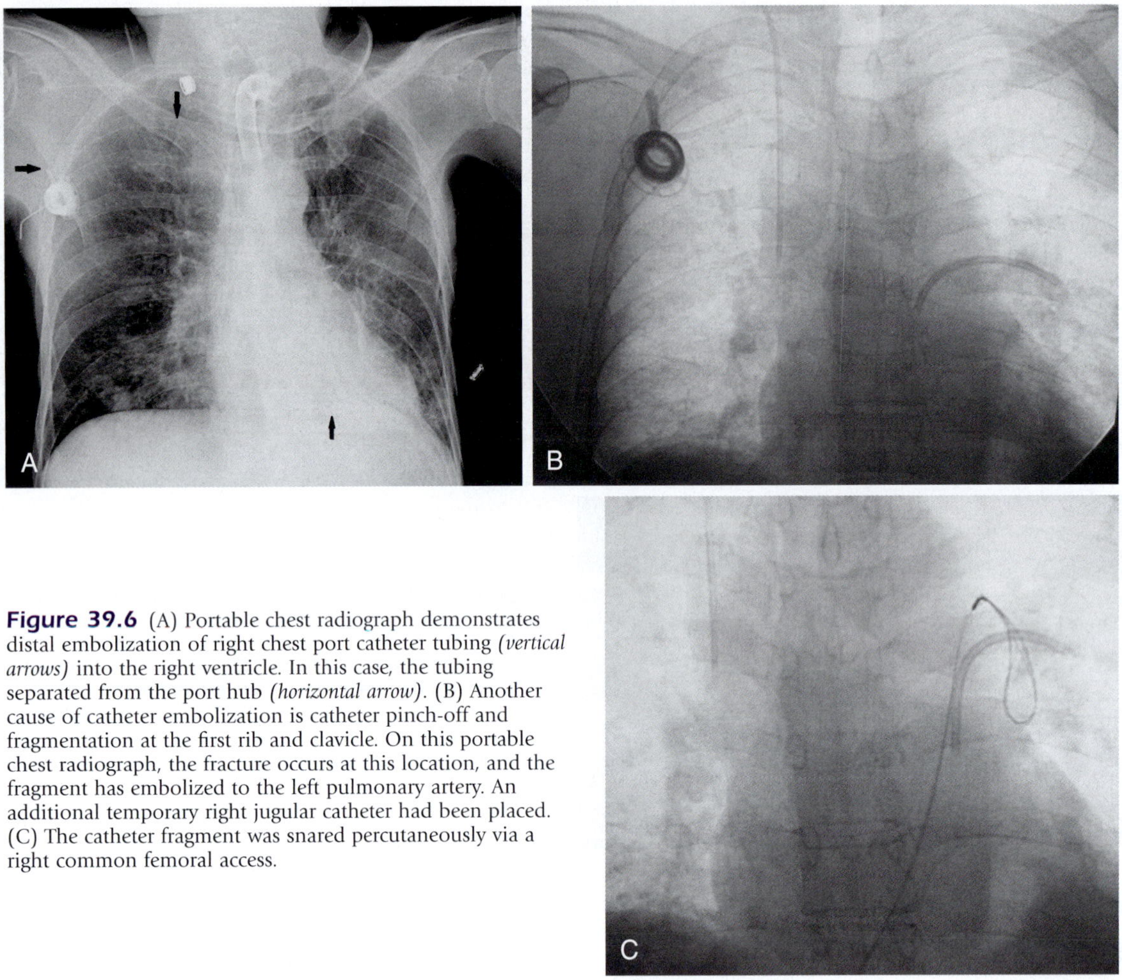

Figure 39.6 (A) Portable chest radiograph demonstrates distal embolization of right chest port catheter tubing *(vertical arrows)* into the right ventricle. In this case, the tubing separated from the port hub *(horizontal arrow)*. (B) Another cause of catheter embolization is catheter pinch-off and fragmentation at the first rib and clavicle. On this portable chest radiograph, the fracture occurs at this location, and the fragment has embolized to the left pulmonary artery. An additional temporary right jugular catheter had been placed. (C) The catheter fragment was snared percutaneously via a right common femoral access.

radiograph. The tip should be within 2 to 4 mm of the epicardial fat pad; further displacement of the tip may suggest myocardial perforation (see Fig. 39.7B and C). A second lead may enter the right atrial appendage. On the frontal view, the lead terminates over the right upper heart border, often with a cranially directed curve. On the lateral view, the lead will follow the smooth anterior curve of the midportion of the heart. A third electrode placed into a coronary vein will traverse the coronary sinus and will be directed upward and laterally. On the lateral radiograph, this lead will course posteriorly.

Distinguishing Between an Implantable Cardioverter-Defibrillator and a Pacemaker

An implantable cardioverter-defibrillator will appear slightly larger and can be identified by the high-voltage defibrillation or shock coils (see Fig. 39.2). Lead fractures may occur at points of stress near the tip, near the pacemaker generator, and at the venous access site. Leadless pacemakers, which can be delivered via a percutaneously inserted catheter, have recently been developed. All the components exist within a cylindric pacemaker (the appearance resembles a AAA battery) residing in the right ventricular apex (see Fig. 39.7D).

Pulmonary Catheters

Ideal Location of a Pulmonary Artery Catheter and Complications That Can Occur With Malposition

Pulmonary catheters are typically inserted for hemodynamic monitoring but may also be used for delivery of medication, such as thrombolytic infusions. These venous catheters are usually inserted via the jugular or subclavian vein from above or the femoral vein from below. The course will traverse the tricuspid and pulmonary valves. The tip should reside centrally within the right or left main pulmonary artery, ideally proximal to the interlobar pulmonary artery. An inflatable balloon at the catheter tip assists in estimating the pulmonary artery pressure. The balloon is usually not radiographically identifiable. When the balloon is inflated, the catheter moves distally, wedging into smaller arterial vessels. This wedge pressure serves as a surrogate for the pulmonary artery pressure. If the catheter is too distal, pulmonary infarction and/or hemorrhage may result, which may manifest as a wedge-shaped peripheral consolidation distal to the catheter (Fig. 39.8). Pulmonary artery pseudoaneurysms can also develop. When the catheters loop back on themselves in the right heart, valvular damage or arrhythmias can occur.

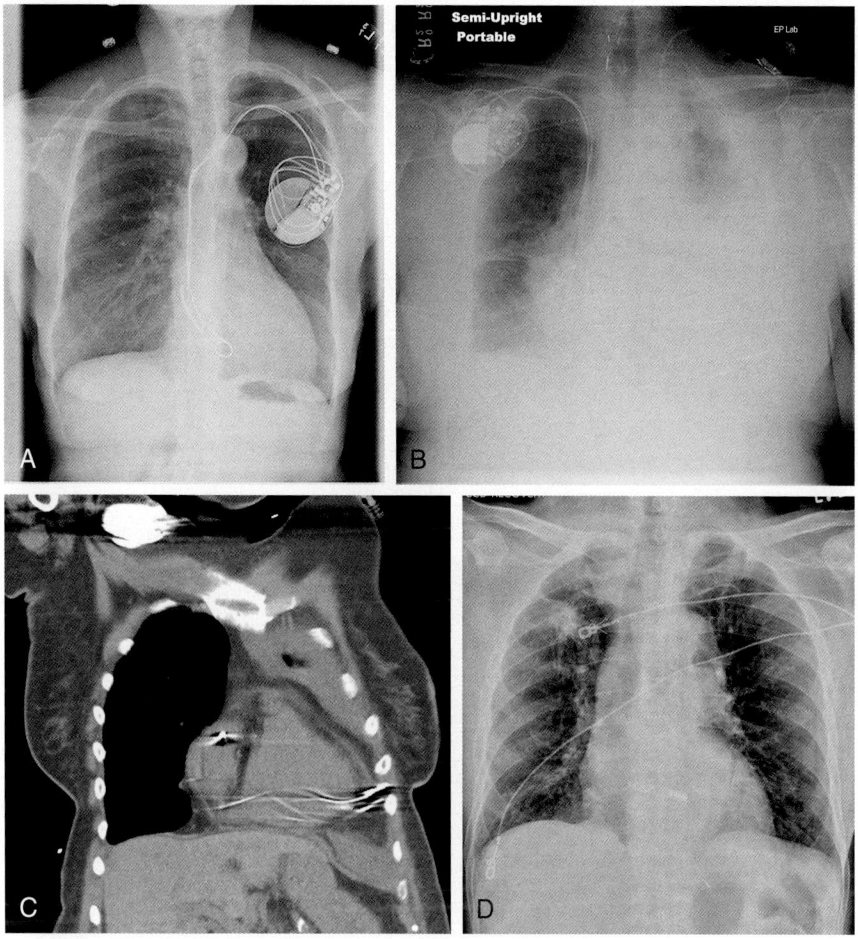

Figure 39.7 (A) Portable chest radiograph demonstrates malposition of the right ventricular (RV) lead of this automatic implantable cardioverter-defibrillator. The tip is short of the RV apex, and the wire is looped near the tricuspid valve. (B) Portable chest radiograph demonstrates an abnormally peripheral course of the RV lead. There is also a left pleural effusion. (C) Myocardial perforation is confirmed on this coronal reformatted noncontrast CT. (D) Portable chest radiograph shows a leadless pacemaker in the right ventricle. There is also a right upper lobe pulmonary nodule.

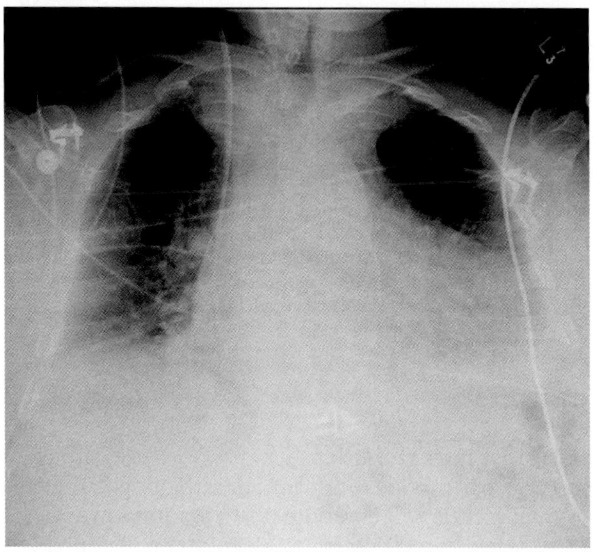

Figure 39.8 Portable chest radiograph demonstrates a malpositioned right jugular Swan-Ganz catheter extending distally into a branch of the right descending pulmonary artery. Distally located catheters put the patient at risk for a pulmonary infarct or pulmonary artery injury, such as a pseudoaneurysm.

Aortic and Cardiac Support Catheters

Types and Location of Arterial Catheters in the Thorax

Intraaortic balloon counterpulsation is used as a temporary therapeutic option in patients with severe hemodynamic compromise from myocardial ischemia. When the balloon inflates during diastole, coronary blood flow may be improved. When the balloon deflates during systole, the afterload is reduced through a vacuum effect. The catheter can be introduced via the femoral or subclavian artery. The tip is identified by a radiopaque marker, optimally just below the superior contour of the aortic knob (just distal to the left subclavian artery). When too proximal (Fig. 39.9A), the origins of the aortic arch vessels may be affected, and cerebral embolism may result. When too distal, myocardial perfusion may be suboptimal (see Fig. 39.9B).

Ventricular assist devices are surgically implanted mechanical circulatory assist devices typically used as a bridge to cardiac transplantation (see Fig. 39.2). They are implanted in the preperitoneal space or in the peritoneum and provide continuous perfusion. An inflow cannula receives blood from the left ventricle, which then circulates blood to the ascending aorta. These conduits are not always radiopaque in their entirety. There are

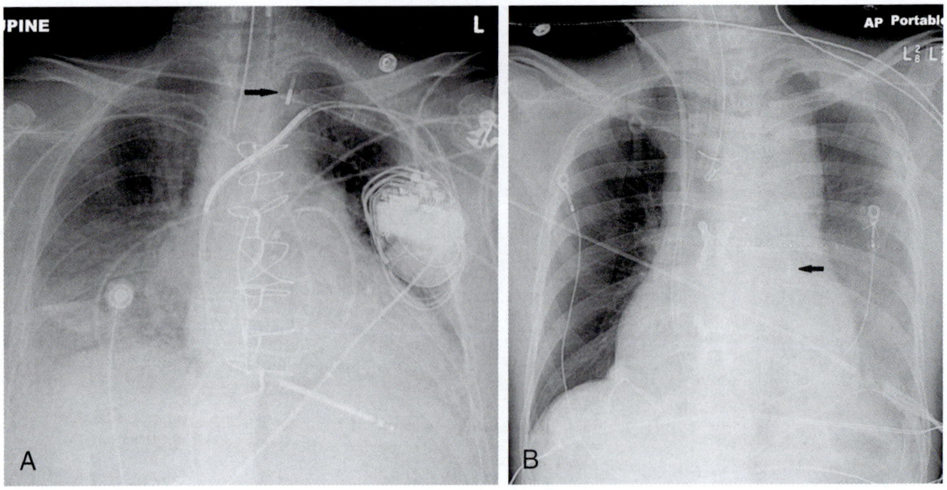

Figure 39.9 (A) Portable chest radiograph demonstrates an intraaortic balloon pump (IABP) marker too cranially and likely within the left common carotid or subclavian artery *(arrow)*. (B) In this portable chest radiograph, the IABP marker is positioned too far caudally *(arrow)*. The cylindric, vertically oriented lucency represents the inflated balloon, indicating that the radiograph was taken during diastole. Note the mediastinal widening due to a mediastinal hematoma and aortic dissection.

also biventricular and right ventricular assist devices. These may run on battery power and are connected to a mechanical driveline. Rarely, the driveline can fracture. Seromas, abscesses, or hematomas may also occur. Smaller pumps can be inserted percutaneously through the femoral artery, into the ascending aorta, and across the aortic valve into the left ventricle. The inlet sits in the left ventricle, and blood is then expelled through the catheter into the ascending aorta (Fig. 39.10).

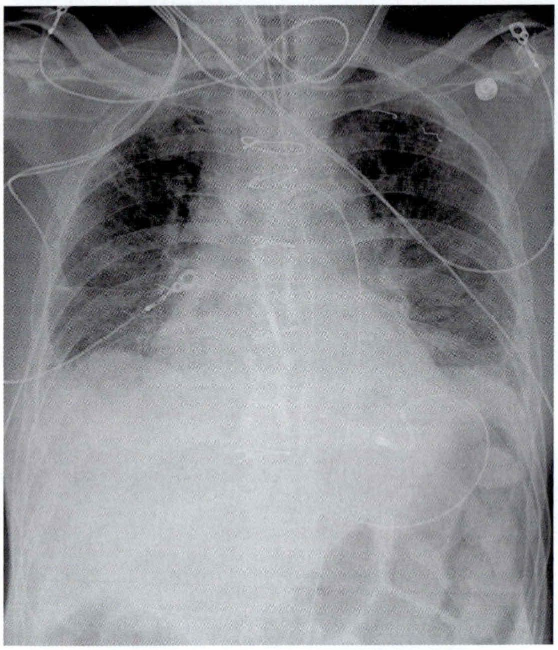

Figure 39.10 Portable chest radiograph shows a percutaneously inserted left ventricular assist device. The device can be tracked from the inferior margin of the image as it courses cranially, crests in the aortic arch, and then descends through the aortic valve into the left ventricular apex.

■ Pulmonary Disease

Atelectasis

Common Locations

Atelectasis is usually seen in the left lower lobe, possibly secondary to compression of the left lower lobe bronchus by the heart. On radiography, this often leads to complete opacification of the normal lung usually seen posterior to the left aspect of the heart, also known as the *ivory heart sign* (Fig. 39.11).

Causes

Any process that reduces alveolar ventilation, including obstruction from a mass or mucus plugging, hypoventilation secondary to general anesthesia, infection, or shallow breathing secondary to pain may cause atelectasis. In the presence of pleural effusions or masses, compressive atelectasis can be seen.

Imaging Characteristics

The hallmark of atelectasis is volume loss; elevation of the hemidiaphragm, displacement of the fissures, crowding of the vasculature, splaying of the vasculature in the nonaffected lobe, mediastinal shift, loss of normal silhouettes, and/or displacement of the main stem bronchi are indicative of atelectasis. The degree of atelectasis ranges from linear bands seen with subsegmental atelectasis to dense homogeneous opacity, with lobar collapse (see Fig. 39.11). In contrast to infection, atelectasis can develop and resolve rapidly.

Aspiration

Imaging Characteristics

Most ICU patients are recumbent or semiupright; therefore, aspirated debris will enter the posterior and lower aspects of the lungs, which are most dependent. The posterior segments of the upper lobes and basal segments of the lower lobes are commonly affected. The material aspirated can lead to different outcomes. For example, aspiration of gastric contents can lead to chemical pneumonitis and noncardiogenic pulmonary edema, whereas bland aspiration may resolve without complications. Radiographs demonstrate perihilar opacification or opacification in the dependent portions of the lung. Persistent opacity suggests the development of pneumonia.

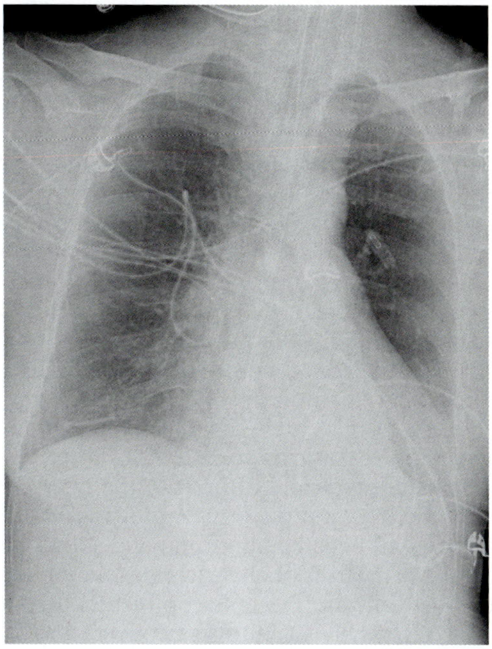

Figure 39.11 Portable chest radiograph shows left lower lobe atelectasis. The silhouette of the diaphragm is lost, and a double density is noted near the left heart border.

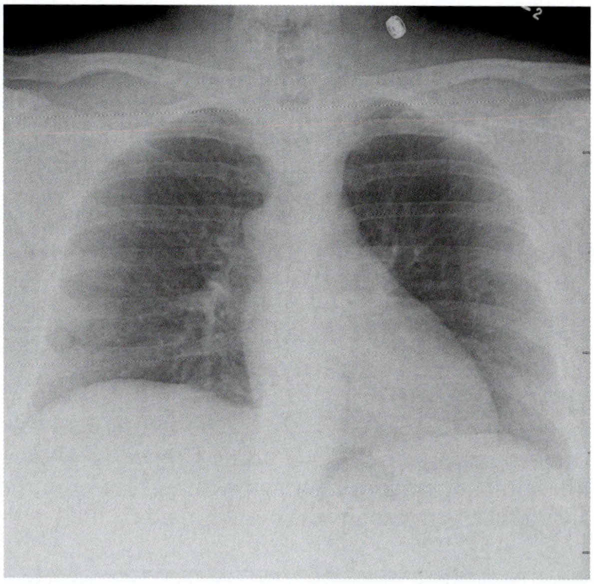

Figure 39.12 Portable chest radiograph shows distention of the azygos vein best seen above the right main bronchus. In this case, azygos distention was due to congenital inferior vena cava interruption. In cases of volume overload, septal lines, cardiomegaly, and pleural effusion are common concurrent findings.

Pneumonia

Common Causes and Patterns of Pneumonia

Nosocomial pneumonia may be caused by a wide variety of pathogens, may be polymicrobial, and may involve multidrug resistant pathogens. It is one of the leading causes of death among hospital-acquired infections. By definition, hospital-acquired pneumonia occurs 48 hours after admission, and ventilator-acquired pneumonia occurs 48 to 72 hours after intubation. Radiologic manifestations of pneumonia overlap with other pulmonary processes. The diagnosis depends on clinical and radiologic findings but should be suspected in patients with fever, leukocytosis, purulent sputum, and/or hypooxygenation who manifest a new air space opacity on chest radiograph.

Pulmonary Edema

Common Imaging Manifestations

When excess intravascular fluid moves into the alveoli, pulmonary edema results. In cardiogenic pulmonary edema, high pulmonary capillary pressures drive this movement. In noncardiogenic edema, other factors, such as an increase in capillary permeability, cause this shift. It is often difficult to separate cardiogenic from noncardiogenic edema, especially radiographically, and a combination of the two can also occur. Signs of heart failure, such as cardiomegaly, septal thickening, and pleural effusions, suggest a cardiogenic cause. Measurement of brain natriuretic peptide level, echocardiography, and right heart catheterization may be necessary to assist in differentiation. Underlying architectural abnormalities (e.g., superimposed emphysema or fibrosis) in the lung may lead to an atypical appearance and distribution.

Early mild pulmonary edema is often not radiographically evident. When pulmonary capillary pressures increases to approximately 15 mm Hg, vascular redistribution of flow is seen. This disproportional enlargement of upper chest nondependent vessels is termed *cephalization.* A ratio greater than 1:1 between the pulmonary artery and adjacent bronchus in the upper lungs suggests increased pulmonary flow. The width of the vascular pedicle is a useful estimate of the patient's overall volume status. The vascular pedicle is represented by the width of the superior mediastinum measured from the right lateral border of the SVC, where it crosses the right main bronchus to the outer border of the left subclavian artery as it arises from the aortic arch. Most range from 38 to 58 mm in diameter, and variability on serial radiographs can be used to estimate changes in fluid status. Another useful indicator of hypervolemia is azygos vein distention greater than 1 cm (Fig. 39.12). When the capillary pressure exceeds 20 mm Hg, interstitial edema is usually seen. Fluid accumulates within the interlobular septa, resulting in fine linear horizontal opacities that extend to the pleural surface (Kerley B lines) or perihilar, central linear opacities (Kerley A lines). In practice, this distinction is typically not made, and the term *septal lines* suffices. With higher pressures, typically in excess of 25 mm Hg, alveolar edema results, with the classic perihilar bat wing distribution of air space opacification (Fig. 39.13).

Limitations on the assessment of cardiac size on portable ICU radiographs must be considered. Classically, a cardiothoracic ratio greater than 50% is indicative of cardiomegaly, although on ICU radiographs this would commonly result in an overestimation of cardiac size. On an anteroposterior portable radiograph, the divergent beam enters anteriorly and the shorter distance between the source and detector results in magnification of the heart. Additionally, radiographs of patients who are critically ill and/or ventilated usually show hypoinflation, which also results in overestimation of the cardiac size because the transverse diameter of the heart widens as the diaphragm moves up. In a relatively lordotic projection, there is greater enlargement of the cardiac silhouette.

Acute Respiratory Distress Syndrome and Acute Lung Injury

Common Causes of Acute Respiratory Distress Syndrome

Acute respiratory distress syndrome (ARDS) is an acute, diffuse inflammatory lung injury with increased pulmonary vascular permeability that results in excess fluid in the interstitium and alveoli. The pathologic hallmark is diffuse alveolar damage. ARDS is associated with an exhaustive list of risk factors and causes; these are grouped together because the pathophysiology and treatment are the same. Sepsis is the most common cause of ARDS. Aspiration, community-acquired pneumonia, severe trauma, blood transfusion, and transfusion-related lung injury are other leading causes. The diagnosis of ARDS is made in patients with acute hypoxemic respiratory failure with bilateral pulmonary opacities consistent with pulmonary edema. The respiratory failure cannot be related to cardiac failure or fluid overload, and the pulmonary opacities cannot be fully explained by pleural effusions, atelectasis, or other pulmonary pathology.

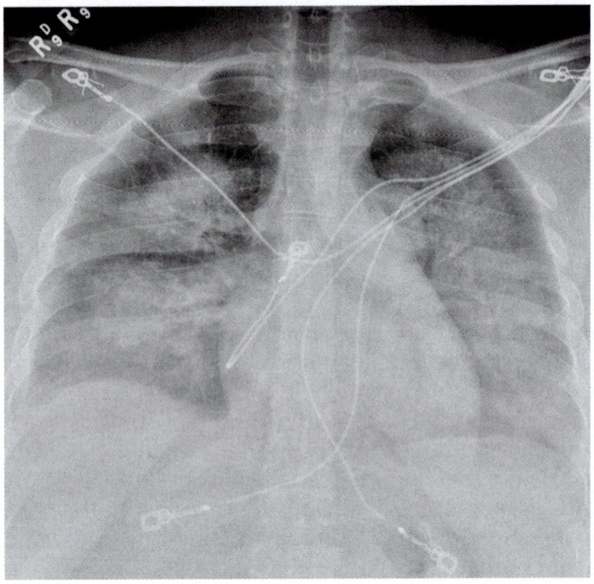

Figure 39.13 Portable chest radiograph demonstrates pulmonary edema with a perihilar distribution of interstitial and air space opacity (bat wing distribution).

Imaging Manifestations in the ICU Patient

Radiographs are typically normal in the first 24 hours after the inciting injury. Days following the injury, radiographs will become abnormal and show bilateral, peripheral patchy areas of air space consolidation, which increase over time and become confluent. The opacities need not necessarily be diffuse or severe to diagnose ARDS. After 7 to 10 days, a proliferative stage develops in which the edema resolves, but type II alveolar cells proliferate, and collagen is deposited. Reticular opacities are more typical in this phase (Fig. 39.14). The progression of opacities suggests superimposed pneumonia, especially if focal. Mechanical ventilation is usually required to maintain oxygenation. High ventilator pressures may lead to barotrauma, with pneumothorax and pneumomediastinum, although this is now less common due to low tidal volume ventilation strategies. Some patients progress to a fibrotic stage, with cyst formation.

Considering the paucity of clinical information typically available to the interpreting radiologist, the following imaging findings should alert the reader to the possibility of ARDS over cardiogenic edema using imaging findings alone:

- Radiologic abnormality is delayed relative to the clinical presentation.
- Heart size is normal.
- Opacities are relatively peripheral.

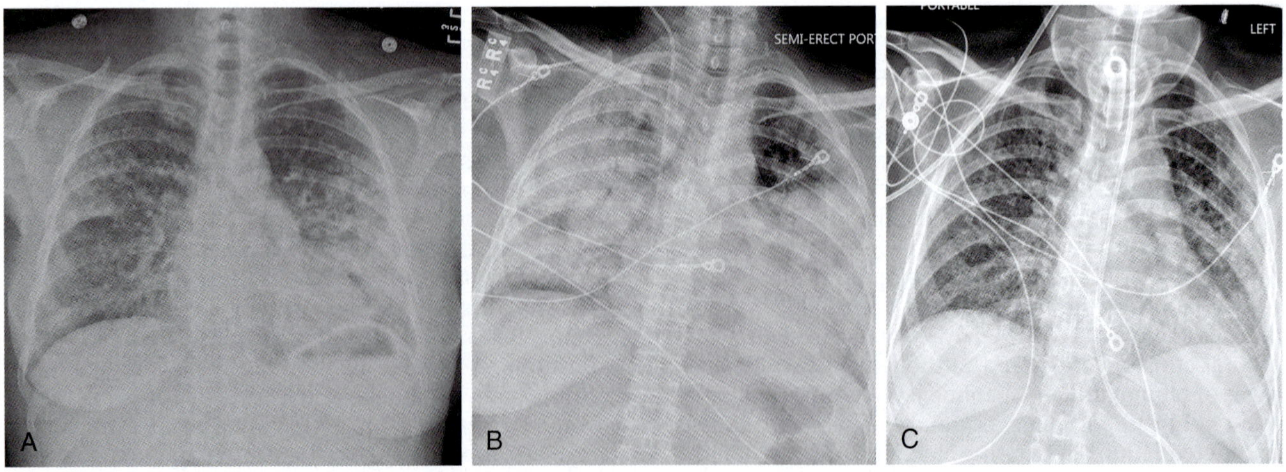

Figure 39.14 (A) Progression of acute respiratory distress syndrome. Initially, peripheral patchy airspace opacities are present. (B) Over a few days, the opacities become confluent. (C) In the proliferative stage, edema resolves but reticular opacities from fibrosis or scarring may become apparent.

- Linear interlobular septal thickening and pleural effusions are absent.
- The appearance changes slowly and persists longer.

Pulmonary Embolism: Imaging Characteristics

Chest radiographs are neither sensitive nor specific for the diagnosis of pulmonary embolism, although abnormalities such as atelectasis, pulmonary parenchymal abnormalities, pleural effusion, or cardiomegaly are frequently seen. In up to 20% of cases, the radiograph is normal. Generally, the radiograph is useful for excluding other diagnoses that may lead to similar clinical symptomatology. Classic findings of the Hampton hump (wedge-shaped peripheral opacity) and Westermark sign (sharp cutoff of the pulmonary vessels, with distal segmental hypoperfusion) are rare.

Abnormal Air Collections

Considerations if Subcutaneous Emphysema Is Seen

Subcutaneous emphysema may be secondary to the percutaneous placement of drains, chest tubes, or other devices. Also, traumatic intubation and barotrauma from positive end-expiratory pressure ventilation may promote dissection of air in the fascial planes of the subcutaneous tissues. Isolated cervical subcutaneous emphysema should raise suspicion for upper airway injury secondary to traumatic intubation or placement of a feeding tube. Subcutaneous emphysema may limit the detection of a pneumothorax.

Imaging Findings of Pneumothorax

Diagnosis of a small pneumothorax on a portable radiograph can be difficult. Pneumothorax can be confidently diagnosed by finding the visceral pleural edge, evident as a fine white line, with a radiolucent collection between the visceral and parietal pleura. No lung markings should be present superiorly and laterally to this line. Air will move to the nondependent portions of the chest. When a patient is upright, the gas will accumulate apicolaterally, and as little as 50 mL can be seen on a radiograph. In a supine radiograph, air will collect along the anterior mediastinal structures and subpulmonically (Fig. 39.15). This will displace the costophrenic angle inferior and create what is known as the *deep sulcus sign*. Much more gas is needed to diagnose a pneumothorax confidently in comparison to upright views.

Hyperlucency of one lung compared to the contralateral side may suggest a pneumothorax. A decubitus view can be obtained to confirm. Although some practitioners find expiratory radiographs useful, most do not use this technique in everyday practice. With coexistent pleural fluid (hydropneumothorax), an air-fluid level may or may not be seen based on projection.

Very common mimics of the pleural line of pneumothorax are skin folds, overlying tubes and lines, and the medial scapular margin (Fig. 39.16). These are better described as edges (a density and lucency) rather than lines (a thin density with lucency on both sides) and will extend beyond the pleural space. The line narrows centrally and fans out

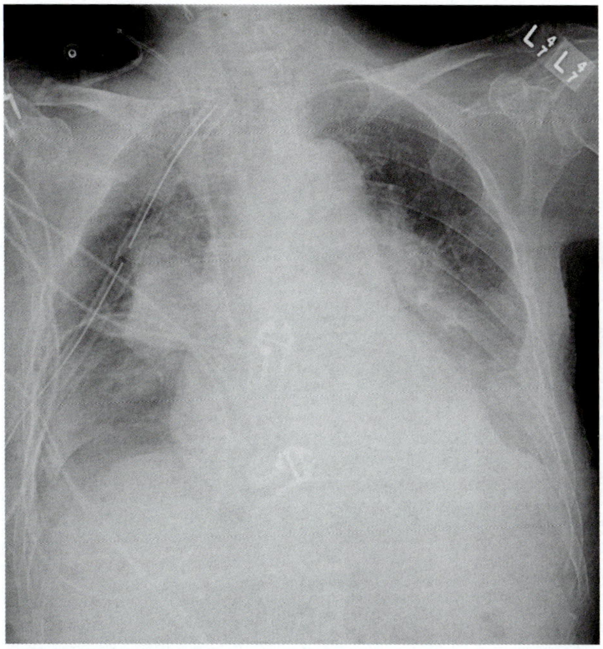

Figure 39.15 Portable chest radiograph shows a right subpulmonic pneumothorax. A right-sided chest tube is directed superomedially. The sidehole is well visualized and within the pleural space.

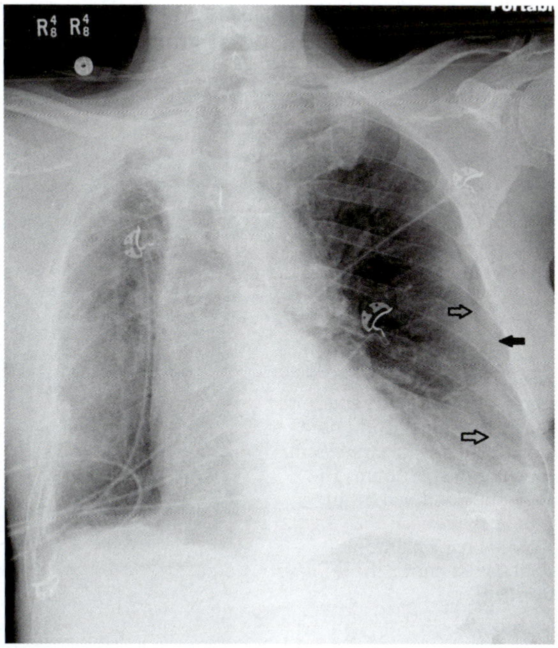

Figure 39.16 Portable chest radiograph demonstrates a left pneumothorax with mediastinal shift. Note the difference in appearance between the visceral pleural line *(black arrow)* and multiple edges of density due to superimposed skin folds *(open arrows)*.

peripherally, and lung markings will extend beyond the line. Multiple parallel edges, sometimes bilaterally, may be seen with skin folds, helping confirm the diagnosis. Additionally, severe apical bullous emphysema can sometimes be impossible to distinguish from a pneumothorax because no distinct markings are seen in the upper chest. Because the appearance can be confusing, even on CT, comparison to prior radiographs is of great value.

Bedside ultrasound has become increasingly used for the rapid diagnosis of pneumothorax. Normally, so-called lung sliding is visible on grayscale ultrasound due to the sliding of the visceral and parietal pleura. When this is absent, a pneumothorax is suggested. Smooth horizontal echogenic lines will demarcate the visceral pleural line. In some studies, the sensitivity of bedside ultrasound has exceeded that of radiography for the detection of pneumothorax.

Significance of Pulmonary Interstitial Emphysema

When air dissects around the pulmonary veins and the lymphatics, pulmonary emphysema is present. It can be detected in ARDS patients and is usually seen with concomitant usual interstitial pneumonitis. Although it is often asymptomatic, this may dissect centrally, leading to pneumomediastinum (Fig. 39.17), air cysts, or pneumothorax. In trauma patients, the Macklin effect—alveolar rupture and air dissection along the bronchovascular sheath, with mediastinal extension—is much more commonly the mechanism responsible for pneumomediastinum than tracheobronchial injury.

Radiographic Evaluation of Pneumomediastinum

Pneumomediastinum appears as radiolucent streaks that outline the contours of mediastinal structures. The thymic sail sign (outlining and elevating the thymus), the tubular artery sign (outlining the major aortic branches), and the double bronchial wall sign (outlining the trachea and proximal bronchi) have all been described. Although most ICU patients do not receive lateral chest radiographs, it should be noted that a well-defined lucency along or surrounding the right pulmonary artery on a lateral chest radiograph is called the *ring around the artery sign*. When air outlines the superior surface of the diaphragm, it is separated from the heart, resulting in the continuous diaphragm sign. The Naclerio V sign (air outlining the descending aorta and extending laterally between the parietal pleural and medial left hemidiaphragm) and the extrapleural sign (air trapped between the parietal pleural and hemidiaphragm) have also been described. On close inspection, the air can be frequently seen extending into the neck. In contradistinction to pneumothorax, the air will not move to nondependent portions because it is tightly contained by fascial planes. It therefore will not change significantly with alterations in patient positioning, as opposed to a pneumothorax.

However, pneumomediastinum and pneumothorax commonly coexist (Fig. 39.18A). Pneumopericardium can sometimes mimic pneumomediastinum. In true pneumopericardium, the air should not be present above the pericardial reflection on the proximal great vascular pedicle, although it will shift on decubitus positioning (see Fig. 39.18B). Isolated pneumopericardium is less common than pneumomediastinum and is seen almost exclusively after surgery in adults and in association with mechanical ventilation in infants. Finally, a Mach band can simulate pneumomediastinum. This describes an optical phenomenon relating to retinal enhancement of a light or dark line on a radiograph where there is a concave or convex interface in a patient (e.g., the heart border). Pneumomediastinum tends to have an overlying opaque line, which represents the pericardium.

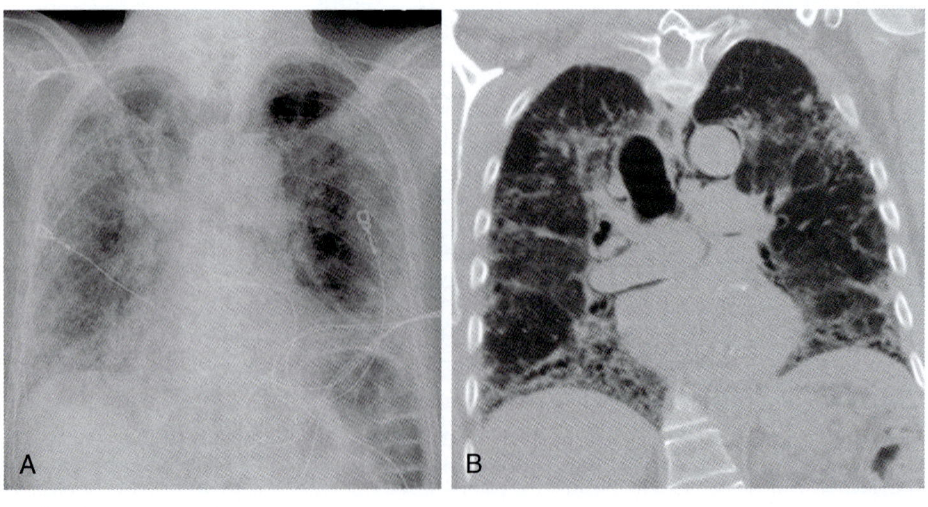

Figure 39.17 (A) Portable chest radiograph demonstrates interstitial lung disease with superimposed pulmonary interstitial emphysema and pneumomediastinum. The aortic knob is outlined by air (known as the *tubular artery sign*). (B) Coronal reformat from a noncontrast CT shows the findings to advantage.

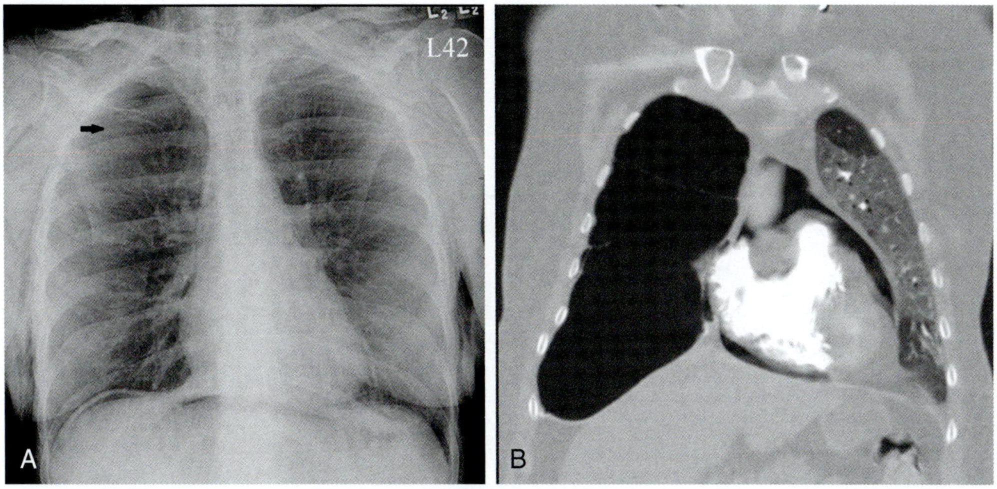

Figure 39.18 (A) The overlying subcutaneous emphysema and pneumomediastinum make the detection of the right pneumothorax more difficult. The arrow denotes the visceral pleural line. Pneumoperitoneum is also present. (B) Coronal reformat from contrast-enhanced CT in a different patient shows pneumopericardium with the air contained by the pericardial reflections.

Bibliography

Amorosa J, Bramwit M, Mohammed T, et al. ACR appropriateness criteria routine chest radiographs in intensive care unit patients. *J Am Coll Radiol*. 2013;10(3):170–174.

Chasen MH. Practical applications of Mach band theory in thoracic analysis. *Radiology*. 2001;219(3):596–610.

Ginat D, Massey H, Bhatt S, et al. Imaging of mechanical cardiac assist devices. *J Clin Imaging Sci*. 2011;1(21).

Godoy M, Leitman B, Groot P, et al. Chest radiography in the ICU: part 1, evaluation of airway, enteric, and pleural tubes. *Am J Roentgenol*. 2012;198(3):563–571.

Godoy M, Leitman B, Groot P, et al. Chest radiography in the ICU: part 2, evaluation of cardiovascular lines and other devices. *Am J Roentgenol*. 2012; 198(3):572–581.

Kalanuria A, Zai W, Mirski M. Ventilator-associated pneumonia in the ICU. *Crit Care*. 2014;18(2):208.

Khan A, Al-Jahdali H, Al-Ghanem S, et al. Reading chest radiographs in the critically ill (part I): normal chest radiographic appearance, instrumentation and complications from instrumentation. *Ann Thorac Med*. 2009;4(2): 75–87.

Khan A, Al-Jahdali H, Al-Ghanem S, et al. Reading chest radiographs in the critically ill (part II): radiography of lung pathologies common in the ICU patient. *Ann Thorac Med*. 2009;4(2):149–157.

Sigakis CJG, Mathai SK, Suby-Long TD, et al. Radiographic review of current therapeutic and monitoring devices in the chest. *Radiographics*. 2018;38:1027–1145.

Vesely TM. Central venous catheter tip position, a continuing controversy. *J Vasc Interv Radiol*. 2003;14(5):527–534.

CHAPTER 40

Cardiac CT for the Evaluation of Acute Coronary Syndrome in the Emergency Department

Christopher G. Brown and Charles S. White

CHAPTER OUTLINE

Introduction

More than 8 million Americans each year present to the emergency department (ED) with acute chest pain. This poses a diagnostic challenge to physicians, who must distinguish patients with life-threatening conditions, including acute coronary syndrome (ACS), aortic dissection, and pulmonary embolism, from those who have chest pain related to more benign causes.

Most patients with chest pain are discharged with a diagnosis of noncardiac origin. Only 12% to 15% of patients with chest pain have ACS, which includes diagnoses such as unstable angina, non-ST elevation myocardial infarction (NSTEMI), and ST elevation myocardial infarction (STEMI).

Routine workup for chest pain is estimated to cost approximately $8 billion each year and often requires admission of patients who ultimately have a non–life-threatening or noncardiac cause of chest pain. Despite advances in diagnostic tools, about 2% to 4% of patients are misdiagnosed and discharged home with ACS, and these patients have twice the mortality rate as those who are admitted and treated with the standard of care. These deficiencies highlight the need for improved algorithms to evaluate patients with acute chest pain. Noninvasive imaging has the potential to rule out ACS in select patients to prevent admission and additional cardiac testing.

Standard Approach in Diagnosing Acute Coronary Syndrome

ACS is a heterogeneous syndrome ranging from unstable angina to myocardial infarction (MI; NSTEMI or STEMI), which is usually caused by a ruptured atherosclerotic plaque and thrombus formation that significantly narrows or occludes a coronary artery. Symptoms arise when the oxygen demand of myocardium exceeds supply delivered by coronary vessels, causing reversible myocardial ischemia (unstable angina) or infarction (NSTEMI or STEMI).

The most common clinical presentation is chest pain, which is relatively nonspecific for ACS. Chest pain can also represent other life-threatening conditions, such as aortic dissection, pulmonary embolism, tension pneumothorax, cardiac tamponade, and mediastinitis, or it can represent more common non–life-threatening conditions such as gastroesophageal reflux disease, musculoskeletal pain, and pneumonia.

On admission, the initial history and physical examination are helpful in identifying factors to increase suspicion of or exclude ACS as the cause of chest pain. Chest pain from myocardial ischemia or MI is often gradual in onset and is described as chest discomfort, and radiation to the left arm or lower jaw is more specific to ACS. Other nonspecific symptoms include diaphoresis, nausea and vomiting, dyspnea, syncope, and palpitations. Caution should be taken with patients who are older, female, or diabetic because they may present with atypical symptoms such as weakness, dyspnea, and abdominal pain, and consequently this population is at higher risk for missed diagnosis and delay in care. Pain that responds to nitroglycerin is often thought to have a cardiac cause (or esophageal spasm), but this is not a reliable indicator to distinguish cardiac pain from noncardiac chest pain. Although the presence of cardiac risk factors or known coronary artery disease (CAD) increases the risk for ACS, it is a poor predictor in an acute setting because chest pain itself has a much higher predictive value for ACS than the presence of cardiac risk factors.

All patients undergo 12-lead electrocardiography to assess for evidence of ischemia or infarction, such as new ST elevation (the most specific finding for ACS) or depression in two anatomically contiguous leads, Q waves >30 ms, and inverted T waves in precordial leads. Ischemic changes may be masked in patients who have baseline electrocardiographic abnormalities from hypertrophy, bundle branch block, or ventricular pacing. In most patients with ACS, the electrocardiogram (ECG) is normal or nondiagnostic, so it is recommended that the patient be placed on telemetry with serial ECGs obtained every 5 to 10 minutes to assess for ongoing ischemia in suspected cases of ACS.

Serum biomarkers are also drawn to assess for myocardial injury. Many serum biomarkers have been studied in the setting of ACS (e.g., troponin, creatine kinase-muscle/brain [CK-MB], natriuretic peptides, C-reactive protein [CRP], myeloperoxidase), but cardiac troponin is the most commonly used biomarker in EDs because it is widely available and is highly sensitive and specific for myocardial injury. However, myocardial injury is not specific to ACS. Troponin levels can be elevated in the setting of trauma, renal failure, sepsis, hypertensive emergency, pulmonary embolism, and other conditions. In the setting of ACS, troponin level elevation may not be detected until 4 to 6 hours after the onset of symptoms, so current guidelines recommend that serial troponin levels be checked every 6 to 8 hours to improve detection of ACS. High-sensitivity troponin assays are being developed to detect infarction earlier in ACS, but this will increase the number of false-positives and potentially lead to unnecessary additional testing.

After obtaining the history, physical, initial ECG, and cardiac biomarkers, the need for further studies—noninvasive or invasive imaging—is determined by risk stratification.

Patient Stratification in the Evaluation of Acute Coronary Syndrome

From a noninvasive imaging perspective, patients can be divided into three groups based on their risk for ACS and need for further evaluation and workup. The first group of patients consists of those who have high-risk or definite ACS based on the physical examination, ECG, and cardiac biomarkers. These patients are admitted and referred for invasive coronary angiography and possible percutaneous or surgical intervention. Noninvasive imaging is unnecessary in these patients because it will not change the need for catheterization.

The second group of patients consists of those who have a clear noncardiac and non–life-threatening diagnosis, with a normal ECG and cardiac biomarkers, in whom ACS can be confidently excluded. These patients can safely be discharged from the ED without the need for observation or cardiac imaging.

The third group of patients is the largest and consists of those who fall in between the two other groups. These patients often have nonspecific or atypical chest pain, normal or nondiagnostic ECG, and normal cardiac biomarkers. This group usually represents the patient population at a low to intermediate risk for ACS, and they require further evaluation to include or reasonably exclude ACS. Patients with unstable angina usually fall into this group because, by definition, they have normal cardiac biomarkers and frequently have normal or nondiagnostic ECGs. Patients in this group are usually admitted to an observation unit for serial ECGs and cardiac biomarkers; additional tests with stress testing or noninvasive imaging techniques are performed, depending on patient characteristics.

Multiple scoring systems have been developed to assess clinical risk after an ACS; they are primarily based on the physical examination, history, electrocardiographic findings, and biomarkers. Two widely used scoring systems include the TIMI (Thrombolysis In Myocardial Infarction), which assesses the risk of 14-day mortality and MI after ACS, and GRACE (Global Registry of Acute Coronary Events), which assesses index hospitalization mortality and 6-month mortality after ACS. Although these risk-scoring systems focus on outcomes and are not designed to diagnose ACS, they are often used as part of risk stratification to guide management in individuals with suspected ACS. Patients who are at a higher risk of mortality will often be immediately referred for invasive coronary angiography.

Role of Noninvasive Imaging in the Conventional Assessment of Acute Coronary Syndrome

Chest Radiography

Most patients with ACS have a nondiagnostic chest radiograph. However, a chest radiograph is obtained in virtually all patients who present to the ED with chest pain because it gives a global survey of chest anatomy and can quickly rule out potentially life-threatening pathologies, such as pneumothorax, which require urgent intervention, and more common nonemergent or non–life-threatening pathologies, such as pneumonia or rib fractures. Other abnormalities may give clues to the underlying diagnosis—a widened mediastinum is observed in about 90% of patients with aortic dissection, a wedge-shaped pulmonary infarct (Hampton's hump) may be present with pulmonary embolism, and pneumomediastinum may be evident with esophageal perforation. Myocardial calcification suggests prior MI (Fig. 40.1), and coronary artery calcification indicates CAD, but these findings are neither sensitive nor specific to ACS.

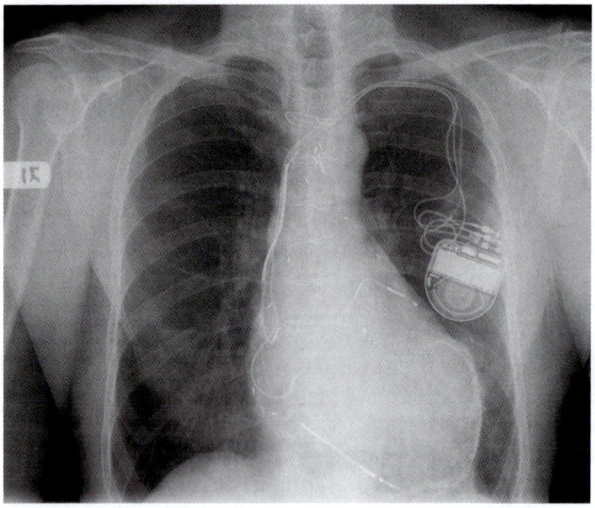

Figure 40.1 Chest radiograph of a 66-year-old male patient with chest pain. This frontal radiograph shows rimlike calcification along the left myocardial margin consistent with prior myocardial infarction.

Exercise Tolerance Test

For many years, the exercise tolerance test (ETT) has been the preferred method in appropriate patients to detect inducible ischemia due to its low cost and wide availability. A standard ETT can be performed on a treadmill or stationary bike, and the ECG is continually monitored to detect ischemic changes as the patient progresses from a resting to a stress state. Although meta-analyses have shown only a modest sensitivity and specificity for detecting CAD, ETT has a negative predictive value greater than 98% for ACS, making it an excellent screening test to rule out ACS. The major limitation of ETT is that a significant number of patients are not suitable candidates because of physical limitations, inability to achieve the necessary heart rate (85% of maximum heart rate), and resting electrocardiographic abnormalities that make ischemic changes difficulty to identify (e.g., ST segment changes, left bundle branch block, arrhythmias). Patients with negative ETT results are usually cleared for discharge, but abnormal or nondiagnostic results require additional cardiac imaging for further evaluation.

Echocardiography

Resting echocardiography can detect ischemia and infarction by visualizing regional wall motion abnormalities, but its usefulness is limited by timing of the examination and size of the ischemic or infarcted myocardium. ACS is a dynamic process and, in the absence of symptoms representing ongoing ischemia or infarction, echocardiography is less likely to visualize wall motion abnormalities. Furthermore, more than 20% of the myocardial thickness must be involved for wall motion abnormalities to appear. Given these limitations, it is not surprising that substantial variability in negative predictive values has been reported, ranging from 57% to 98%. When performed after symptom resolution, echocardiography is a less reliable predictor of future adverse cardiac events and the need for revascularization. Therefore, in the setting of acute chest pain, resting echocardiography is most useful in detecting ACS when the patient is symptomatic or within a few hours of clinical presentation.

Stress echocardiography allows detection of inducible ischemia and can be performed during exercise or, more commonly, using pharmacologic agents (e.g., dobutamine). Multiple studies have found consistently high negative predictive values, ranging from 96% to 100%, which provides support for discharging a patient from the ED with a negative result. Multiple studies have also shown that stress echocardiography gives important prognostic information regarding early and late cardiac events.

Possible advantages of echocardiography include the ability to detect other pathologies such as proximal aortic dissection, large pulmonary embolism, pericarditis, and cardiomyopathy, as well as complications of MI. Echocardiography also provides important cardiac anatomic and physiologic information, including ventricular function, valvular function, and ejection fraction. The use of newer microbubble contrast agents has been shown to improve the ability to detect wall motion abnormalities, which may enhance the sensitivity to detect ACS. Disadvantages include limited availability of sonographers and cardiologists for interpretation during off-hours.

Radionuclide Myocardial Perfusion Imaging

Myocardial perfusion imaging (MPI) assesses the distribution of coronary blood flow, which gives direct evidence of ischemia or infarction and clearly identifies the location and extent of abnormality. Old infarctions typically have the same appearance as new infarctions, but they can be distinguished by the presence or absence of cardiac biomarkers.

To perform MPI, a cardiac specific tracer material is injected, and imaging is acquired using single-positron emission computed tomography (SPECT), which is demonstrated in Fig. 40.2. Technetium tracers have mostly replaced the use of thallium tracers because thallium rapidly redistributes and requires imaging within minutes of injection, whereas technetium allows for imaging up to 2 to 4 hours after injection. The timing of the injection is critical because images that are subsequently acquired reflect blood flow and myocardial perfusion at the time of injection. There is evidence that perfusion abnormalities can persist many hours after resolution of symptoms, but MPI has the highest sensitivity when the patient is symptomatic. Current guidelines recommend that the injection should occur while the patient is symptomatic or within 2 hours of symptom resolution.

Rest MPI has been shown to have a sensitivity of up to 97% for obstructive CAD causing ischemia in patients with ACS and has been recommended with class 1 indications for patients with acute chest pain, a nondiagnostic ECG, and normal cardiac biomarkers. Its negative predictive value is 97% to 100%, which makes ACS extremely unlikely in a patient with a normal rest MPI. Randomized clinical trials (RCTs) have found that

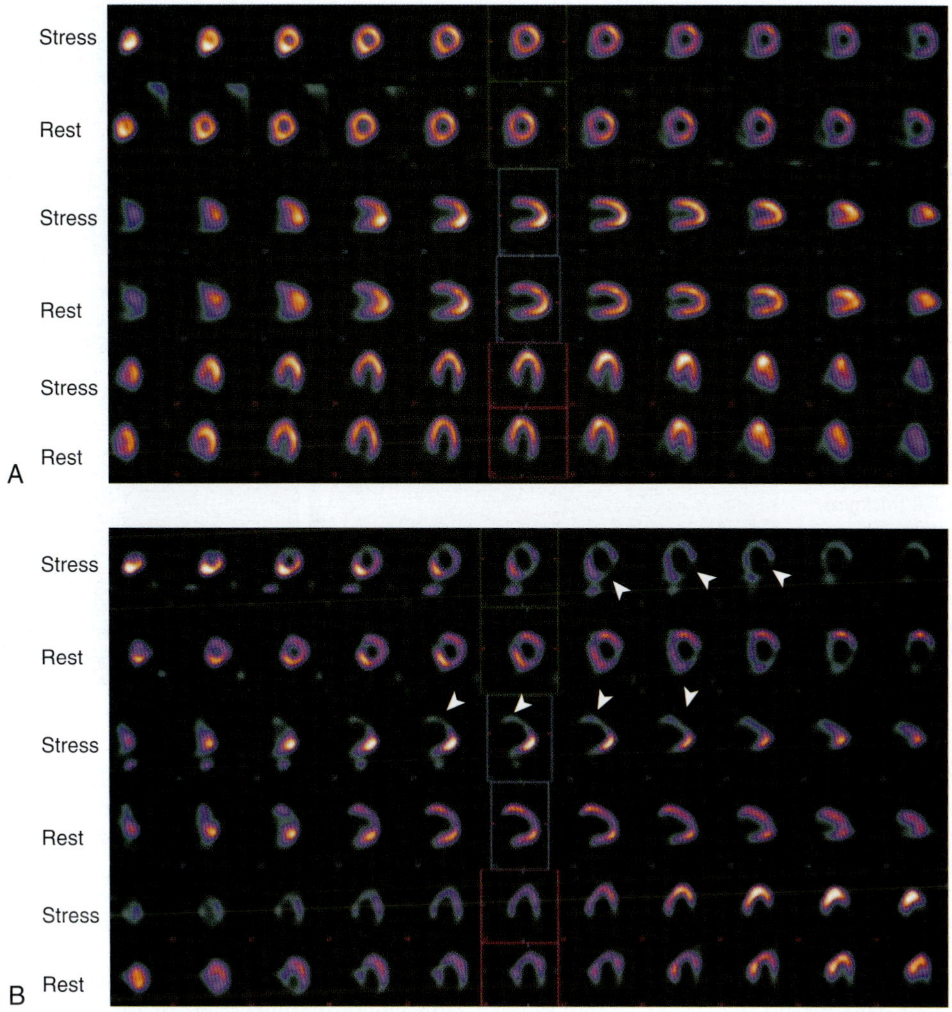

Figure 40.2 Normal and abnormal myocardial perfusion tests. (A) A 16-year-old male patient with chest pain. Following treadmill exercise testing, thallium-201 was given intravenously, and stress tomography imaging was performed. The patient returned to the department 2 hours later, and rest redistribution tomography imaging was performed. Exercise stress myocardial perfusion single-photon emission computed tomography (SPECT) shows no evidence of myocardial ischemia or prior infarction. The patient has normal left ventricular size, wall motion, and systolic function, with a left ventricular ejection fraction (LVEF) of 61%. (B) A 56-year-old female patient with a history of known coronary artery disease and an abnormal electrocardiogram. Following regadenoson pharmacologic stress testing, thallium-201 was given intravenously and stress tomography imaging was performed. The patient returned to the department 2 hours later, and rest redistribution tomography imaging was performed. A myocardial perfusion SPECT scan demonstrated myocardial ischemia in the anterior and anteroseptal regions (left anterior descending vascular territory) and the middle to basal inferolateral region (circumflex vascular territory) of the left ventricle *(arrowheads)*. Globally, hypokinesis, dilated left ventricle with abnormal systolic function, and an LVEF of 24% were noted. (Courtesy Dr. Qi Cao, University of Maryland Medical Center, Baltimore.)

using rest MPI in diagnostic evaluation results in fewer inappropriate admissions for suspected ACS, a shorter hospital stay, and decreased total costs when compared to standard care.

The use of stress MPI with exercise or pharmacologic agents may increase the sensitivity of detecting ACS compared to rest MPI in stable patients whose symptoms have resolved, although studies have yielded mixed results regarding the superiority of stress MPI compared to rest MPI. Alternatively, vasodilators (e.g., dipyridamole, adenosine) can be administered that preferentially dilate the normal coronary arteries and produce relative perfusion deficits in myocardium supplied by diseased vessels.

Disadvantages of MPI include exposure to radiation when performing the SPECT scan. From a technical standpoint, diagnostic value may be limited by soft tissue densities, which can cause attenuation artifacts that mimic or confound the appearance of perfusion defects. Another weakness is that most institutions have a limited availability of nuclear medicine staff to perform and interpret the study after hours.

Magnetic Resonance Imaging

Cardiac MRI has a limited role in the evaluation of acute chest pain. The advantage of MRI is its ability to assess

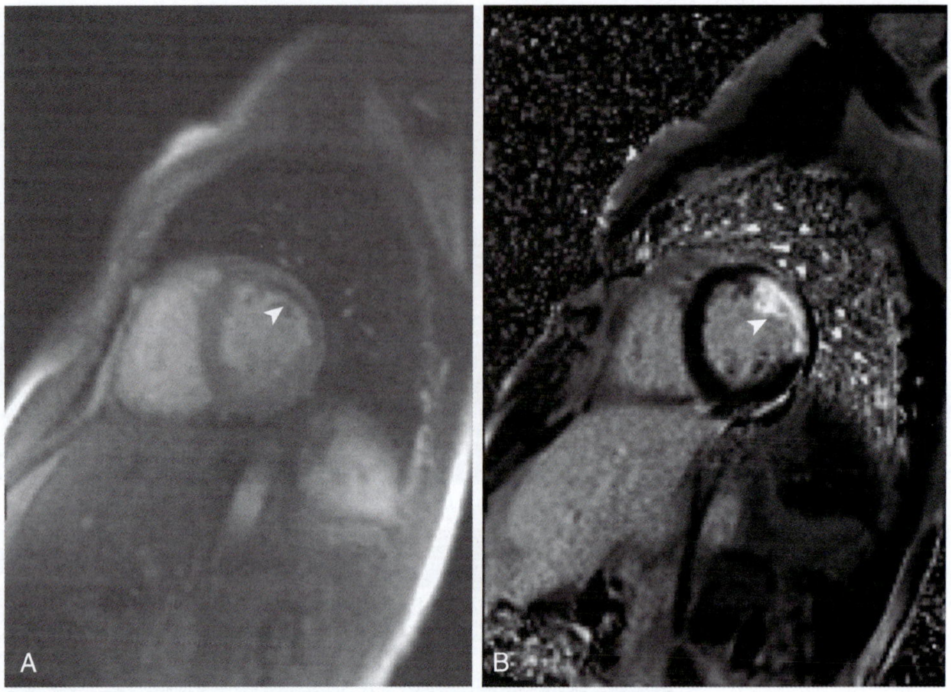

Figure 40.3 Abnormal cardiac magnetic resonance perfusion. (A) Short-axis view of first-pass perfusion imaging after administration of intravenous gadolinium demonstrates a perfusion defect involving the subendocardial anterolateral left ventricular wall *(arrowhead)*. (B) Short-axis view of images obtained 10 minutes after the administration of gadolinium demonstrates marked delayed subendocardial enhancement in the same region of the anterolateral left ventricular wall *(arrowhead)*. The region of delayed myocardial enhancement exceeds 50% of the myocardial thickness, with portions that appear transmural in extent. Cine clips (not shown) revealed marked focal hypokinesis involving the anterolateral left ventricular wall.

cardiac function, perfusion, and tissue characteristics in a single examination. Unlike other imaging modalities, it can identify areas of reversible and irreversible injury and distinguish acute (Fig. 40.3) from chronic infarction. However, cardiac MRI is not recommended in the setting of acute chest pain due to lack of data, the need to remove the patient from the monitored environment of the emergency room, and the longer duration of the study. The few existing studies show encouraging results. In a study by Kwong et al., 161 patients with suspected ACS underwent MRI to assess perfusion, left ventricular function, and gadolinium enhancement. Sensitivity was 84% and specificity was 85% for detecting ACS. In another study, by Cury et al., the addition of T2-weighted imaging increased the accuracy of detection of ACS from 84% to 93% and improved specificity from 84% to 96%. Larger trials are needed to understand fully the utility of cardiac MRI in the setting of acute chest pain.

Computed Tomography Calcium Scoring

Coronary artery calcification (CAC) has a well-established association with cardiovascular disease and mortality. CAC occurs when calcium is deposited in maturing atherosclerotic plaques, and the amount of CAC correlates with the total atherosclerotic plaque burden. In the 1980s, Agatston described a method using electron beam CT to quantify the amount of CAC, which is referred to as the *Agatston score*. This is a summation of values based on the area and highest density of each calcified plaque. An often used interpretation of the Agatston score is as follows: 0 represents no identifiable disease, 1 to 99 represents mild disease, 100 to 399 represents moderate disease, and >400 represents severe disease.

Because the prevalence of CAD varies across different demographic groups, calcium percentile scores are often calculated based on a patient's age and gender. For example, in one study, the 95% percentile without significant stenosis in men <40 corresponded to an Agatston score of 8 or less; in men >70, the equivalent percentile corresponded to an Agatston score of 134 or less. In this regard, the Agatston score is a better marker of the extent of atherosclerosis than the severity of stenosis, which is reflected by its high sensitivity but low specificity for obstructive CAD.

In general, the presence of CAC indicates at least some degree of CAD. As the CAC score increases, so does the total atherosclerotic burden and the likelihood of obstructive CAD and risk for cardiac events (Fig. 40.4). A CAC score of 0 indicates no identifiable atherosclerosis, but this does not rule out CAD because not all atherosclerosis contains calcification (Fig. 40.5). In asymptomatic patients, the CAC score has demonstrated excellent prognostic ability and is a predictor for cardiac events, MI, and all-cause mortality. The absence of CAC in asymptomatic patients predicts a 10-year survival rate of 99%. The 2010 American College of Cardiology/American Heart Association guidelines stated that CAC scanning is reasonable for cardiovascular risk assessment in asymptomatic adults at intermediate risk (10%–20% 10-year risk).

However, there is no consensus yet concerning the utility of CAC score in symptomatic patients with acute chest pain. The limitation in using the CAC score to evaluate for ACS is that unlike traditional noninvasive imaging techniques, it does not provide any direct anatomic or functional information to suggest ischemia or infarction. Rather, the CAC score may be useful in the evaluation of ACS because it can be used as a surrogate marker for obstructive CAD.

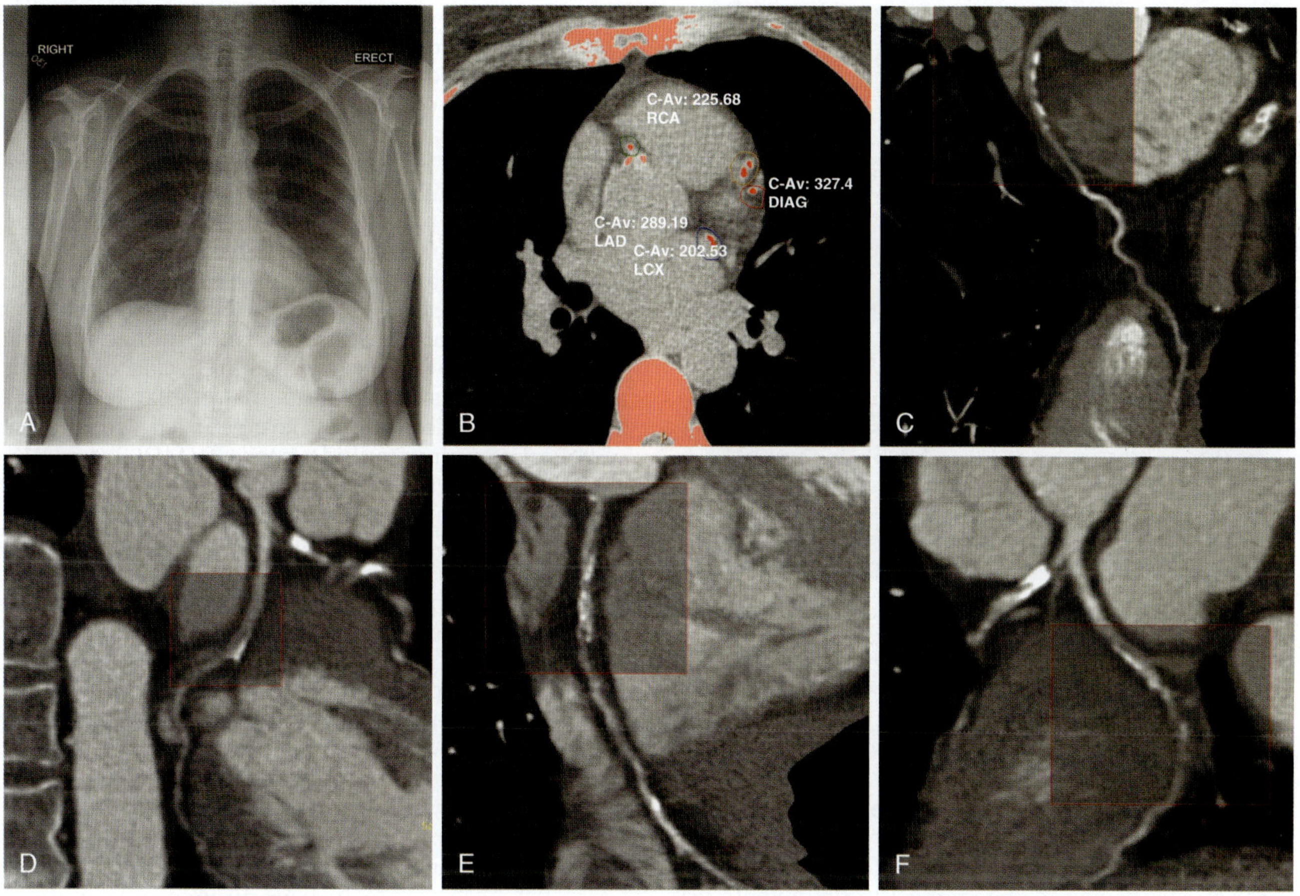

Figure 40.4 A 56-year-old female patient who presented with chest pain. (A) Normal chest radiograph. (B) Computed calcium score by the Agatston method was 1217, thus placing her at the 100th percentile for risk, adjusted for age and gender. (C–F) Curved multiplanar reconstruction views of the coronary vessels demonstrate widespread atherosclerotic disease in the left anterior descending artery (*LAD;* C), left circumflex artery (*LCX;* D), right coronary artery (*RCA;* E), and obtuse marginal artery (F). There was no evidence of pulmonary emboli or acute aortic disease. A subsequent regadenoson pharmacologic stress thallium myocardial perfusion study revealed a reversible perfusion defect in the anteroseptal and inferolateral walls. The patient underwent a cardiac catheterization, and a bare metal stent was placed in the obtuse marginal. *C-Av,* Calcium average; *DIAG,* diagonal artery.

The presence of CAC alone is not particularly useful in evaluating for ACS because it lacks specificity for obstructive CAD, especially in patients who are older or with known CAD, in which CAC is an expected finding. Using a particular cutoff score to triage patients (e.g., 400, which is often interpreted as severe atherosclerotic disease) is an inadequate strategy because sensitivity decreases as specificity increases (for a CAC score of 400, sensitivity for obstructive CAD was 60% and specificity was 88% in one study of asymptomatic patients); this will miss a significant portion of patients with obstructive CAD. The absence of CAC has clinical value in the setting of ACS because it indicates no identifiable atherosclerosis and minimal risk of obstructive CAD, making ACS an unlikely diagnosis. On this basis, CAC scoring can potentially serve as a screening tool to rule out ACS in low-risk patients with a CAC score of 0.

Several studies have confirmed this concept. In a meta-analysis of 13 studies by Tota-Maharaj et al., the absence of CAC had a sensitivity of 94% and negative predictive value of 99.4% for obstructive CAD and cardiac events among 3035 symptomatic patients at low to intermediate risk. These findings support the potential of CAC scoring as a gatekeeper for the need of further cardiac testing. In this approach to evaluate for suspected ACS, low-risk patients with normal or nondiagnostic ECGs, normal biomarkers, and a CAC score of 0 may be safe for discharge. Any CAC above 0 is considered abnormal and warrants further cardiac testing.

The CAC score in symptomatic patients has also shown to have strong long-term prognostic utility. In a study by Georgiou et al., 192 patients who presented with suspected ACS were followed for an average follow-up period of 50 months. Patients with a CAC score of 0 had an extremely low annual event rate of 0.6%. For patients who had CAC, increasing scores and adjusted percentiles were strongly related to the incidence of cardiac events.

Despite these promising results, CAC scoring has not been recommended for the evaluation of ACS because several other studies have shown the presence of functionally significant, obstructive CAD in patients with a CAC score of 0. In one such study, by Rubenshtein et al., 7% of symptomatic patients with CAC scores of 0 had obstructive CAD on both coronary computed tomography

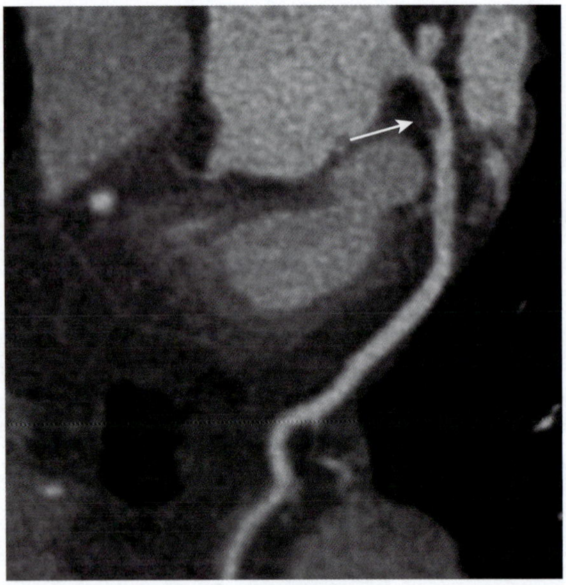

Figure 40.5 A 56-year-old male patient who presented with chest pain. The computed calcium score by the Agatston method was 0. Curved multiplanar reconstruction of the left anterior descending coronary artery shows at least a 50% proximal stenosis resulting from a noncalcified plaque *(arrow)*.

angiography (CCTA) and invasive coronary angiography. These patients all had single-vessel disease, tended to be younger, and were more likely to be female. In another study by Henneman et al., among 13 intermediate-risk patients with suspected ACS and a CAC score of 0, 11 patients (85%) had atherosclerotic plaques and 5 patients (39%) had significant stenosis. The authors of these studies concluded that the absence of CAC cannot reliably exclude the presence of obstructive CAD and should not be used to exclude ACS.

The use of CAC scoring in the evaluation of acute chest pain must still be validated by large multicenter trials before it can be incorporated into routine clinical practice. The observed discrepancies in its ability to rule out obstructive CAD in symptomatic patients are likely due to patient selection. Existing studies have demonstrated that a CAC score of 0 has the highest negative predictive value in low-risk patients, which suggests that the use of the CAC score as a screening tool for ACS is appropriate only in low-risk populations. Because CAC increases with age, this screening method is less beneficial in older populations because fewer patients have a CAC score of 0.

Concerning safety, the use of CAC scoring has advantages when compared to other noninvasive imaging modalities. No contrast is required, and it has a lower radiation dose than SPECT (3 vs. 25 mSv). Its dose compared to CCTA depends on the protocol that is used.

Coronary Computed Tomography Angiography

Although the traditional noninvasive imaging techniques (e.g., ETT, echocardiography, MPI) provide functional information to detect ischemia or infarction, CCTA provides anatomic information about the coronary vessels. Although the gold standard for imaging coronary vessels remains invasive coronary angiography, its use is limited because of associated risks, invasiveness, and costs of the procedure. CCTA is an attractive, noninvasive, alternative modality. Since its introduction, CCTA has been well studied and now plays an important role in the detection of CAD and evaluation of acute chest pain.

CCTA is widely available and can be performed on any modern 64-slice CT scanner (or higher, such as a 256- or 320-slice CT scanner). Early cardiac imaging was developed with electron beam CT, and diagnostic ability was limited by suboptimal spatial resolution. Many technologic advances have occurred with the use of helical scanning, multidetector CT (MDCT; typically 64 rows and up to 320 rows), faster rotating gantries (<300 ms/rotation), and dual-energy applications. Current state of the art CT technology allows imaging coronary arteries with spatial resolution of 0.4 mm and temporal resolution less than 100 ms. Total scan time is usually less than 10 seconds, and can be less than 1 second with some scanners.

In the setting of acute chest pain with suspected ACS, the value of coronary angiography (both CT and invasive) is based on the pathophysiologic cause of ACS, in which a ruptured atherosclerotic plaque thromboses and causes hemodynamically significant coronary stenosis. Coronary angiography directly visualizes the lumen of coronary arteries and identifies the location and severity of stenosis. CCTA has been shown to have an excellent ability to detect coronary stenosis in ACS and CAD. In a 2007 meta-analysis by Abdulla et al., CCTA demonstrated a sensitivity of 97.5% and specificity of 91% in detecting ACS when compared to invasive coronary angiography. In a 2008 meta-analysis by Mowatt, CCTA demonstrated a sensitivity of 98%, specificity of 89%, and negative predictive value of 100% when compared to invasive coronary angiography for the detection of CAD.

Many studies have compared the use of CCTA to traditional protocols in the setting of acute chest pain with suspected ACS. The underlying premise is that patients who have absent or minimal coronary stenosis should have an extremely low risk of ACS and can be safely discharged from the ED (Fig. 40.6). Three major trials RCTs have been conducted to date—the CT-STAT, ACRIN-PA, and ROMICAT-II trials.

The CT-STAT trial was a multicenter RCT consisting of 699 patients with low-risk acute chest pain who were randomized to a strategy involving CCTA or rest-stress MPI. Major inclusion criteria included a normal or nondiagnostic ECG, normal cardiac biomarkers, and TIMI score ≤4, and exclusion criteria included known CAD or cardiomyopathy. In the MPI arm, patients were eligible for discharge to home if MPI was normal; patients with equivocal or abnormal MPI were recommended for invasive coronary angiography. In the CCTA arm, patients were eligible for discharge to home if areas of stenosis were <25% and/or the calcium score was <100 Agatston units. Patients with areas of stenosis >70% were recommended for invasive coronary angiography, and patients with intermediate stenosis were recommended for MPI.

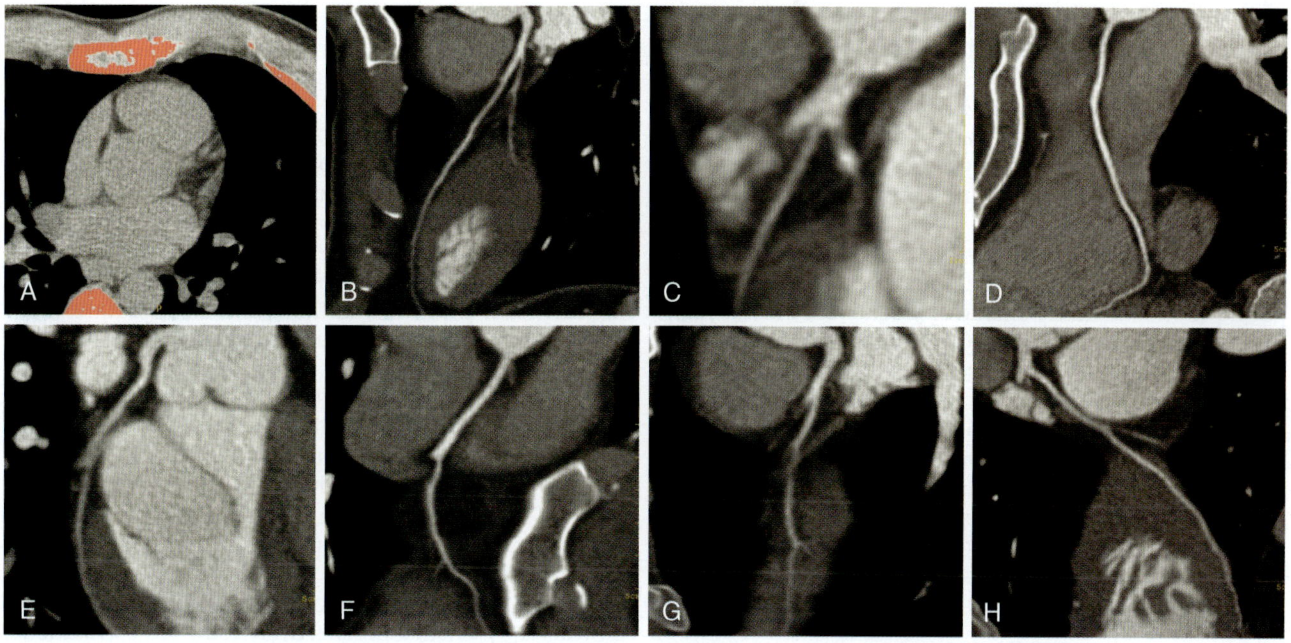

Figure 40.6 A 44-year-old male patient who presented with chest pain and shortness of breath. (A) Computed calcium score by the Agatston method was 0, thus placing the patient below the 25th percentile for risk adjusted for age and gender. (B–H) Curved multiplanar reconstruction views of the coronary vessels demonstrate no evidence of calcified or noncalcified plaque in the left main coronary artery (B), left anterior descending artery, ramus intermedius (C), right coronary artery (D), left circumflex artery (E), acute marginal artery (F), diagonal artery (G), or obtuse marginal artery (H). The patient had no pulmonary emboli or acute aortic disease.

Results from the CT-STAT trial favored the use of CCTA over MPI. Patients who underwent CCTA had a quicker time to diagnosis (2.9 vs. 6.2 hours), decreased total ED costs ($2137 vs. $3458), and lower effective radiation dose (median 11.5 vs. 12.8 mSv). Regarding safety, there was no difference in major adverse cardiac events (MACEs) over a 6-month follow-up period.

The ACRIN-PA trial was a multicenter RCT that consisted of 1370 patients with low to intermediate risk of ACS who were randomized to CCTA or traditional care. Major inclusion criteria consisted of an ECG that did not show signs of ischemia and a TIMI score ≤2. In the traditional group, the method of testing was left to the discretion of the treating physician, and most patients (87%) underwent stress imaging. Clinically significant stenosis on CCTA was defined as >50% of a major coronary artery.

Results from the ACRIN-PA trial showed that patients who underwent CCTA had a higher discharge rate from the ED (49.6% vs. 22.7%), shorter length of stay (median, 18.0 vs. 24.8 hours), and higher rate of diagnosis of CAD (9.0% vs. 3.5%). There was no difference in the rate of invasive coronary angiography or revascularization between the two groups. Interestingly, patients in the CCTA group who were referred for invasive coronary angiography were less likely to have a negative result than those from the traditional care group, suggesting that CCTA was a better predictor of patients who are appropriate for invasive coronary angiography. During the 30-day follow-up period, there were no cardiac deaths in either group, and there were a similar number of MIs (1%). The authors concluded that CCTA was effective in diagnosing ACS and met a safety threshold that most EDs would find acceptable.

The ROMICAT-II trial was a multicenter, randomized controlled clinical trial that consisted of 100 patients with chest pain and suspected ACS who were randomized to CCTA or traditional care. Major exclusion criteria consisted of known CAD, ischemic changes on the ECG, and elevated cardiac troponin levels. Results from the ROMICAT-II trial showed that patients who underwent CCTA had a quicker time to diagnosis with CCTA (10.4 vs. 18.7 hours), higher discharge rate from the ED (47% vs. 12%), and shorter length of stay (median, 8.6 vs. 26.7 hours). No cases of undetected ACS were identified, and the number of MACEs was similar in both groups. Patients in the CCTA group on average received more exposure radiation, but the average radiation exposure from CCTA was less than that from SPECT (11.3 vs. 14.1 mSv). Concerning resource utilization, patients in the CCTA group underwent more diagnostic tests and had higher ED costs, but total costs in the 28-day follow-up period were similar in both groups. The authors concluded that CCTA improved efficiency, with a shorter hospital stay and higher discharge rate, without comprising patient safety.

A meta-analysis was performed by Hulten et al. using the above three RCTs (CT-STAT, ACRIN-PA, and ROMICAT-II), as well as a fourth smaller RCT by Goldstein et al. to assess outcomes after CCTA compared to usual care in the ED. The authors concluded that using CCTA to evaluate for ACS was a safe practice. No differences were observed between CCTA and usual care with regard to the rate of death, MI, return ED visits, and recurrent hospitalizations due to cardiac causes. In each trial, the use of CCTA reduced the length of stay. A notable finding was that CCTA increased the need for invasive coronary angiography and revascularization by 2%, but data were insufficient to analyze the reason for this difference. The authors posited that this likely represented overutilization in the CCTA group or underutilization in the traditional care group.

Long-term follow-up after CCTA for the evaluation of chest pain in the ED has demonstrated that CCTA has good prognostic utility. A study by Schlett et al. analyzed 368 patients from the ROMICAT study (an earlier observational study to assess the usefulness of CCTA in patients with suspected ACS) for a follow-up period of 2 years. Patients who had no CAD on CCTA had an absence of MACEs over the 2-year follow-up, suggesting that patients with normal CCTA are risk-free of MACEs for at least 2 years. Patients who had nonobstructive or obstructive CAD had a higher 2-year risk of MACEs (4.6% and 30.3%, respectively). Patients who had stenosis and regional wall motion abnormalities had the highest 2-year risk of a MACE (62.4%).

In addition to providing a method for accurate noninvasive coronary angiography, CCTA also provides the ability to characterize atherosclerotic plaque morphology. Plaques at risk for rupturing and causing an acute cardiac event are defined as vulnerable or high-risk plaques, and they usually have a necrotic, lipid-rich core, with a thin fibrous cap, whereas more stable plaques have a thicker fibrous cap. Vulnerable plaques are associated with positive vascular remodeling (outward arterial wall expansion), which helps preserve blood flow across an area of stenosis. In comparison, stable plaques are more frequently associated with negative vascular remodeling (arterial wall constriction) and are typically observed in patients with stable angina. These plaque characteristics can be detected on CCTA and help identify patients who are at high risk for ACS.

Motomaya et al. have compared plaque morphology in patients with ACS to those of stable angina and found that plaques in ACS patients had a significantly higher presence of positive vascular remodeling (87% vs. 12%), low-attenuation plaque (79% vs. 9%), and spotty calcification (63% vs. 21%).

In another study, Motomaya et al. examined the relationship between two CT characteristics of vulnerable plaque—low-attenuation plaque and positive vascular remodeling—and the development of acute cardiac events. It was found that 22% of patients with both characteristics subsequently developed an acute cardiac event, compared to 3% of patients with one characteristic, and 0.5% of patients with neither characteristic. Results from the ROMICAT-II trial showed that vulnerable plaques were more frequent in patients with ACS and were a significant predictor of ACS (odds ratio, 8.9) independent of a history of CAD, age, sex, and other cardiac risk factors.

Another CT morphologic characteristic of high-risk plaques has been termed the *napkin ring sign,* which can be seen on cross section of the coronary artery lumen (Fig. 40.7). The napkin ring sign is defined as a structure that narrows the lumen; it consists of a central, low area of attenuation (representing the necrotic core) surrounded by a thin rim of high attenuation (representing the inflamed fibrous cap). Otsuka prospectively followed 895 patients who underwent a baseline CCTA and found that the presence of the napkin ring sign was an independent predictor of future cardiac events, with subsequent development of ACS in 41% of patients with the napkin ring sign.

The use of CCTA is supported by current guidelines from a number of organizations. In 2010, the American College of Cardiology Foundation, Appropriate Use Criteria Task Force, Society of Cardiovascular Computer Tomography, American College of Radiology (ACR), American Heart Association, American Society of Echocardiography, American Society of Nuclear Cardiology, North American Society for Cardiovascular Imaging, Society for Cardiovascular Angiography and Interventions, and Society for Cardiovascular Magnetic Resonance released a document that outlined appropriate use criteria for CCTA. The use of CCTA was deemed appropriate to evaluate a patient who has no known history of CAD, acute symptoms suspicious for ACS, a normal or nondiagnostic ECG, normal cardiac biomarkers, and low to intermediate risk of ACS.

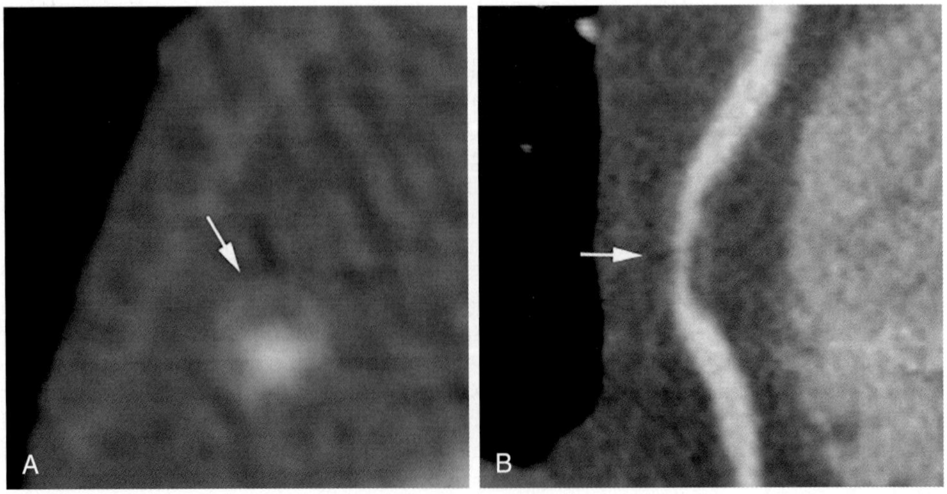

Figure 40.7 A 42-year-old man who underwent screening with coronary CT angiography was found to have vulnerable plaque in the middle segment of the right coronary artery. (A) Cross section demonstrates the napkin ring sign *(arrow)*. (B) Longitudinal reconstruction shows noncalcified plaque with positive vascular remodeling *(arrow)*. Two months later, the patient experienced a non-ST elevation myocardial infarction. (Courtesy Dr. Seung Min Yoo, Department of Diagnostic Radiology, CHA University Bundang Medical Center, Sungnam, South Korea.)

Guidelines from the 2012 ACR Appropriateness Criteria rated the use of CCTA as "usually appropriate" in the evaluation of acute, nonspecific, chest pain with a low probability of CAD. In comparison, resting echocardiography was also rated "usually appropriate," and MPI was rated as "may be appropriate" for the same clinical scenario. In the evaluation of acute chest pain suggestive of ACS, invasive coronary angiography, MPI, and stress echocardiography were rated as "usually appropriate," whereas resting echocardiography and CCTA were rated as "may be appropriate."

There is an alternative MDCT imaging protocol to evaluate patients who present to the ED with acute chest pain. In the so-called triple rule-out protocol, the entire chest is imaged, which allows evaluation of not only the coronary arteries (as in a dedicated CCTA), but also the pulmonary vasculature and great vessels. It is called the triple rule-out protocol because a normal scan can effectively rule out ACS, pulmonary embolism (Fig. 40.8), and aortic dissection (Fig. 40.9). The protocol was developed so that all images could be acquired using a biphasic or triphasic injection of intravenous contrast within a single breath-hold. Importantly, no significant difference has been found in image quality of coronary arteries in both protocols. In addition to ruling out the life-threatening conditions mentioned, the triple rule-out protocol can also identify other pathologies, such as pneumonia, rib fractures, and lung cancer. Compared to CCTA, the main disadvantages of the triple rule-out protocol are higher radiation exposure and a somewhat larger contrast dose.

A study by Takakuwa and Halpern found that in patients with a low to intermediate risk of ACS, the triple rule-out protocol identified a noncoronary diagnosis that explained clinical presentation in 11% of patients. It also identified moderate to severe CAD in 11% of patients, which obviated additional cardiac testing in most of these patients, without any adverse outcomes at 30 days.

A study by Madder et al. has found that the triple rule-out protocol has a similar diagnostic yield of coronary stenosis compared to CCTA (14.3% and 16.3% of patients, respectively) in patients who presented with acute chest

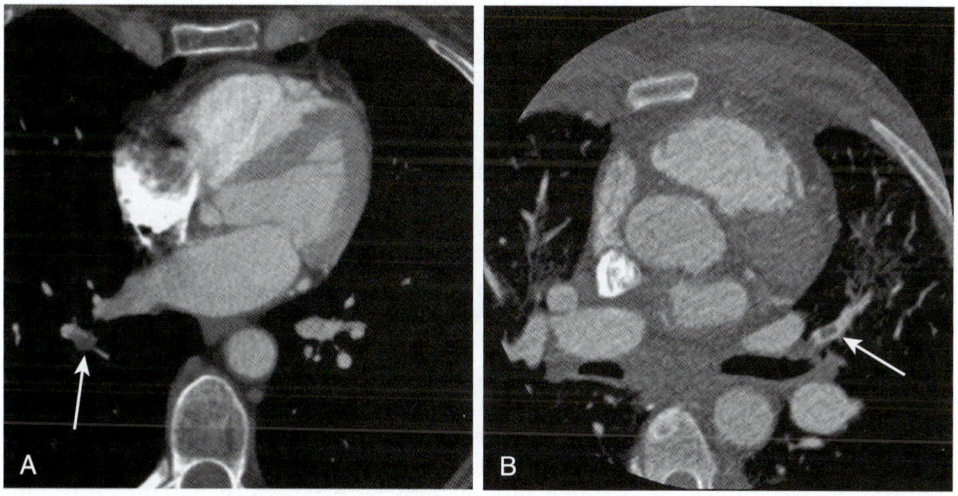

Figure 40.8 Two patients with chest pain with no plaque identified. (A) Right lower lobe acute pulmonary embolus *(arrow)*. (B) Lingular acute pulmonary embolus *(arrow)*.

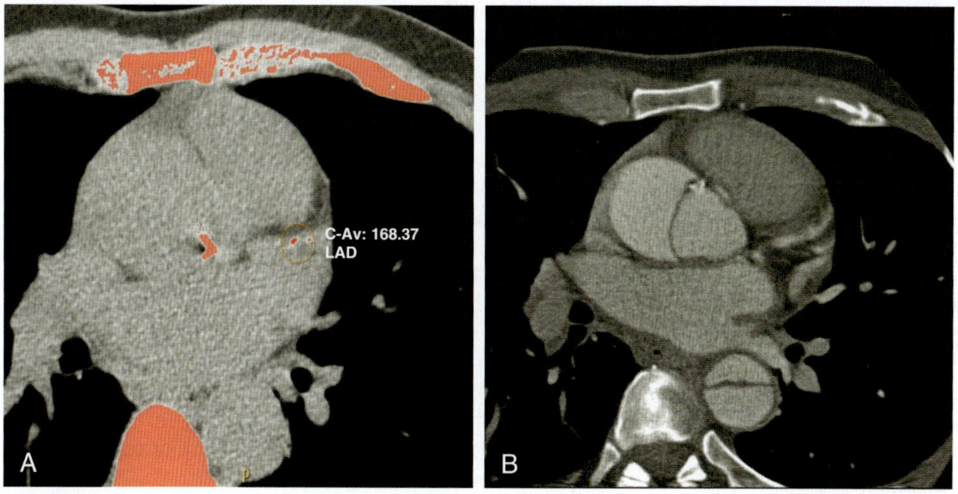

Figure 40.9 A 58-year-old male patient presenting with chest pain. (A) Minimal calcified plaque was identified in the left anterior descending artery *(LAD)*, and the computed calcium score by the Agatston method was 6.6, thus placing the patient between the 50th and 75th percentiles, adjusted for age and gender. (B) Contrast-enhanced CT of the chest in this patient demonstrates a type A aortic dissection, with the intimal flap visualized in the ascending and descending aorta. *C-Av*, Calcium average.

pain, but a lower diagnostic yield for pulmonary embolism (1.1%) and aortic dissection (0%). This suggests that most patients who present with acute chest pain have a low pretest probability of having pulmonary embolism or aortic dissection. The triple rule-out protocol is likely most useful in clinical scenarios in which patients have overlapping presentations of ACS, pulmonary embolism, and aortic dissection. With appropriate patient selection criteria, the triple rule-out protocol may have higher diagnostic yield than CCTA alone due to its additional capabilities.

The use of CCTA has several limitations based on certain patient characteristics. In general, the use of iodinated contrast is contraindicated in patients with contrast allergy or impaired renal function, but several protocols exist to minimize the risk of anaphylaxis or prevent contrast nephropathy if the examination is deemed necessary. To minimize motion artifact due to respiration, patients must be able to hold their breath for the duration of image acquisition (usually <10 seconds). This may be difficult for patients with compromised lung function or patients who are uncooperative, but the problem can be alleviated by the use of advanced CT scanners that have the capability to obtain a full cardiac scan rapidly, sometimes in less than 1 second. To minimize cardiac motion and allow for ECG-gated image acquisition, the patient should have a regular rhythm and heart rate no more than 60 to 70 beats/min, depending on the CT scanner. Most patients are given oral or intravenous beta blockers to reduce the heart rate, but this strategy does not always achieve the desired heart rate reduction, and beta blockers may not be tolerated in some patients with asthma or significant heart block. Nitroglycerin is sometimes given to achieve vasodilation of the coronary arteries, but this should be avoided in patients who are hypotensive or have become hypotensive with prior use.

Other limitations are based on CT imaging characteristics. Patients with extensive CAC or cardiac stents may have suboptimal assessment of the coronary artery lumen due to CT artifact. With current MDCT technology, coronary segments with a diameter <1.5 mm are often difficult to assess accurately.

Radiation is another concern due to the risk of malignancy with increased radiation exposure. The average radiation dose from CCTA has previously been estimated to be 12 mSv, which is about 120 times as much as a chest radiograph. Technologic advancements in CT equipment have greatly reduced the radiation dose from this level with the development of more efficient detectors and dual-energy sources, and protocols have been developed to adjust parameters based on patient body habitus. Another important advancement has been the transition from retrospective ECG gating to prospective ECG gating, which achieves an approximately 75% reduction of radiation dose. With prospective ECG gating, the beam is turned on only during critical periods during the cardiac cycle (diastole). This differs from retrospective ECG gating, in which the beam is turned on continuously to capture multiple cardiac cycles in their entirety, and images corresponding to a specific part of the cardiac cycle are then reconstructed to produce a final image for interpretation. Finally, advances in computational power have allowed the development of sophisticated image reconstruction algorithms that permit use of a smaller radiation dose. Filtered backprojection techniques have been historically used because they were fast and required less computational power. Newer iterative reconstruction algorithms produce images with significantly less noise, thereby allowing the radiation dose to be reduced up to 40% to 50% without sacrificing image quality. By using these techniques with modern CT equipment, the total radiation dose can be potentially reduced by 80% to 90%.

Future directions of CCTA include more widespread use of CT perfusion to visualize areas of ischemia and infarctions directly, as well as calculating fractional flow reserve to assess the hemodynamic significance of plaques causing stenosis. Several investigations have shown promise for these techniques in the outpatient setting to evaluate obstructive CAD, but further studies are needed to evaluate their clinical utility in the setting of acute chest pain.

Overall, there is substantial evidence that CCTA can quickly and reliably evaluate patients who are at low to intermediate risk in the setting of acute chest pain. In the usual algorithm that incorporates CCTA, patients who have no significant stenosis on CCTA (<50%) are considered safe for discharge, whereas patients who have significant stenosis on CCTA are typically admitted and evaluated with MPI or invasive coronary angiography.

Conclusion

Acute chest pain has a broad differential diagnosis that includes potentially life-threatening conditions; a missed diagnosis can have serious consequences with respect to morbidity and mortality. Although there are a variety of techniques to assess chest pain with noninvasive imaging, MDCT has the capability to obtain diagnostic information quickly and accurately to triage patients with acute chest pain. Evidence has shown that select patients with negative CCTA scans can be discharged home safely without further cardiac testing, which may reduce patient costs and improve resource utilization.

The use of CCTA has been validated in the evaluation of acute chest pain with suspected ACS in low- to intermediate-risk patients, but its use in the ED has been variably implemented. Emergency medicine physicians, radiologists, and cardiologists must continue to develop a clear algorithm that outlines specific indications and patient populations that will benefit from CCTA. Further studies are needed before CAC scoring can be recommended for use in the ED.

The increased use of CT has raised concern for radiation-induced complications, including malignancy. However, cardiac CT may lower total cumulative exposure by reducing the need for downstream and future testing, including SPECT and invasive coronary angiography, both of which often have greater radiation exposure than CCTA and CAC scanning. As cardiac CT becomes more widely used in various clinical scenarios, long-term follow-up data will be needed to assess safety, diagnostic utility, and patient outcomes.

Bibliography

Abdulla J, Abildstrom SZ, Gotzsche O, et al. 64-Multislice detector computed tomography coronary angiography as potential alternative to conventional coronary angiography: a systematic review and meta-analysis. *Eur Heart J.* 2007;28:3042–3050.

Cury RC, Shash K, Nagurney JT, et al. Cardiac magnetic resonance with T2-weighted imaging improves detection of patients with acute coronary syndrome in the emergency department. *Circulation.* 2008;118(8):837–844.

Georgiou D, Budoff MJ, Kaufer E, et al. Screening patients with chest pain in the emergency department using electron beam tomography: a follow-up study. *J Am Coll Cardiol.* 2001;38(1):105–110.

Goldstein JA, Chinnaiyan KM, Abidov A, et al. The CT-STAT (coronary computed tomographic angiography for systematic triage of acute chest pain patients to treatment) trial. *J Am Coll Cardiol.* 2011;58(14):1414–1422.

Henneman MM, Schuijf JD, Pundziute G, et al. Noninvasive evaluation with multislice computed tomography in suspected acute coronary syndrome: plaque morphology on multislice computed tomography versus coronary calcium score. *J Am Coll Cardiol.* 2008;52(3):216–222.

Hulten E, Picket C, Bittencourt MS, et al. Outcomes after coronary computed tomography angiography in the emergency department. *J Am Coll Cardiol.* 2013;61:880–892.

Kwong RY, Schussheim AE, Rekhraj S, et al. Detecting acute coronary syndrome in the emergency department with cardiac magnetic resonance imaging. *Circulation.* 2003;107(4):531–537.

Madder RD, Raff GL, Hickman L, et al. Comparative diagnostic yield and 3-month outcomes of "triple rule-out" and standard protocol coronary CT angiography in the evaluation of acute chest pain. *J Cardiovasc Comput Tomogr.* 2011;5(3): 165–171.

Motoyama S, Sarai M, Harigaya H, et al. Computed tomographic angiography characteristics of atherosclerotic plaques subsequently resulting in acute coronary syndrome. *J Am Coll Cardiol.* 2009;54:49–57.

Motoyama S, Sarai M, Narula J, Ozaki Y. Coronary CT angiography and high-risk plaque morphology. *Cardiovasc Interv Ther.* 2013;28:1–8.

Rubenshtein R, Gaspar T, Halon DA, Goldstein J, Peled N, Lewis BS. Prevalence and extent of obstructive coronary artery disease in patients with zero or low calcium score undergoing 64-slice cardiac multidetector computed tomography for evaluation of a chest pain syndrome. *Am J Cardiol.* 2007;99:472–475.

Schlett CL, Banerji D, Siegel E, et al. Prognostic value of CT angiography for major adverse cardiac events in patients with acute chest pain from the emergency department: 2-year outcomes of the ROMICAT trial. *JACC Cardiovasc Imaging.* 2011;4(5):481–491.

Takakuwa KM, Halpern EJ. Evaluation of a "triple rule-out" coronary CT angiography protocol: use of 64-section CT in low-to-moderate risk emergency department patients suspected of having acute coronary syndrome. *Radiology.* 2008;248(2):438–446.

Tota-Maharaj R, McEvoy JW, Blaha MJ, et al. Utility of coronary artery calcium scoring in the evaluation of patients with chest pain. *Crit Pathw Cardiol.* 2012;11:99–106.

CHAPTER 41
Lung and Heart Transplantation

Brett M. Elicker and Karen Ordovas

CHAPTER OUTLINE

■ Lung Transplantation

Since the first lung transplantation was performed in 1963, there have been major improvements in the surgical technique and posttransplantation management of organ recipients. Lung transplantation represents the only effective therapeutic option for many patients with advanced lung disease. Although there continue to be advancements in the understanding of the posttransplantation care of these patients, improvements in long-term survival have been limited by complications, primarily chronic allograft dysfunction. Radiology plays a major role in the detection and characterization of transplantation complications. The goal here is to discuss the imaging findings of these complications and the role of radiology in the multidisciplinary care of lung transplant recipients.

Determining Who Gets a Lung Transplant

In 2013, approximately 1900 lung transplantations were performed in the United States according to the Organ Procurement and Transplantation network. This represents a relatively small number compared to other organs including kidney (~17,000) and liver (~6500). Lung transplantation is performed in patients with advanced lung disease from a variety of causes (Table 41.1). Trends over the past decade have shown increased utilization of lung transplantation in interstitial lung disease patients, primarily idiopathic pulmonary fibrosis, compared to those with chronic obstructive pulmonary disease.

Selection Process

Lung transplant recipients are chosen based on their lung allocation score. This system was developed in 2005 in an attempt to prioritize waiting list candidates based on their need and expected posttransplantation survival. Priority is given to patients who are likely to have a significantly greater 1-year survival with a transplant compared to a patient without a transplant. Some of the variables included in the lung allocation score include age, body mass index, diagnosis, lung function (i.e., forced vital capacity), need for oxygen, P_{CO_2} levels, pulmonary artery systolic pressure, and the presence of comorbidities such as diabetes and renal failure.

Some absolute contraindications to lung transplantation include a history of malignancy (nonskin) in the past 2 years, untreatable nonlung major organ dysfunction, noncurable infection, such as viral hepatitis B, and significant chest wall deformity.

Problem Solving With CT and PET

Radiology is valuable in screening for lung cancer prior to transplantation. Patients with advanced lung disease have a significantly higher incidence of bronchogenic carcinoma compared to the population as a whole. Volumetric CT of the chest is routinely performed in candidates when their lung allocation score predicts a reasonable likelihood of transplantation in the near future. It is important to note that bronchogenic carcinoma may have an atypical radiographic appearance in patients with advanced lung disease because of the significant architectural

TABLE 41.1 Indications for Lung Transplantation, 1995–2011

INDICATION	LUNG TRANSPLANTS (%)
Chronic obstructive pulmonary disease (excluding alpha-1 antitrypsin deficiency)	33.5
Interstitial lung disease	23.7
Cystic fibrosis	16.6
Alpha-1 antitrypsin deficiency	5.8
Idiopathic pulmonary arterial hypertension	3.1
Sarcoidosis	2.5
Connective tissue disease	1.3
Lymphangioleiomyomatosis	1.0

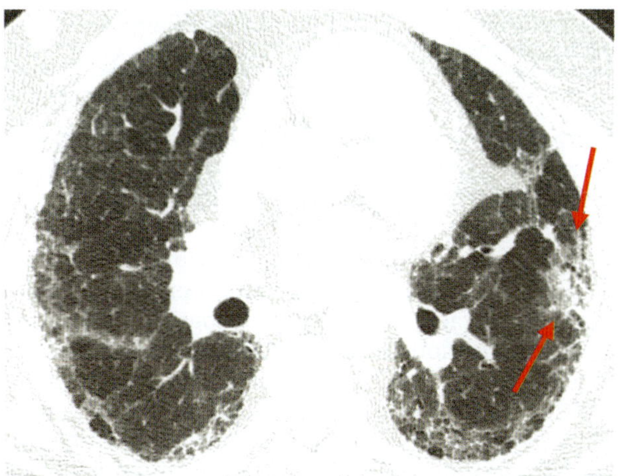

Figure 41.1 Primary bronchogenic carcinoma, pretransplantation. A patient with idiopathic pulmonary fibrosis underwent bilateral lung transplantation. Pathology of the explant revealed a mucinous lung adenocarcinoma that retrospectively was present *(arrows)*, but closely resembles lung fibrosis.

distortion of the lung (Fig. 41.1). Any persistent focal lung opacity should be viewed as possible malignancy. ^{18}F-fluorodeoxyglucose (FDG) PET is useful in patients with indeterminate CT abnormalities and is particularly helpful in distinguishing malignancy from scar in patients with fibrotic lung disease.

How a Lung Transplantation Is Performed

A bilateral or single lung transplantation may be performed. A bilateral transplantation is required for patients with chronic infection, such as those with cystic fibrosis. Bilateral lung transplantation is also preferred at many institutions for all patients because there is evidence to suggest improved survival compared to a single lung transplant. Single lung transplantation is preferred for patients who are at a higher surgical risk, such as older patients. It also may be performed when complications, such as bleeding, necessitate early termination of the surgery.

The surgical procedure is performed one lung at a time. The pulmonary veins, pulmonary artery, and bronchus are divided. These are then reanastomosed to the allograft, typically in reverse order. Of note, the lymphatic, bronchial arterial, and neurogenic connections are not reestablished in the allograft. Cardiopulmonary bypass may be required in selected patients.

Common Surgical Complications

Major postoperative complications have become less common, given advances in technique over the past several decades. The most common complications include postoperative pleural hematomas, sternal dehiscence, and anastomotic issues.

Problem Solving With Chest X-Ray and CT

Postoperative pleural hematomas may be seen in the first few days after surgery and are more common in patients with significant pretransplantation pleural inflammation and adhesion formation, as in patients with cystic fibrosis. Pleural hematomas are usually discovered on chest radiographs and manifest as a significant pleural collection that develops immediately or within the first few days after surgery.

Sternal dehiscence is often the result of infection resulting in weakening of the bone. It usually occurs within the first few months after transplantation. Typical CT findings include separation of sternal fragments, areas of bone lysis, and significant fluid collections adjacent to the sternum. Sagittal and coronal reformats may be helpful in visualizing the distortion of the three-dimensional structure of the sternum.

Anastomotic breakdown usually involves the bronchial connection and is typically seen in the first month after transplantation. Pneumomediastinum and/or pneumothorax may indicate that the anastomosis is not intact. Postoperative air in the mediastinum is a normal finding in the first several weeks after surgery, but a predominance of air around the bronchial anastomosis should raise concern for an anastomotic dehiscence (Fig. 41.2). Additionally, significant mediastinal air after the first few weeks is also suggestive. Extraluminal air should not be confused with the normal finding of a telescoped bronchial anastomosis.

Breakdown of the pulmonary arterial or venous anastomoses is rare, but has a high rate of mortality. This manifests as saccular extraluminal collections of contrast at anastomotic sites. Stenoses may also occur at the vascular anastomoses.

Typical Medical Therapy After Transplantation and Normal Surveillance Regimens

After receiving a lung transplant, recipients are treated with lifelong immunosuppression. The lung is unique because of its constant exposure to infectious agents in the environment; thus immunosuppression is a balance between the risk of infection and rejection. Typical regimens include a combination of a calcineurin inhibitor

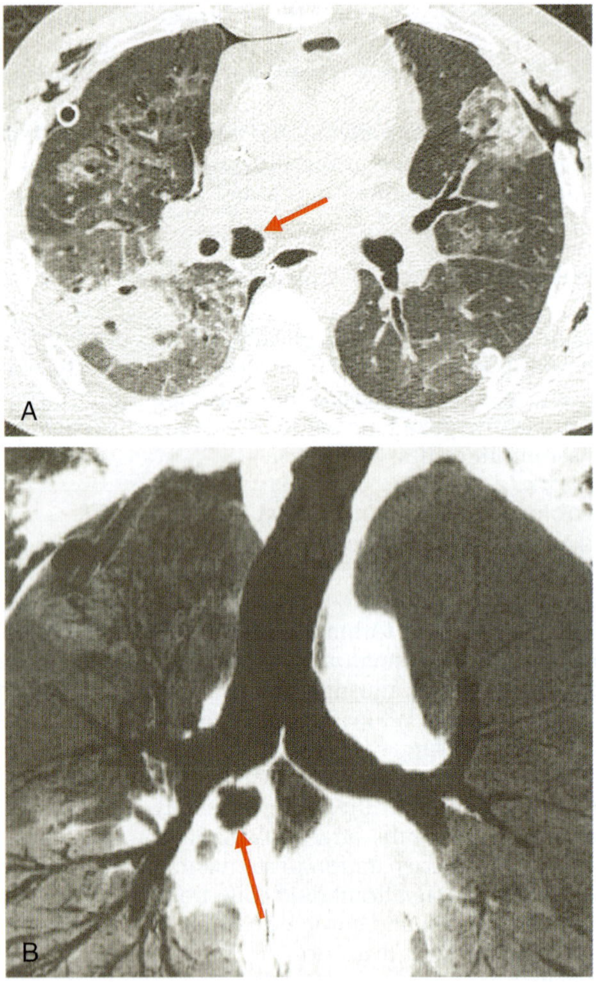

Figure 41.2 Breakdown of bronchial anastomosis. Axial (A) and coronal minimum intensity projection (B) CT images show an extraluminal collection of air adjacent to the right main bronchial anastomosis *(arrows)* 1 month after transplantation. Bronchoscopy confirmed an anastomotic dehiscence.

(e.g., tacrolimus), antimetabolite (e.g., mycophenolate mofetil), and corticosteroids. Asymptomatic patients undergo regular bronchoscopy, pulmonary function tests (PFTs), and CT imaging. This surveillance is most intensive in the first year posttransplantation and then subsequently falls off in regularity. Patients with any symptom will also undergo a similar diagnostic evaluation.

Problem Solving With Chest X-Ray and CT

Routine imaging surveillance may be performed with volumetric CT or axial high-resolution CT (HRCT). Axial HRCT with skipped sections is sensitive for most abnormalities and offers the advantage of imparting a lower radiation exposure. It is appropriate in the surveillance of common complications such as infection, acute rejection, and chronic rejection. Volumetric CT is more sensitive for focal complications, such as bronchial strictures and malignancies of the native lung. At institutions where axial HRCT is the preferred routine imaging test, volumetric CT should be performed periodically to assess for focal abnormalities.

Most Common Complications of Lung Transplantation and the Role of Imaging in Monitoring These Complications

Complications in lung transplantation may be due to the surgery itself, the immunosuppression regimen, or an immune reaction against the allograft. Diagnosis of these complications is a multidisciplinary endeavor that incorporates clinical symptoms, laboratory findings, bronchoscopic findings, pathologic information, and radiology. Radiology is a key component in the detection and characterization of abnormalities. Complications tend to occur at predictable intervals after transplantation, and imaging findings must always be interpreted in this context (Table 41.2). The role of imaging includes the following.

TABLE 41.2 Timing of Complications After Lung Transplantation

TIMING	COMPLICATION	COMMENTS
Postoperative period	Primary graft dysfunction	Most common cause of diffuse opacities within first 72 h
	Hyperacute rejection	Immediate reaction from preformed antibodies; rare
	Venous anastomotic stenosis	Rare
	Pleural hematoma	Significant pleural collection appearing within first few days
Early complications (typically within first year)	Infection	Bacterial and fungal infections peak at 1 month; viral infections peak at 150 days.
	Acute cellar rejection	Initial episode usually in first year, but recurrent episodes may occur for years after
	Anastomotic issues	Stenosis or dehiscence of bronchus, artery or vein
	Bronchial strictures	Usually occurs 2–10 months after transplantation
	Posttransplantation lymphoproliferative disease	Peak incidence at 1 year
Late complications (typically after first year)	Infection	Common cause of abnormalities throughout the life of the transplant
	Chronic rejection	Most common cause of mortality, usually after 1 year
	Recurrence of primary disease	May be early or late
	Complications in native lung (e.g., malignancy or infection)	May be early or late

Role of Imaging

DETECTION

Imaging may detect complications prior to their becoming clinically occult. In some cases, radiology may be more sensitive than clinical symptoms or abnormalities on PFTs. By detecting complications early, treatment can be initiated to prevent further injury.

CHARACTERIZATION

Complications may display overlapping clinical, laboratory, and PFT abnormalities. Radiology adds significant additional information in the determination of which complication is present. For example, both chronic allograft dysfunction and a bronchial stricture may cause dyspnea and airflow obstruction on PFTs; however, these are easily distinguished on imaging.

ASSESSING RESPONSE TO TREATMENT

Radiology is accurate in determining the extent and severity of complications. It provides a global assessment of lung abnormality and thus can determine if there has been an appropriate response to treatment on interval follow-up imaging.

Primary Graft Dysfunction

Primary graft dysfunction (PGD) is a form of acute lung injury that occurs within 72 hours of transplantation. It is a result of multiple factors relating to the harvesting and reimplantation of the graft, including ischemic injury, the preservation process, and reperfusion on reimplantation. PGD replaces previously used terms such as *reperfusion edema, reimplantation edema,* and *primary graft failure.* PGD is seen in 10% to 50% of lung transplant recipients and is the most common cause of early mortality. It also predisposes patients to the development of late complications, namely chronic allograft dysfunction. It is graded (0–3) using two parameters, the oxygenation (ratio of PaO_2/FiO_2) and the presence or absence of radiographic infiltrates consistent with pulmonary edema.

PROBLEM SOLVING WITH CHEST X-RAY AND CT

Typical radiographic or CT features of PGD include diffuse or symmetric bilateral consolidation and/or ground-glass opacities appearing within 72 hours after transplantation (Fig. 41.3). Interlobular septal thickening on CT, representing interstitial edema, is also commonly seen. To make a diagnosis of PGD, other causes of diffuse pulmonary opacities should be excluded, including hyperacute rejection, venous anastomotic obstruction, cardiogenic pulmonary edema, and pneumonia. Abnormalities are most severe within the first 2 weeks after lung transplantation, but typically show significant improvement by at least the 12th week.

Infection

The constant exposure of the allograft to the environment puts lung transplant patients at a particularly high risk of infection. Also, the immunosuppressive regimen they receive is particularly intensive when compared to most other solid organ transplantations. The titration of this regimen is a constant balance between the risks of infection and rejection.

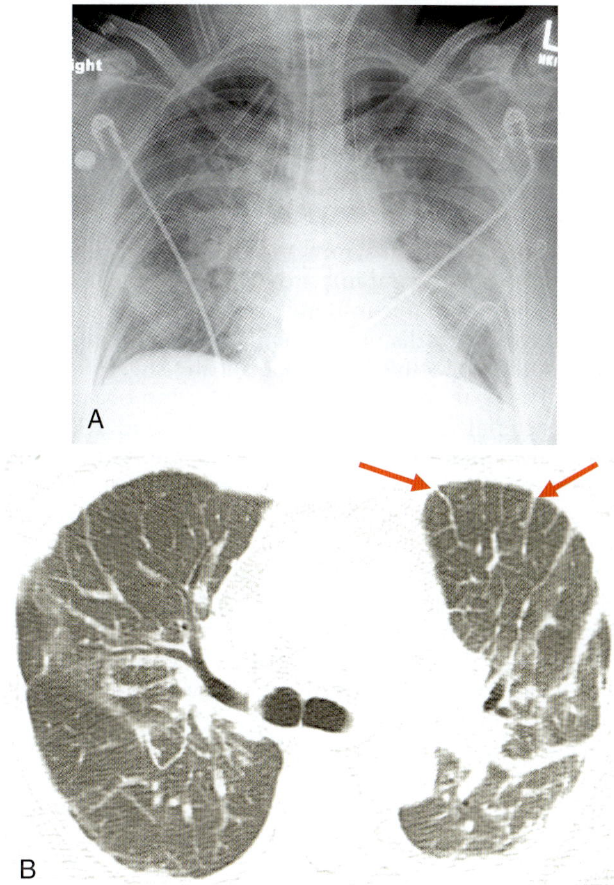

Figure 41.3 Primary graft dysfunction (PGD). (A) Immediately after bilateral lung transplantation for idiopathic pulmonary fibrosis, a patient develops extensive bilateral consolidation consistent with PGD. (B) One month later, only mild interlobular septal thickening *(arrows)* remains on CT.

Other features that may predispose patients to infection include denervation of the graft, causing a diminished cough reflex, impaired lymphatic drainage, and lack of a bronchial arterial supply. Infection is the leading cause of mortality between 31 days and 1 year posttransplantation, but remains a common cause of morbidity and mortality throughout the life of the recipient.

PROBLEM SOLVING WITH CHEST X-RAY AND CT

The radiographic findings of infection mirror those seen in nontransplanted patients. There is significant overlap in the radiographic findings of different organisms, so imaging needs to be interpreted in the context of clinical and laboratory findings. A comprehensive review of the imaging findings of infection is covered in Chapter 16; however, it is important that the radiologist understand issues specific to lung transplant patients and which specific CT patterns are particularly suggestive of certain categories of organisms.

Bacterial infection is the most common infection overall. Its incidence peaks in the early period, approximately 1 month posttransplantation. Unilateral or bilateral asymmetric consolidation, with or without centrilobular nodules and tree-in-bud opacities, is usually due to bacterial infection, particularly when seen in this early period.

Bilateral large nodules or rounded regions of consolidation with irregular margins are most suggestive of fungal infection, particularly *Aspergillus* (Fig. 41.4). Fungal infections are the second most common type of infection and tend to peak early after transplantation, similar to bacterial infections.

Diffuse or bilateral symmetric ground-glass opacities are usually due to viral infection (Fig. 41.5). Consolidation, nodules, and tree-in-bud opacities may also be seen, but the symmetric distribution and presence of significant ground-glass opacity should specifically suggest a viral cause. The peak incidence of viral infection occurs later than bacterial and fungal infections, around 150 days posttransplantation. Viral infections are particularly important given their predisposition to induce chronic allograft dysfunction (bronchiolitis obliterans). Because of this association, many centers will treat an acute viral infection with an increase in the antirejection regimen. It is important to note that viral infection cannot be distinguished from acute cellular rejection (ACS) based on imaging alone. Cytomegalovirus pneumonia is the most common pathogen, although universal prophylaxis against cytomegalovirus has led to a decreased incidence.

Other infections, including mycobacterial, *Pneumocystis jiroveci*, and *Nocardia*, may be seen in lung transplantation patients, but are much less common than the others discussed above. Nontuberculous mycobacterial infections are more common in cystic fibrosis patients. *Mycobacterium abscessus* is a particularly virulent pathogen and is a relative contraindication to transplantation when discovered. Its CT features overlap with those of other nontuberculous mycobacterial infections; these include centrilobular nodules, tree-in-bud opacities, bronchiectasis, and cavities.

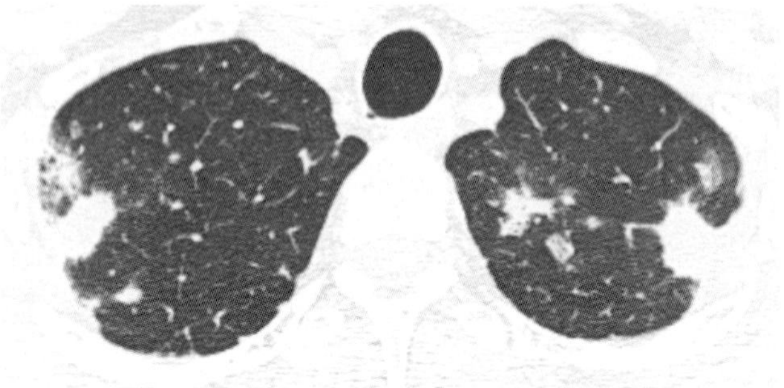

Figure 41.4 Fungal infection. Nodular and masslike regions of consolidation are seen bilaterally in a lung transplant patient with *Aspergillus* pneumonia.

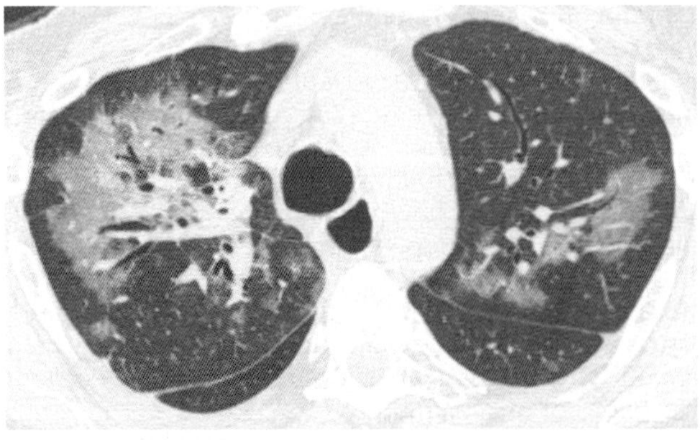

Figure 41.5 Viral infection. Patchy bilateral ground-glass opacities are seen in a transplant patient with cytomegalovirus pneumonia. The bilateral distribution and predominance of ground-glass opacities predominantly suggest viral infection or acute cellular rejection.

Rejection

There are different types of rejection after lung transplantation.

Antibody-Mediated and Hyperacute Rejection

Antibody-mediated rejection (AMR) is rare and occurs when the humoral immune system targets the allograft. This is in contrast to ACS, a predominantly T cell–mediated reaction. When AMR occurs immediately after transplantation, it is due to preexisting antibodies in the recipient and is called a *hyperacute rejection*. The predominant pathologic manifestation is acute lung injury, and loss of the allograft is common. The radiographic manifestations are indistinguishable from PGD and consist of diffuse or symmetric ground-glass opacities and consolidation that develop immediately after transplantation.

AMR may also occur later, often within the first year after transplantation, and is due to the interval development of an antibody response against the graft. Pathology shows diffuse alveolar damage, often with capillaritis. Radiographic manifestations are similar to those of hyperacute rejection, with diffuse or symmetric ground-glass opacities and consolidation. Patients who survive an episode of AMR are at high risk for developing bronchiolitis obliterans syndrome (BOS).

Acute Cellular Rejection

ACS affects more than 50% of lung transplant recipients. Although the first episode of ACS typically occurs within the first year after transplantation, patients may have recurrent episodes long after the initial 1-year period. ACS accounts for less than 5% of the mortality of lung transplantation but is the primary risk factor for the development of BOS. Histopathologically, ACS is characterized by perivascular mononuclear predominant inflammation, often accompanied by a lymphocytic bronchiolitis. The clinical manifestations are varied. It may be detected incidentally on surveillance bronchoscopy in asymptomatic patients or may be seen in patients with profound dyspnea and hypoxemia.

Bronchoscopy is the cornerstone of diagnosis in ACS. Findings on transbronchial biopsy are graded based on the severity of findings (0–4) and the form(s) of rejection present, including ACS (A), lymphocytic bronchiolitis (B), and obliterative bronchiolitis (C). Pulse dose corticosteroids are typically given to patients with mild cellular rejection (A2) or higher.

PROBLEM SOLVING WITH CT

The most common CT findings of ACS are ground-glass opacities, consolidation, and septal thickening (Fig. 41.6).

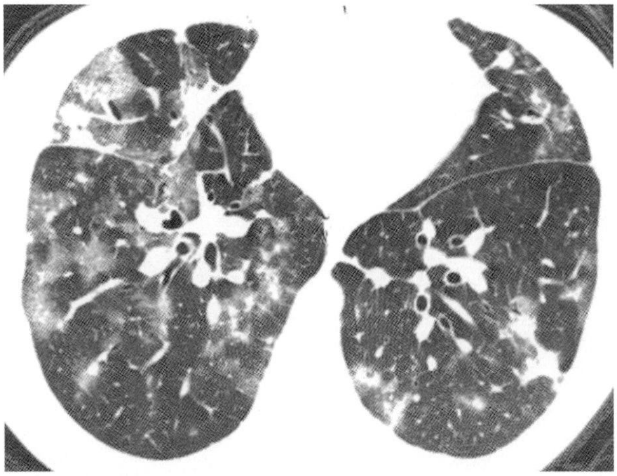

Figure 41.6 Acute cellular rejection (ACS), patchy bilateral ground-glass opacities and consolidation in a patient with ACS. This is indistinguishable from infection, particularly viral infection.

The findings are typically bilateral and symmetric, but may occasionally be unilateral or asymmetric. Pleural effusion may be seen as the only manifestation of ACS or may be seen in association with other findings. These findings overlap significantly with infections, particularly viral infections, so bronchoscopy is the primary diagnostic test used to distinguish them.

Chronic Allograft Dysfunction

BOS is the main pattern of injury associated with chronic allograft dysfunction in lung transplant recipients and the primary cause of long-term mortality. Pathologically, BOS shows concentric fibrosis tissue involving the bronchial wall and peribronchiolar tissues. This results in small airway obstruction and reduced ventilation. BOS is defined as a sustained, nonreversible airflow obstruction on PFTs and the exclusion of alternative causes of this PFT abnormality. This usually occurs after the 1-year posttransplantation period. The main risk factors for BOS are ACS and infection, particularly viral infection. There is no consistently proven and effective treatment for BOS. Changes in the immunosuppressive regimen may be undertaken, and azithromycin has been used with some success.

In addition to BOS, two other unique manifestations of chronic allograft dysfunction have recently been described: restrictive allograft syndrome and acute fibrinous and organizing pneumonia (AFOP). The pathology of restrictive allograft syndrome is identical to that of idiopathic pleuroparenchymal fibroelastosis, a rare cause of disease in nontransplanted patients. AFOP has a subacute onset and typically follows a more fulminant course than BOS, with a rapid decline in lung function and a high mortality rate.

PROBLEM SOLVING WITH CT

CT, and in particular HRCT, is a vital component of the diagnostic evaluation of patients with suspected chronic rejection. The CT findings will vary, depending on the cause of chronic allograft dysfunction. BOS is the most common manifestation. CT is very sensitive in detecting BOS and may be more sensitive than PFTs. CT also is valuable in distinguishing BOS from other causes of airflow obstruction on PFTs. The CT findings of BOS from chronic allograft dysfunction mirror those of bronchiolitis obliterans from other causes. Mosaic perfusion and air trapping are often seen in isolation. Expiratory images should be obtained routinely because they increase the sensitivity for these findings. The extent of abnormality may range from small lobular regions of lucent lung to diffuse lung lucency (Fig. 41.7). Bronchiectasis may develop in severe cases.

Radiology of restrictive allograft syndrome shows progressive, apical, predominant lung fibrosis and pleural thickening. The CT findings of AFOP are bilateral ground-glass opacities, with nodular regions of consolidation that may progress to diffuse lung fibrosis (Fig. 41.8).

Other Complications

These include bronchial strictures, recurrence of primary lung disease, complications in the native lung, and post-transplantation lymphoproliferative disorder (PTLD).

Bronchial Strictures

Central airways stenoses may occur at the main bronchial anastomosis; however, with improvements in surgical technique, this complication has become less common. Stenoses may also occur distal to the anastomosis in the central, lobar, and segmental airways. Their development is likely due to a combination of ischemia and chronic inflammation and/or infection. This complication typically occurs 2 to 10 months after transplantation.

PROBLEM SOLVING WITH CT

Although bronchoscopy is considered the gold standard for the diagnosis of airway stenosis, CT is valuable in the detection and evaluation of this complication (Fig. 41.9). CT may provide a better assessment than bronchoscopy in regard to the length of narrowing and the status of the airways distal to the stenosis. This is important in the planning of treatment, such as dilation and stent placement. Volumetric CT is the imaging test of choice because the skipped sections of HRCT may miss lesions. Air trapping is often seen in the region of lung supplied by the stenosed airway. This air trapping is lobar in distribution, in distinction to BOS, which usually doesn't involve a lobe uniformly.

Recurrence of Primary Lung Disease

Recurrence of the lung disease that predated the transplantation occurs in approximately 1% of patients. Sarcoidosis is the most common disease to recur and may be seen in more than 30% of transplanted patients. Other diseases that may recur include lymphangioleiomyomatosis, Langerhans cell histiocytosis, and pulmonary alveolar proteinosis. Recurrent disease may be radiographically occult and may only be discovered on surveillance bronchoscopy. Additionally, recurrent disease may show different CT manifestations than the pretransplantation imaging.

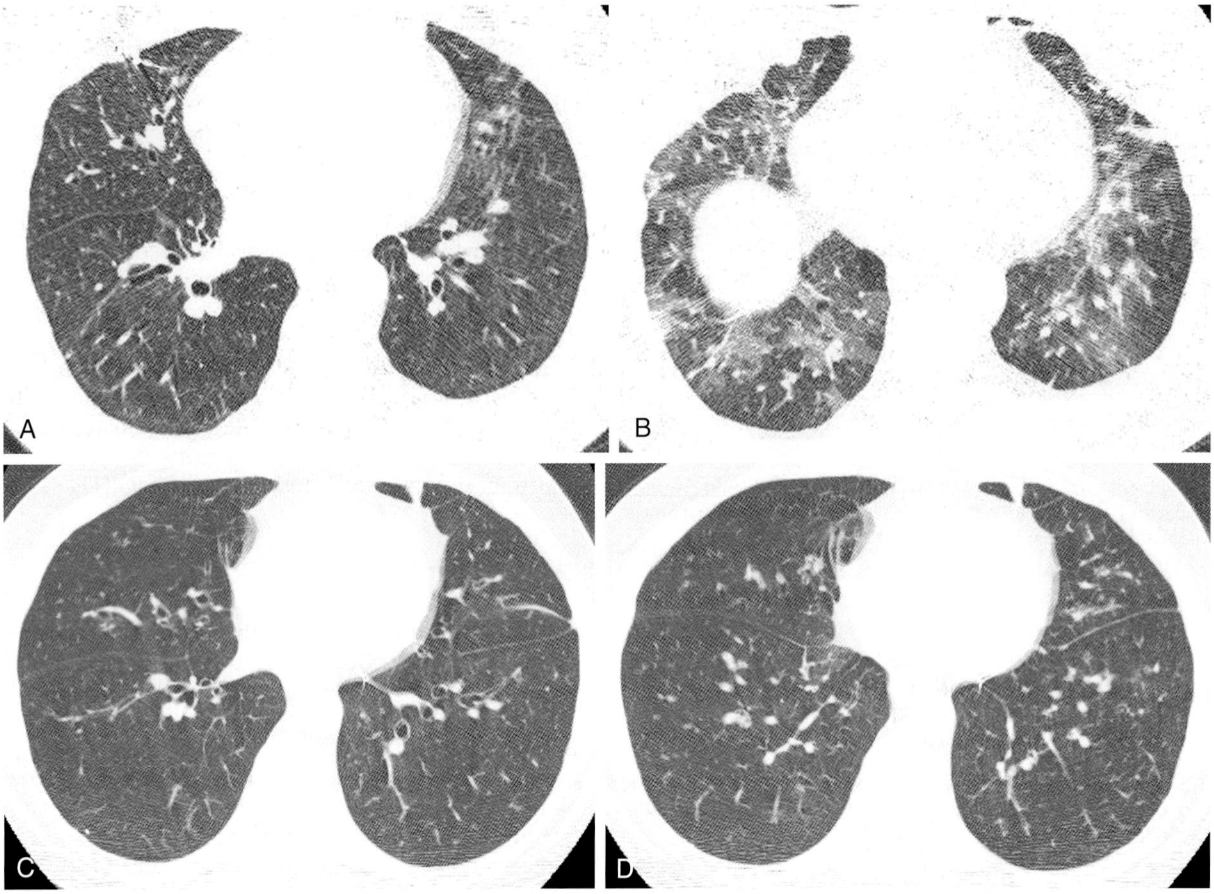

Figure 41.7 Bronchiolitis obliterans syndrome (BOS). Inspiratory (A) and expiratory (B) CT images in a patient with moderate BOS show patchy bilateral areas of air trapping. The inspiratory image is normal. Inspiratory (C) and expiratory (D) CT images in another patient with severe diffuse BOS show diffuse lung lucency and air trapping. Note no change in the density of the lung on the expiratory image.

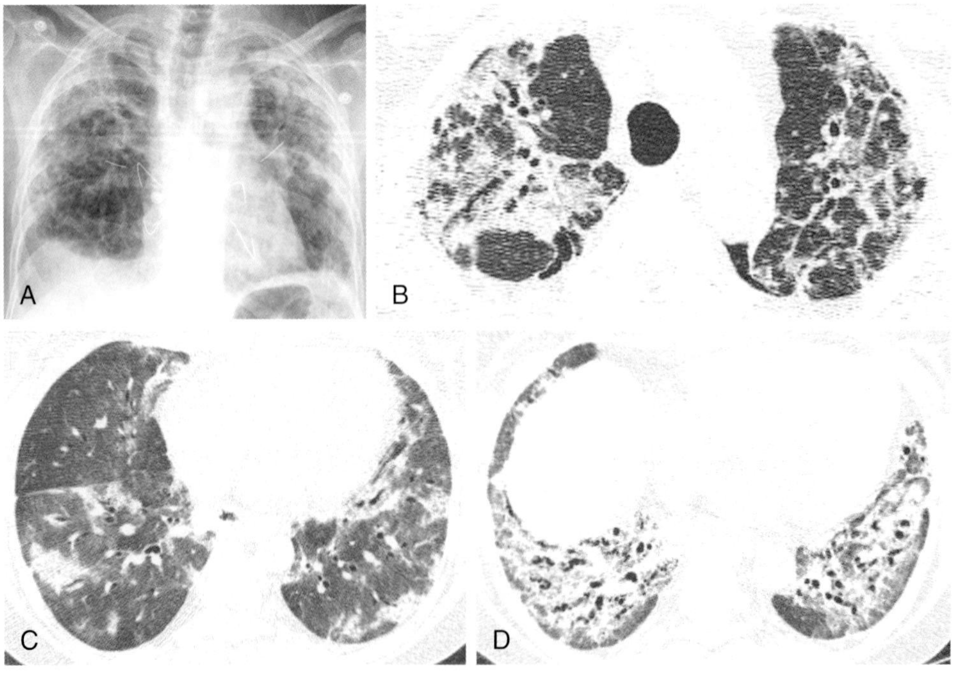

Figure 41.8 Chronic rejection. (A) Radiograph in a patient with restrictive allograft syndrome shows apical predominant pleural thickening and fibrosis. (B) The corresponding CT image shows reticulation, traction bronchiectasis, and architectural distortion in the upper lobes. (C) Acute and fibrinous organizing pneumonia, another manifestation of chronic rejection, demonstrates extensive bilateral ground-glass opacities and nodular areas of consolidation. (D) Two years later, the same patient has developed extensive fibrosis in the same regions.

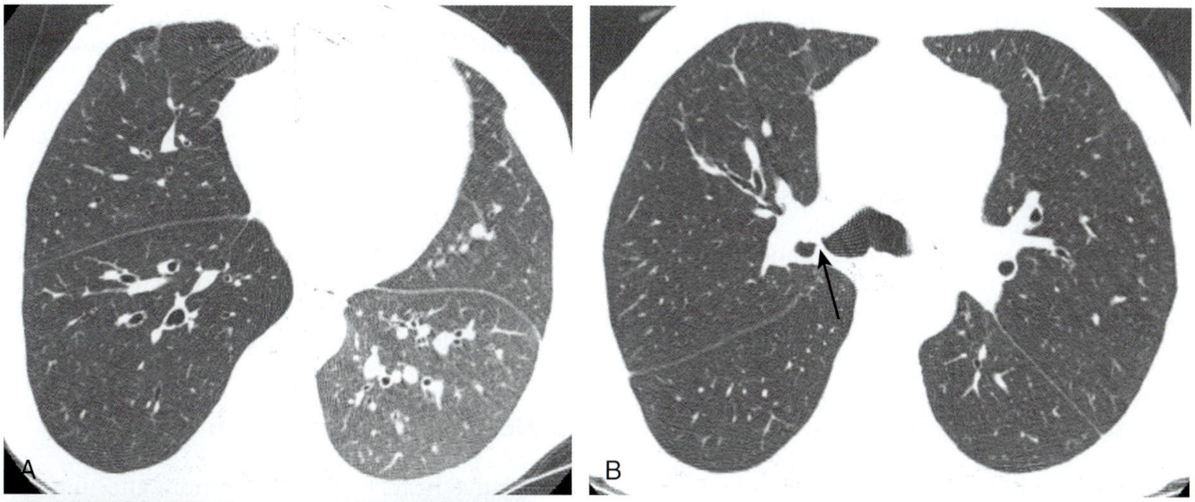

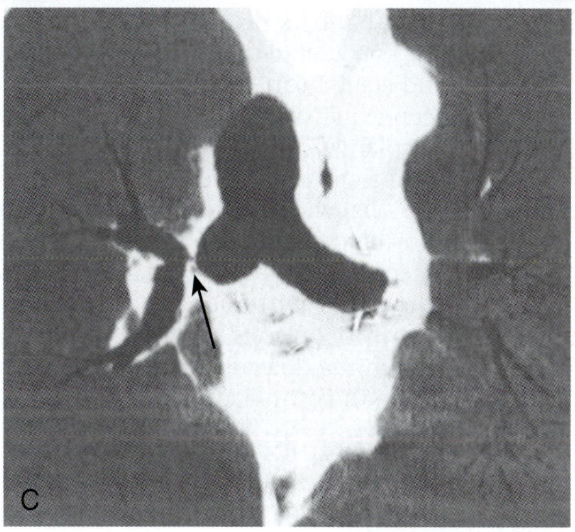

Figure 41.9 Bronchial stricture. (A) Expiratory CT image demonstrates diffuse air trapping in the right middle and lower lobes. A high-grade bronchial stricture *(arrows in B and C)* is seen on the axial (B) and coronal minimum intensity projection (C) images in the distal right main bronchus.

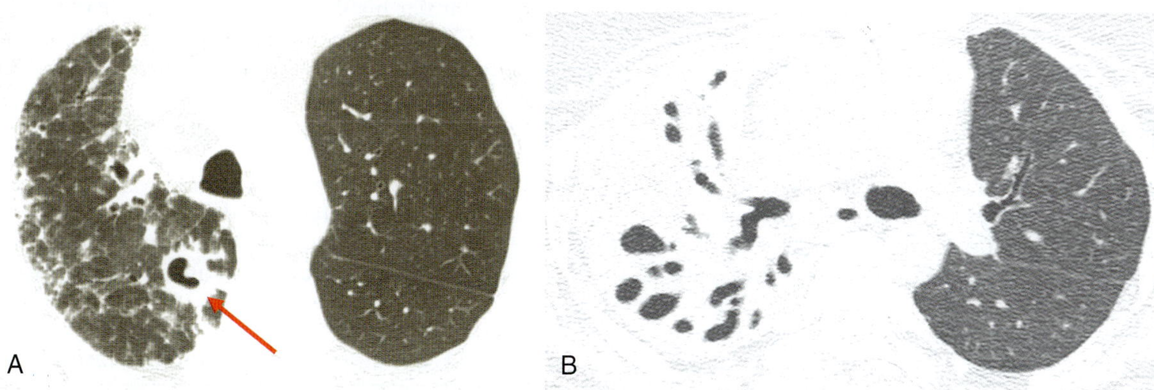

Figure 41.10 Native lung infection. (A) Cavitary lung lesions *(arrow)* are seen in the native lung in a patient with unilateral lung transplant for idiopathic pulmonary fibrosis. Bronchoscopy diagnosed a nontuberculous mycobacterial infection. (B) In another patient with a unilateral lung transplant for end-stage constrictive bronchiolitis, a *Stenotrophomonas* infection caused diffuse consolidation and bronchiectasis in the native lung.

Complications in the Native Lung

Single lung transplant recipients may develop complications in their native lung. This may partly account for the higher mortality of single versus bilateral transplant recipients. The primary abnormalities seen in the native lung include infection (Fig. 41.10) and malignancy. CT is valuable in the surveillance of these complications, particularly because patients may be asymptomatic until the disease becomes advanced.

Posttransplantation Lymphoproliferative Disorder

PTLD ranges in severity from lymphoid hyperplasia to an aggressive lymphoma. It is closely related to Epstein-Barr virus infection. Approximately 3% to 8% of lung transplant patients will be affected, and the incidence peaks at 1 year after transplantation. The incidence is much lower now than it was prior to 2000 because of differences in the immunosuppression regimen. The most common organs involved by PTLD include the lung and gastrointestinal system. Mediastinal and hilar lymphadenopathy is commonly seen. PTLD of the lungs commonly shows multiple large nodules, masses, or masslike regions of consolidation. FDG-PET is particularly helpful in evaluating the extent of disease in PTLD.

What to Look for on Post–Lung Transplantation Imaging

- Different complications occur at different times post–lung transplantation. Abnormalities must be interpreted in the context of when the transplantation was performed.
- Complications that occur immediately after lung transplantation include PGD, AMR, cardiogenic pulmonary edema, and edema from venous anastomotic obstruction. Surgical complications such as pleural hematoma may also occur in this period.
- Complications that occur early (typically within or around the first year) include infection, ACS, bronchial stenoses, and PTLD.
- Complications that occur after the first year include infection and chronic rejection.
- Certain complications may occur at any time (early or late), such as recurrence of the primary disease or complications in the native lung.
- HRCT, using skipped axial sections, may be used for routine surveillance, with the understanding that it shows reduced sensitivity for certain focal abnormalities. Volumetric CT should be performed periodically for the surveillance of abnormalities that tend to be focal, such as bronchial stenosis and malignancy in the native lung.
- PGD is the most common complication to occur immediately after transplant and manifests as bilateral consolidation and/or ground-glass opacities.
- Acute cellar rejection and infection cannot be distinguished from each other based on imaging. Both can show ground-glass opacities, consolidation, and nodules. Tree-in-bud opacities are very suggestive of infection.
- The primary complication to occur after the first year is chronic rejection, primarily BOS.
- The CT findings of BOS include mosaic perfusion, air trapping, and bronchiectasis. CT may detect early disease prior to the development of symptoms or PFT abnormalities.
- Although BOS is the most common manifestation of chronic rejection, two other types have been identified—restrictive allograft syndrome and AFOP.
- Restrictive allograft syndrome manifests as progressive apical predominant fibrosis and pleural thickening.
- AFOP presents in a subacute fashion and shows diffuse ground-glass opacities with focal and nodular regions of consolidation.
- Bronchial strictures not related to the anastomosis involve the proximal bronchi and may cause unilateral or lobar air trapping.
- Recurrence of primary disease in the allograft is most common with sarcoidosis and is often radiographically occult. When imaging abnormalities are seen on CT they may differ from pretransplantation findings.
- In single lung transplant patients, attention should be given to the native lung because this may also develop complications, primarily infection, and malignancy.
- PTLD typically occurs in the first year and may show lymphadenopathy or lung nodules or masses on CT.

■ Heart Transplantation

Congestive heart failure is common, affecting approximately 7.5 million patients in North America. Cardiac transplantation is considered the treatment of choice for patients with end-stage heart failure for whom medical options have been exhausted. The annual mortality rate while on the transplantation waiting list is approximately 14%. This has significantly improved over the last decade, primarily due to the widespread use of implantable cardioverter-defibrillators and cardiac resynchronization therapy. Despite strict patient selection and advances in posttransplantation care, mortality after transplantation is still high, primarily because of rejection. Imaging plays an important role in the detection and characterization of posttransplantation complications.

Determining Who Gets a Heart Transplant

Several cardiac insults and diseases may lead to advanced heart failure. Independent of the cause, patients with advanced heart failure (New York Heart Association Class IV) should be considered for heart transplantation if optimal medical therapy has failed to improve symptoms or arrest the progression of the underlying disease. For patients to be considered a candidate, an advanced heart failure team must determine that there is no reversible or surgically amenable condition. The most common indications for heart transplantation are shown in Table 41.3.

TABLE 41.3 Indications for Cardiac Transplantation

INDICATION	HEART TRANSPLANTS (%)
Nonischemic cardiomyopathy	54
Ischemic cardiomyopathy	37
Valvular heart disease	3
Retransplantation	2
Congenital heart disease	3
Others	2

Data from Stehlik J, Edwards LB, Kucheryavaya AY, et al. The registry of the international society for heart and lung transplantation: 29th official adult heart transplant report—2012. *J Heart Lung Transplant.* 2012;31(10):1052–1064.

How the Procedure Is Performed

Biatrial orthotopic heart transplantation was the initial surgical technique developed and has been in use for many years. In this approach, the donor heart is transected in the mid–left atrium and mid–right atrium. It is subsequently anastomosed to the recipient's posterior left atrial wall, which contains the native pulmonary venous connections, and posterior right atrial wall, which contains both venea cavea. The aorta and pulmonary arteries, including their respective valves, are anastomosed in a supravalvular manner.

An alternative approach, more frequently performed nowadays, is the bicaval orthotopic heart transplantation. This procedure differs from the biatrial approach in that the venea cavae from the recipient are anastomosed separately to the donor's intact right atrium. Recent data have suggested that the bicaval approach has better outcomes because it preserves the electroanatomic structure of the right atrium.

Of note, the surgical technique for connecting the native and donor left atria may simulate an enlarged left atrium (Fig. 41.11) on imaging.

Most Common Complications

Despite advances in the clinical and surgical management of heart transplant patients over the last few decades, the mortality rate remains high, reaching approximately 25% at 5 years. Mortality due to acute postoperative complications is very low (<1% in most centers) and is typically due to primary graft failure. Postoperative complications that benefit from early diagnosis and management are pericardial effusion, mediastinal hematoma, and mediastinitis. Major causes of mortality and morbidity after the acute postoperative stage include ACS and mediastinitis in the first year. Late mortality is usually due to cardiac allograft vasculopathy (CAV) and malignancies (Table 41.4).

Primary Graft Failure

Primary graft failure is the most common cause of death within the first 30 days after transplantation. The diagnosis is based on evidence of ventricular dysfunction (left, right, or both) within the first 24 hours after heart transplantation when other causes of acute graft failure, such as cardiac tamponade and hyperacute rejection, have been excluded. Patients usually present with severe hemodynamic instability and cardiogenic shock.

PROBLEM SOLVING WITH CHEST X-RAY AND CT

Chest radiographs classically demonstrate acute and severe pulmonary edema within 24 hours after transplantation. The main role of CT is to exclude other causes of clinical decompensation, including large pericardial effusions and mediastinal hematoma.

Pericardial Effusion and Hematoma

Pericardial effusion is the most common complication immediately after heart transplantation. Effusions may be asymptomatic in some cases, but significant effusions may cause deleterious hemodynamic effects, particularly when they accumulate rapidly. Echocardiography remains the first-line test for confirmation of a pericardial effusion. However, the ability of echocardiography to differentiate

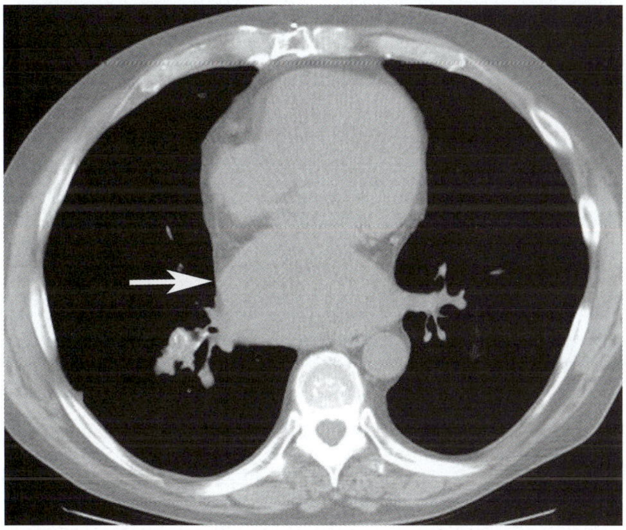

Figure 41.11 Biatrial heart transplant. This axial noncontrast CT image shows apparent enlargement of the left atrium *(arrow)*. This is a normal finding in a patient after heart transplantation with a biatrial approach.

TABLE 41.4 Timing of Complications After Heart Transplantation

TIMING	COMPLICATION	COMMENTS
Postoperative period	Primary graft failure	Most common cause of death within first month after surgery; radiograph shows edema immediately after surgery
	Pericardial effusion	Most common complication; can be hemorrhagic
	Mediastinal hematoma	May require re-intervention; best diagnosed with chest CT
	Mediastinitis	May be challenging to differentiate from normal postoperative appearance
Early complications (typically within first year)	Acute cellular rejection	Initial episode usually in first year, but recurrent episodes may occur for years after; cardiac MRI is promising diagnostic method
	Mediastinitis	Responsible for 30% of mortality in first year posttransplantation
Late complications (typically after first year)	Coronary allograft vasculopathy	Most common overall cause of death after cardiac transplantation; can start as early as 1–3 months after surgery; can be diagnosed with coronary CT angiography
	Malignancies	Increased incidence of multiple malignancies; risk increased with older age, early development of rejection

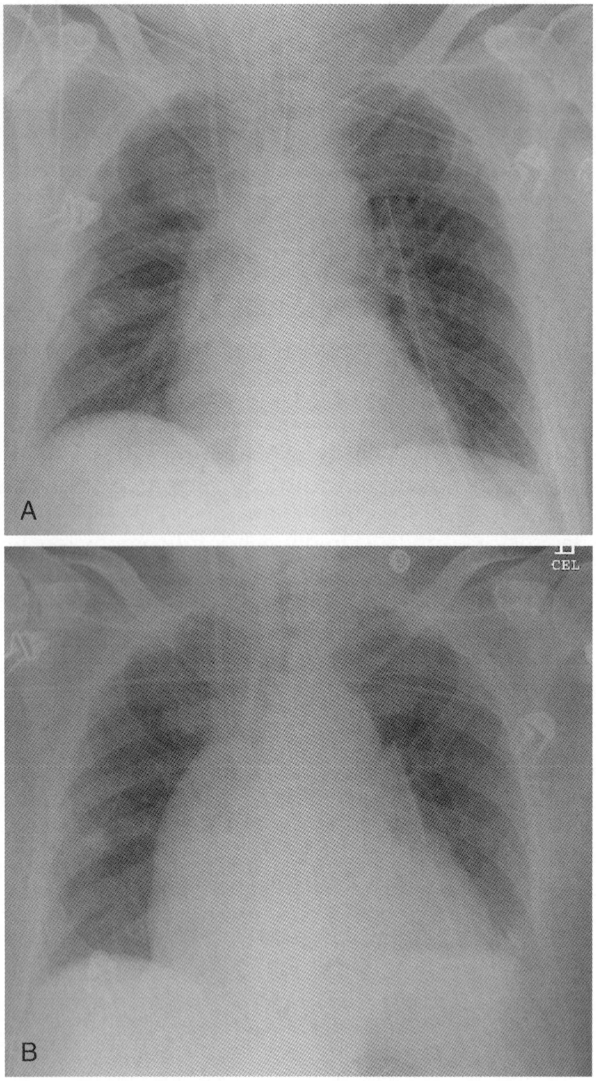

Figure 41.12 Pericardial collection. Frontal portable chest radiograph after heart transplantation on postoperative day 1 (A) and day 3 (B). Note the increase in size of the cardiac silhouette from postoperative day 1 to 3 after the mediastinal drain has been removed. This finding is highly suggestive of a pericardial collection.

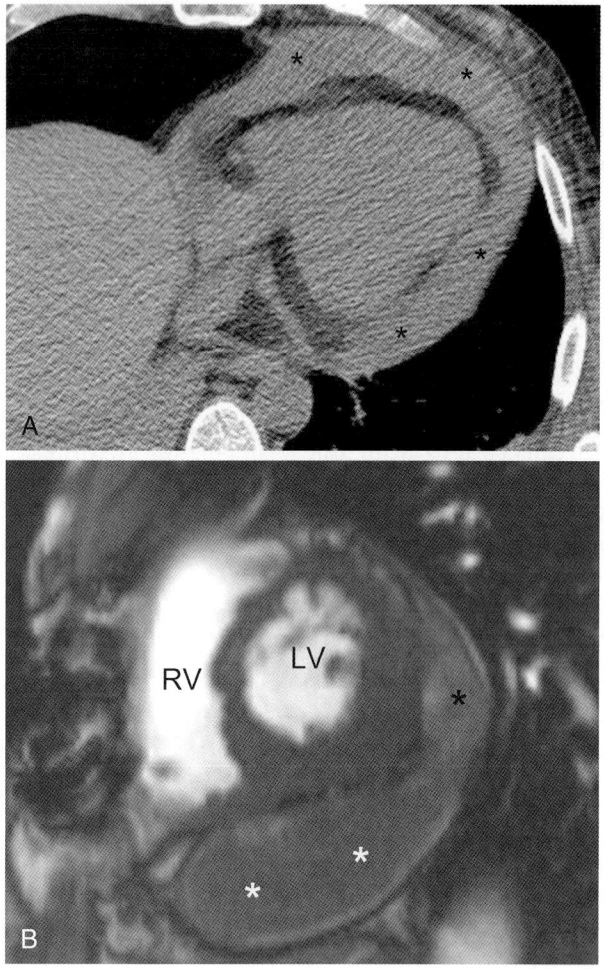

Figure 41.13 Pericardial hematoma. (A) Axial noncontrast CT image of the chest shows a high-density (50-HU) collection in the pericardium *(asterisks)*, consistent with a hematoma. (B) Steady-state free precession MRI scan in the short-axis plane acquired from a different heart transplantation patient shows an intermediate intensity collection in the inferior aspect of the pericardium *(asterisks)*, consistent with a subacute hematoma. *LV,* Left ventricle; *RV,* right ventricle.

a simple pericardial effusion from a complex collection or a pericardial hematoma is limited.

PROBLEM SOLVING WITH CHEST X-RAY, CT, AND MRI

Serial portable postoperative chest radiography is routinely performed in the surveillance of complications immediately after transplantation. Large pericardial effusions may be detected using this modality. The key feature is an increase in the size of the cardiac silhouette on serial examinations (Fig. 41.12). CT and MRI are superior to radiography for the detection of small to moderate-sized effusions and also may be used to characterize a complex pericardial collection further. In addition, complex pericardial effusions with an unusual distribution can be clearly delineated using cross-sectional imaging. This may be necessary in the planning of interventions. On chest CT, a pericardial hematoma is characterized by increased density, with Hounsfield units (HU) approaching 40 to 60 HU (Fig. 41.13A). In most acute posttransplantation patients, pericardial collections are serosanguineous and have a density slightly higher than that of simple fluid. On MRI, the signal characteristics of the pericardial collection depend on the chronicity of the bleeding. In the acute postoperative period, pericardial collections are either high (acute) or intermediate (subacute) in signal on T1-weighted, double inversion recovery turbo field-echo sequences (see Fig. 41.13B).

Mediastinal Hematoma

Mediastinal hematoma is typically suspected when patients are hemodynamically unstable after transplantation. Early detection is important because patients may require reoperation.

PROBLEM SOLVING WITH CHEST RADIOGRAPHY, CHEST CT, AND MRI

Increased size of the mediastinal silhouette on chest radiographs is the most common finding to suggest the presence of hematoma. CT is the method of choice to detect and characterize the nature and distribution of postoperative mediastinal collections. The typical CT appearance of mediastinal bleeding is a high-density

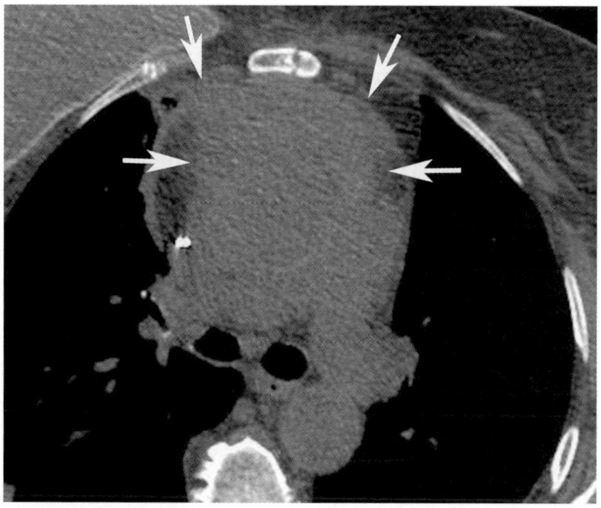

Figure 41.14 Mediastinal hematoma. This axial noncontrast CT image of the chest shows a high-density collection *(arrows)* contiguous with the sternum and the ascending aorta in this patient after heart transplantation, consistent with a mediastinal hematoma.

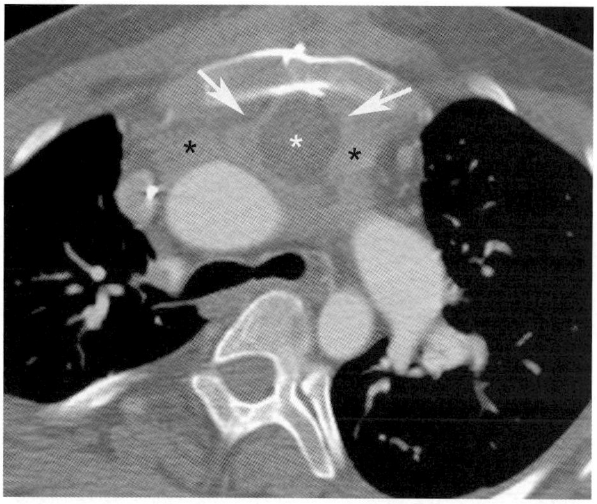

Figure 41.15 Mediastinitis. This contrast-enhanced CT image of the chest demonstrates a rim-enhancing collection *(arrows, white asterisk)* in the anterior mediastinum, contiguous with the sternum, in a patient with mediastinitis after heart transplantation. Note the adjacent high-density collection *(black asterisks)*, consistent with associated hematoma.

collection in contiguity with the heart and great vessels, particularly adjacent to the anastomotic sites. Slow bleeding may have a density that is intermediate between that of hematoma and fluid. Contrast CT with arterial and delayed phases (90 seconds after contrast infusion) is important to identify the source of hemorrhage. Also, increase in density of the mediastinal collection in the arterial or delayed phases, in comparison to noncontrast images, is suggestive of active bleeding (Fig. 41.14).

Mediastinitis

Mediastinitis is responsible for 30% of the mortality of heart transplant recipients within the first year. The most frequent radiologic dilemma in evaluating patients after transplantation by CT is to differentiate normal postoperative findings from mediastinitis. It is important to correlate the imaging findings with the clinical presentation and serial changes (Fig. 41.15). Collections that increase in volume, become more circumscribed, or develop air components are particularly worrisome for mediastinitis. A radiologist must recognize that complex-appearing collections can be seen in the normal postoperative mediastinum up to 20 to 30 days after surgery.

Acute Cellular Rejection

ACS is the most common type of rejection and is usually seen in the first year after the treatment, with an incidence of about 8%. This type of rejection is characterized by myocardial edema and necrosis resulting from a T cell–mediated immune reaction. Transjugular endomyocardial biopsy is the gold standard for diagnosis and can accurately estimate the severity of disease. Because early disease may be asymptomatic, transplant patients undergo a rigorous screening process that involves frequent myocardial biopsies during the first postoperative year.

PROBLEM SOLVING WITH MRI

MRI is a robust technique that allows for myocardial tissue characterization, particularly regarding the presence of myocardial edema. Several MRI variables have shown good correlation to biopsy results, the strongest of which is quantitative T2 assessment, or T2 mapping. Therefore, MRI is a promising tool for noninvasive screening for ACS and may be able to replace invasive procedures for this purpose in the future.

Coronary Allograft Vasculopathy

CAV is the principal cause of late death in heart transplant patients. Previous studies using conventional coronary angiography have documented its presence in up to 10% of patients at 1 year and 50% of patients at 5 years after transplantation. The use of intravascular ultrasound (IVUS) has led to even higher estimates for the presence of disease. Clinically, this disease is insidious in nature and may give no indication as to its presence until the onset of heart failure, myocardial infarction, or death. CAV is a diffuse process of the coronary arteries, with a higher prevalence of concentric and noncalcified lesions compared to atherosclerosis.

The current standard of care involves immunosuppression. Angioplasty may also be performed in selected cases for focal disease. Aggressive screening programs have been advocated for heart transplant patients, including frequent invasive coronary angiography and IVUS in the first few years after transplantation.

PROBLEM SOLVING WITH CT

Recent studies have shown that coronary CT angiography (CTA) has good accuracy for the detection of coronary stenosis after heart transplantation (Fig. 41.16). In comparison to invasive coronary angiography, coronary CTA has good accuracy in the detection of stenoses >50% and can be used as a clinical tool for the detection of such obstructive lesions. An early manifestation of CAV is diffuse concentric coronary wall thickening, which can be identified with IVUS in combination with cardiac catheterization. It has also been shown that there is a good correlation between the coronary vessel wall area measured by CT compared to IVUS.

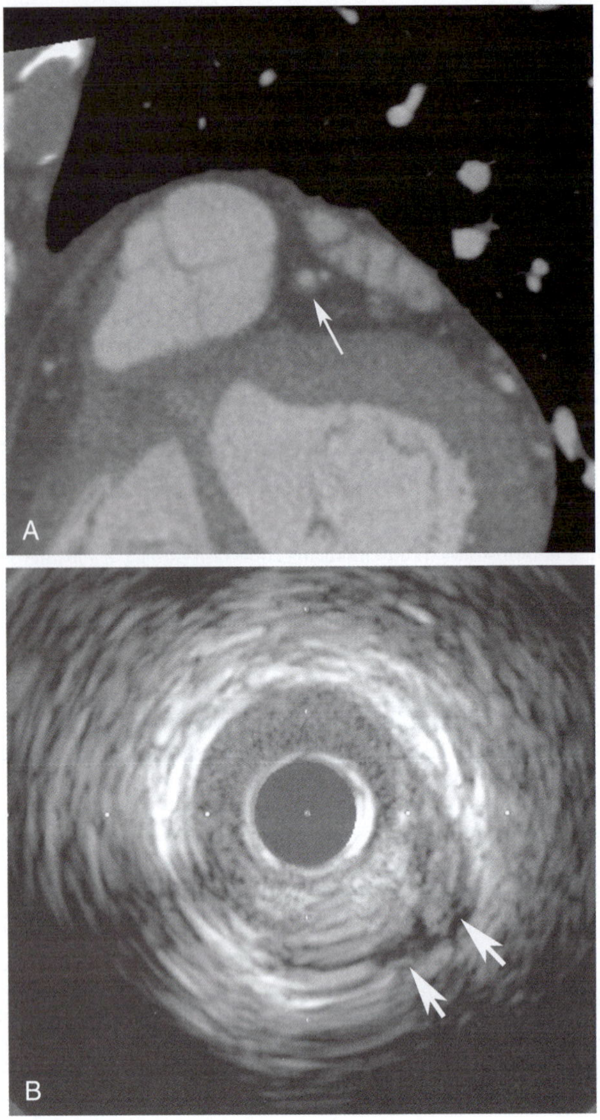

Figure 41.16 Coronary allograft vasculopathy. (A) Cross-sectional image from coronary CT angiography of a patient with coronary allograft vasculopathy shows eccentric, noncalcified wall thickening *(arrow)*. (B) Coronary intravascular ultrasound image of the same patient confirms the presence of wall thickening *(arrows)*.

Malignancies

An increased incidence of malignancies, including PTLD, has been described after heart transplantation. As patient survival from cardiac graft complications improves, post-transplantation malignancies are becoming an important clinical issue in this patient population. The main predictors for the development of malignancy include older age and early development of graft rejection.

Commonly Encountered Abandoned Materials That Can Be Normal After Heart Transplantation

Interpretation of imaging studies after heart transplantation can be complicated by the presence of multiple abandoned lines, wires, and patches. These are commonly present and are a normal finding in this clinical setting. The typical example is the abandoned intravascular pacer lead in the subclavian vein. Pacemaker leads have often been in place for prolonged periods of time prior to transplantation. It is common for surgeons to encounter resistance when trying to remove an intravascular pacer wire during the surgery. Given the potential for vascular injury, these are often left in place and should not cause clinical concern (Fig. 41.17A). It should be noted, however, that the presence of abandoned intravascular pacer wires is currently considered an absolute contraindication for an MRI examination.

Another common abandoned wire that can be seen after heart transplantation is one or more temporary epicardial pacer leads, typically located in a subxyphoid location (see Fig. 41.17B). These very thin wires may be difficult to remove after a long hospital course because of adhesion formation. There is no evidence to suggest an increased risk of infection or other complications associated with the chronic presence of abandoned epicardial leads.

Finally, most patients who undergo heart transplantation have had a temporary left ventricular assist device (LVAD) placed as a bridge to transplantation. Frequently, a Dacron pericardial patch is placed in the previous location of a LVAD and may be confused with abandoned surgical material, particularly a sponge.

What to Look for on Post–Heart Transplantation Imaging

- Different complications occur at different times post–heart transplantation. Abnormalities must be interpreted in the context of when the transplantation was performed.
- Complications that occur immediately after heart transplantation include primary graft failure, pericardial effusion or hematoma, mediastinal hematoma, and mediastinitis.
- Complications that occur early (typically within or around the first year) include ACS and mediastinitis.
- The primary complication that occurs after the first year is CAV.
- Certain complications may occur at any time, including infection and malignancy.
- Primary graft failure will exhibit pulmonary edema within the first 24 hours after transplantation.
- Postoperative pericardial and mediastinal collections are often detected on surveillance radiographs. CT and MRI may be useful to characterize the nature of the fluid further and plan interventions.
- Mediastinitis may be difficult to distinguish from normal postoperative findings. Collections that are well circumscribed, contain air, or are increasing in size on serial imaging suggest mediastinal infection.
- ACS is typically seen in the first year and is evaluated with transjugular myocardial biopsy. MRI may become an important noninvasive screening method in the future.
- CAV is the main cause of late mortality. It is typically assessed using conventional coronary angiography,

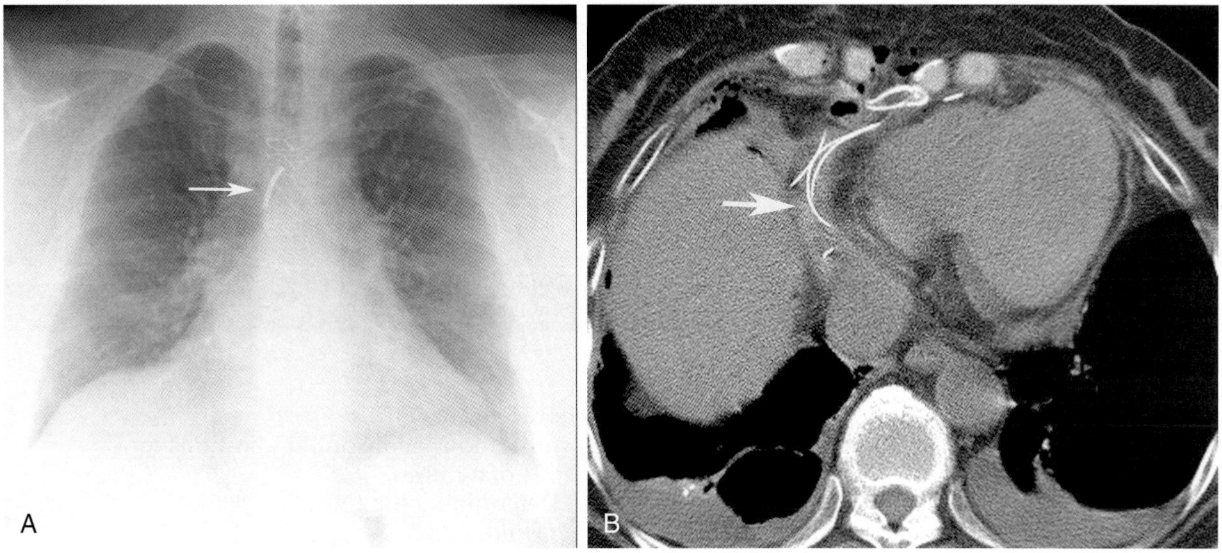

Figure 41.17 Abandoned material after heart transplantation. (A) Frontal chest radiograph of a patient after heart transplantation shows an abandoned intravascular pacemaker wire *(arrow)*. (B) Axial noncontrast CT image of the chest from a different patient shows multiple abandoned epicardial pacer leads *(arrow)*.

but coronary CTA is a noninvasive method of assessment, with good accuracy.

- Abandoned materials are common after heart transplant and should be considered expected findings. These include pacemakers leads in the subclavian vein, epicardial pacer leads, and pericardial patches.

Heart-Lung Transplantation

Heart-lung transplantation is performed rarely. In 2013, approximately 23 procedures were performed in the United States. The most common indications include congenital heart disease (35.7%), pulmonary arterial hypertension (27.6%), cystic fibrosis (14.1%), and acquired heart disease (5.0%). There is reduced survival of heart-lung transplantation compared to lung transplantation alone, particularly in the first year, 63% versus 79%. Of the patients who survive the first year, however, there is an excellent prognosis, with an average survival of 10 years. Patients may develop complications specific to the lung or heart transplantation, but complications related to the lung tend to predominate. For example, at the 5-year point after transplantation, approximately 40% of patients will have evidence of BOS, whereas only 10% of patients will have evidence of coronary artery vasculopathy.

Bibliography

Belperio JA, Weigt SS, Fishbein MC, Lynch JP. Chronic lung allograft rejection: mechanisms and therapy. *Proc Am Thorac Soc*. 2009;6(1):108–121.

Boasquevisque CHR, Yildirim E, Waddel TK, Keshavjee S. Surgical techniques: lung transplant and lung volume reduction. *Proc Am Thorac Soc*. 2009;6(1):66–78.

Burguete SR, Maselli DJ, Fernandez JF, Levine SM. Lung transplant infection. *Respirology*. 2013;18(1):22–38.

Butler CR, Thompson R, Haykowsky M, et al. Cardiovascular magnetic resonance in the diagnosis of acute heart transplant rejection: a review. *J Cardiovasc Magn Reson*. 2009;11(1):7.

Christie JD, Edwards LB, Kucheryavaya AY, et al. The registry of the International Society for Heart and Lung Transplantation: 29th adult lung and heart-lung transplant report—2012. *J Heart Lung Transplant*. 2012;31(10):1073–1086.

Collins J, Hartman MJ, Warner TF, et al. Frequency and CT findings of recurrent disease after lung transplantation. *Radiology*. 2001;219(2):503–509.

Davies RR, Russo MJ, Morgan JA, et al. Standard versus bicaval techniques for orthotopic heart transplantation: an analysis of the united network for organ sharing database. *J Thorac Cardiovasc Surg*. 2010;140(3):700–708.

Gradek WQ, D'Amico C, Smith AL, et al. Routine surveillance endomyocardial biopsy continues to detect significant rejection late after heart transplantation. *J Heart Lung Transplant*. 2001;20:497–502.

Hunt SA, Abraham WT, Chin MH, et al. 2009 focused update incorporated into the ACC/AHA 2005 guidelines for the diagnosis and management of heart failure in adults: a report of the American College of Cardiology Foundation/American Heart Association task force on practice guidelines developed in collaboration with the International Society for Heart and Lung Transplantation. *Circulation*. 2009;119:e391–e479.

Kremer BE, Reshef R, Misleh JG, et al. Posttransplantation lymphoproliferative disorder after lung transplantation: a review of 35 cases. *J Heart Lung Transplant*. 2012;31(3):296–304.

Krishnam MS, Suh RD, Tomasian A, et al. Postoperative complications of lung transplantation: radiologic findings along a time continuum. *Radiographics*. 2007;27(4):957–974.

Lee JC, Christie JD. Primary graft dysfunction. *Proc Am Thorac Soc*. 2009;6(1):39–46.

Lindenfeld J, Miller GG, Shakar SF, et al. Drug therapy in the heart transplant recipient: part I: cardiac rejection and immunosuppressive drugs. *Circulation*. 2004;110:3734–3740.

Lower RR, Shumway NE. Studies on orthotopic homotransplantation of the canine heart. *Surg Forum*. 1960;11:18–19.

Luckraz H, Goddard M, Charman SC, et al. Early mortality after cardiac transplantation: should we do better? *J Heart Lung Transplant*. 2005;24:401–405.

Paraskeva M, McLean C, Ellis S, et al. Acute fibrinoid organizing pneumonia after lung transplantation. *Am J Respir Crit Care Med*. 2013;187(12):1360–1368.

Roger VL, Go AS, Lloyd-Jones DM, et al. Heart disease and stroke statistics—2011 update: a report from the American Heart Association. *Circulation*. 2011;123:e18–e209.

Sato M, Waddell TK, Wagnetz U, et al. Restrictive allograft syndrome (RAS): a novel form of chronic lung allograft dysfunction. *J Heart Lung Transplant*. 2011;30(7):735–742.

Stehlik J, Edwards LB, Kucheryavaya AY, et al. The registry of the International Society for Heart and Lung Transplantation: 29th official adult heart transplant report—2012. *J Heart Lung Transplant*. 2012;31(10):1052–1064.

Yancy CW, Jessup M, Bozkurt B, et al. 2013 ACCF/AHA guideline for the management of heart failure: a report of the American College of Cardiology Foundation/American Heart Association task force on practice guidelines. *J Am Coll Cardiol*. 2013;62:e147–e239.

CHAPTER 42
Thoracic Interventions

Florian J. Fintelmann, Jo-Anne O. Shepard, and Amita Sharma

CHAPTER OUTLINE

■ Introduction

Thoracic interventions are performed for the diagnosis and treatment of focal lesions in the thorax. Image-guided percutaneous biopsy is used to obtain tissue for the diagnosis of benign and malignant conditions. Drainage of fluid or air from the pleural space or mediastinum can aid both diagnosis and therapy, and ablative therapies treat primary or secondary malignancy in lungs and chest wall.

■ Lung and Mediastinal Needle Biopsy

Technical Principles

Tissue from a lesion in lung or mediastinum can be obtained percutaneously using CT guidance. A coaxial technique allows multiple biopsies to be performed with only one pleural puncture, thereby limiting complications. A 19-gauge introducer needle, in combination with a 22-gauge needle for aspirates, and a 20-gauge automatic, spring-loaded core needle provide adequate tissue for lung biopsies, but a larger gauge needle such as a 17-gauge introducer is advised for mediastinal biopsies, especially if lymphoma is suspected. Whenever possible, moderate sedation should be used because it will minimize respiratory motion and maximize patient comfort and immobility, without the need for breathing instructions. If the patient is cooperative, these biopsies can also be performed using local anesthesia only.

Indications and Contraindications for Lung and Mediastinal Biopsy

Indications for biopsy include establishing a diagnosis of infection and neoplasm and enabling the referring physician to determine the optimum management of a lesion.

In a nonoperative patient, biopsy can be performed to justify radiotherapy or demonstrate the feasibility of image-guided thermal ablation. In cases of known lung cancer, tissue analysis allows molecular testing for targeted chemotherapy and identification of mechanisms for resistance to targeted therapy. Mediastinal lesions can be biopsied to differentiate a thymic epithelial neoplasm from lymphoma because the latter requires chemotherapy rather than resection. Lung biopsy can also be performed to confirm a benign process, such as a hamartoma, and therefore save the patient from a surgical resection.

Severe cardiorespiratory compromise, uncorrectable coagulopathy, and an uncooperative patient are absolute contraindications. Relative contraindications include pulmonary hypertension with a right ventricular systolic pressure >50 mm Hg, prior pneumonectomy, severe emphysema, or interstitial lung disease with a forced expiratory volume in 1 second (FEV_1) <35% predicted. Patients on continuous positive airway pressure (CPAP) therapy for obstructive sleep apnea can undergo lung biopsy if they are able to manage without their CPAP machine and maintain adequate ventilation during the procedure and for 24 hours afterward.

Determining Which Patients Would Benefit From Alternative Means of Obtaining Tissue Rather Than Lung Biopsy

In patients with suspected lung cancer and extrapulmonary findings, the lesion that would result in the highest stage should be biopsied. Such lesions include masses in the adrenal glands and liver and mediastinal lymphadenopathy. For centrally located lung masses, endobronchial ultrasound or bronchoscopy is recommended. Navigational bronchoscopy can be used to sample more peripheral lung lesions, especially in emphysematous patients. In high-risk patients such as those with severe emphysema and a highly suspicious lung lesion, definitive therapy such as radiotherapy can be considered, even without tissue confirmation. Interval growth between CT scans and fluorodeoxyglucose (FDG) uptake is helpful in determining the probable cause. If infection is suspected, the patient is best served by a short-interval follow-up CT (Fig. 42.1) after empiric treatment for community-acquired pneumonia.

Diagnosis of diffuse lung disease is best established with video-assisted thoracoscopic surgery wedge resection because limited tissue from a percutaneous needle biopsy is usually not adequate.

How to Determine if Biopsy Is Technically Feasible

Needle biopsy of a mediastinal lesion is technically feasible if a needle can be directed into the lesion without causing injury to adjacent critical structures, particularly the internal mammary arteries, aorta, and heart. A parasternal approach with the needle directed away from the heart and aorta is usually safe (Fig. 42.2).

The feasibility of lung biopsy depends on lesion size, location, and any concurrent lung disease, such as emphysema and interstitial lung disease. As a general rule, lesions larger than 1 cm are amenable to CT-guided needle biopsy. However, if a nodule lies in a particular location, such as the lung bases, respiratory motion may preclude successful biopsy. This explains why a small nodule located in the apex or superior segment of a lower lobe is easier to biopsy than if the same lesion were located at the lung base. A central lesion may not be accessible because of intervening vessels, airways, and fissures.

Preprocedure Checks Required for a Lung or Mediastinal Biopsy

Medications, platelet count, and coagulation parameters need to be reviewed to assess bleeding risk. Although low-dose aspirin is permissible, patients would ideally have stopped all anticoagulation in time for the effects to wear off at the time of biopsy. Specialty society recommendations include lung biopsy among procedures with moderate bleeding risk, for which a platelet count >50,000/μL is sufficient, but we prefer to biopsy patients with a platelet count >100,000/μL. The previous medical history needs to be reviewed for relative contraindications to moderate sedation, such as left ventricular ejection

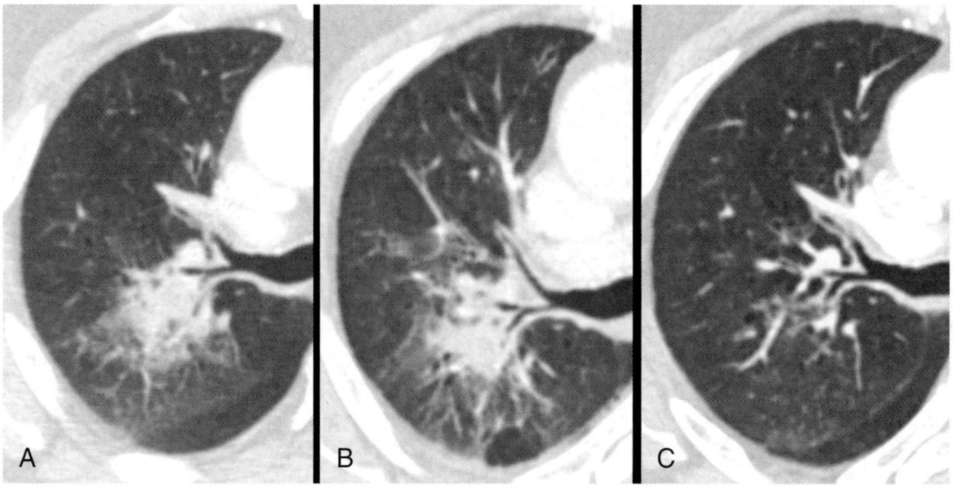

Figure 42.1 (A) Axial contrast-enhanced CT images show a consolidative right upper lobe opacity abutting the major fissure, surrounded by ground-glass opacity. (B) Three weeks later, the lesion has decreased in size, and bronchoscopy yielded *Pneumococcus.* (C) With treatment, the infection completely resolved at 3 months.

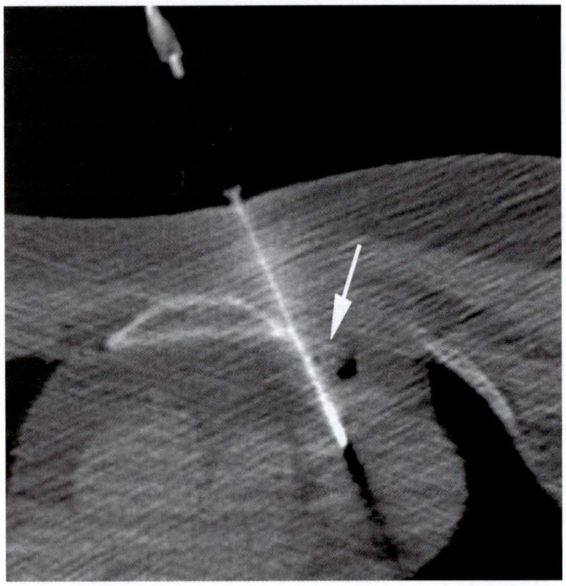

Figure 42.2 Axial noncontrast enhanced CT demonstrates a left parasternal approach for biopsy of an anterior mediastinal mass. The introducer courses between the lateral sternal cortex and internal mammary artery *(arrow)*.

fraction <30%, recent myocardial infarction, or severe stenosis of the aortic valve or carotid arteries. Renal or liver failure would be another reason to consider not using moderate sedation. If moderate sedation is used, the patient needs to have had nothing by mouth for at least 8 hours and have an escort to accompany him or her home after the procedure. While obtaining informed, written consent, the operator should check whether somebody is available to stay with the patient overnight after the procedure in case a delayed pneumothorax develops.

How a Lung Biopsy Is Performed

The patient should be positioned comfortably on the CT table, and sedation should be started. A grid with radiopaque markers is positioned on the patient's skin. Preliminary CT images are obtained with quiet respiration to assess for a clear path between the skin and the biopsy target (Fig. 42.3).

Gantry angulation may be necessary to demonstrate a clear path between the skin and target. Angling the gantry may also be helpful to access an upper lobe nodule located just anterior to the fissure through a more superior intercostal interspace. Sagittal and coronal reformats can be helpful in conceptualizing how this maneuver could move ribs, fissures, and large vessels out of the biopsy path (Fig. 42.4).

The skin overlying the target is then cleaned, and a sterile field is set up. Local anesthesia is administered to the skin with a 25-gauge needle, and the needle is left in place. Repeat imaging is performed to assess whether the skin entry site marked by the lidocaine needle can be lined up with the target and the distance between skin and pleura and skin to target lesion (Fig. 42.5).

Local anesthesia is administered in the thoracic soft tissues. Subsequently, the introducer needle is advanced

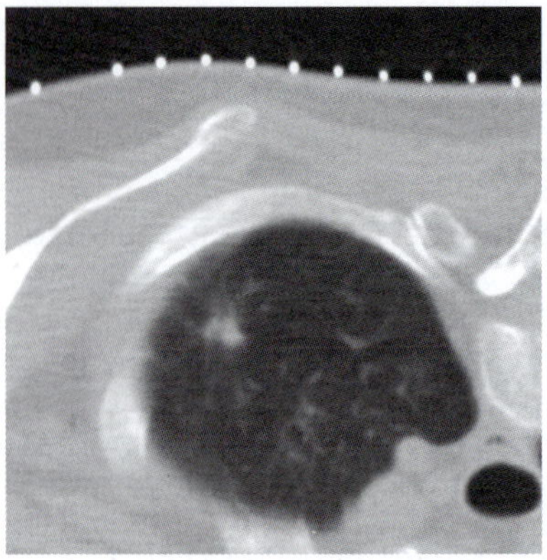

Figure 42.3 Axial noncontrast CT image shows the biopsy target, a left apical nodule. The patient is prone and the biopsy grid lies on the skin of the upper back. Note that a rib blocks the path from the skin to the target.

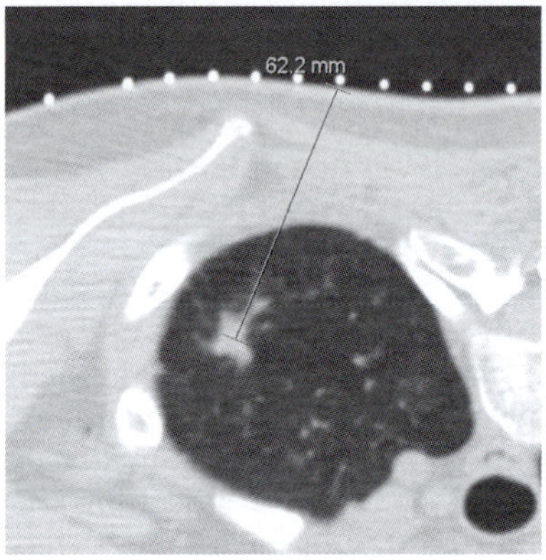

Figure 42.4 Axial noncontrast CT image obtained after angulating the gantry by 10 degrees cephalad shows a clear path to the biopsy target. The distance from skin to target is 6.2 cm, and the operator can choose the appropriate length of introducer needle at this time.

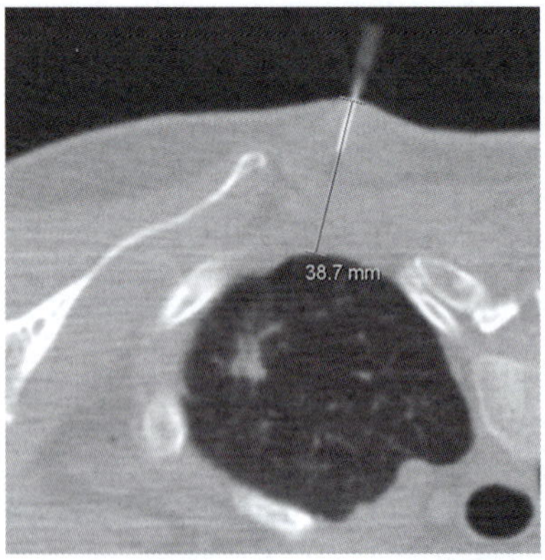

Figure 42.5 Axial noncontrast CT image shows a clear path between the skin entry site, marked by the local anesthesia needle and biopsy target. Note that the distance to pleura measures 3.7 cm.

in parallel to the CT gantry. Care is taken to advance less than the distance from skin to pleura to avoid a pneumothorax (Fig. 42.6). Repeat imaging is performed, as necessary, to check for alignment of the needle with the imaging plane and to measure the residual distance from the needle tip to pleura. If the introducer is no longer in plane, one can adjust either the orientation of the

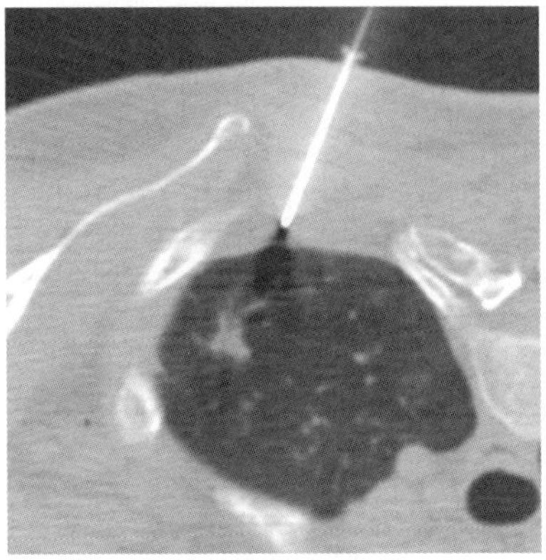

Figure 42.6 Axial noncontrast CT image shows the introducer needle well anchored in the soft tissues, with the tip just short of the pleura. The introducer needle is well aligned with the biopsy target.

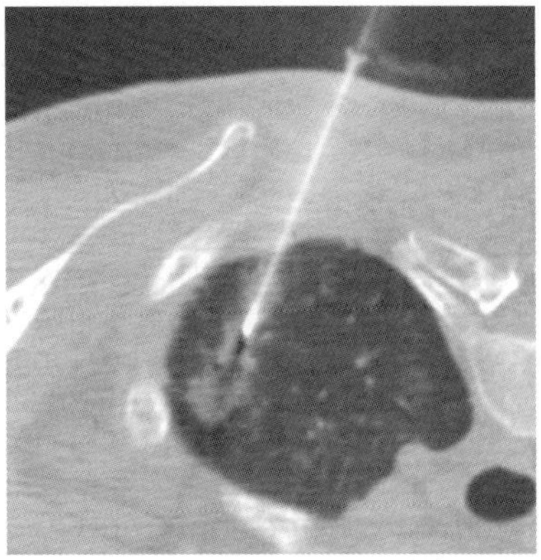

Figure 42.8 Axial noncontrast CT image shows the introducer needle in the target. New ground-glass opacities around the target reflect a small amount of hemorrhage, expected after fine-needle aspiration.

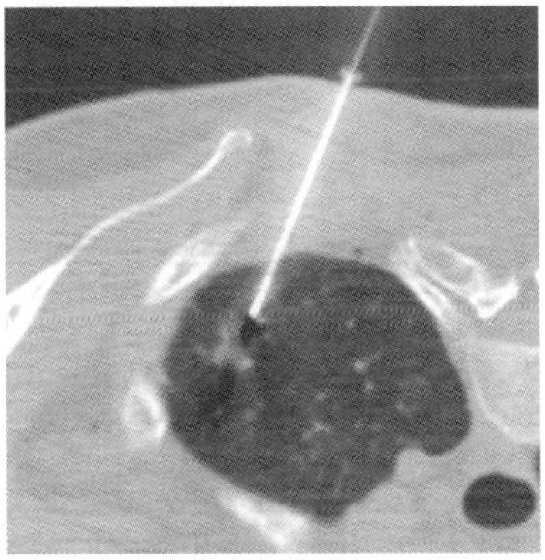

Figure 42.7 Axial noncontrast CT image shows the introducer in the lung parenchyma short of the lesion. Note the air bubble adjacent to the parietal pleura, indicating that pleural anesthetic was injected into the intended plane.

needle or the gantry angulation to achieve alignment of the introducer and target in chest wall soft tissues. It is key to align the introducer and target in chest wall soft tissues prior to puncturing the pleura. Injecting 1% lidocaine through the introducer needle once the tip is close to the parietal pleura anesthetizes this sensitive structure prior to the puncture.

Pleural puncture should only be done once the alignment between introducer and target in chest wall soft tissues has been confirmed to avoid having to pull out of the lung and risk additional pleural punctures. Deliberate advancement of the introducer by 2 to 3 cm will puncture the pleura (Fig. 42.7). One may feel the pleura give way with a subtle pop.

The introducer is advanced incrementally into the lesion. Fine-needle aspirates are obtained while taking care not to advance the fine needle beyond the distal edge of the lesion. Filling the coaxial needle with saline will potentially protect against the risk of air embolism during needle exchanges. Repeat imaging should be performed to assess for complications such as pneumothorax, significant bleeding, and air embolus and confirm needle position. A small amount of blood products around the biopsy target can be expected (Fig. 42.8).

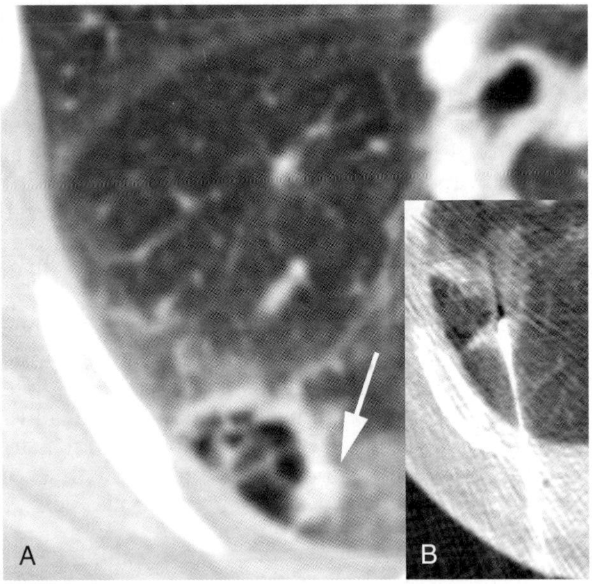

Figure 42.9 (A) Axial contrast-enhanced CT image shows a cystic right lower lobe lesion with a dominant wall nodule *(arrow)*. (B) Biopsy of the nodule revealed adenocarcinoma. Ground-glass opacities around the target represent an expected small amount of biopsy-related hemorrhage.

Maximizing the Yield of Lung and Mediastinal Biopsy

Prior to the procedure, the most recent contrast-enhanced CT and/or positron emission tomography (PET)-CT examinations should be reviewed. Enhancement and/or FDG avidity indicate high-yield areas that should be targeted first. If the biopsy target is cystic, cavitary, or necrotic, viable cells are more likely present in the wall of the lesion than in the center (Fig. 42.9). A trajectory should be chosen that shows a direct path from the skin into the lesion, clear of ribs, bulla, fissures, and vessels (especially those with a diameter larger than 5 mm).

Approaching lung lesions through the back, with the patient in the prone position, is advantageous because the patient does not see the needle and can recover in the supine position. Most patients are not comfortable lying in a prone position for several hours without moving. The posterior approach also minimizes respiratory motion and allows access to the intercostal spaces that are wider compared to an anterior approach while avoiding subclavian vessels and costal cartilages. This is why the posterior approach is preferred over the anterior approach for apical lesions, even though the trajectory may be longer. However, the anterior approach may be necessary for lesions in the anterior upper lobes, right middle lobe, and lingula to avoid crossing the major fissures.

Selection of the appropriate introducer needle length is important. Ideally, the introducer is at least 3 to 5 cm longer than the expected needle trajectory to provide the operator with enough needle length to account for gantry angulation, allow for needle repositioning, and guarantee that the nodule can be reached in the case of a pneumothorax. Positioning the patient at an angle may reduce the length of the biopsy tract, especially for central lesions (Fig. 42.10).

Optimum sedation involves administration of incremental doses of narcotic and anxiolytic to achieve consistent, low-excursion respiratory motion and patient immobility. Excessive sedation can cause significant atelectasis, which may obscure the lesion or cause it to move out of the selected path. It can also lead to erratic deep respirations. Local anesthetic administered through the introducer needle just prior to crossing the pleura prevents pain and sudden patient movement.

Rapid on-site evaluation by a pathologist has been proven to decrease the rate of nondiagnostic lung biopsies. This can confirm that diagnostic material has been sampled and can help guide redirecting the introducer needle, if necessary. Based on this intraprocedural assessment, the radiologist can decide to proceed with a core biopsy to obtain more solid tissue or obtain dedicated fine-needle aspirates for microbiologic analysis, special stains, or flow cytometry. Tissue cores increase the chances of establishing the specific diagnosis of neoplasm and provide material for additional molecular analysis and subtyping. As a general principle, tissue cores should be obtained whenever it is safe, especially if no pathologist is available for preliminary interpretation during the procedure and if a benign entity is suspected, such as a hamartoma or granuloma.

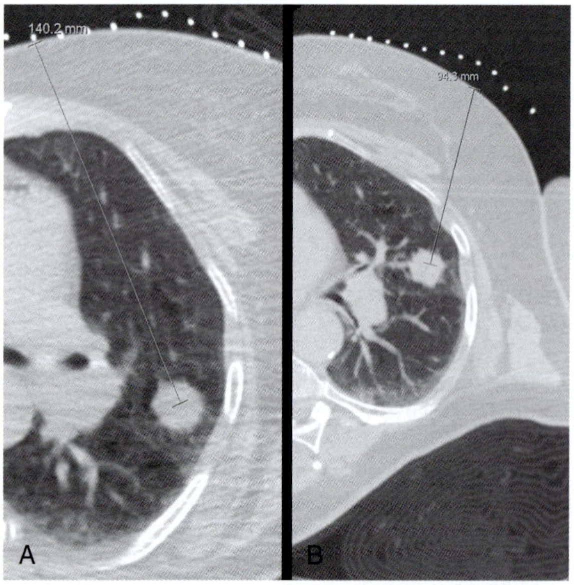

Figure 42.10 Axial noncontrast enhanced CT images demonstrate an anterior approach to a left upper lobe nodule located anterior to the major fissure. (A) With the patient supine, the path was longer and came closer to larger vessels compared to the patient tilted obliquely by 45 degrees (B) using a rolled-up blanket.

Complications and Management of Lung and Mediastinal Biopsy

Complications associated with lung biopsy and their likelihood of occurrence are listed in Table 42.1. A pneumothorax incurred prior to positioning the introducer needle close to the biopsy target poses a challenge because partially deflated lung will move away from the chest wall and will be difficult to puncture. In this case, a small chest tube can be placed to aspirate the air to continue the procedure (Fig. 42.11). If an introducer needle crosses the pleura but is malpositioned and cannot be redirected, this needle should be left in the lung, and a second introducer needle should be placed. The first needle serves as an anchor while the biopsy is performed through the second needle, and both introducer needles can be removed at the end of the procedure.

Pneumothorax evident at the end of the procedure can be aspirated through the introducer needle as it is removed. In addition, 10 mL of the patient's own coagulated blood injected through the introducer at the end of the procedure (blood patch) has been shown to decrease the likelihood of significant pneumothorax, which requires chest tube placement. A small pneumothorax detected on a postprocedure chest radiograph should trigger another chest radiograph 1 to 2 hours later. No intervention is required, provided that the patient

TABLE 42.1 Complications of Lung Biopsy by Likelihood

COMPLICATION	LIKELIHOOD (%)
Pneumothorax	20
Pneumothorax requiring chest tube placement	5
Hemoptysis	5
Hemothorax	1.5
Tract seeding	0.6
Death	0.15
Air embolism	0.06–0.4

Modified from Manhire A, Charig M, Clelland C, et al. Guidelines for radiologically guided lung biopsy. *Thorax.* 2003;58(11):920–936; Wu CC, Maher MM, Shepard J-AO. Complications of CT-guided percutaneous needle biopsy of the chest: prevention and management. *AJR Am J Roentgenol.* 2011;196(6):W678–W682; Wiener RS, Wiener DC, Gould MK. Risks of transthoracic needle biopsy: how high? *Clin Pulm Med.* 2013;20(1):29–35.

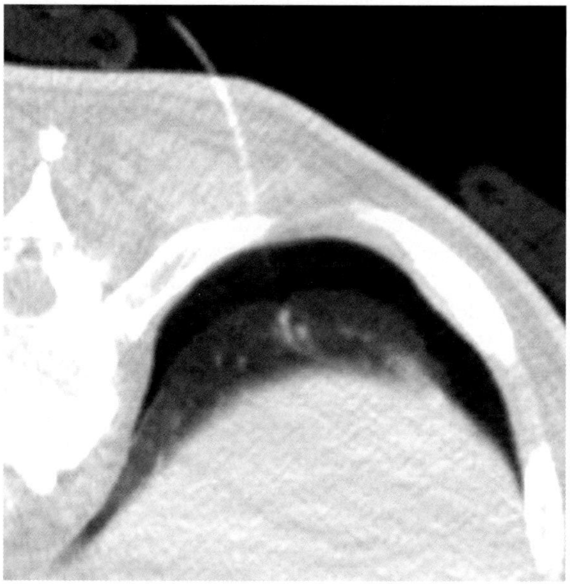

Figure 42.11 Axial noncontrast enhanced CT image shows a 5-Fr catheter used to aspirate a small left pneumothorax during a lung biopsy (introducer needle not shown).

remains asymptomatic, and the pneumothorax does not enlarge. With rest and oxygen by nasal cannula, the body will eventually absorb a small, nonenlarging pneumothorax, and the patient can be discharged, accompanied by an escort.

If hemoptysis occurs during the procedure, the operator should temporarily stop the procedure until it resolves. Even small amounts of blood can irritate the airway, and such irritation can be reduced with intravenous fentanyl. The oral cavity should be inspected and suction provided to help evacuate blood products. If hemoptysis continues, the procedure should be stopped, the needle removed, and the patient positioned with the biopsied side down to prevent aspiration of blood into the contralateral lung. The patient should be encouraged to cough and clear the airway. Whereas mild hemoptysis is self-limiting, severe and prolonged hemoptysis should trigger surgical consultation. In cases of prolonged hemoptysis, contrast-enhanced CT and evaluation for coil embolization should be considered. In significant hemoptysis, bronchoscopy to clear the airways of clots may be required. A bronchial blocker insertion can isolate the bleeding site and protect the contralateral lung from aspiration of blood.

Air embolism is a rare complication and is diagnosed by air in the left-sided chambers of the heart and systemic arteries during the procedure; it can manifest as seizure activity or myocardial infarction. Treatment involves placing the patient in a left lateral decubitus position with the head down to prevent air from entering the systemic circulation, and 100% oxygen should be administered via a nonrebreather mask. A hyperbaric oxygen chamber may be required.

Decreasing the Risk of Complications

The risk of pneumothorax is minimized by puncturing the pleura only once and by not crossing fissures. Not traversing aerated lung significantly reduces the risk of pneumothorax. Previous surgery can be protective due to pleural adhesions. Crossing areas of abnormal lung, such as foci of emphysema, should be avoided whenever possible. A blood patch has been reported to reduce the rate of significant pneumothorax and subsequent chest tube placement. Immediately after removing the introducer needle, the patient should be positioned with the biopsy side down for 3 hours to induce atelectasis in this area and apposition of the pleural layers.

Choosing a needle trajectory away from medium and large-sized vessels, in addition to correcting any bleeding diathesis and avoiding medications that alter hemostasis, minimizes the risk of hemorrhage. Of note, even though specialty society recommendations include lung biopsy among procedures with moderate bleeding risk, we prefer to biopsy patients with a platelet count >100,000/μL. In patients who do not have normal platelet function or number, extreme caution should be exercised and biopsy performed only once the risks have been discussed and minimized with the use of platelet transfusions. Anticoagulation should not be resumed until the day after the procedure.

Instructing the patient not to talk or cough during the procedure minimizes the risk of air embolism. If a coaxial technique is used, the introducer should be sealed by dripping saline into the hub prior to and during needle exchanges to prevent air from entering the thoracic cavity through the coaxial needle.

Optimal Postprocedure Patient Care

The patient should be positioned with the dependent side down, with instructions not to cough, talk, or move, and observed in a monitored recovery unit for 3 hours. Oxygen should be provided per nasal canula. Radiographs are obtained 1 and 3 hours postprocedure to assess for pneumothorax and hemorrhage. Once the observation period is completed and no complications have developed, the patient is discharged, accompanied by an escort, with firm instructions not to engage in strenuous activity for the next 48 hours and to seek medical attention if she or he becomes symptomatic. In case of severe chest pain, shortness of breath, or significant hemoptysis, patients should immediately proceed to the nearest emergency room. Patients are advised to follow up with the referring physician to discuss biopsy results.

Special Considerations After Lung and Mediastinal Biopsy

Patients who live alone and are at high risk for complications are best served with overnight hospital admission for observation. If a pneumothorax is documented during or after the procedure, the patient should be instructed not to travel by air, because the decrease in atmospheric pressure at a high altitude can result in expansion of a previously asymptomatic pneumothorax during the flight. As per the British Thoracic Society, patients should be able to fly 2 weeks after resolution of a traumatic pneumothorax has been documented on a chest radiograph.

Thoracentesis

Thoracentesis describes the removal of fluid from the pleural space using a needle or catheter. No catheter is left at the end of the procedure.

Indications and Contraindications for Thoracentesis

Thoracentesis is used to provide symptomatic relief for patients with shortness of breath and to investigate the cause of pleural fluid. Thoracentesis is not possible if the patient is uncooperative or has an uncorrectable coagulopathy. Thoracentesis is considered a procedure with a low bleeding risk, and consensus guidelines suggest that coagulopathy be evaluated and managed as outlined in Table 42.2.

Determining the Cause of Pleural Fluid

Pleural fluid is classified as exudate or transudate using Light's criteria, which rely on comparing levels of cholesterol, lactate dehydrogenase, and protein in pleural fluid with serum levels. For this purpose, a sample of removed pleural fluid should be sent to the biochemistry laboratory. In addition, a separate sample should be sent to the microbiology laboratory with a request for Gram staining and cultures with sensitivities. If a malignant pleural effusion is suspected, a third sample should be sent to pathology with a request for cell count. A negative cell count does not exclude a malignant pleural effusion, and repeat thoracentesis may be necessary to confirm the diagnosis of malignancy.

TABLE 42.2 Periprocedural Management of Coagulation Status and Hemostasis Risk in Image-Guided Interventions With a Low Bleeding Risk[a]

PARAMETER	GUIDELINES
Preprocedure testing	INR—routinely recommended for patients receiving warfarin anticoagulation or with known or suspected liver disease aPTT—routinely recommended for patients receiving intravenous unfractionated heparin Platelet count—not routinely recommended Hematocrit—not routinely recommended
Management	INR >2.0—threshold for treatment (e.g., FFP, vitamin K) PTT—no consensus Hematocrit—no recommended threshold for transfusion Platelets—transfusion recommended for counts <50,000/μL Clopidogrel—withhold for 5 days before procedure Aspirin—do not withhold LMWH (therapeutic dose)—withhold one dose before procedure

[a]Society of Interventional Radiology Consensus Guidelines.
aPTT, Activated partial thromboplastin time; *FFP,* fresh frozen plasma; *INR,* international normalized ratio; *LMWH,* low-molecular-weight heparin; *PTT,* partial thromboplastin time.

How Thoracentesis Is Performed

When obtaining informed, written consent, possible complications to discuss include pain, bleeding, and infection, as well as pneumothorax, with or without the need to place a chest tube and reexpansion pulmonary edema.

Thoracentesis can be performed at the bedside or in the interventional radiology suite using ultrasound guidance. Ideally, the patient should be sitting on the side of the bed leaning over a side table to increase the space between the ribs. If the patient cannot sit upright, the procedure can be performed in the lateral decubitus position, with the fluid-filled side down. A sagittally oriented, curved, 3.5-MHz probe is used to visualize the largest fluid pocket, and the overlying skin is marked to identify the entry point (Fig. 42.12). The trajectory should be above the rib to avoid injury of the intercostal neurovascular bundle. After sterilizing the field, local anesthesia is provided to skin and parietal pleura using up to 20 mL of 1% lidocaine. If there is insufficient fluid to accommodate a catheter, a 20-gauge needle is advanced into the fluid under direct visualization using an ultrasound probe with a sterile cover. Large pleural fluid collections can be accessed without direct visualization, using an 8-Fr pigtail catheter.

The catheter is introduced over a guidewire (Seldinger technique) or mounted on a stylet (trocar technique). The catheter is connected to a vacuum bottle after the guidewire or stylet is withdrawn. The catheter is secured by hand and held in position. As soon as fluid starts flowing, samples should be obtained for analysis. After removing more than 500 mL, the patient is likely to experience the urge to cough as the lung starts to expand. Slowing down the flow of fluid until coughing subsides will decrease the risk of pneumothorax. Uncontrollable coughing is a sign to stop and remove the catheter. Rapid removal of large fluid volumes (>1 L) may result in

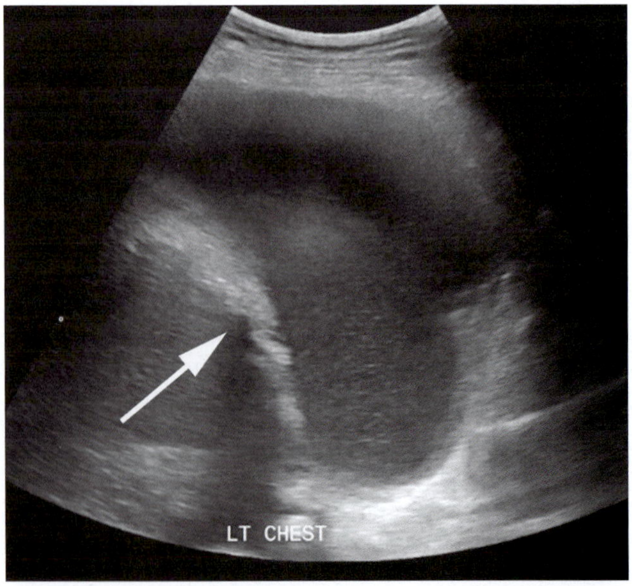

Figure 42.12 Sagittal ultrasound image of the left hemithorax shows atelectatic lung *(arrow)* surrounded by a moderate amount of pleural fluid. Note pleural thickening due to malignancy.

unilateral reexpansion pulmonary edema. Following catheter removal, a frontal chest radiograph should be obtained to evaluate for pneumothorax, residual fluid, and adequate lung expansion.

■ Pleural Drainage

Pleural drainage differs from a thoracentesis because the catheter is left in the pleural space to allow continued drainage.

Indications and Contraindications for Pleural Drainage

Pleural drainage is indicated for pneumothorax, loculated pleural fluid, hemothorax, especially when infection of the pleural space is suspected, and recurrent large pleural effusions—for example, after cardiac surgery (Fig. 42.13).

Leaving a catheter in the pleural space allows subsequent manipulation over a wire, such as replacement with a larger drain (known as *upsizing*), injection of contrast to evaluate change in size of the space, and administration of tissue plasminogen activator (tPA) and deoxyribonuclease (DNase) to break up protein, thereby facilitating evacuation of residual fluid.

The contraindications for pleural drainage are the same as for thoracentesis.

How Pleural Drainage Is Performed

When obtaining informed, written consent, possible complications to discuss include the fact that a drain will be placed for an unknown period of time, in addition to the risks detailed for thoracentesis. Drainage of large pleural effusions can be performed at the bedside or in the interventional radiology suite using ultrasound guidance in a similar fashion as thoracentesis. Loculated small effusions or multiple pockets are best drained using CT guidance to minimize the risk of placing a catheter into lung parenchyma. By keeping the access path away from the posterior paravertebral area, one can minimize injury to the intercostal arteries, which are found halfway between the ribs in this location. It is important to prepare the water seal of a chest drainage system prior to setting up the sterile field. When choosing the catheter, one has to consider that although larger catheters cause more discomfort, they are able to more easily evacuate thicker fluid. Usually, the choice of catheter will range from 10 or 12 Fr to evacuate a pneumothorax, and up to 16 Fr to evacuate blood products or an empyema.

Local anesthesia is administered into the skin and parietal pleura using 1% lidocaine. The catheter is introduced using the Seldinger or trocar technique and immediately connected to the drainage system to prevent an iatrogenic pneumothorax. The catheter is secured to the skin with silk sutures, and the site is covered with an airtight dressing. Subsequently, the connections of the catheter to the chest drainage system are secured with cloth tape to preclude inadvertent disconnection, which would lead to a large pneumothorax. The chest drainage system is set to water-seal and kept below the patient to facilitate evacuation of fluid. A frontal chest radiograph should be obtained to evaluate for iatrogenic pneumothorax, residual fluid, or air and to document tube position at baseline.

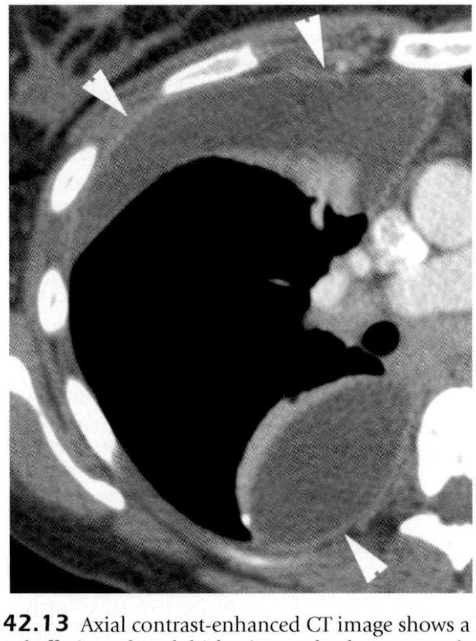

Figure 42.13 Axial contrast-enhanced CT image shows a loculated right pleural effusion, pleural thickening, and enhancement *(arrowheads)* consistent with a split pleura sign. Complete evacuation requires at least one chest tube placement and tissue plasminogen activator.

Complications of Pleural Drainage

In addition to pneumothorax, pleural drain placement can result in airway injury if the tube is advanced into the lung parenchyma. This would manifest as an air leak, despite tight tubing connections. A bright red output should raise concern for vessel injury and trigger monitoring of the patient's vital signs and hemoglobin level, as well as a contrast-enhanced CT with delayed images.

Management

There are various options for treatment.

Treatment of a Pleural Drain

On the floor, the chest drainage system should be connected to wall suction at 20 cm H_2O (30 cm H_2O in case of air leak). Tubing should be flushed with 20 mL of sterile saline every shift to prevent clogging. Output needs to be recorded, and daily chest radiographs should be obtained to assess for tube migration and residual fluid or air.

Dwell time depends on the reason for tube placement (Fig. 42.14) and should be minimized to prevent the introduction of infection into the thorax via the tube. Removal can be done at the bedside after cutting the retention sutures while the patient is exhaling or humming. The site should be covered with an airtight dry dressing. It is prudent to obtain a chest radiograph after drain removal to document the absence of a pneumothorax.

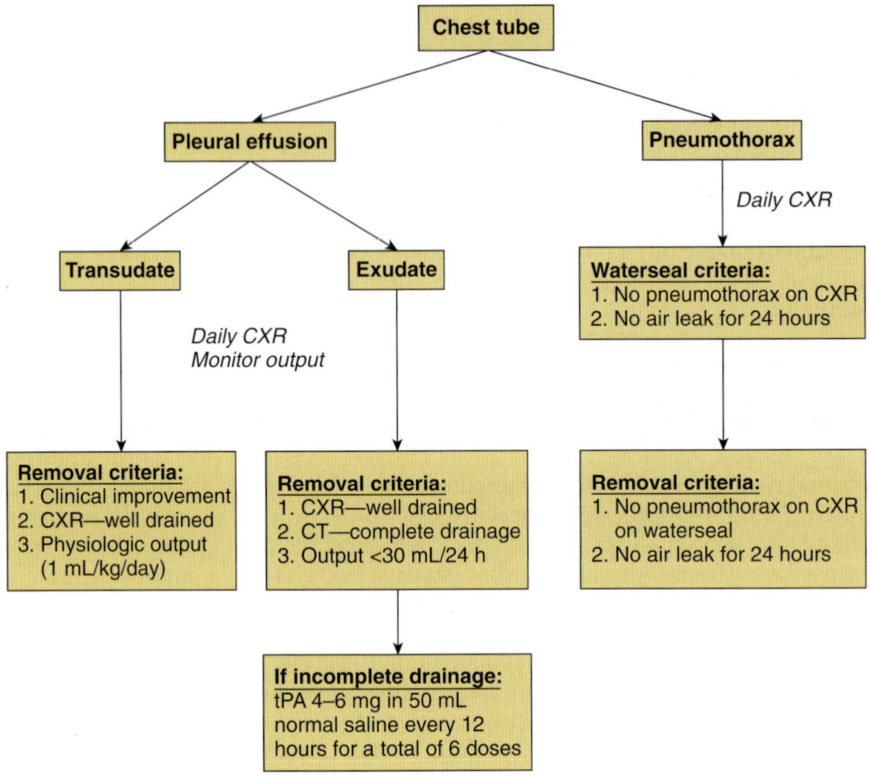

Figure 42.14 Chest tube management algorithm. *CXR*, Chest radiograph; *tPA*, tissue plasminogen activator. (From McDermott S, Levis DA, Arellano RS. Chest drainage. *Semin Intervent Radiol.* 2012;29:247–255.)

Options if Pockets of Pleural Fluid Persist After Pleural Drain Placement

As a first step, a course of tPA and DNase injected into the pleural space using the existing drain has been shown to be effective in improving drainage of loculated effusions not drained with catheters alone. Whereas prophylactic systemic anticoagulation does not increase bleeding risk after the intrapleural administration of tPA, therapeutic anticoagulation is associated with a significantly increased risk of pleural hemorrhage in this setting. Fluid pockets refractory to this treatment can be drained by placing additional catheters using CT guidance.

■ Drainage of Lung and Mediastinum

The indications for percutaneous drainage of lung and mediastinum include lung and mediastinal abscesses that failed antibiotic treatment and esophageal anastomotic leaks. Drain placement in the lung and mediastinum is not possible if the patient has an uncorrectable coagulopathy because these procedures are considered to be associated with a moderate bleeding risk. Consensus guidelines suggest that coagulopathy be evaluated and managed as outlined in Table 42.3.

TABLE 42.3 Periprocedural Management of Coagulation Status and Hemostasis Risk in Image-Guided Interventions With a Moderate Bleeding Risk[a]

PARAMETER	GUIDELINES
Preprocedure testing	INR—recommended aPTT—recommended for patients receiving intravenous unfractionated heparin Platelet count—not routinely recommended Hematocrit—not routinely recommended
Management	INR—correct to <1.5 PTT—no consensus Hematocrit—no recommended threshold for transfusion Platelets—transfusion recommended for counts <50,000/μL Clopidogrel—withhold for 5 days before procedure Aspirin—do not withhold LMWH (therapeutic dose)—withhold one dose before procedure

[a]Society of Interventional Radiology Consensus Guidelines.
aPTT, Activated partial thromboplastin time; *INR*, international normalized ratio; *LMWH*, low-molecular-weight heparin; *PTT*, partial thromboplastin time.

How Drainage of Lung and Mediastinum Is Performed

Catheters are usually inserted using CT guidance and with moderate (procedural) sedation. Both the tandem trocar and Seldinger technique are effective methods. Normal lung should be avoided as much as possible to minimize the risk of an infected bronchopleural fistula, pyopneumothorax, and bleeding.

■ Lung Ablation

Lung ablation is focused application of energy through one or more percutaneously introduced probe(s) to achieve cell death. Cells are destroyed by heat created by alternating electric currents (radiofrequency), electromagnetic waves (microwave energy), or by cold created by rapidly expanding gas (cryotherapy).

Indications and Contraindications for Lung Ablation

There are various indications and contraindications for lung ablation.

Indications

In general, an interdisciplinary tumor board should identify candidates for ablation. The procedure can be considered for patients with early-stage primary lung cancer who are not surgical candidates due to medical comorbidities or limited pulmonary reserve and either do not qualify or desire to undergo radiation therapy. Patients who present with new or recurrent tumors in the lung, pleura, or chest wall after surgery and/or radiation may also benefit from ablation. In addition, patients with oligometastatic disease from extrathoracic cancers may benefit from ablation over resection.

Absolute and Relative Contraindications

The contraindications are similar to those for lung and mediastinal biopsy. However, unlike biopsies, ablation should not be performed without moderate sedation because the procedure is longer and potentially more painful. Moderate sedation ensures patient comfort and immobility, thereby reducing the risk for complications.

Considerations if the Patient Has a Pacemaker or Automatic Implanted Cardioverter-Defibrillator

Only radiofrequency ablation (RFA) and microwave ablation (MWA) interfere with these devices. A cardiology consult should be obtained prior to the procedure. As a precaution, pacers should be set to automatic mode, and defibrillators should be turned off for the duration of the procedure. Pacing and defibrillator systems should be available on standby. Reassessment of the implanted device by the electrophysiology laboratory is recommended after the procedure has been completed.

How Lung Ablation Is Performed

Prior to the procedure, the operator has to decide whether RFA, MWA, or percutaneous cryotherapy (or cryoablation) is the best technique to treat the lesion(s) at hand. Lesion size and location, as well as operator experience with a particular technique, are all involved in the selection. In general, ablation is best suited for tumors located in the peripheral two-thirds of the lung parenchyma, entirely surrounded by lung and not in contact with large vessels, pleural surfaces, or mediastinal structures. Ablation of central lesion can also be considered. Vessels larger than 3 mm in diameter in close proximity to the ablation target are likely to result in heat dissipation during the application of thermal energy. This phenomenon is known as *heat* (or *thermal*) *sink* and can result in incomplete ablation. Structures such as the chest wall, nerves, bones, esophagus, pericardium, and bronchi can be damaged. Table 42.4 compares the perceived advantages and disadvantages of the different techniques in more detail.

Treatment probes are referred to as *electrodes* in RFA, *antennae* in MWA, and *cryoprobes* in cryoablation. CT guidance allows exact placement of probes in the lung, and ultrasound can be used to target chest wall lesions. It is critical to refer to manufacturer instructions to understand where a particular probe emits energy. This active part should be positioned ideally within or as close as possible to the target lesion(s). Once position is confirmed, energy is applied. For RFA and MWA, the ablation zone depends on the number of probes, as well as the frequency (MHz) and generator power (in watts) used, in addition to the geometry of the active part in relation to the target (Fig. 42.15). For cryoablation, the ablation zone depends on the number of probes, relationship of the active part of the probes to the target, and

TABLE 42.4 Comparison of Perceived Advantages and Disadvantages of Lung Ablation Techniques

	TECHNIQUE		
PARAMETER	**RADIOFREQUENCY**	**MICROWAVE**	**CRYOABLATION**
Compatibility with pacer-AICD and surgical clips	No	Some issues	No issues
Risk of thermal sink	+++	+	++
Risk of pain	+++	++	+
Risk of bleeding	++	+	+++
Risk of bronchial damage	+++	++	+
Ability to cover lesions ≤3 cm	+++	+++	+++
Ability to cover lesions >3 cm	+	+++	++
Suitability for lung lesions ≤1.5 cm from pleura	+ (pain)	+ (air leak)	+++
Suitability for chest wall lesions	+	++	+++
Suitability for mediastinal lesions	+	+	++

AICD, Automatic implanted cardioverter-defibrillator; +, rare; ++, occasional; +++, common.

freeze-thaw protocol used (Fig. 42.16). It is important to monitor the size of the treatment zone during the procedure frequently.

Complications of Lung Ablation

Complications include those that can occur during a lung biopsy, as outlined in Table 42.1. In addition, there is a risk for nerve and rib injury, depending on the distance of the treated lesion to the chest wall and the path of the probe in relationship to chest wall and mediastinal nerves. Bronchopleural fistulas may occur after treatment of very peripheral lung lesions. Incomplete treatment and the need for retreatment may be possible outcomes and could be considered a complication. Finally, the patient should be prepared for experiencing malaise in the first week after the ablation as part of the postablation syndrome.

In addition to the postprocedure care that would be provided after lung biopsy, patients are often admitted for overnight observation, with special attention to pain control.

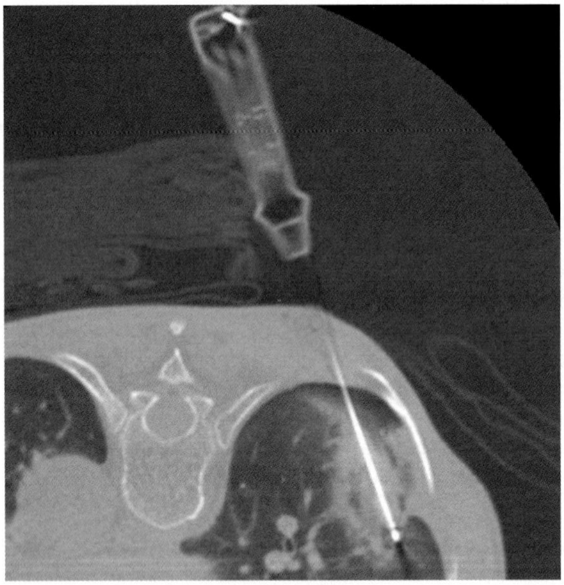

Figure 42.15 Axial noncontrast-enhanced CT image shows a radiofrequency ablation probe in a right lower lobe lung nodule. The ground-glass opacities around the shaft of the probe indicate that treatment has started. Note the small pneumothorax.

Discharge and Follow-Up Instructions After Lung Ablation

Patients are instructed to not engage in strenuous activity and not to use CPAP for 1 month to minimize the risk of complications. At 1 week, patients should be followed up with chest radiography and a phone call or clinic appointment to assess for delayed complications. Chest CT should be performed at 1 month, with contrast if possible and with dual energy if available. Thereafter, FDG PET-CT is performed at 3 months and thereafter every 6 months (alternating with CT alone performed every 6 months) until 2 years postablation. The ablation zone may increase in size during the first week postablation due to acute inflammation, edema, and hemorrhage. Whereas the ablation zone may be larger than the original tumor 1 month postablation, it is expected to decrease in size with time (Fig. 42.17). Imaging features suggestive of residual or recurrent disease

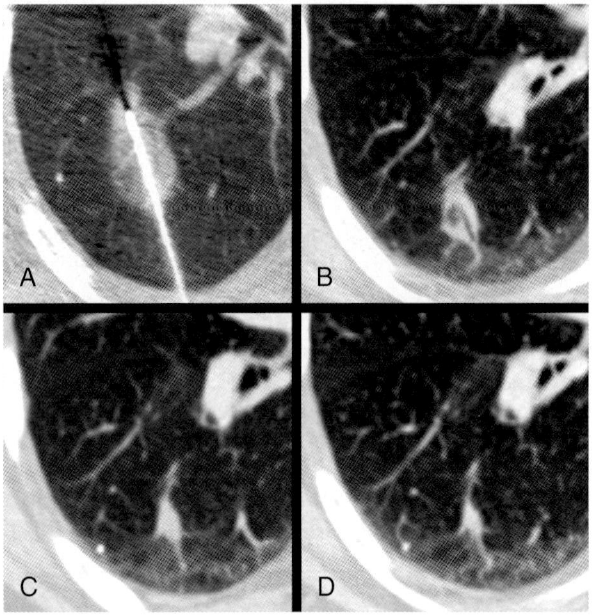

Figure 42.17 Composite of serial axial CT images demonstrates the expected involution of an ablation zone. (A) Intraprocedural image with the ablation probe in place demonstrates an ablation zone, which extends beyond the tumor to create a safety margin. The ablation zone decreases in size at 1-month (B), 6-month (C), and 12-month (D) follow-up.

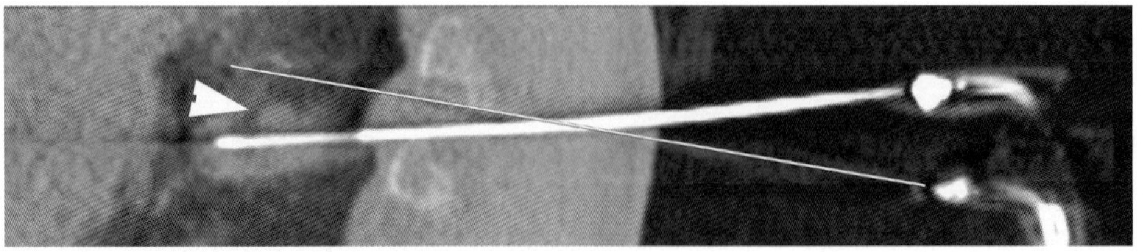

Figure 42.16 Sagittal reformat of a noncontrast-enhanced CT image shows a nodule targeted by two cryoablation probes using the chopstick technique. The active part of the probe with the inferiorly oriented tip is along the nodule *(arrowhead)*. The white line indicates the path of the partially imaged probe with the superiorly oriented tip. Note that the nodule is encompassed by ground-glass opacities and consolidative opacities corresponding to treatment-induced ice and blood products.

include increasing enhancement of the ablation zone and more contrast material uptake in the ablation zone than prior to treatment. Peripheral enhancement around the ablation zone may be present for up to 6 months, but it should be smooth and decrease in thickness over time. Irregular nodular peripheral enhancement measuring >10 mm, growth of the ablation zone after 3 months postablation, and enlargement of regional or distant lymph nodes after 6 months is highly suspicious for residual or recurrent disease. FDG activity should not increase after 2 months' postablation, and no focal FDG uptake should be demonstrated in the location of the treated lesion, usually the center of the ablation zone.

Bibliography

Abtin FG, Eradat J, Gutierrez AJ, et al. Radiofrequency ablation of lung tumors: imaging features of the postablation zone. *Radiographics*. 2012;32(4):947–969.

Ahmedzai S, Balfour-Lynn IM, Bewick T, et al. Managing passengers with stable respiratory disease planning air travel: British Thoracic Society recommendations. *Thorax*. 2011;66(suppl 1):i1–i30.

Chheang S, Abtin F, Guteirrez A, et al. Imaging features following thermal ablation of lung malignancies. *Semin Intervent Radiol*. 2013;30(2):157–168.

Dewhurst C, O'Neill S, O'Regan K, Maher M. Demonstration of the course of the posterior intercostal artery on CT angiography: relevance to interventional radiology procedures in the chest. *Diagn Interv Radiol*. 2012;18(2):221–224.

Dupuy DE. Image-guided thermal ablation of lung malignancies. *Radiology*. 2011;260(3):633–655.

Gervais DA, Levis DA, Hahn PF, et al. Adjunctive intrapleural tissue plasminogen activator administered via chest tubes placed with imaging guidance: effectiveness and risk for hemorrhage. *Radiology*. 2008;246(3):956–963.

Malone LJ, Stanfill RM, Wang H, et al. Effect of intraparenchymal blood patch on rates of pneumothorax and pneumothorax requiring chest tube placement after percutaneous lung biopsy. *AJR Am J Roentgenol*. 2013;200(6):1238–1243.

Manhire A, Charig M, Clelland C, et al. Guidelines for radiologically guided lung biopsy. *Thorax*. 2003;58(11):920–936.

McDermott S, Levis DA, Arellano RS. Chest drainage. *Semin Intervent Radiol*. 2012;29(4):247–255.

Patel IJ, Davidson JC, Nikolic B, et al. Consensus guidelines for periprocedural management of coagulation status and hemostasis risk in percutaneous image-guided interventions. *J Vasc Interv Radiol*. 2012;23(6):727–736.

Pereira PL, Masala S, Salvatore M. Standards of practice: guidelines for thermal ablation of primary and secondary lung tumors. *Cardiovasc Intervent Radiol*. 2012;35(2):247–254.

Rahman NM, Maskell NA, West A, et al. Intrapleural use of tissue plasminogen activator and DNase in pleural infection. *N Engl J Med*. 2011;365(6):518–526.

Sharma A, Abtin F, Shepard J-AO. Image-guided ablative therapies for lung cancer. *Radiol Clin North Am*. 2012;50(5):975–999.

Wiener RS, Wiener DC, Gould MK. Risks of transthoracic needle biopsy: how high? *Clin Pulm Med*. 2013;20(1):29–35.

Wilcox ME, Chong CAKY, Stanbrook MB, et al. Does this patient have an exudative pleural effusion? *JAMA*. 2014;311(23):2422.

Wu CC, Maher MM, Shepard J-AO. Complications of CT-guided percutaneous needle biopsy of the chest: prevention and management. *AJR Am J Roentgenol*. 2011;196(6):W678–W682.

Wu CC, Maher MM, Shepard J-AO. CT-guided percutaneous needle biopsy of the chest: preprocedural evaluation and technique. *AJR Am J Roentgenol*. 2011;196(5):W511–W514.

CHAPTER 43

Imaging of Thoracic Trauma

Saurabh Agarwal, Constantine Raptis, and Sanjeev Bhalla

CHAPTER OUTLINE

Introduction

Thoracic injury is a common sequela of acute trauma and is the third most common injury in trauma patients, after head and extremity injuries. The overall mortality rate approaches 25%, with acute aortic, tracheobronchial, and cardiac injuries often having an even worse prognosis. Given the high mortality rate and the impact on clinical management, rapid and accurate assessment of thoracic trauma imaging is imperative.

Appropriateness of Imaging Modalities and Technique

When CT Should Be Performed

There are conflicting data in the literature on whether routine chest CT should be performed in all cases of thoracic trauma. Chest CT is much more accurate than chest radiography in evaluating thoracic trauma, with at least 50% of pneumothoraces, rib fractures, and pulmonary contusions missed on routine anteroposterior chest radiographs. Some studies have shown that CT changes management in a significant proportion of patients, and potentially fatal injuries such as aortic laceration could be missed. Other studies have shown that with appropriate clinical assessment and use of other radiographic and demographic data, patients can be selected for whom chest CT would be more likely to identify injuries, thus saving cost and radiation. The American College of Radiology Appropriateness Criteria for blunt thoracic trauma in 2014 have suggested that CT should be strongly considered in patients with "high-mechanism injury, abnormal chest radiographs, altered mental status, distracting injuries, or clinically suspected thoracic injuries. CT angiogra[phy] should be routinely used in patients with suspected acute aortic laceration."

Appropriate Imaging Protocol

Unless contraindicated due to allergy or renal failure, contrast should be used in all CT scans of thoracic trauma. This allows for much more accurate assessment of vascular injury, which is a significant cause of morbidity and mortality in thoracic trauma. In most cases, precontrast images are not necessary. It is also important to choose a reconstruction algorithm with some degree of overlap. This allows for high-quality multiplanar reconstructions, which can be very helpful in the detection of certain types of thoracic injury.

Abnormal Gas and Fluid Collections

In the setting of trauma, gas and fluid can accumulate in different thoracic spaces, with different causes and clinical significance. It is important to be aware of each

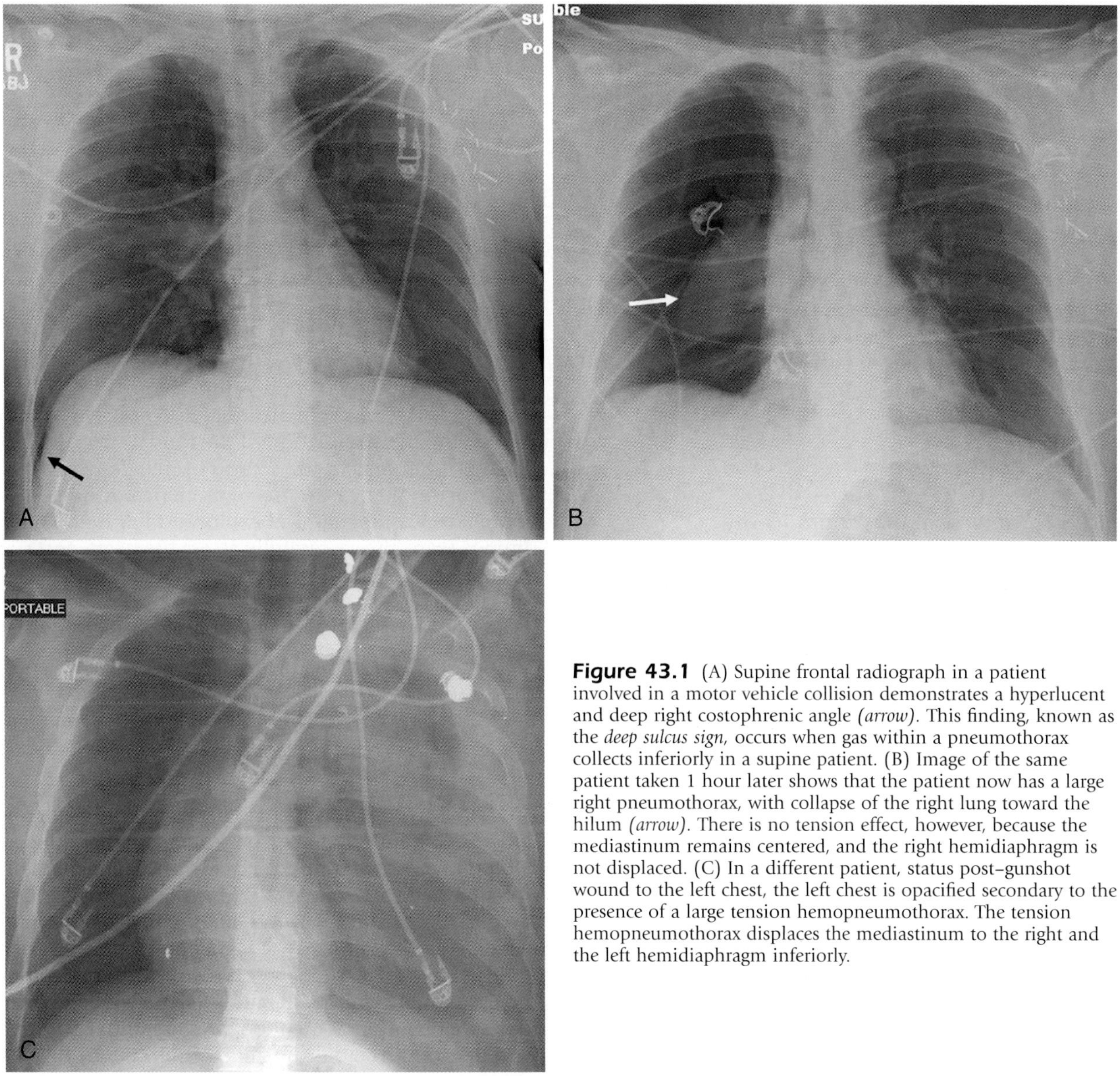

Figure 43.1 (A) Supine frontal radiograph in a patient involved in a motor vehicle collision demonstrates a hyperlucent and deep right costophrenic angle *(arrow)*. This finding, known as the *deep sulcus sign,* occurs when gas within a pneumothorax collects inferiorly in a supine patient. (B) Image of the same patient taken 1 hour later shows that the patient now has a large right pneumothorax, with collapse of the right lung toward the hilum *(arrow)*. There is no tension effect, however, because the mediastinum remains centered, and the right hemidiaphragm is not displaced. (C) In a different patient, status post–gunshot wound to the left chest, the left chest is opacified secondary to the presence of a large tension hemopneumothorax. The tension hemopneumothorax displaces the mediastinum to the right and the left hemidiaphragm inferiorly.

of these to direct the appropriate management of the trauma patient.

Pneumothorax

Incidence of Pneumothorax in Trauma; Occult Pneumothorax

Pneumothorax or air within the pleural space occurs in up to 20% to 40% of blunt trauma patients presenting to the emergency department. Up to 50% of pneumothoraces may be missed with portable radiography (Fig. 43.1A). These are termed *occult pneumothoraces* and are rarely symptomatic. However, in the setting of positive end-expiratory pressure mechanical ventilation, they can significantly enlarge, and therefore are often drained with a chest tube.

Pitfalls in Diagnosis

On a chest radiograph, one should be careful not to mistake a skin fold for a pneumothorax. The pleural line in a pneumothorax is seen as a thin white line, with no lung markings beyond it, whereas a skin fold is often less dense, has lung markings beyond it, and can be seen projecting into the soft tissues. Mach bands, which are due to an optical illusion resulting in incorrect perception of density at the borders, of varying shades of gray, can also simulate pneumothorax on chest radiograph. On chest CT, use of a sharp kernel such as with a bone algorithm can result in an artifact mimicking pneumothorax.

Determining if There Is Tension Physiology

One of the most important findings to assess is whether there are signs of tension physiology because this can be lethal to the patient. Signs of tension in the pleural space from pneumothorax or hemothorax include contralateral mediastinal shift, flattening or inversion of the ipsilateral hemidiaphragm, and a hyperexpanded ipsilateral chest (see Fig. 43.1B and C). If these signs are seen, emergent decompression is warranted because cardiovascular collapse can occur.

Associated Injuries

Rib fractures are commonly associated with pneumothorax, and careful attention should be given to the ribs when a pneumothorax is seen in the setting of trauma. Multiple contiguous segmental rib fractures are termed *flail chest,* which has a high (≈50%) association with injuries requiring surgical treatment and prolonged mechanical ventilation.

Pneumomediastinum

Cause of Pneumomediastinum in the Traumatic Setting

Most cases of pneumomediastinum in blunt thoracic trauma are due to the Macklin effect, which is alveolar rupture resulting in gas dissecting along the bronchovascular sheath into the mediastinum (Fig. 43.2). This is typically due either to barotrauma or increased pressure against a closed glottis.

Associated Injuries

In the setting of trauma, one should always carefully assess the esophagus and tracheobronchial tree because direct injury to these structures can result in pneumomediastinum.

Pneumopericardium

Importance of Pneumopericardium and Associated Injuries

Pneumopericardium, or air within the pericardial space, implies a defect in the pericardium and is unusual after blunt thoracic trauma. Pneumopericardium in the setting of penetrating trauma, however, can be enough to warrant surgical exploration to assess for cardiac injury. When encountered, one should carefully assess for any pericardial defect and look for signs of cardiac injury. CT cannot exclude cardiac injury because the right ventricular free wall, the most anterior portion of the heart, is only 2 to 3 mm thick, and lacerations are often not seen.

Hemothorax

Signs of Hemothorax

Hemothorax is blood within the pleural space. In the setting of trauma, one should always measure the attenuation of fluid in any space including the pleura, because this can direct management (Fig. 43.3A). Blood generally measures between 30 and 70 Hounsfield units. One should also assess for any focal areas of high attenuation close to a blood pool, which may represent pseudoaneurysm or active extravasation, because these may require surgical or intravascular treatment (see Fig. 43.3B). Most hemothoraces will require chest tube placement to prevent the development of constrictive fibrothorax.

Massive Hemothorax

Drainage can also help guide management. This is because a massive hemothorax (initial drainage >1 L, or rapid drainage, 100 mL/h for 5 hours) can indicate the need for surgical exploration.

Hemopericardium

Signs of Hemopericardium and Associated Injuries

Hemopericardium is blood within the pericardial space. If fluid is seen in the pericardial space, it is important to measure the attenuation of the fluid, especially in the setting of trauma. In the setting of penetrating trauma, like pneumopericardium, hemopericardium can be enough to warrant surgical exploration. If hemopericardium is seen, always carefully assess the heart, aorta, and great vessels to look for a potential source. Often a source cannot be readily determined.

Extrapleural Hematoma

Signs of Extrapleural Hematoma and Associated Injuries

The extrapleural space is the potential space that exists between the parietal pleura and the body wall, diaphragm, and mediastinum. When blood accumulates in this space, it is known as *extrapleural hematoma.* This is relatively uncommon in the setting of trauma occurring in approximately 7% of cases; however, if seen, it is almost always associated with rib fractures and commonly associated with hemothorax (see Fig. 43.3C). The morphology of the hematoma can help guide management because biconvex hematomas are thought to be due to the higher pressure of arterial bleeding and require surgical decompression more often.

Localizing Abnormal Gas Collections on Chest Radiography and CT

Pneumothorax and pneumopericardium are caused by air within true potential spaces, whereas pneumomediastinum is air within a false space. Because of this, on chest radiography, if the patient changes position, pneumothorax and pneumopericardium will change location to the most nondependent area, whereas pneumomediastinum will generally not move. On chest CT, one can differentiate these entities because pneumomediastinum, being within a false space, will have multiple webs interspersed between the air collection, as opposed to pneumopericardium and pneumothorax, which generally do not.

Determining Signs of Tamponade

Cardiac tamponade refers to a clinical syndrome caused by the accumulation of air or fluid in the pericardial space resulting in hemodynamic compromise. Signs of cardiac tamponade on imaging include collapse of the heart chambers, flattening of the anterior border of the

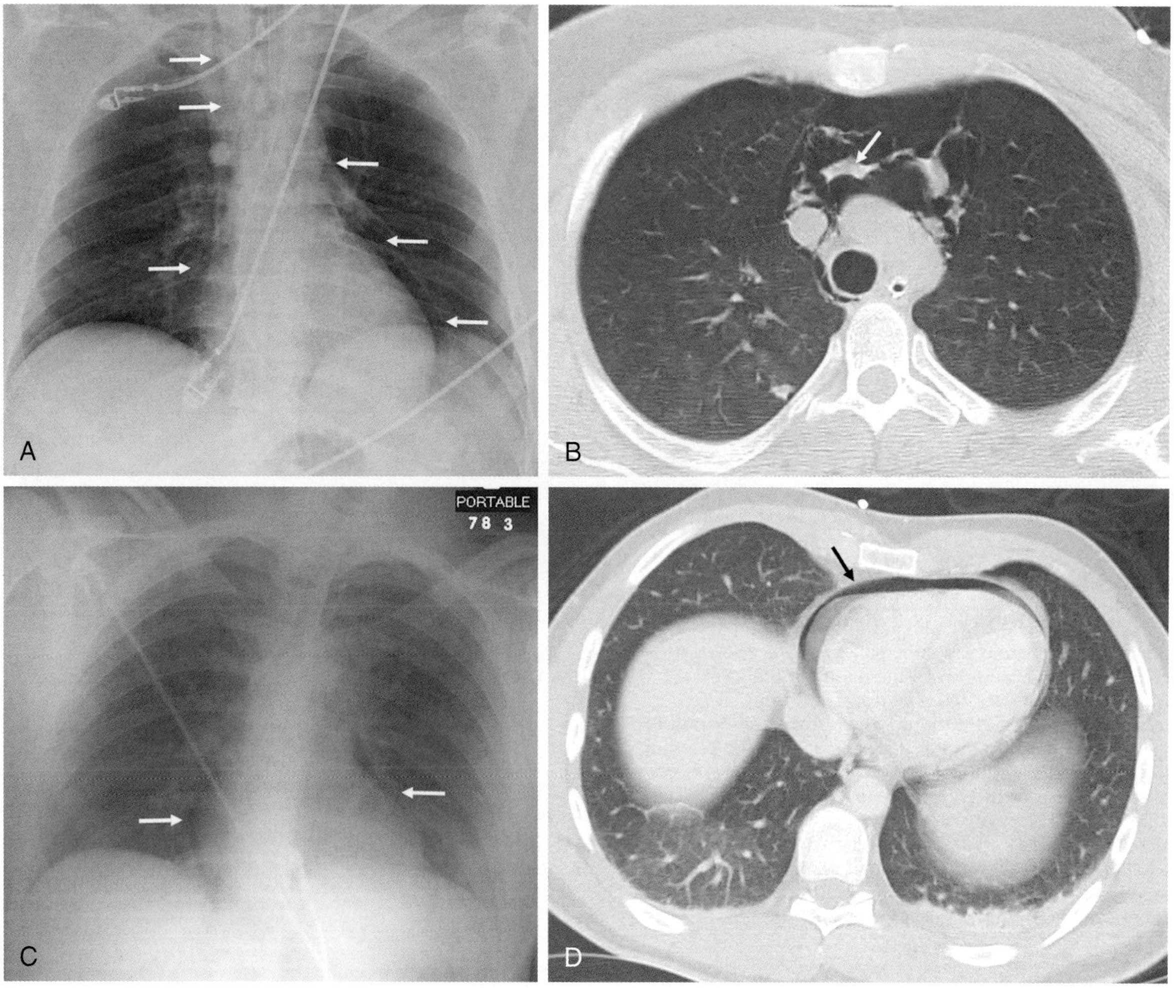

Figure 43.2 (A) Supine radiograph in a patient status post–motor vehicle collision shows vertical lucencies about the mediastinum *(arrows)*, consistent with pneumomediastinum. Note that the left heart border is outlined with gas, which has tracked inferiorly and can be difficult to distinguish from pneumopericardium. (B) An image from the CT of this patient confirms the presence of pneumomediastinum in the anterior mediastinum. Note that the gas in pneumomediastinum is insinuating among the mediastinal fat, which can be seen as displaced islands of increased density *(arrow)*. (C) Image in a different patient who was stabbed in the chest also shows gas outlining the heart *(arrows)*, but note the absence of gas more superiorly in the mediastinum. (D) An image from the CT scan of this patient shows gas in the pericardium *(arrow)*, consistent with pneumopericardium. Note that in contrast to the gas shown in (B), which was present in the potential space of the mediastinum, this gas is present in a true space (the pericardial space) and does not have islands of fat or strands of tissue within it. Given the presence of pneumopericardium, the patient underwent surgical exploration, which found a pericardial defect but no evidence of myocardial injury.

heart, and distention of the inferior vena cava on CT. On frontal chest radiograph, what is known as the *small heart sign* has been described when there is a sudden decrease in the size of the cardiac silhouette.

■ Lung Parenchymal Injury

Contusion

Imaging Appearance of Pulmonary Contusion

Pulmonary contusion is the most common lung injury occurring in blunt thoracic trauma. It is due to traumatic alveolar hemorrhage, but without significant alveolar injury. It can occur at the site of injury or sometimes opposite the site of injury in a contrecoup pattern. CT signs include nonsegmental patchy air space opacity and consolidation. Subpleural sparing may also be observed because this can mimic centrilobular nodules. Pulmonary contusions often do not respect normal anatomic borders and can cross fissures (Fig. 43.4A and B).

Laceration

Imaging Appearance of Pulmonary Laceration

Pulmonary laceration represents disruption of the lung parenchyma, with the elastic recoil of the lung resulting in a space that can fill with air, fluid, or both. This can persist for much longer periods of time. When a pulmonary laceration is encountered, one should carefully look for any high areas of attenuation, which suggest active bleeding (see Fig. 43.4C).

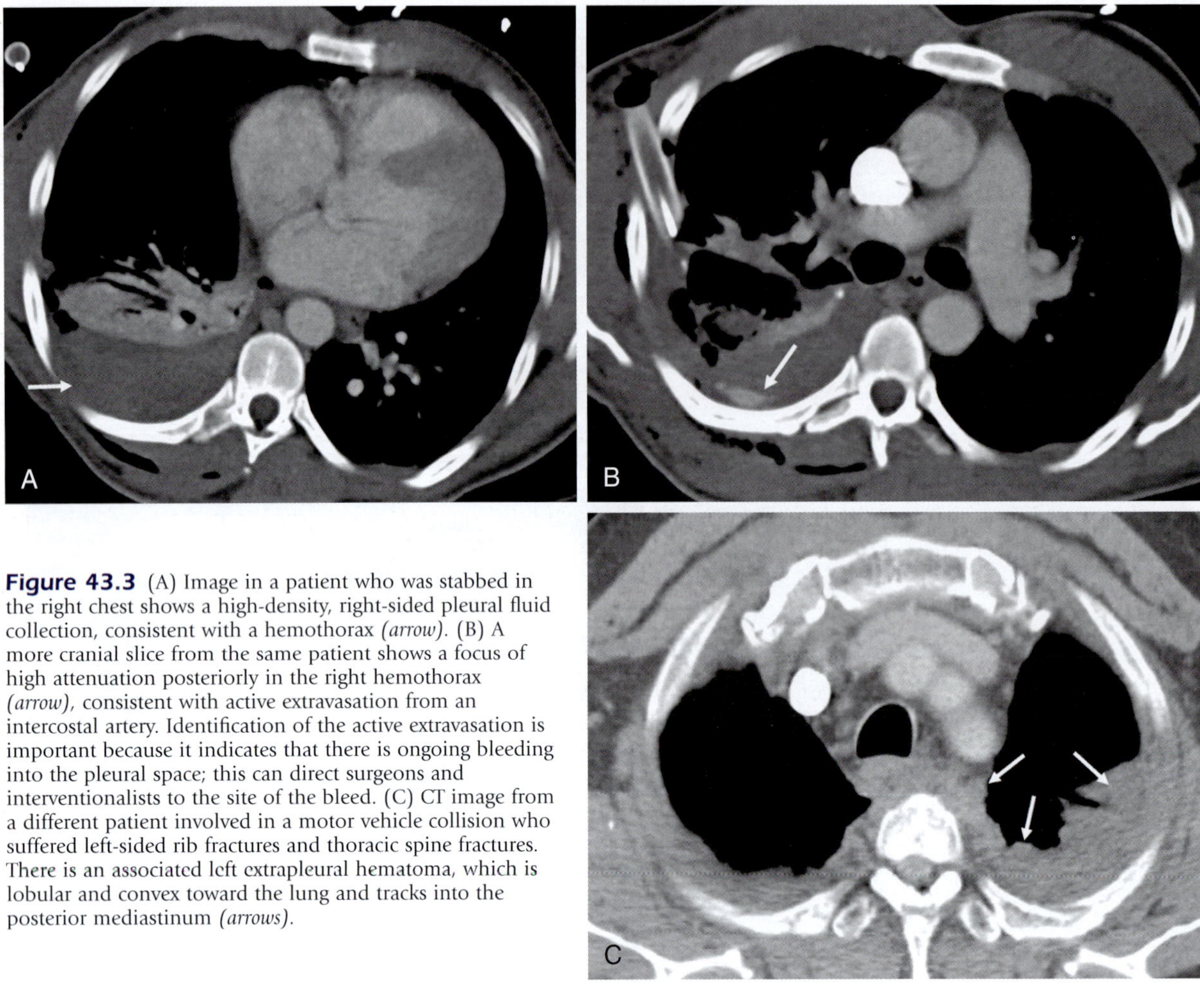

Figure 43.3 (A) Image in a patient who was stabbed in the right chest shows a high-density, right-sided pleural fluid collection, consistent with a hemothorax *(arrow)*. (B) A more cranial slice from the same patient shows a focus of high attenuation posteriorly in the right hemothorax *(arrow)*, consistent with active extravasation from an intercostal artery. Identification of the active extravasation is important because it indicates that there is ongoing bleeding into the pleural space; this can direct surgeons and interventionalists to the site of the bleed. (C) CT image from a different patient involved in a motor vehicle collision who suffered left-sided rib fractures and thoracic spine fractures. There is an associated left extrapleural hematoma, which is lobular and convex toward the lung and tracks into the posterior mediastinum *(arrows)*.

Distinguishing These Entities From Aspiration, Pneumonia, and Other Processes

Timing of a contusion can help differentiate it from other entities, such as aspiration or pneumonia. Pulmonary contusion peaks within 6 to 12 hours and begins to clear after 24 hours. If one encounters new air space opacity on chest radiography or CT scans after 24 hours, one should consider aspiration, pneumonia, or other processes, such as fat embolism in the appropriate clinical setting (e.g., extensive long bone fractures). Pulmonary contusion also occurs in relation to the trauma in a nondependent fashion, which may help differentiate it from aspiration, and is often nonsegmental, with subpleural sparing, which may help distinguish it from pneumonia (see Fig. 43.4D).

■ Mediastinal Injury

Aortic and Great Vessel Injury

Thoracic aortic injury is usually fatal, with most patients not surviving before reaching the hospital. Approximately 50% of patients who initially survive may not survive past 1 week without appropriate treatment. Therefore, it is important for the radiologist to be able to detect these injuries in a timely manner to direct treatment. The most common location of emergent aortic injury from blunt trauma is the aortic isthmus.

Direct and Indirect Signs of Vascular Injury

Understanding the concept of indirect and direct CT signs of vascular injury can be very helpful. An indirect sign of vascular injury refers to effacement of the fat plane of a suspected injured vessel by adjacent hematoma. When this sign is present, care must be taken to look for any direct signs of vascular injury because this is very sensitive for detecting injury, but not very specific. Direct signs of vascular injury include visualization of an intimal or intimomedial flap, an outpouching from the contour of the vessel, intimal irregularity or eccentric thrombus, intramural hematoma, change in vessel caliber, and extravasation of contrast (Fig. 43.5A–C).

Minimal Aortic Injury

Aortic injury has usually required treatment via open or endoluminal repair. With recent advances in imaging technology, patients with minimal intimal irregularity or minimal aortic injury have been found. This usually occurs in the descending aorta and manifests as a focal

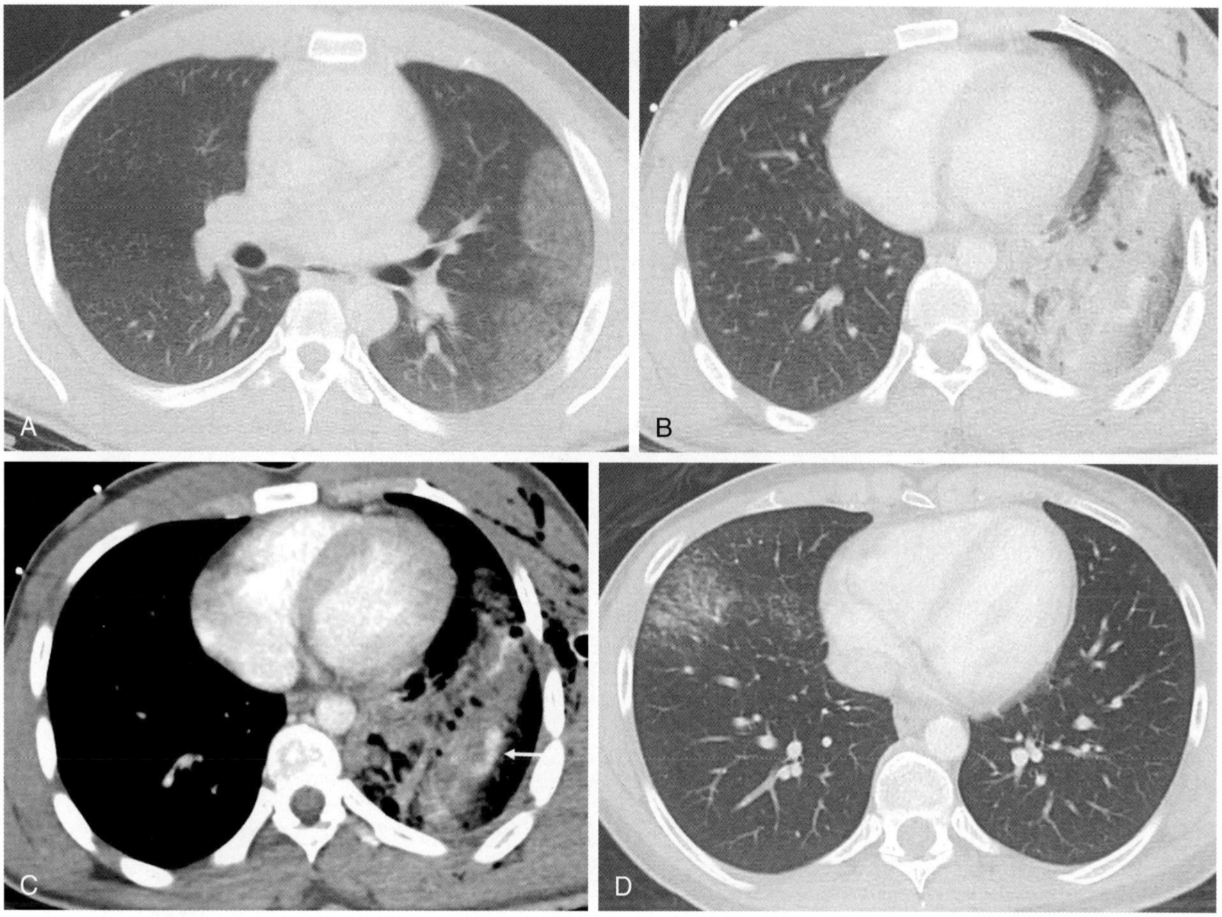

Figure 43.4 (A) Image from a patient involved in a motor vehicle collision shows centrilobular nodular ground-glass opacities in the left upper and lower lobes that cross the major fissure, consistent with contusion. The nodular ground-glass opacities represent blood accumulating in the alveoli. The contiguous extension beyond one lobe and into the adjacent lobe, without respect for the fissure, is characteristic of pulmonary contusion. (B) A CT image on lung windows of a different patient who was shot in the anterior left chest shows a linear opacity extending through the left lung. (C) On soft tissue windows, multiple areas of high attenuation *(arrow)* are seen, consistent with active extravasation in this patient with a pulmonary laceration. Note that in a pulmonary laceration, the lung architecture is disrupted or torn. (D) In a different patient involved in a motor vehicle collision, there is a cluster of small nodular opacities in the anterior right lower lobe, with some showing a tree-in-bud distribution. These dependent small nodular opacities are characteristic of aspiration. Although aspiration can be difficult to distinguish from pulmonary injury, respect for anatomic borders and its dependent location typically favor aspiration.

rounded or triangular intraluminal filling defect. In this subset of patients, medical management with blood pressure control and anticoagulation has been shown to achieve excellent results.

Most Common Great Vessel Injury

Great vessel injury is less common than aortic injury. The innominate artery is the most commonly injured of the great vessels. The concept of indirect and direct signs of vascular injury can also be helpful for detecting great vessel injury. When examining a chest radiograph in the setting of trauma, predominantly high and right-sided mediastinal widening should raise suspicion for a great vessel injury (see Fig. 43.5D and E).

Finding Subtle Vascular Injury

Looking for the above-mentioned indirect and direct signs of vascular injury can help with the detection of a subtle vascular injury. If hematoma is seen effacing the fat plane of a suspected injured vessel, without direct sign of injury, consider repeat CT in 24 hours to see if vascular injury has manifested itself.

Differentiating Artifact From Dissection Flaps and Other Signs of Injury; Decreasing Artifacts

Pulsation artifact can mimic dissection flaps and can pose a diagnostic dilemma when evaluating for vascular injury. When trying to distinguish between these, it is helpful to look for other signs of vascular injury, such as a mediastinal hematoma. Another tip is to see if the flap extends into adjacent structures, such as the cardiac chambers, which may suggest pulsation artifact. In cases where it is not possible to determine this and clinical management will be affected, consider obtaining a gated CT scan, which should eliminate most pulsation artifacts.

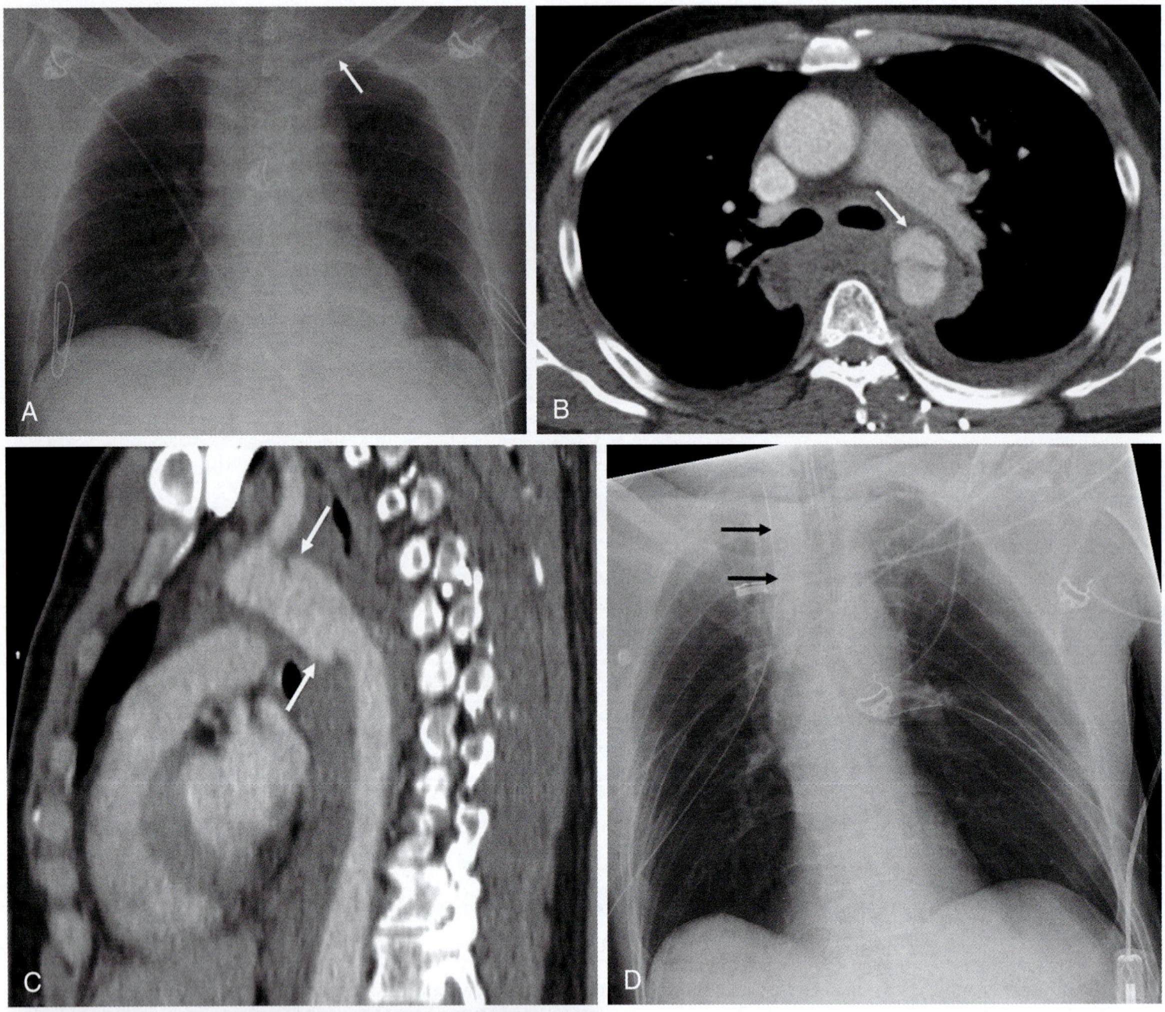

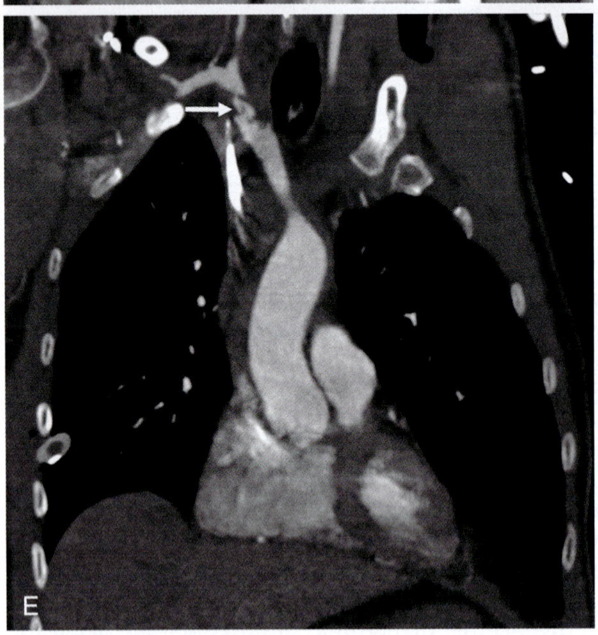

Figure 43.5 (A) Supine radiograph in a patient involved in a motor vehicle collision shows widening of the mediastinum and loss of the normal descending aortic contour, findings worrisome for an underlying mediastinal hematoma and acute traumatic aortic injury (ATAI). In addition, there is opacity extending over the left apex, consistent with blood tracking in an extrapleural fashion along the left subclavian artery reflection *(arrow)*. The trachea is displaced to the right, and the left main stem bronchus is displaced inferiorly, findings also suggestive of an underlying hematoma. (B) An axial CT image from this patient confirms the presence of a mediastinal hematoma (indirect sign of aortic injury), which manifests as increased density replacing the normal mediastinal fat. There is also a lobular outpouching from the aorta *(arrow)*, which is a direct sign consistent with an ATAI. (C) A sagittal reconstruction of the CT scan confirms these findings and shows that there is aortic disruption anteriorly and posteriorly *(arrows)* in this patient, who was found to have an aortic transection. (D) A chest radiograph from a different patient involved in a motor vehicle collision shows predominantly right-sided mediastinal widening *(arrows)*. When the mediastinal widening on a chest radiograph is high and right, a great vessel injury should be suspected. (E) A coronal reconstruction from the CT scan of this patient confirms the presence of an innominate artery injury. The innominate artery is disrupted and markedly irregular *(arrow)*.

Esophageal Injury

Sites of Esophageal Injury and Associated CT Findings

Esophageal injury usually occurs where it transitions from being mobile to fixed, which is at the cervical and thoracic junction. Because the esophagus is well protected in the mediastinum, injury is quite rare. A significant amount of force is required to cause esophageal injury in cases of blunt thoracic trauma. Associated CT findings include lower cervical and upper thoracic spine fractures, pneumomediastinum, air-fluid levels in the mediastinum, and air space disease suggesting aspiration.

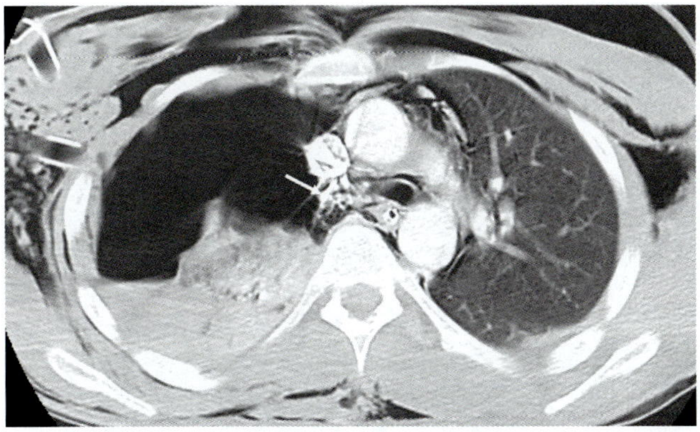

Figure 43.6 An axial CT image from a patient involved in a motor vehicle collision shows extensive subcutaneous gas, pneumomediastinum, and a large right pneumothorax. Given that a chest tube was already in place, the large persistent pneumothorax should raise the suspicion of an underlying bronchial injury. The right main stem bronchus abruptly cuts off *(arrow)*, and the right lung is displaced posteriorly from the bronchus. The posterior displacement of the right lung is known as the *fallen lung sign* and is concerning for a bronchial injury. A bronchial injury was confirmed at surgical exploration.

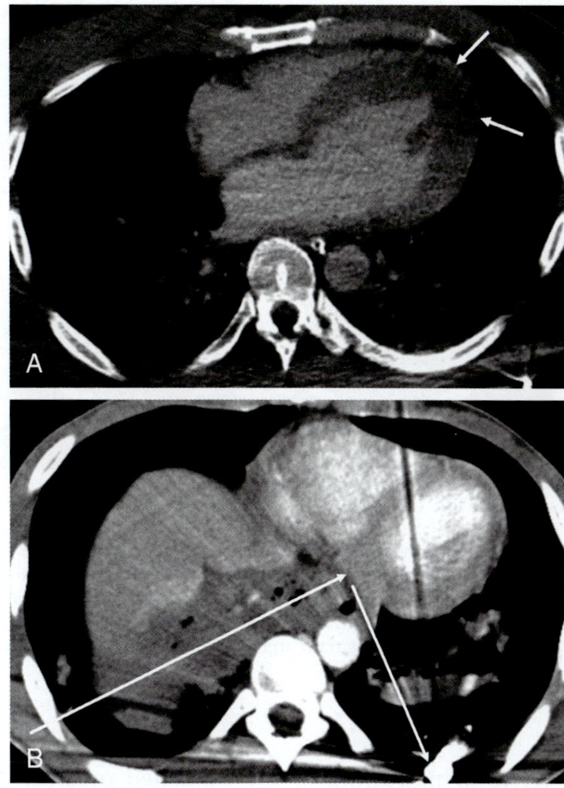

Figure 43.7 (A) An axial CT image from a patient who ran into a post while playing basketball shows a geographic area of hypoattenuation, with sharp margins involving the left ventricular apex *(arrows)*. This was concerning for a blunt cardiac injury, which was confirmed in this patient who had elevated cardiac enzyme levels, normal coronary arteries by catheterization, and an acutely depressed ejection fraction, which later recovered. Although not always seen, focally decreased attenuation in the myocardium is a direct finding suggestive of blunt cardiac injury. (B) An axial CT scan from a different patient who was shot in the right back shows a liver laceration, with the bullet located in the posterior left chest (*arrows* define the bullet tract). Although no direct findings of cardiac injury were found, the tract itself was concerning for possible myocardial injury. The patient went on for surgical exploration, and a pericardial and left ventricular injury was found.

Tracheobronchial Injury

Suspecting Tracheobronchial Injury and Associated CT Findings

Injury to the tracheobronchial tree is rarely imaged because most patients will die at the site of trauma due to their inability to ventilate adequately. Bronchial injuries are more commonly seen than tracheal injuries and usually occur close to the carina. CT findings include direct visualization of a defect and a large amount of pneumomediastinum. Tracheobronchial injury should also be suspected if there is a persistent pneumothorax in the presence of an adequately placed chest tube (Fig. 43.6). Another sign of tracheobronchial injury is what is called the *fallen lung sign*, where the lung distal to the transection collapses away from the mediastinum in contradistinction to atelectasis, which collapses toward the mediastinum.

■ Cardiac Injury

Cardiac injuries are among the most lethal of thoracic injuries. The heart should be part of a routine search pattern when evaluating trauma patients.

Detecting Cardiac Injury

Signs of cardiac injury include decreased attenuation of the myocardium suggesting contusion, hemopericardium, contrast extravasation, pneumopericardium, or, rarely, cardiac herniation. The right ventricle is most commonly injured due to its anterior location. Often cardiac injury cannot be directly visualized, but electrocardiographic abnormalities or elevated cardiac enzyme levels may suggest the diagnosis (Fig. 43.7).

Suspecting and Detecting Coronary Artery Injury

Coronary artery injury should be suspected when ischemic or infarct changes are seen in the myocardium or electrocardiogram, or clinical laboratories suggest that this may be present. In patients with suspected coronary artery injuries, the test of choice is catheter angiography.

■ Diaphragmatic Injury

Signs of Diaphragmatic Injury on Chest Radiography and CT

Diaphragmatic injury is fairly uncommon in blunt thoracic trauma and is seen in less than 5% of cases. Because the diaphragm is a thin structure traveling in the transaxial plane, coronal and sagittal multiplanar reconstructions can be very helpful in the detection of diaphragmatic injury. Signs of diaphragmatic injury on chest radiography include abnormal elevation of a hemidiaphragm or visualization of the intraabdominal contents in the chest. Signs on chest CT include direct visualization of a diaphragmatic defect and what is called the *collar sign*, which has many other named iterations;

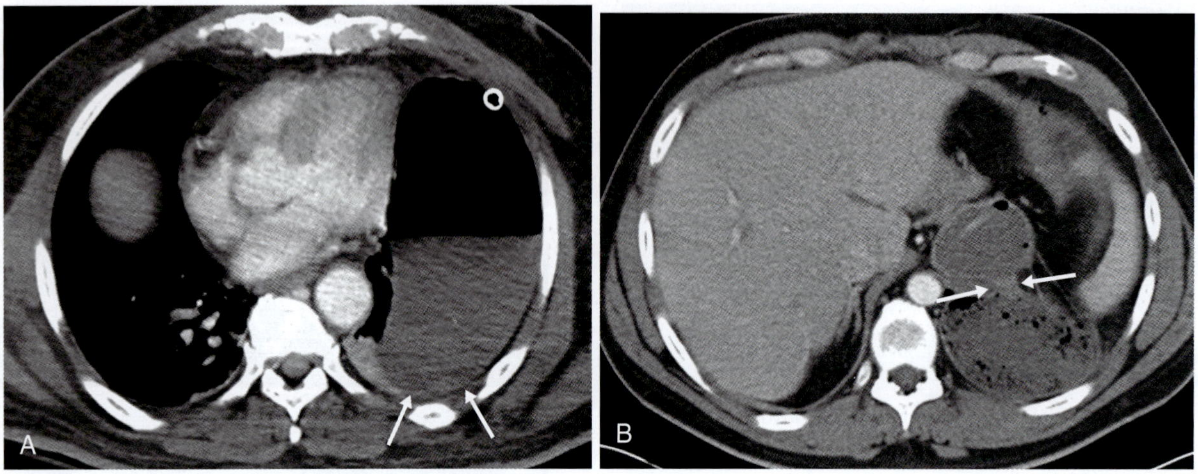

Figure 43.8 (A) An axial CT image from a patient involved in a motor vehicle collision demonstrates elevated left-sided abdominal organs, including the stomach *(arrows)*. The stomach is displaced against the posterior left ribs, a finding known as the *fallen organ sign*, and is indicative of diaphragmatic injury. A left-sided diaphragmatic injury was confirmed on surgical exploration. (B) An axial CT scan from a different patient involved in a motor vehicle collision shows what is known as the *collar sign*, compression of the stomach as it extends through the left diaphragmatic defect *(arrows)*. This patient also had a diaphragmatic injury, which was confirmed on surgical exploration.

this refers to narrowing of the herniated organ as it traverses the diaphragmatic defect. The terms *dependent viscera* or *fallen organ sign* have also been described, referring to the herniated organ falling against the posterior chest wall on axial CT images (Fig. 43.8).

Differentiating Eventration From Diaphragmatic Injury

Detection of a focal defect and visualization of an abdominal organ herniating into the chest can help differentiate eventration from diaphragmatic injury. This can be very hard to determine on axial images; routine assessment of multiplanar reconstructions should be performed in the setting of trauma to assess for diaphragmatic injury.

■ Conclusion

Understanding common injury patterns in thoracic trauma, pitfalls in diagnosis, and problem-solving techniques can greatly aid in the appropriate clinical management of thoracic trauma patients.

Bibliography

Ball CG, Kirkpatrick AW, Laupland KB, et al. Incidence, risk factors, and outcomes for occult pneumothoraces in victims of major trauma. *J Trauma*. 2005;59:917–924.

Barrios C Jr, Pham J, Malinoski D, et al. Ability of a chest x-ray and an abdominal computed tomography scan to identify traumatic thoracic injury. *Am J Surg*. 2010;200:741–744.

Brink M, Deunk J, Dekker HM, et al. Added value of routine chest MDCT after blunt trauma: evaluation of additional findings and impact on patient management. *AJR Am J Roentgenol*. 2008;190:1591–1598.

Brink M, Deunk J, Dekker HM, et al. Criteria for the selective use of chest computed tomography in blunt trauma patients. *Eur Radiol*. 2010;20:818–828.

Chung J, Carr R, Stern E. Extrapleural hematomas: imaging appearance, classification, and clinical significance. *J Thorac Imaging*. 2011;26:218–223.

Chung JC, Cox CW, Mohammed TH, et al. ACR appropriateness criteria blunt chest trauma. *J Am Coll Radiol*. 2014;11:345–351.

Cohn SM. Pulmonary contusion: review of the clinical entity. *J Trauma*. 1997;42:973–979.

Cummings K, Javidan-Nejad C, Bhalla S. MDCT on non-osseous trauma. *Semin Roentgenol*. 2014;49(2):134–142.

Exadaktylos AK, Sclabas G, Schmid SW, et al. Do we really need routine computed tomographic scanning in the primary evaluation of blunt chest trauma in patients with "normal" chest radiograph? *J Trauma*. 2001;51:1173–1176.

Gunn ML, Lehnert BE, Lungren RS, et al. Minimal aortic injury of thoracic aorta: imaging appearances and outcome. *Emerg Radiol*. 2014;21:227–233.

Ho AS, Ahmed A, Huang JS, et al. Multidetector computed tomography of spontaneous versus secondary pneumomediastinum in 89 patients: can multidetector computed tomography be used to reliably distinguish between the 2 entities? *J Thorac Imaging*. 2012;27(2):85–92.

Kaewlai R, Avery LL, Asrani AV, et al. Multidetector CT of blunt thoracic trauma. *Radiographics*. 2008;28:1555–1570.

Lee WA, Matsumura JS, Mitchell RS, et al. Endovascular repair of traumatic thoracic aortic injury: clinical practice guidelines of the society for vascular surgery. *J Vasc Surg*. 2011;53(1):187–192.

Macklin CC. Transport of air along sheaths of pulmonic blood vessels from alveoli to mediastinum: clinical implications. *Arch Intern Med*. 1939;64:913–926.

Mayberry JC. Imaging in thoracic trauma: the trauma surgeon's perspective. *J Thorac Imaging*. 2000;15:76–86.

Miller LA. Chest wall, lung, and pleural space trauma. *Radiol Clin North Am*. 2006;44:213–224.

Mirvis SE, Shanmuganathan K. Diagnosis of blunt traumatic aortic injury 2007: still a nemesis. *Eur J Radiol*. 2007;64:27–40.

Rashid M, Wikström T, Ortenwall P. Nonmenclature, classification, and significance of traumatic extrapleural hematoma. *J Trauma*. 2000;49:286–290.

Restrepo CS, Gutierrez FR, Marmol-Velez JA, et al. Imaging patients with cardiac trauma. *Radiographics*. 2012;32(3):633–649.

Wagner RB, Crawford WO Jr, Schimpf PP. Classification of parenchymal injuries of the lung. *Radiology*. 1988;167:77–82.

Wintermark M, Schnyder P. The Macklin effect: a frequent etiology for pneumomediastinum in severe blunt chest trauma. *Chest*. 2001;120:543–547.

Young CA, Menias CO, Bhalla S, Prasad SR. CT features of esophageal emergencies. *Radiographics*. 2008;28(6):1541–1553.

INDEX

Page number followed by *t*, *f*, or *b* indicates table, figure, or box, respectively.

E

F

U